the complete DAVID BOWIE

THE COMPLETE DAVID BOWIE

REVISED AND EXPANDED THIRD EDITION

NICHOLAS PEGG

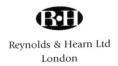

Reynolds & Hearn Ltd
London

Front cover: A Reality Tour at Wembley Arena, 26 November 2003
(photograph by Tabatha Fireman © Redferns)

Back cover (top): the Station To Station tour, 1976
(photograph by Roger Bamber © Rex Features)

Back cover (bottom): performing 'Rebel Rebel' on Dutch television, 1974
(photograph by Roger Bamber © Rex Features)

First published in 2004 by
Reynolds & Hearn Ltd
61a Priory Road
Kew Gardens
Richmond
Surrey TW9 3DH

Reprinted 2004

A CIP catalogue record for this book is available from the British Library.

ISBN 1 903111 73 0

Designed by Chris Bentley.

Printed and bound in Great Britain by Biddles Ltd.

contents

INTRODUCTION:
THE MUSIC IS OUTSIDE

"The piece of work is not finished until the audience come to it and add their own interpretation – and what the piece of art is about is the grey space in the middle."
David Bowie, December 1999

On 8 January 1947 Elvis Presley celebrated his twelfth birthday and Stephen Hawking his fifth. In New York, Jackson Pollock made his first drip-painting. In London the day began with a portent, when freezing conditions caused the Lambeth Town Hall clock to strike thirteen times at midnight. Less than half a mile away, at 40 Stansfield Road, Brixton, Peggy Burns gave birth to a baby boy.

This book is about that boy, but it is not a biography. It's a reference work which, it is to be hoped, will satisfy the enthusiast and inform the newcomer. To both I implore: if you want to enjoy David Bowie's work to the full, keep an open mind. What makes Bowie such a supremely fascinating artist is that his career presents an implicit challenge to conventional notions of creative continuity. He has repeatedly confounded attempts to pigeon-hole him as this or that kind of artist, and the result has been one of rock music's longest and most successful careers. "People would like artists to be expendable, to fit into one generation or another," said Bowie's painter friend Julian Schnabel in 1997. "They don't like it when somebody keeps going." Bowie himself is fond of quoting a maxim of Brian Eno's, as he did on Radio 2's *Golden Years* documentary in March 2000: "In art you can crash your plane and walk away from it. If you have that chance, you should take it. The worst thing would be to maintain a particular kind of celebrity and commercial success for the entire career, and then look back and think of all the things that one could have

tried and could have done, and think – why didn't I do that?"

There will always be those who mistrust Bowie because he borrows other people's ideas. Serious glam-rockers will state a preference for Marc Bolan, advocates of synthesizer minimalism will go straight to Kraftwerk, soul-boys grimace at *Young Americans*, drum'n'bass aficionados have no time for *Earthling*. Bowie's ability to remake his music, his appearance and even his personality has prompted some to accuse his work of a kind of fundamental dishonesty. The charge frequently levelled against Bowie throughout his career is that he is a dilettante, a style vampire who has his finger on the pulse but never his hand on his heart. "Some people say Bowie is all surface style and second-hand ideas," said Brian Eno in 1999, "but that sounds like a definition of pop to me. It's a folk art. It's only in the conceited fine arts that we're supposed to be totally original and pretend that it came out of nowhere, straight from God to us. In pop music, everyone is listening to everyone else." A decade earlier Bowie had told *Melody Maker* that "There's no point in just ripping something off, but if you hear something and think, 'I like what that guy is doing; I know what I can do with that', it's like having a new colour to paint with, and I think it depends very much on what you do with that colour once you've found it."

The not uncommon hypothesis that the Ziggy Stardust period is Bowie's only true moment of relevance is based on the circumstantial fact that that's when the public at large happened to start buying him. "I know that they were decisive years for me," David said in 1998, "because for the first time I had a real audience. But at the same time, I really worked hard before 1970." Glam rock was merely the latest idiom of an artist who had already worked though the guises of R&B frontman, Mod, psychedelic balladeer, Dylanesque protest singer and embryonic prog-rocker. Bowie has attributed the long years of his pre-fame struggle to the very fact that he was unwilling to nail his colours to one stylistic mast: "At that point, particularly, it wasn't 'right' to have an interest in all areas," he said in 1999. "It was make-your-mind-up time. You were either a folk singer or a rock singer or a blues guitarist ... I felt: well, I don't wanna be like this. I wanna keep my options open; there's lots of things I like." In 2003 he described his creative principle as "an undiminished idea of variability. I don't think there's one truth, one absolute. It's an idea that I have always felt instinctively, but it was reinforced by the first thing I read on postmodernism, a book by George Steiner called *In Bluebeard's Castle*. That book just confirmed for me that there was actually some kind of theory behind what I was doing with my work – realizing that I could like artists as disparate as Anthony Newley and Little Richard, and that it was not wrong to like both at the same time. Or that I can like Igor Stravinsky *and* The Incredible String Band, or The Velvet Underground *and* Gustav Mahler. That all just made sense to me." Commercially *Ziggy Stardust* was of massive significance, but artistically it was just another milestone on the meandering road of discovery. Bowie may not have invented glam, but the point is that he conquered it. Unlike Bolan, he then escaped it. A few years later he repeated the same pattern with synthesizer pop, dropping a few classic albums our way and leaving behind another trail of imitators who failed to move on. That's what makes him David Bowie.

And that's why, despite the occasional commercial jackpot, Bowie's music has never been wholly accepted in America, where honesty and denim and Bruce Springsteen are what rock music is all about: "I'm not a guy that gets on stage and tells you how my day's just gone," he once remarked. Bowie's work is about artifice, about allusion, about signifying the enactment of rock music. "I feel like an actor when I'm on stage, rather than a rock artist," he told *Rolling Stone* in 1972. Twenty-five years later he informed another interviewer that "Bertolt Brecht believed that it was

impossible for an actor to express real emotion in a natural form every night. Instead, you portray the emotion symbolically. You don't try to draw the audience into the emotional content of what you're doing, but give them something to create their own dialogue about what you're portraying. You play anger or love through stylistic gesture. The voice doesn't rise and fall and the face doesn't go through all the gambits you would portray as a naturalistic actor. I've done that an awful lot throughout my career. A lot of what is perceived as mannered performance or writing is a distancing from the subject matter to allow an audience to have their own association with what I'm writing about."

This sort of assertion creates a problem only for those who consider theatre to be somehow synonymous with insincerity. Working within an art form which jealously guards its stylistic boundaries and stigmatizes those who fail to define their artistic allegiances, David Bowie has made a career out of playing counter to the unwritten rules of rock. Many of the major artists he has professed to admire – people like Lou Reed, Bob Dylan, Iggy Pop and Joni Mitchell – have won respect precisely because they have stuck to their guns, devoting whole careers to the meticulous exploration of a carefully defined musical landscape. By contrast, Bowie delights in presenting a moving target. Making no attempt to conceal his own short attention span and his assimilation of new enthusiasms, he constantly challenges our complacency as consumers, writing and rewriting the parameters of his work on the *tabula rasa* he calls David Bowie. "Sometimes I don't feel like a person at all," he said in 1972, "I'm just a collection of other people's ideas." Warning against autobiographical readings of his 1999 album *'hours...'*, he told Q that "I am only the person the greatest number of people believe I am. So little of it has anything to do with me, so I just have to do the best I can with what I've got [a close paraphrase of the album's opening line] – knowing that it has a complete second life by the time it leaves me."

Undoubtedly, a crucial part of Bowie's enduring appeal is his ability to shed skins: "I find that I am a person who can take on the guises of different people that I meet," he told Russell Harty in 1973. "I can switch accents in seconds of meeting someone ... I've always found that I collect. I'm a collector, and I've always just seemed to collect personalities and ideas." In 1997 he reflected that "I create something out of my enthusiasms of that particular moment. I get re-enthused by something else, and suddenly I don't see that any more, and I'm over here. And that's the way I am. I have no apology."

Any attempt to pry beneath the theatrical guises would be hugely missing the point, but it does not follow that Bowie's music is therefore without substance or continuity. Collaborators, influences, hairstyles and even accents have come and gone, but as far as the essence of the work is concerned, rather too much has been made of Bowie's "changes". There's an obvious blood relation between *Hunky Dory*, *Low* and *1.Outside*, or any other random batch of albums you care to pick. "The reinvention thing, I don't buy into that at all," said David in 1997. "I think there's a real continuity with what I do, and it's just about expressing myself in a contemporaneous fashion." In the same interview he mocked the facile commentaries all too frequently trotted out about his career: "I'm probably the chameleon of rock because what I do is all about ch-ch-changes! The clichés are a stack high." (Meaningless comparisons between David Bowie and a certain genus of polychromatic lizard will not be a feature of this book. "It's a piece of lazy journalism, for several reasons," Bowie himself pointed out in 2003. "One reason, of course, is that the chameleon is always trying to blend into his surroundings, and I don't think that's exactly what I'm known for.")

There are, however, deeper resonances at play. Central to Bowie's habit of dismantling his music and himself, and reassembling them in unexpected ways, is the recurring motif of a quest for the authentic self. His lyrics disclose an abiding preoccupation with burrowing through the layers of pretence to discover who is, in the words of 'Wild Eyed Boy From Freecloud', "really you and really me". In 'Changes' he "turned myself to face me" only to find that to do so was to "turn and face the strange". There are encounters with sinister *doppelgängers* in countless songs. Bowie's constant refrain in interviews throughout the 1970s and 1980s was that each new album or tour was about to unveil "the real me". It's a subject that has clearly concerned David throughout his career: "I'm not sure if that's really me coming through in the songs," he said in 1972. "They come out and I hear them afterward and I think, well, whoever wrote that really felt strongly about it. I *can't* feel strongly. I get so numb."

The constantly shifting "me", like the masks and mirrors that litter his lyrics, videos and concerts, are all part of Bowie's galvanizing restlessness. As he said in 1976, "The minute you know you're on safe ground, you're dead. You're finished. It's over. The last thing I want is to be established." Twenty years later he commented that "not knowing where you're going is what makes it exciting for me. It leaves a permanently open landscape." As he proved so (un)spectacularly with Tin Machine, Bowie is at his least interesting when he abandons the quest and tries to ape the rootsy authenticity of the rock'n'roll band. In 1997 the *NME*'s Stephen Dalton summed up the situation succinctly if hyperbolically: "Hating Bowie in 1997 means hating everything overblown, theatrical, pretentious, pseudo-intellectual and jarringly progressive in the past 25 years of pop. In other words, everything *great* about pop. It also means hating yourself."

Bowie's early manager Kenneth Pitt wrote in his memoir that those who judge Bowie and "take as their yardstick rock and roll, fail to understand that David never was a devotee or exponent of rock and roll. Whenever he rocked and rolled he did so in the context of theatre, as an actor. It has been his most successful role to date." The accepted wisdom of the rock fan – and of many Bowie fans – is to cast the eyes skyward and groan with embarrassment at *Labyrinth* and the Bing Crosby duet and all those silly early songs about gnomes and bombardiers, because they don't fit in with our narrow preconception of what a credible rock singer should be doing. Why do we punish ourselves like this? *Station To Station* is a great rock album, but that doesn't stop *Labyrinth* being a great children's movie. They are different things, and Bowie excels at doing different things. No other artist of his stature straddles and thereby defies the conflict between the opposing camps of "rock" and "pop". Bowie enjoys the rare ability to appeal to fans of both Led Zeppelin and ABBA, of both Frank Zappa and Duran Duran. Those who take their "rock" too seriously have a problem with this, but it's a problem of their own making; Bowie challenges the tribalism of such allegiances. "I never, ever wanted to be regarded as the leader or the forefront of any movement," he said in 1983. "Never wanted it. I did want to be regarded as an individualist. But that's about it." Leading by example, his career actively encourages his followers to reject uniforms and movements, to shed their skins, to revel in the transience of musical and sartorial fashion. In so doing he has cannily avoided locking his own fan base into an ephemeral time frame, but more significantly it has enabled his music to defy categorization: was there ever a better example than *Ziggy Stardust* of an album that is simultaneously pure rock and pure pop?

It is perhaps this sense of individualism, as much as Bowie's native charisma, which has always made his music seem so personal both to him and to his audience. On stage he is blessed by the ability to make every individual in a stadium audience feel as if he is singing directly to him or her, and his songs have always struck an intensely intimate chord with devotees. "I felt that his records had been made with me in mind," recalled The Cure's Robert Smith in 2003. "He was blatantly different, and everyone of my age remembers the time he played 'Starman' on *Top Of The Pops*. The school was divided between those who thought he was a queer and those who thought he was a genius. Immediately, I thought: this is it. This is the man I've been waiting for. He showed that you could do things on your own terms; that you could define your own genre and not worry about what anyone else is doing, which is I think the definition of a true artist."

In any case, Bowie's muse operates outside rock's accustomed frames of reference. We can and must point to Little Richard, Lou Reed, Kraftwerk, Marc Bolan and countless other crucial role-models from within the world of rock, but to form a proper understanding of what makes Bowie tick as a creative artist it is equally important to consider the influences of an altogether different sphere. The fusion of rock music with pantomime, science fiction and nursery rhyme, which remains a constant from 'The Laughing Gnome' to 'Thursday's Child' and from 'Space Oddity' to 'Looking For Satellites', is inextricably linked with the imaginative framework of Bowie's childhood universe. "He is the only person who I have met who brings nursery rhymes and fairy stories to the foreground of my mind," wrote one of his earliest profilers for *Chelsea News* in 1967, and it remains a perceptive observation. Time and again Bowie's music has raised the ghosts of his suburban childhood in the 1950s and 1960s: fairy stories like *Snow White* and *Aladdin*, radio comedies like *The Goon Show* and *Hancock's Half Hour*, nursery rhymes like 'Inchworm', 'Lavender Blue' and 'London Bridge Is Falling Down', popular television classics like *Quatermass*, *Doctor Who*, *Not Only…But Also* and, as repeatedly quoted in interviews, *The Flowerpot Men*. The rock critic who pooh-poohs such texts as being beneath the dignity of his subject or of himself will never get to the bottom of David Bowie's work.

If one element above all others recurs throughout Bowie's career, it is the ongoing sci-fi *shtick* that infuses his most celebrated characters, from Major Tom and Ziggy Stardust to *The Man Who Fell To Earth* and *Earthling*. He has always professed to believe firmly in the existence of extraterrestrial life, and his fascination with everything from UFO sightings to Ridley Scott's *Blade Runner* is well documented. Even so, as Bowie has often insisted, the alien characters of his early songs merely exploit outer space as a metaphor for his own inner space: "They were metaphysically in place to suggest that I felt alienated," he explained in 1997, "that I felt distanced from society and that I was really in search of some kind of connection."

This distance – the "otherness", contrived or otherwise, that has defined so much of Bowie's work – is perhaps the keynote in any attempt to appreciate his creative priorities. Time and again it is the vessel which articulates an apparent dread of time, mortality and oblivion that runs like a seam through Bowie's songwriting. It's detectable in the Blakeian cries for lost childhood that riddle his earliest compositions, it's there in the chilling mortal angst of *Scary Monsters*, and it's there in the middle-aged regret and spiritual anguish that infuse the melancholic musings of *'hours…'*, *Heathen* and *Reality*. Perhaps most obviously it rampages through his early 1970s work, a darkening force that looms over a whole parade of famous songs.

Hand in hand with this nagging existential anxiety comes Bowie's endlessly complex relationship with spirituality and religion. Much of the soul-searching that has characterized his work has its roots in the traditions and vocabulary of a typical middle-class Church of England upbringing – indeed, he has often cited the BBC's Sunday radio broadcasts of Mendelssohn's 'O For The Wings Of A Dove' as his earliest musical memory. But it was an upbringing that would be fragmented and cast into doubt by his fascination with other faiths and with a parade of underground or outsider lifestyles. David's youthful dabblings in Buddhism are well documented, as are his unhealthy interests in more arcane spiritual systems such as Aleister Crowley's teachings and MacGregor Mathers's *The Kabbalah Unveiled* during the 1970s. In more recent years the liberal, intellectual, left-leaning autodidact Renaissance Man would seem to bear all the hallmarks of a confident atheist, but Bowie has instead remained, if not quite a believer, then certainly a committed doubter.

Ground Control's memorable injunction to

"Check ignition, and may God's love be with you" perfectly encapsulates these two counterbalancing aspects of Bowie's creative imagination. The spacemen and extraterrestrial visitors who crop up repeatedly in his work offer an illuminating counterpoint to the preoccupation with priests, heaven, hell, churches, prayers, angels, devils, gods and Messiahs which have positively littered his lyrics over the past forty years. Bowie's earliest songs often revolve around provincial lives timidly hidebound by religion ("Remember when we used to go to church on Sunday?", "Tiny Tim sings prayers and hymns", "I saw a photograph of Jesus and I asked him if he'd make me five", "God knows I'm good"), later giving way to an explosion of false Messiahs, sci-fi gods and risqué excursions into doubt and blasphemy ("They called it The Prayer, its answer was law", "God is just a word", "God did take my logic for a ride", "The church of man, love, is such a holy place to be", "Praying to the light machine", "Till there was rock, you only had God"). Then comes the desperate spiritual surrender of *Station To Station* ("Each night I sit there pleading", "Lord I kneel and offer you my word on a wing, and I'm trying hard to fit among your scheme of things"), and the bleak quasi-redemptions of the Berlin period ("Thank God heaven left us standing on our feet", "Seemed like another day I could fly into the eye of God on high", "Strung out in heaven's high"). Even *Let's Dance*, *Tonight* and *Never Let Me Down* have their dark spiritual undertones ("God and man, no religion", "Prayers, they hide the saddest view", "I could not take on the church", "You've seen who's in heaven, is there anyone in hell?"), while the Tin Machine albums articulate an uneasy relationship with the almighty ("God's the one we pick to curse us", "I'm a young man at odds with the Bible, but I don't pretend faith never works"). Then comes the resignation of the early 1990s ("Now you're looking for God in exciting new ways", "God is on top of it all – that's all", "Don't tell God your plans", "Prayer can't travel so far these days"), the ostentatious Christian imagery of *'hours...'*, and the intimations of a final loss of faith on *Heathen* and *Reality* ("I demand a better future, or I might just stop loving you", "I lost God in a New York minute").

These examples represent the merest tip of the iceberg in this most recursive element of Bowie's songwriting; whatever other changes may be afoot from one album to another, certain themes remain constant. "I don't keep changing just for the sake of it, but there is a desire to change, even though the subject matter remains much the same from album to album," David said in 2003. "I don't think I write about a terribly wide range of subjects. My excitement is in finding a new way of approaching that same subject, and at heart I think that is what most writers do. They have, maybe, only a small basket of subjects that they write about, but they re-approach those subjects differently every time, and that's what I tend to do as a writer. I invariably deal with the same senses of isolation and lack of communication and all these kinds of negatives, and I'll probably deal with them to the end of my life. There'll be certain spiritual questionings and all that, and it won't change very much, because it never has, it appears, from Major Tom to *Heathen*. It really is all about the same thing, and obviously my big four or five questions are in there somewhere."

Much of Bowie's methodology as an artist derives not from music or theatre, but from a third art form that has long informed his creative sensibility. "I see the whole of what I do in terms of painting," he once explained. "I've always thought they were very close. A lot of the songs I've written are, for me, paintings in words. A lot of the more embellished pieces, the ones really loaded with sound, where there are lots of things to listen to on repeated play, came from the idea of building up layers of paint so that you see something new each time." Inevitably, just as rock music jealously guards the battlements of its fragile edifice, so too does the rarefied world of fine art. The attempts of a rock musician to be taken seriously as a painter are ripe for attack by the snob element within both establishments, and Bowie has been predictably ridiculed by those who believe that he should only be permitted to be one or the other. The notion that he could be both, or neither, is apparently just too complicated to consider.

The assimilation of different media is at the heart of Bowie's creative pursuit. His best music is often organically and inextricably linked to his painting, his writing, his stage presentations and his trailblazing video work. In 1996 he told an interviewer that "because I didn't have any real training in any [artistic media] it didn't occur to me that you were supposed to only stay in one of them. So for me it was quite appropriate that if I'm doing music, then I should also actually design some scenery for the stage and probably the costumes, and I'll do some paintings while I'm at it. And it just never stopped."

In the recording studio, Bowie has little interest in

adhering to the accepted grammar of rock music. His best work is founded on the pursuit of unlikely juxta-positions and unorthodox frictions in style, instru-mentation and tempo. He delights in demolishing his own musical vocabulary and thrives on the uncertain-ty of the new idea. He has a penchant for collabora-tors who are prepared to scrap the rule-book and establish alternative methodologies, whose very rejec-tion of conventional notions of "efficiency" creates the necessary stimulus: Tony Visconti, Mike Garson, Brian Eno, Robert Fripp, Reeves Gabrels and many others. Even among more conventional players he has always favoured those whose technical dexterity and melodic instincts are matched by a willingness to step off the creative brink: Earl Slick, Herbie Flowers, Carlos Alomar, Gail Ann Dorsey, Mick Ronson. "That's what I do as a producer," Bowie told *Guitar Player* in 1997. "I'm good at opening musicians to areas of their own technique or creativity that they might not have looked at before." In the same inter-view he offered a precise summary of his creative pri-orities: "A girl wearing a red dress in a forest will be some strange vision of unexpected eroticism, but a girl wearing a red dress on a catwalk will be highly pre-dictable."

Bowie's career has been defined by a series of pen-dulum-swings and shifting compromises, and he has systematically surrounded himself with colleagues who exert conflicting gravitational pulls on his own strongly vaudevillean instincts. Figures like Iggy Pop, Pete Townshend and Tin Machine's Sales brothers have popped up over the years to inject into Bowie's work the kind of authentic rock'n'roll street cred he has often craved, while the likes of Eno, Fripp and Gabrels have empowered his avant-garde ambitions. Bowie is blessed with the rare ability to synthesize what he wants from two necessarily confrontational approaches: it is his particular triumph that he is nei-ther Lou Reed nor John Cale, but a bit of both.

There are certain challenges and pitfalls attendant on the Bowie chronicler. It is a venerable cliché that history is written by the winning side, but in the case of biographies of the rich and famous, the opposite tends to be true. Anyone who has read an unautho-rized life of a successful actor, politician or rock star will be familiar with the parade of forgotten school-mates, ex-lovers and fired colleagues who line up, not always in a spirit of generosity, to clutch at their moment of fame. Whenever a true story is told and re-told at second hand, a consensus begins to crystallize

which can quickly distort the reality, as witnessed in some of the silly, hyperbolic mythologies that have been built up around Bowie's life and career. In par-ticular, many of the key figures during David's break-through period – people like Kenneth Pitt, Tony Defries and Angela Bowie – have been painted in such brash primary colours over the years that they have been reduced to a series of grotesque caricatures that are unspeakably injurious to the individuals in ques-tion and entirely unhelpful to seekers of the truth. One only has to look at Todd Haynes's 1998 film *Velvet Goldmine* to see how reality has been transmut-ed into a colourful fantasia. The truth is less polarized, less sensational, and far more interesting.

Most unhappily of all, the misfortunes of David's family have often been cast in a nastily melodramatic light, a succession of darkly-whispered asylum secrets from some third-rate Hammer horror. The most sen-sitive and contentious element in any study of Bowie's work is the question of how far his songwriting is informed by his family history, in particular the men-tal illness of various relatives. These are deep waters, and have occasionally tempted biographers to write unpleasantly inflammatory and profoundly silly things. David has long since confirmed that much of his early writing was indeed concerned with such anx-ieties: "One puts oneself through such psychological damage in trying to avoid the threat of insanity," he said in 1993. "You start to approach the very thing that you're scared of. It had tragically afflicted particu-larly my mother's side of the family. There seemed to be any number of people who had various mental problems and varying states of sanity. There were far too many suicides for my liking, and that was some-thing I was terribly fearful of … I felt that I was the lucky one because I was an artist and it would never happen to me. As long as I could put these psycho-logical excesses into my music and into my work, I could always be throwing it off." The challenge con-fronting the responsible writer is that it would be prig-gish and precious to ignore the subject entirely, but the worst kind of gutter-sniping to start casting around for gory details. I have tried very hard to steer the right path between the two.

The fascination inspired by Bowie's often impene-trably cryptic songwriting has sparked an unending search for pattern and meaning in his work. The arch media-manipulator is famous for his ability to disarm journalists just when they believe they're on the point of getting a fundamental answer out of him. "He invariably agrees with opinions," wrote Scott Isler, who interviewed David for *Musician* magazine in 1987. "Like James Dean, one of his idols, Bowie prefers to mirror an interviewer rather than open a window to his own personality." When, on the *Tonight* show in 1979, Valerie Singleton attempted a probing question about whether David still felt there was anything he really *wanted*, he replied with absolute solemnity, "Yes, a train ticket to Penge."

The elusive charm of Bowie under interview conditions remains one of his most endearing and enjoyable talents. Sometimes, both frustratingly and amusingly, he is content to assimilate the prevailing critical opinion of his own history, praising and condemning exactly the same albums and tours as everyone else, despite what he may have said at the time. "When I think about the past these days it's through other people's eyes," he said in 1999, adding that his personal history "doesn't really exist. It's just circumstances that are vaguely remembered, often incorrectly, by both myself and other people."

By being such a slippery customer, Bowie has remained a past master at manipulating the cultivated mystery that surrounds his work. In 1973 he told *Rolling Stone* that fans "...will send me back their own kind of write-ups of what I'm talking about, which is great for me because sometimes I don't know." But it would be a mistake to assume that Bowie's songwriting is not precious to him. "My songs are all from the heart, and they are wholly personal to me and I would like people to accept them as such," he said in 1969. "I dearly want to be recognized as a writer, but I would ask them not to go too deeply into my songs. As likely as not, there's nothing there but the words and music you hear at one listening." Thirty years later, he gave perhaps his most cogent analysis of his own craft: "Let me say that my songs are a construction," he told *Uncut* in 1999. "It's very rare that they inherently have a particularly deep 'meaning'. Or if they do, it's a very

personal thing which I wouldn't expect other people to perceive or understand. That's not why I write songs. I like the idea that they're vehicles for other people to interpret or use as they will. It's a device. That's what I do with songs, with art generally. Yes I have an interest in how an artist works, but I don't need to know what it's 'about'. I'm quite capable of reading the ciphers and symbols for myself. I think a lot of people these days have ended up cobbling together a belief system that works for them."

Ultimately, no book of this kind can achieve an adequate appreciation of music, which is not a form of expression to be broken down into its constituent parts by anything so clumsy as words. They, to quote the sizzlingly overheated sleeve-notes that appeared on RCA's reissue of *Space Oddity*, "cannot speak of music; they cannot elucidate nor illuminate. Both sounds enter through the ears, but only music travels throughout and animates the whole body. David Bowie has always known this." A book of this kind will always run the risk of over-emphasizing the lyrics at the expense of the music, and as Bowie told the *NME* in 1980, "music does have an implicit message of its own; it makes its case very pointedly. If that were not the case, then classical music would not have succeeded to the extent that it did ... It makes me very angry ... when people concentrate only on the lyrics because that's to imply there is no message stated in the music itself, which wipes out hundreds of years of classical music. Ridiculous."

Bearing that in mind, together with Bowie's more recent observation that "the image and the sound of a word hold as much inherent information as its dictionary meaning", it must be conceded that no amount of close textual analysis will ever provide an adequate or even a coherent alternative to the process of listening to the music itself. But then, that was never my intention. I just wanted to pull together the history behind David Bowie's work. Here it is.

HOW to USE this BOOK

Chapter 1 catalogues Bowie's songs in alphabetical rather than chronological order, so as to obviate the need for an additional index and to overcome the obvious problems presented by songs such as 'I Feel Free', which from Bowie's point of view belongs chronologically in 1972, 1980 and 1993. The remainder of the book arranges albums, tours, films and so on in chronological order, and with the assistance of Chapter 10 some judicious hopping between chapters will allow for a chronological overview of Bowie's career.

Key figures in Bowie's work are introduced with a thumbnail biography at the point of their first significant collaboration; for example, Tony Visconti is introduced in Chapter 1's entry on 'Let Me Sleep Beside You', and Brian Eno in Chapter 2's entry on *Low*.

Chapter 1 uses the abbreviations set out below. Cross-referencing with Chapter 11's discography will yield full details of single releases.

The date (month/year) of each single release is followed where applicable by the highest UK chart placing in square brackets. "Compilation" listings are only given if this was the first official release of the track, or if the version in question is otherwise unavailable on a major album release. Likewise soundtrack albums are only cited in Chapter 1 if they contain exclusive material. "Bonus" listings refer to the extra tracks included on EMI/Rykodisc's 1990-1992 reissues of the albums from *Space Oddity* to *Scary Monsters*, and Virgin's 1995 reissues of the albums from *Let's Dance* to *Tin Machine*. EMI's more recent multi-disc anniversary reissues of albums like *Ziggy Stardust*, *Aladdin Sane*, *Diamond Dogs* and *Black Tie White Noise* are referred to in Chapter 1's abbreviations as *Ziggy (2002)*, *Aladdin (2003)* and so on. Songs available on commercial video releases are also included, subdivided into "Video" and "Live Video".

SAMPLE ENTRY

MOONAGE DAYDREAM
• A-Side: 5/71 • Album: *Ziggy* • Live: *David, Motion, SM72* • Bonus: *Man, Ziggy (2002)* • B-Side: 2/96 [12] • Live Video: *Ziggy*

This tells us that 'Moonage Daydream' was released, in chronological order, as (i) a single A-side in May 1971, which did not chart; (ii) an album track on *Ziggy Stardust*; (iii) live versions on *David Live*, *Ziggy Stardust: The Motion Picture* and *Santa Monica '72*; (iv) a bonus track on the Rykodisc reissue of *The Man Who Sold The World* and the 2002 EMI reissue of *Ziggy Stardust*; (v) the B-side of a February 1996 single which peaked at number 12 in the UK chart; (vi) and, finally, a live version can be seen on the video/DVD release *Ziggy Stardust And The Spiders From Mars*.

ABBREVIATIONS USED IN CHAPTER 1

Studio Albums

Bowie	*David Bowie*
Oddity	*Space Oddity*
Man	*The Man Who Sold The World*
Hunky	*Hunky Dory*
Ziggy	*The Rise and Fall of Ziggy Stardust and the Spiders From Mars*
Aladdin	*Aladdin Sane*
Pin	*Pin Ups*
Dogs	*Diamond Dogs*
Americans	*Young Americans*
Station	*Station To Station*
Low	*Low*
"Heroes"	*"Heroes"*
Lodger	*Lodger*
Scary	*Scary Monsters (And Super Creeps)*
Dance	*Let's Dance*
Tonight	*Tonight*

Never	*Never Let Me Down*
TM	*Tin Machine*
TM2	*Tin Machine II*
Black	*Black Tie White Noise*
Buddha	*The Buddha of Suburbia*
1.Outside	*1.Outside*
Earthling	*Earthling*
'hours…'	*'hours…'*
Heathen	*Heathen*
Reality	*Reality*

Live Albums

David	*David Live*
Stage	*Stage*
Motion	*Ziggy Stardust: The Motion Picture*
Oy	*Tin Machine Live: Oy Vey, Baby*
SM72	*Santa Monica '72*
liveandwell.com	*liveandwell.com*
Beeb	*Bowie At The Beeb (bonus disc)*

Compilations

Early	*Early On (1964-1966)*
Manish	*The Manish Boys/Davy Jones and the Lower Third*
Rare	*Bowie Rare*
Tuesday	*Love You Till Tuesday*
S+V	*Sound + Vision*
S+V (2003)	*Sound + Vision [expanded 2003 reissue]*
SinglesUK	*The Singles Collection*
SinglesUS	*The Singles 1969 to 1993 [US version of the above]*
Rarest	*RarestOneBowie*
BBC	*BBC Sessions 1969-1972 (Sampler)*
Deram	*The Deram Anthology 1966-1968*
69/74	*The Best Of David Bowie 1969/1974*
74/79	*The Best Of David Bowie 1974/1979*
Beeb	*Bowie At The Beeb*
Saints	*All Saints: Collected Instrumentals 1977-1999*
Ziggy (2002)	*The Rise and Fall of Ziggy Stardust and the Spiders From Mars [2002 reissue]*

Best Of Bowie	*Best Of Bowie*
Aladdin (2003)	*Aladdin Sane [2003 reissue]*
Black (2003)	*Black Tie White Noise [2003 reissue]*
Club	*Club Bowie*
Dogs (2004)	*Diamond Dogs [2004 reissue]*

Video & DVD

Tuesday	*Love You Till Tuesday*
Ziggy	*Ziggy Stardust And The Spiders From Mars*
EP	*David Bowie Video EP*
Moonlight	*Serious Moonlight*
Ricochet	*Ricochet*
Glass	*Glass Spider*
Oy	*Oy Vey, Baby – Tin Machine Live At The Docks*
Black	*Black Tie White Noise*
Collection	*The Video Collection*
Best Of Bowie	*Best Of Bowie*
Reality	*Reality (Tour Edition DVD)*

A NOTE ON THE TEXT

Where spellings and stylings of song and album titles vary over the years, I have favoured the earliest official release: hence, for example, 'It's No Game (No. 1)', rather than 'It's No Game (Part 1)'. I have preserved various grammatically challenging offerings ('The Hearts Filthy Lesson', 'Thru' These Architects Eyes') as on the official releases, and have remained faithful to such vagaries as the three different variations of "rock and roll" to be found in the correct spellings of 'Rock'n'Roll Suicide', 'Rock'n Roll With Me' and 'You Belong In Rock N'Roll'.

The one exception is my decision to refer to Bowie's 1969 album as *Space Oddity* throughout this book. Originally released in Britain as *David Bowie* and in America as *Man Of Words/Man Of Music*, it was renamed *Space Oddity* in 1972. I have opted for the latter, its official title for more than three decades, simply to avoid confusion with 1967's *David Bowie*.

1 the songs from a to z

This chapter covers songs written, recorded, covered, produced or played live by David Bowie, either by himself or for other artists. Except in cases of exceptional interest, I have restricted myself to material from 1964 – i.e. The King Bees – onwards. Some Bowie books have cited long lists of numbers mooted for Bowie's 1968 cabaret act; I have restricted myself to those David actually rehearsed,

omitting the many that never went further than Kenneth Pitt's notebook. Where appropriate, prominent cover versions of Bowie's songs are mentioned, but I make no attempt to include every last one; among those I have elected to ignore are covers found on "tribute albums" recorded by obscure bands.

ABDULMAJID
• Bonus: *"Heroes"* • Compilation: *Saints*

Mixed in 1991 for release as a bonus track, this Eastern-influenced instrumental (dating either from the *Low* or *"Heroes"* sessions) was renamed in honour of Bowie's fiancée Iman Muhammid Abdulmajid. Its original title, if there was one, is unknown. 'Abdulmajid' provides the basis for the second movement of Philip Glass's 1997 *"Heroes" Symphony*.

ABSOLUTE BEGINNERS
• A-Side: 3/86 [2] • Soundtrack: *Absolute Beginners* • Bonus: *Tonight* • Live: *Beeb* • Video: *Collection, Best Of Bowie* • Live Video: *Glass*

In June 1985 a group of session musicians working with Thomas Dolby at Abbey Road received letters from EMI inviting them to work on a session with "Mr X". This unorthodox overture turned out to be from David Bowie, who had approached producers Alan Winstanley and Clive Langer with the demo of 'Absolute Beginners'. Former Prefab Sprout guitarist Kevin Armstrong, for whom this was the beginning of a sporadic ten-year working relationship, explained that Bowie "came in with the song 'Absolute Beginners' half written. The whole band helped out, whether it was a missing chord or a rhyme for the last verse. Over an afternoon it evolved into the backing track, which we recorded. That's how Bowie operated

– from the germ of an idea, which the group polished up into the master. Once he saw what we could do, he relaxed. We fitted."

'Absolute Beginners', the title song for the film then in pre-production, was completed at a breakneck pace. "David liked to work at top speed," recalled ex-Soft Boys and Thompson Twins bassist Matthew Seligman. "He said he loved the Abbey Road session, which reminded him of *"Heroes"*." Laid down during the same sessions were Bowie's other contributions to the *Absolute Beginners* soundtrack, 'Volare' and 'That's Motivation'.

Blasted along in a breezy 1950s doo-wop style with some exhilarating swoops of guitar, pounding piano from *Hunky Dory* veteran Rick Wakeman ("Rachmaninov-style," in his words), and a triumphant saxophone sound that Bowie spent much time failing to capture elsewhere during the mid-1980s, 'Absolute Beginners' isn't merely an above-average effort from a lean period; it's one of the all-time great Bowie recordings. When it was released in March 1986 it shot up the chart to number 2, denied pole position by Diana Ross's 'Chain Reaction' but staying in the top ten for a month. It remains David's biggest hit since 'Let's Dance'.

Julien Temple's video, shot in monochrome on Westminster Bridge and the Thames Embankment, is a pastiche of the 1950s "You're never alone with a Strand" cigarette commercial. Cutting a dash in trench-coat and fedora, Bowie runs out of "Zebra" cigarettes and makes for the nearest slot-machine, only to find his movements shadowed by a foxy dancer decked out in zebra-striped make-up. He chases her down to the Thames and they kiss, only for the girl to disappear and leave just a burning cigarette stub. Interspersed are colour images from *Absolute Beginners* itself. The eight-minute cut of the video was used to trail the movie in British cinemas, sparking a few complaints from cinemagoers alarmed by the riot scenes towards the end. This is the version that appears on *Best Of Bowie*.

In addition to the 7" edit, the excellent full-length version of 'Absolute Beginners' was released on 12" and CD, an instrumental 'Dub Mix' forming the B-side of all formats. The film itself features different edits from those released on disc: the main title is only 2'18" while the closing version runs to 6'56". Meanwhile a re-orchestrated instrumental version, which appears on the soundtrack album as 'Absolute Beginners (Refrain)', was performed by Gil Evans. Bowie performed 'Absolute Beginners' throughout the Glass Spider tour, and resurrected the number for his summer 2000 concerts and the Heathen tour. A superb live version recorded at the BBC Radio Theatre on 27 June 2000 appears on the *Bowie At The Beeb* bonus disc.

ACROSS THE UNIVERSE (*Lennon/McCartney*)
• Album: *Americans*

Bowie's blue-eyed soul reworking of the Beatles number (from their 1970 album *Let It Be*) was recorded at New York's Electric Lady Studios in January 1975, with John Lennon contributing vocals and guitar. Recorded on the same day as 'Fame' it was apparently intended as a warm-up track but, bowled over by the Lennon collaboration, David made room for it on *Young Americans* by dropping other numbers. "I thought, great," said Lennon later, "because I'd never done a good version of that song myself. It's one of my favourite songs, but I didn't like my version of it." David concurred, rather immodestly telling the *NME* in 1975 that The Beatles' original version "was fabulous, but very watery in the original, and I hammered the hell out of it. Not many people like it. I like it a lot and I think I sing very well at the end of it."

In 1997 Bowie chose The Beatles' original version as one of his all-time favourite recordings in an article for *Guitar Player*. "It's a portrait of the spiritual heart of where Lennon was at, really," he explained, "the por-

trait of a spiritually confused but incredibly philanthropic man. Just a spectacular mind at work there. A genuine intellectual who didn't talk in the vocabulary of an intellectual." Bowie has never played 'Across The Universe' live, although in 1983 he briefly considered performing the song on the last night of the Serious Moonlight tour as a tribute to Lennon, who had died three years earlier to the day. In the event, he decided to go the whole hog and sing 'Imagine'.

AFRAID
• Album: *Heathen*

Originally recorded for inclusion on *Toy* and later revamped for *Heathen*, 'Afraid' received its first public airing on 2 November 2000 when David and Mark Plati performed a live version during a BowieNet webcast. Unlike its fellow *Toy* casualty 'Slip Away', which was entirely re-recorded during the *Heathen* sessions, 'Afraid' makes use of the original *Toy* backing track recorded and produced by Bowie and Plati, although in David's words the recording was extensively "groomed" to suit the style of the new material. "I had always liked the version of 'Afraid' that I did with Mark Plati," he explained in 2002, "so Tony and I got him to do a little more work on his guitar parts so that it would be more in line with the rest of the album, Tony again playing bass. Then Tony mixed it."

Setting an energetic New Wave rhythm backing against a trademark Tony Visconti string arrangement and a retro-1970s 'Popcorn' synthesizer break, 'Afraid' is one of *Heathen*'s more upbeat numbers. It's a familiar meditation on personal insecurity and the fear of individuality, with a lyric that strongly recalls 'I Can't Read' (in particular the 1997 re-recording, whose reworded lyrics are echoed in the final chorus: "If I can smile a crooked smile / If I can talk on television / If I can walk an empty mile"). It also features one of Bowie's occasional John Lennon paraphrases, as he removes the "don't" from Lennon's 'God' to insist that "I believe in Beatles".

"I guess it's supposed to be an ironic song," David explained. "It's, 'Well, if I do everything I'm told to do, and I do it the way everybody expects things to be done, then I won't be afraid of anything.' He doesn't really want to do things like that." In this respect the song revisits the themes of 'Jump They Say', which David had once described as being about "whether you should stay with the crowd", but despite its obvious empathy with earlier compositions Bowie suggested that 'Afraid' was "probably the one song on the album that I don't see as being representative of me," explaining that the protagonist "believes that his security will be bought if he plays the game, so to speak … it's an interesting deceit, but it's not mine."

In November 2001 America's XM Radio ran an advertisement featuring an excerpt from 'Afraid', which was subsequently performed throughout the Heathen and A Reality tours.

AFRICAN NIGHT FLIGHT (Bowie/Eno)
• Album: *Lodger*

In February 1978 Bowie went on safari to Kenya with his six-year-old son Joe. His meeting with the Masai tribespeople sparked an immediate interest in the music of the subcontinent and, as he told an American interviewer shortly afterwards, "I intend going back. I haven't finished there … I wanted to understand what I was seeing and what I was dealing with before I was presumptuous enough to start recording anything."

In Mombasa Bowie was fascinated to meet maverick German fighter pilots who drank away their hours in local bars and felt unable to return to the fatherland. "You've got a good idea why they are there in the first place," he said, "but they live strange lives, flying about in their Cessnas over the bushland, doing all kinds of strange things. They're very mysterious characters, permanently plastered and always talking about when they are going to leave. The song came about because I was wondering exactly what they were doing there and why they flew around."

The instrumental backing of 'African Night Flight' was recorded at Mountain Studios in September 1978, forming the beginning of *Lodger*'s quirky musical journey through ethnic diversity. Over a backing of eccentric clattering percussion, warbling keyboards, Swahili chanting and ambient safari sounds (Brian Eno, whose 1975 album *Another Green World* provides an obvious template, is memorably credited on this track with "cricket menace"), Bowie's quickfire vocal is a bizarre, almost rap-like patter of disconnected barroom thoughts: "Getting in mood for a Mombasa night flight, pushing my luck, gonna fly like a mad thing, Bare-strip take-off, skimming over rhino…" He later explained that the musical backing was based around Dale Hawkins's 1957 song 'Suzie Q', played

backwards: "Then Brian decided to put prepared piano on it. He put pairs of scissors and all kinds of metal things on the strings of the piano." The result is terrifically weird, and weirdly terrific.

AFTER ALL
• Album: *Man*

Far removed from the hard rock sounds that permeate much of its parent album, 'After All' is a whispering fairground waltz, awash with hallucinatory overdubs paying obvious homage to The Beatles' 'Being For the Benefit of Mr Kite!'. The lyric covers familiar early Bowie territory – paranoia, inadequacy and isolation – in an intensely withdrawn style reeking of suburban repression. When he advises us to "forget all I've said, please bear me no ill" it's as though he's disowning the idealistic posture of his previous album, and it takes no great leap of the imagination to read the line "we're painting our faces and dressing in thoughts from the skies" as a rallying-call for Bowie's disillusioned hippy aftermath to forge a new society of glammed-up pretty things.

There are echoes of the closeted innocence of Bowie's early song 'There Is A Happy Land', although this time "paradise" has a darker twist: "some sit in silence, they're just older children, that's all." The pondering on "rebirth" and "impermanence" recalls the Buddhist themes of his earlier work, but here the effect is chilling rather than revelatory. The line "live till your rebirth and do what you will" bridges Bowie's journey between Buddha and Aleister Crowley, whose credo of "Do what thou wilt shall be the whole of the law" was his justification for the dissolution of universal morality.

The multi-octave chorus of cartoon voices chanting "oh by jingo" is another dark reprise of the more experimental tracks from the Deram period, also resembling the sinister vocal effects deployed on 'All The Madmen' and 'The Bewlay Brothers'. Like them it's an outstanding song, and certainly one of Bowie's most underrated recordings.

Unusually, the recording began with David's acoustic guitar and vocals, followed later by the rhythm track and bassline. Tony Visconti revealed that he and Mick Ronson hijacked 'After All' during the mixing stage: "The basic song and the 'oh by jingo' line were David's ideas. The rest was Ronno and me vying for the next overdub. I love that track."

'After All' has been covered by Human Drama (on their 1993 album *Pin Ups*, whose sleeve photo apes that of Bowie's *Pin Ups* and also features a cover of 'Letter To Hermione'), and by Tori Amos on the B-side of her 2001 single 'Strange Little Girl'.

AFTER LIGHTS *(Ralphs)* : see **READY FOR LOVE**

AFTER TODAY
• Compilation: *S+V*

Two versions of 'After Today' were taped during the *Young Americans* sessions at Sigma Sound in August 1974, one of which was eventually released on *Sound + Vision*. "There was a completely different take of that song," confirmed Rykodisc's Jeff Rougvie, "Very slow, like a soul ballad – but we preferred the one we used." The released take of 'After Today' (which, unlike the completed "ballad" version, required mixing by Rykodisc), is a buoyant soul-disco number distinguished by an outrageously ambitious falsetto vocal, at the end of which David chuckles, "I was getting into that!" It's a great song, albeit rough-edged alongside the highly polished album from which it was dropped.

AIN'T NO SUNSHINE *(Withers)*

The 1971 Bill Withers single (a hit the following year for a young Michael Jackson) was included in David's medley with the host of *The Cher Show* in November 1975.

AL ALBA : see **DAY-IN DAY-OUT**

ALABAMA SONG *(Brecht/Weill)*
• A-Side: 2/80 [23] • Bonus: *Scary, Stage*

Originally from the 1930 Brecht/Weill opera *The Rise and Fall of the City of Mahagonny* (not, as often claimed, from *The Threepenny Opera*), 'Alabama Song' was immortalized by Weill's wife Lotte Lenya, the Austrian actress and singer whose famously expressionless rendition patented the song's burned-out sense of decadence and alienation. The song was later popularized in English translation by The Doors.

Long before Bowie's performance in *Baal*, Bertolt Brecht had assumed a significant position among his creative influences; in 1978 there was even talk of David starring in a film remake of *The Threepenny Opera*. 'Alabama Song' first entered his repertoire on the 1978 tour, from which a live version appeared on the 1992 reissue of *Stage*. On 2 July 1978, the day after the tour's European leg ended, Bowie's magnificent studio version of 'Alabama Song' was recorded at Tony Visconti's Good Earth Studio in London. "It had been such a hit on the tour that David wanted to do it as a single," explained pianist Sean Mayes, who also recalled that "David had some new ideas for the drumming. He wanted Dennis [Davis] to play very freely against the rhythm to give an unstable, insane atmosphere to the track. When we tried to do this it proved hilariously difficult so we finally laid the backing down without drums then Dennis overdubbed his demolishing attack when his efforts couldn't disturb the beat."

The studio version was eventually released as a single in 1980, by which time *Lodger* had come and gone and Bowie was already working on *Scary Monsters*. Boasting a fold-out poster sleeve and backed by the new acoustic rendering of 'Space Oddity' heard on *Kenny Everett's New Year's Eve Show*, the single reached number 23, no mean achievement for one of the most defiantly uncommercial, discordant and aggressive recordings Bowie has ever released. The message "Ta Kurt" was scratched into the single's play-out vinyl. The studio version later appeared on *Bowie Rare* and, misleadingly, on 1992's reissue of *Scary Monsters*.

'Alabama Song' was resurrected for the Sound + Vision and Heathen tours, a fine performance appearing in the BBC radio session of 18 September 2002.

ALADDIN SANE (1913-1938-197?)
• Album: *Aladdin* • Live: *David*

Usually documented without the parenthesis, 'Aladdin Sane (1913-1938-197?)' was inspired by Evelyn Waugh's 1930 novel *Vile Bodies*. David wrote the song in December 1972, en route to London aboard the RHMS *Ellinis* at the end of his first US tour – in keeping with the album's style, the label appends "RHMS *Ellinis*" alongside the title. "The book dealt with London in the period just before a massive, imaginary war," Bowie explained in 1973. "People were frivolous, decadent and silly. And suddenly they were plunged into this horrendous holocaust. They were totally out of place, still thinking about champagne and parties and dressing up. Somehow it seemed to me that they were like people today." The dates in brackets, alluding to the years prior to the outbreak of the world wars and pointing ominously to the imminence of the next, place the song firmly in Bowie's milieu of eschatological sci-fi. He explained that it tackled "feelings of imminent catastrophe which, at the point in America when I was writing, I felt."

The defining feature is Mike Garson's stunning, deranged piano solo, which hints at Gershwin's *Rhapsody in Blue* as it does battle with Trevor Bolder's relentless bassline. Garson described the solo as "dissonant, rebellious, atonal, and very *outside*," an interesting choice of adjective to which Bowie himself would return more than once. Garson's early attempts at the solo involved more traditional structures – a blues motif, then a Latin one – but Bowie rejected both and asked him to let rip in the style of the avant-garde jazz clubs Garson had played in the 1960s. In his contemporary review of *Aladdin Sane*, Ben Gerson of *Rolling Stone* summed up the complementary effect on Bowie's "images of earlier, more romantic wars. The impatient chug of the machine (the electric guitar) gently clashes with the wilder, more extreme flailings of a dying culture (the piano)." The collision of signifiers is heightened by Bowie's interpolation of a line from the old Lieber/Stoller/Weill standard 'On Broadway' just as Garson's solo moves into top gear. Garson later recalled his contribution, which was recorded in one take, as "a strange, dissonant solo, one of those streaks of luck and magic. I had difficulty trying to imitate it on the road later."

'Aladdin Sane' received its live premiere in February 1973 with the start of Bowie's second American tour. It became a more frequent fixture on the following year's Diamond Dogs tour, from which a fine version appears on *David Live*. Thereafter the song remained unheard until 1996 when, with Garson once more on board to recreate the piano solo, it was added to the set for the Summer Festivals tour. Bassist Gail Ann Dorsey shared vocal duties with Bowie on the tour renditions and on the pared-down acoustic version later unveiled at the Bridge School benefit shows in October 1996, while a new studio recording, also featuring Dorsey on vocals, was recorded for the *ChangesNowBowie* BBC session.

Emergency Broadcast Network's 1996 album *Telecommunication Breakdown*, featuring guest keyboardist Brian Eno, included a track called 'Homicidal Schizophrenic (A Lad Insane)' which used samples from the original Bowie track.

ALADDIN VEIN : see ZION

ALI (Bowie/Deacon/May/Mercury/Rogers/Taylor) : see COOL CAT

ALL DAY AND ALL OF THE NIGHT (Davies)

During performances of 'Aladdin Sane' on the 1996 Summer Festivals tour (notably at the Loreley Festival on 22 June), Bowie would occasionally interpolate a snatch of The Kinks' 1964 hit.

ALL SAINTS (Bowie/Eno)
• Bonus: *Low* • Compilation: *Saints*

A driving, sinister instrumental out-take probably dating from the *Low* sessions, 'All Saints' was mixed in 1991 for release as a bonus track. Like 'Abdulmajid', the track was left untitled at the time of recording, and was named 'All Saints' after Brian Eno's record label. It should be noted, however, that the composition is believed to hark back to David's attempt to score *The Man Who Fell To Earth* in 1975, the year of cocaine madness in which he became temporarily fixated on the idea that he was going to be attacked by witches on All Saints' Eve. *All Saints* subsequently became the title of an ultra-rare compilation of instrumental tracks compiled by Bowie in 1993 as a Christmas present for friends and colleagues, a revised version of which received an official release in 2001.

ALL THE MADMEN
• Album: *Man* • US Promo: 12/70 • Soundtrack: *Mayor Of The Sunset Strip*

With its menacing alternation of soft-spoken whimsy and explosive rock guitar, 'All The Madmen' declares its subject matter via musical schizophrenia as much as through its haunting lyric. It's commonly accepted that the narrator is inspired by Bowie's half-brother Terry Burns, who by 1970 was confined to south London's Cane Hill Hospital, the forbidding edifice recalled in the "mansions cold and grey" of the song's opening lines and portrayed on the cover artwork of the album's American release. David would confirm in 1972 that the song was "written for my brother and it's about my brother." The quietly chilling spoken section, in which Bowie asserts that "a nation hides its organic minds in a cellar," directly echoes a comment he had made in an interview for the *Times* a year earlier about mental illness being hidden away "in the servants' quarters".

But despite its horror-comic trappings, Bowie's lyric significantly concludes that "all the madmen" are "just as sane as me". He would rather stay and play with them than with "the sadmen roaming free", once more aligning himself with society's non-conformists, outcasts and lost boys. David has often cited Jack Kerouac's 1957 beat classic *On The Road* as a seminal influence introduced to him by his brother, and the similarity with one of the book's key passages can be no coincidence: "The only people for me are the mad ones, the ones who are mad to live, mad to talk, mad to be saved, desirous of everything at the same time, the ones who never yawn or say a commonplace thing, but burn, burn, burn like fabulous yellow Roman candles." So 'All The Madmen' is not only a horror story about social exclusion, but a virtual mission statement for the creative and spiritual frenzy of Bowie's muse in the early 1970s.

In common with much of the parent album, the arrangements are largely the work of Mick Ronson, who plays both synthesizer and guitar. Despite rumours of a second cut mixed at Trident in August 1970, featuring different percussion and omitting the song's central spoken passage, the so-called alternate version that has appeared on bootlegs is almost certainly a fake. In December 1970 a heavily edited promo single was pressed by Mercury for circulation in America prior to Bowie's first promotional visit, during which he gave impromptu solo performances of the song on acoustic guitar; an atrociously recorded extract of one such rendition has appeared on bootlegs, and was later segued with the original studio version on the 2004 soundtrack album of the Rodney Bingenheimer biopic *Mayor Of The Sunset Strip*. A US single backed by 'Janine' was also pressed in December 1970, but this was withdrawn and is now extremely rare.

The song's unhinged closing chant of "Zane, Zane, Zane, Ouvrez le chien" was reprised 23 years later in Bowie's throwback song 'Buddha Of Suburbia'. A giant mobile reading "Ouvrez le Chien" hung over the stage on the 1995 Outside tour, although 'All The Madmen' wasn't on the set-list. Its only major live outing was for 1987's Glass Spider tour, although sadly it fails to appear on the video release.

ALL THE YOUNG DUDES
• Compilation: *Rarest, 69/74* • Bonus: *Aladdin (2003)*
• Live: *Motion, David* • Live Video: *Ziggy, The Freddie Mercury Tribute Concert*

'All The Young Dudes' was Bowie's gift to Mott The Hoople, a small-time rock outfit who had emerged in 1969 when Guy Stevens, the manager of a Herefordshire band called Silence, replaced their original vocalist with pianist/singer Ian Hunter. Re-named Mott The Hoople after a novel by Willard Manus, the band scraped the lower reaches of the chart with a string of albums, but despite a loyal following on the live circuit they failed to make a substantial breakthrough. Even an appearance on *Top Of The Pops* in late 1971 failed to push their 'Midnight Lady' single into the charts, and the band was on the point of splitting when it crossed paths with Bowie in March 1972.

Although he was already on the road with the Ziggy Stardust tour David's own breakthrough was still far from guaranteed. He was continuing to tout new compositions around other artists, and had sent Mott The Hoople a demo of 'Suffragette City' earlier in the year. Mott's bassist Pete "Overend" Watts recalled: "He'd scrawled on the box, 'This might be of some use to you, would you like to cover it?' We played it and didn't think it was quite right." Watts called Bowie "and said, 'Thanks very much for the tape, we won't be needing it because we've split up. And he sounded genuinely upset ... He called me back two hours later and said he'd spoken to Tony Defries, his manager at MainMan, who would try to get us out of the position we were in. He said, 'Also, I've written a song for you since we spoke, which could be great.'" David met Watts a few days later. "Bowie played me this song, 'All The Young Dudes', on his acoustic guitar. He hadn't got all the words but the song just blew me away, especially when he hit the chorus." Watts wasted no time introducing Bowie to the rest of the band, and while Defries set about negotiating a new deal with

CBS, Bowie introduced them to 'All The Young Dudes'. "We couldn't believe it," said drummer Dale Griffin. "In the office at Regent Street he's strumming it on his guitar and I'm thinking, he wants to give us that? He must be crazy! We broke our necks to say yes! You couldn't fail to see it was a great song."

'All The Young Dudes' was to become not only the saviour of the band but a standard-bearer for Bowie's own brand of rock. Mott The Hoople's definitive version, produced by Bowie and Mick Ronson, was recorded at Olympic Studios on 14 May 1972. "It was a high," said Ian Hunter of the session, "Because we knew we were singing a hit." He was right: the single was released in August and peaked at number 3 in the UK chart in early September, a fortnight before Bowie released 'John, I'm Only Dancing'. It went on to provide the title of the group's fifth album, produced by Bowie and Ronson at Trident during the summer. Both The Spiders and Mott The Hoople toured the US during the autumn of 1972, and Bowie boosted Mott's profile by introducing their gig and joining them for the number at the Tower, Philadelphia on 29 November. This performance was released on the 1998 Mott compilation *All The Way From Stockholm To Philadelphia*.

'All The Young Dudes' is invariably glossed as the definitive glam anthem, a three-minute glorification of the new generation's hot-tramp aesthetic, personified by the boy in the lyric who "dresses like a queen, but he can kick like a mule" while his "brother's back at home with his Beatles and his Stones". There's an obvious echo of The Who's 'My Generation' in the line "Don't want to stay alive when you're twenty-five", making 'All The Young Dudes' a rallying-cry for the disaffected children of Heath's Britain, a newly reactionary landscape of anti-permissive values and moral rearmament. The less frequently quoted line following the one about the Beatles and the Stones is even more explicit in its joyous trashing of the 1960s: "We never got it off on that revolution stuff / What a drag, too many snags."

Released at the height of Bowie's "bisexual" period, the song has also been read as a gay-lib manifesto, a shot across the bows of the bigots' belief that homosexuality has no meaning beyond the physical act itself: "We can love, we can really love", it admonishes, and Ian Hunter admitted that the song was seized as an anthem "by the closet gays". But according to Bowie 'All The Young Dudes' was a darker affair, bound up in the apocalyptic sci-fi parable of *Ziggy*

Stardust. Outlining the plot for *Rolling Stone* in 1973, David explained that the bulletin of imminent Armageddon revealed by the "news guy" in 'Five Years' was the same news carried by the Dudes: "'All The Young Dudes' is a song about this news. It is no hymn to the youth as people thought. It is completely the opposite."

During the *Aladdin Sane* sessions Bowie recorded his own studio version, curiously restrained and in every way inferior to Mott's (Bowie had written a great song, but it was Mott The Hoople's embellishments, in particular Hunter's delicious spoken outro, that made the single a classic). Although shortlisted for *Aladdin Sane* this version didn't see the light of day until 1995's *RarestOneBowie*, in a different mix from the one that has appeared on bootleg releases. This version subsequently appeared on *The Best Of David Bowie 1969/1974* and the 2003 reissue of *Aladdin Sane*. Meanwhile Bowie's original 3'58" guide demo for Ian Hunter has appeared on bootlegs and, remixed with the backing track of Mott The Hoople's finished version, was released in the 1998 box set *All The Young Dudes: The Anthology*.

Bowie added 'All The Young Dudes' to The Spiders' live set at the Earls Court gig on 12 May 1973, incorporating it into a medley with 'Wild Eyed Boy From Freecloud' and 'Oh! You Pretty Things'. The song reappeared on the Diamond Dogs tour, from which a version appears on *David Live*. The chorus melody of 'All The Young Dudes' was later incorporated into Peter Frampton's guitar rendition of 'Time' on the Glass Spider tour, and the song was resurrected in its entirety on the 1996 summer tour. "It is a trigger for all the real, fabulous unity that used to be a part of the late Ziggy shows," said David at the time, "and it does sort of come flooding back." It came flooding back once again for the June 2000 live shows, and the song made numerous reappearances on A Reality Tour.

For Mott The Hoople, 'All The Young Dudes' was a mixed blessing. It revived their fortunes, kick-started their chart career and bought them their place in the annals of rock, but in doing so it utterly overshadowed anything else they achieved. "I remember going to get a pizza with David Bowie while we were recording the album at Trident," recalled keyboardist Verden Allen. "His record 'Starman' was on the jukebox while we were waiting, and he said, 'Yours will be on there soon.' I said, 'Yeah, great, but for some reason I'm not as excited as I would have been if it had come from the band.' And he said, 'I know what you mean.'" Then again, without 'All The Young Dudes' few would ever have heard of Mott The Hoople. "We owe a big debt to David, because without it, I think we'd have been finished," said Ian Hunter many years later. "You can say it might have had an adverse effect on the band's image, but without it there wouldn't have been a band: simple as that."

Mott, and latterly Ian Hunter, continued to play the song in concert; versions appear on various live albums. For sheer nostalgia value, the greatest live performance was the one that reunited Bowie, Ronson and Hunter for the Freddie Mercury Tribute concert at Wembley Stadium on 20 April 1992. This rendition later became the closing track on Ronson's posthumous solo album *Heaven And Hull*, and Hunter performed the number once again at 1994's Mick Ronson memorial concert.

One of the most influential Bowie compositions, 'All The Young Dudes' has been covered by numerous acts including The Damned, Billy Bragg, The Skids (on their 1979 single 'Working For The Yankee Dollar'), the Chanter Sisters (on 1976's *First Flight*), Morgan Fisher (on 1984's *Ivories*), Catherine's Cathedral (on *Equilibrium*), Bruce Dickinson (on 1990's *Tattooed Millionaire*), Carl Wallinger (for the soundtrack of the 1995 movie *Clueless*) and Travis, whose live version appeared on the B-side of their 2001 single 'Side'. Oasis blatantly lifted the unmistakable syncopated chorus bar for their 1997 hit 'Stand By Me', while Marvelous 3's 'Cigarette Lighter Love Song', a track on their 2000 album *ReadySexGo*, reused sections of 'All The Young Dudes' and duly gave Bowie a songwriting credit.

ALL YOU NEED IS LOVE *(Lennon/McCartney)*

The Beatles classic was included in Bowie's ill-fated 1968 cabaret package.

ALMOST GROWN *(Berry)*
• Live: *Beeb*

Chuck Berry's 1959 hit made a one-off live appearance for Bowie's BBC radio session on 3 June 1971, in a recording which now appears on *Bowie At The Beeb*. The performance saw David sharing vocals with his old schoolmate Geoffrey Alexander, later to make his mark on the Bowie canon under the names Geoffrey

MacCormack and Warren Peace. 'Almost Grown' was dropped from Bowie's repertoire in favour of Berry's 'Round And Round' as the *Ziggy Stardust* sessions loomed large.

ALWAYS CRASHING IN THE SAME CAR
• Album: *Low* • Live: *Beeb*

Recorded at Hansa in November 1976, 'Always Crashing In The Same Car' was a late addition to the *Low* set. Tony Visconti recalled that "David spent quite a while writing the melody and lyrics, and even recorded a verse in a quasi-Dylan voice. But it was too spooky (not funny, as intended), so he asked me to erase it and we started again."

The lyrics make direct reference to an unfortunate incident in which David drunkenly wrote off his 1950s Mercedes while recklessly negotiating an underground parking-lot in Berlin (according to the song, "I was just going round and round the hotel garage, must have been touching close to 94"). But on a wider scale the song operates as a metaphor for Bowie's convulsive career swings, lifestyle changes and obsessive travelling ("every chance that I take, I take it on the road"). As metaphors go it's a succinct one, consisting of a mere two verses; typically of *Low*, Bowie's sense of his own underachievement provides a sharp contrast with the sublime accomplishment of the track itself, a beautifully crafted and spine-chilling slice of self-doubt and paranoia.

'Always Crashing In The Same Car' made its live debut twenty years later on the American leg of the Earthling tour, during which a stripped-down acoustic guitar version was performed for a number of US radio sessions. The song was revived in an atmospheric rearrangement for guitars and piano on some of the summer 2000 dates and again on the Heathen and A Reality tours. An excellent live version recorded at the BBC Radio Theatre on 27 June 2000 was included on the *Bowie At The Beeb* bonus disc.

AMAZING *(Bowie/Gabrels)*
• Album: *TM* • Live: *Oy*

One of the better songs on the first Tin Machine album and certainly the most underrated, 'Amazing' is a simple, laid-back love ballad (perhaps addressed to David's then girlfriend Melissa Hurley) on which a rare absence of cacophonous drumming allows for a lush build-up of textured guitar atmospherics, including some wonderfully evocative seagull-like squeals in the opening bars. The mood is one of unabashed optimism ("Since I found you, my life's amazing"), and it's delivered in winning style. 'Amazing' was performed live during both Tin Machine tours, on the first of which it was usually the opening number. A live version appears on *Oy Vey, Baby*.

AMERICA *(Simon)*
• Live: *The Concert For New York City* • Live Video: *The Concert For New York City*

On 20 October 2001, Bowie opened the epic-length World Trade Centre benefit concert at Madison Square Garden with a fragile and appropriately resonant performance of Simon and Garfunkel's meditation on the American dream, originally found on their 1968 album *Bookends*. "I was looking for something which really evoked feelings of bewilderment and uncertainty," David later explained, "because for me that's how that particular period really felt. And I really thought that Paul Simon's song in this new context really captured that." The performance, which surely ranks as one of Bowie's most evocative live moments, is now available on the CD and DVD of the event. On 30 May 2002 David reprised 'America', this time to the accompaniment of a pre-recorded backing track, at a charity auction at Manhattan's Javits Center on behalf of the Robin Hood Foundation.

AMERICAN DREAM *(Combs/Bowie/Winans/ Gibson/Cioffe/Ross/Curry/Metheny/Mays)*
• Soundtrack: *Training Day*

Bowie recorded his vocal for P Diddy's radical reworking of 'This Is Not America' at Daddy's House Studio, New York, in July 2001. See 'This Is Not America' for further details.

AMLAPURA *(Bowie/Gabrels)*
• B-Side: 8/91 [33] • Album: *TM2* • Live Video: *Oy*

For the gentlest moment on *Tin Machine II* Bowie revisits Indonesia, but with very different results from 1984's 'Tumble And Twirl'. Amlapura, a region of Bali

he had visited on a holiday just prior to the sessions, was the location of a catastrophic volcanic eruption in 1963. Here Bowie softly evokes the region's ancient sites ("golden roses round a rajah's mouth … a princess in stone") and its tragic history ("all the dead children buried standing"). The slow acoustic strum is strongly reminiscent of the 1971 version of 'The Supermen', while Reeves Gabrels contributes a wistful, Moody Blues-style electric solo. It's a slight song that would benefit from a stronger melody, but it offers a welcome expansion of Tin Machine's accustomed territory.

Producer Tim Palmer tells David Buckley that he recalls Bowie "re-singing the lead vocal slightly flat, very intentionally, to get a sad-sounding performance. That control of pitch really impressed me." An alternative Indonesian vocal version of 'Amlapura' was included on single formats of 'You Belong In Rock N'Roll', and the song was performed on the It's My Life tour.

AMSTERDAM *(Brel/Shuman)*
• B-Side: 9/73 [3] • Bonus: *Pin, Ziggy (2002)* • Live: *Beeb*

Via the trailblazing cover versions recorded by his hero Scott Walker, Bowie was drawn in the late 1960s to the work of the Belgian singer-songwriter Jacques Brel, whose bittersweet ballads have remained a favourite with artists as diverse as Alex Harvey, Dusty Springfield, Nina Simone and Marc Almond. When the Broadway stage revue *Jacques Brel Is Alive And Well And Living In Paris* came to London in 1968, Bowie was in the audience. He later remarked that "By the time the cast, led by the earthy translator and Brooklynite Mort Shuman, had gotten to the song that dealt with guys lining up for their syphilis shots ['Next', soon to appear in the Feathers repertoire], I was completely won over. By way of Brel, I discovered French chanson a revelation. Here was a popular song form wherein poems by the likes of Sartre, Cocteau, Verlaine and Baudelaire were known and embraced by the general populace."

Jacques Brel Is Alive And Well And Living In Paris would become a significant source of inspiration for Bowie, directly influencing his songwriting – most obviously in 'Rock'n'Roll Suicide' – and yielding two of his pivotal cover versions. The first was 'Amsterdam' (referred to as 'Port of Amsterdam' in some Bowie documents), a bittersweet tale of hard-drinking sailors, prostitutes and broken dreams that was added to David's live repertoire in 1969. A tremendously passionate live version was included in the BBC radio session recorded on 5 February 1970 (it now appears on *Bowie At The Beeb*), and another excellent BBC recording was made on 21 September 1971. Bowie continued to perform 'Amsterdam' with The Spiders well into the summer of 1972, before it was edged out of the repertoire in favour of the even more melodramatic Brel composition 'My Death'.

Bowie's official studio rendition of 'Amsterdam' was recorded at Trident in the summer of 1971, preceded by a similar but rougher three-minute demo (on which David sings an octave lower for most of the song) which has appeared on bootlegs. As late as 15 December 1971 'Amsterdam' was still slated as the closing track on side one of *Ziggy Stardust*, but was ultimately replaced by 'It Ain't Easy'. The track remained unused until it became the B-side of 'Sorrow' in 1973. Latterly it appeared on RCA's cash-in *Bowie Rare*, complete with a hilariously inaccurate lyric sheet that made mincemeat of the already free Mort Shuman translation. In 1990 'Amsterdam' appeared as a bonus track on Rykodisc's reissue of *Pin Ups*, and at the same year's London press conference to announce the Sound + Vision tour David unexpectedly launched into the song's opening lines, a trick he repeated at the Brussels concert on 21 April. The studio recording of 'Amsterdam' resurfaced once again on the 2002 reissue of *Ziggy Stardust*, and in 2004 it was included on the various artists compilation *Next: A Tribute To Jacques Brel*.

AND I SAY TO MYSELF

• B-side: 1/66 • Compilation: *Early*

For this rather likeable B-side, which finds him trying to shake off an unwanted girlfriend, Bowie brazenly adapts the chord structure and call-and-response vocals of Sam Cooke's 'Wonderful World' – but in the style of The Righteous Brothers, who had struck gold in 1965 with their most famous pair of hits.

ANDY WARHOL

• Album: *Hunky* • B-Side: 1/72 • Live: *SM72, BBC, Beeb*

Most of *Hunky Dory*'s second side is devoted to Bowie's tributes to American influences, and 'Andy Warhol' is perhaps the best known. The artist had played an important role in David's creative development ever since Kenneth Pitt arrived back from America in 1966 with an acetate of *The Velvet Underground and Nico*. With its quirky intro, eavesdropping on studio banter ("This is 'Andy Warhol', and it's take one," announces Ken Scott, only to have his pronunciation corrected by Bowie), through the sophisticated twin acoustic guitar work to the ragged applause at the end, the track has long been a cult favourite. The lyric celebrates Warhol's appropriation of the Wildean dictum that "One should either be a work of art or wear a work of art", and thus the wilful blurring of the division between artist and artifice. "If you want to know all about me," Warhol once said, "just look at the surface of my paintings and films, and there I am. There's nothing behind it." This is entirely in keeping with Bowie's own preoccupations in 1971 as the long gestation of Ziggy Stardust neared its conclusion.

In his portrait of Warhol as "a standing cinema" and "a gallery" who is indistinguishable from the silver screen and wants to "put you all inside my show", Bowie anticipates his own assumption of the role of a blank canvas onto which rock stardom would be written. "It wasn't *why* he painted a Campbell's soup can, it was 'What kind of man would paint a Campbell's soup can?'" said Bowie later. "That's what aggravates people. That's the premise behind anti-style, and anti-style is the premise behind me."

'Andy Warhol' was originally written for Bowie's long-time friend Dana Gillespie, who took lead vocal during his free-for-all BBC session on 3 June 1971. In an effusive introduction David described Gillespie as "another friend of mine who lives in London, and she's a very very very very very very excellent songwriter, and she hasn't been recorded as yet with her own compositions, and needless to say tonight is no exception, ha ha! She's doing one of my things that I wrote for her, and it's called 'Andy Warhol'." Gillespie's own studio version was recorded the same year with a hard-rocking guitar break from Mick Ronson, while David provided backing vocals and acoustic guitar. An early mix appeared on the Bowie/Gillespie promo album pressed by Tony Defries in August 1971, but otherwise Gillespie's version remained unreleased until 1974, when it appeared as a single and on her album *Weren't Born a*

Man.

In September 1971, during Bowie's trip to New York to sign his RCA contract, the fabled first meeting of the two great artificers took place. "Andy was never a talker," recalled Tony Zanetta, who had arranged the meeting at Warhol's Factory studio. "Andy waited for other people to do things around him. So did David." This would account for the stilted encounter that has entered the annals of Bowie lore. David played the newly-minted acetate of 'Andy Warhol' to his hero, who reacted by leaving the room. "He absolutely hated it," Bowie recollected in 1997. "He was cringing with embarrassment. I think he thought that I really put him down in the song, and it really wasn't meant to be that – it was kind of an ironic *hommage* to him. He took it very badly, but he liked my shoes. I was wearing a pair of shoes that Marc Bolan had given me – brilliant canary yellow, semi-wedge heel, semi-point rounded toe. He liked those because he used to design shoes, so we had something to talk about." Warhol is said to have returned with his Polaroid to take several pictures of David's shoes, and also shot some film footage of David performing a couple of Lindsay Kemp mime staples (this footage surfaced at a Tate Modern Warhol retrospective in 2001, where vistors could view the long-haired David miming his insides falling out, followed by the "trapped in a glass box" routine he would later perform during 'The Width Of A Circle' in the Ziggy concerts). After discussing the finer points of footwear, Warhol ended the interview by saying, "Goodbye, David. You have such nice shoes." Bowie said that he found the meeting "fascinating" because Warhol had "nothing to say at all, absolutely nothing".

The two were later seen together on numerous occasions, although David commented in 1999 that "we never particularly got on." Warhol was at Bowie's breakthrough American gig at Carnegie Hall in September 1972, and attended the Broadway opening of *The Elephant Man* in 1980. He was later to say that "David always tried out combinations that no-one else would have dreamt of." In 1995, eight years after Warhol's death, Bowie took their bizarrely artificial relationship to its logical extreme when he played the role of Warhol himself in Julian Schnabel's film *Basquiat.*

In addition to the BBC radio version performed by Dana Gillespie, David recorded 'Andy Warhol' for two subsequent BBC sessions on 21 September 1971 and 23 May 1972; the former appears on the *BBC Sessions* *1969-1972* sampler, while the latter is included on *Bowie At The Beeb.* In 1972 the original album version was issued as the B-side of the 'Changes' single, on the American release of which the studio chatter was edited out. Yet another BBC version was recorded for the 1997 birthday broadcast *ChangesNowBowie*, this time with a flamenco-style acoustic guitar break.

'Andy Warhol' made regular live appearances in 1972 as part of an acoustic sequence along with 'Space Oddity' and 'My Death'. Thereafter it remained absent from the concert repertoire until receiving a vigorous electric makeover for the Outside and 1996 Festival tours. Bowie's demented accompanying dance routine was self-consciously avant-garde, more than a little pretentious, and absolutely marvellous – not unlike the song itself.

In the 1970s Nick Cave regularly played the song with his original outfit Boys Next Door, while another notable cover was performed by the Stone Temple Pilots during their 1993 MTV *Unplugged* set. Former S Club 7 singer Rachel Stevens used the 'Andy Warhol' guitar riff on the title track of her amusingly titled top ten album *Funky Dory*. Released as a single, 'Funky Dory' reached number 26 in the UK singles chart in December 2003. Bowie considered the song, which not only filched the tune of 'Andy Warhol' but also paraphrased its lyric, to be "quite nice".

ANDY'S CHEST *(Reed)*

Co-produced by Bowie for Lou Reed's *Transformer*, the surreal gem 'Andy's Chest' was resuscitated from an old Velvet Underground song inspired by the 1968 attempt on Andy Warhol's life by Valerie Solanas. The Velvets originally recorded it in 1969, but the definitive 1972 *Transformer* version is based around a jauntier, more acoustic arrangement. Bowie provides prominent backing vocals in probably the only rock song to contain the phrase "dentured ocelot".

ANGEL ANGEL GRUBBY FACE

Information is scarce about this Bowie composition slated for the planned second Deram album in 1968. A demo version appeared at a Christie's auction in 1993 on a two-sided acetate with 'London Bye Ta Ta', which suggests it was recorded in March 1968.

ANYWAY, ANYHOW, ANYWHERE
(Townshend/Daltrey)
• Album: *Pin*

Bowie covers The Who's second hit, a top ten in 1965, with greater panache than his version of 'I Can't Explain'. Subjected to the *Pin Ups* treatment 'Anyway, Anyhow, Anywhere' becomes a test-drive for David's burgeoning soul mannerisms – soon to be adopted to greater effect on *Diamond Dogs* and *Young Americans* – while Aynsley Dunbar contributes some tremendous drumming.

At his Bridge School benefit performance on 19 October 1996, Bowie launched into the opening line of the song in affectionate tribute to Pete Townshend, who had played some Who numbers earlier the same evening.

APRIL IN PARIS *(Duke/Harburg)*

During Tin Machine's It's My Life tour, David occasionally added a few lines from the jazz standard to 'Heaven's In Here'. While on the same tour he serenaded Iman with a suitably modified 'October In Paris' by way of making his marriage proposal, and at Brixton Academy the following month the lyric became the decidedly less poetic "November in Brixton".

APRIL'S TOOTH OF GOLD

This little-known demo dates from early 1968. The strumming guitar riff is reminiscent of 'Baby Loves That Way', but the quasi-hippy lyrics point in a psychedelic, Beatle-influenced direction whose transcendental theme has more in common with compositions like 'Karma Man' and 'Silly Boy Blue': "See the child with hair of blue, the one the boys are talking to, I can smell the spring in her mind / Friends of mine are red and green, I see you don't know what I mean and I'm sad / Look at the man with the pretty balloons, be dazzled by April's tooth of gold." Together with 'Mother Grey' and 'Ching-a-Ling', the song later became the subject of a copyright dispute. In May 1973 Essex Music International claimed that under a 1967 agreement they owned the copyright on the three numbers, and that Bowie was in breach of contract by signing them over to Chrysalis.

ARE YOU COMING ARE YOU COMING

One of a handful of song titles (also including 'Cyclops', 'Shilling The Rubes', 'Wilderness' and, bizarrely, a cover of the Johnny Cash country classic 'The Ballad Of Ira Hayes') which have been attached by collectors to Bowie's proposed 1973 stage version of *Nineteen Eighty-Four*. Other than 'Cyclops' there is no confirmation that any of these tracks were recorded, and their provenance remains dubious. The fact that 'Shilling The Rubes' was also a mooted title for *Young Americans* suggests that wires have been crossed.

AROUND AND AROUND *(Berry)* :
see **ROUND AND ROUND**

ART DECADE
• Album: *Low* • Live: *Stage* • B-Side: 11/78 [54]

Explaining that *Low* was his "reaction to certain places", Bowie said in 1977 that 'Art Decade' was about West Berlin, "a city cut off from its world, art and culture, dying with no hope of retribution." Hence the obvious pun, for Bowie's perception of West Berlin is of "art decayed". It's a hauntingly sparse instrumental distinguished by the beautiful cello playing of Hansa engineer Eduard Meyer. Tony Visconti, who scored the cello part, had originally intended to play it himself until Meyer revealed himself to be a cellist. 'Art Decade' was performed throughout the 1978 tour (from which the *Stage* version was released on the 'Breaking Glass' EP), and reappeared many years later on the Heathen tour.

AS THE WORLD FALLS DOWN
• Soundtrack: *Labyrinth* • Bonus: *Tonight* • Video: *Collection, Best Of Bowie*

This undemanding but very pretty love ballad works beautifully in the context of *Labyrinth*, accompanying a dream sequence in which Bowie, head to foot in ravishing glamour, whisks a Cinderella-like Jennifer Connelly through admiring crowds at a decadent masked ball that puts Adam And The Ants' 'Prince Charming' video to shame. Out of context it veers dangerously close to the Chris de Burgh school of soft-smooch romance; indeed, given the massive success of 'The Lady In Red' earlier that year, it's hardly surprising that 'As The World Falls Down' was slated for a Christmas 1986 single release. The track was edited to 3'36" and a video was shot by Steve Barron, splicing clips from *Labyrinth* with monochrome "performance" footage and a storyline about photocopies of Bowie enchanting a girl in a deserted office (shades of Barron's earlier promo for A-ha's 'Take On Me'). The single, however, was shelved at the last minute. One suspects it might have been a big hit, but perhaps Bowie had elected to clear the decks in preparation for the comparatively harder sound of the forthcoming *Never Let Me Down*.

Trivia buffs will note that the track features backing vocals by Robin Beck, who would enjoy her moment of fame two years later with the Coca-Cola commercial and international chart-topper 'First Time'. 'As The World Falls Down' was bafflingly added to the 1995 reissue of *Tonight*, while the previously unreleased video was included on *The Video Collection* and *Best Of Bowie*. That David still regards the song with affection is indicated by the fact that he included it on the five-track CD of romantic numbers packaged with the initial release of his wife's 2001 autobiography *I Am Iman*.

ASHES TO ASHES

• A-Side: 8/80 [1] • Album: *Scary* • Live: *Beeb* • Video: *Collection*, *Best Of Bowie* • Live Video: *Moonlight*

Even without its obvious historical interest this is one of the all-time great Bowie tracks. Lush layers of synthesized sound, ska backbeats and funk guitar consolidate all Bowie's late 1970s experimentation in one classic piece of pop, while David Mallet's outstanding promo redefined rock video and jump-started the New Romantic movement. "It's certainly one of the better songs that I've ever written," was Bowie's considered judgement in 1999. All this, and it's a sequel to 'Space Oddity' too.

Eleven years after Major Tom's lift-off, Ground Control receives a message from the ether which transmutes into an articulation of numbness, isolation and personal insecurity, larded with cryptic references to Bowie's ongoing struggle against his drug habit and the oppressive weight of his past career. In an interview for the *NME* in 1980, David called the song an "ode to childhood, if you like, a popular nursery rhyme … about spacemen becoming junkies!" He

cited the lyric "I've never done good things, I've never done bad things, I never did anything out of the blue" as representing "a continuing, returning feeling of inadequacy over what I've done." Expanding on the song's heritage, he explained, "When I originally wrote about Major Tom, I was a very pragmatic and self-opinionated lad that thought he knew all about the great American dream and where it started and where it should stop. Here we had the great blast of American technological know-how shoving this guy up into space, but once he gets there he's not quite sure why he's there. And that's where I left him. Now we've found out that he's under some kind of realization that the whole process that got him up there had decayed, was born out of decay; it has decayed him and he's in the process of decaying. But he wishes to return to the nice, round womb, the earth, from whence he started." Elsewhere he added weight to the sense of narrative closure found throughout *Scary Monsters* by describing the song as "long overdue – the end of something", and more recently he explained that "I was wrapping up the seventies really for myself, and that seemed a good enough epitaph for it – that we've lost him, he's out there somewhere, we'll leave him be."

Given Bowie's declaration that *Scary Monsters* was an attempt to "accommodate" his "pasts" ("you have to understand why you went through them"), there is a persuasive case for reading 'Ashes To Ashes' as an autobiographical note about the process that had sent him "up there" and "decayed" him in the mid-1970s – and not just because of the obvious drug references, which he admitted were fun to smuggle past the radio censors. The "Action Man" who has fallen so low might well parallel the former "Main Man" whose music went from "funk to funky" in 1975 as he became "a junkie" in the City of Angels ("strung out in heaven's high"), before hitting the depths during *The Man Who Fell To Earth* ("I ain't got no money and I ain't got no hair"), and relocating to Europe for creative and spiritual rebirth ("hitting an all-time *Low*"), but still yearning to demolish the frozen emotions and paranoiac isolation to which he had fallen victim ("Want an axe to break the ice, I wanna come down right now"). If 'Space Oddity' was in part a metaphor of space travel as celebrity as drug-taking as sensory isolation, then 'Ashes To Ashes' represents the pay-off.

Melodically the song is indebted to one of Bowie's very earliest influences, the Danny Kaye number 'Inchworm', which hails from the 1952 musical *Hans*

Christian Andersen. "I was seven or eight when that came out," David recalled, not entirely accurately, in 2003. "The chords were some of the first I learned on a guitar. They're remarkable chords, very melancholic. 'Ashes To Ashes' is influenced by that. It's childlike and melancholic in that children's story way."

The queasy Wurlitzer effect underpinning the rhythm track was achieved by feeding the sound of a grand piano through a gadget rejoicing in the name of the Eventide Instant Flanger. "We wanted a Wurlitzer but couldn't wait for a hire company to deliver one," explained Tony Visconti. "I tried my best to turn an ordinary piano into one, but settled with feeding it to the Eventide and setting it at maximum wobble, which everyone preferred to the Wurlitzer which never arrived." Meanwhile the rhythmic back-beat gave Bowie's percussionist a few headaches. "I'm sure Dennis Davis won't mind me saying this," said David a few years later, "but when we did 'Ashes To Ashes', that beat was an old ska beat, but Dennis had an incredibly hard time with it, trying to play it and turn the beat backwards, and in fact we worked through the session and it wasn't turning out at all well, so I did it on a chair and a cardboard box and he took it home with him and learnt it for the next day. He really found it a problem."

RCA stressed the continuity between 'Ashes To Ashes' and 'Space Oddity' by releasing a 12" promo in America which faded one into the other. In Britain the edited single came in a choice of four different picture sleeves, each accompanied by a sheet of adhesive stamps, marking RCA's belated adoption of the craze for limited-edition collectables that had swept the 7" market in the late 1970s. Trail-blazed by the famous video it was a huge hit, entering the chart at number 4 and knocking ABBA's 'The Winner Takes It All' off the top spot the following week to become Bowie's fastest-selling single yet. It was his second number one – the first, ironically enough, had been the reissued 'Space Oddity'.

The superb video, perhaps Bowie's best, used the new-fangled Paintbox technique to turn skies black and seas pink, and premiered one of his best-remembered looks. The sad-faced clown wandering up a lonely beach, pursued by a bulldozer and harangued by his ageing mother, is a resonant image that reaches back across Bowie's career. It's redolent of his white-faced mime period in the late 1960s (photos of David from Lindsay Kemp's *Pierrot In Turquoise* are startlingly similar), of the "love-machine" that "lumbers

through desolation row" in 'Cygnet Committee', of the original sleeve artwork for the *Space Oddity* album, of his 1971 estimation of rock as "the clown, the Pierrot medium", of his later denunciation of rock as "a toothless old woman", and of his own perennial predicament, jumping through hoops at the centre of the industry's three-ring circus. The trio of characters Bowie enacts in the video's unsettling, dreamlike juxtapositions – clown, asylum inmate and spaceman – are staples of his work from its earliest days, again fuelling the notion that 'Ashes To Ashes' is a comprehensive exorcism of his past.

The closing refrain of "My Mama said, to get things done / You'd better not mess with Major Tom" is another of David's darkling nursery-rhymes, paraphrasing the traditional skipping-game: "My mother said, I never should / Play with the gypsies in the wood." In view of the video it's worth noting that the poem continues "I went to the sea – no ship to get across", and concludes: "Sally tell my mother I shall never come back". The video's incongruous cardigan-clad mother (not, as some believed, David's own) has been interpreted as a reaction to the embarrassingly public family strife highlighted by the *NME*'s famous 1975 interview with Peggy Jones ("A MOTHER'S ANGUISH – DAVID NEVER COMES TO SEE ME!"). In the years since that article David had repaired his relationship with his mother – "I think the recognition of the frailty of age makes one more sympathetic to the earlier strains of the child-parent relationship," he said. "It's a shared responsibility and you get more mature about it." All the same, Bowie's work has always clung to the fantasy of a flight from parental dominance and suburban domesticity.

"Although it looked pretty po-faced, it was a riot making it!" he later recalled of the 'Ashes' video, shot at Beachy Head and Hastings in May 1980 on a budget of £25,000, making it the most expensive pop video of its day. Bowie storyboarded the promo himself, drawing it shot by shot and dictating the editing process. "I brought my drawings to David Mallet and said, look, I'd like to have a crack at this. Some of the images were kind of violent – the plough following the figures is an image of oncoming violence which I find very scary, and there's something very religious about the four other characters in the video, an ominous quality that's rooted quite deeply." One of these exotically attired figures was the up-and-coming New Romantic icon Steve Strange, shortly to enjoy chart success with his own group Visage. His costume and make-up in 1981's 'Fade To Grey' video exactly mimic Bowie's Pierrot, but the inspiration was a two-way process. David had recruited Strange and the other extras after a visit to The Blitz, the Bowie-worshipping nightclub that was home to the rapidly emerging New Romantic scene. Among those disappointed to be passed over for the 'Ashes' video were Blitz regulars Marilyn and long-time Bowie fan George O'Dowd.

The Italian Pierrot costume was designed by Natasha Kornilof, an occasional collaborator since the days of *Pierrot In Turquoise*, who had most recently worked with David as costume designer on the Stage tour. The sequences depicting Bowie in a padded cell and, bizarrely, as an anaesthetised astronaut sitting in an exploding kitchen, were developed from the elaborate performance of 'Space Oddity' shot by Mallet for *Kenny Everett's New Year's Eve Show* the year before. The shots of David in a spacesuit linked to his ship by umbilical lifelines were, he explained, "intentionally" derivative of H R Giger's famous production designs for *Alien*, released the previous year. "It was supposed to be the archetypal 1980s ideal of the futuristic colony that has been founded by the earthling," said David, "and in that particular sequence the idea was for the earthling to be pumping out himself and to be having pumped into him something organic. So there was a very strong Giger influence there: the organic meets hi-tech." Of the video as a whole, he explained that it conveyed "some feeling of nostalgia for a future. I've always been hung up on that; it creeps into everything I do, however far away I try to get from it ... The idea of having seen the future, of somewhere we've already been, keeps coming back to me."

'Ashes To Ashes' would define rock video for the early 1980s, its techniques and effects aped by countless early promos from the likes of Adam Ant, Duran Duran and The Cure among many others. Neil Tennant of the Pet Shop Boys, whose state-of-the-art promos would set the pace during the 1990s, described 'Ashes' as "an amazing video." One shot – the stricken Pierrot-Bowie submerged up to his chest in water – was lampooned in the notorious 'Nice Video, Shame About the Song' sketch on *Not The Nine O'Clock News*, and was later appropriated by Peter Gabriel for 'Shock The Monkey'. Marilyn Manson's video for 'The Dope Show' is particularly influenced by the 'Ashes' promo, and Manson is evidently a fan; in 'Apple Of Sodom' he sings "I'm dying, hope you're dying too".

In 1992 Tears For Fears recorded a slavish cover of 'Ashes To Ashes' for the *Ruby Trax* charity album; it later appeared on *David Bowie Songbook*. Covers have also been recorded by Uwe Schmidt and The Mike Flowers Pops, while in 2000 Samantha Mumba's number 3 hit 'Body II Body' extensively sampled Bowie's original.

According to Tony Visconti, 'Ashes To Ashes' was originally entitled 'People Are Turning To Gold', and in October 2000 he treated viewers of Channel 4's *Top Ten: 1980* documentary to a snatch of an early demo in which Bowie sings a "la la" vocal along to the backing track. Rumours persist that a 13-minute original version, featuring an extra verse and a lengthy instrumental passage, resides in the archives (the twelve-minute version that has appeared on bootlegs merely splices and re-splices already familiar verses, and is almost certainly a fake). Only once during 1980 did David perform 'Ashes To Ashes' live, on 5 September for NBC's *The Tonight Show With Johnny Carson*. Despite being a particularly challenging song to reproduce live, 'Ashes to Ashes' made successful transitions to the stage for the Serious Moonlight, Sound + Vision, 1999-2000, Heathen and A Reality tours. An excellent live version recorded at the BBC Radio Theatre on 27 June 2000 was included on the *Bowie At The Beeb* bonus disc.

AWAKEN 2 (*Bowie/Gabrels*)

An instrumental track recorded by Bowie with Reeves Gabrels in 1999 for exclusive use in the *Omikron* computer game.

BAAL'S HYMN (*Brecht/Muldowney*)
• A-Side: 2/82 [29] • Compilation: *S+V (2003)*

The first track on the *Baal* EP cobbles together Brecht's 'Hymn Of Baal The Great', which appears in the play as a series of disconnected verses between the vignetted scenes of Baal's life. It's an unsentimental account of Brecht's hard-hearted romantic and his amoral philosophies, peppered with images of the overarching sky that inspires, nourishes and oppresses him.

BABY *(Pop/Bowie)*

Produced and co-written by Bowie for Iggy Pop's *The Idiot*, 'Baby' appeared on the B-side of Iggy's unsuccessful singles 'Sister Midnight' and 'China Girl' in 1977. 'Baby' has also been documented as an alternative title for Bowie's unrelated 1965 demo 'That's A Promise'.

BABY CAN DANCE

• Album: *TM* • B-Side: 10/89 • Live: *Best Of Grunge Rock*

'Baby Can Dance' partially redeems the tiresome second half of *Tin Machine* with some excellent lead guitar and one of the best tunes on the whole record. Bowie seems to be calling the shots here; he wrote the track alone and it recalls older compositions, with a guitar intro building on the 1988 version of 'Look Back In Anger' and a rhythmic verse structure reminiscent of 'Modern Love'. There's even a reminder of an obscure 1971 out-take as he declares "I'm the shadowman, the jumping jack, the man who can and don't look back." Even the title, for once, is pure Bowie. Unfortunately, as with so many Tin Machine recordings, 'Baby Can Dance' over-eggs its pudding with, to mix one's muso-culinary metaphors, an excessive jam session. Reeves Gabrels and Hunt Sales slip their moorings and the album grinds to a halt with yet another overdose of pointless feedback and prattling drums.

'Baby Can Dance' featured on both Tin Machine tours. A 1989 live version recorded in Paris appeared on the B-side of the 'Prisoner Of Love' single while another, from Hamburg in 1991, was released exclusively on the US compilation *Best Of Grunge Rock*.

BABY, IT CAN'T FALL *(Pop/Bowie)*

Co-written and co-produced by Bowie for Iggy Pop's *Blah-Blah-Blah*, 'Baby, It Can't Fall' was released as the B-side of the 'Shades' single.

BABY LOVES THAT WAY

• B-Side: 8/65 • Compilation: *Early* • B-Side: 9/02 [20]

The B-side of David's first single with The Lower Third was, he admitted, a homage of sorts to Herman's Hermits, whose singer Peter Noone would later enjoy success with his cover of 'Oh! You Pretty Things'. The lyric, about a girl who "treats me good each and every night" but "fools around" with other men "who treat her like a worn-out toy", hints at the sleazy sexuality of his later work. The backing vocals were apparently meant to suggest monastic chanting, perhaps the earliest intimation of a Buddhist motif in David's music. The group was joined in the chanting by two studio engineers, producer Shel Talmy and manager Les Conn who, according to drummer Phil Lancaster, was "really out of tune".

An excellent new version of 'Baby Loves That Way' was recorded during the *Toy* sessions in 2000, eventually seeing release two years later as a B-side of the Japanese 'Slow Burn' CD and the European single 'Everyone Says 'Hi''.

BABY PLEASE DON'T GO *(Morganfield)* : see **HEAVEN'S IN HERE** and **THE JEAN GENIE**

BABY UNIVERSAL *(Bowie/Gabrels)*

• Album: *TM2* • A-Side: 10/91 [48] • Live Video: *Oy*

Driven by Tin Machine's rock'n'roll fundamentalism but packed with retroactive gestures toward Bowie's early 1970s music, the opening track of *Tin Machine II* is one of the band's finest achievements. The previous album's deliberately grotty production style is swept away by a sophisticated multi-track mix, blending a trademark Bowie double-octave vocal with a lead guitar reminiscent not only of Tin Machine favourites Pixies, but also of Mick Ronson's work on the *Ziggy Stardust* version of 'Holy Holy'. The lyric, too, tips a wink at the visionary sci-fi apocalypse of 'Starman' or 'Oh! You Pretty Things': "Hallo humans, can you feel me thinking / I assume you're seeing everything I'm thinking / Hallo humans, nothing starts tomorrow…" The track provides a template for later solo projects; the lyric ("chaos", "dust", "hallo humans") would be heavily recycled for 'Hallo Spaceboy', while the underscoring vocal mantra is revisited in 'Looking For Satellites'.

'Baby Universal' became Tin Machine's final single in October 1991. Like its predecessor the CD came in a round tin, while the 12" included a pull-out reproduction of the censored US album sleeve. Both formats featured tracks from Tin Machine's BBC session – including a new version of 'Baby Universal' – recorded on 13 August. The video mingled archive shots with live footage from Tin Machine's Los Angeles Airport gig on 25 August. The single barely scraped the top 50, despite a live preview on BBC1's *Paramount City* on 3 August and a memorable appearance on *Top Of The Pops*, which was then going through a much-publicized phase of compulsory live performance. If nothing else this allowed Tin Machine to demonstrate their live credentials at a time when many chart bands were making fools of themselves; it also allowed a clueless presenter to introduce the song as 'Baby Unusual'.

In 1992 the song appeared in the soundtrack of *Hellraiser III: Hell On Earth*. That Bowie regards 'Baby Universal' as worthy of greater exposure was confirmed in 1996 when it featured on the Summer Festivals tour, becoming one of the few Tin Machine numbers to earn itself a place in his solo repertoire. In the same year a new studio version was taped during the *Earthling* sessions. "I thought 'Baby Universal' was a really good song and I don't think it got heard," said David. "I didn't really want that to happen to it, so I put it on this album … I think this version is very good." Plans changed, however, and the *Earthling* version remains unreleased.

BABY WHAT YOU WANT ME TO DO *(Reed)* : see THE JEAN GENIE

BACK TO WHERE YOU'VE NEVER BEEN

Recorded at Trident on 24 October 1968, this number was to be the B-side of the proposed Feathers single 'Ching-a-Ling', taped the same day. Sadly, the track never saw the light of day and is now a notable rarity; it has never appeared on the bootleg circuit and remains something of a mystery. It's worth noting that the 1970 demo 'Tired Of My Life' includes the remarkably close paraphrase "so I'm leading you away, home where you've never been" – but there is no direct evidence that the songs are connected.

BACKED A LOSER

Co-produced and arranged by Bowie for Dana Gillespie's 1974 album *Weren't Born A Man*, the unremarkable 'Backed A Loser' is often listed as a Bowie composition despite some uncertainty surrounding its authorship.

THE BALLAD OF IRA HAYES *(LaFarge)* : see ARE YOU COMING ARE YOU COMING

BALLAD OF THE ADVENTURERS
(Brecht/Muldowney)
• B-Side: 2/82 [29]

The third track on the *Baal* EP is a bitterly aggressive song sung by Baal in a public bar just before he stabs his friend Eckart to death. "Another bucket of sentiment for the coal merchant" is the script's cruelly Brechtian opinion of the number. Infused with Baal's customary sky-imagery, it is in part a meditation on his dead mother, doubtless fuelled by the fact that Brecht's own mother died while he was writing the play.

BANG BANG *(Pop/Kral)*
• Album: *Never* • US Promo: 1987 • Live Video: *Glass*

Never Let Me Down closes with the last in Bowie's long line of 1980s Iggy Pop covers. 'Bang Bang' was written with former Patti Smith collaborator Ivan Kral for inclusion on Iggy's 1981 album *Party*, from which it was culled as a single in the same year. Bowie's version isn't a patch on the original, substituting a dull AOR arrangement in place of Iggy's energetic rock-out, but it's fun to hear David's full-on vocal impersonation of his friend ("Y'all ought to be in pictures!"). If nothing else, 'Bang Bang' meshes successfully with *Never Let Me Down*: "angels" have already turned up on 'Day-In Day-Out' and there's a reprise of the synthesized sitar from 'Zeroes', while the arch adolescent symbolism matches the album's prevailing style of dumb rock-'n'roll ("Rockets shooting up into space / Buildings they rise to the skies"). Ultimately, though, this is a drab cover which ends the album not with a bang but a whimper.

'Bang Bang' was performed throughout the Glass

Spider tour, and a live version recorded in Montreal on 30 August 1987 appeared on a limited edition US promo CD.

BARS OF THE COUNTY JAIL

• Compilation: *Early*

Despite verging on the whimsical, this mid-1965 acoustic demo offers a significant early instance of a Bowie lyric that jettisons R&B's standard boy-meets-girl subject matter. It's the serio-comic tale of a man wrongly accused of murder who will face the gallows at dawn, and although it's hardly 'Wild Eyed Boy From Freecloud' it suggests an awakening interest in the idea that a song could be rooted elsewhere than in the mundanity of suburban romance. The demo itself is unimpressive, with ragged backing vocals and mist-imed handclaps aplenty, but the combination of a folksy sound with an almost vaudevillian sensibility is another signal that Davy Jones was already growing impatient with the derivative nature of his released recordings to date.

BATTLE FOR BRITAIN (THE LETTER)

(Bowie/Gabrels/Plati)
• Album: *Earthling* • Live: *liveandwell.com*

Bowie's traditional songwriting sensibilities here lock horns with the strident drum'n'bass habitat of 'Little Wonder', scattering drum-loops and bursts of guitar over an otherwise old-fashioned Bowie melody – stripped of the ultra-modern production it would be easy to imagine this as one of his late 1960s compositions. In *Strange Fascination* co-producer Mark Plati reveals that the germ of the song was his "attempt to do a jazz-tinged jungle track" which Bowie radically rewrote, changing the chord structure into what Plati considered "our first real 'Bowie' song." There are some quirky piano syncopations from Mike Garson (Bowie had asked him to adopt the style of a Stravinsky octet) and, at one point, a simulation of the sound of a jumping CD – a digital-age variation on the stuck-needle playout of *Diamond Dogs*.

While the lyric defies scrutiny, it appears to confront Bowie's ambiguous feelings about his national identity. "It's another cut-up," he explained, "But it probably comes from a sense of 'Am I or am I not British?', an inner war that rages in most expatriates.

I've not lived in Britain since 1974, but I love the place and I keep going back." *Earthling* marks an upswing in Bowie's apparent sense of his own Britishness, and here as on 'Little Wonder' he dusts down his best Anthony Newley for the occasion. 'Battle For Britain' was performed at the fiftieth birthday concert and throughout the Earthling tour (a version recorded in New York on 15 October 1997 later appeared on *liveandwell.com*), and was revived six years later for A Reality Tour.

BE MY BABY *(Barry/Greenwich/Spector)* : see **THE JEAN GENIE**

BE MY WIFE

• Album: *Low* • A-Side: 6/77 • Live: *Rarest* • Video: *Collection, Best Of Bowie*

Cranked up by Roy Young's barrelling bar-room piano, 'Be My Wife' is a cry for help among the suicidal indulgences of *Low*'s first side. Bowie reflects on his occupational rootlessness and inability to settle down ("I've lived all over the world, I've left every place"), in a frighteningly candid confession of loneliness – although who exactly is addressed by the title is open to debate. "It was genuinely anguished," David later said, "but I think it could have been about anybody." Some have claimed that he was still attempting to resuscitate his ailing marriage during the *Low* sessions, while Tony Visconti later recalled having to break up a fight between Bowie and Angie's new boyfriend in the Château d'Hérouville's dining room.

Despite its predecessor's success, 'Be My Wife' failed to chart as *Low*'s second single, becoming Bowie's first new-release flop since the pre-Ziggy days. The video, Bowie's first since Mick Rock's Ziggy-era clips, was shot in Paris by Stanley Dorfman and featured David ghoulishly made up like Joel Grey's Emcee in *Cabaret*, strenuously hamming away at his guitar against a white backdrop. Alternative edits of the video circulate among collectors.

'Be My Wife' was performed throughout the Stage tour, from which a fine recording made at Earls Court later appeared on *RarestOneBowie*. It was later revived for the Sound + Vision, Heathen and A Reality tours.

BEAT OF YOUR DRUM

• Album: *Never*

One of the better *Never Let Me Down* tracks, 'Beat Of Your Drum' attempts a mainstream, rootsy sound along the lines of 'Blue Jean'. Unfortunately, like so much of the album, it collapses under superfluous layers of guitars and saxophones. There are signs of imagination in the lyric, in which Bowie juxtaposes a Warholian photographic motif with images of transience ("fashions may change … colours may fade … seasons may change … negative fades … follow the pack"), comically over-reacts to his own ageing by casting himself as Dracula ("Sweet is the night, bright light destroys me"), and then forgets that he's growing long in the tooth and plumps instead for a trusty metaphor of rock'n'roll as sex: "I'd like to blow on your horn, I'd like to beat on your drum."

In 1987 David explained rather disconcertingly that "It's a *Lolita* number! Reflection on young girls – Christ, she's only fourteen years old, but jail's worth it!" A more wholesome claim to fame, if not the greatest boast a song could hope to make, is that both musically and lyrically ("I like the smell of your flesh, I like the dirt that you dish") it's the direct ancestor of Tin Machine's 'You Belong In Rock N'Roll'.

'Beat Of Your Drum' was performed live during the Glass Spider tour.

BEAUTY AND THE BEAST

• Album: *"Heroes"* • A-Side: 1/78 [39] • Live: *Stage* •
US Promo: 12/77

'Beauty And The Beast' opens with sporadic blips of percussion and synthesizer, building rapidly via a thumping piano and Bowie's crescendo howl to kick the *"Heroes"* album into life. With its woozy bassline, discordant wailings and melodramatic vocal it's a tremendously sinewy performance of a strong composition.

Although Bowie has never discussed the lyric at any length, it seems likely that 'Beauty And The Beast' operates in part as a recantation of the ugly underside of his Thin White Duke phase, and an exploration of the undesirable inner character unleashed during his drink and drug binges: "There's slaughter in the air, protest in the wind, someone else inside me, someone could get skinned … I wanted to believe me, I wanted to be good". In the light of his later remark that Berlin

"brought me back in touch with people" and "got me back on the streets", the song might also be interpreted as an expression of gratitude and relief at his escape from Los Angeles: "Nothing will corrupt us, nothing will compete / Thank God heaven left us standing on our feet." However, the song offers a salutary lesson in the danger of over-analysing Bowie's lyrics. The line "someone fetch a priest", which it would be tempting to interpret as a confessional impulse or a testimony of spiritual rebirth, actually derives from "someone fuck a priest", Tony Visconti's favourite expletive during the *"Heroes"* sessions.

'Beauty And The Beast' proved a little too outré for the singles chart, managing a modest number 39. In America and Spain a five-minute edit appeared on a 12" promo; although labelled the 'Disco Version', it was merely an early instance of that forthcoming bane of the 1980s, the extended remix. 'Beauty And The Beast' was performed throughout the Stage tour.

BECAUSE YOU'RE YOUNG

• Album: *Scary* • B-Side: 1/81 [20]

In contemporary interviews Bowie dedicated 'Because You're Young' to his nine-year-old son, and like much of *Scary Monsters*, the song finds David seemingly preoccupied by his impending mid-thirties and assessing his role as guru to a new generation. But this is no catalogue of wisdom dispensed Polonius-like from father to son. Bowie's anguished portrait of "love back to front and no sides" makes no bones about the potential for unhappiness in affairs of the heart. "Hope I'm wrong, but I know", he ponders morosely, telling the young addressee that "you'll meet a stranger some night" and "a million dreams" will become "a million scars". An autobiographical element seems unavoidable: "She took back everything she said, left him nearly out of his mind" is a painfully stark observation from a man whose divorce has only just come through.

'Because You're Young' is also notable for a guest appearance by Pete Townshend on guitar. It was a collaboration that had long been on the cards; Bowie, who had covered The Who's first two hits on *Pin Ups* and supported them in concert with The Lower Third in 1965, was a long-standing admirer. While recording 'Because You're Young', Townshend apparently behaved in the studio exactly in the style of his famous stage act, jumping into the air and performing his trademark windmill. Tony Visconti remembered it as "...a very bizarre session. Pete's from the old school of breaking the guitar against the amplifier, playing loud chords and getting extremely drunk on a session. Now, he didn't do that. He wasn't rowdy or anything, he was extremely polite ... But he couldn't quite understand what we were about, because we're not, David and I are not rock and rollers ... Pete was very surprised to see us two sober, little old men sitting in the studio. He was ready for a right rave-up and he felt like playing guitar all day and night."

Despite immaculate production and a successful symbiosis of Townshend's guitar with some dramatic rhythm-synth from Roy Clark (conspicuously indebted to the style of Blondie's Jimmy Destri, who had accompanied Bowie on keyboards on *Saturday Night Live* shortly before the *Scary Monsters* sessions), 'Because You're Young' remains perhaps the weakest track on the album. The markedly different 4'52" demo that has appeared on bootlegs suggests that the song may have been over-worked to its detriment. 'Because I'm Young', as it was at this stage, features a significantly different lyric (the opening "Look in my eyes, nobody home" was clearly too close to the first verse of 'Scary Monsters' to pass muster) together with a cleaner, less cluttered backing arrangement.

'Because You're Young' was rehearsed for the Glass Spider tour but dropped from the set-list before the show opened. It has yet to be performed live.

BELIEVE TO MY SOUL *(King)*

Albert King's number was played live by The Manish Boys.

A BETTER FUTURE

• Album: *Heathen* • Bonus: *Heathen*

This terrific track is one of *Heathen*'s catchiest numbers, marrying a deceptively simple melody with richly textured production, hypnotic rhythms and an arrangement which recalls both the electronic minimalism of the Berlin period and the catchy synthesizer pop of *The Buddha Of Suburbia*'s 'Dead Against It'. Bowie's multi-tracked vocal has a sing-song nursery-rhyme quality which, accompanied by a descending synth phrase borrowed from the Bacharach/David standard 'Do You Know The Way To San José?', con-

spires to give the song a playful edge belying the stark spiritual demands of the lyric. "'A Better Future' was really for my daughter," David explained. "It's a very simple song that says 'God, if you don't change things, I'm not gonna love you any more.' There's no skirting around the issue – it's like, 'What are you doing to us? Why have you allowed my daughter to come into a world of such chaos and despair? I demand a better future or I'm not gonna like you any more.' It's a threat to God! There are a few threats to God on this album, actually, but a lot of them sound like they could just be love songs."

A remix by Air was included on the bonus disc issued with initial pressings of *Heathen*. 'A Better Future' was performed live on the first two dates of the Heathen tour.

BETTY WRONG *(Bowie/Gabrels)*

• Soundtrack: *The Crossing* • Album: *TM2* • Live Video: *Oy*

Recorded in Australia in late 1989, 'Betty Wrong' first surfaced in the soundtrack of the 1990 Australian film *The Crossing*. This version was superseded by the superior mix of the same recording featured on *Tin Machine II*. Although blessed with an excellent melody and a chunky bassline borrowing heavily from 'Changes', it's effectively a return to the sound of the less inspiring space-fillers on the band's first album, recalling both 'Run' and 'Working Class Hero'. Still, Bowie's lyric – an avowal of love in the face of mortality – displays a stark muscularity often absent from his work during the period. "I was carved from a hand nurtured on grime, good-will and screams" is a line that would sound more at home on *Scary Monsters* or *1.Outside*, and there are some neat percussion effects anticipating the woodblock atmospherics of 'Seven Years In Tibet'. A reworked version, complete with languorous saxophone interludes from David, was performed during the It's My Life tour.

BEWITCHED, BOTHERED AND BEWILDERED *(Rodgers)*

A synthesized instrumental of the 1937 Richard Rodgers standard from *Babes In Arms* forms the backing of 'Future Legend', the opening track on the *Diamond Dogs* album.

THE BEWLAY BROTHERS

• Album: *Hunky* • Bonus: *Hunky*

Probably the most cryptic, mysterious, unfathomable and downright frightening Bowie recording in existence, 'The Bewlay Brothers' has defied commentary for more than three decades. Vocally it finds Bowie pushing *Hunky Dory*'s Dylan affectation to its logical extreme, pulling off a creditable cross between his own rapidly emerging vocal trademarks and Bob's "sand and glue" rasp. Instrumentally, the acoustic strum that forms the foundation-stone of many great Bowie compositions is augmented by a rising wall of sinister sound effects and chattering demons, recalling the multi-tracked vocals and synthesizer experiments of *The Man Who Sold The World*. Much of the song's impact lies in the grace with which it combines the best of both albums, matching the simplicity and melodic power of 'Quicksand' with the shivering menace of 'All The Madmen' to achieve an even more striking result than either. Interestingly, producer Ken Scott recalls that unlike the rest of *Hunky Dory*, 'The Bewlay Brothers' was a last-minute addition to the album and was not demoed prior to recording: "Arrangements were worked out in the studio, but no writing."

The wilfully obscure lyric, which Bowie once claimed was written with an American audience in mind so that they might "read whatever in hell they want to read into it", has provoked innumerable, intriguing, and often desperately shaky interpretations. Many have found a gay agenda in the song – notably Tom Robinson, who once remarked that "until then all pop music was boy meets girl. Suddenly, you heard 'The Bewlay Brothers' and you felt, that's me!". Many more have read it as an account of David's relationship with his schizophrenic half-brother Terry Burns, contending that it confronts the fear of congenital madness that Bowie has admitted was a factor in his early work. Neither topic is particularly unusual among his early 1970s recordings, and in a rare moment of candour David confirmed in 1977 that the song was "very much based on myself and my brother." On Radio 2's *Golden Years* documentary in 2000 he described it as "another vaguely anecdotal piece about my feelings about myself and my brother, or my other *doppelgänger*. I was never quite sure what real position Terry had in my life, whether Terry was a real person or whether I was actually referring to another part of me, and I think 'Bewlay

Brothers' was really about that."

With very few facts to impede the full flow of the imagination, various commentators have taken it upon themselves to provide ingenious but dodgy explanations of 'The Bewlay Brothers'. George Tremlett posits a fantastically flimsy theory that the song relates the disastrous outcome of a séance held by David and Terry "at a time when Terry's incipient insanity was only just becoming clear." Other writers have gone so far as to conflate Terry's misfortunes with the gay reading to suggest that 'The Bewlay Brothers' is a fantasy of sexual consummation between David and his half-brother.

There's certainly no difficulty in winkling a gay subtext out of the lyric, which deploys the coded slang of the Greenwich Village ghetto after the fashion of the same album's 'Queen Bitch'. In this interpretation the emphasis is on the "real cool traders" who lurk "in the crutch-hungry dark", forced to maintain a closeted existence by day ("they wore the clothes, they said the things to make it seem improbable, the whale of a lie..."), hanging up their dresses while make-up is "woven on the edging of my pillow". By this reading the song's unforgettable image of the lifeless brother, otherwise believed to be a vision of Terry insensible after a schizophrenic seizure, might just as easily be post-coital. And it is undeniable that the line "I was stone and he was wax so he could scream and still relax" might well be, as the Gillmans rather primly propose in their book, "a precise description for successful homosexual intercourse" – albeit a description conveyed via the characteristically skewed image of the children's game of stone, scissors and paper.

And yet, as with all Bowie's finest songs, the more one tries to grab at the lyric, the more elusive it proves. For all its enticing clues, the entire gay reading is dark and insubstantial, almost as though it might be a red herring. There are just as many images among the hallucinatory whole to suggest a drug-fixated subtext ("dust would flow through our veins … shooting up pie in the sky … we were so turned on in the Mind-Warp Pavilion"). Other images are familiar elsewhere on *Hunky Dory* – the observation that "the solid book we wrote cannot be found today" recalls the lost poems in 'Song For Bob Dylan' and the "books … found by the golden ones" in 'Oh! You Pretty Things', while the line about "fakers" takes us back to 'Changes' at the start of the album. It has been noted, persuasively, that the mannequin-like image of the lifeless body, reduced to the status of "chameleon, comedian, Corinthian and caricature", coincides with Bowie's decision at the end of *Hunky Dory* to efface his own artistic personality and create instead the *tabula rasa* onto which the face of Ziggy Stardust would be painted. If this reading holds water, then it's amusing to note that Bowie had called himself a "chameleon" long before rock journalists seized the word and turned it into the ultimate Bowie cliché.

Even the song's title has been hotly debated. Charles Shaar Murray and Roy Carr suggest that the unexplained Bewlay Brothers may be a reference to the gods of classical mythology, while others have conjectured that "Bewlay" is a corruption of "Beulah" or even of "Newley", as in Anthony. The reality is more prosaic – it's a little-known fact that "Bewlay Bros." was the name of a tobacconist's shop in Brixton High Street (not in Soho, as Ken Scott has said) at the time of the *Hunky Dory* sessions.

Bowie has never discussed 'The Bewlay Brothers' in detail, and when he has mentioned it at all, he has only succeeded in obfuscating it even further. "I can't imagine what the person who wrote that had on his mind at the time," he once remarked. In 1971 he described the song as "Another in the series of David Bowie confessions – *Star Trek* in a leather jacket," whatever that may mean. Ken Scott says that Bowie told him during recording that "the lyrics make absolutely no sense." And yet the song clearly meant enough to Bowie to provide the name, years later, for his music publishing company Bewlay Bros Music. Perhaps even this was a calculated move to add to the song's mystique. Perhaps it also explains the appearance of a rather pointless and almost identical 'Alternate Mix' on the 1990 reissue of *Hunky Dory*. And perhaps it explains why, for over 30 years, Bowie declined to perform the song live. 'The Bewlay Brothers' finally made its long-awaited concert debut at the BBC session recorded in London on 18 September 2002. "I have never, ever performed this in my life until this minute," David told the audience. "One of the reasons, probably," he added wryly as he unfurled a lyric sheet, "is that there are more words in this than there are in Tolstoy's *War and Peace*." The magnificent performance that followed didn't disappoint. 'The Bewlay Brothers' made just two more appearances, at concerts in Hammersmith and Brooklyn the following month, before disappearing from the repertoire.

Ultimately, to try to unravel the enigma of 'The Bewlay Brothers' is to miss the point entirely. The very proliferation of different readings should be evidence enough that the song doesn't need to be "about" homosexuality or schizophrenia or drugs or religion, when it can embrace them all among a multiplicity of possibilities. Hearing Bowie at the peak of his powers wailing darkly about "the Goodmen of Tomorrow", "the crust of the sun", "flashing teeth of brass" and "the grim face on the cathedral floor", it's hard *not* to impose one's own reading. We shouldn't really care whether it's a meticulously precise puzzle-box or a surreal nightmare conceived in the aftermath of some ghastly heroin experiment – or something in between. Regardless of all that, both musically and lyrically it's a strong contender for the accolade of Bowie's greatest song, and the slow fade of sinister cartoon voices chortling "Please come away" provides one of the finest and most unsettling endings to any album in rock history.

BIG BOSS MAN *(Smith/Dixon)*

Jimmy Reed's blues standard, probably brought to David's attention as the B-side of The Pretty Things' single 'Rosalyn', was among The Manish Boys' live repertoire.

BIG BROTHER
• Album: *Dogs* • Live: *David*

Although the title announces its origins in Bowie's abandoned *Nineteen Eighty-Four* adaptation, 'Big Brother' is a logical continuation of concerns found throughout his early albums, stretching as far back as 1970's 'Saviour Machine' or even 1967's 'We Are Hungry Men'. Once again the theme is the dangerous charisma of absolute power, and the facility with which societies succumb to totalitarianism's final solutions. Big Brother is "someone to claim us, someone to follow", but also "someone to fool us, someone like you": the glamour of dictatorship is balanced with the banality, reminding us that anyone with a mind to it could be a Hitler – as, raddled with cocaine and alcohol, Bowie would ill-advisedly begin to claim a year or two later.

Given the portentous menace of the finished track, replete with space-age synthesizers and distorted saxophones, 'Big Brother' betrays a surprisingly mixed parentage. On the one hand the lyric recalls earlier

Bowie tracts – the opening phrase about "dust and roses" echoes the "dead roses" of 'Aladdin Sane', while the soft falsetto section and the "glass asylum with just a hint of mayhem" both revisit 'All The Madmen' – but on the other hand the chording and lyrics of the chorus are inescapably reminiscent of the Bonzo Dog Band's burlesque 1969 entreaty to "follow Mr Apollo" (*Diamond Dogs* drummer Aynsley Dunbar had played with the Bonzos in 1969, but this is probably mere coincidence).

'Big Brother' was performed during the Diamond Dogs tour and was revived in 1987 for the Glass Spider show. Interestingly the chorus melody is quoted note-for-note (and almost word-for-word: "Someone to pray for"), in the same year's *Never Let Me Down* track 'Shining Star (Makin' My Love)'; perhaps it was this minor piece of self-plagiarism that prompted David to revive the original.

A BIG HURT
• Album: *TM2* • B-Side: 10/91 [48]

Activated by an energetic punk riff indebted to the Sex Pistols/Buzzcocks legacy, *Tin Machine II*'s only solo Bowie composition is a turgid thrash-up recalling the less imaginative portions of the band's debut album. Shouty vocals, squealing guitars, relentless drumming and a sexist lyric (including a bizarre reference to "a glass eye in a duck's ass") add up to very little. A re-recorded version from Tin Machine's 1991 BBC session appeared on the 'Baby Universal' 12", and the song was performed throughout the It's My Life tour.

BLACK COUNTRY ROCK
• B-Side: 1/71 • Album: *Man*

This is a jaunty, tightly-played number with a similar chord sequence to the previous year's 'Unwashed And Somewhat Slightly Dazed', and as on that track David drops into an almost actionable impersonation of Marc Bolan's trademark electro-warble. Tony Visconti later recalled that "David spontaneously did a Bolan vocal impression because he ran out of lyrics. He did it as a joke, but we all thought it was cool, so it stayed. In fact, we re-recorded it to get it right, and I thinned out David's voice with equalisation to get it to sound more like Bolan's."

Although the melody was already written at the start of the album sessions, the words were apparently a last-minute job after a frustrated Tony Visconti demanded some input from the apathetic Bowie. Perhaps this explains the rather minimal lyric – a single repeated two-line verse and chorus – which nonetheless crystallizes the travelling/climbing quest motif which recurs throughout the album.

THE BLACK HOLE KIDS

Described by Bowie in 2000 as "fascinating", this unfinished song from the Ziggy period was among the half-dozen fragments then being reworked with a view to release in 2002 to mark the thirtieth anniversary of the *Ziggy Stardust* album. The project was shelved and the song remains unheard. Judging by its title, it may originally have been written for the aborted 1973 stage show (see 'Starman' for more on Bowie's interest in black holes).

BLACK TIE WHITE NOISE
• Album: *Black* • A-Side: 6/93 [36] • Bonus: *Black (2003)* • Video: *Black, Best Of Bowie*

On 29 April 1992, Bowie and his new wife Iman arrived in Los Angeles to begin house-hunting. On the same day the acquittal of four policemen in the Rodney King case triggered the city's worst ever race riots. A curfew was imposed, and from the safety of their hotel window the newlyweds watched shops being looted and buildings set alight. "It was an extraordinary feeling," David told *Record Collector*. "I think the one thing that sprang to our minds was that it felt like a prison riot more than anything else. It felt as if innocent inmates of some vast prison were trying to break out – break free from their bonds."

Bowie's eyewitness experience of the Los Angeles riots would infuse much of *Black Tie White Noise*, most tangibly on the title track, an edgy plea for mutual respect of ethnic identity that tries very hard to avoid the banalities attendant on the genre. "I didn't want it to turn into an 'Ebony And Ivory' for the nineties," he told *Rolling Stone*. To his credit, it doesn't. 'Black Tie White Noise' sees Bowie ripping and re-wrapping in his best mid-1970s style, incorporating a quotation from Marvin Gaye's 'What's Going On' alongside a blatant reworking of the backing vocals from 'Fame', a song whose savage, streetwise cynicism is here revisited: Bowie cocks a snook at the fatuity of corporate race-relations ("Getting my facts from a Benetton ad, looking through African eyes") and simplistic idealism ("Reach out over race and hold each other's hand, walk through the night thinking 'We Are The World'"). The reference to USA For Africa's mealy-mouthed charity hit suggests an altogether different Bowie from the all-round entertainer who had wowed the masses at Live Aid eight years earlier. "We're far too keen, as white liberals, to suggest to black people how they should improve their lot," he told the *NME*. "I don't think they actually wanna hear it any more. They've got their own ideas of how they can improve their lot, and they couldn't give a fuck what we think. They don't want our advice." In another interview he added that "If we can start recognizing and appreciating the differences between ourselves, and not look for white sameness within everybody, then we have a much better chance of creating a real and meaningful integration. I wanted to get some of that in the song."

On the subject of America's ongoing racial struggle Bowie was even more forthright. "It won't be gained easily," he opined in *Record Collector*, "And it won't be gained by singing 'We Are The World' or 'We Shall Overcome'. Those elements of coming together should be foremost in our minds, but it's not going to be like that in actuality. There's going to be an awful lot of antagonism before there's any real move forward." The song reaffirms this belief, as the black and white voices of Bowie and guest vocalist Al B Sure! uneasily conclude that "There will be some blood, no doubt about it, but we should come through."

Thankfully though, 'Black Tie White Noise' isn't ponderously worthy. It's slick and funky, with wah-wah guitars and bursts of Lester Bowie's trumpet laid over an atmospheric gramophone crackle. David lets Al B Sure! take the first verse and the lion's share of the vocal duties. "I've never worked longer with any artist than with Al B," laughed Bowie later. "I had a particular thing that I wanted to do with this song, and he spent a long time working through it … It was often quite punishing for both of us. However, out of those kind of punishments, jewels often appear." It is believed that Bowie's first choice for duettist was the unavailable Lenny Kravitz, who later guested on 'Buddha Of Suburbia'.

'Black Tie White Noise' was released as the album's second single, credited to "David Bowie featuring Al B Sure!". It barely scraped the UK top 40, and in America, not even a mind-boggling barrage of club remixes could trigger any chart action. The excellent and undervalued video, directed by Mark Romanek, is a deft bricolage of images against the backdrop of an urban ghetto: Bowie and Al B appear alongside despondent black children roaming the rubble and alternately displaying toy guns and Bowie's saxophone (a motif borrowed from Kate Bush's 'Army Dreamers' video); a black child looks at a picture of a white Jesus; a black face retreats into a white hood. A mimed studio version appeared on the *Black Tie White Noise* video release, and Bowie also performed the song twice on US television, appearing with Al B on *The Arsenio Hall Show* and *The Tonight Show With Jay Leno* in May 1993.

BLACKOUT

• Album: *"Heroes"* • Live: *Stage*

Typical of the darkly exhilarating sonic schizophrenia of the *"Heroes"* album, 'Blackout' would work perfectly well as a straightforward rock and roll song – the basic riff is not dissimilar to 'Suffragette City' – but as it is, it's one of the more left-field noises even on *"Heroes"*. Swathes of squealing synthesizers are punctuated by crazed percussion breaks and spliced loops of background noise, topped off by the vocal "Bowie histrionics" for which the title track is so noted. The lyric is an elliptical cut-up of fractured images returning to the album's preoccupation with alcohol: "Too high a price to drink rotting wine from your hands … Get me to a doctor's, I've been told someone's back in town, The chips are down, I just cut and blackout, I'm under Japanese influence and my honour's at stake!" Contemporary reviewers assumed it was an account of Bowie's much-publicized collapse at the end of the *Low* sessions in November 1976 (according to this reading "get me to a doctor" speaks for itself, while "someone's back in town" might refer to Angela, who arrived from the airport just in time for the crisis) – but David denied this, claiming the song was about the great New York power blackout of July 1977, an event on which jazz musician Lionel Hampton did indeed base an album called *Black Out*. The song was performed on the 1978 tour, from which an excellent live version appears on *Stage*.

BLAH-BLAH-BLAH *(Pop/Bowie)*

Co-written and co-produced by Bowie for Iggy Pop's album of the same name, this excellent experiment in sonic montage is one of the few genuinely ground-breaking songs of Bowie's mid-1980s period. A live version, also co-produced by David, appeared on the B-side of 1987's 'Fire Girl' single.

BLEED LIKE A CRAZE, DAD
• Album: *Buddha*

Further evidence of Bowie's self-sampling can be found on this track, which sets a creditable Robert Fripp guitar impression against *Lodger*-style percussion and a bassline ripped straight from 'Sister Midnight' via 'Red Money'. With Mike Garson free-wheeling on piano and a lyric quoting Shirley And Company's 1975 hit 'Shame Shame Shame' (often said, incorrectly, to have inspired 'Fame'), it's a kaleidoscopic reshuffle of Bowie's past over which he delivers a quickfire white rap, referring at one point to "where the dead man walks", reminding us that his habit of self-recycling is an ongoing process.

BLOWIN' IN THE WIND *(Dylan)* :
see **THE JEAN GENIE**

BLUE JEAN
• Album: *Tonight* • A-Side: 9/84 [6] • Video: *Jazzin' For Blue Jean, Collection, Best Of Bowie* • Live Video: *Glass*

Tonight's uneasy fusion of R&B basics with trick-shot percussion, all-pervading saxophones and plonking marimba finally comes good on 'Blue Jean', arguably the album's most successful number. It's a great throwaway single in the 1950s-throwback tradition of 'The Jean Genie', a track recalled by the title. Based on the classic Eddie Cochran riff found on hits like 'Somethin' Else' and 'C'mon Everybody' (and thus a replay of Bowie's inspiration for 'Hang On To Yourself'), it's also an obvious result of the R&B homework David undertook before the *Let's Dance* sessions eighteen months earlier. "It was inspired from that Eddie Cochran feeling," he said, "but that of course is very Troggs as well … it's quite eclectic, I suppose. What if mine isn't?" Elsewhere he described 'Blue

Jean' as a "sexist piece of rock'n'roll," pretty much summing up the lyric which is little more than a paean to a passing rock-chick.

As *Tonight*'s lead-off single 'Blue Jean' went top ten on both sides of the Atlantic – number 6 in Britain, 8 in America – propelled by the most elaborate video of Bowie's career (see Chapter 5 for details of *Jazzin' For Blue Jean*). A few days after shooting finished on *Jazzin' For Blue Jean*, Julien Temple filmed a second, less elaborate video at Soho's Wag Club for a one-off screening at New York's MTV Awards on 14 September 1984. Sporting an alarmingly naff print jacket from Culture Shock and clutching an acoustic guitar, Bowie introduced the song to camera as though it were a live performance (it wasn't; the same backing extras used in *Jazzin' For Blue Jean* were in attendance, although this time their live vocals were mixed in for the choruses). He introduced his band as "The Aliens" and dedicated the number to "all our friends in the American Empire". This version appeared as a concealed "Easter Egg" on the *Best Of Bowie* DVD, as did the full-length *Jazzin' For Blue Jean* film.

'Blue Jean' was played throughout the Glass Spider and Sound + Vision tours, and made a few reappearances on A Reality Tour.

BLUE MOON *(Rodgers/Hart)*

The Rodgers & Hart standard was included in David's medley with Cher on CBS's *The Cher Show* in November 1975.

BOMBERS
• Bonus: *Hunky* • Live: *Beeb*

Tight, *Ziggy*-style production and unlikely bassman backing vocals combine on this out-take from the *Hunky Dory* sessions. Not the finest song of its time, and certainly not up to the prevailing standards of the album, it's a frenetic piece of hippy-flavoured satire in which a nuclear bomb test accidentally leads to all-out war. Bowie called it "a kind of skit on Neil Young", and he may also have borrowed from Joni Mitchell's 'Woodstock' ("I dreamed I saw the bombers riding shotgun in the sky…"). Considering that this lyric is contemporaneous with some of his most multi-textured masterpieces it's hard not to smile at vaudeville lines like "the pilot felt quite big-time as the bomb sailed through the air", but then, the fact that Bowie's music-hall streak has never fully deserted him is one of the keys to his greatness. Even here there are echoes of *Hunky Dory*'s more substantial concerns, including a "crack in the world" to mirror the "crack in the sky" found in 'Oh! You Pretty Things' (it's worth pointing out, too, that *Crack In The World* was the title of a rather corny 1965 sci-fi movie, in which scientists drilling into the earth's crust nearly bring about the planet's destruction).

Bowie accompanied himself on piano for the rough 2'52" demo of 'Bombers' which has appeared on bootlegs, and again for a BBC session on 3 June 1971; the latter recording, which now appears on *Bowie At The Beeb*, offers an alternative ending which presses home *Hunky Dory*'s bookish preoccupation with religious texts and eschatological themes: "Except a man, dear Lord, who looked like you / Used to look / In my holy book". The full studio version (with the revised final couplet "Floating high / Up in the sky") came soon afterwards during the *Hunky Dory* sessions, and for a while 'Bombers' was slated to open the album's second side; a marginally different mix from the rare August 1971 promo LP, whose extended fade-out segues into 'Andy Warhol', has surfaced on bootlegs. Even after it was dropped from *Hunky Dory* 'Bombers' was being considered for future use, but *Ziggy Stardust* material it wasn't.

BOOM BOOM (*Hooker*) :
see **HEAVEN'S IN HERE**

BORN OF THE NIGHT

In May 1965 Davie Jones and The Lower Third recorded several demos at Denmark Street's Central Sound Studios, of which David's composition 'Born Of The Night' is the only confirmed title. It was touted as a single by Davie himself in a brazenly confident press release he typed at home and sent to dozens of agents, bookers and promoters: "THE LOWER THIRD – THE group to watch this year. Gaze on, as their record, *BORN OF THE NIGHT* (released shortly) rushes up the charts. Stand astounded at their brilliant backings for Davie. TEA-CUP on lead. DEATH on bass. LES on drums." The press release went on to claim that Davie was about to reappear on BBC2's *Gadzooks! It's All Happening*. He wasn't; 'Born Of The Night' was reject-

ed by producer Shel Talmy, and went no further than the demo stage.

BOTH GUNS ARE OUT THERE

This semi-instrumental funk out-take (the title is far from official) was recorded by Bowie with his former *Space Oddity* guitarist Keith Christmas, who tells Christopher Sandford that he was called to a session in Hampstead a year after he had pulled out of the Diamond Dogs tour. This seems unlikely, as Bowie was in America throughout 1975; perhaps it was in May 1976, during the UK leg of the Station To Station tour. According to Christmas, Bowie later "nicked" the riff for *Black Tie White Noise*.

BOYS KEEP SWINGING (*Bowie/Eno*)
• A-Side: 4/79 [7] • Album: *Lodger* • Video: *Collection, Best Of Bowie*

Interpreted by some as a message of optimism for Bowie's seven-year old son Joe, by others as a tongue-in-cheek assault on male chauvinism, and by everyone as evidence of an enduring preoccupation with blurring the boundaries of gender (the line "When you're a boy, other boys check you out" is open to a variety of readings), 'Boys Keep Swinging' was a particular favourite with the critics on its release. *Smash Hits*, which in April 1979 was only a few months old and still a serious-minded magazine specializing in new wave music, called it "his best in ages". In an effort to suggest "young kids in the basement just discovering their instruments", Bowie famously made his musicians swap roles on the track: drummer Dennis Davis plays bass, while guitarist Carlos Alomar moves to percussion, with deliciously garage-like results. As for Bowie himself, 'Boys Keep Swinging' offers the first significant showcase of a vocal style that would dominate his recordings well into the 1980s: the mockingly butch faux-Elvis baritone later deployed to such explosive effect on tracks like 'Let's Dance' (and, when unwisely transmuted into an all-out croon, to such toe-curling embarrassment on the likes of 'God Only Knows').

'Boys Keep Swinging' is remembered as much for its video as for the song itself. The first of Bowie's many collaborations with director David Mallet, it's the earliest substantial specimen of his espousal of rock video which, during the early 1980s, would become an inextricable part of his creative process. Mallet, a restless pioneer of cutting-edge video technology who had made his name on innovative American TV shows like *Hullabaloo* and *Shindig*, was directing Thames Television's *The Kenny Everett Video Show* when Bowie appeared to perform 'Boys Keep Swinging' on the 23 April 1979 edition. The show was renowned in industry circles for Everett's outrageous experiments with techniques like chromakey and Quantel, as well as for his anarchically disrespectful behaviour towards the big-name guests he invariably attracted. On this occasion Everett's "Angry of Mayfair" character (an apoplectic bowler-hatted city gent whose rear view revealed a penchant for women's lingerie) chased the hapless Bowie around the studio yelling, "Look at you, you lily-livered mincer! I was in the war, but I didn't see you there. I fought for people like you – and I never got one!"

The lasting legacy of Bowie's appearance on the Everett show was his decision to hire Mallet for the 'Boys Keep Swinging' promo, which was recorded back-to-back with the Everett performance. Both starred a fresh-faced schoolboy Bowie in a 1950s Mod-style suit, but it was the video that added the three glamorous lady backing singers who, through the magic of split-screen, each turn out to be David in drag. At the end of the clip the first two approach the camera in turn, remove their wigs and ferociously smear their make-up in the style David had observed at Romy Haag's Berlin nightclub. "That was a well-known drag act finale gesture which I appropriated," he said. "I really liked the idea of screwing up [the] make-up after all the meticulous work that had gone into it. It was a nice destructive thing to do – quite anarchistic." Variations on the lipstick-smearing motif appear in many later Bowie videos, including 'China Girl' and 'Jump They Say'. The final figure, a dowdy and severe lady in tweeds (intended, Bowie confessed, to lampoon his *Just A Gigolo* co-star Marlene Dietrich), merely glares at the camera and blows a kiss. Incidentally, five years later David Mallet was responsible for rock's even more famous megastars-in-drag video, Queen's 'I Want To Break Free'.

The publicity drive, which also included a guest DJ spot on Radio 1's *Star Special*, pushed 'Boys Keep Swinging' to number 7 after it had already begun falling, giving Bowie his biggest hit since 'Sound And Vision'. But the gender-bending video and dodgy lyric proved too much for the poor souls at RCA America,

who decided against a US release – an exact repeat of the 'John, I'm Only Dancing' fiasco seven years earlier. Considering the transatlantic enormity of Village People's less than heterosexual smash 'YMCA' only a few weeks earlier, it seems almost incredible.

'Boys Keep Swinging' was among the numbers performed in Bowie's famous 1979 *Saturday Night Live* appearance; surprisingly, its only other live outing was for 1995's Outside tour. Struggling Dundee hopefuls The Associates released an exuberant cover version in October 1979 in a deliberate attempt to infringe copyright and get themselves noticed; the ploy worked and led to the band's first contract. Susanna Hoffs of The Bangles included a cover on her 1991 solo album *When You're a Boy*; this version now appears on *David Bowie Songbook*. Damon Albarn described Blur's heavily indebted 1997 single 'M.O.R.' as a tribute to 'Boys Keep Swinging', and latterly, following legal rumblings, releases have credited it to Blur/Bowie/Eno.

BREAKOUT *(Knight/Bernstein)*

This 1966 US hit for Mitch Ryder and the Detroit Wheels was performed live by The Buzz.

BREAKING GLASS *(Bowie/Davis/Murray)*
• Album: *Low* • Live: *Stage* • A-Side: 11/78 [54] • Australian A-Side: 1977 • Live Video: *Moonlight*

Little more than a bizarre song-fragment, and in its original form one of the shortest Bowie tracks, 'Breaking Glass' epitomizes the experimental nature of the *Low* project. According to Tony Visconti, Bowie suffered from acute writer's block during the *Low* sessions. Encouraged by Brian Eno to turn every circumstance to good advantage, he ended up with songs like this, less than two minutes long and with only the sketchiest lyric. "The feeling around was that we'd edit it together," explained Eno, "and turn it into a more normal structure, and I said, 'No, don't – leave it abnormal, leave it strange, don't normalize it.'" So 'Breaking Glass' makes a virtue of its brevity, etching out a sharp, disturbing portrait of a half-demented lover before imploding in a blast of synthesizers. Of particular note is the simultaneous menace and absurdity of the line "Don't look at the carpet, I drew something awful on it" – initially farcical, the image twists nastily in the light of David's unwholesome preoccupation with Kabbalistic symbols like the Tree of Life (which he was photographed drawing on the floor a few months earlier – see the rear sleeve of Rykodisc's *Station To Station* reissue). Asked about the line following the publication of this book's first edition, Bowie confirmed that "it is a contrived image, yes. It refers to both the Kabbalistic drawings of the Tree of Life and the conjuring of spirits."

The song is among the *Low* tracks celebrated in 'I Love The Sound Of Breaking Glass', a top ten hit for Nick Lowe in 1978. Flagrantly borrowing the bassline of 'Sound And Vision' and the tinkling piano of 'Be My Wife', Lowe pays enjoyable homage to Bowie's new-wave pioneering but never goes quite so far as plagiarizing it. Ever the wag, Lowe had reacted to the release of *Low* in 1977 by issuing an EP called *Bowi*.

A rare 2'47" version of the original studio track was released as a single in Australia in 1977. Bowie performed 'Breaking Glass' on the Stage, Serious Moonlight, Outside, Heathen and A Reality tours; the excellent *Stage* version was released as an EP single.

BRILLIANT ADVENTURE *(Bowie/Gabrels)*
• Album: *'hours…'*

The avant-rock numbers that close *'hours…'* are punctuated by this frail instrumental which, like 'New Angels Of Promise', is instantly evocative of *"Heroes"*. In this case the models are the doomy melody of 'Sense Of Doubt' and the fragile koto of 'Moss Garden', forming the basis of a haunting Eastern melody of beguiling simplicity.

BRING ME THE DISCO KING
• Soundtrack: *Underworld* • Album: *Reality* • Live Video: *Reality*

Originally essayed during the *Black Tie White Noise* sessions, and re-recorded as a potential *Earthling* track four years later, 'Bring Me The Disco King' was finally brought to fruition on *Reality*. "That was written in 1992 and it was going to be part of *Black Tie White Noise*," Bowie confirmed in 2003, "but I wanted it to sound cheesy and kitschy, and be a kind of real uptempo, disco-y kind of slam at late seventies disco. And the trouble is, it *sounded* cheesy and kitschy, ha ha! It just didn't work. It didn't have any weight to it. I tried it again in the mid-nineties, and it still didn't

work. So I thought, 'Well, I know there's something good about this song, but I'm not quite sure what it is.' So Garson and I just stripped it down completely, with the intention of building the arrangement back up again when we'd gotten to the essential song itself. But once we'd put down the song against Garson tinkering away, it didn't need any more. That was the song. It worked so much better just like that."

Following hard upon the raucous guitar-led assault of *Reality*'s title track, 'Bring Me The Disco King' initially seems incongruous, but its stately presence succeeds in binding the album together. It's one of the most idiosyncratic and strikingly dramatic numbers in the entire Bowie songbook, and it is not difficult to see why David bided his time with it. The earlier versions remain unreleased; re-recorded for *Reality* it finds its natural home, confidently taking its place among Bowie's classic album-closers.

Running to nearly eight minutes, it is also one of Bowie's longest studio tracks: a leisurely, confident excursion into a sophisticated New York jazz sound which allows pianist Mike Garson to take centre-stage in a dazzling display of what he does best, rivalling even 'Aladdin Sane' as a masterclass in his particular talent. "It is pointless to talk about his ability as a pianist – he is exceptional," Bowie observed in 2003. "However, there are very, very few musicians, let alone pianists, who naturally understand the movement and free thinking necessary to hurl themselves into experimental or traditional areas of music, sometimes, ironically, at the same time. Mike does this with such enthusiasm that it makes my heart glad just to be in the same room with him." Garson's performance on 'Bring Me The Disco King' is inspired, the audaciously sparse production allowing it to inhabit and define the song. The remaining instrumental backing consists merely of Matt Chamberlain's echoing snare drums and an ambient, rhythmic hiss, as if of a smoke-machine periodically exhaling in a deserted club.

Remarkably, the arrangement came together in the most roundabout of ways, beginning not with the piano but with the percussion, which was in fact recorded during the *Heathen* sessions for an entirely different number. "That's the only track on the album where we utilise the drumming of Matt Chamberlain, even though he was playing to a completely different song," Tony Visconti explained. "The way that he played was so seductive, so melodic and so beautiful, that we just recorded 'Disco King' over the loops that

I'd made of his performance."

Only after recording his vocal over the drum loops did Bowie enlist Mike Garson to complete the track. "He called me in," explained Garson, "and all he played for me was a drum loop and his voice, and he said, 'Show me the chords and play the piano over that,' and I came up with this whole arrangement." As on 'The Loneliest Guy', Garson then re-recorded the part in his home studio, although on this occasion Bowie elected to use the original Looking Glass recording: "I took the MIDI file home, recorded onto my piano, and ultimately he decided he liked the synth sound better – the Yamaha S-90 keyboard," explained Garson, "so that's what's on there."

'Bring Me The Disco King' blends perfectly with the themes that run throughout *Reality*, offering an elegiac twist on the album's now familiar meditations on creeping age, squandered opportunities, thwarted lives and impending dissolution. The fragmentary images conjure up a time of wasteful, superficial glamour: there's precious little rosy nostalgia in Bowie's chilly recollections of "killing time in the seventies" with "good-time girls", spending "cold nights under chrome and glass" and seeing "damp morning rays in the stiff bad clubs".

The opening line, "You promised me the ending would be clear / You'd let me know when the time was now", revives the title track's weary acceptance of life's chaotic disorder, and also its morbid anticipation of mortality. Again like the title track, the lyric offers an immediate echo of 'My Death': Jacques Brel's "But whatever lies behind the door / There is nothing much to do" here becomes Bowie's "Don't let me know when you're opening the door". There are other echoes too: the repeated refrain of "Don't let me know we're invisible" and the cry of "Soon there'll be nothing left of me" both revive the depressive anxiety of earlier songs like 'Conversation Piece' ("I'm invisible and dumb, and no-one will recall me").

As if recognizing its pivotal significance in the Bowie oeuvre, many press reviews of *Reality* singled out the track for particular praise. *Rolling Stone* hailed it as "another of Bowie's ambivalent farewells to the era in which he wreaked such havoc 'in the stiff bad clubs / Killing time in the seventies'. The difference is he now knows that time is killing him, and all of us, and that the Disco King, that master of revels who promised eternal life on the dance floor, is nowhere to be found."

Bowie's vocal is perhaps his finest on the album,

delivering a polished, evocative lyric with depth and conviction. As he slides through the spine-tingling succession of images there's a palpable sense that this song means a great deal to him, and the result is a magnificently dramatic creation: luminous, sinister, intriguing and ultimately uplifting. From lyrics to production to performance, this is quintessential Bowie: the kind of recording that no other artist could ever come close to delivering.

'Bring Me The Disco King' became the first *Reality* song to be released, albeit in a radically different form. Two weeks ahead of the album, the so-called 'Loner Mix' appeared on the soundtrack CD of the chic, *Matrix*-indebted horror movie *Underworld*. Heavily reworked under the auspices of the film's music supervisor, Nine Inch Nails guitarist Danny Lohner (hence, presumably, 'Loner Mix'), the *Underworld* version discards Mike Garson's piano in favour of a lush rearrangement for strings, guitars and keyboards. Lead guitar is played by John Frusciante of the Red Hot Chili Peppers, while keyboards are courtesy of erstwhile Bowie sessioner Lisa Germano. Most startlingly, and least successfully, some passages of Bowie's vocal are re-sung by Maynard James Keenan, who performs elsewhere on the film's soundtrack. Despite these unlikely blandishments the 'Loner Mix', although lacking the purity and drama of the *Reality* version, is undeniably impressive, and it's a pity that its appearance in the movie itself is restricted to a few bars of the intro.

'Bring Me The Disco King' was a regular highlight of A Reality Tour, opening the encores on most of the initial European dates.

BUDDHA OF SUBURBIA
• Album: *Buddha* • A-Side: 11/93 [35] • Video: *Best Of Bowie*

Bowie's theme song for the BBC's adaptation of *The Buddha Of Suburbia* was conceived as a pastiche of his early 1970s sound, but the result transcends mere self-parody to become the first truly great composition of his 1990s renaissance. The lyric approaches the serial's subject matter from a characteristically oblique angle, becoming a piece of Bowie nostalgia as well as a signature for *Buddha*'s central character Karim. With suggestively autobiographical overtones David sings of "Englishmen going insane" and a youngster "screaming along in south London, vicious but ready to learn" as he dallies with sexual experimentation ("Sometimes I fear that the whole world is queer, sometimes but always in vain … Down on my knees in suburbia, down on myself in every way") and swaps personae in classic style ("with great expectations I change all my clothes"). There's even a superbly cheeky realignment of William Blake's *Jerusalem* for the rock'n'roll generation ("Elvis is English and climbs the hills"). Amid the new androgyny and studied narcissism of "Britpop", David Bowie had come home.

Earlier in 1993, in a joint interview for *NME*, Suede's Brett Anderson had told David that his band consciously "ripped off" the "octave lower vocals" favoured by Bowie twenty years earlier – a technique strongly in evidence on early Suede singles like 'The Drowners' and 'Metal Mickey'. Listening to 'Buddha Of Suburbia' one can't help wondering whether Brett deserves credit for reminding Bowie of the trick, because the split-octave vocals and acoustic guitars instantly evoke memories of tracks like 'The Bewlay Brothers', 'Andy Warhol' and in particular 'All The Madmen'. The latter's opening and closing lines ("Day after day … Zane Zane Zane, Ouvrez le chien") are co-opted for the playout, while the acoustic guitar tag from 'Space Oddity' is cheekily incorporated into the solo. Topped off with a quintessential Bowie saxophone break, the result is what *Q*'s David Cavanagh described as "a kind of historical double-bluff" and "probably his best song since 'Loving The Alien'."

A second mix of 'Buddha Of Suburbia', identical save for a pointless guitar break from Lenny Kravitz which interferes with the textured pastiche of the original, was included at the end of the album. Similar mixes of both cuts (the Kravitz version now dubbed the 'Rock Mix') appeared on the CD single which, saddled with the same feeble publicity as the album, scraped a paltry number 35. The video, featuring footage from the series intercut with shots of David vamping to the song in the middle of St Matthew's Drive, Bromley, was handled by the BBC serial's director Roger Michell and was prepared in two edits after US networks objected to the terrifying sight of Bowie smoking a cigarette. As if to prove that America is not alone in prudishness, BMG pressed a limited run of ten censored CD singles for use by UK radio stations, on which Bowie's voice was thrown into reverse for the duration of the word "bullshit". This preposterous rarity is now valued by collectors at around £200.

BUNNY THING

Little is known about this 1966 out-take except that it was occasionally performed live by The Buzz, and that a studio version was recorded during the *David Bowie* sessions. Blocked from inclusion on *The Deram Anthology 1966-1968*, like the equally mysterious 'Your Funny Smile' and 'Pussy Cat', it remains in the Decca archives and in the hands of a few private collectors.

BUS STOP *(Bowie/Gabrels)*
• Album: *TM* • B-Side: 9/89 [48] • Bonus: *TM* • Live Video: *Oy*

This is one of the more throwaway Tin Machine tracks and, perhaps for that very reason, also one of the best. It's a short, sharp joke about "a young man at odds with the Bible" who finds religion at a bus stop, set to an enjoyable Buzzcocks-style riff. Bowie resurrects his best Anthony Newley "mockney" for the occasion, inviting comparisons with that other great comedy-bus-stop-mentioning-cod-punk classic 'Jilted John'. "The song felt so English," David commented. "It's almost vaudeville. I don't know if the others feel very American or whatever by comparison, but that felt very English."

The first verse of 'Bus Stop' appeared as part of the Tin Machine medley filmed by Julien Temple in 1989, segueing into 'Video Crime'. Pursuing the song's cross-cultural sense of fun, Bowie re-styled it for the 1989 tour in a twanging Country & Western setting, throwing cries of "Good God, hallelujah!" into the mix. A live version recorded in Paris appeared on the 'Tin Machine' CD single. Bowie has often cited Country & Western as the one musical style he regards with total antipathy, and the mocking 'Live Country Version' (retitled 'Country Bus Stop' on 1995's *Tin Machine* reissue) offers ample evidence of this. The song was also played in more conventional form on both Tin Machine tours.

BUZZ THE FUZZ *(Rose)*

This little-known number, penned by Biff Rose of 'Fill Your Heart' fame and originally found on his 1968 album *The Thorn In Mrs Rose's Side*, appeared in Bowie's live repertoire during 1970 and 1971. On 5 February 1970 'Buzz the Fuzz' was captured during a live BBC session. Rose's tongue-in-cheek hippy ditty tells the story of "a rookie cop" in "the land of the free and the home of the hip", who is corrupted by the drug-taking "Alice Dee" (geddit?); it reaches a low with the disastrous lyric "Love is so sensational / When you fall in love with eyes dilational". Perhaps mercifully, David appears not to have recorded a studio version.

CACTUS (Francis)
• Album: *Heathen*

Since the early days of Tin Machine Bowie had often sung the praises of the Bostonian alt-rock band Pixies, and had even covered their 1989 track 'Debaser' on Tin Machine's It's My Life tour. In 1997 the band's now solo singer Frank Black (formerly Black Francis) joined David to perform 'Scary Monsters' and 'Fashion' at his fiftieth birthday concert, and five years later Bowie once again tipped his hat to Francis when he contributed to the Pixies documentary *Gouge* and recorded an energetic cover version of 'Cactus' for inclusion on *Heathen*. Hailing originally from Pixies' 1988 debut album *Surfer Rosa*, 'Cactus' boasts a typically gritty Francis lyric, written from the perspective of a prison inmate who entreats his lover to rub her dress with sweat, food and blood before sending it to him as a keepsake.

Featuring David on guitar, drums and keyboards, and backed by the distorted wobble of Tony Visconti's pile-driving bass, Bowie's raw-edged but tightly produced version is a sophisticated piece of garage rock which makes much of the song's obvious debt to T Rex's 'The Groover', even inserting a tongue-in-cheek cry of "D-A-V-I-D!" into the instrumental break in tribute to the "T-R-E-X!" which opens the Bolan number. 'Cactus' was performed throughout the Heathen and A Reality tours, clocking up a number of recordings for TV shows including *Top Of The Pops* and *Late Night With Conan O'Brien*, and featuring in the live BBC radio session of 18 September 2002.

CAMERAS IN BROOKLYN :
see **UP THE HILL BACKWARDS**

CAN I GET A WITNESS (Holland/Dozier/Holland)

Marvin Gaye's seminal single was covered live by The King Bees in 1964. Bowie has cited the Kon-rads' unwillingness to perform 'Can I Get A Witness' as a reason why he left his earlier outfit, although the date of Gaye's single (October 1963) casts doubt over this recollection.

CAN YOU HEAR ME
• Album: *Americans* • B-Side: 11/75 [8]

'Can You Hear Me' began life as a composition for the Lulu album Bowie was intending to produce after her successful cover of 'The Man Who Sold The World'. The pair had collaborated on the abandoned 'Dodo' during the *Diamond Dogs* sessions, and in April 1974 they convened at RCA's New York studios to record 'Can You Hear Me'. Among the musicians was Puerto Rican guitarist Carlos Alomar, a regular RCA sessioner; it was Bowie's first encounter with one of his most loyal and significant collaborators.

In the run-up to the Diamond Dogs tour Bowie was still enthusing to journalists about Lulu. "I'd like to take her to Memphis and get a really good band like Willie Mitchell's and do a whole album with her, which I will do," he told *Rock* magazine in April 1974. "Lulu's got this terrific voice and it's been misdirected all this time, all these years. People laugh now, but they won't in two years' time, you'll see! I produced a single with her, 'Can You Hear Me', and that's more the way she's going. She's got a real soul voice, she can get the feel of Aretha." Neither album nor single ever happened, and Lulu's version of 'Can You Hear Me' remains one of the lost grails of Bowie fans.

'Can You Hear Me' was revived for *Young Americans* at Sigma Sound in August 1974, from which a 5'24" demo version has appeared on bootlegs. The finished track, benefiting from an elegant Visconti string arrangement, is one of the album's highlights, prefiguring the majestic ballad style Bowie would hone to perfection on *Station To Station*. In 1975 he told an interviewer that 'Can You Hear Me' was "written for somebody, but I'm not telling you who it is. That is a real love song. I kid you not." It's usually assumed that the song is addressed to David's then girlfriend Ava Cherry.

It is worth noting that the line "it's harder to fall" echoes the title of Humphrey Bogart's last movie, a boxing melodrama called *The Harder They Fall* which appeared in 1956, the same year as the similarly-themed *Somebody Up There Likes Me*, which of course gave its title to another *Young Americans* track. From shadow-boxing on stage in 1974 to his appearance on the sleeve of *Let's Dance* and the lyrics of 'Shake It' nine years later, Bowie has maintained an interest in the cinematic image of a sport which, like so much of his music, functions on the unsettling meeting-point between violence and glamour.

On 23 November 1975 David performed 'Can You Hear Me' as a duet with Cher on CBS's *The Cher Show*.

CANDIDATE

• Album: *Dogs* • Live: *David* • Bonus: *Dogs, Dogs (2004)*

There are two distinct Bowie songs called 'Candidate', and although both hail from the *Diamond Dogs* sessions they're sufficiently different to warrant separate discussion. The more familiar version forms the central section of the 'Sweet Thing/Candidate/Sweet Thing' sequence which dominates the first side of *Diamond Dogs*. This 'Candidate' is musically and lyrically inseparable from the rest of the nine-minute medley and is discussed in this book under 'Sweet Thing'.

The other 'Candidate' was unknown until it appeared as a bonus track in 1990, subsequently resurfacing on 2004's anniversary edition of *Diamond Dogs*. Although originally labelled a "demo version" it is in fact an entirely different song, with only the solitary line "pretend I'm walking home" to connect it with the later version. Led by Mike Garson's piano and bumped along by some jaunty swing-band percussion and rasping guitar, the song dabbles with two of Bowie's favourite mid-1970s topics, self-image and Messianic megalomania: "I make it a thing when I gazelle on stage to believe in myself / I make it a thing to glance in window panes and look pleased with myself." There's a hint of the abortive *Nineteen Eighty-Four* project in the Orwellian reference to "the correction room", while Bowie serves alarming notice of his Thin White Duke period when he announces "I'm the Führerling". As lyrics go, it's also one of Bowie's most sexually suggestive, with an opening couplet guaranteed to raise eyebrows. One of the finest tracks unearthed during Rykodisc's reissue programme, this original 'Candidate' offers a valuable glimpse into the genesis of a classic album and is entirely worthy of attention.

CAN'T HELP THINKING ABOUT ME

• A-Side: 1/66

In the autumn of 1965, The Lower Third and their newly renamed singer David Bowie struck a deal with Pye records and producer Tony Hatch, who had been introduced to David's manager Ralph Horton by a mutual acquaintance, Denny Laine of The Moody Blues. Hatch, who had revived Petula Clark's career a year earlier with the monumental hit 'Downtown', would later make his mark on cultural history as the composer (with his wife Jackie Trent) of the theme tunes to *Crossroads* and *Neighbours*. Legend has it that at Pye's Marble Arch Studios, Hatch handed Bowie the tambourine used on 'Downtown' with the words, "I hope this brings you luck." Many years later, Hatch recalled that David was "good to get on with and excellent in the studio. His material was good, although I thought he wrote too much about London dustbins. Those were his formative years and he hadn't reached maturity, but he was unusual, unique." The Lower Third's first recording with Hatch was an early take of David's composition 'The London Boys', rejected by Pye on lyrical grounds.

On 14 January 1966, David Bowie with The Lower Third released 'Can't Help Thinking About Me', Bowie's first Hatch-produced single on Pye. As well as featuring Petula Clark's lucky tambourine, the session was marked by an incident in which Hatch is said to have berated the band's backing vocals as sounding "like a Saturday night at the old Bull and Bush". A launch party for the single was held at the Victoria Tavern in Strathearn Place, financed by Bowie's sponsor Raymond Cook and attended by all manner of minor celebrities including, surreally, John Lennon's father. Apparently David was steered among the press while the rest of the band were ignored, fuelling the discontent already in the air after the singer had been flown back from their recent Paris gigs while the band tagged behind in their converted second-hand ambulance.

The release of 'Can't Help Thinking About Me' sees arguably the earliest full-blown evidence of the darker and more abstruse elements of songwriting which would distinguish David's later career, and this, as much as the rejected 'London Boys', is surely at the root of Tony Hatch's "dustbins" comment. The standard fodder of the R&B lyric – heartless girlfriend doesn't fancy singer – here surrenders to familiar Bowie themes of solipsistic self-withdrawal and emotional alienation, in an obscure narrative about the singer leaving town for an imagined "never-never land" after having mysteriously "blackened the family name". The lyric is also notable for featuring the singer's name ("My girl calls my name – Hi, Dave"), a distinction it shares only with 'Teenage Wildlife' and Bowie's cover version of 'Cactus'.

Bowie later laughingly referred to the title of 'Can't Help Thinking About Me' as "an illuminating little piece". Bearing in mind its position in his career – as the last single for many years that he would release as a band frontman rather than a solo singer – it's worth speculating on the wider implications of lines like "I've got a long way to go, I hope I make it on my own". Long years of struggling and disappointment lay ahead, but already the motif of lonely travelling as a metaphor for the creative quest, later surfacing in tracks like 'Black Country Rock', 'Be My Wife' and 'Move On', was becoming evident. In his first *Melody Maker* interview, in February 1966, Bowie revealed that "Several of the younger teenagers' programmes wouldn't play 'Can't Help Thinking About Me', because it is about leaving home. The number relates several incidents in every teenager's life – and leaving home is something which always comes up." It would be daft to make any claims, but The Beatles came up with their classic 'She's Leaving Home' not so very long afterwards.

Like its predecessors the single was a flop, and this despite a desperate attempt at chart-rigging. Using £250 borrowed from Cook, Ralph Horton contrived to push 'Can't Help Thinking About Me' into the *Melody Maker* chart at number 34. Notwithstanding a curt review in *Record Retailer* ("Original song about teenage trouble. Words worth listening to but arrangement not all that original"), it failed to appear in that periodical's chart or in any other. A forthcoming booking on Associated Rediffusion's *Ready, Steady, Go!* wasn't enough to keep the band together, and the failure of the single spelled the end of David's association with The Lower Third. Heavily in debt, the group elected to disband – not without acrimony if some accounts are to be believed – before a gig at the Bromel Club on 29 January.

The performance of 'Can't Help Thinking About Me' on *Ready, Steady, Go!* went ahead on March 4,

with Bowie's new outfit The Buzz miming along to a backing track they had pre-recorded the day before. David, who sang live vocals, wore a white suit which caused problems for the cameras, bathing him in an unearthly glow. Appearing in the same edition were The Yardbirds and The Small Faces, whose vocalist Steve Marriott apparently disrupted proceedings by shouting to David, "Leap about, you're on TV!"

In May 1966 'Can't Help Thinking About Me' became David's first US release, issued on the Warner Brothers label. Needless to say this too was a flop. Later the same year the track apeared on a Pye compilation called *Hitmakers Volume 4*, making it the first Bowie recording to be released on an album.

More than 30 years later David unexpectedly launched into a snatch of the number during a 1997 gig in San Francisco. Even then, few were prepared for its full-scale revival on the *'hours…'* tour. Unveiling 'Can't Help Thinking About Me' at his *VH1 Storytellers* concert in August 1999, David grinningly proclaimed that the "Hi, Dave" section amounted to "two of the worst lines I've ever written." The revival was executed with real gusto: a superb version was included in Bowie's BBC session two months later, and a new studio recording was made during the following year's *Toy* sessions.

CAN'T NOBODY LOVE YOU (Burke)

The Solomon Burke number was among David's live repertoire with The Manish Boys.

CASUAL BOP : see MADMAN

CAT PEOPLE (PUTTING OUT FIRE)
(Bowie/Moroder)
• A-Side: 4/82 [26] • B-Side: 3/83 [1] • Album: *Dance*
• Live Video: *Moonlight, Best Of Bowie*

In 1981 Bowie was approached by Paul Schrader, the screenwriter-turned-director whose previous credits included writing *Taxi Driver* and directing *American Gigolo*, with a view to collaborating on his remake of Jacques Tourneur's 1942 thriller *Cat People*. Giorgio Moroder had already composed the music, and Bowie was invited to provide and sing the lyrics for the title song. The result, co-produced by Bowie and Moroder (who had first met in 1976 during the recording of Iggy Pop's *The Idiot*), was recorded at Mountain Studios in Montreux in July 1981. It was during this session that Bowie bumped into Queen, a meeting that resulted in 'Under Pressure'.

Among the finest of Bowie's recordings of the 1980s, the original cut of 'Cat People (Putting Out Fire)' is a brooding monolith of a song that finds Bowie in fine vocal fettle; the pure adrenaline rush as the sepulchral intro detonates on the line "I've been putting out fire – *with gasoline!*" is among the most thrilling moments he's ever committed to tape. The lyric is quintessential Bowie material, drawing on imagery previously explored in 'Sound And Vision' and 'It's No Game': "Those who feel me near / Pull the blinds and change their minds" (a line paraphrased by Suede's 1999 track 'Down'). The relevance to Schrader's movie is fleeting at best, although the opening "See these eyes so green / I can stare for a thousand years" evokes the ancient line of feline lycanthropes.

Running to nearly seven minutes, the full-length 12" edit (later on the US release *The Singles 1969 To 1993*) remains the best of the various different versions. The 7" edit, which took the single to number 26 in the UK chart (and number 67 in America), later appeared on several non-UK editions of 2002's *Best Of Bowie*. Both single formats were originally backed by 'Paul's Theme' from Moroder's *Cat People* soundtrack. The single, incidentally, was released on MCA records for contractual reasons relating to Moroder; Bowie, whose relationship with his own label had reached rock bottom, was doubtless happy with the arrangement.

Completists should note that a 3'18" mix appeared on a US promo single, while a longer 9'20" edit featured on the Australian 12". The version in the movie itself is a 4'55" mix with added panther roars. The opening titles feature an instrumental version of the intro, over which Bowie hums the melody; this appears on the soundtrack album as 'The Myth'.

Unfortunately 'Cat People' was later subjected to a decidedly wet re-recording for inclusion on *Let's Dance*, the massive sales of which guaranteed that this drastically inferior take has since become the better-known version. It was supposedly re-recorded because David felt the original lacked punch, which is ironic: the subtle menace and pulsing synthesisers of Moroder's arrangement are usurped by an irritating keyboard motif, Stevie Ray Vaughan contributes an alarmingly Knopfleresque guitar solo, and the slow, chugging intro is dispensed with altogether. This version became the B-side of the 'Let's Dance' single.

The *Let's Dance* version was performed throughout the Serious Moonlight tour, while Bowie's ubiquitous mid-1980s mucker Tina Turner gave a live performance on Channel 4's *The Tube* in 1984, sticking to the preferred Moroder-type arrangement. A cover version by Waldeck, from his album *The Night Garden Reflowered*, was released as a single in 2003.

A CERTAIN GIRL (Neville) :
see **HEAVEN'S IN HERE**

C'EST LA VIE

Bowie demoed this number in October 1967, and it was offered without success to Chris Montez (best known, amusingly enough, for a song called 'Let's Dance'). Nothing more was heard of the song until 1993, when an acetate of Bowie's demo was sold to a German collector at Christie's.

CHANGES
• Album: *Hunky* • A-Side: 1/72 • B-Side: 9/75 [1] • Live: *David, Motion, S+V, SM72, Beeb* • Live Video: *Ziggy*

Regarded for three decades as Bowie's musical manifesto, 'Changes' has become one of his pivotal recordings, seldom omitted from greatest hits compilations even though it never charted in its own right. As Bowie's first single for RCA it was an unmitigated flop, despite becoming (apparently to David's distress) Tony Blackburn's record of the week. When the pleasures of *Hunky Dory* were belatedly discovered in the wake of its follow-up's success, 'Changes' rapidly became a turntable favourite, embedding itself deep in the pop-culture psyche. John Hughes's 1985 brat-pack film *The Breakfast Club* – a cinematic anthem for a new generation of young dudes – opened with a quotation from the song, and as recently as 2000 an episode of *The Simpsons* featured Homer changing the oil in his car while singing, "time to change the oil, ch-ch-changes, don't wanna be a greasy man…" Now that's immortality.

Although every clapped-out rock hack has at one

time or another churned out a Bowie retrospective called 'Changes', only at the most superficial level does the song truly set the template for Bowie's own role-hopping. Stripped of its retrospective resonance the lyric seems rather to be a meditation on the twentysomething Bowie's frustrated attempts to create work of a lasting value, set against the relentless march of time and the incursions of younger minds; in this respect it's very much of a piece with its bedfellows 'Quicksand' and 'Oh! You Pretty Things'. As early as 1972, Bowie described the lyric as "very neurotic".

As many have noted, the song's lurching fluctuations in tempo and key neatly reflect its theme. While time is "running wild" and all around is "impermanence" (a crucial word in Bowie's vocabulary at the time, cropping up on the previous album and reappearing in several interviews of the period), Bowie reflects that his career has taken him down "a million dead-end streets, and every time I thought I'd got it made it seemed the taste was not so sweet." He ponders his familiar 1970s preoccupations about identity and the perception of an artist by his followers: the line "I turned myself to face me" echoes David's encounter with himself in 'The Width Of A Circle', while his anxiety about being perceived as a "faker" is tempered by the knowledge that he is "much too fast" to be affected by how others perceive him. For a seemingly innocuous piece of pop, 'Changes' advances a remarkably sophisticated thought process: Bowie appears to be holding a mirror to his face on the eve of his own stardom. Time for self-confrontation; time to "turn and face the strange".

"I guess it was me being sort of arrogant," David mused in 2002. "It's sort of baiting an audience, isn't it? It's saying, 'Look, I'm going to be so fast you're not going to be able to keep up with me'. It's that kind of perky arrogance of youth. You think you can get away with anything when you're young."

The famous stammering chorus conflates The Who's 'My Generation' (for "hope I die before I get old", read "pretty soon now you're gonna get older") with Dylan's 'The Times They Are A-Changin'' ("time may change me, but I can't trace time"), as Bowie speaks up for *his* generation, angrily berating his elders and demanding to know "Where's your shame? You've left us up to our necks in it!" It's a sentiment that can be traced back to an interview he gave in 1968: "We feel our parents' generation has lost control, given up, they're scared of the future," he told the *Times*. "I feel it's basically their fault that things are so

bad."

A rough 3'33" demo, featuring Bowie accompanying himself on piano with more enthusiasm than accuracy and adding some breathy "hah's" to a marginally different lyric ("now I place myself to face me ... the weeks still seem the same"), has appeared on bootlegs. The *Hunky Dory* version, recorded at Trident, substitutes a superb Rick Wakeman piano performance alongside one of David's earliest saxophone solos – recorded, he later said, "when I was still going through ideas of using melodic saxophone." A further rendition was taped for a BBC radio session on 22 May 1972, and was later included on *Bowie At The Beeb*.

In 2003 'Changes' was performed by Tony Hadley on ITV's talent show *Reborn In The USA*, while the following year a cover version by Butterfly Boucher appeared in the soundtrack of *Shrek 2*. Bowie performed 'Changes' on the Ziggy Stardust, Diamond Dogs, Station To Station, Sound + Vision, 1999-2000, Heathen and A Reality tours. A live version recorded in Boston on 1 October 1972 appeared on the *Sound + Vision Plus* CD, and on the 2003 reissue of *Aladdin Sane*.

CHANT OF THE EVER CIRCLING SKELETAL FAMILY
• Album: *Dogs* • Live: *David*

Diamond Dogs reaches its apocalyptic climax as the death-throes of 'Big Brother' melt into a hypnotic guitar loop in a repeating six-bar pattern alternating between 5/4 and 6/4 time, backed by sinister swishing maracas and a relentless chant that culminates in a stuck-needle effect as the first syllable of "brother" repeats over and over until it echoes into silence. "That was an accident," explained Bowie many years later. "I wanted to have the machine say 'Brother', but it got stuck and kept repeating 'Bro-' which sounded much better!" The effect is, of course, indebted to the end of *Sgt Pepper's Lonely Hearts Club Band*, but here the tone is nightmarish rather than playful, and indeed it's difficult to imagine a darker conclusion to this bleakest of albums. In giving such a stark piece of music an almost absurdly melodramatic title, Bowie deftly sketches in the final image of an emaciated tribe dancing around a fire in some post-holocaust wasteland.

The song was recreated on stage during the

Diamond Dogs tour, augmented by a skittering saxo-phone solo from David Sanborn, and appears at the end of 'Big Brother' on *David Live* despite being uncredited on the track-listing. The backing-tape providing the stuck-needle effect on stage was unreliable, as witnessed in *Cracked Actor* when it makes an unscheduled reappearance during 'Time'. The song returned on the Glass Spider tour.

One of the unlikeliest Bowie tracks ever to have been covered by another artist, 'Chant Of The Ever Circling Skeletal Family' was recorded by The Wedding Present as the B-side of 'Loveslave', the September release in their one-single-a-month gimmick of 1992.

CHILLY DOWN

• Soundtrack: *Labyrinth*

This is the least engaging of Bowie's *Labyrinth* songs, but sparing his blushes is the fact that he doesn't actually sing lead vocals. In the film, 'Chilly Down' is performed by the Fire Gang, five ultra-hip, jive-talking Muppet creations who enjoy dismantling their bodies to play football with their own heads and limbs, but fail to understand that humans can't do the same. It's every bit as daft as it sounds and is probably the movie's weakest sequence. The song, which revisits the Gospel styling of 'Underground', is within a whisker of being a grotesque retread of Iggy Pop's 'Success'. Lead vocals are by voice artists Charles Augins, Richard Bodkin, Kevin Clash (best known as the voice of Elmo in *Sesame Street*) and Danny John-Jules (later to find fame as *Red Dwarf*'s Cat). The 1986 documentary *Into The Labyrinth* featured footage of the puppeteers rehearsing to a different mix of the song, in which Bowie's backing vocals were far more prominent.

CHIM CHIM CHEREE *(R M Sherman/R B Sherman)*

This is not a joke. A popular number in Bowie's live repertoire with The Lower Third in 1965 was a rock-heavy version of the Sherman brothers' Oscar-winning song 'Chim Chim Cheree' from the previous year's Walt Disney movie *Mary Poppins*. The song was among the numbers played by The Lower Third at their unsuccessful BBC audition on 2 November 1965. "A Cockney type, but not outstanding," was one of the comments recorded by the talent selection group, which makes one wonder what they thought of Dick Van Dyke. Tragically, no studio version appears to have been recorded, although some of The Lower Third's Saturday concerts at the Marquee were broadcast live by the pirate station Radio London, so it's just possible that tapes might exist. If so, they'd blow 'The Laughing Gnome' out of the water.

CHINA GIRL *(Pop/Bowie)*

• Album: *Dance* • A-Side: 5/83 [2] • Live: *VH1 Storytellers* • Compilation: *Club* • Video: *Video EP, Collection, Best Of Bowie* • Live Video: *Moonlight, Glass*

Originally produced and co-written by Bowie for Iggy Pop's *The Idiot*, 'China Girl' would go on to become a huge international hit for David when re-recorded for *Let's Dance* six years later. Iggy Pop's original, a flop single in May 1977, later appeared on *David Bowie Songbook*. It's markedly tougher and less poppy than Bowie's version, and Iggy's angrily growling vocal makes better sense of the lyric's forebodings about cultural imperialism and despoliation. "My little China girl, you shouldn't mess with me, I'll ruin everything you are," Iggy warns, before raising the old 1976 Bowie/Pop chestnut of Nazi delusion: "I stumble into town just like a sacred cow, visions of swastikas in my head, plans for everyone…"

All these elements are there in Bowie's *Let's Dance* version, but the addition of an Oriental guitar motif and cute backing vocals (the original has none of that "oh-oh-oh-oh, little China girl" stuff) softens the genuinely sinister side. It was Nile Rodgers who devised the guitar riff, and he tells David Buckley that playing it to Bowie was "the most nervous moment I had in my entire career … I thought I was putting some bubblegum over some great artistic heavy record. I was terrified. I thought he was going to tell me that I'd blasphemed, that I didn't get the record and that I didn't get him, and that I'd be fired. But it was exactly the opposite. He said it was great!" It's a testament to Rodgers's judgment, and to the sheer melodrama of Bowie's bellowing vocal, that the *Let's Dance* version remains a tremendously effective slice of hardcore pop, delivered with gusto and forming a cornerstone for the album's underlying themes of cultural identity and desperate love.

The lengthy album cut was edited for release as the second *Let's Dance* single, peaking at number 2 in June

1983 while the Police held the top spot with 'Every Breath You Take'. In America it made number 10. The great talking point of 'China Girl' was David Mallet's MTV-award-winning video, shot back-to-back with the 'Let's Dance' clip in Australia in February, and featuring an actress called Jee Ling. "She was a lovely girl," Bowie said later. "I went out with her for a while. After that shoot she became a girlfriend of mine." Of the video itself, he explained that it was "a vignette of my continuing fascination with all things Asian. One thing that I'd been surprised by when I was in Australia was the large Chinese population ... so I based this whole piece of work around that particular community."

The video plays up the theme of clashing cultural perspectives, juxtaposing the couple's playful frolics with a sequence in which Jee Ling is transformed into a Westerner's vision of an exotic Chinese goddess, while the animated flashes of barbed wire that frame the shots press home the totalitarian undertones. But at the time, any such subtleties were overshadowed by the closing sequence in which David and Jee Ling recreated *From Here To Eternity*'s famous Burt Lancaster/Deborah Kerr beach scene, only this time without recourse to bathing suits. Predictably, the press foamed at the mouth with excitement (one tabloid weighed in with the classic headline "MY ROMP WITH NAKED BOWIE IN SURF"). *Top Of The Pops* initially banned the video, and subsequently played an expurgated version that kept everything in long-shot and clumsily inserted slow-motion edits to spare us the sight of David's enviably well-toned bottom. Irritatingly, it is this bowdlerized cut that now appears on *Best Of Bowie*.

Long before recording his own version, Bowie played keyboards on 'China Girl' during Iggy Pop's 1977 tour. He latterly included the song in many of his live sets, performing it on the Serious Moonlight, Glass Spider and Sound + Vision tours. A semi-acoustic version featured in his Bridge School benefit set on 20 October 1996. The following year he was taken to task by the host of *The Rosie O'Donnell Show* because he never played the number any more; he responded with an impromptu acoustic rendition, suitably re-titled 'Rosie Girl'. The song returned to the live repertoire in the *'hours...'*, 2000, Heathen and A Reality tours, with Mike Garson occasionally adding a sentimental cabaret-style opening which gave way to a bass-heavy version more reminiscent of Iggy Pop's original. A live version recorded on 23 August 1999

appears on the *VH1 Storytellers* compilation. A year earlier in 1998, Bowie's original version appeared in the soundtrack of *The Wedding Singer*, while an uncredited cover version provided the backing in trailers for the same year's animated Disney feature *Mulan*. More notable cover artists include Nick Cave's early band Boys Next Door, who added the song to their live act as early as 1978, while a live version by James was included on the 1998 reissue of their anthemic hit 'Sit Down'.

In 2003 a radical Far Eastern reworking of Bowie's original appeared in the form of 'China Girl (Club Mix)', which overlaid Chinese instrumentation including the plaintive ehru, a two-stringed bowed instrument. The track accompanied the more widely heard 'Let's Dance (Club Bolly Mix)', later appearing on *Club Bowie* and the 2003 US reissue of *Best Of Bowie*; for further information on the Asian remixes, see 'Let's Dance'.

CHING-A-LING
• Compilation: *Tuesday, Deram* • Video: *Tuesday*

This whimsical acoustic piece, the closest Bowie ever came to Marc Bolan's elves-and-unicorns phase, was a staple in the 1968-1969 Feathers repertoire. Although it would rapidly be consigned to history, the play-out riff was to come in handy a couple of years later when Bowie re-used it to greater effect on 'Saviour Machine'.

The studio version was recorded by Feathers with Tony Visconti on 24 October 1968. Financed by Essex Music in the aftermath of Bowie's split from Decca, the session marked David's first recording at Trident Studios in Wardour Street, later the birthplace of *Hunky Dory* and *Ziggy Stardust* among others. Trident's reputation as a state-of-the-art venue was growing rapidly; the previous July it had become the first studio in London to boast eight-track recording, and its reputation as the venue for The Beatles' recent number 1 'Hey Jude' was a badge it wore with pride.

The full-length 'Ching-a-Ling' featured three verses sung in turn by Bowie, Hermione Farthingale and John Hutchinson. The latter did not enjoy the session: "Visconti wanted me to sing much higher, in a way I wasn't used to," he recalled. "I found him very awkward and didn't get on with him very well." 'Ching-a-Ling' was mooted as a single, possibly to be credited to Feathers, but nothing came of this. An edited version of the recording, excising Bowie's opening verse (and thus sadly removing the reference to "the doo-dah horn"), was used for the 1969 film *Love You Till Tuesday*, and it is this truncated version which is now available on *The Deram Anthology 1966-1968*. The full-length version has only ever appeared on the 1992 CD of the *Love You Till Tuesday* soundtrack; the vinyl version has the edited cut.

The film clip accompanying 'Ching-a-Ling', featuring the three singers cross-legged on cushions strumming at their guitars, was shot at Clarence Studios on 1 February 1969. After Hermione Farthingale's departure, Bowie and Hutch recorded a further, rather ponderous 3'02" acoustic demo around April 1969. "This is a duo version," David explains apologetically on the tape, before digressing to reveal that Hermione has departed for America.

'Ching-a-Ling' later became the subject of a copyright dispute with Essex Music (see 'April's Tooth Of Gold').

CIGARETTE LIGHTER LOVE SONG
(Walker/Bowie) : see **ALL THE YOUNG DUDES**

COLOUR ME *(Ronson/Morris)*

Together with Def Leppard's Joe Elliott, Bowie provides backing vocals for this track on Mick Ronson's posthumously released *Heaven And Hull*.

COLUMBINE

Written and performed by David as part of Lindsay Kemp's mime production *Pierrot In Turquoise*, 'Columbine' survives as a 1'32" demo made for the 1970 TV adaptation *The Looking Glass Murders*. Like its companion pieces 'Threepenny Pierrot' and 'The Mirror', the song concerns the eternal triangle of the *commedia dell'arte* figures of Harlequin, Pierrot and Columbine.

COME AND BUY MY TOYS
• Album: *Bowie*

Of a piece with 'There Is A Happy Land', this Blakeian evocation of innocence taps into the nostalgia for an illusory Edwardian childhood that was an essential

ingredient in the British psychedelia scene. Accompanied only by a folksy twelve-string guitar, Bowie paints a bucolic idyll of "smiling girls and rosy boys" with "golden hair and mud of many acres on their shoes", whose carefree years will soon be over: "you shall work your father's land, but now you shall play in the market square till you be a man." The song was offered without success to Judy Collins and to Peter, Paul and Mary, already legendary for their version of 'Blowing in the Wind'. Bowie's version was recorded on 12 December 1966.

COME BACK MY BABY :
see **IT'S GONNA BE ME**

COME SEE ABOUT ME *(Holland/Dozier/Holland)*

The Supremes' 1965 hit was played live by The Buzz in 1966.

COMME D'HABITUDE *(François/Thibault/Revaux)* :
see **EVEN A FOOL LEARNS TO LOVE**

COMMERCIAL

In 1995 Bowie recorded a 60-second synth/sax realignment of '"Heroes"', reminiscent of Thomas Dolby's Live Aid makeover, for a Kodak Advantix television commercial screened in various countries the following year. Athough also referred to as 'Kodak', it appears that 'Commercial' is the track's thrilling official title.

COMPANIES OF COCAINE NIGHTS :
see **MADMAN**

CONVERSATION PIECE
• B-Side: 3/70 • Bonus: *Oddity, Heathen, Heathen* (SACD)

This overlooked and melancholy 1969 number features a lovely melody and an emotive lyric covering familiar Bowie topics of alienation and social exclusion. The self-portrait of a misunderstood and unappreciated young writer struggling to achieve something worthwhile from his London bedsit ("I'm invisible and dumb, and no-one will recall me") acutely matches the image, suggested by countless contemporary accounts, of David himself on the eve of his first success.

The 3'07" acoustic demo, recorded with John Hutchinson around April 1969, is introduced on the tape by Bowie as "a new one". This, together with a fumbled start and an apologetic closing mutter of "A bit rough, but there you are," dates the composition immediately prior to the recording of *Space Oddity*. The finished studio cut, recorded at Trident during the album sessions, was later released as the B-side of the 1970 single 'The Prettiest Star'. Kenneth Pitt considered 'Conversation Piece' "one of David's most underrated and little-known compositions", citing the line "my essays lying scattered on the floor fulfil their needs just by being there" as a perfect evocation of "the atmosphere of his room at [my] flat and perhaps every room he has lived and worked in."

The delayed release of 'Conversation Piece' has led to erroneous conclusions that it might hail from a later session, but its unmistakable Tim Renwick guitar line places it firmly with the *Space Oddity* recordings, and it is only the subsequent pairing with 'The Prettiest Star' that gave rise to the false rumour that Marc Bolan plays guitar on the track. Tales of a 1972 re-recording are almost certainly untrue, but thirty years later the song was revived during 2000's *Toy* sessions. This stately recording, taken at a slower pace, sung an octave lower and much benefiting from a sumptuous string arrangement by Tony Visconti, was later included on the bonus disc issued with initial pressings of *Heathen* – whose liner notes claimed erroneously that it was recorded in 2002.

COOL CAT *(Mercury/Deacon/Taylor/May)*

Recorded alongside 'Under Pressure' during the brief Bowie/Queen collaboration in Montreux in July 1981, an early version of 'Cool Cat' (subsequently remixed for Queen's *Hot Space*) features some rudimentary backing vocals from Bowie. Often incorrectly described as a demo, this version is in fact an early mix of the album recording and even appeared on some early promo pressings. Bowie is understood to have requested at a late stage that his vocals be removed.

The performing rights organization BMI lists a further three song titles credited to David Bowie and various members of Queen: these are 'Ali', 'It's Alright' and 'Knowledge'. Other than their titles, these songs remain a mystery.

COSMIC DANCER *(Bolan)*

On 6 February 1991 Bowie made a surprise appearance during the encores of a Morrissey concert in Los Angeles to duet on Marc Bolan's 'Cosmic Dancer', originally from the 1971 T Rex album *Electric Warrior*. A clip from this performance appeared in Channel 4's 2003 documentary *The Importance Of Being Morrissey*.

COUNTRY BUS STOP : see BUS STOP

CRACK CITY
• Album: *TM* • B-Side: 10/89 • Live Video: *Oy*

With a drum figure and guitar riff blatantly borrowed from Jimi Hendrix's reading of The Troggs' classic 'Wild Thing', and a lyric of unabashed finger-wagging didacticism, 'Crack City' epitomizes the Tin Machine paradigm – so direct as to be verging on the crass, but somehow pulling off a touch of visceral excitement all the same. The subject (and hence, clearly, the adoption of the Hendrix setting) is the urban drug apocalypse blighting America and elsewhere, with the newcomer of the late 1980s – crack cocaine – taking centre stage. Fifteen years on from his own descent into the maelstrom, Bowie rages with unmitigated disgust on 'Crack City', without doubt the most unambiguous song he's ever written. He dismisses rock stars who glorify drug abuse as "icon monsters" who are "corrupt with shaky visions," and lays a curse on "the master dealer".

Nobody could doubt the integrity of the intention, but 'Crack City' is ill served by its hoary rock'n'roll pretensions and a ridiculous outburst of swearing (pardon me for coming over all Mary Whitehouse, but this is the track on which you can hear David Bowie shouting "piss", "whore", "assholes", "buttholes" and "fuckheads" – the cumulative effect is sadly not the desired result of appearing mature and serious). There are leaden attempts at drug-related puns: "They'll bury you in velvet and place you underground," he sings at one point. "This is not a slight on Lou because Lou is clean," Bowie explained to *Q* at the time. "The sound that one associates with that particular lifestyle is very much personified by the early Velvets. I had hoped that I gave that away in those two lines." But despite its one-dimensional rage, 'Crack City' does its work. The evocation of Hendrix and the memory of Bowie's own past make for a powerful enough ride, and it's not as if Bowie was under any illusions that this was a multi-faceted work of art: "I don't wanna go on preaching but I've only heard a couple of anti-drug songs," he told *Melody Maker*. "Frankly, I don't think many people are writing them, but I've not heard one that's effective because they're all intellectual, they're all literate, and they're written for other writers."

A 'Crack City' excerpt was included in Julien Temple's 1989 Tin Machine film, and the song was performed on both of the band's tours. A live version recorded in Paris appeared on extended formats of the 'Prisoner Of Love' single, and in 1996 a cover version was released by Spacehog.

CRACKED ACTOR
• Album: *Aladdin* • Live: *David, Motion, Beeb* • B-Side: 10/83 [46] • Live Video: *Ziggy, Moonlight*

Bowie's harmonica and Mick Ronson's dirty blues guitar reaffirm *Aladdin Sane*'s "Ziggy in America" manifesto in this sleazy tale of a superannuated film star paying for sex in a tinseltown back-room. Thematically it's this album's 'Rock'n'Roll Suicide', but the dignity, melodrama and even optimism of that song have been usurped by the jaundiced reality of a superstar's seedy decline. The hollow gratification of meaningless celebrity is exposed by the punning juxtapositions of movie stardom with kinky sex and drug dependency: "show me you're real" can also be "show me your reel", while lines like "I'm stiff on my legend", "smack, baby, smack" and "you've made a bad connection" speak for themselves. The faded grandeur of Beverly Hills and Sunset Boulevard, where half-remembered screen stars struggle to maintain a grotesque parody of glamour as they totter towards death, has rarely been so savagely exposed.

'Cracked Actor' was performed live throughout the 1973 tour. For the following year's Diamond Dogs show Bowie became a cod Hamlet, donning a Shakespearean doublet and singing the song to a skull. It was a great image: not only did the Yorick

affectation provide instant shorthand for everything actorish, but it reinforced the song's terror of ephemerality with Hamlet's own: "let her paint an inch thick, to this favour she must come." The song was dropped from the Philly Dogs show (one of the last performaces was filmed for the BBC documentary which took the song's title), but 'Cracked Actor' returned nine years later, complete with the skull routine, for the Serious Moonlight tour. It was revived once again for the 1999-2000 concerts, from which a live version recorded at the BBC Radio Theatre on 27 June 2000 was included on the *Bowie At The Beeb* bonus disc.

Among the many covers of 'Cracked Actor' are versions by Big Country (on their 1993 CD single 'Ships (Where Were You)'), Duff McKagan (on 1993's 'Believe In Me') and Marry Me Jane (on 1995's 'Misunderstood').

CRIMINAL WORLD *(Godwin/Browne/Lyons)*
• Album: *Dance*

'Criminal World' was originally released as a single in 1977 by Metro, an early synth-pop duo fronted by Peter Godwin. The single was banned by the BBC, who fled in terror from its bisexual propositions. By 1982, when young pretenders like Boy George and Marc Almond were reinventing Ziggy Stardust's decade-old androgyne chic with the new buzzword "gender-bending", it was fitting that Bowie should appropriate one of his lesser-known imitators and quietly slip a cover version like 'Criminal World' in among the ostentatious heterosexuality of *Let's Dance*.

Musically Bowie's version bears no great surprises, conforming to the smooth dance-floor backbeats of *Let's Dance*, although the tight guitar solo is Stevie Ray Vaughan's finest moment on the album. By comparison with Metro's original it's a rather polite sound, but perhaps David is consciously putting one over on a mainstream audience who'd need to stop dancing and listen to the words before noticing anything amiss. 'Criminal World' became the B-side of the overseas 'Without You' single.

CRY FOR LOVE *(Pop/Jones)*

Co-produced by Bowie for Iggy Pop's *Blah-Blah-Blah* and released as the album's first single. A demo, featuring backing vocals from David, has appeared on bootlegs.

CRYSTAL JAPAN

• B-Side: 3/81 [32] • Bonus: *Scary* • Compilation: *Saints*

Originally entitled 'Fuje Moto San', this instrumental made its first appearance in a 1980 Japanese television commercial for a sake drink called Crystal Jun Rock. Bowie himself appeared in the ad, and when asked why he had taken this unexpected career move, he gave three sensible reasons: "No one has ever asked me to do this before. And the money is a useful thing. And the third, I think it's very effective that my music is on television twenty times a day. I think my music isn't for radio."

Although recorded in 1980 during the *Scary Monsters* sessions, 'Crystal Japan' is more in tune with the second side of *"Heroes"*, its melody strongly reminiscent of the earlier out-take 'Abdulmajid'. Dropped from *Scary Monsters* (it would apparently have ended the album before David opted to reprise 'It's No Game' instead), it was released as a single in Japan only, before appearing in other territories as the B-side of 'Up The Hill Backwards'.

CYCLOPS

'Cyclops' was among the titles included in a set of reel-to-reel recordings sold at Sotheby's in 1990. It has been suggested that 'Cyclops', along with 'The Invader', might hail from the aborted *Nineteen Eighty-Four* stage show, but Tony Visconti has indicated an earlier date, citing them as working titles for 'The Supermen' and 'Saviour Machine' respectively.

CYGNET COMMITTEE

• Album: *Oddity* • Live: *Beeb*

This lengthy and intricate composition, developed from the 1969 demo 'Lover To The Dawn', is considered by many to be one of Bowie's first true masterpieces. The theme, set in a Dylanesque environment of Vietnam-era rage, is David's disillusion with the idle sloganeering and sell-out values of the hippy movement, and perhaps specifically the Beckenham-

based "arts laboratory" he had helped to establish in 1969. Four years earlier Dylan had issued his famous warning not to "follow leaders", and here Bowie pursues the point, warning his listeners not to follow alternative leaders either. His mistrust and rejection of guru figures (a topical enough stance in the aftermath of The Beatles' recent experiences) is an undercurrent that continues throughout Bowie's early 1970s lyrics. Incorporating lyrical references to Dylan's 'Desolation Row' and a Beatle-esque "Love is all we need", 'Cygnet Committee' builds in intensity and anger before imploding in a cautiously optimistic chant of "I want to live" over a relentless 5/4 beat. The cynical yell of "I will fight for the right to be right, and I'll kill for the good of the fight for the right to be right" echoes the sentiments expressed in 'I Kill For Peace', a track on The Fugs' third LP which Kenneth Pitt had given David in late 1966. Meanwhile, the anguished cry of "Screw up your brother or he'll get you in the end" has been seized on as evidence of Bowie's growing preoccupation with his half-brother's schizophrenia; Terry was regularly visiting David from Cane Hill at the time of the *Space Oddity* sessions.

In November 1969 Bowie told George Tremlett that 'Cygnet Committee' was the best song on the album, and would have been released as a single but for the record company: "They say it's too long, nine-and-a-half minutes as opposed to the usual three ... but that's a song in which I had something I wanted to say. It's me looking at the hippy movement, saying how it started off so well but went wrong when the hippies became just like everyone else, materialistic and selfish." In *Music Now!* he explained that 'Cygnet Committee' was "one way of using a song" to attack those who "don't know what to do with themselves. Looking all the time for people to show them the way. They wear anything they're told, and listen to any music they're told to. People are like that." In the same interview Bowie warned – for the first time evoking ideas that would return to plague him in years to come – that "This country is crying out for a leader. God knows what it is looking for, but if it's not careful it's going to end up with a Hitler. This place is so ready to be picked up by anybody who had a strong enough personality to lead." In the light of these remarks 'Cygnet Committee' emerges as a savage exploration of the dangerous and tormented relationships between fashion, charisma, celebrity, Messianism and extremist politics which would later infuse many of Bowie's most famous works – not, as an irresponsible minority of journalists once tried to suggest, as an extension of any personal manifesto, but as a dire warning that the alternative to self-empowerment is likely to be totalitarianism.

Bowie performed 'Cygnet Committee' with ferocious gusto as a cornerstone of his live shows in the months following the album's release. A vigorous live version recorded at the BBC session on 5 February 1970 now appears on *Bowie At The Beeb*.

D.J. *(Bowie/Eno/Alomar)*
• Album: *Lodger* • A-Side: 6/79 [29] • Video: *Collection, Best Of Bowie*

Kicking off the cynical snapshots of Western consumerism that occupy side two of *Lodger*, 'D.J.' is Bowie's wry investigation of the vicarious celebrity and unreal lifestyle of that rising late-1970s icon, the disc jockey. "This is somewhat cynical but it's my natural response to disco," he said. "The DJ is the one who is having ulcers now, not the executives, because if you do the unthinkable thing of putting a record on in a disco not in time, that's it. If you have thirty seconds' silence, your whole career is over."

Bowie was not alone in his distaste for the cult of the DJ. In October 1978 Elvis Costello's bitter diatribe 'Radio Radio' ("radio is in the hands of such a lot of fools trying to anaesthetize the way that you feel") led to all-out war when Tony Blackburn dismissed Costello on air as a "silly little man". When Blackburn found himself introducing the song live on the following week's *Top Of The Pops*, Costello changed the line "such a lot of fools" to "silly little men" and shook a fist at the off-screen presenter. 'D.J.' is less confrontational but just as dramatic, featuring Bowie in top histrionic form ("You think this is easy, realism?") over a wonderfully queasy synthesizer backing and demented violin from Simon House. Adrian Belew's squalling guitar part is also of note, composed from numerous takes so that, as Belew explains in *Strange Fascination*, it "goes through a whole mismatch of different guitar sounds almost like you're changing channel on the radio and each channel has a different guitar solo on it."

'D.J.' is fantastically uncommercial though, and was a questionable choice as a follow-up single to 'Boys Keep Swinging'. Available initially on limited-edition green vinyl, the edited single only just made the top 30. David Mallet's fine video featured

unrehearsed sequences filmed on the Earl's Court Road – Bowie nonchalantly strides along as genuinely surprised passers-by recognize and follow him, and there's a startling moment when he is passionately kissed by a burly man. These naturalistic reflections on celebrity are intercut with scenes of Bowie as a tortured DJ (the initials, of course, are also his own), who smashes up his studio and re-enacts the famous closing scene of David Lean's *Great Expectations*, ripping down the curtains to let the light come flooding in.

'D.J.' was played live for the first time on the 1995 Outside tour.

DA DOO RON RON *(Spector/Greenwich/Barry)*

Phil Spector's classic, originally a hit for the Crystals in 1963, was included in David's medley on *The Cher Show* in November 1975.

DANCE, DANCE, DANCE

"I don't think it's the Beach Boys song but one of mine," Bowie wrote in an Internet post in 1999, having discovered that a mysterious number called 'Dance, Dance, Dance' was in The Buzz's live repertoire in 1966.

DANCE MAGIC : see **MAGIC DANCE**

DANCING IN THE STREET
(Hunter/Stevenson/Gaye)
• A-Side: 8/85 [1] • Compilation: *Best Of Bowie* • Video: *Collection, Best Of Bowie*

"There was absolutely nothing premeditated about it," said Bowie of his celebrated duet with his old sparring partner Mick Jagger, which evolved from initial plans for a transatlantic conjuring trick at the Live Aid concert. "We had intended to do a live satellite thing where Mick would sing in New York and I would sing in England," he explained. "Then we found out that the half-second time delay really screwed that up. Technically there was no way around it." Instead it was decided to make a pre-recorded video for exclusive screening at Live Aid. The first choice, Bob

Marley's 'One Love', was dropped in favour of the 1964 Martha And The Vandellas classic.

Bowie, who was working on the *Absolute Beginners* soundtrack at Abbey Road, recruited most of the same personnel for the session, which took place at the end of a recording day in June 1985. Co-producer Alan Winstanley recalls that band rehearsals began only an hour before Mick Jagger's arrival, and that the results were "fuckin' awful" until Jagger appeared – at which point "Suddenly the whole band picked up. We already had a mike set up in the booth next to Bowie. At this point Bowie was singing on his own. Jagger went into the booth, started singing with Bowie, and it was one take." Drummer Neil Conti recalled Jagger "being 'on' the whole time … strutting around and trying to upstage David. It was a huge ego-trip for him." Apparently Bowie was happy with the first takes, but Jagger wanted various instrumental re-dubs.

Having completed the recording and a rough mix in barely four hours, Bowie and Jagger left with David Mallet to shoot the video in London's docklands. The entire session from studio recording to completion of the video was accomplished in just over twelve hours: "We started work at seven o'clock in the evening, and we finished the record by 11.30," said Bowie. "Then we rushed down to the docks and started work at about a quarter past twelve, and we rolled through to eight o'clock the next morning." The video is testament to the frantic and apparently alcohol-fuelled exuberance of the night's work: Jagger and Bowie send each other up relentlessly, Mick campily imitating David's favourite point-the-arm-and-drop-to-the-floor-manoeuvre.

Jagger took the master tapes to New York, where overdubs were added by guitarists Earl Slick and G E Smith (the latter had previously appeared in Bowie's 'Fashion' video and at the *Saturday Night Live* and *Tonight Show* performances in 1979 and 1980), and members of David's recent horn sections. Full credits for the track are: Kevin Armstrong (guitar); G E Smith (guitar); Earl Slick (guitar); Matthew Seligman (bass); John Regan (bass); Neil Conti (drums); Pedro Ortiz (percussion); Jimmy Maclean (percussion); Mac Gollehon (trumpet); Stan Harrison (saxophone); Lenny Pickett (saxophone); Steve Nieve (keyboards); Helena Springs, Tessa Niles (backing vocals).

Although 'Dancing In The Street' was originally conceived as a one-off for the big day, plans soon changed. The video was shown twice during Live Aid, the second time as a filler when The Who's reunion

was beset with sound problems. The response was overwhelming and there was immediate talk of a Band Aid single release. Sure enough 'Dancing In The Street' was issued at the end of August, entering the chart at number 1 where it remained for four weeks – ironically, it was toppled by Band Aid's co-founder Midge Ure with 'If I Was'. The single version, now on *Best Of Bowie*, is half a minute longer than the original 2'50" video mix.

On 20 June 1986, a year after Live Aid, Bowie and Jagger performed 'Dancing In The Street' live at The Prince's Trust Concert at Wembley Arena. Although David has never reprised the song since, the trumpet intro was later worked into the Glass Spider tour arrangement of 'Fashion'. The original Bowie/Jagger recording was among the songs played during the Golden Jubilee fireworks display at Buckingham Palace on 3 June 2002.

DANCING WITH THE BIG BOYS
(Bowie/Pop/Alomar)
• Album: *Tonight* • B-Side: 9/84 [6]

Tonight's final track offers a taste of things to come on the critically mauled *Never Let Me Down*. There's a tough bassline and a big, brassy arrangement for trumpets and saxes, while Bowie's vocal (augmented by a very audible Iggy Pop) is refreshingly rough-edged by comparison with the rest of the album. The 'Ricochet'-esque lyric of societal meltdown is decent enough, but the lack of any strong melodic hook leaves an impression of overproduced meandering.

Bowie cited the track as the best example of what he was striving for on *Tonight*. "There's a particular sound I'm after that I haven't really got yet and I probably won't drop this search until I get it," he said in 1984. "I'll either crack it on the next album or just retire from it. I think I got quite close to it on 'Dancing With The Big Boys' … That was quite an adventurous bit of writing in the sense that we didn't look for any standards. I got very *musical* over the last couple of years; I stayed away from experimentation … but in 'Big Boys' Iggy and I just broke away from all that for the one track. That came nearer to the sound I was looking for than anything. I'd like to try maybe one more set of pieces like that." Cue *Never Let Me Down*.

'Dancing With The Big Boys' became the B-side of the 'Blue Jean' single; an Arthur Baker remix, widely considered superior to the original, appeared on the

12" version. The song was later performed on the Glass Spider tour.

DAVID BOWIE'S REVOLUTIONARY SONG : see REVOLUTIONARY SONG

DAY-IN DAY-OUT
• A-Side: 3/87 [17] • Album: *Never* • Video: *Day-In Day-Out, Collection, Best Of Bowie* • Live Video: *Glass*

Everything that's initially promising but ultimately infuriating about *Never Let Me Down* is encapsulated in its opening track and debut single. Somewhere in there is a concerted attempt to reclaim Bowie's former territory of guitar-based rock'n'roll, but 'Day-In Day-Out' suffers badly from over-elaboration: it's a slab of 1980s soft-rock which now sounds incredibly dated by comparison with much of Bowie's earlier work. Echo-laden Robert Palmeresque power percussion, zapping trumpets and a distressing guitar solo seal its fate.

What's infuriating is that 'Day-In Day-Out' is actually a pretty fine song, announcing *Never Let Me Down*'s serious-minded manifesto with an excoriating portrait of urban deprivation in Reagan's America – David explained that it was an "indictment of an uncaring society". The fragmentary narrative about a young woman drawn into prostitution and drug addiction is leavened by pleasing flashes of Bowie's traditional lyric-sampling habit, something prevalent throughout this album. Opening with a wink to Oscar Wilde ("She was born in a handbag!") he goes on to paraphrase a Beatles classic ("She's got a ticket to nowhere, she's gonna take a train ride..."). The overall impression of liberal rage carries more weight than the ponderous pronouncements later entrusted to Tin Machine.

Although several previous singles had spawned 12" versions, 'Day-In Day-Out' marked Bowie's first major incursion into the brave new world of multi-format releases and endless remixes. The single did middling business in both Britain (number 17) and America (number 21), notwithstanding the short-lived notoriety of Julien Temple's video. The new-look mullet-haired Bowie, resplendent in studded black leathers a good six months before Michael Jackson unveiled a similar and equally 'Bad' image, was seen travelling through Los Angeles and its seedy Pacific Grand Hotel, gliding past on conveyor belts and roller-skates while harsh scenes unfolded around him. Most of the 200 extras were recruited from the city's homeless population and choreographed by members of the City Stage street theatre group. "There's an amazing amount of courage and dignity that they hold," said Bowie. "It's quite numbing that they're treated in such a shabby way – billions are spent on armaments, on getting a few guys back from the Middle East, when just a few dollars would help out so much. But I suppose that's the difference between social care and wanting to be re-elected."

The resulting video is no classic, but worthy of attention as one of Bowie's most blatant anti-American statements: the elaborate climax as armoured police vehicles ram-raid the woman's home is remarkable. The video was censored by several television stations to remove the sequence in which the protagonist is dragged into a car and raped, while a scene showing her baby playing with building-bricks was shot in two different forms – in the proper version, the child spells out the words "Mom", "Food", and "Fuck", a bleak summation of its cycle of dependency, while in the bowdlerized version the bricks spell "Mom", "Look" and "Luck", which rather loses the point. Needless to say the latter version received the most airplay, but even this was banned by the BBC. "I've seen such a lot of banning going on," commented David at the time, "and it's coming up with quite a puritanical face at the moment. I was pissed off because it was for the wrong reasons." He pointed out that the clip for Madonna's number 1 'La Isla Bonita' passed without comment at the same time: "It's a mesmerising video, but basically seems to be about Madonna having an affair with Jesus ... I find that has something a lot more perverse about it than anything in my video. Mine was very straight-ahead street violence and it was quite obvious. There's nothing titillating about what was happening on that screen. It certainly wasn't done for its sexual overtones, so I think that they have a morality problem at the BBC." The banning of the 'Day-In Day-Out' video prompted its release as a video EP in 1987, while the censored version appears on *The Video Collection* and *Best Of Bowie*.

'Day-In Day-Out' was performed live throughout the Glass Spider tour. To drum up publicity for his first ever Spanish concerts Bowie recorded a Spanish vocal version, variously referred to as 'Al Alba' and 'Dia Tras Dia', which received a one-off radio transmission in Spain. The master was apparently destroyed thereafter, although copies of the broadcast circulate among collectors.

A DAY IN THE LIFE (Lennon/McCartney) : see YOUNG AMERICANS

THE DAY THE CIRCUS LEFT TOWN
(Leigh/Thomas)

This whimsical standard about a childhood disappointment and the loss of innocence, popularized in the late 1950s by Eartha Kitt (an occasional if oft-ignored influence throughout Bowie's career – see also 'Just An Old Fashioned Girl' and 'Thursday's Child'), was included in David's 1968 cabaret show. A likely influence on Bowie's own Deram-era compositions, the song is incorrectly cited by Kenneth Pitt as 'When The Circus Left Town'.

DAY TRIPPER (Lennon/McCartney)

The Beatles' 1965 hit was included in David's November 1975 medley with Cher on The Cher Show.

DAYS
• Album: Reality • Live Video: Reality

Among Reality's often oblique lyrics this beautifully melodic track stands as a surprisingly direct and uncomplicated love song, albeit one that maintains the album's prevailing air of weary retrospection and ageing regret. 'Days' operates rather like a sadder, less rose-tinted variation on the famous Kinks song of the same name: where Ray Davies's lyric wistfully celebrates a past relationship, Bowie's nakedly brings to account the narrator's shortcomings and selfishness in a confessional apology for "all the days I owe you". The regret-laden line "All I've done, I've done for me" stands in diametric opposition to the swaggering boast of "Everything I've done, I've done for you" which Bowie had belted out in Labyrinth's self-deluding love song 'Within You' seventeen years earlier. 'Days' is a modest reversal of such sentiment: rather than a grandstanding imposition, it's a simple and poignant plea for forgiveness, appropriately delivered

in the fragile, unadorned vocal style already showcased in 'The Loneliest Guy'.

The arrangement and production are as sophisticated as the rest of Reality, but the chosen style is deliberately simple: a faux-naif arrangement of low-tech synthesizers and twanging guitars against a jogging beat, which conspire to give 'Days' a charming retro ambience, recalling the early 1980s style of Soft Cell or Depeche Mode. Like the rest of the album, 'Days' was performed throughout A Reality Tour.

DEAD AGAINST IT
• Album: Buddha • B-Side: 11/93 [35]

Most of The Buddha Of Suburbia harks back to various points in the 1970s, and in this case it's the new wave pop that emerged at the end of that decade and went on to define the next. With a buzzing riff, tinny electronic percussion and zaps of space-age synthesizer reminiscent of early XTC, OMD or Depeche Mode, Bowie pays homage to a movement that had owed more than a little to Low in the first place. The track became the B-side of the 'Buddha Of Suburbia' single.

DEAD MAN WALKING (Bowie/Gabrels)
• Album: Earthling • A-Side: 4/97 [32] • Live: Live From 6A, 99X Live XIV, WBCN: Naked Too • Video: Best Of Bowie

Just as 'Seven Years In Tibet' has no direct connection with the 1997 movie adaptation, so 'Dead Man Walking' shares only its title with the 1995 picture that netted an Oscar for Susan Sarandon. In 1982 Bowie had described Sarandon, then co-starring with him in The Hunger, as "pure dynamite", and was widely reported to be dating her during filming; two decades later, on 5 May 2003, David and Iman would be among the guests who gathered at New York's Lincoln Center to honour Sarandon's career at The Film Society's Gala Tribute. During the Earthling sessions in 1996, 'Dead Man Walking' began life as a tribute to the actress. "My initial idea was to write a paean to Susan Sarandon," David explained, "but then I went over to do Neil Young's benefit for the Bridge School, and watching Neil and Crazy Horse working on stage was really special. There's something sage-like about Young, this grand old man of American rock, a pioneer loaded with integrity, and disarmingly charming as a man; and watching him work with these, let's call them older men, there was a sense of grace and dignity about what they were doing, and also an incredible verve and energy. It was very moving..."

Hence, in the final lyric of 'Dead Man Walking', "Three old men dancing under the lamplight / Shaking their sex in their bones, and the boys that they were." In common with the rest of *Earthling* the song is a cut-and-paste of impressionistic moments, but what emerges is the touching testimony of another grand old man of rock who finds himself at fifty ("And I'm gone, now I'm older than movies / Let me dance away, now I'm wiser than dreams"), but still eager to "fly while I'm touching tomorrow." 'Dead Man Walking' is a confident, exuberant slice of modern rock, incorporating the programmed spangles of techno acts like Underworld, but based on a riff originally used in 1970's 'The Supermen' – a song revived, almost certainly for this reason, on the Earthling tour. Mark Plati recalled that 'Dead Man Walking' took five days to mix, working in a progression whereby "It begins completely programmed and by the time it's finished it's completely live."

The track is probably *Earthling*'s most commercial offering, and it came as no surprise when it followed 'Little Wonder' as a single in April 1997. The seven-minute 'Moby Mix' marked the beginning of Bowie's association with producer/performer Moby, later to achieve global success with his album *Play*. The video, shot in Toronto in March 1997 by Floria Sigismondi, pushes further into the mutant *Eraserhead* chic of her 'Little Wonder' promo, featuring the same rapidly shifting focus and flailing choreography. Tod Browning-style extras dangle from puppet-strings and pull lumps of raw meat through the *Doktor Caligari* sets, while a straitjacketed Bowie dances with Gail Ann Dorsey, who is demonically attired with cloven hoofs, horns and tail. On 25 April the band mimed to the number on *Top Of The Pops*, Gail resplendent in her demon outfit and David in his Union Jack coat. The single went on to collect a Grammy nomination for Best Male Rock Vocal Performance.

'Dead Man Walking' was performed in all its electric glory on the Earthling tour, and also underwent a radical acoustic reworking that became a feature of several television and radio appearances at the time. The performance on NBC's *Late Night With Conan O'Brien* on 10 April 1997 was given an American release on the compilation album *Live From 6A*, while

the version recorded on 8 April for WNNX Atlanta was included on *99X Live XIV*, a small-circulation release of the station's session recordings. Boston's WBCN released an album of live performances called *WBCN: Naked Too*, including yet another version recorded on the very same day. Meanwhile the original studio version appeared on the US soundtrack album of *The Saint*.

DEAD MEN DON'T TALK (BUT THEY DO)

Michael Apted's 1997 documentary *Inspirations* includes a sequence filmed at Looking Glass Studios during preparations for Bowie's fiftieth birthday concert, in which David and the *Earthling* band improvise a short piece called 'Dead Men Don't Talk (But They Do)'. Apted's film examines different aspects of the creative process, and here he concentrates on Bowie assembling a lyric out of cut-ups from the *New York Times*.

DEATH TRIP *(Pop/Williamson)*

Mixed by Bowie for Iggy And The Stooges' 1973 album *Raw Power*.

DEBASER *(Francis)*

Boston's Pixies were often cited as an influence by Bowie during his Tin Machine period, and the opening track of their 1989 album *Doolittle* was performed live during the It's My Life tour.

DIA TRAS DIA : see DAY-IN DAY-OUT

DIAMOND DOGS
• Album: *Dogs* • A-Side: 6/74 [21] • Live: *David* • Compilation: *The Best Of Bowie* • Bonus: *Dogs (2004)*

Consciously subverting Ziggy Stardust's swansong with an opening yell of "This ain't rock'n'roll – this is *genocide!*", the title track of *Diamond Dogs* introduces us to Bowie's new persona, Halloween Jack, "a real cool cat" who "lives on top of Manhattan Chase" in the urban wasteland of the album's dystopian future.

From his rooftop hideout Halloween Jack rules the Diamond Dogs, a synthesis of the street-gangs Bowie had found so evocative in the works of writers like Burroughs, Burgess and Dickens: "I had in my mind this kind of half *Wild Boys, Nineteen Eighty-Four* world," David explained in 1993's *The David Bowie Story*, "and there were these ragamuffins, but they were a bit more violent than ragamuffins. I guess they staggered through from *Clockwork Orange* too. They'd taken over this barren city, this city that was falling apart. They'd been able to break into windows of jewellers and things, so they'd dressed themselves up in furs and diamonds, but they had snaggle teeth – really filthy, kind of like violent Oliver Twists. It was a take on, what if those guys had gone malicious? If Fagin's gang had gone absolutely ape-shit?"

Bowie has often recalled that the Diamond Dogs' rooftop habitat was drawn in part from a story told to him by his father, who had worked for Dr Barnardo's, about Lord Shaftesbury's account of destitute children living on rooftops in London slums. "That always stayed in my mind as being an extraordinary image, all these kids living on the roofs of London," he explained, "So I had the Diamond Dogs as living on the streets. They were all little Johnny Rottens and Sid Viciouses really. And, in my mind, there was no means of transport, so they were all rolling around on these roller-skates with huge wheels on them, and they squeaked because they hadn't been oiled properly. So there were these gangs of squeaking, roller-skating, vicious hoods, with Bowie knives and furs on, and they were all skinny because they hadn't eaten enough, and they all had funny-coloured hair. In a way it was a precursor to the punk thing."

The fractured lyric spreads its net wide, drawing in references to the surrealist painter Salvador Dali (sometime lover of Amanda Lear, one of David's liaisons during the *Diamond Dogs* sessions), Tarzan (Halloween Jack is imaged as the vine-swinging hero, reaffirming Hunger City as the ultimate urban jungle), and most evocatively film director Tod Browning, the man behind the notorious 1932 exploitation shocker *Freaks*, in which a cast of genuine circus freaks wreak their revenge on the able-bodied villainess. Banned in several countries and disowned by MGM on grounds of taste, *Freaks* is a significant reference-point for David's growing interest in all manner of schlock, grotesquerie and gothic controversy – it clearly provides the basis for the *Diamond Dogs* sleeve artwork.

The sound of a screaming audience at the beginning of 'Diamond Dogs' was mixed in from The Faces' live album *Coast To Coast – Overture And Beginners*. If you listen carefully, the sample includes Rod Stewart shouting "Hey!" a couple of seconds after the guitar riff begins. This is almost certainly the origin of the unsubstantiated rumour that Stewart actually plays uncredited somewhere on the album.

'Diamond Dogs' provides a notable showcase for Bowie's lead guitar playing which, together with some excellent percussion, delivers a sophisticated and raunchy piece of garage rock. Both the riff and David's yodelling vocals are plainly indebted to the Rolling Stones' 'It's Only Rock'n'Roll', which was recorded simultaneously in the next-door studio while Bowie was completing *Diamond Dogs* at Ludolf; David occasionally added the line "It's only rock'n'roll but I like it" to the song during the 1976 tour. Another likely inspiration is The Stooges' 1969 single 'I Wanna Be Your Dog', later covered on the Glass Spider tour.

'Diamond Dogs' proved an unlikely single, limping to number 21 in Britain and failing to chart in America (not that the latter was anything unusual at the time), making it the most disappointing performance by a new Bowie single since his breakthrough with 'Starman'. A different 4'37" edit appeared on the 1980 compilation *The Best Of Bowie* and was later included on the 2004 reissue of *Diamond Dogs*.

Unsurprisingly the song formed a mainstay of the Diamond Dogs tour, and continued into the Philly Dogs and Station To Station shows. It was included in rehearsals for the Sound + Vision tour, the lyrics even appearing in the souvenir brochure, but the song was dropped before the concerts began and didn't reappear until the 1996 Summer Festivals tour. In the same year an amusingly conversational cover version ("This ain't rock'n'roll, this is genocide, ladies and gentlemen") was included in the Mike Flowers Pops' 'Bowie Medley', found on their CD single 'Light My Fire'. Duran Duran included a bonus version of 'Diamond Dogs' on the Japanese edition of their 1995 covers album *Thank You*. A radical makeover was recorded by Beck for the soundtrack of Baz Luhrmann's 2001 film *Moulin Rouge*, making only a fleeting appearance in the film itself (in which the Parisian nightclub dancers are introduced as "the Diamond Dogs"). Beck has susequently performed his version live.

DID YOU EVER HAVE A DREAM
• B-Side: 7/67 • Compilation: *Deram*

Recorded on 24 November 1966 during the *David Bowie* sessions, 'Did You Ever Have A Dream' was relegated to B-side status before turning up on various repackages over the years. It's a mystery why this particularly jaunty number was left off an album whose commercial chances it might well have improved – even in America, a *Cash Box* review of the 'Love You Till Tuesday' single made special mention of its "brilliant" B-side.

Typical of Bowie's Deram period, the lyric is a paean to "the magic wings of astral flight" that unfetter the imagination in dreams, a playful fantasy juxtaposing wild ambition with suburban drudgery in the outrageous couplet: "It's a very special knowledge that you've got, my friend / You can walk around in New York while you sleep in Penge". The spiky bar-room piano includes a faint but unmistakable figure later repeated in Roy Bittan's play-out on 'Station To Station'.

Bowie performed 'Did You Ever Have A Dream' on the German TV show *4-3-2-1 Musik Für Junge Leute* in February 1968.

DIRT *(The Stooges)*

A Stooges number performed during the 1977 Iggy Pop tour with Bowie on keyboards. A live version featuring Bowie can be heard on Iggy's *TV Eye* and *Suck On This!*

DIRTY BLVD. *(Reed)*

Lou Reed's blistering exposé of urban degradation, originally from his 1989 album *New York*, was the only unfamiliar number to feature at Bowie's fiftieth birthday concert on 9 January 1997. David shared lead vocals with Lou for the song, considered by many to be one of Reed's finest; and it's one which chimes well with the sentiments more figuratively expressed in Bowie's 'I'm Afraid Of Americans'.

DIRTY OLD MAN *(Sanders/Kupferberg)*

The Fugs' 1966 number was played live by The Riot Squad.

THE DIRTY SONG *(Brecht/Muldowney)*
• B-Side: 2/82 [29]

The last track on the *Baal* EP is a short, crude number in which Baal humiliates his lover Sophie on stage in a seedy cabaret. In the BBC version Bowie performed the song practically unaccompanied and drowned out by the jeering of the crowd; on the subsequent studio recording it is given a full German pit orchestra arrangement.

DO ANYTHING YOU SAY
• A-Side: 4/66 • Compilation: *Early*

On 22 February 1966 David and his new backing group The Buzz demoed his latest composition 'Do Anything You Say' at Regent Sound Studios. At Pye on 7 March they recorded the finished track with producer Tony Hatch. Released on 1 April, it has the distinction of being the first record to be credited simply to "David Bowie". Sadly this is about all that distinguishes this unimaginative R&B jilted-love song, which betrays little promise by comparison with some of Bowie's other 1966 material. The call-and-response harmonies are blatantly nicked from The Who's 1965 hit 'Anyway, Anyhow, Anywhere', while the opening line ("Two by two they go walking by, hand in hand they watch me cry") would be echoed by David's later composition 'Conversation Piece'.

The track was performed live by The Buzz during 1966, but 'Do Anything You Say' failed to perform any better than David's previous singles. Change, however, was in the air: two weeks after its release he met his future manager Kenneth Pitt, whose belief and investment would prove instrumental in helping the young singer take his next step forward.

DO THE RUBY

In the *Mirabelle* diary dated 21 December 1974, "David" reveals that he has just recorded a demo for his friend Bette Midler, a supporter of his American career in the mid-1970s. "Can you believe it?" goggles the diary. "Me getting into the field of disco music! Well, anyway, I've done the demo and I've named it

'Do The Ruby'! I'm counting on 'The Ruby' to sweep all over the world as soon as Bette and I figure out what all the steps that go with it will be! Bette wants to record 'Do The Ruby' and put it on one of her albums, too!" Presumably *Mirabelle* ghostwriter Cherry Vanilla hadn't bothered going to any of her employer's recent gigs if she was that amazed by the concept of Bowie getting involved in disco music, but it seems likely that there is some basis to the story. Even so, 'Do The Ruby' was never heard of again.

DO THEY KNOW IT'S CHRISTMAS? *(Geldof/Ure)*

Famed as the fastest-selling single in British history (at least until a certain Elton John recording in 1997), Band Aid's 'Do They Know It's Christmas?' was record-ed in London on 25 November 1984 as a reaction to the BBC's coverage of the Ethiopian famine. Bob Geldof rallied many of the hottest chart acts of the day, but among those unable to make the recording was Bowie, who was originally invited to sing the opening line. Instead, along with other unavailable artists like Paul McCartney and Holly Johnson, he recorded a spoken message for the instrumental B-side 'Feed The World'. His message ran: "This is David Bowie. It's Christmas 1984, and there are more starving folk on the planet than ever before. Please give a thought for them this season and do whatever you can, however small, to help them live. Have a peaceful New Year."

At Live Aid the following year, David was able to take a more active involvement in the number. "I think you know the next song," deadpanned Bob Geldof to a deafening cheer as the Wembley stage filled with famous faces for the final encore. "It might be a bit of a cock-up, but if you're going to cock it up you may as well do it with two billion people watching you. So let's cock it up together." Bowie obliged with a slightly but forgivably fluffed rendering of the opening line, before passing his microphone to George Michael and dancing his way through the rest of the number.

DODO

- Compilation: *S+V* • Bonus: *Dogs, Dogs (2004)*

Originally entitled 'You Didn't Hear It From Me', 'Dodo' was composed in 1973 for David's planned adaptation of *Nineteen Eighty-Four*. The jaunty melody is undercut by a darkly paranoid lyric in which brainwashed children inform on their parents in a totalitarian state: "Can you wipe your nose, my child, without them slotting in your file a photograph? / Will you sleep in fear tonight, wake to find the scorching light of neighbour Jim who's come to turn you in?"

The only official airing of 'Dodo' came as part of a live medley with an embryonic version of '1984' in *The 1980 Floor Show*, recorded at the Marquee in October 1973. A more elaborate studio version of the medley was cut the same month at Trident, and this recording, eventually released on *Sound + Vision* and later on 2004's *Diamond Dogs* reissue, is by far the best extant version of the song.

During the *Diamond Dogs* sessions at Olympic Studios, Bowie revamped 'Dodo' with the intention of releasing it as a duet with Lulu. The bonus version included on the 1990 and 2004 reissues of *Diamond Dogs* is the subject of some dispute among collectors: it is either a guide vocal for Lulu (which would explain why Bowie's singing is rather lacklustre), or else it's the actual duet version with Lulu's contribution removed by Rykodisc. A longer 4'31" version featuring both David and Lulu has appeared on bootlegs, and despite some differences in the backing mix, Bowie's vocal is the same one that appears on the *Diamond Dogs* bonus track. Lulu's performance is also fairly non-committal, suggesting that this is another try-out rather than a finished track. Whatever the story, 'Dodo' was destined to go no further.

DON'T BE AFRAID

This Bowie composition, demoed in 1971, is also referred to as 'Oh Darling'. Two versions have appeared on bootlegs, neither featuring Bowie on vocals. A completed 2'40" version was broadcast along with another out-take, 'Bombers', on US radio in January 1972 during an interview with David about the forthcoming *Ziggy Stardust* album. It's a tightly-produced if undemanding slice of guitar pop, owing something to the easygoing anthems of The Lovin' Spoonful or even The Beach Boys, with an uncompli-cated love lyric which appears to skim lightly over the subject matter of some of Bowie's weightier composi-tions of the period: "Don't be afraid to reveal what you know / Don't be afraid to conceal what you show / Oh darling, don't be afraid."

DON'T BRING ME DOWN *(Dee)*
• Album: *Pin*

The second of two numbers on *Pin Ups* originally recorded by The Pretty Things, 'Don't Bring Me Down' was the group's biggest hit, taking them to number 10 in 1964. Of all the *Pin Ups* tracks 'Don't Bring Me Down', with its pulsing bass and blues harmonica, represents the most spirited return to the rootsy R&B sound favoured by Bowie during his earliest recordings. Nowhere are his influences more clearly on show than here, and it's no coincidence that The Pretty Things' live repertoire included Johnny Kidd's 'Shakin' All Over' and Muddy Waters's 'I'm A King Bee', two songs which exerted a similar influence on David: the first as an occasional live number, the second giving its name to one of his early bands.

DON'T LET ME DOWN & DOWN *(Tarha/Valmont)*
• Album: *Black* • Bonus: *Black (2003)*

The most obscure of the four covers on *Black Tie White Noise* was brought to Bowie's attention by his wife Iman, who had heard the original recording by her friend Tarha, a Mauritanian princess, on a visit to Paris in 1992. Tarha composed both the music and the original Arabic lyrics, which had undergone a free English translation by her French producer Martine Valmont. According to a friend of Valmont, "You'd have to hear the original version to comprehend the immense input that Bowie put into the song!"

'Don't Let Me Down & Down' provides one of the quieter moments on *Black Tie White Noise*, with breathy backing vocals and shimmering synth flourishes recalling the romantic balladeering of mid-1970s tracks like 'Win' and 'Can You Hear Me'. In common with those numbers, the fragility of Bowie's strangely mannered vocal in the early minutes is blown away when he suddenly lets rip, reminding us what a great singer he really is.

An edited 2'32" version appeared on a US promo CD in advance of the album. The track was briefly scheduled for release as an American single in 1993 until the bankruptcy of Savage Records put paid to the idea. In Singapore, the *Black Tie White Noise* CD included an Indonesian vocal version entitled 'Jangan Susahkan Hatiku', which later appeared as a bonus track on the 2003 reissue of the album. On 8 May 1993 a mimed performance was filmed at the Hollywood Center Studios for the *Black Tie White Noise* promotional video, but failed to make the final edit.

DON'T LOOK DOWN *(Pop/Williamson)*
• Album: *Tonight* • B-Side: 5/85 [19]

Iggy Pop's passing parade of New York life, originally featured on 1979's *New Values*, was reworked for *Tonight* with an unlikely but curiously convincing reggae treatment. After toying with reggae on 'Yassassin' a few years earlier Bowie had intimated that he didn't intend trying it again, but changed his mind during the *Tonight* sessions almost by accident. "I think it was the drum machine," he explained. "I was trying to rearrange 'Don't Look Down' and it wouldn't work. I tried it as a march, and then I just hit on an old ska-sounding beat, and it picked up life. Taking energy away from the musical side of things reinforced the lyrics and gave them their own energy. I think working with Derek Bramble really helped a lot, because he played proper reggae bass lines … where Derek can succeed is that he will leave a lot of spaces. He's not scared *not* to play a note." Bowie would go on to subject Iggy's 'Tonight' to a similar reggae styling. 'Don't Look Down' boasts the album's other trademarks of tricksy percussion and zappy brass interludes, but both are reined in with admirable restraint.

An instrumental remix was used as background music in Julien Temple's film *Jazzin' For Blue Jean*, and further remixes later appeared on single formats of 'Loving The Alien'.

DON'T SIT DOWN
• Album: *Oddity*

A throwaway piece of studio tomfoolery (anticipating the background chat later incorporated into various *Hunky Dory* tracks), this begins with Bowie singing the memorable lyric "Yeah yeah baby yeah", before dissolving into laughter after a few seconds. It was removed from the album's re-release in 1972 and remained absent until the Rykodisc reissue.

DON'T START ME TALKIN' *(Williamson)* :
see **THE JEAN GENIE**

DON'T THINK TWICE, IT'S ALRIGHT *(Dylan)*

David sang Bob Dylan's 1963 song (from *The Freewheelin' Bob Dylan*) live in 1969.

DON'T TRY TO STOP ME

Among David's live repertoire with The Manish Boys.

THE DREAMERS *(Bowie/Gabrels)*
• Album: *'hours…'*

The final track on *'hours…'* is melancholic even by this album's standards, with a Scott Walkeresque lyric conjuring up an ageing, forlorn traveller whose glory days are behind him in a world of "shallow men": "He's always in decline, no-one heals any more … Just a searcher, a lonely soul, the last of the dreamers." Links with the *Nomad Soul* computer game notwithstanding, this is heart-plucking stuff. The musical cues hail from disparate pages in Bowie's songbook: the Eastern windchime intro recalls the second side of *"Heroes"*, the techno-dance backing revisits 'No Control' before shifting into a synthesized version of the Bo Diddley rhythms he had favoured in the early 1970s, and the rhythm break near the end is straight from his 1983 cover 'Criminal World'. Finally 'The Dreamers' builds to a classic Bowie chorus, its swooping guitars and vocal harmonies bringing *'hours…'* to a stately conclusion. A so-called "easy listening" version, slightly longer than the album cut, appears in *Omikron: The Nomad Soul.*

DRINK TO ME : see MOVING ON

DRIVE IN SATURDAY
• Album: *Aladdin* • A-Side: 4/73 [3] • Bonus: *Aladdin (2003)* • Live Video: *Best Of Bowie*

Not only is it arguably the finest track on *Aladdin Sane*, 'Drive In Saturday' is also the great forgotten Bowie single. A huge hit in edited form, its relative obscurity since 1973 can only be attributed to the fact that it failed to appear on any greatest hits compilation until nearly twenty years later.

The 1950s records of Bowie's childhood are heard nowhere stronger than on this album, and 'Drive In Saturday' fuses a nostalgic doo-wop style with The Spiders' futuristic soundscape – here beefed up by zaps and gurgles of phased synthesizer – to convey an impression of fractured time in yet another portrait of post-holocaust humanity. The inspiration came during a long overnight train journey in November 1972: unable to sleep as the train sped through the barren landscape somewhere between Seattle and Phoenix, Bowie later explained that he saw "the moon shining on seventeen or eighteen enormous silver domes. I couldn't find out from anyone what they were. But they gave me a vision of America, Britain, and China after a nuclear catastrophe. The radiation has affected people's minds and reproductive organs, and they don't have a sex life. The only way they can learn to make love again is by watching films of how it used to be done." The result would become one of Bowie's most haunting lyrics: "Perhaps the strange ones in the dome can lend us a book, we can read up alone / And try to get it on like once before / When people stared in Jagger's eyes and scored, like the video films we saw…"

As well as name-checking Jagger – a ubiquitous figure on *Aladdin Sane* – the song tips its hat to Marc Bolan ("try to get it on") and even drops in a mention of swinging London's original supermodel Twiggy. In her autobiography Twiggy recalls hearing 'Drive In Saturday' on the radio for the first time: "When the chorus came around, there it was again, Twig the Wonder Kid, and I thought, blimey. I remember being absolutely bowled over and of course I rushed out and bought it." The song also contains a passing mention of "the Astronette", a name Bowie had originally given to Lindsay Kemp's dancers during his Rainbow Theatre shows in August 1972, and would later ascribe to the group fronted by his girlfriend Ava Cherry.

A fan who attended the Phoenix gig on 4 November 1972 has insisted that 'Drive In Saturday' was performed there, although official Bowie lore has it that the song received its stage premiere in Fort Lauderdale on 17 November. On that night (one of the few 1972 US gigs to be bootlegged), David told the audience that "this takes place probably in the year 2033," before performing the number alone on acoustic guitar to thunderous applause. A similar acoustic version recorded a few days later, in Cleveland on 25 November, was included on the 2003 reissue of *Aladdin Sane*.

'Drive In Saturday' was immediately offered to

Mott the Hoople (also touring the States in November 1972) as a possible follow-up to 'All The Young Dudes'; they turned it down in favour of 'Honaloochie Boogie', which they would successfully take to number 12. "I never understood that because I always thought that would've been a great single for them, perfect," David said in 1998. "I do know that Ian [Hunter] hates owing anything to anyone and he found the idea of singing another David Bowie song exasperating." This account doesn't entirely square with the recollection of Mott's drummer Dale Griffin: "[Bowie] said that 'Drive In Saturday' would be our next single but then he changed his mind. But it was great that we now had to come up with something from within the group." In any case 'Drive In Saturday' was promptly repossessed by Bowie, who took it into the studio on his return to Britain and pre-viewed it on LWT's *Russell Harty Plus* on 17 January 1973, as the *Aladdin Sane* sessions neared completion. This performance was later included on the *Best Of Bowie* DVD. An instrumental backing track, allegedly from the Trident sessions, has appeared on bootlegs, but its authenticity is dubious.

'Drive In Saturday' is a favourite track of Bowie's old friend Morrissey, who performed it on his 1999-2000 tour. The song made the occasional reappearance in David's own repertoire during the 1973 Ziggy tour, while on the initial leg of the Diamond Dogs show it was performed in stripped-down acoustic form, with Bowie on guitar and David Sanborn on saxophone. Dropped from the set after a month or so, it remained in obscurity until 1999, when Bowie resurrected it for the *'hours...'* promotional tour, including fine versions in his *VH1 Storytellers* set and the 25 October BBC session – a welcome return for one of Bowie's most underrated classics.

DROWN IN MY OWN TEARS *(Glover)* : see **YOUNG AMERICANS**

THE DROWNED GIRL *(Brecht/Weill)*
• B-Side: 2/82 [29] • Compilation: *S+V (2003)*

The only *Baal* track with music by Brecht's famous collaborator Kurt Weill, 'The Drowned Girl' is arguably the highlight of the EP, ghoulishly relating the Ophelia-like suicide of Johanna, one of Baal's under-age conquests. Weill's setting comes from a later work

called *The Berlin Requiem*. In the BBC play, the song is performed by Bowie looking straight into camera on the left hand side of a split screen, while to the right is a freeze-frame of the dead Johanna, played by Tracey Childs.

A simple black-and-white video was shot by David Mallet, back-to-back with the clip for 'Wild Is The Wind', again featuring Bowie sitting on a stool and surrounded by his backing musicians.

DUKE OF EARL *(Edwards/Williams/Dixon)* : see **HELLO STRANGER**

DUM DUM BOYS *(Pop/Bowie)*

Lyrically a tribute to Iggy Pop's former band The Stooges, 'Dum Dum Boys' was produced and co-written by Bowie for *The Idiot*, and also features David on guitar and backing vocals. "When David plays guitar he gets nuts," Iggy once recalled. "You know that little part on 'Dum Dum Boys', that 'Boweeewaaaah'? That's his part, that's David doing that. He struggles with that thing when he plays!"

Typically of *The Idiot*, the song was a collaborative effort: "I only had a few notes on the piano, I couldn't quite finish the tune," Iggy explained in 1997. "Bowie said, 'Don't you think we could make a song with that? Why don't you tell the story of the Stooges?' He gave me the concept of the song and he also gave me the title ... Then he added that guitar arpeggio that metal groups love today. He played it, and then he asked Phil Palmer to play the tune again because he didn't find his playing technically proficient enough."

EARLY MORNING : see **ERNIE JOHNSON**

EIGHT LINE POEM
• Album: *Hunky* • Live: *Beeb*

On *Hunky Dory*'s most overlooked number, Bowie gives a virtuoso vocal performance against a gentle piano and an almost tongue-in-cheek Country & Western guitar line from Mick Ronson. Asked about the song at the time of *Hunky Dory*'s release, David remarked cryptically that "The city is a kind of high-life wart on the backside of the prairie." The lyric is an impressionistic snapshot of a city room, in which a cat has just knocked over a spinning mobile while a cactus sits enigmatically in the window. Swamped by the big production numbers surrounding it, 'Eight Line Poem' is quiet, mysterious and strangely magnificent; Bowie's future friend William Burroughs considered the lyric reminiscent of *The Waste Land*. A second version, featuring a different vocal and some very minor lyrical variations, appeared on the seven-track *Hunky Dory* sampler pressed in August 1971 by Tony Defries. The song was given only one more performance, during a BBC session recorded on 21 September 1971, and this excellent rendition was later included on *Bowie At The Beeb*.

'87 AND CRY

• Album: *Never* • B-Side: 8/87 [34]

Of the last five tracks on *Never Let Me Down* only "87 And Cry' rises above the mire to offer something with a bit of punch, and like 'New York's In Love' it's also a clear prefiguring of Tin Machine. According to Bowie, "It started off when I was originally writing it as a kind of indictment of Thatcher's England, but then it took on all these surreal qualities of a pushy person eating the energies of others to get to where they wanted and leaving the others behind: 'It couldn't be done without dogs'. It was a Thatcherite statement made through the eyes of a potential socialist, because I always remained a potential socialist, not an active one."

But on closer inspection, it's tempting to speculate on whether the "pushy person eating the energies of others" has a more precise nature. If Bowie is railing against "a one-dollar secret, a lover's secrets in the UK", and "just the ghost of a story", adding "you can't make love with money," and "only you whisper these things aren't true", he's doing so at the very moment that his personal life has been invaded by an upsurge of intrusive kiss-and-tell copy. Just prior to the *Never Let Me Down* sessions, Peter and Leni Gillman's *Alias David Bowie* was published, dredging up for the first time a parade of half-forgotten relatives and lovers eager to stake their claim on Bowie's past. After preview extracts appeared in the *Sunday Times*, Bowie launched a counterblast in *Today* against biographers who "drag out long-lost aunts to supply all the details, aunts I've had absolutely no contact with for maybe twenty years – who have no knowledge of me – and

absolutely unbelievable, blatant lies are told". While there's no proof that "87 And Cry' sets out to address these concerns, the resonance is certainly there.

The song later became a B-side and featured throughout the Glass Spider tour.

THE ENEMY IS FRAGILE : see THE 'LEON' TAPE

ERNIE BOY : see ERNIE JOHNSON

ERNIE JOHNSON

Although mentioned in Kenneth Pitt's memoir *The Pitt Report*, Bowie's unrealized 1968 "rock opera" remained an almost complete mystery until a tape of it came up for auction at Christie's in 1996. It went unsold and has yet to see the light of day, but details of the ten songs emerged in the pages of *Record Collector* at around the same time.

Under the collective title *Ernie Johnson*, the linking narrative seems every bit as tenuous as the "non-linear gothic drama hyper-cycle" of *1.Outside*, and its colourful parade of characters bears a superficial similarity to the style of the rock opera projects devised by Bowie's sometime idols The Who. The story, such as it is, runs something like this: Ernie Johnson, nineteen, invites friends to a party at which he intends to commit suicide. One of the guests, Tiny Tim, describes it as a "most exquisite party, darlings. Everyone was there. They busted me for masquerading as a man!" Ernie reminisces about past loves and has a racist conversation with a tramp; he addresses himself in a mirror; and he takes a trip to Carnaby Street to purchase a tie in which to kill himself.

The individual songs begin with 'Tiny Tim', apparently borrowing heavily from The Searchers' 'Sweets For My Sweet' (it's uncertain whether this Tiny Tim is supposed to be the novelty performer then renowned for his appearances on *Rowan & Martin's Laugh-In*; it's worth noting that a character called Tiny Tim had already appeared in Bowie's 'There Is A Happy Land'). 'Where's The Loo' is said to prefigure 'Queen Bitch', while the lyric anticipates the vapid chit-chat of Lou Reed's 'New York Telephone Conversation': "Where's the loo? What crappy chairs, what fabby clothes, is it true? / That after tonight there's no more you? And can we watch? Is it true? / Knock knock, who's there? It's all the rest / One's got tattoo marks on his chest…"

The songs continue with 'Season Folk', 'Just One Moment Sir' (the racist tramp song), and a suite under the collective title 'Various Times Of Day', individually titled 'Early Morning', 'Noon-Lunchtime' and 'Evening'. The last three songs are 'Ernié Boy' (a monologue in which Ernie addresses himself in the mirror while smoking a joint, including a surprising foretaste of 'Modern Love' in its spoken introduction: "I'm not running away, I know who I am, I know what I'm made of"), 'This Is My Day', and a final untitled number.

The 35-minute *Ernie Johnson* tape, probably dating from February 1968, was accompanied by a five-page manuscript detailing camera shots and stage-directions, suggesting that Bowie envisaged the project as a film or television play. Recorded on David's four-track home equipment, the tape apparently features surprisingly sophisticated multi-track recording with layered vocal overdubs and expansive instrumentation. *Ernie Johnson* clearly offers compelling evidence that Bowie's consistent preoccupation with theatrical acts of self-immolation did not begin with 'Rock'n'Roll Suicide'.

EVEN A FOOL LEARNS TO LOVE
(François/Thibault/Revaux/Bowie)

In February 1968, while David's Decca career was beginning to stall, Kenneth Pitt busied himself finding work for his client writing English lyrics for overseas music publishers. One of the songs that fell in Bowie's lap was 'Comme D'Habitude' by Claude François, Gilles Thibault and Jacques Revaux. As he began putting English lyrics to the song, in Pitt's words "it was becoming clear that he was writing a song that could and should be his next single."

Bowie's English version, 'Even A Fool Learns To Love' (a "pitifully awful title", he laughed many years later), was committed to a rough-and-ready demo which merely involved David singing over the original Claude François recording. Bowie's lyrics owed much to his then involvement with Lindsay Kemp's mime company, and perhaps a little to his new girlfriend Hermione Farthingale, telling how the easy laughter won by a clown is subjugated by the sudden arrival of love: "The clown turned around and saw her smile, oh how she loved me / She'd clap her hands and beg me

stay / To make her laugh, to make her life gay / Who wants the love of all the world when here was love in the eyes of just one girl / That day, that precious day / When even a fool learns to love."

On 9 February Pitt took the demo to his publishers at Essex Music and later to Decca, but plans for David to record the single were dashed when the French publisher raised an objection. As Essex Music's affiliate Geoffrey Heath recalled, "Their attitude was that they wanted a star to record the song, not this yobbo from Bromley." Not long afterwards Paul Anka's American translation immortalized the self-same song as none other than 'My Way'. An extract of Bowie's demo was later aired in BBC2's *Arena* documentary about the number that became Frank Sinatra's signature tune.

Referred to in some documentation under the alternative title 'Reprise', 'Even A Fool Learns To Love' was included in Bowie's abortive 1968 cabaret show. David later paid tribute to 'My Way' and its most famous interpreter with his classic composition 'Life On Mars?', a reworking of the same chord sequence that was, in the words of *Hunky Dory's* sleeve-notes, "inspired by Frankie".

EVENING : see ERNIE JOHNSON

EVERYONE SAYS 'HI'
• Album: *Heathen* • A-Side: 9/02 [20] • US Promo: 1/03 • Compilation: *Hope*

A lush and nostalgic arrangement dominated by acoustic and rhythm guitars (the latter courtesy of David's long-time sideman Carlos Alomar), paired with an ostensibly cheerful lyric apparently addressed to a loved one abroad, led many reviewers of *Heathen* to assume that 'Everyone Says 'Hi'' was addressed to David's grown-up son, and as such should be regarded as a sequel of sorts to 'Kooks'. This, however, was a complete misreading. As Bowie explained at the time, the song is in fact a meditation on bereavement. "When my father died in 1969, I couldn't actually believe that he was not going to come back again," David recalled. "I kind of thought that he'd just put his raincoat and his cap on, and that he'd be back in a few weeks or something. And I felt like that for years. It really took a long time for me to be able to take in the fact that I wouldn't see him again. So this one was just a little simplistic reference to that, about how it always feels like somebody has gone on a holiday of some kind. And there's something sad about ships as well. That's why this person in this song doesn't go on a plane. A ship took them away – I guess that's the boat that took people over the river Styx, isn't it?"

Once this reading is understood, not only does the superficial cheeriness of the lyric dissolve into melancholy and yearning, but it also suggests a touch of black comedy in the reference to "the guy upstairs" (not to mention the narrator's hope that "the weather's good and it's not too hot"). Understood as a lyric of bereavement and denial, 'Everyone Says 'Hi'' is surely one of Bowie's most emotionally affecting songs. The melancholy overtones are pressed home by the mournful chord changes, and there are even some evocative 'Absolute Beginners'-style doo-wop backing vocals in the closing choruses as, in the only moment that's truly evocative of 'Kooks', David sings "If the money is lousy, you can always come home / We can do all the old things". But whereas 'Kooks' was full of optimism for the future, here the protagonist knows that it's too late.

'Everyone Says 'Hi'' was performed live throughout the Heathen tour. Originally scheduled for a June 2002 single release in European territories, the 3'31" single edit eventually appeared on 16 September (coincidentally the 25th anniversary of Marc Bolan's death, which seemed oddly apposite) in a three-CD set which included several bonus tracks from the *Heathen* and *Toy* sessions. The single, which reached number 20 in the UK chart, was supported by a little-seen live video shot at the Cologne concert on 12 July 2002 (its few appearances included a screening during BBC2's coverage of the Mercury Music Awards, which conveniently fell in the week of the single's release). There were several television performances during Bowie's autumn 2002 tour, including a memorable rendition on BBC1's *Parkinson*, while *Top Of The Pops* screened the live performance Bowie had recorded for them the previous June. The song also featured in the BBC radio session of 18 September 2002.

In January 2003 a horrible seven-minute remix by dance producers METRO (alias Brian Rawling and Gary Miller, who had also produced the original *Heathen* version) appeared as a 12" vinyl promo in America. An "interactive" version of this creation was subsequently included in the 2003 Sony PlayStation 2 music-mixing game *Amplitude*, while the shorter radio edit appeared on the same year's War Child charity compilation album *Hope*.

EVERYTHING IS YOU

This Bowie composition was demoed in May 1967 and offered, without success, to Manfred Mann's producer John Burgess. The demo has yet to resurface and it seems unlikely that David ever recorded a full version, although on 27 April 1968 he did contribute backing vocals to a cover recorded by The Beatstalkers at CBS Studios. This was released as the B-side of their June 1968 single 'Rain Coloured Roses'.

EVERYTHING'S ALRIGHT

(Crouch/Konrad/Stavely/James/Karlson)
• Album: *Pin*

Originally a number 9 hit for The Mojos in 1964, 'Everything's Alright' boasts some of the tightest ensemble playing on *Pin Ups*, with splendid turns from Mike Garson, Aynsley Dunbar and Bowie himself on honking sax and histrionic vocals. An energetic live version, complete with fantastically cheesy backing-vocalist choreography from the Astronettes, was recorded at the Marquee on 19 October 1973 for NBC's *The 1980 Floor Show*.

EXALTED COMPANIONS : see MADMAN

FALL DOG BOMBS THE MOON

• Album: *Reality* • Live Video: *Reality*

Here is *Reality*'s most inscrutable lyric, not to mention its most baffling title. There's nothing new about Bowie's penchant for using dogs as a lyrical symbol of animalistic destructiveness (they're to be found not just in 'Diamond Dogs', but also in 'We Are The Dead', 'Wild Eyed Boy From Freecloud', 'Life On Mars?', ''87 And Cry', 'Fun', 'Gunman', 'I Pray, Olé' and 'We All Go Through', to name but a few), but 'Fall Dog Bombs The Moon' presents a more than usually cryptic challenge.

The key on this occasion is the fearful predicament of global politics at the time of the *Reality* sessions. The album was recorded during the preamble to, and the prosecution of, the Iraq war, and it's impossible to hear lyrics like "I don't care much, I'll win anyway ... I'm goddamn rich, an exploding man / When I talk in the night, there's oil on my hands" without pondering their most obvious resonance. It wouldn't be particularly extravagant to surmise that the 'Moon' of the title suggests the Crescent Moon of Islam, thereby narrowing down the candidates for 'Fall Dog' fairly decisively. At the time of *Reality*'s release, Bowie confirmed the song's political intent and revealed that the title was a kind of assonant joke: "It came from reading an article about Kellogg Brown & Root, a subsidiary of Halliburton, the company that Dick Cheney used to run. Basically, Kellogg Brown & Root got the job of cleaning up Iraq. What tends to happen is that a thing like an issue or a policy manifests itself as a guide. It becomes a character of some kind, like the one in 'Fall Dog'. There's this guy saying, 'I'm goddamn rich.' You know, 'Throw anything you like at me, baby, because I'm goddamn rich. It doesn't bother me.' It's an ugly song sung by an ugly man. So it was definitely about corporate and military power."

Thus 'Fall Dog Bombs The Moon' revives the pseudo-protest tradition that occasionally creeps into Bowie's songwriting: it's a lament for the circumstances that have brought us to "these blackest of years", cocking a contemptuous snook at the increasing predilection of political parties to find "someone to hate" while jumping into bed with business corporations. This is a song for the brave new world of Bush and Blair: married on stage with such loaded selections as 'Fantastic Voyage', 'Loving The Alien' and 'I'm Afraid Of Americans', the implications became ever clearer.

As is so often the case, Bowie's ideas were translated onto paper very rapidly; he later recalled that the lyric for 'Fall Dog Bombs The Moon' was written in about half an hour. Musically, the number is a close cousin of the rhythms and riffs of 'New Killer Star', distinguished by Earl Slick's emotive lead guitar line. The song was performed throughout A Reality Tour, during which a roadie would occasionally contribute to the proceedings by assisting a large cuddly dog to dance in the background (the capering canine can be spotted on the Riverside Studios DVD). The AOL session recorded on 23 September 2003 included an unusual acoustic version of the number.

FALL IN LOVE WITH ME
(Pop/Bowie/H.Sales/T.Sales)

The closing track of Iggy Pop's *Lust For Life* is co-written and co-produced by Bowie, who also plays keyboards.

FAME *(Bowie/Lennon/Alomar)*
• Album: *Americans* • A-Side: 8/75 [17] • Live: *Stage, Beeb* • Compilation: *The Best Of Bowie* • A-Side: 3/90 [28] • Video: *Collection, Best Of Bowie* • Live Video: *Moonlight, Ricochet, Glass*

In January 1975, while mixing *Young Americans* in New York, Bowie summoned members of his tour band for an impromptu recording session with John Lennon at Electric Lady. After taping 'Across The Universe', the band renewed their attempts to lay down a studio version of The Flare's 'Footstompin'', a staple in the previous autumn's tour repertoire. However, the song which had worked so well in concert proved lacklustre in the studio, and Bowie elected instead to discard 'Footstompin'' and salvage the writhing guitar riff created by Carlos Alomar. According to Alomar, "David recorded my chord changes and riff, and he hated it. He took out the lyrics and ended up with the music and cut it up on the master so that it would have classic R&B form. He's a perfectionist and experiments with the original tape, running it backwards, cutting it up, doing things on the master as opposed to recording them live. 'Fame' was totally cut up. When he had the form of the song he wanted, he left. I stayed behind and overdubbed four or five different guitar parts on it. He listened to it and said, 'That's it'."

Alomar denies the apocryphal claim that 'Fame' was based on Shirley And Company's 'Shame Shame Shame', a story originating in Tony Zanetta's less-than-eyewitness account in his book *Stardust*. But like so many of the iconic Bowie classics, 'Fame' was clearly the product of a happy collision of accidents and methodologies. John Lennon later suggested another source, telling an interviewer in 1980 that "We took some Stevie Wonder middle eight and did it backwards, you know, and we made a record out of it! I like that track."

"With John Lennon in the studio it was more the influence of having him that helped," said Bowie. "There's always a lot of adrenalin flowing when John is around, but his chief addition to it all was the high-pitched singing of 'Fame!' The riff came from Carlos and the melody and most of the lyrics came from me. But it wouldn't have happened if John hadn't been there. He was the energy, and that's why he got a credit for writing it. He was the inspiration."

'Fame' is an immaculately produced slice of bump-and-grind funk that cuts to the quick of Bowie's (and indeed Lennon's) very immediate disaffection with the trappings of stardom: money-grabbing managers, mindless adulation, unwanted entourages and the meaningless vacuity of the limousine lifestyle. Only three years after the wide-eyed aspirations of 'Star', Bowie had lived that song's dream and tasted it turn sour. Having spent most of 1974 simultaneously touring America and fighting with his manager over control of his finances and career, David was singing from the heart. There's nothing abstract about lines like "what you need you have to borrow", which precisely articulate David's predicament in the dying days of the MainMan empire. Much of the lyric seems to be addressed directly to Tony Defries. "There was a degree of malice," Bowie later agreed. "I'd had very upsetting management problems and a lot of that was built into the song." On another occasion he recalled that he and Lennon had "spent hours talking about fame, and what it's like not having a life of your own any more. How much you want to be known before you are, and then when you are, how much you want the reverse: 'I don't want to do these interviews! I don't want to have these photographs taken!' We wondered how that slow change takes place, and why it isn't everything it should have been. I guess it was inevitable that the subject matter of the song would be about the subject matter of those conversations."

Despite its intensely personal nature, Bowie was initially unenthusiastic about 'Fame'. "That was my least favourite track on the album," he recalled in 1990, "even though John had contributed to it and everything, and I had no idea, as with 'Let's Dance', that that was what a commercial single is. I haven't got a clue when it comes to singles. I just don't know about them, I don't get it, and 'Fame' was really out of left-field for me." Ironically given its lyric, 'Fame' was the Bowie single that finally broke America and propelled him into the full glare of Stateside celebrity. It became a US number 1 in the summer of 1975 before David had ever topped the chart in his home country, where the single managed a more modest number 17. The 3'30" single edit, incidentally, has only ever appeared on one compilation, 1980's The Best Of Bowie.

Two early studio mixes, timing at 3'53" and 4'17" respectively and both distinguished by a prominent flute line, have appeared on bootlegs. On 4 November 1975 David gave a mimed performance of 'Fame', together with his latest single 'Golden Years', on ABC TV's Soul Train. A fortnight later on November 23 he performed the song again (this time with a live vocal and a sax-heavy backing mix) on CBS's The Cher Show. This clip, shot against a backdrop of twinkling Vegas lights, would subsequently become the unofficial "video" for 'Fame', despite being shot a good two months after the single's chart success.

In January 1976 James Brown, one of Bowie's long-standing idols, released a single called 'Hot' – followed two months later by an album of the same name – which was a blatant and un-sanctioned cover of 'Fame' with a few different lyrics. Apparently Bowie was flattered to have his work recorded by one of his heroes, yet at the same time dismayed by what he considered plagiarism; according to Carlos Alomar, he decided that "If it charts, then we'll sue him." However, in common with many of Brown's mid-1970s offerings 'Hot' failed to chart, and all was forgotten. (Garbled reports of this episode have led several Bowie books to claim that Bowie covered a James Brown composition called 'Hot' during his days with The Spiders, but this was of course 1971's 'Hot Pants', an entirely different number.)

In March 1990 a barrage of 'Fame 90' remixes by the likes of Arthur Baker and Jon Gass were released to spearhead the ChangesBowie album and the Sound + Vision tour. "It covers a lot of ground, 'Fame'," Bowie explained, "it stands up really well in time. It still sounds potent. It's quite a nasty, angry little song. I quite like that." This time the single only reached number 28 in Britain and failed to chart in America, despite the additional publicity of featuring in the Pretty Woman soundtrack. 'Fame 90' was by no means an improvement on the original, smothering its slinky funk sounds with gunshot percussion and fashionable scratch-mix effects. The numerous subsidiary remixes, which have all dated more rapidly than the 1975 original, range in palatability from the amusing 'House Mix' to the truly ghastly 'Queen Latifah's Rap Version'. Innumerable re-edits of 'Fame 90', together with other versions like the 'Acapulco Rap Mix' and the terrifying 19-minute 'Dave Barratt 12" Uncut Version', continue to infest the collectors' circuit.

The Cher Show performance was one of several

archive clips used for Gus Van Sant's 'Fame 90' video, in which miniature screens relaying past glories framed new footage of Bowie vogueing with Sound + Vision tour dancer Louise LeCavalier. 'Fame' featured on the Station To Station, Stage, Serious Moonlight, Glass Spider, Sound + Vision, Earthling, summer 2000, Heathen and A Reality tours, making it one of Bowie's hardiest perennials. He has often adapted and augmented the number on stage: in 1983 he added a lengthy call-and-response sequence with the audience, while in 1987 he incorporated snatches of the Edwin Starr/Bruce Springsteen hit 'War' ("Fame – what is it good for? Absolutely nothing!"), the traditional folk-songs 'London Bridge Is Falling Down' and 'Lavender Blue' ("I will be king, dilly dilly, you can have fame!") and, bizarrely, 'Who Will Buy?' from Lionel Bart's *Oliver*. During the early leg of the Sound + Vision tour 'Fame' segued into a live rendering of the 'Fame 90 House Mix'. In a similar spirit the Earthling shows developed the line "Is it any wonder?" into a new drum'n'bass workout which soon acquired a life of its own (see 'Fun'), and when the original 'Fame' was revived on the same tour, splendidly dirty blasts of fuzzy guitar and spooky synthesized strings finally transformed the song from a rinky-dinky "greatest hit" back into the prowling monster it had once been. This is the version that has reappeared on subsequent tours, from which a live version recorded at the BBC Radio Theatre on 27 June 2000 was included on the *Bowie At The Beeb* bonus disc.

'Fame' has been covered by innumerable artists, among them God Lives Underwater (for the soundtrack of the 2001 film *15 Minutes*), Tommy Lee (on his 2002 album *Never A Dull Moment*), Dr Dre (on 1996's *Dr Dre Presents The Aftermath*) and Duran Duran, whose 1983 B-side version can now be heard on *David Bowie Songbook*. Among those who have performed the song live are Pearl Jam, George Michael, Iggy Pop, the Dave Matthews Band, The Feelies, Jean Meilleur and comedian Bob Downe (who spliced the song with Irene Cara's 'Fame', no doubt with hilarious consequences). House Of Pain's 1992 single 'Shamrocks And Shenanigans (Boom Shalock Lock Boom)' uses a sample from Bowie's original, as does 'Put It On You', a track from MC Lyte's 1998 rap album *Seven On Seven*. Vanilla Ice, best known for sampling 'Under Pressure' for 'Ice Ice Baby', reworked 'Fame' on his 1994 album *Mind Blowin'*. Bowie's original version reappeared on the soundtrack albums of

the 1998 film *A Soldier's Daughter Never Cries*, and 2000's *Next Friday: Old School*.

FANTASTIC VOYAGE *(Bowie/Eno)*
• Album: *Lodger* • B-Side: 4/79 [7] • B-Side: 10/82 [3]

After the forbidding musical architecture of *Low* and *"Heroes"* the opening track of *Lodger* is surprisingly serene, spurred gently along by Sean Mayes's lilting piano and the trio of Simon House, Adrian Belew and Tony Visconti strumming on mandolins borrowed from a Montreux music shop. 'Fantastic Voyage' is a heartfelt plea for sanity amid the nuclear escalation of the Carter/Brezhnev stand-off in the late 1970s, and as such it's Bowie's first "protest" lyric in many a long year. "It's a pretty straightforward song about how I feel in a very old-fashioned romantic fashion," he said. "One feels constantly that so many things are out of our own control, and it's just this infuriating thing that you don't want to have their depression ruling your life or dictating how you will wake up each morning."

It's a touching song that offers a less bombastic anti-nuclear prayer than the later 'When The Wind Blows'. The tone is wearily fatalistic ("We'll get by, I suppose") and suspicious of the motives of nationalism ("loyalty is valuable, but our lives are valuable too"), making for an unequivocal rejection of the Thin White Duke's more contentious proclamations. The track is melodically reminiscent of 'Word On A Wing' and, as Visconti pointed out, it has "the exact same chord changes and structure, even the same key" as 'Boys Keep Swinging' – "just the tempo and instrumentation are different".

'Fantastic Voyage' became the B-side of two different UK singles, and went on to make an impressive live debut some 24 years later on A Reality Tour. In 2003 Bowie described it as a song "which I've always liked and I've never done, so it's rather thrilling to do." It was a good choice politically as well as aesthetically: in the global climate of the Iraq war and its aftermath, the sentiments expressed in 'Fantastic Voyage' had never seemed more appropriate.

FASCINATION *(Bowie/Vandross)*
• Album: *Americans*

As well as being the most unabashed homage to

Gamble and Huff's "Philly" sound to be found on *Young Americans*, 'Fascination' deserves a footnote in the history of black music as the first published credit for a then unknown young soul singer called Luther Vandross. The two met at Sigma Sound in August 1974. "I was visiting my schoolmate Carlos Alomar in the studio," Vandross later recalled. "David overheard me singing a vocal idea of mine and immediately put me on the microphone. It was my first experience of recording and it cemented my desire to pursue a career in music." Vandross, who sang backing vocals on the album and went on to accompany David on tour, receives a co-writing credit for 'Fascination', a direct re-working of his own composition 'Funky Music (Is A Part Of Me)', which he sang in the Garson Band's support set on the Philly Dogs tour and later included on his 1977 album *Luther*.

Fat Larry's Band, later to enjoy a massive hit with 'Zoom', released a cover version of 'Fascination' as a single in 1976. Like most of *Young Americans* the song has remained absent from Bowie's live sets, although in 1985 it was shortlisted for his Live Aid show. Ultimately – and apparently against David's wishes – it lost out to the more obviously crowd-pleasing 'Modern Love'.

FASHION

• Album: *Scary* • A-Side: 10/80 [5] • A-Side: 11/02 • Compilation: *Club* • Video: *Collection, Best Of Bowie* • Live Video: *Moonlight, Glass*

The second *Scary Monsters* single was, according to Tony Visconti, the last track to be completed during the sessions; it had developed from a basic riff under the title 'Jamaica', a name that highlights its hardcore fusion of funk and reggae. Although the bassline and some of the melody were lifted straight from Bowie's earlier hit 'Golden Years' (you can hum the one along to the other with no problem at all), the addition of a classic deadpan lyric and Robert Fripp's trademark guitar squeals gave 'Fashion' an edge all its own. It became a popular choice for catwalk fashion shows, where the scornful irony of the lyric presumably went unnoticed. "I do think that fashion is funny, really funny," David said. "It's so nonsensical. We don't have to do it." The ridiculous exclusivity of the London and New York club scenes at the turn of the 1980s provides the springboard, but 'Fashion' has a wider constituency, cocking a snook at the transient ephemera

not only of music and dance, but implicitly of politics and power. The "turn to the left, turn to the right" chorus and the "listen to me, don't listen to me" middle eight both reflect Bowie's shifting fortunes as a celebrity demagogue and style guru over the preceding decade.

In 1980 David explained that the song was "to do with that dedication to fashion. I was trying to move on a little from that Ray Davies concept of fashion; to suggest more of a gritted teeth determination and an unsureness about why one's doing it. But one has to do it, rather like one goes to the dentist and has the tooth drilled … I must say I did feel it when I was in London. I was taken to one extraordinary place by Steve Strange … Everybody was in Victorian clothes. I suppose they were part of the new new wave or the permanent wave or whatever." Apparently oblivious to the track's lambasting of their own "gritted teeth determination", London's Blitz kids adopted the track as their signature tune, while further evidence that the lyric was falling on deaf ears could be found in the hilariously un-ironic "interpretation" of the number undertaken in November 1980 by resident *Top Of The Pops* dance troupe Legs & Co.

It seems entirely likely that Bowie's "talk to me, don't talk to me, dance with me, don't dance with me" lyric owes a debt to the Boomtown Rats' huge 1978 hit 'Rat Trap' ("walk, don't walk, talk, don't talk"), but if anything David was returning a tip of the hat. 'Rat Trap' was Britain's first new wave number 1, famously ending the seven-week residency of 'Summer Nights' with the spectacle of Bob Geldof ripping up a photo of John Travolta on *Top Of The Pops*. Geldof was a big fan – he had even blagged his way backstage to meet David during the Station To Station tour – and with its Bowie-esque sax solo and angsty narrative about a suicidal boy called Billy, 'Rat Trap' was a post-punk 'All The Young Dudes': a bittersweet soundtrack for teenagers betrayed by Callaghan's Britain and disaffected by the cultural ascendancy of disco. In 1979 Bowie's director David Mallet had shot the Rats' most feted video, 'I Don't Like Mondays'; and interestingly, given the reggae basis of 'Fashion', Tony Visconti's next production after *Scary Monsters* was the Rats' 1980 album *Mondo Bongo*, whose reggae-styled single 'Banana Republic' gave an already waning band its last top ten hit.

Nearly five minutes long on *Scary Monsters*, 'Fashion' was edited for its single release and reached a respectable number 5 in the UK chart (yet again

ABBA were at the top spot, this time with 'Super Trouper'), although in America it limped to number 70. Owing to Bowie's *Elephant Man* commitments, David Mallet's video was shot in Manhattan, partly at the Hurrah nightclub also used in the film *Christane F. Wir Kinder Vom Bahnhof Zoo*. Alongside Carlos Alomar, the musicians miming in the video included Hall & Oates guitarist G E Smith and The Rumour's drummer Stephen Goulding, both of whom had recently played with Bowie on *The Tonight Show With Johnny Carson*. Depicting David and his backing musicians as gum-chewing hard men, intercut with shots of rehearsing dancers and a bizarre parade of New Romantic freaks queuing at a skid-row soup kitchen (they include John Lennon's sometime girlfriend and Tony Visconti's future wife May Pang, who provides a "Beep beep" to camera), the video crystallizes the song's anxiety about misplaced idolatry and style-leadership. In the first "listen to me/don't listen to me" sequence the camera cuts rapidly between Bowie on stage and an immobile, expressionless and by implication mindless audience. In the second we see Bowie both as performer (shot from below) and as fan (shot from above), enacting the dialogue with his own *alter ego* – an idea he would take further in his 'Blue Jean' promo. More subtly, the wilfully ludicrous dance moves David performs towards the beginning of the clip (nose-twitching, face-rubbing, a curious sort of kangaroo-hop, and an adaptation of the expansive drop-to-the-floor-while-arching-the-arm gesture previously seen in the 'Ashes To Ashes' clip) have all, by the end of the video, been adopted and assimilated by the dancers in the cutaway shots, as if spread by some baleful infection. The implication is clear: the icon has only to twitch his nose and the fans will follow suit. Bowie's distaste of precisely this phenomenon is one of the pervasive themes of *Scary Monsters*.

The 'Fashion' video won plaudits every bit as warm as those bestowed on its predecessor 'Ashes To Ashes'. Speaking of both, the *New York Times* commented on "the brilliant way they are edited and how they expand on the music itself, rather than merely accompanying it or even contradicting it. These little shorts are genuine music theatre in a new and modern guise ... The real hero of the rock-video revolution so far is that perennial pioneer David Bowie." In Britain the readers of *Record Mirror* concurred, voting 'Ashes To Ashes' and 'Fashion' the best videos of 1980.

'Fashion' made live appearances on the Serious Moonlight, Glass Spider, Sound + Vision, Earthling,

Heathen and A Reality tours, and featured as a duet with Frank Black at Bowie's fiftieth birthday concert. The 1997 version was of particular note, stripped of any "greatest hits" connotations by an aggressively visceral bassline and a shocking set of skin-flick back-projections. Less impressive was 'Fashion 98', a feckless rap version which gave Glamma Kid a minor UK hit in 1998. In November 2002 a radical dance remix by the London-based producer Solaris, re-titled 'Shout' (after the line "You shout it while you're dancing", which it repeats ad nauseam), was released as a 12" single. Credited to "Solaris vs Bowie", it failed to repeat the chart success of the same year's Scumfrog remix of 'Loving The Alien', and subsequently reappeared on *Club Bowie*. Another sample from the original 'Fashion' appeared in 'I Am A Scientist', a track on The Dandy Warhols' 2003 album *Welcome To The Monkey House*, for which Bowie duly received a co-writing credit.

FEED THE WORLD *(Geldof/Ure)* :
see **DO THEY KNOW IT'S CHRISTMAS?**

FEVER *(Davenport/Cooley)* :
see **HEAVEN'S IN HERE**

FILL YOUR HEART *(Rose/Williams)*
• Album: *Hunky*

The only non-Bowie composition on this most song-writerly of albums is the work of American singer/songwriter Biff Rose and collaborator Paul Williams. The original version hails from Rose's 1968 LP *The Thorn In Mrs Rose's Side*, but it's more than likely that Bowie first came across the song in the form of the cover version backing Tiny Tim's infamous novelty single 'Tiptoe Through The Tulips'. Biff Rose, described by Bowie as "a flower-power Randy Newman", was also responsible for the whimsical 'Buzz The Fuzz' which David performed live at around the same time. Bowie later asserted that "Biff Rose is reflected a lot in the style of songwriting" on *Hunky Dory* as a whole.

One of the more up-tempo offerings on *Hunky Dory*, 'Fill Your Heart' was in Bowie's live repertoire as early as 1970, although the jaunty piano-led album arrangement is considerably more sophisticated than the acoustic guitar accompaniment of the earlier live renditions. Interestingly, the guitar intro of the live version (as immortalized by two BBC sessions in 1970 and 1971) is practically identical to the intro of Bowie's forthcoming classic 'John, I'm Only Dancing'.

'Fill Your Heart' replaced 'Bombers' as *Hunky Dory*'s side two opener at a late stage in the album's development. The song sits happily enough alongside the post-hippy whimsy of 'Kooks', and its paean to positive thinking and the folkloric evocation of "dragons" strikes a chord with earlier Bowie compositions. Despite lacking the lyrical and musical depth of the album's highlights, it provides a cogent counterpoint to the angst of 'Quicksand' and 'Changes' with its cautionary warnings: "don't play the game of time" and "forget your mind and you'll be free". The track is likely to be best remembered, however, for David's pleasing saxophone break and the spectacular dexterity of Rick Wakeman's piano solo.

'Fill Your Heart' featured prominently in the soundtrack of the 1993 BBC serial *The Buddha Of Suburbia*, alongside Bowie's specially composed music.

A FLEETING MOMENT :
see **SEVEN YEARS IN TIBET**

FINGERTIPS *(Cosby/Paul)* :
see **YOUNG AMERICANS**

FIRE GIRL *(Pop/Bowie)*

Co-written and co-produced by Bowie for Iggy Pop's *Blah-Blah-Blah*, and released as a single in 1987. A demo, featuring backing vocals from David, has appeared on bootlegs.

FIRST TIME I MET THE BLUES *(Montgomery)* :
see **YOUNG AMERICANS**

FIVE YEARS
• Album: *Ziggy* • Live: *Stage, SM72, Beeb* • Live Video: *Best Of Bowie*

The slow-quick-quick drumbeat that begins *Ziggy*

Stardust has earned a place in rock history as one of the all-time classic album openings. 'Five Years' gradually builds from wistful inevitability to apocalyptic terror as the news breaks that the end of the world is five years hence. The half-sung, half-spoken vocal style is indebted to Lou Reed, the gathering omens of doom are passingly reminiscent of *Julius Caesar*, but the violent images of societal breakdown are straight from *The War of the Worlds* and *Day of the Triffids*, signalling the essence of Bowie's new subject matter: human longing and bruised relationships, expressed in the poignantly tacky idiom of British sci-fi. Once again the theatrical process of dissimulation echoes Bowie's own sense of alienation: on *Hunky Dory* he was "living in a silent film", and now he feels "like an actor" as, Frankenstein-like, he breathes life into his new creation: "your face, your race, the way that you talk / I kiss you, you're beautiful, I want you to walk". The spirit of Ziggy has arrived, and in one of the album's finest songs.

As elsewhere on the album, the vocabulary is precise and revealing in its deployment of an American slang that rings consciously alien through Bowie's frail London vowels. His adulation of "the way that you talk" reaffirms the album's fantasies of Americana: here are a "news guy" and a "cop" (both more jarringly American in 1972 than now), and the adoption of the American abbreviation "TV" (rather than "telly") allows a submerged pun on "transvestite" to accompany the song's other outsiders: "the black", "the priest" and "the queer". With a flock of misfits and minorities gathering around him, Bowie's final exhortation "I want you to walk" acquires a second, Messianic resonance: here is Ziggy raising the crippled and the dead. It's a classic example of the dexterity and economy of Bowie's best songwriting: with its scant few lines 'Five Years' drips with implication.

The track was completed at Trident on 15 November 1971. Bowie recorded his vocal in two separate takes, the better to shift gear into the manic climax of the final chorus. "David starts very quietly," explained Ken Scott, "And so in order to get the best sound I had to crank the level, but as you know he eventually becomes a power-house and so I had to change all the settings. The vocal range was quite different for the second half of the song, and so we had to adjust the levels to compensate for that." A similar ploy would be used by Tony Visconti for the recording of '"Heroes"' five years later.

In his November 1973 interview for *Rolling Stone*,

Bowie extrapolated on the scenario established in 'Five Years': "It has been announced that the world will end because of lack of natural resources. Ziggy is in a position where all the kids have access to things that they thought they wanted. The older people have lost all touch with reality and the kids are left on their own to plunder anything. Ziggy was in a rock'n'roll band and the kids no longer want rock'n'roll. There's no electricity to play it. Ziggy's adviser tells him to collect news and sing it, 'cause there is no news. So Ziggy does this and there is terrible news." Although relatively coherent by comparison with some of Bowie's utterances of the period, this account seems to raise more questions than it answers. Later in the 1970s, in response to a question about his much-publicized fear of flying, David claimed that the original inspiration for the song had been a dream in which his father's ghost had warned him never to fly again, adding that he had only five years to live. An even more surprising source is Roger McGough's poem 'At Lunchtime – A Story Of Love', which Bowie had included in his cabaret act in 1968. It's a tragicomic tale of the sexual abandon that breaks out on a bus when news arrives that the world will end at lunchtime, and includes several images Bowie would adapt for 'Five Years': at one point the bus stops suddenly "to avoid / damaging a mother and child in the road", while the bus conductor "struck up / some sort of relationship with the driver."

'Five Years' was included in the BBC session recorded on 18 January 1972 (this recording appears on *Bowie At The Beeb*), and a further version graced Bowie's *Old Grey Whistle Test* set on 8 February, later appearing on the *Best Of Bowie* DVD. The song featured throughout the Ziggy Stardust and Station To Station tours (a superb rendition appeared on *The Dinah Shore Show* on 3 January 1976), and surfaced once again on the Stage tour. In 1985 'Five Years' was due to be featured in Bowie's Live Aid set, but David volunteered to drop the number in favour of introducing an appeal film. 'Five Years' would not be performed again until 2003, when it made a triumphant reappearance on A Reality Tour.

Among the artists who have covered 'Five Years' are former Marillion frontman Fish, who included versions on his 1993 covers album *Songs From The Mirror* and 1994's live release *Sushi*. Frank Sidebottom covered 'Five Years' on *Frank's Firm Favourites*, and the song has been played live by Low Max, Golden Smog, Aslan and The Polyphonic Spree, whose BBC session

recording was included on their 2002 single 'Hanging Around'.

5.15 THE ANGELS HAVE GONE
• Album: *Heathen*

This mournful song of dashed hopes and emotional isolation was one of Bowie's favourite tracks from *Heathen*. Over an icy backing of percussion and a simple, repetitive guitar phrase, he sings a sparse lyric of disappointment and rejection ("I'm changing trains, this little town let me down … I'm jumping tracks, I'm changing towns … cold station, all of my life, forever, I'm out of here forever"), recalling the image of the despondent loner packing up and leaving town who is a recurring figure throughout Bowie's songwriting, from early numbers like 'Can't Help Thinking About Me' and 'Little Bombardier' to later compositions like 'Be My Wife' and 'Move On'. In this instance the occasion of the character's disappointment appears to be lost love ("We never talk any more / Forever I will adore only you … Angels like them, thin on the ground") but, as ever, the possibilities run deeper. "A man who could once see his angels – hopes and aspirations, maybe – can't see them any more," David explained, "and he blames the crushing dumbness of life for it." Like all of the album, '5.15 The Angels Have Gone' was performed throughout the Heathen and A Reality tours, appearing in the BBC radio session of 18 September 2002 and also on the edition of *Later… With Jools Holland* recorded two days later. The 5.1 remix on the *Heathen* SACD is some 24 seconds longer than the CD version.

FLY
• Bonus: *Reality*

Released on the limited-edition bonus disc that came with initial pressings of *Reality*, this spirited out-take from the album sessions features a contribution from Bowie's veteran guitarist Carlos Alomar, who provides the powerful but jaunty riff (melodically, rhythmically, and in all likelihood unintentionally reminiscent of ABBA's 1980 number 'On And On And On') after an opening salvo of distortion and feedback.

Lyrically, 'Fly' revisits the domestic American angst already witnessed in tracks like 'New Killer Star' and 'She'll Drive The Big Car'; this time the focus is on the catalogue of anxiety and depression eating away at a middle-class family man, perhaps a more sympathetic relative of the protagonist in songs like 'Repetition' and 'I'm Afraid of Americans'. "I'm crying in my car", he confesses, confiding that although "The kids are alright" (once again Pete Townshend casts his shadow over a Bowie lyric), "The boy's on a charge but his mother doesn't know / I never got around yet to telling her so / It would only make her crazy". The only escape is of a desperate and fantastical kind: "I'll be fine / I'm only screaming in my head / I can fly / I close my eyes and I can fly". It's a dark, depressive variation on the fantasy of "astral flight" explored by 1967's tongue-in-cheek 'Did You Ever Have A Dream'. Nearly four decades later 'Fly' is another song of dreams, but they're dreams of an altogether more fearful and delusional kind.

A FOGGY DAY IN LONDON TOWN
(G. Gershwin/I. Gershwin)
• Compilation: *Red Hot + Rhapsody*

Bowie's moody cover of the Gershwin standard (from the 1937 film musical *A Damsel In Distress*) was recorded in 1998 in collaboration with *Twin Peaks* composer Angelo Badalamenti, and released on the Gershwin centenary tribute album *Red Hot + Rhapsody*.

FOOTSTOMPIN' *(Collins/Rand)*
• Live: *Rarest*

During the 1974 Philly Dogs tour, David augmented his *Young Americans* material with a hard-edged funk medley of The Flare's 1961 single 'Footstompin'' and the ancient 'Wish I Could Shimmy Like My Sister Kate', as performed by the 1930s New Orleans jazz diva Blue Lu Barker. Two attempts were apparently made to record a studio version of 'Footstompin'' in the autumn, and it was with a view to a third that Bowie entered Electric Lady studios in January 1975 for the session that would instead produce 'Fame', founded on Carlos Alomar's 'Footstompin'' riff.

On 2 November 1974 Bowie and his band performed the 'Footstompin''/'Sister Kate' medley on Dick Cavett's *Wide World Of Entertainment*. This recording later appeared on *RarestOneBowie*.

FRIDAY ON MY MIND *(Young/Vanda)*
• Album: *Pin*

A number 6 hit for The Easybeats in 1966, 'Friday On My Mind' opens side two of *Pin Ups* with the band on top form, while Bowie delivers a curiously unsteady vocal performance, veering between his Aladdin Sane falsetto and his finest Anthony Newley.

FUJE MOTO SAN : see CRYSTAL JAPAN

FUN
• Album: *liveandwell.com*

Originating on the Earthling tour as the extended drum'n'bass workout 'Is It Any Wonder' (see 'Fame'), this elusive 1997 composition was later radically redeveloped in the studio. Having gained a new set of lyrics the track was initially referred to by Reeves Gabrels in various interviews as 'Funhouse', but was later re-titled 'Fun'. Both the darkly funky bass-driven beat and the techno-trance lyrics recall the Iggy Pop tracks 'Funtime' and 'Fun House' ("Back into the funhouse, music is sublime … We'll show you a really good time, we all lie in the funhouse…"). The 3'09" 'Clownboy Mix' appeared on a CD-ROM offered to BowieNet subscribers in 1998, and a 'Live Version' hailing from the Amsterdam gig on 10 June 1997 later became downloadable for them. The otherwise unavailable 'Dillinja Mix' later appeared on *liveandwell.com*.

FUNKY DORY *(Brammer/Clark/Bowie)* :
see ANDY WARHOL

FUNKY MUSIC (IS A PART OF ME) *(Vandross)* :
see FASCINATION

FUNNY SMILE : see YOUR FUNNY SMILE

FUNTIME *(Pop/Bowie)*

'Funtime' was produced and co-written by Bowie for Iggy Pop's *The Idiot*. The robotic backing and burned-out, joyless vocals (David's are almost as prominent as Iggy's) offer a chilling backward glimpse at the pair's hedonistic excesses in Los Angeles, an ironic dissection of the pursuit of pleasure in which "fun" has long since evaporated. "He had the music and I brought the lyrics to it," Iggy later recalled. "He told me to sing it like Mae West, like a bitch who wants to make money." Bowie's characteristically off-the-wall injunction gave the song a fresh dimension, making it, in Iggy's words, "informed of other genres, like cinema. Also, it was a little bit gay. The vocals there became more menacing as a result of that suggestion."

A live version from Iggy's 1977 tour, featuring Bowie on keyboards, appears on *TV Eye* and *Suck On This!*. 'Funtime' has long been a favourite with other artists; among those who have covered the song are Blondie, Duran Duran, REM, Boy George, The Cars, That Petrol Emotion and Peter Murphy.

FUTURE LEGEND
• Album: *Dogs*

The opening track of *Diamond Dogs* aggressively heralds David's latest vision. A ghostly *Hound of the Baskervilles* howl fades into a nightmarish synthesized rendition of 'Bewitched, Bothered and Bewildered', over which Bowie's narration sketches in the post-apocalyptic hell of Hunger City, where "the last few corpses lay rotting in the slimy thoroughfare" and, in a manner sure to terrify Orwell's Winston Smith, "fleas the size of rats sucked on rats the size of cats". The influence of William Burroughs is never clearer than in Bowie's image of "ten thousand peoploids split into small tribes coveting the highest of the sterile skyscrapers, like packs of dogs" which, as David Buckley notes, paraphrases *The Naked Lunch* with its "baying pack of people". The surrealistic tone-poem style pays homage to Burroughs and acknowledges David's own systematic "ripping and re-wrapping" of himself and his music.

During some dates of the Diamond Dogs tour a pre-recorded tape of 'Future Legend' preceded the title song, although surprisingly this was never the opening number. The backing tapes were often abandoned due to technical difficulties, and were scrapped altogether for the Philly Dogs tour.

GET REAL *(Bowie/Eno)*
• B-Side: 11/95 [39]

This *1.Outside* out-take appeared only as a B-side and on the Japanese release of the album, later cropping up as a bonus track on the 2004 US reissue. It's a far more conventional pop-rock composition than anything on the album, bouncing along to a rhythm track borrowed from 'Modern Love' and dipping briefly into the melody of 'Dead Against It'. Bowie reels off an uninspired *1.Outside*-by-numbers sort of lyric: "It happens in the tunnel when I let myself feel … The dazzle of life, the rape of life, the seed, the curse, the jazz of life, get real." It's less intriguing than its fellow *1.Outside* rarity 'Nothing To Be Desired', but it's an appealing glimpse into the wealth of extra material recorded during the sessions.

GET UP, STAND UP *(Marley/McIntosh)*

Bob Marley's classic, a single for The Wailers from their 1973 album *Burnin'*, formed the closing number at the Tibet House Benefit Concert on 28 February 2003. As in previous years, Bowie joined in the singalong.

GIMME DANGER *(Pop/Williamson)*

Mixed by Bowie for Iggy And The Stooges' *Raw Power*, 'Gimme Danger' appeared on the 1977 Iggy Pop tour; a version featuring Bowie appears on *Suck On This!*.

GIRLS
• B-Side: 6/87 [33] • Bonus: *Never*

Bowie wrote 'Girls' for Tina Turner, who recorded it for her 1986 album *Break Every Rule* and later included a live version on some formats of 1988's *Live In Europe*. Bowie's own version was cut during the *Never Let Me Down* sessions but relegated to B-side status. The full-length recording appeared on the 12" 'Time Will Crawl' single, with a shorter edit appearing on the 7" format. A further Japanese version was included on a second 12" release and on the Japanese issue of the album.

Although something of a curate's egg, the wildly eclectic 'Girls' is an improvement on several of the tracks that made it onto *Never Let Me Down*. It starts in melodramatic torch-song mode, with a wistful guitar riff swiped from 'Andy Warhol' and a piano line recalling, of all things, Ennio Morricone's famous TV theme 'Chi Mai'. Sadly it degenerates into a standard *Never Let Me Down* sax-and-guitar romp, complete with a rehash of the 'Criminal World' bassline and a blatant melodic steal from Rita Coolidge's *Octopussy* theme 'All Time High'. The lyrics, believe it or not, borrow from Ridley Scott's *Blade Runner*. Bowie: "My heart suspended in time, like you vanish like tears in the rain"; *Blade Runner*: "I've seen things you people wouldn't believe … all those moments will be lost in time, like tears in rain". It was a quotation Bowie had previously adapted on his funeral wreath for his half-brother Terry in 1985 which read: "You've seen more things than we could imagine but all these moments will be lost, like tears washed away by the rain".

GLAD I'VE GOT NOBODY
• Compilation: *Early*

Unreleased until 1991's *Early On*, this rejected mid-1965 recording by Davy Jones and The Lower Third was almost certainly recorded during the same session as 'Baby Loves That Way' and the unreleased 'I'll Follow You'. Unlike most of Bowie's 1960s rarities, these two are finished tracks featuring full arrangements. Musically, 'Glad I've Got Nobody' is unremarkable beyond confirming The Lower Third's hero-worship of The Who.

GLASS SPIDER
• Album: *Never* • Live Video: *Glass*

Forever tarred by association with the critically derided tour to which it gave its name, 'Glass Spider' is actually one of *Never Let Me Down*'s better tracks. Purposely written as a live curtain-raiser (it opened every show on the 1987 tour), it has a daring sense of theatre sorely missing elsewhere on the album, but it's let down by indifferent production. The spoken monologue – another of the album's many references to *Diamond Dogs* – has great potential, but by contrast with the gothic relish of 'Future Legend' Bowie's delivery is deadpan and timid. The song doesn't take flight until the splendid guitar riff kicks in and the lyric heaps new images onto the initial narrative.

"The pivotal song on the album is 'Glass Spider'," David said in 1987. "Spiders keep coming up in my references all the time. I don't know what the Jungian aspects of it are but I see them as some kind of mother figure." In another interview he added, "I was fascinated by the fact that the black widow spider does lay out its victims' skeletons on a web. I found that out a few months ago; it came up in some documentary on television … I always saw spiders as being a maternal thing, and I wanted to have an all-encompassing motherhood song: how one is released from the mother and then left on one's own, and you have to get by on your instincts. I wanted to develop the fable of the black widow spider, transform it. The reference to glass obviously fitted. Putting the two together, 'glass spider', reminds me of castles and something almost Chinese. Imagine this layer of webs like a castle; it moves from room to room and has a kind of altar at the top. It's fabricating a mock mythology. The subtext for that one was motherhood, being abandoned by one's mother, which is inevitable."

The tumbling images of mass migration ("Come along before the animals awake / Run, run, we've been moving all night, rivers to the left / If your mother don't love you then the riverbed might") are vaguely reminiscent of 'African Night Flight', but here they echo the Fall of Man, abandoned to fend for himself in a desert of moral uncertainty. This is such a good song. He really ought to re-record it.

GLORIA *(Morrison)*

Them's 1964 number made a one-off appearance on Iggy Pop's 1977 *Idiot* tour, and was later resurrected by Bowie for some of the later Sound + Vision shows: at a Cleveland gig on 20 June 1990 David segued into 'Gloria' during 'The Jean Genie' and was joined on stage by Bono to sing the number, which was frequently incorporated into 'The Jean Genie' at subsequent concerts.

GO NOW *(Banks/Bennett)*
• Live: *Ruby Trax* • Live Video: *Oy*

An unusual addition to Tin Machine's repertoire during the It's My Life tour was Bessie Banks's 'Go Now', a number 1 single for The Moody Blues in 1964. Bassist Tony Sales took lead vocal, and a live recording made in Japan appeared on the *Ruby Trax* charity album in 1992.

GOD KNOWS I'M GOOD
• Album: *Oddity* • Live: *Beeb*

One of the lesser tracks on *Space Oddity*, this bizarre Dylanesque protest song about a hapless shoplifter tackles the customary hippy-era targets of capitalism and "national concern". Bowie explained that it was a diatribe against social mechanization. "Communication has taken away so much from our lives that now it's almost totally involved in machines rather than ordinary human beings," he said in 1969. "There's nobody to talk your troubles over with these days, so this track is about a woman who steals a can of stew, which she desperately needs but can't afford, from the supermarket and gets caught. The machine looks on, 'shrieking on the counter' and 'spitting by my shoulder'."

Guitarist Keith Christmas recalls David weeping "in floods" when listening to a playback of the track during the *Space Oddity* sessions (but it must be added that Angela Bowie offers a very similar recollection regarding 'Cygnet Committee', which somehow seems more likely). Although Bowie regarded 'God Knows I'm Good' as something of a throwback, describing it in 1969 as "more like my earlier songs", he included it in the BBC session recorded on 5 February 1970. This version now appears on *Bowie At The Beeb*.

GOD ONLY KNOWS *(Wilson/Asher)*
• Album: *Tonight*

The Beach Boys classic, a number 2 hit in 1966, was originally mooted for inclusion on *Pin Ups* in 1973 before being consigned to the aborted Astronettes project later the same year. "Nothing came of that. I still have the tapes, though," Bowie revealed in 1984. "It sounded such a good idea at the time and I never had the chance to do it with anybody else again, so I thought I'd do it myself." Sadly, the Val Doonican-esque *Tonight* version is a three-minute masterclass in every pitfall that awaited him in the heady wake of *Let's Dance*. Mired in a baleful morass of turgid strings and awful saxophones, Bowie croons his way haplessly through perhaps the worst track he has ever record-

ed. Nevertheless, in 2001 the song's lyricist Tony Asher cited Bowie's recording of 'God Only Knows' as his favourite cover version of the *Pet Sounds* material.

The 1973 Astronettes version, which finally appeared on 1995's *People From Bad Homes*, keeps to a similarly languourous tempo but boasts a superior and soulful arrangement by Tony Visconti, with emphasis on mandolins and a rather impressive sax solo from David.

GOING BACK TO BIRMINGHAM *(Penniman)* : see YOUNG AMERICANS

GOING DOWN

Together with 'Everything Is You' and a lost track called 'Summer Kind Of Love', this number was demoed in May 1967 and sent, without success, to Manfred Mann's producer John Burgess. The demo emerged in 1996 on the 'Ernie Johnson' tape.

GOLDEN YEARS
• A-Side: 11/75 [8] •Album: *Station* • B-Side: 11/81 [24] • Compilation: *74/79, Best Of Bowie* • Live Video: *Moonlight*

Just as 'Rebel Rebel' had offered a furtive farewell to glam and an unrepresentative preview of *Diamond Dogs* in early 1974, so the immaculate funk of 'Golden Years', preceding the release of its parent album by two months, is more of a piece with *Young Americans* than with the steelier musical landscape of *Station To Station*. Co-producer Harry Maslin recalled that 'Golden Years' was "cut and finished very fast. We knew it was absolutely right within ten days. But the rest of the album took forever." Early in the sessions the album itself was to be called *Golden Years*.

David would later say that the track had been written for, and turned down by, Elvis Presley. Angela Bowie claims that David wrote it in her honour and sang it over the telephone to her, "just the way, all those years before, he'd sung me 'The Prettiest Star'. It had a similar effect. I bought it." The refrain of "angel" certainly suggests that she might be the addressee, although the "walk tall, act fine" optimism and the vow to "stick with you baby for a thousand years" sits ill with what we now know about a marriage already in terminal decline.

On 4 November 1975 Bowie mimed to 'Golden Years' on ABC's *Soul Train*. This appearance came to be regarded as the unofficial video and was used to promote the single worldwide. 'Golden Years' consolidated David's commercial stock in America, reaching number 10; in Britain, hard on the heels of the chart-topping 'Space Oddity' reissue, it made number 8.

'Golden Years' made a few rare appearances on the Station To Station tour before becoming a regular Serious Moonlight fixture. It later reappeared in some of the early Sound + Vision concerts, and was revived once again in 2000. The song has been widely covered by artists including Pearl Jam, Loose Ends, Nina Hagen, and even Marilyn Manson for the 1998 film soundtrack *Dead Man On Campus*. An instrumental version of Bowie's original appeared over the closing credits of the American TV movie *Stephen King's Golden Years*, while the original track was ingeniously remixed by Tony Visconti for use in Brian Helgeland's 2001 film *A Knight's Tale*: as a key ingredient of the picture's tongue-in-cheek synthesis of musical anachronisms, a courtly farandole develops into a disco freak-out as 'Golden Years' gradually supplants the medieval soundtrack.

GOOD MORNING GIRL
• B-Side: 4/66 • Compilation: *Early*

This catchy jazz-tinged track, complete with a scat-singing chorus from David, was recorded with The Buzz on 7 March 1966 and performed live in the same year. It would probably have made a better single than 'Do Anything You Say', to whose B-side it was relegated.

GOODBYE MR. ED *(Bowie/H.Sales/T.Sales)*
• Album: *TM2* • Live: *Oy* • Live Video: *Oy*

Tucked away at the end of that least regarded of albums *Tin Machine II*, 'Goodbye Mr. Ed' is perhaps Bowie's most underrated song, certainly ranking alongside 'I Can't Read' as one of Tin Machine's more valuable legacies. From an acoustic intro the track builds like the opening bars of 'Red Sails' into a superbly structured metronomic arrangement, over which Bowie intones a catalogue of casual atrocities blighting the American Dream. The melody snatches a repetitive figure from Acker Bilk's 1961 hit 'Stranger

On The Shore', while the lyric is a richly allusive composite of classical mythology, paraphrased nursery-rhymes and bourgeois vulgarity, its ironies sharpened by the absurdist reference to the speaking horse in the moralistic all-American sitcom *Mr. Ed*. Alongside Icarus, Bruegel and The Sex Pistols we have, among other things, "four and twenty black kids, some of them are blind" and "Andy's skull enshrined in a shopping mall near Queens." David adopts the off-hand drone previously perfected on 'Repetition', and the cumulative effect is everything that 1987's overblown 'Day-In Day-Out' should have been. Keeping Tin Machine's tendency to sonic self-destruction firmly in check, 'Goodbye Mr. Ed' is an unconsidered gem. It was performed throughout the It's My Life tour.

GOODNIGHT LADIES *(Reed)*

Co-produced by Bowie, this laid-back New Orleans jazz pastiche makes an unlikely but delightful conclusion to Lou Reed's *Transformer*.

THE GOSPEL ACCORDING TO TONY DAY
• B-Side: 4/67 • B-Side: 9/73 [6] • Compilation: *Deram*

Recorded on 26 January 1967 during the *David Bowie* sessions, this B-side is one of the period's more outré numbers, sketching a cynical portrait of various (presumably fictional) acquaintances over a droning background of oboe and bassoon – two instruments much in evidence on 'The Laughing Gnome', recorded the same day. Bowie effectively mimics Tony Hancock when he closes with the exasperated mutter: "Who needs friends? Waste of flipping time! Take a look at my life and you'll see." The song's nearest relation is probably 'Please Mr Gravedigger', and it makes for equally left-field listening. An excellent cover version by Edwyn Collins appeared on *Uncut*'s 2003 compilation *Starman*.

GOTTA GET A JOB :
see **YOU GOT TO HAVE A JOB (IF YOU DON'T WORK – YOU DON'T EAT)**

THE GOUSTER

It is rumoured that a song called 'The Gouster' was recorded during the August 1974 sessions for *Young Americans*, which went by the same title itself during recording.

GOT MY MOJO WORKING (*Morganfield*)

Muddy Waters's 1957 classic was played live by The King Bees.

GROWIN' UP (*Springsteen*)
• Bonus: *Pin, Dogs* (2004)

Despite initially appearing in 1990 as a bonus track on *Pin Ups*, this Bruce Springsteen cover (originally hailing from his 1973 debut *Greetings From Asbury Park, N.J.*) was in fact recorded at Olympic in November 1973 during the early stages of the sessions for *Diamond Dogs*, the album to which it was more appropriately appended on 2004's 30th anniversary reissue. The rumour that Ron Wood makes an uncredited appearance on *Diamond Dogs* almost certainly derives from this track, on which he does indeed play lead guitar. The choice of song steers the emphasis of Bowie's earlier 1973 covers away from swinging London and in the direction of American rock, while vocals, piano and even percussion offer a distinct taste of things to come, as he throws caution to the wind with a full-blown *Diamond Dogs* croon punctuated by bursts of *Young Americans* falsetto.

GROWING UP AND I'M FINE

Written by David for Mick Ronson's 1974 debut *Slaughter On 10th Avenue*, this little gem remains entirely overlooked. The lyric is straight from the Ziggy/Aladdin songbook ("Always got caught by the squad car lights", "somebody's messed with my brain"), and with its piano-led verses and glammed-up choruses, packed with handclaps and falsetto backing vocals, the track sounds like a 1972 Bowie outtake – a feeling rammed home by Ronson's flagrant mimicry of David's vocal mannerisms. Recommended.

GUNMAN (*Bowie/Belew*)

This collaboration from Adrian Belew's 1990 album *Young Lions* features David on lead vocal in a convincing throwback to the ambient Euro-funk of the Berlin era. Bowie delivers a strident performance reminiscent of 'Joe The Lion' as he chants a deadpan lyric which aims a little higher than the previous year's 'Crack City', despite covering similar ground: "Gunman, a trader in arms, the kids on the street are buying your charms … You're more solid than a rock, a rock of cocaine or crack or ice or death."

HALLO SPACEBOY (*Bowie/Eno*)
• Album: *1.Outside* • A-Side: 2/96 [12] • Live: *Phoenix: The Album, liveandwell.com, Beeb* • Video: *Best Of Bowie*

In its original form 'Hallo Spaceboy' is probably the downright noisiest Bowie track to be found outside the work of Tin Machine, a hardcore miasma of sci-fi noise, hypnotic high-speed drumming and an insistent, speaker-hopping four-note guitar riff. Developed from a Reeves Gabrels instrumental called 'Moondust', it combines the darkest elements of Pixies, *Pornography*-era Cure, and 1990s Bowie cheerleaders Nine Inch Nails and Smashing Pumpkins (who released a track called 'Spaceboy' in 1993). Drawing on the lyrics of 'Baby Universal', and raising the ghost of the girl/boy conundrum proposed by 'Rebel Rebel' and restated by Blur's 1994 hit 'Boys And Girls', Bowie hits the jackpot of *1.Outside*'s millennial angst with an anguished howl of "This chaos is killing me!"

In April 2003, several years after his departure from the Bowie camp, Reeves Gabrels told readers of his website that he had mixed feelings about Bowie's appropriation of 'Moondust'. According to Gabrels, the genesis of the track went back to his second visit to Montreux in 1994, to record some supplementary material with Bowie after the main improvisational sessions that yielded the *Leon* album: "One afternoon, near the end of that month-long stay in Switzerland, I wrote an ambient piece which David then recited the words 'moon dust…' etc over," Gabrels recalled. "The words were from a poem written by a poet whose name escapes me (might be John Giorno), but David was reading that poem when I re-entered the control room after recording some of what became the 'Moondust' track. At that point he decided adding that to my idea."

It appears that Gabrels's recollections of this episode are not entirely accurate: Bowie's spoken line "If I fall, moondust will cover me" (unheard on the finished 'Hallo Spaceboy', but later resurfacing in the opening bars of the Pet Shop Boys remix) originates not from John Giorno but from Bowie's long-time muse Brion Gysin, the poet and multi-media artist whose cut-up and "permutation" techniques, developed with William Burroughs, David had long admired. They are in fact reputed to be the last words spoken by Gysin on his Paris deathbed in 1986. "The third time I was in Montreux to work on the *Outside* record," continued Gabrels, "I asked David about the track and he said he didn't feel there was anything special going on with that piece and that he'd pretty much forgotten about it. I still have a rough mix of the original and it's got its own charm, I think."

Nothing more was heard of the track until the New York sessions several months later. Brian Eno's diary reports how 'Hallo Spaceboy' emerged from 'Moondust' in the studio on 17 January 1995, when Bowie, Carlos Alomar and drummer Joey Barron set about "stripping it right down to almost nothing. I wrote some lightning chords and spaces (knowing I wouldn't get long to do it), and suddenly, miraculously, we had something. Carlos and Joey at their shining best. Instantly D. came up with a really great vocal strategy (something about a Spaceboy), delivered with total confidence and certainty." Work continued on the track the following day, when Eno records that a delighted Bowie was already insisting, "Don't change anything."

'Hallo Spaceboy' was performed live on the Outside tour, initially with Nine Inch Nails on the US leg and thereafter as the preferred closing number. In February 1996 it became *1.Outside*'s third single, albeit in a radically different form. Long-time fan Neil Tennant was approached with the idea of remixing the track, and later recalled telephoning David from the studio to explain that he was adding lines from 'Space Oddity' to the remix: "There was this long silence, and then he said, 'I think I'd better come over.'" Tennant got his way, however, and the remixed 'Hallo Spaceboy' arrived complete with a regulation Pet Shop Boys disco beat and a series of cut-ups from 'Space Oddity' sung by Tennant himself: "Ground to Major, bye bye Tom / Dead the circuit, countdown's wrong." David Mallet's brilliant video combined shots of Bowie and the Pet Shop Boys in shafts of stark light with retroactive images from 1950s sci-fi and monster movies, stars, planets, girls, boys, space-rockets, guillotine blades, graveyards, embryos and skeletons. The trio subsequently performed the song at the Brit Awards on 19 February and again on *Top Of The Pops* on 1 March. The remix later replaced 'Wishful Beginnings' on the reissued album *1.Outside Version 2*.

The 'Hallo Spaceboy' CD included live tracks from the Outside tour and a reissue of 'The Hearts Filthy Lesson' (now billed "as featured in the motion picture *Seven*"). The single was a success in many European territories (it topped the chart in Latvia!) and reached number 12 in the UK, Bowie's best placing since 'Jump They Say'. It might have done better but for a piece of unfortunate timing, being released as Babylon Zoo's ersatz-'Starman' hit 'Spaceman' was notching up its fourth week at number 1 – ludicrously, some reviewers suggested that Bowie's single was the copycat of the two.

'Hallo Spaceboy' continued to feature in Bowie's live sets throughout 1996 and 1997, and was resuscitated for the summer 2000 dates and the Heathen and A Reality tours. A live version recorded at the BBC Radio Theatre on 27 June 2000 appeared on the *Bowie At The Beeb* bonus disc. An earlier version recorded at the Phoenix Festival on 18 July 1996 was included on the BBC release *Phoenix: The Album* and on a French promo release, while another live cut, this time from Rio de Janeiro on 2 November 1997, appeared on *liveandwell.com*. The Pet Shop Boys performed their own version during their live residency at London's Savoy Theatre in 1997.

HAMMERHEAD (Bowie/H.Sales)
• B-Side: 8/91 [33] • Album: *TM2*

This insubstantial rocker from the *Tin Machine II* sessions became a B-side, while a minute-long instrumental excerpt appeared as the album's unlisted final track. It's standard pseudo-sexist Tin Machine fare, allowing Bowie to revisit some of his favourite lyrical phrases ("sweet thing" crops up) and tip his hat to an erstwhile collaborator ("She's so fabulous, just like Cher!") before bowing out to an extended guitar and sax workout.

HANG ON TO YOURSELF
• B-Side: 5/71 • Album: *Ziggy* • A-Side: 8/72 • B-Side: 9/72 [12] • Live: *Stage, Motion, SM72, BBC, Beeb* • Bonus: *Man, Ziggy (2002)* • Live Video: *Ziggy*

"Strap the guitar on and thrash it to death, basically," is how Mick Ronson later recalled the nightly challenge of recreating the furious 'Hang On To Yourself' riff, which owes more than a passing debt to The Velvet Underground's 'Sweet Jane' and in particular to Eddie Cochran's 1958 hit 'Summertime Blues', a cover of which had backed Marc Bolan's breakthrough hit 'Ride A White Swan' in 1970. Also indebted to Bolan is Bowie's breathy, panting vocal style, but the crackling duel between his acoustic guitar and Ronson's searing electric solos belongs solely to the *Ziggy Stardust* phenomenon. Although running to a mere handful of lines, the lyric constructs a complex and ever-shifting metaphor in which rock music elides into sex, ambition, fulfilment, self-control and back to sex again, with the multiple innuendo of the central thesis ("If you think we're gonna make it / You better hang on to yourself") conflating the abandon of sexual climax with the attainment of rock stardom – while prefiguring Ziggy's own downfall.

The *Ziggy Stardust* version was recorded at Trident on 8 November 1971 but, like 'Moonage Daydream', the song had begun life several months earlier. During his American trip in February 1971, Bowie was introduced by record producer Tom Ayers to one of his heroes, the legendary rock'n'roller Gene Vincent. "One night, at the recording studio, Tom asked whether I would like to jam or sing something with Gene," Bowie wrote in 2002's *Moonage Daydream*. "At that point, I had already written 'Moonage Daydream', 'Ziggy Stardust' and 'Hang On To Yourself'. We settled on 'Hang On To Yourself' and made a ghastly version of it which is floating around somewhere on eBay, I expect." The Los Angeles demo has indeed appeared on bootlegs, but Gene Vincent is nowhere to be heard. "I can't hear a trace of Vincent anywhere on it," Bowie concedes, "though Tom's son (who sent it to me) assures me that his dad swore Gene was on it." Vincent, who died in October of the same year, would be responsible for another Ziggy trademark. In the 1960s, Bowie had seen Vincent perform in concert with one leg in a brace following a car accident: "It meant that to crouch at the mike, as was his habit, he had to shove his injured leg out behind him, to what I thought great theatrical effect," Bowie

observed. "This rock stance became position number one for the embryonic Ziggy. Mick Rock captured that well on many occasions, the best version appearing on the back of the *Pin Ups* album."

A more familiar early take of 'Hang On To Yourself' is the recording made at London's Radio Luxembourg Studios in April 1971 by Bowie's undercover project Arnold Corns (see *Hunky Dory* in Chapter 2). This cut was twice released as a single by B&C Records, but mercifully and understandably, both flopped. Saddled with a turgid tempo and a plodding arrangement for guitar and tambourine, the uninspiring prototype lyrics contain none of the song's later references to stage performance, groupies or The Spiders From Mars themselves, although the line "And me I'm in a rock-'n'roll show" confirms the debt to 'Sweet Jane' ("And me I'm in a rock'n'roll band"). Topped off by a ghastly, dissonant guitar solo, the Arnold Corns version reveals little sign of the *Sturm und Drang* that would soon guarantee the song its status as a milestone of glam.

'Hang On To Yourself' went on to inspire another defining moment in 1970s rock, as The Sex Pistols' Glen Matlock later explained: "We got a lot of stuff from The Spiders – that riff in 'God Save the Queen' didn't come from Eddie Cochran, it came from Ronno."

The song was included in three BBC sessions in 1972, on 11 and 18 January and 16 May; the last two recordings were both included on *Bowie At The Beeb*. It appeared throughout the Ziggy Stardust and Stage tours, and cropped up again for the first few Serious Moonlight dates, making more regular appearances 20 years later on A Reality Tour.

HANGIN' ROUND *(Reed)*

Co-produced by Bowie for Lou Reed's *Transformer* and based on a riff that starkly betrays 'Suffragette City''s debt to Reed, 'Hangin' Round' benefits from Mick Ronson's superbly tight guitar playing and boogie-woogie piano, and boasts the mind-boggling line: "Cathy was a bit surreal, she painted all her toes / And on her face she wore dentures clamped tightly to her nose."

A HARD DAY'S NIGHT *(Lennon/McCartney)* : see THE JEAN GENIE

A HARD RAIN'S A-GONNA FALL *(Dylan)* :
see **HEAVEN'S IN HERE** and **THE JEAN GENIE**

HARD TO BEAT *(Pop/Williamson)* :
see **YOUR PRETTY FACE IS GOING TO HELL**

HARLEM SHUFFLE *(Relf/Nelson)*

Bob & Earl's 1963 single was played live by The Buzz.

HAVING A GOOD TIME

Produced by Bowie during the 1973 Astronettes sessions, and included on 1995's *People From Bad Homes*, this attempt at a Phil Spector-style "wall of sound" production features multi-layered vocals from Jason Guess and Geoffrey MacCormack. The best thing about the track is the opening snippet of studio banter in which a laughing Bowie is clearly heard to enquire "I beg your sodding pardon?" The song's authorship remains in doubt.

HE WAS ALRIGHT : see **LADY STARDUST**

HE'S A GOLDMINE : see **VELVET GOLDMINE**

HEARTBREAK HOTEL *(Axton/Durden/Presley)* :
see **THE JEAN GENIE**

THE HEARTS FILTHY LESSON
(Bowie/Eno/Gabrels/Garson/Kizilcay/Campbell)
• A-Side: 9/95 [35] • Album: *1.Outside* • B-Side: 2/96 [12] • French Promo: 2/97 • B-Side: 4/97 [32] • Live: *Earthling In The City, liveandwell.com* • Video: *Best Of Bowie*

Released ahead of its parent album in September 1995 and rapidly establishing itself as a strong item in Bowie's live repertoire, 'The Hearts Filthy Lesson' (the lack of apostrophe is apparently deliberate) was a perverse but strangely magnificent choice of lead-off single. To the uninitiated it's a tuneless din described by *Vox* as "dire, chug-chug pop … which runs out of

steam very quickly." To the converted, it's a stunning slab of industrial techno-rock, providing a towering backdrop over which Mike Garson lays eccentric jazz-piano figures while Bowie wheezes a deranged lyric about detective Nathan Adler's relationship with body-parts jeweller Ramona A. Stone. Bowie later described the lyric as "a montage of subject matter, bits from newspapers, storylines, dreams and half-formed thoughts … Overall it became quite powerful and a forbidding piece of work that still disturbs. But I'm buggered if I know what it means." The sinister collision of nursery-room innocence and ultra-violence ("what a fantastic death abyss!") lands implausibly somewhere between Laurie Anderson and early Stooges, managing to be at once hilarious and spine-chilling. When the rhythm track stops for Bowie's demented, childlike query "Paddy, who's been wearing Miranda's clothes?", he scores his first genuinely magic moment in many a long year.

The suitably confrontational video was directed by Sam Bayer, best known for Nirvana's 'Smells Like Teen Spirit' promo. MTV refused to screen the original edit and even the re-cut version proved alarming enough: a sepia-tinted succession of ominous images as Bowie and his followers, in tattered vests and overalls, embark on a ritualistic orgy of suggestive acts in an artist's studio, writhing in dust, daubing themselves in paint, hanging themselves, breaking down walls, displaying body-piercings, dismembering and decapitating mannequins to build a Minotaur. It's a descendant of the Glass Spider tour's abstract choreography, but here the three-ring circus gives way to an X-rated nightmare: there are cutaway shots of skulls, gibbets, candles and gruesome objects in pickling jars, while all the time a skeletal string-puppet drummer thrashes out the rhythm. Like the single it was brilliant, frightening, and unlikely to woo the mass market. In Britain 'The Hearts Filthy Lesson' reached number 35, while in America it limped to 92. But the point had been made: Bowie repeatedly told interviewers that he wanted *1.Outside* to be judged on artistic merit rather than chart potential, and if he'd wanted a short-term hit he knew full well that there were far more obvious candidates on the album. 'The Hearts Filthy Lesson' wasn't just a single; it was a statement.

Trent Reznor of Nine Inch Nails, who supported the US leg of the Outside tour, was responsible for the 'Alt. Mix' available on the single formats, while the original version was used as the closing title music for David Fincher's uncannily *1.Outside*-like film thriller

Seven. A live version from the 1996 Phoenix Festival appeared on a sampler CD issued with early French pressings of *Earthling*, and a live recording from Bowie's fiftieth birthday gig later appeared on the limited-edition *GQ* magazine CD *Earthling In The City*. 'The Hearts Filthy Lesson' featured throughout the Outside and Earthling tours, and a version recorded at the Phoenix Festival on 19 July 1997 later appeared on *liveandwell.com*.

HEATHEN (THE RAYS)

• Album: *Heathen*

"The song 'Heathen' came together quite early on in the making of the album," Bowie revealed in 2002. "The words were literally tumbling out for it. I was very alone, very isolated up in the studio, as is my wont, at five or six o'clock in the morning. I was up in the studio on my own, waiting for everybody else to get up, and I was kind of putting the day's work together. And this thing started appearing before me. I'd already written a melody that I very much liked, and the words started appearing out of nowhere, and I just couldn't control them. And I realized what it was that it was about, and I really didn't want to write it, because I didn't feel sure that I really wanted to voice or articulate those particular thoughts at this time. But it just wouldn't stop, and I had to write it, and I was in tears by the end of the thing. It was a traumatic moment for me. Possibly it was an epiphany. I don't know, I'll have to go and look at 'epiphany' in the dictionary and see if it was an epiphany. I think it was a traumatic epiphany!"

Indeed, even by the grim standards of *Heathen*, the subject matter of the song that became its title track is among the bleakest and most disturbing that Bowie has ever addressed. "'Heathen' is about knowing you're dying," he explained. "It's a song to life, where I'm talking to life as a friend or lover. I virtually couldn't change a word the moment I sung it into a tape recorder." When asked about the significance of the word "heathen", he explained: "It's not a dialogue between a man and his god. It's a dialogue between a man and life itself, so it's almost pagan in some respects, but it definitely has a heathen propensity in that way. It's a man confronting the realization that life is a finite thing, and that he can already feel it, life itself, actually going from him, ebbing out of him, the weakening of age. And I didn't want to write that! You

know, I didn't want to know that I do feel that. Who does?" Hence, as on several of the album's songs, the language of a straightforward love lyric disguises a darker subject: "You say you'll leave me / And when the sun is low and the rays high / I can see it now, I can feel it die."

Musically, too, 'Heathen (The Rays)' offers a culmination of the album's styles, with a slowly building arrangement echoing the ambient menace of the opening track, and a return of the multi-layered backing vocals which are one of the album's trademarks. The threatening wall of synthesizers recalls the doom-laden tones of Berlin-era tracks like 'All Saints' and 'Sense Of Doubt', while the final fade ends the album on a suitably inconclusive dying ebb.

'Heathen (The Rays)' was performed live throughout the Heathen and A Reality tours, featuring in the BBC radio session of 18 September 2002 and on the edition of *Later… With Jools Holland* recorded two days later. At 2003's Tibet House Benefit Concert David fronted a beautiful acoustic rearrangement for guitar and strings orchestrated by Tony Visconti, who accompanied him alongside Gerry Leonard and the Scorchio Quartet.

HEAVEN'S IN HERE

• Album: *TM* • US Promo: 1989 • B-Side: 10/91 [48]
• Live: *Oy* • Live Video: *Oy*

After the disappointments of the mid-1980s, *Tin Machine*'s first track seems to promise more in its opening bars than *Never Let Me Down* had achieved in an album's worth of songs. The lolloping blues riff, bursts of gunshot percussion and thrilling dynamics bode well, while the lyric impresses with a religious re-styling of *Let's Dance*'s pugilistic motif ("I'm taking a swing at this shadow of mine, crucifix hangs and my heart's in my mouth…"). But, like *Tin Machine* in general, 'Heaven's In Here' fails to live up to its initial promise, degenerating into an unwieldy blustering racket and seriously outstaying its welcome. Plans to release the track as a four-minute single in 1989 went no further than the promo stage, although a posed "performance" video was shot by Julien Temple in the standard 1989 Tin Machine style.

'Heaven's In Here' was Tin Machine's first major public performance, at the International Music Awards in New York on 31 May 1989. Thereafter it featured throughout both tours, a live BBC version being taped on 13 August 1991 and a bloated twelve-minute rendition appearing on *Oy Vey, Baby*. During the It's My Life tour Bowie often interpolated lines from other songs into the hushed middle section, including his *Absolute Beginners* cover 'Volare', Peggy Lee's signature song 'Fever', the *West Side Story* number 'Somewhere', Roxy Music's 'In Every Dream Home A Heartache', Muddy Waters's 'I'm A King Bee' and 'Baby Please Don't Go', The Yardbirds' 'A Certain Girl', John Lee Hooker's 'Boom Boom', Cream's 'I Feel Free', Johnny Kidd's 'Shakin' All Over', Sly & The Family Stone's '(You Caught Me) Smilin'', Cole Porter's 'You Do Something To Me', Kraftwerk's 'Radioactivity', Bob Dylan's 'A Hard Rain's A-Gonna Fall', The Troggs' 'Wild Thing', Sonny & Cher's 'I Got You Babe', the Steam/Bananarama hit 'Na Na Hey Hey (Kiss Him Goodbye)', the traditional 'You And I And George', and even the jazz standard 'April In Paris'. The 'Heaven's In Here' guitar intro resurfaced on some dates of the Earthling tour as a prelude to 'The Jean Genie'.

"HELDEN" : see "HEROES"

HELLO STRANGER *(Lewis)*

On 6 October 1964 The Manish Boys made their first recording for Decca. Produced by Mike Smith (or possibly Mickie Most) at Regent Sound Studios in Denmark Street, the session comprised Barbara Lewis's 'Hello Stranger', Gene Chandler's 'Duke Of Earl', and Mickey & Sylvia's 'Love Is Strange', all of which the band had been playing live. The first number was mooted as single material but scrapped because the vocal styles of David and bassist John Watson were thought to be mismatched. 'Love Is Strange' was apparently abandoned because the group had little faith in the song itself. "We all had mixed feelings whether it would work," saxophonist Woolf Byrne told the Gillmans. "A few months later The Everly Brothers had a massive hit with it." These unreleased recordings have never come to light.

HENRY AND THE H-BOMB : see SWEET JANE

HERE COMES THE NIGHT *(Berns)*
• Album: *Pin*

A number 2 hit for Van Morrison's Them in 1965 (and a number 50 flop for Bowie's future collaborator Lulu in 1964), 'Here Comes The Night' receives a full-blooded *Pin Ups* makeover, with a marvellously theatrical Bowie vocal punctuated by blasts of Ken Fordham's baritone sax. "We were particularly pleased with that," enthused David at the time. "We got a real Atlantic horn sound."

HERE TODAY, GONE TOMORROW
(Bonner/Satchell/Jones/Webster/Middlebrooks/Robinson)
• Bonus: *David*

Bowie's beautifully soulful live cover of the Ohio Players number (originating on their 1968 album *Observations In Time*, where it was originally entitled 'Here Today And Gone Tomorrow') was included on the Rykodisc reissue of *David Live*, which inaccurately credits the songwriting to David himself. 'Here Today, Gone Tomorrow' offers a clear indication of the direction in which Bowie's interests were moving a month prior to the *Young Americans* sessions. Quite why it was left off the original cut of *David Live* is a mystery, as it's one of the finest recordings from the show; perhaps the reason is David's split-second fluff as he momentarily begins the chorus instead of repeating the second verse.

Some sources insist that 'Here Today, Gone Tomorrow' was never played at the 1974 Philadelphia concerts, leading many to surmise that the recording hails from a soundcheck rather than from an actual gig – although Bowie's announcement on *David Live* before 'Knock On Wood' that "We're gonna put in some extras tonight, some silly ones," may suggest otherwise. Whether the song was taken into the studio during the *Young Americans* sessions remains similarly uncertain, although more than one of the so-called "Sigma Kids" have claimed that it was indeed among the raw studio cuts that David played to them in August 1974. Whatever the case, its lifespan in Bowie's repertoire was certainly short, and it is not known to have been performed at any other dates on the tour – although another unsubstantiated claim has it that the song was played as an encore at the Tampa gig on 2 July 1974.

"HEROES" *(Bowie/Eno)*
• Album: *"Heroes"* (different versions on
French/German pressings) • A-Side: 9/77 [24]
(different versions on French/German pressings) •
Soundtrack: *Christiane F.* • Live: *Stage, The Bridge
School Concerts Vol. 1, The Concert For New York City* •
Compilation: *Rare, S+V, Club* • A-Side: 6/03 [73] •
Video: *Collection, Best Of Bowie, Bing Crosby's Merrie
Olde Christmas* • Live Video: *Moonlight, Ricochet,
Glass, The Freddie Mercury Tribute Concert, The Concert
For New York City*

"He got up and sang in the microphone at the top of
his lungs," recalled Tony Visconti of the day Bowie
laid down the vocal for this classic track. "You can
hear on '"Heroes"' what he calls his 'Bowie histrionics', his own peculiar style of yelling and screaming."
David's virtuoso performance, building over six minutes from a soft croon to a throaty shriek, is the icing
on the cake of one of his most exhilarating recordings.
"There was no mistaking the sound," said Tony
Visconti later. "We had a feeling on tape immediately,
and I carried that sound throughout every overdub.
There's a kind of clanging metallic sound which is
David or I hitting a big metal ashtray." Robert Fripp's
soaring guitar line is a perfect complement to the pulsating bass (which is clearly indebted to The Velvet
Underground's long-time Bowie favourite 'Waiting
For The Man'), while the shimmering background
effects are, according to Visconti, "Eno magic" devised
on the keyboard-less EMS synthesizer often seen in
vintage Roxy Music performances: "its *pièce de resistance* was a little joystick that you find on arcade
games. He would pan that joystick around in circles
and make the swirling sounds you heard on that
track."

Apparently the vocal was practically an afterthought; the backing track was laid down early in the
"Heroes" sessions and for a time it seemed possible
that it might remain an instrumental. David recorded
his vocal after most of the musicians had left Berlin,
and Brian Eno later revealed that although the backing "sounded grand and heroic" and "I had that very
word – heroes – in my mind", he had no idea what
the lyric would be until he heard the finished track.

To capture David's vocal, Visconti devised an
experimental system that made full use of the unusually spacious dimensions of Hansa Studios: "We had a
microphone about the customary nine inches from
his face, then we had another microphone about

twenty feet from himself, then we had another microphone about fifty feet away." Each microphone was
rigged with an electronic gate, of which only the nearest would open while David sang the quieter early
passages. "If he sang a little louder, the next microphone would open up with the gate, and that would
make sort of this big splash of reverb, and then if he
really sang loud, the back microphone would open up,
and it would just open up this enormous sound." The
lead vocal took two hours to record, after which Bowie
and Visconti added the vocal backings together.

David famously recounted that '"Heroes"' was
inspired by a pair of young lovers he used to watch
from the window of Hansa Studios as they met by the
Berlin Wall: "I thought of all the places to meet in
Berlin, why pick a bench underneath a guard turret on
the Wall? And I – using license – presumed that they
were feeling somewhat guilty about this affair and so
they had imposed this restriction on themselves,
thereby giving themselves an excuse for their heroic
act. I used this as a basis." Tony Visconti later
explained that this was in fact a fanciful interpretation
of a fling he was having at the time with *"Heroes"*
backing singer Antonia Maass. "It was us," he told the
Gillmans. "Coco [Schwab] was sitting up in the control room with David, and both he and Coco said, 'We
saw you walking by the wall,' and that's where he got
that idea from." More recently, Visconti has pointed
out that Bowie's version of the story was as much an
act of diplomacy as anything else: "Because I was married at the time, David protected me all these years by
not saying that he saw Antonia and me kiss by the
wall." This was later confirmed by Bowie himself:
"Tony was married at the time, and I could never say
who it was," he admitted in 2003. "I think possibly
the marriage was in the last few months, and it was
very touching because I could see that Tony was very
much in love with this girl, and it was that relationship which sort of motivated the song."

Another inspiration was a painting in Berlin's
Brücke museum, where David and Iggy Pop had spent
many hours, even adapting the pose of Erich Heckel's
painting *Roquairol* for the sleeve photographs of *The
Idiot* and *"Heroes"*. A work much admired by David
was Otto Mueller's 1916 painting *Lovers Between
Garden Walls*, which depicted a couple locked in a passionate embrace between two looming walls representing the carnage of the Great War.

In the foreword of his wife's 2001 book *I Am Iman*,
Bowie reveals yet another source for the song in the

form of a little-known short story called *A Grave For A Dolphin*, written in 1956 by an Italian Duke, Alberto Denti di Pirajno. The story concerns the doomed love affair between an Italian soldier and a Somalian girl during the Second World War: the girl's destiny seems inextricably linked with that of a dolphin she swims with, and when she dies, so too does the dolphin. "I thought it a magical and beautiful love story," David wrote, "and in part it had inspired my song '"Heroes"'.

These images of doomed love and fragile optimism in the face of adversity are instructive, for '"Heroes"' is by no means the feelgood anthem it's often been taken for. Like the album whose name it shares, the title is embraced by quotation marks to express what Bowie called "a dimension of irony", and despite its serenely uplifting chord sequence and the delirious abandon of the vocal, '"Heroes"' certainly has its dark side. There are hints at David's ongoing marital traumas, alongside other biographical confessions: "I wish I could swim" is no mere aspirational image, for David genuinely couldn't until ten years later. "I couldn't swim a stroke until last year," he said in 1987, "Now I can do a couple of lengths of the pool." (In 2000 he revealed that "I've never swum again. I swam once, it was quite enough for me.") More ominous are the references to the binge-drinking that temporarily took the place of cocaine in Berlin. "I became an alcoholic," he said later. "I knew I had to pull away from that drug addiction, but what the body does is it lets itself open for any other kind of addiction. You replace one with another and in my case I went straight to whisky and brandy and stuff like that."

'"Heroes"' sets its cautious optimism in the face of just such human frailties. "You can be mean, and I'll drink all the time" is hardly the most promisingly heroic sentiment, and the repeated acknowledgement that "nothing will keep us together" presses home the point that time is short. It's surely significant that the reiterated "just for one day" harks directly back to one of David's most darkly personal lyrics, 'The Bewlay Brothers'. The only way to be heroes "for ever and ever" is to "steal time" and enter a fantasy of immortality, but this is a never-land which he now rejects, finally content to be what 'Quicksand' had long ago described as "a mortal with potential of a superman". The real triumph is to be heroes "just for one day", and by conferring heroism on the everyday rather than on the extraordinary Bowie was entering a territory far removed from his early 1970s *Übermenschen*.

In doing so, he was also notably adopting a favourite theme of many of the twentieth-century painters he had begun most closely to admire.

'"Heroes"', then, is a painfully compassionate song that grasps at an optimistic future in a present full of disillusion. As Bowie explained, the song was about "facing reality and standing up to it", about achieving "a sense of compassion" and "deriving some joy from the very simple pleasure of being alive."

The edited single version of '"Heroes"' became the subject of a publicity push unrivalled since the days of 'Space Oddity'. In September 1977 Bowie performed the song for Granada TV's *Marc* (see 'Sleeping Next To You') and *Bing Crosby's Merrie Old Christmas* (see 'Peace On Earth'), while 19 October saw his first *Top Of The Pops* appearance since 1972. Here he laid down a new live recording of '"Heroes"', with Tony Visconti on bass and new recruit Sean Mayes, whose group Fumble had supported Bowie back in 1973, on keyboards. For the actual show Bowie mimed to the new recording with none of the band present, and in one of pop's amusing coincidences, in the very same week The Stranglers' anthemic 'No More Heroes' peaked at number 8. In the same month Bowie sang '"Heroes"' on the Dutch show *Top Pop* and the Italian programmes *Odeon* and *L'Altra Domenica*.

Shot in Paris, Nick Ferguson's promotional video featured a simple series of shots of David, in the bomber-jacket he wore on the *"Heroes"* album cover, backlit in white light. The effect closely resembles 'Maybe This Time', Liza Minnelli's showstopper on a very similar theme, from the Berlin-based 1972 film *Cabaret*. Despite all the frantic publicity '"Heroes"' was never more than a minor UK hit, climbing no higher than number 24. In America it didn't even chart, only later achieving recognition as a Bowie classic ("This is a strange phenomenon that happens with my songs Stateside," David remarked in 2003, "Many of the crowd favourites were never radio or chart hits, and '"Heroes"' tops them all"). Confirming his new-found European allegiances, Bowie recorded special vocals in French ('"Héros"') and German ('"Helden"', with lyrics translated by Antonia Maass) for release as singles; these vocals were also grafted onto the opening English verses for the respective countries' album releases. The full-length '"Helden"' later appeared on the *Christiane F.* soundtrack album and on *Bowie Rare*, while a 1989 remix was included on *Sound + Vision*.

A perennial live favourite, '"Heroes"' featured on the Stage, Serious Moonlight, Glass Spider, Sound +

Vision, 1996 Summer Festivals, Earthling, 2000, Heathen and A Reality tours. The Serious Moonlight version began with a rather touching rendition of the traditional folk-song 'Lavender Blue' ("Lavender Blue, dilly dilly, lavender green, I will be king, dilly dilly, you will be queen", whereupon the '"Heroes"' melody burst into life). On some 1990 dates David sang the '"Helden"' lyrics. There were rousing revivals at Live Aid, the Freddie Mercury tribute concert, Bowie's fiftieth birthday show and, in an unusual semi-acoustic form, at the 1996 Bridge School benefits, from which a live recording made on 20 October appeared on the US release *The Bridge School Concerts Vol. 1*. Five years later to the day, Bowie sang '"Heroes"' at the Concert For New York City at Madison Square Garden, a performance later included on the CD and DVD of the event. He also performed '"Heroes"' at the 2001 Tibet House Benefit concert at Carnegie Hall.

Philip Glass used the song as the basis for the first movement of his 1997 *"Heroes" Symphony*, and in the same year Aphex Twin grafted Bowie's original vocal onto the Glass version for a 3" CD single included with the Japanese release. This remix was later included on Aphex Twin's 2003 compilation *26 Mixes For Cash*.

Unsurprisingly, '"Heroes"' comes a close second to 'Rebel Rebel' as the most widely covered song in the Bowie canon. Among the dozens of artists who have covered it on stage or in the studio are Nico (who once made the utterly insupportable claim that Bowie actually wrote the song for her), The Wallflowers (for the closing credits of the 1998 fim *Godzilla*), Oasis, Smashing Pumpkins, Travis, P J Proby, Iva Davies, Goodbye Mr MacKenzie, Jon Bon Jovi, Ed Harcourt, Joe Jackson and Blondie, whose 1980 live version, featuring Robert Fripp on guitar, now appears on *David Bowie Songbook*. In 2000 King Crimson, boasting two former Bowie guitarists in Robert Fripp and Adrian Belew, introduced '"Heroes"' into their live repertoire. The song was even performed by Liberal Democrat leader Charles Kennedy in a January 2002 edition of BBC1's *Johnny Vaughan Tonight* (a long-time Bowie fan, Kennedy told *Mojo* in 2000 that he had watched David's Glastonbury performance from the side of the stage, and informed the *Mirror* the following year that his favourite album was *Station To Station*. In 2003 he even included 'Young Americans' in his selection of *Desert Island Discs* on Radio 4). At a New York concert in January 2003 the Scorchio Quartet, who had played for Bowie at the Tibet House Benefit concerts and on

Heathen, premiered a string orchestration of the song called *"Heroes" Variations* which had been written for them by Tony Visconti.

Bowie has allowed '"Heroes"' to be used in several advertising campaigns over the years, and its profile was raised once again in 2001 by its prominent appearance in two motion pictures: it forms part of the love medley performed by Nicole Kidman and Ewan McGregor in Baz Luhrmann's *Moulin Rouge* (and appears as such on the accompanying soundtrack album), while Steve Coogan leads the cast in a mass knees-up to Bowie's original recording as the credits roll on John Duigan's comedy *The Parole Officer*.

Following similar ventures by The Scumfrog and Solaris, in 2003 a profoundly irritating dance bootleg by David Guetta featuring samples from Bowie's original track was approved for official release. Credited to "David Guetta vs Bowie", 'Just For One Day (Heroes)' duly appeared in June 2003 and scraped the lower reaches of the Top 75. The extended version later appeared on *Club Bowie*, while both this and the video (directed by Joe Guest, and consisting of shots of loved-up partygoers at an all-night rave) were included on the bonus DVD supplied with the 2003 American reissue of *Best Of Bowie*.

"HÉROS" : see "HEROES"

HEY JUDE *(Lennon/McCartney)* : see JANINE

HEY MA GET PAPA *(Ronson/Bowie)*

The only composition ever co-credited to David Bowie and Mick Ronson is this track on Ronson's debut album *Slaughter On 10th Avenue*. Ronson later explained that it "really was me asking if he could put some words to the music. I was never really a writer, I was always more of a performer." The result is a glam stomper poised somewhere between 'Velvet Goldmine' and late Beatles; like the same album's 'Growing Up And I'm Fine', it has Bowie's fingerprints all over it.

HIDEAWAY *(Pop/Bowie)*

Co-written and co-produced by Bowie for Iggy Pop's

Blah-Blah-Blah.

HIGHWAY BLUES *(Harper)*

Originally from Roy Harper's 1973 album *Lifemask*, 'Highway Blues' was covered by the Astronettes and produced by Bowie at Olympic Studios in late 1973, eventually appearing on 1995's *People From Bad Homes*.

HOLD ON, I'M COMING *(Hayes/Porter)*

Sam & Dave's hit was played live by The Buzz.

HOLE IN THE GROUND

Said to have been recorded during the *Toy* sessions, this unreleased track remains a mystery.

HOLY HOLY
• A-Side: 1/71 • B-Side: 6/74 [21] • Bonus: *Man, Ziggy (2002)*

Some confusion surrounds the two studio versions of this Bolanesque slow-rocker, not least because of some misleading text on Rykodisc's reissue of *The Man Who Sold the World*. The first version was recorded at Trident in June 1970 in the aftermath of that album's sessions, and features Herbie Flowers (who also produced the track) alongside the familiar Ronson and Woodmansey. It's a lethargic rendition, vastly inferior to the subsequent version, and it's not difficult to see why it failed to trouble the charts when released as a single in January 1971. Nonetheless, it was this recording that secured David his publishing contract with Chrysalis, whose executive Bob Grace considered it "fantastic". Bowie promoted the single on Granada TV on 20 January 1971, wearing a Mr Fish dress and accompanying himself on acoustic guitar.

Lyrically, 'Holy Holy' offers a revealing early example of Bowie's fascination with the writings of Aleister Crowley, soon to inform much of the writing on *Hunky Dory*. When Bowie likens himself to "a righteous Brother", he's referring not to the popular 1960s singing duo but to an Everyman figure who appears in the texts of Freemasonry and was later adopted in the

terminology of the Golden Dawn. In this light, the line "I don't want to be an angel, just a little bit evil, feel the devil in me" surely marks a journey into the arcane pseudo-religious sexual practices of Crowley's highly suspect "Sexmagickal" system.

The second take of 'Holy Holy', taken at a faster pace and benefiting from Mick Ronson at his shimmering best, was recorded in the late summer of 1971 and briefly slated for inclusion on the *Ziggy Stardust* album. In the end it remained in the vaults until it was served up as a B-side three years later, and it's this version, not the original, which later appeared on *Bowie Rare* and the reissue of *The Man Who Sold the World*. Contrary to what it says on the latter's sleeve-notes, the single version hasn't been released in any format since 1971.

HONKY TONK WOMEN *(Jagger/Richards)*

Bowie played saxophone and sang backing vocals on Mott The Hoople's live encore of The Rolling Stones' 1969 hit, in Philadelphia on 29 November 1972. This performance can be heard on the 1998 compilation *All The Way From Stockholm To Philadelphia*.

HOOCHIE COOCHIE MAN *(Dixon)*

Willie Dixon's classic, famously covered by Muddy Waters in 1954, was played live by The King Bees and The Manish Boys.

HOP FROG *(Reed)*

Bowie recorded his vocal contribution to this track on Lou Reed's album *The Raven* in November 2001. Released over a year later, the album develops the soundtrack of Reed's theatrical collaboration with director Robert Wilson at Hamburg's Thalia Theatre in 2000, based on the work of the nineteenth-century fantasist Edgar Allan Poe. Originally published in 1849, *Hop-Frog* is one of Poe's nastier short stories, relating the dark tale of a court jester's vengeance on his cruel master; it provided the dramatic climax of the Hamburg production.

"I played him some of the songs and he picked 'Hop Frog'," Lou Reed explained in 2003. "That's the one he wanted to sing. Who knows why? I was happy he was gonna do anything. So he came and did it. I was very pleased, I like what David does. Specially when he's doing background vocals and starts singing up high, I like that." 'Hop Frog' does indeed feature some exuberant backing vocals from Bowie which, set against Reed's characteristic turbo-charged guitar sound, effortlessly recall the good old days of *Transformer*. It's a short number, running to less than two minutes, and offers little in the way of narrative or incident, serving merely as a prelude to the audio dramatization of the story (featuring Willem Dafoe and Amanda Plummer) which follows. Slight the song may be, but the sound of Bowie and Reed duetting once again with such unrestrained gusto is a positive joy.

HOT *(Brown)* : see **FAME**

HOT PANTS *(Brown/Wesley)*

The title track of James Brown's 1971 album (and a hit single in the US in the same year) formed the second half of the James Brown medley performed by The Spiders during some of the early Ziggy gigs in 1972. See 'You Got To Have A Job (If You Don't Work – You Don't Eat)' for further details.

HOW COULD I BE SUCH A FOOL *(Zappa)*

Originally from the 1969 Mothers Of Invention album *Cruising With Ruben & The Jets*, this was one of the covers produced by Bowie for the abandoned Astronettes project in 1973. Among the better Astronettes recordings, it eventually appeared on 1995's *People From Bad Homes*.

HOW LUCKY YOU ARE

Probably recorded in April 1971, the first attempt at 'How Lucky You Are' (also known as 'Miss Peculiar' after a phrase in the chorus) survives on bootlegs as a rough 3'35" demo on which Bowie is backed by piano, drums and bass, with additional vocals provided by Mickey King of 'Rupert The Riley' fame. The song, a swaggering waltz vaguely foreshadowing the pit-band style of Bowie's Kurt Weill phase, includes a

"la la la" outro clearly anticipating 'Starman'. It's evidently work in progress, the lyric repetitive and unfinished, but what exists is a deliciously dumb piece of chauvinistic preening ("When you speak, you speak to me / When you sleep, you sleep by me / When you wake, you wake with me / When you walk, you follow two steps behind … Take a look at how lucky you are!"). A second, more polished version, recorded at the time of the *Hunky Dory* sessions and almost certainly featuring Rick Wakeman on piano, has also appeared on bootlegs.

HUNG UP ON THIS GIRL

The performing rights organization BMI lists this title as a Bowie composition published by the Embassy Music Corporation. It seems likely that this is the same song as 'Hung Up', occasionally performed live by David's 1966 outfit The Buzz.

HURT *(Reznor)*
• Live Video: *Closure (Nine Inch Nails)*

A track from Nine Inch Nails' 1994 album *The Downward Spiral* which Bowie performed live with the band during the US leg of the Outside tour.

I AIN'T GOT YOU *(Carter)*

The Yardbirds' 1964 B-side was among The Manish Boys' live repertoire.

I AM A LASER

Recorded by the Astronettes at Olympic Studios in 1973, and eventually released on 1995's *People From Bad Homes*, 'I Am A Laser' is known to Bowie fans as an early prototype of the *Scary Monsters* track 'Scream Like A Baby'. Although the melody is identical, the finger-clicking arrangement owes more to the funkier tracks on *Diamond Dogs*, while the lyric is entirely different: "I am a laser, burning through your eyes / And I know what kind of man you are, and I long to hold you tight". Although the lyric is as impenetrable as most of Bowie's compositions of the period, the general idea appears to be the singer's predilection for kinky sex: there's a thoroughly suspect section in the second verse in which Ava Cherry sings: "I'm going to turn my beam on, if only for an hour / You'll know I've switched the heat on when you feel my golden shower." The rumour that Bowie recorded his own version of 'I Am A Laser' during the Astronettes sessions remains unconfirmed.

I AM A ROCK (Simon) : see **THE JEAN GENIE**

I AM A SCIENTIST (Taylor-Taylor/Bowie) : see **FASHION**

I AM DIVINE

Originally recorded during the Astronettes sessions in a funky '1984'-style arrangement for wah-wah guitar, cowbell percussion, piano and strings, 'I Am Divine' was heavily reworked in 1974 for *Young Americans* as 'Somebody Up There Likes Me'. Although there are similarities between the two songs (notably Ava Cherry's "so divine" backing vocals), the most interesting lyric from 'I Am Divine' sounds more like David boasting to Iggy Pop – "I'm the Main Man in my city / Hey Jim, I'm in control!" – further evidence of Bowie's preoccupation with self-discipline and the conflicting impulses he had already embodied in 'The Jean Genie' ("let yourself go!") and 'The Man Who Sold The World' ("I never lost control"). The track was finally released on 1995's *People From Bad Homes*, whose US edition includes a sleeve-note claiming, entirely erroneously, that Bowie sings the lead vocal. He doesn't.

I AM WITH NAME
(Bowie/Eno/Gabrels/Garson/Kizilcay/Campbell)
• B-Side: 9/95 [35] • Album: *1.Outside*

This incantatory track, narrated by the *1.Outside* character Ramona, reprises the multi-layered atmospherics of the album's opening. The babble of voices and ominous percussion are vaguely reminiscent of 1983's 'Ricochet', juxtaposing Ramona's repetitive chant with Nathan Adler's mutterings about "anxiety descending" and being (or perhaps turning) "left at the crossroads between the centuries". It's frankly unintelligible, but

as an experiment in pure atmosphere and approaching menace it succeeds wonderfully. Despite being labelled 'Album Version', the B-side is in fact a longer remix. An elaborate ten-minute version of 'I Am With Name' was among the unreleased 1994 material leaked onto the Internet in 2003 (see 'The *Leon* Tape' for details).

I CAN'T EXPLAIN (Townshend)
• Album: *Pin*

The hit that launched The Who, taking them to number 8 in 1965, was occasionally played live by The Spiders in 1972 and later reworked for *Pin Ups* in an unlikely piano and sax-driven arrangement. In October 1973 a live version was included in *The 1980 Floor Show*, and ten years later the song reappeared for the early leg of the Serious Moonlight tour.

I CAN'T READ (Bowie/Gabrels)
• Album: *TM* • B-Side: 9/89 [48] • Live: *Oy* • A-Side: 2/98 [73] • Live Video: *Oy*

Widely and deservedly considered the finest track on Tin Machine's debut album, 'I Can't Read' defies all the usual criticisms aimed at the band. The lyric is oblique and evocative, the arrangement steers away from Tin Machine's usual indiscriminate clatter, and Bowie eschews his unpalatable Robert Palmer-isms in favour of the emotionally numb, burned-away vocal style perfected on his Berlin albums. The themes of introspection, inadequacy and underachievement also echo his late 1970s work, here expressed by a frustrated couch-potato flicking between television channels and ruminating on a celebrated pronouncement of Bowie's one-time muse: "Andy, where's my fifteen minutes?" The refrain of "I can't read shit anymore" sounds uncannily like "I can't reach it anymore" which, coupled with the next line "I just can't get it right," becomes an almost embarrassingly direct reflection on David's ongoing struggle to get back on the artistic rails. Reeves Gabrels achieves a cutting-edge guitar sound redolent of the more experimental tracks on *Lodger*, and the only uncertain note is struck, as usual, by the drumming of Hunt Sales, who almost spoils everything by carpet-bombing the choruses with unnecessary din.

The album version of 'I Can't Read' was recorded

live in one take and mixed in less than an hour during the Compass Point sessions in Nassau. It was an immediate favourite of both Bowie and Gabrels, who admired its "freer jazz spirit". A remixed excerpt was featured in Julien Temple's 1989 promotional video medley, for which David prudently sang "I can't read it" instead of "I can't read shit". The song went on to become one of the band's concert highlights. A live version recorded in Paris on 25 June 1989 appeared as a B-side, while another from the It's My Life tour appeared on *Oy Vey, Baby*.

In subsequent years, Bowie has often cited the song as a vindication of the Tin Machine project. Accosted about Tin Machine in 1995, he advised an *NME* interviewer to "listen to a tune called 'I Can't Read', listen to that one, will you? I don't ask you to listen to any of the rest, just listen to that one song because I think that song is one of the best I have ever written."

'I Can't Read' finally came of age when it was re-recorded during the *Earthling* sessions. Drastically reworked with a soft acoustic guitar and synthesizer backing, it was initially mooted for inclusion on the album before becoming the closing music of Ang Lee's superb 1998 movie *The Ice Storm*, which fitted the re-tooled lyrics like a glove ("Can I see the family smile, can I reach tomorrow, can I walk a missing mile, can I feel, can I please?"). It was released as a single the same year, by which time further revisions had been performed at the Bridge School benefit concerts in October 1996, for *ChangesNowBowie*, and at Madison Square Garden on 9 January 1997, where Bowie recorded a performance backstage for inclusion in the pay-per-view broadcast of his fiftieth birthday concert.

I DIDN'T KNOW HOW MUCH (Wills/Edwards) : see **I NEVER DREAMED**

I DIG EVERYTHING
• A-Side: 8/66 • Compilation: *Early*

On 6 June 1966 David Bowie and The Buzz recorded a demo of their next single, 'I Dig Everything', at Pye Studios. Tony Hatch, who had produced David's previous two singles, was unimpressed by The Buzz and unceremoniously dumped them from the subsequent studio session on 5 July. In their place Hatch elected

to use session musicians whose identities are not recorded. Whoever they were, they provide an unusually perky background of washboard percussion and jaunty Hammond organ for David's lyric, a cynical celebration of a layabout lifestyle on London's transient teen-scene. The cheeky tone (as in the devastating couplet "I've got more friends than I've had hot dinners / Some of them are losers but the rest of them are winners") marks this out as a transitional moment between the R&B stylings of David's previous singles and his more idiosyncratic Deram work. Both the arrangement and the Sam Cooke-style backing vocals are a reminder that The Buzz were reluctantly dipping their toes into soul in the second half of 1966.

Released on 19 August, the single was yet another flop. *Ready, Steady, Go!*, which had featured Bowie earlier in the year, turned it down after receiving an advance dub copy. It was David's last recording for Pye, and despite not playing on the single, The Buzz continued to back him live on this song and others until early December. By then, David had a new deal on a new label, and was recording his first album.

'I Dig Everything' received a shock revival in Bowie's summer 2000 repertoire, and a new studio version was recorded during the same year's *Toy* sessions.

I FEEL FREE (Bruce/Brown)
• Album: *Black* • Live: *Rarest* • Video: *Black*

Cream's 1966 hit first entered Bowie's repertoire during the early Ziggy concerts in 1972. It was shortlisted for a studio recording at the following year's *Pin Ups* sessions but dropped from the final selection. In 1980 an instrumental backing was cut during the *Scary Monsters* sessions in New York, but by the time David recorded his vocals in London the idea had been abandoned, and this version was never completed.

'I Feel Free' was finally taken into the studio in 1992 and subjected to an unlikely but thrilling techno-funk treatment for *Black Tie White Noise*, complete with a joyous guitar break from Mick Ronson – back in the studio with Bowie for the first time since 1973, following their stage reunion at April's Freddie Mercury Tribute. "The dear old thing plays great," David enthused the following January, by which time Ronson's battle with cancer was public knowledge. "He's got the will-power of all time." For his part, Ronson declared that "I hope David's album does well. He's put everything into it. I speak to him often.

He sounds so positive."

Sadly Ronson lost his fight on 29 April 1993, just weeks after the release of *Black Tie White Noise*. In the studio "performance" shot only a few days later for the *Black Tie White Noise* video, Ronson's solo was mimed by Wild T Springer. "I was fortunate enough to know Mick right until the end of his life," said Bowie, "and in the last year of that life I'd gotten back very closely with him." At around the same time David revealed that 'I Feel Free' held another, older memory for him, this time related to his half-brother Terry: "I took him to see a Cream concert in Bromley, and about halfway through – and I'd like to think it was during 'I Feel Free' – he started feeling very, very bad … I remember I had to take him out of the club because it was really starting to affect him." Interesting, then, that Bowie should revive the number on *Black Tie White Noise*, which elsewhere addresses Terry's troubles in some depth.

An early live version of 'I Feel Free', recorded at Kingston Polytechnic on 6 May 1972 and unfortunately blighted by appalling sound quality, appears on *RarestOneBowie*, showcasing a guitar solo later adapted by Mick Ronson for live renditions of 'The Width Of A Circle'. The 4'40" *Scary Monsters* instrumental out-take, startlingly similar to the *Black Tie White Noise* rendition, has appeared on bootlegs. During Tin Machine's It's My Life tour, David occasionally sang a few lines from 'I Feel Free' during the extended rendition of 'Heaven's In Here'.

I FEEL SO BAD (Willis)

On 16 August 2002, the final date of the Area: 2 tour, Bowie marked the 25th anniversary of Elvis Presley's death by opening his encores with a one-off performance of 'I Feel So Bad'. Originally recorded in 1954 by its author Chuck Willis, the song provided a number 4 UK hit for Presley in 1961, as a double A-side with 'Wild In The Country'. Bowie followed this unexpected excursion into rock music's roots with a rendition of Presley's rather more familiar hit 'One Night'.

I GOT YOU BABE (Bono/Cher)

"This isn't anything very serious, it's just a bit of fun – we've hardly rehearsed it!" proclaimed Bowie as he and Marianne Faithfull launched into a ropey rendi-tion of the 1965 Sonny & Cher classic for *The 1980 Floor Show* on 19 October 1973. Faithfull, then appearing in *A Patriot For Me* at Watford's Palace Theatre, later attributed her husky vocal to "too many cigarettes". During Tin Machine's It's My Life tour two decades later, David occasionally sang a few lines from 'I Got You Babe' during the extended rendition of 'Heaven's In Here'.

I HAVE NOT BEEN TO OXFORD TOWN
(Bowie/Eno)
• Album: *1.Outside*

After *1.Outside*'s opening salvo of uncompromising avant-rock, 'I Have Not Been To Oxford Town' quietens the pace with an edgy funk treatment and the dextrous, instantly recognizable rhythm guitar of Carlos Alomar, although bursts of electric bass and weird Eno-noises are never far away. Within the album's loose narrative the song is "to be sung by Leon Blank", now in prison on suspicion of murder but protesting his innocence (hence the title) and implying that he's been framed by Ramona. Again the *fin de siècle* theme hangs heavy: "And the wheels are turning and turning, as this twentieth century dies / If I had not ripped the fabric, if time had not stood still…" The sing-song "Toll the bell … all's well" chorus offers one of the most sublimely catchy hooks in Bowie's 1990s work.

The track began life as 'Trio' on 17 January 1995 when Eno, Alomar and drummer Joey Barron were waiting for Bowie to arrive at the studio. Two days later Eno recorded in his diary that the track "really burst into life today when David heard it. Bizarre: he sat down and started writing the song on the first hearing, listening once more and said, 'I'll need five tracks.' Then he went into the vocal booth and sang the most obscure thing imaginable – long spaces, little, incomplete lines … he unfolded the whole thing in reverse, keeping us in suspense for the main song. Within half an hour he'd substantially finished what may be the most infectious song we've ever written together – currently called 'Toll The Bell'."

Harmonically the song borrows from 1993's 'Miracle Goodnight', and like that track it might have been a big hit if given a full publicity push as a single. As it was, 'I Have Not Been To Oxford Town' remained an album track and was performed throughout the Outside tour. A cover version by Zoë Poledouris, with a fresh set of lyrics which updated the century and altered the title to 'I Have Not Been To Paradise', featured in Paul Verhoeven's 1996 blockbuster *Starship Troopers*. The recording was omitted from the soundtrack album but has since appeared on the collectors' circuit.

I KEEP FORGETTIN' *(Lieber/Stoller)*
• Album: *Tonight*

Bowie's throwaway cover of Chuck Jackson's 1959 chestnut is an inoffensive but uninteresting makeover in the *Tonight* house style: stop-start percussion, zappy trumpets, helter-skeltering marimba and a vapid guitar solo. "I've always wanted to do that song," Bowie said at the time.

I KNOW IT'S GONNA HAPPEN SOMEDAY
(Morrissey/Nevin)
• Album: *Black* • Video: *Black*

"I always thought of Morrissey as a sort of sexual Alan Bennett," said Bowie in 1993, "because of his attention to detail. He'll take a small subject matter and make a very grandiose statement of it." His peripheral relationship with Morrissey, whose narcissistic kitchen-sink melodramas had long inherited aspects of Bowie's legacy, began when the two met backstage at David's Manchester gig in August 1990. The following February David joined Stephen on stage in Los Angeles to perform an encore of Marc Bolan's 'Cosmic Dancer', while 1992 saw the release of Morrissey's pseudo-glam album *Your Arsenal*, produced by none other than Mick Ronson. As David later recounted, "It occurred to me … that [Morrissey] was possibly spoofing one of my earlier songs, and I thought, I'm not going to let him get away with that. I do think he's one of the best lyricists in England, and an excellent songwriter, and I thought his song was an affectionate spoof."

The song in question was 'I Know It's Gonna Happen Someday', co-written by Morrissey and ex-Fairground Attraction guitarist Mark E Nevin. Morrissey's version, which echoes any number of Bowie's early 1970s ballads, culminates in a blatant lift from the climax of 'Rock'n'Roll Suicide', although in a characteristically perverse twist this is the one element Bowie chose to excise from his own version.

Instead, as he explained, "I thought it would be fun to take that song and do it the way I would have done it in 1974-ish." The result is a breathtakingly overblown gospel treatment, complete with heavenly choir and big-band climax. It's an endlessly incestuous joke: Bowie covers Morrissey parodying *Ziggy Stardust* in the style of *Young Americans*. "A window-rattling rendition,' wrote Q's David Sinclair, "which Bowie takes over so completely that it's hard not to think of it as one of his own compositions." Interestingly, the *Black Tie White Noise* video includes studio footage of Mick Ronson playing the riff from the original Morrissey arrangement.

"There's something terribly affectionate about the idea of the lyric," said Bowie. "You know, don't worry, somebody will come along if you wait long enough. I mean, it's very weepy and silly, so I did it very grandly with a gospel choir and horns … It's a bit silly, but it's done with affection." In the *NME* he revealed that when he played his recording to Morrissey, "it brought a tear to his eye and he said, 'Oooh, it's sooo grand!'" Suede's Brett Anderson, meanwhile, found Bowie's rendition "very fifties, very Johnny Ray."

'I Know It's Gonna Happen Someday' features a plangent guitar solo by Wild T Springer, a Trinidadian blues player who met Bowie in Canada during the second Tin Machine tour. "I think he got quite a surprise when I called him up and asked him if he'd come down to New York and do a session," said Bowie. "He was an absolute delight." Describing Springer's playing as "sort of a lilting take on Hendrix's guitar style", Bowie revealed that Wild T's "real name is Anthony. I find it very hard to call him Wild T."

A mimed studio performance was recorded by David Mallet for the *Black Tie White Noise* video. Bowie mimed the song alone before a set of curtains and Christmas lights, holding a cigarette lighter aloft, Barry Manilow-style, in the pursuit of what he described as "a *totally* camp" cover version.

I LOST MY CONFIDENCE

This little-known Bowie composition was tried out and discarded by The Lower Third in 1965.

I NEED A LITTLE SUGAR IN MY BOWL
(Brymn/Small/Williams) : see **YOUNG AMERICANS**

I NEED SOMEBODY (*Pop/Williamson*)

Mixed by Bowie for Iggy And The Stooges' *Raw Power*, 'I Need Somebody' was performed on Iggy's 1977 tour. A version featuring Bowie appears on *Suck On This!*.

I NEVER DREAMED (*Jones/Ferris/Dodds*)

In the summer of 1963 Eric Easton, the agent who had signed The Rolling Stones to Decca, called David's early group the Kon-rads to an audition after one of his assistants had seen the band perform in Bromley. By the time of the audition 16-year-old David had already left Bromley Tech and was on the point of parting company with the Kon-rads, but the chance of an audition strengthened the band's resolve. It was decided that they should play one of David's own songs at the audition, which took place on 30 August 1963 at Decca's studios in Broadhurst Gardens, West Hampstead. Drummer Dave Hadfield tells the Gillmans that the song was a piece David had written based on a news report about an air crash, but singer Roger Ferris remembers differently, telling *Mojo Collections* in 2001 that 'I Never Dreamed' was "a typically upbeat love song of the era" and that he, not David, had written the lyrics: it seems highly likely that more than one song is being recalled in these accounts, although whether both were recorded at the audition is anyone's guess. After running through 'I Never Dreamed' the band stood listening to the playback and watching the faces in the control room. "We smiled a bit and felt like pictures we had seen of the Beatles listening to their playbacks," Hadfield told the Gillmans. "We thought this is it, it's tremendous. But it never materialized." David, apparently, was the most upset. "He had set his sights on it ... That sparked the point where he realized he wasn't going to get anywhere with us." The Kon-rads continued for a while without David, and although fame never beckoned they enjoyed a stint touring as support for The Rolling Stones in 1965, releasing a single called 'Baby It's Too Late Now' on the CBS label in the same year.

Whether nor not he wrote the lyrics, David provided backing vocals and saxophone on this, his earliest known studio recording. A few scratchy acetate copies are understood to have survived, and 'I Never Dreamed' has become the Bowie fan's holy grail. In 2002 a Kon-rads tape apparently containing several takes of the song was advertised for auction at Christie's, but failed to find a buyer.

To confuse matters, in 2001 an undated and previously unknown Kon-rads single called 'I Didn't Know How Much', apparently released only in the US and Canada, surfaced on the Decca label despite baffled band members remaining adamant that Decca never signed the group or released any of their recordings. This intriguing turn of events has led some Bowie collectors to conclude that, despite the songwriting credit going to fellow Kon-rads Neville Wills and Tony Edwards, 'I Didn't Know How Much' may feature David and may date from the August 1963 session. If so, Decca must have released the single overseas without the band's knowledge – hardly an unheard-of occurrence in the 1960s, but highly irregular all the same. There remains no proof that this rare single (Decca 32060), backed by a cover of Ralph Freed's 'I Thought Of You Last Night', really does feature Bowie – but if it does, its place in history is assured.

In 2002 the plot thickened yet again when another studio tape by the Kon-rads, featuring six tracks including 'I Didn't Know How Much' and 'Baby It's Too Late Now' (the others were 'The Better I Know', 'Now I'm On My Way', 'I'm Over You' and 'Judgement Day'), leaked onto the bootleg circuit. This session is understood to date from 1965 and definitely does not feature Bowie, which in turn casts doubt on his presence on the Decca single.

I PITY THE FOOL (*Malone*)
• A-Side: 3/65 • Compilation: *Manish, Early*

Following The Manish Boys' tour supporting The Kinks in December 1964 (see Chapter 3), an introduction to American record producer Shel Talmy offered a significant step in David Bowie's slow rise to success. Talmy was already producing The Kinks (hence the introduction), The Who, Manfred Mann and The Bachelors, who had enjoyed five top ten hits in 1964 alone. "I really liked David," Talmy said many years later, "because of the fact that he was, I thought, ahead of the game."

'I Pity the Fool', originally a hit in 1961 for its American writer Deadric Malone under the name Bobby "Blue" Bland, was selected for The Manish Boys by Talmy himself. "I don't think he would have recorded us otherwise," organist Bob Solly told *Record Collector*. "We thought it was OK because it incorporated saxes and was what we'd call a 'builder' … So we started work on that discordant sax/organ harmony."

The Manish Boys' version was recorded on 8 February 1965 at IBC Studios in Portland Place. As well as showcasing the band's up-front saxophone sound and the young David's finest blues-singer impression, it features the unknown session player Jimmy Page on lead guitar. "He'd just got a fuzzbox and he used that for the solo," recalled Bowie in 1997. "He was wildly excited about it." The session found little favour with the other Manish Boys, whose guitarist Paul Rodriguez told the Gillmans that Shel Talmy "ignored some of the best bits in the original which was *tragic*, and we thought the way he did the whole bass riff was crude in the extreme. It had a counter-riff which Shel destroyed and it sounded crude and tasteless compared to the original." Bob Solly concurs, recalling that "I wasn't pleased with the record. None of us were. It was great to have a record out, but as an artistic achievement, and having Jimmy Page sit in with us, it was a cop-out."

Two different vocal takes were recorded; the single version later appeared on the compilation *The Manish Boys/Davy Jones And The Lower Third*, while the unreleased cut appears on *Early On*.

The intention had been to release the single on the Decca label, but after some delay Talmy leased it to Parlophone, allegedly as part of his personal campaign to win attention as a potential producer for The Beatles. Despite a performance on March 8 for BBC2's *Gadzooks! It's All Happening* (marked by a stage-managed controversy over the length of David's hair – see Chapter 3), the single was a flop. "It was a total non-starter, just not commercial at all," says Bob Solly. "Those saxes were overpowering." This, and David's unhappiness over billing – against his wishes the single had been credited simply to The Manish Boys – spelt the end of his association with the group. Within a month he was fronting The Lower Third.

I PRAY, OLÉ

• Bonus: *Lodger*

This *Lodger* out-take sounds alarmingly like something off *Tin Machine II* – perhaps because it was mixed in 1991. With Bowie on jangly lead guitar, plenty of raucous drum-banging and a fairly forgettable lyric ("It's a god-eat-god world", offers David rather desperately), it's hardly the most glorious thing

he's ever recorded, and its melodic similarity to the vastly superior 'Look Back In Anger' accounts for its original omission from *Lodger*.

I TOOK A TRIP ON A GEMINI SPACESHIP

(Legendary Stardust Cowboy)
• Album: *Heathen* • US Promo: 1/03

In interviews over the years Bowie has often mentioned his semantic debt to the Legendary Stardust Cowboy, an obscure novelty artist who enjoyed a brief period of notoriety in the late 1960s. Born Norman Carl Odam in Lubbock, Texas, "The Ledge" specialized in an indescribable fusion of tuneless space-age rockabilly and stand-up comedy, boasting the slogan: "A legend in his own time – no other time would have him." When asked what subjects interested him, he once replied: "The Old West and space exploration. Everything in between is all garbage, and I'm not interested."

Bowie first became aware of The Ledge during his maiden trip to America in February 1971. "He was a stablemate of mine on Mercury Records," David explained. "A chief executive there called Ron Oberman quietly and conspiratorially put these three singles in my hand and said, 'Hey Dave, you like weird shit, don't you?' And I said, 'Yeah, I love weird shit,' and he said, 'Well, this is the weirdest shit we've got!' And he gave me these wonderful, anarchic singles by this artist, the Legendary Stardust Cowboy, and I completely fell in love with him. I thought he was just terrific."

One of the singles in question was 'I Took A Trip On A Gemini Spaceship', whose cartoonish lyrics Bowie later cited as an influence of sorts on the space-age jargon of the *Ziggy Stardust* album. "Some of the gooniness you hear on *Ziggy* came from him," he said in 2002. "'Freak out in a moonage daydream' is sort of his 'I shot my space gun, boy did I feel blue / I pulled down my sun visor and thought of you.' Now that's a couplet to kill for! Such wonderful lyrics!"

It would be fair to say, however, that The Ledge could hardly be described as a musical influence. "Not really!" David laughed. "Have you heard the records? They are *out there* – he really is solidly outside!" Nevertheless, as he told Jonathan Ross in another 2002 interview, "It's got, inherently, so much integrity. Come hell or high water, this guy was gonna make himself heard! The first thing he put out, 'Paralyzed', was a minor hit in America, like a Texan hit, you know. And he went on *Laugh-In*, the comedy show, in all seriousness, and was laughed off – and he just stormed off in disgust because people just laughed at him. I related to that so much. And I took his name 'Stardust' for Ziggy Stardust. And then I read his site last year – he's got an Internet site – two pages! I think it's one of the slimmest sites on the Internet! And he said, 'One thing ah know is an English guy called David Boo-ie, he took mah name for his Ziggy Stardust character, and ah think he owes me some-thin'.' So I immediately got huge pangs of guilt and recorded one of his songs on the new album."

Those fortunate enough to have attended The Ledge's entirely remarkable performance at Bowie's Meltdown Festival on 15 June 2002 will appreciate that David's sparkling treatment of 'I Took A Trip On A Gemini Spaceship' is only fleetingly reminiscent of the free-form yodelling insanity of the original. Over a sophisticated speed-funk backdrop of drums, gui-tars and saxophones, Bowie piles up layer upon layer of tongue-in-cheek sci-fi clichés: there are crackling wah-wah guitars reminiscent of *Space: 1999*, and a wailing Theremin straight out of *Star Trek*. David's breathy close-to-the-mike vocal capitalizes on the ironic potential of the cod-Elvis croon previously heard on tracks like 'You Belong In Rock N'Roll', ensuring that the innuendo of lines like "I shot my space gun" isn't wasted. The overall effect is com-pletely ridiculous and extraordinarily wonderful; Bowie even manages to imbue the lyric with a 'Space Oddity'-esque sense of melancholy and isolation which simply isn't there in the original. During its few live appearances on the Heathen tour David's enjoy-ment of the number was palpable, and at the time of the album's release he even revealed that 'Gemini Spaceship' was his daughter's favourite track on *Heathen*.

In January 2003 the eight-minute 'Deepsky's Space Cowboy Remix' appeared as the B-side of the US promo 12" of 'Everyone Says 'Hi' (METRO Remix)'. Deepsky, alias Los Angeles-based producers Scott Giaquinta and Jason Blum, were best known for their dance hit 'Stargazer'.

I WALK THE LINE *(Cash)* :
see **THE JEAN GENIE**

I WANNA BE YOUR DOG *(The Stooges)*
• Live Video: *Glass*

This number from The Stooges' 1969 debut album was performed during the 1977 Iggy Pop tour, from which two different versions featuring Bowie appear on *TV Eye* and *Suck On This!*. David later revived it as an encore number during the latter part of the Glass Spider tour, and occasionally segued into it during 'The Jean Genie' on the Sound + Vision tour.

I WANT MY BABY BACK
• Compilation: *Early*

Pre-dating his inglorious cover of 'God Only Knows' by nearly twenty years, this frail demo sees Davy Jones paying direct tribute to The Beach Boys. Particularly reminiscent of 'Don't Worry Baby', it was recorded in 1965 around the time of 'You've Got A Habit Of Leaving', and features David accompanying himself on acoustic guitar with backing vocals probably by The Lower Third's Denis Taylor.

I WISH YOU WOULD *(Arnold)*
• Album: *Pin*

The Yardbirds' debut single, itself a cover version of a song by Billy Boy Arnold, was the first of two of the band's numbers to be recorded for *Pin Ups*. It's not a great highlight of the album, with Mick Ronson's mechanical recreation of a rather irritating guitar riff matched by a pretty phoney R&B vocal from David.

I WOULD BE YOUR SLAVE
• Album: *Heathen*

'I Would Be Your Slave' was one of the first *Heathen* tracks to receive an airing when it was premiered at the Tibet House Benefit concert at Carnegie Hall on 22 February 2002. With its avant-garde and curiously sinister arrangement of mournful strings set against a metronomic sequence of drum loops, it's a stark, min-imalist addition to the album, prefiguring 'A Better Future' with its ambiguous dialogue between a trou-bled protagonist and his mysterious interlocutor, who may be a lover but is probably a God. Bowie described the lyric as "an entreaty to the highest being to show himself in a way that could be understood." The protagonist is clearly uncertain of his status in the relationship: "Give me peace of mind at last / Show me who you are," Bowie implores in a voice both weary and anxious. The lyric echoes the language of countless Christian hymns, although Bowie's tone takes a more direct and questioning line: the final stanza, for example, seems to paraphrase the common conceit expressed in hymns like Christina Rossetti's 'In The Bleak Midwinter' ("What can I give him, poor as I am? … Yet what I can, I give him / Give my heart"), when Bowie declares: "I would give you all my love / Nothing else is free / Open up your heart to me / And I would be your slave". The song was performed during the Heathen tour.

I'D RATHER BE CHROME :
see THE 'LEON' TAPE

I'LL FOLLOW YOU
• Compilation: *Early*

Dating from mid-1965, this rarity is a derivative Beatles-style workout. See 'Glad I've Got Nobody' for details.

I'M A HOG FOR YOU BABY *(Lieber/Stoller)*

Bowie launched into a jokey rendition of The Coasters' 1959 hit during his acoustic set at the Bridge School benefit on 19 October 1996.

I'M A KING BEE *(Moore)*

This blues classic, performed by Muddy Waters and Slim Harpo before being popularized by the cover version on the Rolling Stones' debut album, gave its name to the band with which Bowie released his first single in 1964. Nearly thirty years later, on Tin Machine's It's My Life tour, David occasionally sang a few lines from the number during 'Heaven's In Here'.

I'M AFRAID OF AMERICANS *(Bowie/Eno)*
• Soundtrack: *Showgirls* • Album: *Earthling* • US A-Side: 10/97 • B-Side: 7/00 [32] • Live: *liveandwell.com, Beeb* • Video: *Best Of Bowie*

Described by Bowie as "one of these stereotypical 'Johnny' songs: Johnny does this, Johnny does that", this terrific track takes corporate America to task about its philistine domination of global culture. "The face of America that we have to put up with is the MacDonald's/Disney/Coke face," Bowie told *Mojo*, "This really homogenous, bland cultural invasion that sweeps over us – which is unfortunate, because the aspects of America that are really magical to us are the things it seems to reject, like black music or the Beat poets."

The song began life during the latter *1.Outside* sessions in January 1995, at which a prototype version was recorded featuring different lyrics (it's "Dummy" instead of "Johnny", and in the chorus David is "afraid of the animals"). Originally entitled 'Dummy', this version was intended for the soundtrack to the film *Johnny Mnemonic*, but was eventually consigned to the equally dire *Showgirls*. The darker, funkier *Earthling* re-recording is the preferred version, laying a percussive vocal sample over a synthesized rhythm track to form the foundations of a rising edifice of industrial sound, falling away only for the final resigned conclusion that "God is an American".

In 1997 the track was subjected to six remixes for release as a maxi-single in the US. The project was masterminded by Trent Reznor of Nine Inch Nails, who had supported Bowie during the Outside tour and said of the song "I tried to make it a bit darker." Additional guests included Ice Cube and Photek – Bowie's favourite drum'n'bass exponent – and according to David the forty-minute result was "not just a remix. It almost becomes an album piece in itself. I was absolutely knocked out when I heard what [Reznor] had done. It was great."

The video, also featuring Reznor, was shot in New York in October 1997 between Bowie's Earthling tour commitments. It was directed by the fashionable duo Dom and Nic (later famed for Robbie Williams's award-winning 'She's The One') who, as Bowie explained, were "making very interesting, quite hard-edged British videos at the moment. I felt it was important that it retained that outsider's perspective of America, you know." Reznor plays a menacing Yankee character who threatens Bowie's paranoid

English gent in the streets of New York. "They wanted a kind of *Taxi Driver* feel to the whole thing," explained Reznor. "That's kind of what it's based on. That's why I'm in my Travis Bickle outfit!" The clip won a nomination in the Best Male Video category at the 1998 MTV Video Music Awards, while the single reached number 66 in the American chart – hardly spectacular, but Bowie's best US placing in a decade.

Sonic Youth guested on 'I'm Afraid Of Americans' at Bowie's fiftieth birthday concert, and the song subsequently featured throughout the Earthling tour. It is interesting to observe that Bowie's only other "stereotypical 'Johnny' song" is 1979's 'Repetition', which in the immediate wake of the *Earthling* sessions was unexpectedly exhumed for live performance. It seems more than likely that the one was prompted by the other. 'I'm Afraid Of Americans' has reappeared regularly on every subsequent Bowie tour, while the video appeared on CD formats of the 'Seven' single before its inclusion on *Best Of Bowie*. A version recorded in New York on 15 October 1997 appeared on *liveandwell.com*, while a live performance from the BBC Radio Theatre concert on 27 June 2000 was included on the *Bowie At The Beeb* bonus disc.

I'M DERANGED (*Bowie/Eno*)
• Album: *1.Outside* • B-Side: 4/97 [32] • Soundtrack: *Lost Highway* • Live: *liveandwell.com*

All the familiar *1.Outside* trademarks are present and correct here – Eno's layered synthesizer backings, Mike Garson's demented piano interludes, Carlos Alomar whirling away on rhythm guitar – and with one of the album's best vocal performances the sweeping, epic chorus really takes flight. It is "to be sung by the Artist/Minotaur", and the pseudo-*Waste Land* lyrics have been well and truly chewed by Bowie's computer: "And the rain sets in, it's the angel-man, I'm deranged … Big deal Salaam, Be real deranged Salaam, Before we reel I'm deranged."

Melodically the song looks both forward and back, borrowing phrases from 'Real Cool World' and anticipating the drum'n'bass stylings of the next album. 'I'm Deranged' was performed on a few early dates of the Outside tour and later revamped for the Earthling show, from which a version recorded in Amsterdam on 10 June 1997 later appeared on *liveandwell.com*. In 1997 two exclusive remixes appeared on the soundtrack of David Lynch's *Lost Highway*.

I'M IN THE MOOD FOR LOVE (*McHugh/Fields*)

The Astronettes' cover of the old jazz standard was shelved with the rest of the project, but the song was later performed by Ava Cherry during the Philly Dogs support set. The Bowie-produced studio version, featuring some insanely overwrought scat-style backing vocals from Geoffrey MacCormack, eventually appeared on 1995's *People From Bad Homes*.

I'M NOT LOSING SLEEP
• B-Side: 8/66 • Compilation: *Early*

This forgettable B-side, on which David turns the other cheek to a treacherous friend ("I can get my satisfaction knowing you won't get reaction" he sings, echoing The Rolling Stones' year-old hit) was recorded at Pye Studios on 6 June 1966. As with the A-Side 'I Dig Everything', producer Tony Hatch hired unknown session musicians in place of The Buzz, who nonetheless performed it live in the same year.

I'M NOT QUITE : see LETTER TO HERMIONE

I'M SO FREE (*Reed*)

Co-produced by Bowie for Lou Reed's *Transformer*, 'I'm So Free' features prominent backing vocals from David and a superbly controlled guitar from Mick Ronson.

I'M TIRED : see NEVER LET ME DOWN

I'M WAITING FOR THE MAN :
see WAITING FOR THE MAN

I'VE BEEN WAITING FOR YOU (*Young*)
• Album: *Heathen* • Live Video: *Oy*

Neil Young's aspirational love song dates from his eponymous 1969 debut album: "When I got that album in 1969, I was dazzled by the overall complexity of sound," Bowie recalled in 2002. "It was so majestic, aloft and lonely-sounding at the same time.

A real yearning. And I'd always wanted to do that song on stage or someplace." He first fulfilled the wish on Tin Machine's It's My Life tour, during which Reeves Gabrels took lead vocal on the number. Interestingly enough, only a year earlier 'I've Been Waiting For You' had also been covered by Bowie favourites Pixies (as the B-side of their 1990 single 'Veloria'), which perhaps accounts for its addition to the Tin Machine repertoire.

Ten years later Bowie elected to cover the song on *Heathen* alongside his version of Pixies' 'Cactus'. Boasting typically smart Tony Visconti production and a bellowing solo from guest guitarist Dave Grohl, it's a strong and direct rendition, if perhaps the least essential of the album's three cover versions. The 5.1 remix on the *Heathen* SACD is marginally longer than the CD version. 'I've Been Waiting For You' was performed live throughout the Heathen tour and made the occasional reappearance on A Reality Tour. In September 2002 it was released as a single in Neil Young's homeland of Canada.

I'VE GOT LIGHTNING :
see **LIGHTNING FRIGHTENING**

IAN FISH, U.K. HEIR
• Album: *Buddha*

Like the same album's 'The Mysteries', this is a low-key piece of ambient sound created by slowing down the original backing track, this time augmented by gramophone static of the kind Bowie had used on 'Black Tie White Noise' a few months earlier. In his sleeve notes for *The Buddha Of Suburbia*, Bowie writes that "The real discipline is … to pare down all superfluous elements, in a reductive fashion, leaving as near as possible a deconstructed or so-called 'significant form', to use a 30's terminology." As an exercise in pure texture without theme, 'Ian Fish' stands as perhaps Bowie's most minimalist track of all, accompanied only by a hesitant acoustic guitar that picks out a few phrases which develop into snatches of the 'Buddha Of Suburbia' melody itself. The title, incidentally, has no arcane connotations: it's simply an anagram of "Hanif Kureishi".

IF I'M DREAMING MY LIFE *(Bowie/Gabrels)*
• Album: *'hours…'*

The longest track on *'hours…'* explores the album's motif of the dream state on a shifting sand of rhythmic patterns, as the lyric attempts to recall a half-remembered relationship that may be only a fantasy ("Was she ever there? … All the lights are fading now if I'm dreaming all my life"). The basis appears to be the Jungian paradox about falling asleep and dreaming one is someone else, and thereafter being unable to tell whether the waking state is any more "real", or just the next part of the dream. The relationship with Bowie's shedding of successive identities – not to mention the intellectual inversion of early compositions like 'When I Live My Dream' – is evident.

As with 'Something In The Air' there are fleeting recollections of past glories, in this case an 'All The Young Dudes' guitar break 3'50" into the track, and a slowly building outro reminiscent of 'Memory Of A Free Festival'. Overall, however, it's one of the less satisfactory experiments on *'hours…'*, a rather turgid interlude between the melodic beauty of 'Survive' and 'Seven'.

IF THERE IS SOMETHING *(Ferry)*
• Album: *TM2* • B-Side: 10/91 [48] • Live: *Oy* • Live Video: *Oy*

Having covered a John Lennon protest lyric on their first album, Tin Machine turn their hard-rock guns on a less suitable target for their second. This characteristically complex number from Roxy Music's 1972 debut is all but demolished by the usual Tin Machine symptoms: drums too loud, guitar too messy, irony disastrously bypassed. The image of Bowie, against a backing of industrial noise, yelling that he's going to "sit in the garden, grow potatoes by the score," simply beggars description. There were rumoured to be plans to re-record the track as a duet with Bryan Ferry, but this came to nothing. The song was performed on the It's My Life tour, with versions included at the BBC session on 13 August 1991 (later appearing as a B-side of 'Baby Universal') and on *Oy Vey, Baby*.

IF YOU DON'T COME BACK *(Lieber/Stoller)*

The Drifters' 1963 B-side was played live by The

Manish Boys.

IMAGINE *(Lennon)*

Bowie performed a one-off live version of John Lennon's classic in Hong Kong on the final date of the Serious Moonlight tour, marking the third anniversary of Lennon's death. It's a passionate if idiosyncratic saxophone-led rendition which has found its way onto bootlegs.

IN EVERY DREAM HOME A HEARTACHE
(Ferry) : see **HEAVEN'S IN HERE**

IN THE HEAT OF THE MORNING
• Compilation: *World, Deram* • Live: *Beeb*

'In The Heat Of The Morning' made its studio debut as part of Bowie's first BBC radio session on 18 December 1967, in an embryonic form quite different from the subsequent studio version. The original BBC recording lacks the familiar opening riff, instead substituting a delicate arrangement for strings and woodwind over the opening chord sequence. The lyric, too, is markedly different, with a rather woolly opening verse: "My memory keeps me turning round, turning around / Looking down the valley of years / Where cunning magpies steal your name / I'm watching your face appear on a cloud drifting by". When, three months later on 12 March 1968, the more familiar version was produced by Tony Visconti at Decca Studios as part of Bowie's final session for Deram, this opening gambit had been rewritten to rather more striking effect: "The blazing sunset in your eyes will tantalize / Every man who looks your way / I watch them sink before your gaze / Senorita sway, dance with me before their frozen eyes".

Following the rejection of 'When I Live My Dream', 'In The Heat Of The Morning' was also turned down as a single, prompting David's departure from Deram the following month. As a result the track remained unreleased until the 1970 compilation *The World of David Bowie*, by which time yet another recording, this time closely in keeping with the Deram version, had been aired as part of a second BBC session recorded on 13 May 1968. This version later appeared on *Bowie At The Beeb*.

'In The Heat Of The Morning' is one of the more sophisticated tracks of the Deram period, distinguished by a Doors-style fusion of guitar and pixiephone (courtesy of Steve Peregrine Took, the less fêted half of Visconti stablemates Tyrannosaurus Rex), and a sweeping and instantly recognizable Visconti string section of the kind later heard on tracks like '1984' and 'It's Hard To Be A Saint In The City'. Amid its rather torrid romanticism there are hints that David is recycling earlier Deram out-takes (he is "like a little soldier catching butterflies"), but he has now abandoned his Anthony Newley voice in favour of a cod American drawl. Like 'Let Me Sleep Beside You', whose subject matter it practically photocopies, it's a significant step towards the *Space Oddity* sound.

The so-called demo that has appeared on bootlegs is identical to the finished track except that the final fade-out comes a few seconds earlier. In 2000 a new version was recorded during the *Toy* sessions, but this remains unreleased.

THE INVADER : see **CYCLOPS**

IS IT ANY WONDER : see **FAME** and **FUN**

IS THERE LIFE AFTER MARRIAGE?

Little is known about this unfinished track from the *Scary Monsters* sessions – rumoured in some quarters to feature Iggy Pop – although studio documentation confirms its existence. Considering Bowie's private affairs at the time, it's quite possibly a tongue-in-cheek working title, possibly for a song we know by another name. The instrumental released on bootlegs under this title is in fact the backing track for the abandoned *Scary Monsters* version of 'I Feel Free'.

ISN'T IT EVENING (THE REVOLUTIONARY)
(Slick/Bowie)

Bowie co-wrote and sang vocals on this track from Earl Slick's 2003 album *Zig Zag*, produced by Mark Plati and recorded in tandem with the *Reality* sessions. According to Earl Slick, the composition was in embryonic form when Bowie "came up with the lyrics and fleshed out the melody and turned it into this killer song." 'Isn't It Evening' carries David's unmistakeable stamp in its chord changes, harmonics and split-octave vocals, and the lyric, too, covers familiar territory, sketching a portrait of forlorn souls and broken lives which recollects several of the *Heathen* lyrics (the phrase "nothing remains" even crops up). There are echoes, too, of far older compositions, including a distinct taste of 'After All' in the lines: "Some stand in the sun / Some are blind / One puts his hand in mine / One disappears, his name isn't written down / One dies on the lawn / His face turned away from it all."

"David sounds amazing on the song," said Earl Slick in 2003. "I remember being in the studio when he recorded the vocals and thinking, 'This is weird. For once, I'm on the other side of the glass and he's playing on a track for me. He nailed his vocals in one or two takes and it came out great – that's the beauty of working with David."

ISOLATION *(Pop/Bowie)*

Co-written and co-produced by Bowie for Iggy Pop's *Blah-Blah-Blah*, 'Isolation', which also features David on backing vocals, was released without success as the album's fifth single in 1987.

IT AIN'T EASY *(Davies)*
• Album: *Ziggy* • Live: *Beeb*

Often wrongly attributed to Ray Davies, this American white-blues number in fact derives from the pen of the late American singer-songwriter *Ron* Davies, originating on his 1970 LP *Silent Song Through The Land*. It's been suggested that Bowie was introduced to 'It Ain't Easy' by Mick Ronson (rumour has it that the song was already part of The Rats' repertoire), but by the time of the *Ziggy* sessions the song was by no means obscure. Covers had already been recorded by Three Dog Night in 1970 and Long John Baldry in 1971 – in both cases the parent albums were named after the track – and Dave Edmunds cut a version for *Rockpile*, released in June 1972, the same month as *Ziggy Stardust*. (Interestingly, the song later went on to become the opening track of *Phew*, a 1973 album by Claudia Lennear, the American singer who is said to have inspired Bowie's 'Lady Grinning Soul'.)

The song was originally picked up by Bowie around the time of the Arnold Corns sessions, and his

interpretation received its first live hearing as the closing number of his BBC concert session on 3 June 1971; this recording was later included on *Bowie At The Beeb*. Cut at Trident on 9 July, the subsequent studio version has the distinction of being the first *Ziggy Stardust* track to be recorded; initially mooted for inclusion on *Hunky Dory*, it was among the tracks on the ultra-rare promo album pressed by Tony Defries in August that year.

As the only cover on *Ziggy Stardust*, 'It Ain't Easy' has been understandably marginalized by critics, which is a pity as it features some of Ronson's most searing slide guitar and some of Bowie's most acrobatic vocals. Production is immaculate and David is clearly relishing his cod-American act against a riotous backing chorus (boosted by Dana Gillespie, who received a belated credit for backing vocals on the album's 1999 reissue). The lyric is by no means incongruous, dovetailing perfectly with the travelling/climbing/searching metaphor already prevalent in Bowie's writing: the opening line, "When you climb to the top of the mountain, look out over the sea", is practically a rewrite of 'Black Country Rock', while "you jump back down to the rooftops" would later be echoed in 'Diamond Dogs'. The imprecation to "think about all of the strange things circulating round" is suggestive of both 'Five Years' and 'Starman', and the lyrical nod to The Rolling Stones' 'Satisfaction' suits Bowie's methodology to a tee. The devotional aspect of the obvious blues clichés ("With the help of the good Lord, we can all pull on through ... sometimes He'll take you right up and sometimes down again") acquires a darker twist in the context of *Ziggy Stardust*'s Messianic overtones and its reiterated dismissals of a religious establishment.

All the same, in the final analysis it remains mystifying that 'It Ain't Easy' was favoured above 'Velvet Goldmine' and 'Sweet Head' for inclusion on the album. The song never featured in the Ziggy tour sets and hasn't been performed since.

IT CAN'T HAPPEN HERE *(Zappa)*

The Mothers of Invention's second single, released in 1966, was performed live by Bowie's short-lived outfit The Riot Squad the following year.

IT DOESN'T MATTER ANYMORE *(Anka)*

Buddy Holly's posthumous 1959 hit was played live by The Buzz.

IT HAPPENS EVERY DAY :
see **TEENAGE WILDLIFE**

IT'S A LIE

The title of a radio jingle for Puritan recorded by The Lower Third in May 1965 (see Chapter 3).

IT'S ALRIGHT : see **SWEET JANE**

IT'S ALRIGHT *(Bowie/May/St Gian/Warren)* :
see **COOL CAT**

IT'S GETTING BACK

A long-forgotten Bowie composition included in The Buzz's repertoire.

IT'S GONNA BE ME
• Bonus: *Americans*

Recorded at Sigma in August 1974 under the working title 'Come Back My Baby', this is one of Bowie's overlooked masterpieces. It's a languid soul ballad in the Aretha Franklin style, featuring one of David's most brilliant vocal performances against a virtuoso Mike Garson piano line and full-bodied gospel-choir backing. Astonishingly it was one of the numbers David elected to drop from *Young Americans* to make room for the two Lennon collaborations, and as a result 'It's Gonna Be Me' was denied an official release until 1991. That he was able to reject material like this says a lot about the quality of his 1974 output.

'It's Gonna Be Me' graced the live circuit for a while, featuring throughout the Philly Dogs tour prior to the release of *Young Americans*. Tony Visconti has confirmed that a more heavily orchestrated mix exists from the Sigma sessions, "with a full string section, but I have no idea why it was never released. It's gorgeous."

IT'S GONNA RAIN AGAIN

Nothing is known about this unfinished track except that it was demoed during the *Ziggy Stardust* sessions at Trident, probably around September 1971.

IT'S HARD TO BE A SAINT IN THE CITY
(Springsteen)
• Compilation: S+V, 74/79

Like Bowie's earlier cover 'Growin' Up', this tough-talking portrait of urban America hails originally from Bruce Springsteen's 1973 debut *Greetings From Asbury Park, N.J.*, an album that had a considerable impact on David at the time. When playing a selection of his favourite records on Radio 1's *Star Special* some years later in 1979, David included Springsteen's 'It's Hard To Be Saint In The City', remarking that "after I heard this track I never rode the subway again … That really scared the living ones out of me."

While working on his own version during the Sigma *Young Americans* sessions in August 1974, Bowie received an unexpected visit from the Boss himself. As he recalled many years later, "A Philadelphia DJ who was quite a supporter of mine said, 'You're doing these Springsteen numbers, do you want me to get Bruce down?' He brought Bruce down, and I was out of my wig. I just couldn't relate to him at all. It was a bad time for us to have met. I could see what he was thinking, 'Who is this weird guy?', and I was thinking, 'What do I say to normal people?' There was a real impasse. But I still think he was one of the better American songwriters around in those early days." The rumour that Springsteen contributed to Bowie's version of 'It's Hard To Be A Saint In The City' is almost certainly untrue. "I remember chickening out of playing it," David said. "I didn't want to play it to him because I wasn't happy with it anyway."

For many years the track remained unreleased, languishing in the vaults until finally appearing on *Sound + Vision* and latterly *Best Of 1974/1979*. Both these releases list it as a *Station To Station* out-take, and although rumours persist that a second version was indeed cut at Cherokee in 1975, the available version undoubtedly contains elements of the *Young Americans* cut, confirmed by the unmistakable piano of Mike Garson and a shimmering string arrangement which has Tony Visconti's fingerprints all over it. The evidence would suggest that, rather than a brand new version being recorded during the *Station To Station* sessions, what actually happened was that fresh over-dubs were added to the *Young Americans* version at Cherokee before the track was once again abandoned. Whatever its provenance it's a fine, robust rendition of one of Springsteen's better compositions, with Bowie on spectacular vocal form.

IT'S NO GAME (NO. 1)

• Album: *Scary*

The two versions of 'It's No Game' which book-end the *Scary Monsters* album are adapted from 'Tired of My Life', a song Bowie had demoed as early as 1970 and reputedly wrote when he was just sixteen. The uncompromisingly raucous 'It's No Game (No. 1)' weds David's histrionic scream of a vocal to Robert Fripp's crazed guitar loops (Bowie explained that he asked Fripp "to imagine he was playing a guitar duet with B B King where he had to out-B B B B, but do it in his own way"). The most striking feature, however, is Michi Hirota's aggressive narration of the lyric's Japanese translation by Hisahi Miura. According to Tony Visconti, the original idea was that Bowie should sing it himself, and Hirota was "a Japanese actress from the London production of *The King And I* who was hired to coach David. She discovered that the lyrics were literal and not poetic, therefore they couldn't synchronize with the melody. It was David's idea for her to narrate parts of the song instead." Bowie explained that he conceived the idea "to break down a particular kind of sexist attitude about women and I thought the Japanese girl typifies it where everybody sort of pictures her as a geisha girl – sweet, demure and non-thinking. So she sang the lyrics in a macho, Samurai voice." The track was subsequently released as a single in Japan.

With a characteristically twisted sense of nostalgia, a reference to Eddie Cochran's 'Three Steps To Heaven' here becomes a sinister intimation of mortality. The line "Put a bullet in my brain / And it makes all the papers", deriving from the earlier 'Tired Of My Life', offers compelling evidence of Bowie's ongoing preoccupation with the vulnerability of fame and the prurient glamour of sudden death as the ultimate media sensation. He has always been acutely conscious of the dark underside of "the papers" who once asked Major Tom whose shirts he wore, and during the 1970s Bowie occasionally mentioned that he lived in

fear of being shot on stage. Tragically such anxieties were put to the test less than three months after the release of *Scary Monsters*, when John Lennon was shot dead only a few blocks from where Bowie was performing in *The Elephant Man*.

'It's No Game (No. 1)' was the most obvious target in a contemporary lampoon by the BBC comedy team the HeeBeeGeeBees, who included young comedians Philip Pope and Angus Deayton. Their 1981 album *439 Golden Greats* included the skit 'Quite Ahead of My Time' by "David Bow-Wow", a cruel but brilliant parody which teased the art-house pretensions of Bowie's *Scary Monsters* period. While an aggressive Oriental voice intoned the names of Japanese motor-cycle manufacturers, Pope affected an uncanny imitation of Bowie's most histrionic yell to deliver lines like "Ooh, I'm an elephant / Look what I've just gone and done" with hugely portentous sincerity. Some artists responded to the HeeBeeGeeBees' parodies (Stewart Copeland of the Police congratulated 'Too Depressed To Commit Suicide' as the only successful recreation of his drumming he'd ever heard, while the Bee Gees, renowned for their ability to laugh at themselves, were apparently livid about 'Meaningless Songs In Very High Voices'), but Bowie's reaction is sadly not recorded.

Although 'It's No Game' has yet to be included in a live set, the closing moments of 'No. 1' were recreated for the melodramatic curtain-raiser of the Glass Spider show, as Carlos Alomar's manic guitar was interrupted by an amplified cry of 'Shut up!' from the unseen Bowie.

IT'S NO GAME (NO. 2)

• Album: *Scary*

A gentler, more melodic revision of the above, the closing track on *Scary Monsters* dispenses with the pulsing guitars and screeching Japanese vocals, offering new lyrics and a meditative and earnest vocal in which, after years of uncomfortable speculation about the star's political beliefs, he lashes out at "Fascists" with all the weary venom of the left-wing radical which much of his early 1980s output suggests Bowie had now become.

A 3'52" demo of 'No. 2' has appeared on bootlegs, featuring a more basic arrangement with Bowie evidently test-driving his vocal rather than going for a take. The finished version was the first *Scary Monsters* track to be completed, and the only one for which

David recorded his vocal at New York's Power Station. The remainder of the album's vocals were added in London two months later.

The Nine Inch Nails song 'Pinion' (from their 1992 'Broken' EP) is apparently concocted from extracts of 'It's No Game (No. 2)' played in reverse and slowed down.

IT'S ONLY ROCK'N'ROLL *(Jagger/Richards)*

During the Philly Dogs and Station To Station tours David occasionally sang the title of The Rolling Stones' 1974 hit in his rendition of 'Diamond Dogs', a song clearly indebted to it. Rumours persist that Bowie made an uncredited contribution to the Stones' original version, or even that he co-wrote it with Ron Wood despite its official Jagger/Richards credit. It was certainly recorded in Hilversum while David was there putting the finishing touches to *Diamond Dogs*, and Keith Richards has since confirmed that the song was developed from a jam session in which David participated, but it remains uncertain whether he actually appears on the finished track.

IT'S SO EASY *(Holly/Allison/Petty/Mauldin)*

The Crickets' 1958 single (their last with Buddy Holly) was covered live by The Buzz.

JAILHOUSE BLUES
(Goss/Madigan/Marien/Sheridan) :
see **YOUNG AMERICANS**

JAMAICA : see **FASHION**

JANGAN SUSAHKAN HATIKU :
see **DON'T LET ME DOWN & DOWN**

JANGIR *(Bowie/Gabrels)*

An instrumental track recorded by Bowie with Reeves Gabrels in 1999 for exclusive use in the *Omikron* computer game.

JANINE
• Album: *Oddity* • Live: *Beeb*

The jauntiest number on this prevailingly morose album, 'Janine' was Tony Visconti's favourite track from the *Space Oddity* sessions. Although it's apparently a playful admonition of a girl who is "too intense" and in danger of "standing on my toes", other lines suggest more complex undercurrents. For those who like to see Bowie's mask-wearing and play-acting as a mechanism against confronting his own personality, lines like "I've got to keep my veil on my face", "I've got things inside my head that even I can't face", and "if you take an axe to me you'll kill another man, not me at all", suggest that 'Janine' offers a substantial early example of the fictive self-distancing that was to acquire legendary proportions in the following decade.

The 3'32" demo recorded with John Hutchinson around April 1969 is notable for some minor lyrical differences but mainly for its unexpected segue into the closing refrain of The Beatles' 'Hey Jude'. On the demo tape Bowie reveals that Janine is "the girlfriend of a guy called George who does very nice album covers." This can only be his long-time friend George Underwood, and the following October David told *Disc & Music Echo* that the song was "...a bit hard to explain without sounding nasty. It was written about my old mate George and is about a girl he used to go out with. It's how I thought he *should* see her."

'Janine' was briefly mooted as a follow-up single to 'Space Oddity', even being announced as such in the *NME* in November 1969, but this plan was dropped. Two BBC session versions were recorded on 20 October 1969 and 5 February 1970, of which the former now appears on *Bowie At The Beeb*. Thereafter 'Janine' disappeared from the Bowie repertoire, although the album version was included on the rare unreleased US single of 'All The Madmen'. Many years later it cropped up again on the soundtrack album of the 1998 movie *Whatever*.

THE JEAN GENIE
• A-Side: 11/72 [2] • Album: *Aladdin* • Live: *David, SM72, Aladdin (2003)* • B-Side: 4/94 • Bonus: *Aladdin (2003)* • Video: *Collection, Best Of Bowie* • Live Video: *Glass*

'The Jean Genie' was the first *Aladdin Sane* song off the

starting-blocks, written during the early days of Bowie's 1972 US tour, recorded at RCA's New York studios on Sixth Avenue on 6 October, and mixed in Nashville the following month. The story goes that the song started life as 'Bussin'', an impromptu jam on the tour's chartered Greyhound between the first two concerts in Cleveland and Memphis, when Mick Ronson began picking out the chugging Bo Diddley-style riff on his new Les Paul guitar. Thirty years later Bowie would describe 'The Jean Genie' as "a smorgasbord of imagined Americana" and "my first New York song", revealing that he wrote the lyric to entertain Cyrinda Foxe, a key figure in the Warhol crowd and an occasional girlfriend during his 1972 US tour. "I wrote it for her amusement, in her apartment," David explained. (Foxe, who later married David Johansen of the New York Dolls and subsequently Steve Tyler of Aerosmith, sadly died in 2002).

Juggling appropriate Genie/Aladdin references with overt phallic imagery and whoops of wild abandon, 'The Jean Genie' encapsulates all Bowie's 1972 pet subjects in one slice of perfect glam-pop. In early live introductions on the US tour, David announced that the number was "about a guy who lives in New York" and, more explicitly, "for a friend of ours, Iggy Pop". In 1996 he described the song as "focused around Iggy, an Iggy-type character to be fully fair. It wasn't *actually* Iggy," and he later called the character a "white-trash, kind of trailer-park kid thing – the closet intellectual who wouldn't want the world to know that he reads." Of particular note is the line "Keeps all your dead hair for making up underwear", which appears to be an early indication of the unhealthy interest in voodoo magic which would later grip Bowie during the depths of his 1975 Los Angeles period (Angela Bowie and others have claimed that David became obsessed with preserving his hair-trimmings and nail-clippings for fear that witches might use them in magic rituals, a precaution advised in one of Aleister Crowley's "secret teachings"). As for the oft-cited Jean Genet pun, Bowie initially denied that it was intentional. "It was very, very subconscious, but I think it's probably there, yes," he said in 1973. "Lindsay Kemp did the most fantastic production of [Genet's] *Our Lady Of The Flowers* a couple of years ago, and it's always been in the back of my mind." Of the recording itself, he added that he "wanted to get the same sound the Stones had on their very first album on the harmonica. I didn't get that near to it, but it had a feel that I wanted – that sixties thing."

'The Jean Genie' received its live premiere in Chicago on 7 October – the day after the studio recording was completed – while a version recorded a fortnight later survives on *Santa Monica '72*. The following month's single only reached number 71 in America, but at home it climbed to number 2 to become Bowie's biggest hit so far – tragically it was kept off the number 1 spot by no less a record than Little Jimmy Osmond's 'Long-Haired Lover From Liverpool'. In other territories 'The Jean Genie' encountered mixed fortunes, becoming a huge hit in Japan but getting itself banned in Rhodesia, where the authorities considered it "undesirable".

By the time 'The Jean Genie' peaked in the UK chart in mid-January 1973, its irresistibly catchy guitar riff had already been replicated by Sweet's huge hit 'Blockbuster!', which promptly sailed past it to succeed Jimmy Osmond with five weeks at number 1. Some controversy surrounded this turn of events, although 'Blockbuster!' co-writer Nicky Chinn later insisted that it was an "…absolute coincidence. The ridiculous thing was, of course, they were both on the same record label. But I know we had never heard Bowie's 'Jean Genie' and to the best of my knowledge he hadn't heard 'Blockbuster!'. There was a lot of fuss about it at the time." On another occasion, Chinn remarked that "Because Bowie was hipper than Sweet, the tendency was to infer that we'd ripped off Bowie. I remember being introduced to Bowie at Tramp at that very time, and he looked at me completely dead-pan and said, 'Cunt!' And then he got up and gave me a hug and said, 'Congratulations…'" In reality, of course, the 'Jean Genie' riff already had its antecedents in The Yardbirds' version of Bo Diddley's 'I'm A Man' and, by the same route, their own delta-blues classics like 'Over Under Sideways Down'.

To promote the single at home, Mick Rock's video was shot in San Francisco on 27 and 28 October 1972, featuring snatches of concert footage interspersed with shots of The Spiders posing moodily in and around the appropriately-named Mars Hotel while Bowie, a post-glam Warhol, sizes up a blonde dancer through a film director's finger-frame. "It looks sort of Beatle-y now," said David in 1986. "It was very new in terms of the way it was dressed. We wanted to get a very graphic, white, almost *Vogue* look – big faces, big bits of faces, eyes against stark white backdrops, and to throw in an environment, so we found a place called the Mars Hotel in California somewhere and we stuck the band in there." The model who dances in the video, often mistakenly identified as Angela Bowie, is in fact Cyrinda Foxe. "Wanting it to locate Ziggy as a kind of Hollywood street-rat," David explained in *Moonage Daydream*, "it became important to me that he had a consort of the Marilyn brand. So I telephoned Cyrinda Foxe back in New York and asked her if she was into playing the role. She was, quite rightly, as no-one could have done it better, and she flew in immediately." The Mars Hotel sequences were shot early on 27 October, while the live footage of the band performing 'The Jean Genie' was filmed the following night at the second of two shows at San Francisco's Winterland.

Among other things, 'The Jean Genie' video commemorates one of Bowie's favourite stage gestures of the Ziggy period: framing his eyes with the forefingers and thumbs of his upside-down hands to create an "alien eyes" effect. "I don't know where the funny little Ziggy finger-mask came from," he wrote in 2002, "but it caught on like crazy with the front row and could be prompted at will." He has continued to reprise the gesture on stage over the years, usually heralding the performance of a Ziggy number.

An early monitor mix of 'The Jean Genie', featuring Mick Ronson's guitar even higher in the mix, has appeared on bootlegs. Meanwhile both the *Santa Monica '72* live cut and the original single mix, which is only marginally different from the album version, were both included on 2003's *Aladdin Sane* reissue.

A close contender with 'Rebel Rebel' for the accolade of the most frequently performed number in Bowie's entire repertoire, 'The Jean Genie' has featured in every major solo outing since late 1972 with the exceptions of the Outside, 'hours...' and Heathen tours. For the final Ziggy Stardust concert on 3 July 1973, Jeff Beck joined The Spiders on stage for the number, while a tight live take was recorded at the Marquee on 19 October 1973 for NBC's *The 1980 Floor Show*. For this version, Ken Scott mixed Bowie's vocal to achieve a close-to-the-mike glam timbre in the style of Marc Bolan or Brian Connolly.

Over the years the song has been the basis of much on-stage experimentation, and the incorporation of other rock'n'roll standards into often lengthy guitar breaks has become something of a concert tradition. In 1973 (notably during the Jeff Beck performance), 'The Jean Genie' segued into The Beatles' 'Love Me Do', complete with David on harmonica. The Beck/Ronson duet in that final concert also slipped briefly into The Yardbirds' 'Over Under Sideways

Down'. For the Diamond Dogs show the song was reincarnated in a slow cabaret style, to which the 'Love Me Do' interlude was occasionally added during the Philly Dogs tour. It was this version that provided the blueprint for the curtain-raiser of the first half of the Serious Moonlight tour, when Bowie strolled on stage to croon the opening lines before snapping into 'Star' (the full 'Jean Genie' came later in the encores). The Station To Station concerts used 'The Jean Genie' as the final encore, often spinning the number out to epic length with guitar jams, false endings and ecstatically abandoned ad-libbed vocals from the frequently sloshed Thin White Duke. The Glass Spider tour had Peter Frampton and Carlos Alomar embarking on an epic guitar duet incorporating The Rolling Stones' 'Satisfaction', while for the Sound + Vision tour the song shifted gear into a huge variety of numbers, most commonly Van Morrison's 'Gloria', but also incorporating such occasional rarities as Bowie's Iggy Pop covers 'Tonight' and 'I Wanna Be Your Dog', The Beatles' 'A Hard Day's Night', Bob Dylan's 'A Hard Rain's A-Gonna Fall' and 'Blowin' In The Wind', Elvis Presley's 'Baby What You Want Me To Do' and 'Heartbreak Hotel', Muddy Waters's 'Baby Please Don't Go', Sonny Boy Williamson's 'Don't Start Me Talkin'', Paul Simon's 'I Am A Rock', Johnny Cash's 'I Walk The Line', George Clinton's 'Knee Deep', Jimi Hendrix's 'Purple Haze', the *West Side Story* classic 'Maria', The Ronettes' 'Be My Baby', and even the Ronnie Spector single 'Try Some, Buy Some', which David would later record for *Reality*. In October 1996 Bowie unveiled an unusual acoustic version at the Bridge School benefit shows, while the Smashing Pumpkins' Billy Corgan duetted on a more conventional rendition at David's fiftieth birthday concert. The Earthling tour offered a slow, bluesy first verse, usually augmented by a few lines from an ever-changing selection of hoary blues standards, before picking up speed for a storming chorus.

Not surprisingly 'The Jean Genie' has attracted its share of cover artists, including Van Halen, the Hothouse Flowers, Camp Freddy, Shed Seven (on the B-side of their 2001 single 'Step Inside Your Love'), and Bowie favourites The Dandy Warhols (on the B-side of 2003's 'Plan A'). Stadium giants Simple Minds have explained on more than one occasion that they named themselves after the "so simple-minded" line in Bowie's lyric. In 2000 the original version appeared on the soundtrack album of Julien Temple's Sex Pistols film *The Filth And The Fury*.

JEEPSTER *(Bolan)*

The 1971 T Rex hit, culled from *Electric Warrior*, is based on a circular guitar riff from Howlin' Wolf's 1962 classic 'You'll Be Mine'. On their 1989 tour Tin Machine recycled the riff for their live makeover of Bob Dylan's 'Maggie's Farm', to which David occasionally added a few lyrics from 'Jeepster'.

JENNY TAKES A RIDE *(Little Richard/Willis)*

This 1966 single by Mitch Ryder and the Detroit Wheels was covered live by The Buzz.

JERKIN' CROCUS *(Hunter)*

Produced by Bowie for Mott The Hoople's *All The Young Dudes*.

JEWEL *(Gabrels/Black/Bowie/Plati)*

Together with Frank Black and Dave Grohl, Bowie co-wrote the lyrics and provided vocals on this track from Reeves Gabrels's 1999 album *Ulysses (della notte)*. It's a rambling, dissonant rocker in the Tin Machine style, in which Gabrels sings a chorus about being "the king of cruelty" in between verses provided by his guest vocalists. Dave Grohl would later recall Bowie writing the lyrics on sheets of paper spread across the studio floor.

JOE THE LION
• Album: *"Heroes"* • Bonus: *"Heroes"*

An early instance of the fascination with self-mutilating performance art that would inform the dark landscape of *1.Outside* nearly twenty years later, 'Joe The Lion' is Bowie's tribute to artist Chris Burden, who publicly nailed himself to the roof of a Volkswagen in Venice, California in 1974. According to Tony Visconti the song was composed on mike in the studio, with David "writing the melody and lyrics and singing the final vocal at the same time. It took less than an hour." Bowie later recalled: "I would put the headphones on, stand at the mike, listen to a verse, jot down some key words that came into mind, then take. Then I would

repeat the same process for the next section. It was something that I learnt from working with Iggy, and I thought a very effective way of breaking normality in the lyric."

Restating the alcoholic leitmotif of *"Heroes"*, 'Joe The Lion' considers the artist as visionary and the revelatory symbolism of crucifixion ("A couple of drinks on the house and he was a fortune-teller, he said 'Nail me to my car and I'll tell you who you are'"), ponders the blurred division between states of waking and dreaming ("You will be like your dreams tonight, you get up and sleep"), and hints at the urban-gypsy characterization of the long-lost Halloween Jack ("You slither down the greasy pipe, so far so good, No-one saw you hobble over any freeway").

'Joe The Lion' was performed live on the opening two Serious Moonlight dates, and more frequently during the US leg of the Outside tour. Rykodisc's reissue of *"Heroes"* included a superfluous 1991 remix.

JOHN, I'M ONLY DANCING
• A-Side: 9/72 [12] • A-Side: 4/73 • B-Side: 12/79 [12] • Live: S+V, SM72, Aladdin (2003) • Bonus: Ziggy, Ziggy (2002), Aladdin (2003) • Compilation: S+V, SinglesUK, 69/74, Best Of Bowie • Video: Collection, Best Of Bowie

Recorded at Olympic Studios on 26 June 1972 and released as the follow-up to 'Starman', this landmark *Ziggy*-era single pushed back the frontiers of David's dalliance with sexual ambiguity and – give or take a little local trouble over *The Man Who Sold the World*'s sleeve artwork – saw his first brush with censorship. Considering it caused such a fuss at the time, 'John, I'm Only Dancing' now seems remarkably innocuous. It's by no means a foregone conclusion that the singer is addressing his boyfriend (he could just as easily be a straight man reassuring the girl's lover), but despite its chart success in Britain the song was considered too alarming by RCA in America, where it remained unreleased until *ChangesOneBowie* later in the decade.

In Britain the single boasted David's first bona fide video, directed by Mick Rock on a budget of £200 during rehearsals at the Rainbow Theatre on 18 August 1972. Intercutting moodily side-lit shots of The Spiders with a pair of androgynous dancers from the Lindsay Kemp company, the film was considered too suggestive by *Top of the Pops*, who ironically replaced it with a film of butch motorcycle riders. The anchor motif painted on Bowie's cheekbone was inspired by an unusual source, as David recalled 30 years later: "When the TV series *Bewitched* went into colour in the late 1960s, for some strange reason Samantha occasionally wore tiny tattoos on her face. I thought it looked really odd, but inspired. So I used a little anchor on my face myself for the 'John, I'm Only Dancing' video."

'John, I'm Only Dancing' exists in three distinct versions which share a rather complicated history. First came the 26 June 1972 single recording, released in September. On 20 January 1973 The Spiders recorded a second take at Trident for possible inclusion as the final track on *Aladdin Sane*, featuring tighter guitar playing and saxophone from Ken Fordham. This recording, sometimes referred to as the "sax version", was rather confusingly released as a single in April 1973, bearing exactly the same catalogue number and B-side as the previous version. It was later inadvertently included on the first 1000 pressings of 1976's *ChangesOneBowie*, before being again replaced by the 1972 cut. Finally, the original 1972 version was remixed in 1979 as the B-side of 'John, I'm Only Dancing (Again)', reducing the echo on Bowie's vocal and pushing it higher in the mix. All three versions have since appeared on CD: the original single is on various compilations including *ChangesBowie*, *The Singles 1969-1993* and the 2002 reissue of *Ziggy Stardust*, while the 1979 remix appears as a bonus track on the 1990 reissue of *Ziggy Stardust*. Meanwhile the 1973 "sax version", considered the best by many, appears on *The Best Of David Bowie 1969/1974*, *Sound + Vision* and the 2003 reissue of *Aladdin Sane*. The last two also feature a live version recorded in Boston on 1 October 1972. Just to complicate matters further, most editions of *Best Of Bowie* include the "sax version", but some substitute the original instead.

'John, I'm Only Dancing' was added to Bowie's live set in July 1972, when he was already introducing it as his new single. It was dropped after the 1973 Japanese leg and remained unperformed until the Sound + Vision tour. The song has been covered by The Chameleons and The Polecats, whose 1981 version was a minor UK hit and later appeared on *David Bowie Songbook*.

JOHN, I'M ONLY DANCING (AGAIN)
• A-Side: 12/79 [12] • Bonus: *Americans* • Compilation: 74/79

This radical funk reworking of 'John, I'm Only Dancing' is a seven-minute track culled from a two-hour jam during the *Young Americans* sessions at Sigma in August 1974. The new lyric is easily as risqué as the original ("It's got you reelin' and rockin', won't you let me slam my thang in?"), and boasts one of David's most accomplished soul vocals against an infectious James Brown groove.

'John, I'm Only Dancing (Again)' was added to the live set for the opening night of the Philly Dogs tour in Los Angeles, as Bowie nonchalantly announced, "This is something to dance to, anyway. It's an old song." (To American audiences, denied a release of the original version, it was in fact anything but.) A snippet of this first performance was captured on film for the closing moments of Alan Yentob's documentary *Cracked Actor*. The song was performed for the remainder of 1974, but never thereafter.

Although originally track-listed for *Young Americans* the studio version remained unreleased until 1979, when it appeared as a single backed by a remix of the 1972 original. The 7" edit subsequently turned up on *Bowie Rare*, while the full-length version was included on *ChangesTwoBowie*, the 1991 reissue of *Young Americans*, and *The Best Of David Bowie 1974/1979*.

JOIN THE GANG
• Album: *Bowie*

This entertainingly cynical snapshot of a vacuous London clique – the spiritual successor of 'I Dig Everything' and a distant ancestor of 'Fashion' – was recorded on 24 November 1966. It features Bowie's most explicit references yet to drug-taking ("acid" and "joints" supplant the coy "pills" of 'The London Boys'), and introduces a parade of wounded characters of the kind who would later populate entire albums. The swinging London archetypes include Molly, "the model in the ads", Arthur the inebriate rock singer, and Johnny the existentialist, heralded by a crazed sitar paying tongue-in-cheek homage to the Eastern influences then being popularized by George Harrison. "I love the sitar at the front," Gus Dudgeon told David Buckley, "it's totally manic, bloody brilliant!" The transience of musical fads is stressed by another moment of melodic wit: just after the line "This club's called the Web, it's this month's pick", Bowie inserts the bassline of the Spencer Davis Group's hit 'Gimme Some Loving', which peaked at number 2 the very same week that 'Join The Gang' was recorded.

'Join The Gang' was played live by The Buzz, and like several other Bowie compositions of the period it was offered unsuccessfully to Peter, Paul and Mary. Contrary to some reports, however, it was never recorded by Oscar of 'Over The Wall We Go' notoriety.

JULIE
• B-Side: 3/87 [17] • Bonus: *Never*

A strong contender for the most mundane title ever given to a Bowie song, this *Never Let Me Down* outtake was demoted to B-side status, despite being arguably one of the best tracks from the whole session. It's a pleasingly melodic pop throwaway, structured on the same chords and phrasing as Iggy Pop's 'Bang Bang', and addressed to an unattainable girl ("Julie, pretend for me that I'm someone in your life…"). It might even have given Bowie a decent hit single.

JUMP THEY SAY
• A-Side: 3/93 [9] • Album: *Black* • B-Side: 1/97 [14]
• Bonus: *Black (2003)* • Video: *Black, Best Of Bowie*

On 16 January 1985, Bowie's 47-year-old half-brother Terry walked out of Cane Hill Hospital in South London and took his life on the railway track at Coulsdon South station. The tabloid press had a predictably prurient field-day, and David elected not to allow the funeral at Elmers End cemetery to become a media circus. He stayed in Switzerland, sending a wreath and a message but otherwise remaining silent on the subject.

Eight years later, 'Jump They Say' finally confronted Bowie's feelings about his brother's life and death. "It's the first time I've felt capable of addressing it," he told *Rolling Stone* in 1993, adding in another interview that his childhood relationship with Terry had never been easy, affected not only by his brother's incipient schizophrenia but by the ten-year age gap and Terry's periodic ousting from the family home: "I saw so little of him and I think I unconsciously exaggerated his

importance. I invented this hero-worship to discharge my guilt and failure, and to set myself free from my own hang-ups."

The jittery, perversely catchy 'Jump They Say', bristling with distorted bursts of guitar, trumpet and reversed sax, deploys characteristically abstruse lyrics to consider the pressures driving a man to desperate straits. Those seeking a detailed confessional about Terry will not find it in this song, which is even less lyrically direct than 'All The Madmen' or 'The Bewlay Brothers'. Bowie explained to *NME*'s Steve Sutherland that it was "semi-based on my impression of my stepbrother [sic] and, probably for the first time, trying to write about how I felt about him committing suicide. It's also connected to my feeling that sometimes I've jumped metaphysically into the unknown and wondering whether I really believed there was something out there to support me, whatever you want to call it; a God or a life-force. It's an impressionist piece – it doesn't have an obvious, cohesive narrative storyline to it, apart from the fact that the protagonist in the song scales a spire and leaps off." In the *Black Tie White Noise* documentary he added that the song was about "when you're living on the edge of life, and when you really want to explore areas that haven't been explored or places that you're not supposed to go, whether you're really right to do that, whether you should stay with the crowd."

'Jump They Say' was released ahead of its parent album in March 1993, accompanied by an unforgettably graphic Brit Award-nominated video directed by newcomer Mark Romanek (now famous for state-of-the-art promos like Missy Elliot's 'She's A Bitch' and Michael & Janet Jackson's 'Scream'). The success of the video lies in its evocative tumble of non-linear images, juxtaposing shots of Bowie poised to leap from a skyscraper with scenes of his broken body on the street below, intercut with sinister medical orderlies spying through telescopes and restraining Bowie in some sort of nightmarish sensory-deprivation apparatus. Shot at London's Mayfair Studios, the clip is an exercise in cinematic reference, with obvious quotes from Fritz Lang's *Metropolis*, Kubrick's *2001*, the paranoid identity-theft thrillers of John Frankenheimer, and Hitchcock's *The Birds*, *Vertigo* and *Rear Window*. Perhaps more significantly it reshuffles many of Bowie's past characterizations, including the business-suited executive of 'Let's Dance', the wired-up asylum patients of 'Ashes To Ashes' and 'Loving The Alien', and the spreadeagled corpse of the *Lodger* sleeve. Rivalling the classic 'Ashes' clip as one of Bowie's finest, 'Jump They Say' assembles an allusive *bricolage* of executive stress, peer pressure, conformity, mental illness, spying, voyeurism, brainwashing, vertigo, desperation and ultimately suicide.

Bowie's estranged aunt Pat, who had proved an eager participant in the public trashing of her famous nephew when Terry was alive, was moved by the 'Jump They Say' video to offer a further outpouring to Britain's tabloids. "Now he is using [Terry's] tragic death to put his record in the charts and I find that not only macabre but pathetic," she told the *Sun* on 31 March 1993. "The picture of David with his face scarred so much upset me terribly. There is a real resemblance. David looks just like Terry did when he became schizophrenic…"

The single shot to number 9 in the UK, Bowie's best placing since 'Absolute Beginners' seven years previously. It performed equally well across Europe, but despite the additional exposure of a playback performance on *The Arsenio Hall Show* on 6 May 1993 the American market failed to bite. In addition to the numerous remixes on single formats, an inferior 'Alternate Mix' was included on CD and cassette formats of *Black Tie White Noise* itself. In 1994 the song became the central focus of *Jump* (see Chapter 8), a CD-ROM which included a reworked 'Lift Music' version. 'Jump They Say' became a live highlight of the Outside tour.

JUST AN OLD FASHIONED GIRL *(Fisher)*

As bootlegs reveal, Bowie toyed with the idea of adding Eartha Kitt's signature tune to the middle of 'Changes' during rehearsals for the Station To Station tour.

JUST FOR ONE DAY (HEROES) :
see **"HEROES"**

JUST ONE MOMENT SIR :
see **ERNIE JOHNSON**

JUST WALKING IN THE RAIN
(Bragg/Killen/Riley) : see **YOUNG AMERICANS**

KARMA MAN
• Compilation: *World, Deram* • Live: *Beeb*

'Karma Man' was recorded at Advision on 1 September 1967 with David's new producer Tony Visconti. With its central figure "cloaked and clothed in saffron robes" it's a prime example of the growing interest in all things Buddhist and Tibetan that had surfaced in 'Silly Boy Blue' some months earlier, and its meditations on "the Wheel of Life" and perpetual reincarnation ("I see my times and who I've been") coincide with the point at which Bowie and Visconti both joined the Tibet Society.

Originally touted as a B-side for the rejected singles 'Let Me Sleep Beside You' and 'When I Live My Dream', 'Karma Man' remained unreleased until 1970's *The World Of David Bowie*. By this time the song had been aired in two BBC sessions recorded on 13 May 1968 and 5 February 1970, the first of which, featuring a lush string arrangement and prominent backing vocals from Tony Visconti and Steve Peregrine Took, now appears on *Bowie At The Beeb*. An allegedly different studio mix that has appeared on bootlegs is merely an adulterated version of the original.

The "Slow down, slow down" chorus appears to have been a source of some inspiration for Bowie fan Brett Anderson: Suede's 1992 single 'The Drowners' begins its chorus with the same words (sung practically to the tune of 'Starman') and there's a strong melodic echo of 'Karma Man' in the outro of their 1996 single 'Beautiful Ones'. The song has evidently remained precious to Bowie, who recorded a new version of 'Karma Man' during the *Toy* sessions in 2000.

THE KING OF STAMFORD HILL *(Gabrels/Bowie)*

Before Tin Machine got off the ground in the summer of 1988, Bowie and his new collaborator Reeves Gabrels toyed with the idea of an album based on Steven Berkoff's 1983 cockney melodrama *West*. The project was abandoned but the only completed demo, 'The King Of Stamford Hill', was salvaged for Gabrels's 1995 solo album *The Sacred Squall Of Now*. "Most of the track was re-recorded in 1995," he told *Record Collector*, "…with the exception of David's vocal, which I took off the demo and then manipulated and altered in a variety of ways." With Berkoffian obscenities aplenty and a cockney "running commentary" provided by David's *Basquiat* co-star Gary

Oldman, the result sounds like a punked-up variant of Blur's 1994 hit 'Parklife', replete with customary chains of squealing guitar sound from Gabrels. Dispensable.

KINGDOM COME (Verlaine)
• Album: *Scary*

The only cover version on *Scary Monsters* (indeed the first on any Bowie album since *Station To Station*) was penned by former Television vocalist Tom Verlaine, whose original version appeared on his eponymous solo debut in 1979. Bowie's choice of such an obscure number demonstrates his strengthening affiliation with America's East Coast new wave, and of Verlaine's song he remarked that "it was simply one of the most appealing on his album. I'd always wanted to work with him in some way or another, but I hadn't considered doing one of his songs. In fact Carlos Alomar, my guitarist, suggested that we do a cover version of it since it was such a lovely song." Given a *Scary Monsters* makeover 'Kingdom Come' fits seamlessly among David's own compositions and is one of the unlikely highlights of the album, distinguished by an extraordinary vocal performance for which Bowie mingles an almost ridiculous vibrato with falsetto swoops and an affected glottal attack borrowed from Buddy Holly via Elvis Costello.

An interesting 3'59" demo, devoid of Robert Fripp and the backing vocalists and featuring a far more restrained Bowie vocal, has appeared on bootlegs. An unconfirmed rumour has it that Verlaine himself was to have played lead guitar throughout *Scary Monsters*, but that test sessions with Bowie had failed to yield satisfactory results. Over twenty years later Bowie's links with Verlaine were reaffirmed when Television were included on the bill of the 2002 Meltdown Festival.

KNEE DEEP (Clinton/Wynn) :
see THE JEAN GENIE

KNOCK ON WOOD (Floyd/Cropper)
• A-Side: 9/74 [10] • Album: *David*

"We're gonna put in some extras tonight, some silly ones," declares Bowie on *David Live* as the band launches into an enthusiastic rendition of Eddie Floyd's 1967 Stax hit. The inclusion of such an off-the-cuff number was an indication not only of David's growing soul affiliations but also his increasing impatience with the tightly scripted Diamond Dogs show. A top ten hit in the UK (*Top Of The Pops* made its own unofficial video to accompany the number), 'Knock On Wood' reappeared occasionally during the Philly Dogs tour.

KNOWLEDGE (Bowie/Deacon/May/Harris/Taylor) :
see COOL CAT

KODAK : see COMMERCIAL

KOOKS
• Album: *Hunky* • Live: *Beeb*

Duncan Zowie Haywood Jones was born on 30 May 1971 and, according to legend, David wrote 'Kooks' the very same day. He certainly must have been quick off the mark, because the song was premiered at his BBC session on 3 June. "I'd been listening to a Neil Young album and they phoned through and said that my wife had a baby on Sunday morning, and I wrote this one about the baby," David told the studio audience, before warning them that he wasn't sure of the words yet. This performance, later included on *Bowie At The Beeb*, is notable for including an extra line: "And if the homework brings you down / Then we'll throw it on the fire and take the car downtown / And we'll watch the crazy people race around". It was to be the song's only live airing, although a further recording was made for a BBC session on 21 September.

A three-minute studio demo, featuring David accompanying himself on acoustic guitar and including some slight lyrical variations, has appeared on bootlegs. The *Hunky Dory* version itself, much enhanced by Mick Ronson's string arrangement and Trevor Bolder's trumpet, was recorded at Trident around July 1971, while a slightly different mix appeared on the rare promo album pressed in August.

Dedicated to "Small Z" on the *Hunky Dory* sleeve-notes, 'Kooks' is an endearing pledge from a new father and, as David's remark suggests, it bears a resemblance to some of Neil Young's lighter moments. "The baby was born," said David at the time of the album's release, "and it looked like me and it looked like Angie, and the song came out like – if you're gonna stay with us you're gonna grow up bananas." Although it's unashamedly lightweight alongside tracks like 'Quicksand' and 'Life On Mars?', 'Kooks' nevertheless carries a hint of *Hunky Dory*'s pre-occupation with the compulsion to fictionalize life, as Bowie invites his son to "stay in our lovers' story".

"Zowie", incidentally, was pronounced like the girl's name Zoe, intended as a masculine version of the Greek word for "life" – it therefore rhymes with the correct pronunciation of "Bowie". By the end of the 1970s David's son was known as Joey or Joe, and nowadays he answers to his given name of Duncan. As for 'Kooks': "He likes it," said David in 1999. "Yeah, he's got a fondness for it. He knows full well that it was written for him."

'Kooks' has been covered by The Smashing Pumpkins, Tindersticks (on their limited-edition 1993 'Unwired' EP), Danny Wilson (whose 1987 B-side version can now be found on *David Bowie Songbook*) and even Robbie Williams (on his 1997 single 'Old Before I Die'). The Smiths' 1987 hit 'Sheila Take a Bow' finds Morrissey affectionately paraphrasing Bowie's lyric: "Throw your homework onto the fire / Come out and find the one you love".

A LAD IN VEIN : see ZION

LADY GRINNING SOUL
• Album: *Aladdin*

The closing track of *Aladdin Sane* is one of Bowie's most underrated recordings, and quite unlike anything else he has ever done. Written and recorded in London towards the end of the Trident sessions, it was conceived as a paean to the American soul singer Claudia Lennear, already the inspiration of the Rolling Stones' 1971 hit 'Brown Sugar'. As Bowie paints his portrait of a sensuous seductress, the Stateside flavour of the album gives way to a torrid Latin torch style, with European influences to the fore in Mike Garson's rippling piano and Mick Ronson's stunningly perfect flamenco guitar break. "There was a very romantic piano on that," Garson later recollected, "a Chopin, Liszt type of attitude of the late 1800s." Bowie rises to the occasion with a Scott Walker-esque croon of spine-tingling depth and intensity. After

Aladdin Sane's succession of ravaged vignettes, here at last is an overwhelming serenity, the paranoia of the opening track ("he's only taking care of the room") subjugated to a surrender of the senses ("don't be afraid of the room").

'Lady Grinning Soul' became a B-side in various European territories in 1973, and the following year it backed the US version of 'Rebel Rebel'. To this day Bowie has never performed it live. Suede appear to draw on the song both lyrically and melodically for their startlingly similar 1994 track 'My Dark Star'.

LADY MIDNIGHT *(Cohen)*

Leonard Cohen's number, from 1969's *Songs From A Room*, was performed by Feathers.

LADY STARDUST
• Album: *Ziggy* • Bonus: *Ziggy, Ziggy (2002)* • Live: *Beeb*

Mick Ronson's underrated piano skills open *Ziggy Stardust*'s second side in this wistfully melodic recollection of the star's charismatic stage act. Again the lyric thrives on a glut of wide-eyed Americanisms ("awful nice", "outta sight"), but the content of 'Lady Stardust' is a very British affair. Bowie hints at a Wildean fall from grace via a paraphrase of Lord Alfred Douglas's most famous utterance ("I smiled sadly for a love I could not obey"), but the key inspiration is thought to be Bowie's friend and rival Marc Bolan who, with "long black hair" and "make-up on his face", had already pointed the way for David's reincarnation as Ziggy. Bolan's face was projected on the backcloth when 'Lady Stardust' opened Bowie's shows at the Rainbow Theatre in August 1972, among the few instances when he has played the song live.

The young David's fascination with what he perceived as the glamorous idiom of streetwise American youth has been well documented, and interestingly the description of Ziggy as "outta sight" can be traced back to the first American fan letter he ever received. Kenneth Pitt records in *The Pitt Report* that a letter arrived from New Mexico in September 1967 from a young fan describing David's first album as "outasite" and "so neat". According to Pitt, "David added some Americanese to his vocabulary. For a couple of weeks everything he saw was, paradoxically, outasite."

The album version of 'Lady Stardust' was recorded at Trident on 12 November 1971, while an edited version of the demo, cut at Haddon Hall the previous spring under the alleged working titles 'He Was Alright (The Band Was All Together)' and 'A Song For Marc', appeared on the 1990 and 2002 reissues of *Ziggy Stardust*.

Bowie recorded two performances for BBC radio on 11 January and 23 May 1972, of which the latter now appears on *Bowie At The Beeb*. A new version, with a stately bassline and additional backing vocals by Gail Ann Dorsey, was taped at David's semi-acoustic session for *ChangesNowBowie* in January 1997. "This, I think, is a really lovely song," he said on the show. "It sounds really good even today."

LADYTRON *(Ferry)*

A cover of this classic track from Roxy Music's 1972 debut album is rumoured to have been demoed during the *Pin Ups* sessions.

LAND OF A THOUSAND DANCES
(Kenner/Domino)

Cannibal & The Headhunters' 1963 single was played live by The Buzz.

LASER : see I AM A LASER

LAST NIGHT

This band composition, described by organist Bob Solly as "a surging 50s-style instrumental", opened many of David's gigs with The Manish Boys.

THE LAST THING YOU SHOULD DO
(Bowie/Gabrels/Plati)
• Album: *Earthling*

Recorded towards the end of the *Earthling* sessions and originally intended as a B-side, this track replaced the re-recorded 'I Can't Read' when Bowie decided it was stylistically more in keeping with the rest of the album. "All my grand advice!" is how he described the

cut-up lyric. "I think it's a cautionary tale … It gives you quite a lot of room for speculation: it could be about drugs, promiscuity, any number of the modern 'don'ts', but it's not particularized." Certainly the lyric suggests an edge of joylessness ("Nobody laughs any more, it's the worst thing you can do") and post-AIDS austerity ("Give the last kiss to me, it's the safest thing to do"). After 'Little Wonder' and 'Battle For Britain' this is the third and final assault on the jungle sound often over-attributed to *Earthling*. At his fiftieth birthday gig Bowie performed the song with The Cure's Robert Smith, and it was subsequently reworked for the Earthling tour.

THE LAUGHING GNOME
• A-Side: 4/67 • A-Side: 9/73 [6] • Compilation: *Deram*

In many eyes this infamous song epitomizes the aimless and embarrassing dilettantism of Bowie's pre-'Space Oddity' career. Love it or loathe it, 'The Laughing Gnome' isn't going to go away, so let's at least credit it with self-awareness. It's *funny*, and moreover it's meant to be. It isn't 'Warszawa', but it's probably been played at more parties and the world would be a duller place without it.

For the uninitiated, 'The Laughing Gnome' is a jaunty bassoon-led ditty in which David meets the chucklesome title character and his brother Fred, whose mirthful interjections are laced with appalling puns on the word "gnome". The "Ha ha ha, hee hee hee" chorus is borrowed from the traditional jazz standard 'Little Brown Jug'.

The track was recorded on 26 January 1967 during the *David Bowie* sessions, apparently veering between 2'30" and 3'30" during successive studio cuts. The Pinky & Perky-style voices of the two gnomes were provided by David himself and studio engineer Gus Dudgeon, later to produce 'Space Oddity'. "I remember we sat around for ages, trying to come up with those ghastly jokes," recalled Dudgeon in 1993. "I haven't had the courage to play the record at half-speed, because if I did I'd hear my actual voice. We had a good laugh."

The single, released on 14 April, was the latest in a long line of flops. A year later Bowie included the song in his ill-fated cabaret audition, performing it with the assistance of a glove-puppet gnome. Also in 1968 Ronnie Hilton, who had enjoyed several hits in the previous decade and charted in 1965 with 'A Windmill In Old Amsterdam', recorded a cover version in his broadest Yorkshire brogue which had no more success than the Bowie single.

Infamously, however, 'The Laughing Gnome' was reissued in September 1973 at the height of Bowie's first flush of stardom, shortly before the release of *Pin Ups*. This time it reached number 6, and would return to torment its creator regularly thereafter: "It just shows you it doesn't pay to be cool, man!" chortled Marc Bolan in *Melody Maker* a few years later, "'Rock'n'Roll Suicide' hit the dust and the laughing gnomes took over." In 1990, when it was announced that the set-list for the Sound + Vision tour would be determined by a telephone survey, the *NME* launched a "Just Say Gnome" campaign – T-shirts and all – urging readers to jam the switchboard with requests for the song. "I'll tell you what," Bowie told *Melody Maker* as the tour got under way, "I was thinking of doing 'Laughing Gnome' and was wondering how to do it, maybe in the style of the Velvets or something, until I found out that all the voting had been a scam or something, perpetrated by another music paper. I mean, that was an end to it. I can't pander to the press, now can I?"

As recently as 1998 Queen's Roger Taylor name-checked the song in his solo track 'No More Fun', while Buster Bloodvessel's hilarious techno reworking, surely one of the most unlikely Bowie covers of all, was included on the 2001 compilation *Diamond Gods*. In 1999 incredulous suggestions began to circulate that Bowie would be performing 'The Laughing Gnome' at the BBC's Comic Relief extravaganza on 12 March. The rumours proved to be exaggerated: Bowie's pre-recorded insert, which he introduced as 'Requiem For A Laughing Gnome', involved him tootling tunelessly on a descant recorder and making nonsensical interjections, while the BBC flashed messages promising to stop it if viewers phoned in with their pledges.

LAVENDER BLUE (*Traditional*) :
see **FAME** and **"HEROES"**

LAW (EARTHLINGS ON FIRE) (*Bowie/Gabrels*)
• Album: *Earthling*

Earthling's final track is perhaps its weakest moment, a stab at club credibility that welds a succession of synthesizer effects to a zappy dance-floor bassline reminiscent of Squeeze's 1978 hit 'Take Me I'm Yours'. It's a descendant of 1993's 'Pallas Athena', using a similar distortion effect on Bowie's growled vocal samples. "I used what I believe is a Bertrand Russell quote," David explained, "'I don't want knowledge, I want certainty,' which appealed to me 'cos that's how we feel some of the time … To me, it's the avenue of insanity to presume that if you keep studying you'll find the answers … it actually lightens the load when you realise there are no certainties." The exact Russell quotation, from *The Listener* in 1964, is "What men really want is not knowledge but certainty." Bowie's relentless chant of "With this sound, mark the ground" hints at the sinister allure of false "certainties" by recalling the conflations of music, black magic and totalitarianism that had informed *Station To Station* twenty years earlier.

The song's existential concerns are further hinted at by another line in the lyric: "In a house a man drops dead / As he hits the floor he sighs 'What a morning'". This is surely an obscure reference to the sudden death of Samuel Beckett's father, whose final words after suffering a stroke were, according to the famously mordant playwright, "What a morning".

THE 'LEON' TAPE
(*Bowie/Eno/Gabrels/Garson/Kizilcay/Campbell*)

Ever since gaining full control of his business affairs following his split from Tony Defries in the mid-1970s, Bowie has remained understandably protective of his recordings, keeping a tight rein on the fate of demos, out-takes and other unreleased rarities. However, no system is ever watertight, as witnessed by the appearance on the bootleg circuit of items like the *Scary Monsters* demos and various tour rehearsal tapes. In March 2003 there occurred perhaps the most substantial archive "leak" of Bowie's post-MainMan career, when a private collector released onto the Internet a series of MP3 files taken from a fully mixed tape of the unreleased *Leon* album – the product of the 1994 Montreux sessions which would later be re-edited and augmented with new recordings before eventually seeing the light of day as *1.Outside* (see Chapter 2 for full details of this saga).

Given the fluid and non-linear nature of the *Leon* recordings, and the additional complication that the leaked material consists of a series of MP3s which are spliced together at the whim of the collector with arbitrary beginnings and endings and the occasional repetition, it is difficult to make a definitive assessment of how many "tracks" are included in the approximately 30 minutes of music. Asked about the find on his website, guitarist Reeves Gabrels described the original 1994 mix of the album as a "three hour plus improvised opus".

Besides a wealth of ambient sequences and spoken interludes (many of which take the form of lengthier, unexpurgated versions of the segues that survive on *1.Outside*), four distinct "songs" are discernible on the leaked *Leon* tape. They make for fascinating listening, casting considerable illumination on the nature of the original album. Stripped of the generally more upbeat and commercial numbers that were added at the 1995 New York sessions (such as 'Outside', 'Hallo Spaceboy', 'I Have Not Been To Oxford Town', 'No Control', 'We Prick You', 'Thru' These Architects Eyes' and 'Strangers When We Meet'), *1.Outside* already looks like a very different proposition, and it comes as no surprise that the numbers on the *Leon* tape bear a closer resemblance to the more avant-garde Montreux tracks on the final album, such as 'A Small Plot Of Land', 'The Motel' and 'I Am With Name'. An expansive ten-minute version of 'I Am With Name' is indeed among the tracks on the *Leon* tape, augmented by a lengthy, almost rap-like middle section as Bowie chants a dizzying litany of barely comprehensible snippets ("They won't smell this, she can't tell it, I won't be there, he should eat me, he said tell it," and on and on in the same vein). Reworked variations on this vocal sequence appear in some of the other leaked tracks, and indeed this sense of repetition and re-wrapping is a hallmark of the *Leon* tape in general: it appears that the original album would have been characterized by an aspect not unlike the "permutation poetry" of Brion Gysin, in which key words and phrases reappear throughout in varying configurations and against new backgrounds: on the *Leon* tape phrases like "blood-red sky", "Laugh Hotel", "we'll creep together" and "chrome" crop up repeatedly. The ten-minute 'I Am With Name' draws to a close with more elaborate (and more profane) versions of *1.Outside*'s Nathan Adler and Ramona A Stone segues, here spoken over the rhythm track and culminating in Ramona's surreal observation that "you could think of me as a 'syllannibal' – someone who eats their own words."

The *Leon* tape's most melodic piece is a full-length cut of 'We'll Creep Together', of which a short snippet had previously appeared on the *1.Outside* EPK back in 1995. Bowie adopts his finest Jacques Brel chanson style to deliver an impassioned vocal over Mike Garson's rippling piano, punctuated by a series of twisted sci-fi sound effects: the lyric is characteristically impenetrable ("Way back in the Laugh Hotel I'll reel out of the window / You die for diamonds but you won't live for love"), and the overall impression is sweetly mysterious and somewhat in the style of 'My Death' (and, interestingly enough, of Bowie's subsequent recording of 'Nature Boy' for the *Moulin Rouge* soundtrack).

The prowling, catchy number known unofficially as 'I'd Rather Be Chrome' (a phrase repeated several times in the lyric) is sung in Ramona's familiar cyborg drone against a pounding bass and percussion track. 'The Enemy Is Fragile' (a title confirmed by Reeves Gabrels) revisits the rhythmically insistent patterns of 'A Small Plot Of Land', as Bowie tops the clattering drum patterns, guitar squeals and piano runs with a series of outrageous vocal swoops, alternating between menacing spoken sections, hammy over-enunciations and preposterous falsetto howls: his opening gambit is "Hallo Leon, would you like something really fishy?", before going on to paraphrase Henry II ("Who will rid me of this shaking head?") and cracking a sort of metaphysical pun around a sinister *Silence Of The Lambs* image: "There's something in her mouth – something mysterious ... I bet it is a speech". The appearance of the word "permutation" in the final mantra ("You are a permutation, you are a patois, You are Chinese poetry, You are something mysterious ... You are something really fishy") points to the lyrics' obvious debt to Brion Gysin, and brings the proceedings to a splendidly bewildering climax.

In addition to several further tracks that are inauthentically cobbled together from different sequences (the piece labelled by bootleggers as 'OK Riot' is stitched together from parts of 'I'd Rather Be Chrome' and other numbers), the remaining material includes a short instrumental piece overlaid with some further Nathan Adler narration ("Last time I saw him he was standing by a pile of cantaloupes under the lamp, and I looked up at the blood-red sky, and I saw the words 'Ramona A Stone'"), and, finally, a hypnotic drum, piano and guitar sequence lasting nearly seven minutes, which utilizes various spoken segments, again including radically different mixes of some of the *1.Outside* segues, in what bears a passing resemblance to a courtroom scene. We hear witness testimonials from Nathan Adler ("I says to myself, wow, *quelle courage*, what nerve!"), Ramona ("I was sittin' there in the Laugh Hotel the other night looking for window demons, when in comes this Leon!") and Algeria Touchshriek ("I met Leon once – bit of a dark spiral with no end, I thought"). These monologues alternate with a reprise of Bowie's deranged chants from the extended 'I Am With Name' track, and a new selection of manic declarations ("Some day the Internet may become an information superhighway – do not make me laugh! ... A nineteenth-century railroad that passes through the badlands of the old West!"). The overall effect is not unlike some sort of Brechtian or Kafkaesque theatre piece, and every bit as unsettling.

On several occasions since the release of *1.Outside*, Bowie has intimated that he hopes one day to make more of the Montreux recordings officially available. The leaking of the *Leon* material, in all its fascinating but infuriatingly chopped-up brilliance, only reinforces the impression that this is indeed a consummation devoutly to be wished.

LEON TAKES US OUTSIDE
(Bowie/Eno/Gabrels/Garson/Kizilcay/Campbell)
• Album: *1.Outside*

1.Outside opens with an ambient instrumental in which guitars twang fitfully over layers of slow-building synthesizers and distant voices while Bowie, in the guise of murder suspect Leon Blank, intones snatches of half-heard names and dates. It's an atmospheric introduction to the David Lynch-like setting of Oxford Town and the cracked sonic landscape we're about to enter. One can't help thinking that this is exactly what the beginning of 'Glass Spider' should have sounded like back in 1987, and the resemblance to the opening of U2's *Zooropa* (also co-produced by Brian Eno) is unlikely to be a coincidence.

LET IT BE *(Lennon/McCartney)*

At Live Aid Bowie joined the likes of Bob Geldof, Pete Townshend and Alison Moyet to provide backing vocals for Paul McCartney's rendition of the 1970 Beatles classic.

LET ME SLEEP BESIDE YOU
• Compilation: *World*, *Deram* • Live: *BBC*, *Beeb* • Video: *Tuesday*

Together with 'Karma Man', recorded the same day, 'Let Me Sleep Beside You' enjoys the distinction of being the first Bowie track to be produced by David's long-time collaborator Tony Visconti. The two were brought together when Kenneth Pitt proposed a change of producer following the commercial failure of the Mike Vernon-produced Deram recordings. Pitt's initial suggestion, Denny Cordell, was unwilling to accept David's material and suggested his assistant, a young New Yorker called Tony Visconti who had arrived in England at the end of 1966. Teamed with Cordell, Visconti had already distinguished himself with a sharply commercial ear and a flamboyant taste for elaborate orchestral backings. He suggested the addition of the woodwind section on The Move's September 1967 hit 'Flowers In The Rain', and scored the string arrangement for 'Cherry Blossom Clinic' on their eponymous debut album.

In future years Visconti would win acclaim for his production of Marc Bolan's glam hits, but it is his intermittently fruitful partnership with David Bowie that has been his most substantial legacy to date. In 1967 commercial success lay several years ahead, but the combination of Bowie's rapidly maturing songwriting and Visconti's fiercely clever production would soon turn out to be a marriage made in heaven. Many still regard Tony Visconti as Bowie's most brilliant producer.

'Let Me Sleep Beside You' and 'Karma Man' were recorded on 1 September 1967 at Advision Studios in New Bond Street (another first – at its relocated Gosfield Street premises Advision would later be home to some of *The Man Who Sold The World*'s sessions). Both tracks were apparently the fruit of David's decision "to write some top ten rubbish." Uncertainty surrounds the identity of the session players hired for these recordings, but it is known that they included guitarist John McLaughlin, subsequently to find fame with his Mahavishnu Orchestra, and drummer Alan White, later a member of Lennon's Plastic Ono Band and Yes. Visconti is understood to have hired guitarist Mick Wayne (later of 'Space Oddity' fame) for some of Bowie's Decca sessions, but exact details are elusive.

The two songs were promptly turned down by Decca as a proposed follow-up to the three singles so far released. It's possible that the rejection was on the grounds of the song's risqué title which Decca had already requested be changed to 'Let Me Be Beside You'. The lyric, in which Bowie urges a young lover to put away childish things and receive education in the ways of the flesh, was probably equally terrifying to Decca's selection board, but it may be that the label was simply losing confidence in its costly and thus far unsuccessful protégé. The song remained in the vaults until 1970's *The World Of David Bowie*.

Although neither top ten nor rubbish, 'Let Me Sleep Beside You' represents a vital moment of transition between the Deram material and the rockier sounds of the *Space Oddity* album. "It might have been influenced by Simon and Garfunkel, but gone a little heavier," Bowie suggested many years later. "I still thought I might have a chance of being a romantic songwriter, which never actually proved to be my forte." Visconti's production lends the recording an edge and a maturity quite new to Bowie's sound, and like 'Karma Man' it was one of the few Deram numbers Bowie was still performing in 1969. He recorded a fine version at his BBC session on 20 October, later included on 1996's *BBC Sessions 1969-1972* sampler and also on *Bowie At The Beeb*.

The song was featured in one of the less imaginative segments of the *Love You Till Tuesday* film, in which David mimed to a remix of the Deram version while brandishing a dummy guitar and pulling off some creditable Mick Jagger gyrations. On 29 January 1969 a German vocal was recorded at Trident with lyrics translated by Lisa Busch, in anticipation of a German release for the film. This never transpired and the German version remained under wraps. An early mix of the original Deram recording, including some different vocal overdubs, has appeared on bootlegs. Thirty years later, a new version was recorded during the *Toy* sessions.

LET'S DANCE

• A-Side: 3/83 [1] • Album: *Dance* • Live: *Beeb* • Compilation: *Club* • Video: *Collection, Best Of Bowie* • Live Video: *Moonlight, Glass, Tina Live – Private Dancer Tour (Tina Turner)*

The rest of the album may be of variable quality, but the title track of *Let's Dance* – the first to be recorded during the sessions – justifies the price of admission on its own. Bowie's collaboration with Nile Rodgers reaps its most brilliant reward with one of his finest recordings of the 1980s and undoubtedly one of the all-time great pop singles.

"Frankly, the song 'Let's Dance' didn't start out to be anything more than just another track on the album," David admitted later. "It was Nile Rodgers who took it and structured it in such a way that it had incredible commercial appeal." Rodgers recalled on Radio 2's *Golden Years* that when Bowie first played him the song on acoustic guitar it was "very reminiscent of a folky kind of song … I thought it was really bizarre, but he was convinced it could be a hit, and I just kept working on it." At the time of the album's release, Rodgers suggested that "everybody is gonna think I wrote 'Let's Dance' because it has that Chic feel with Bernard [Edwards] playing a real walking bass – the bassline is, in fact, very much like the one in 'Good Times'." Another obvious Chic connection is what Rodgers calls the "breakdown" on the full-length album and 12" version, in which the lead instruments cut out one by one, leaving just bass and drums before building back to the full arrangement. "On a song like Chic's 'Good Times', the most important part was the breakdown," Rodgers explains to David Buckley. "Whenever the band would go to the breakdown the audience would scream."

Also crucial to 'Let's Dance' is the controlled ferocity of Stevie Ray Vaughan's brilliant guitar solo, which lends the track an extra weight by superimposing an edgy blues-inflected sound over the smooth Chic-style dance groove. "After his blistering solo on the title song," Bowie recalled many years later, "he ambled into the control room and with a cheeky smile on his face, shyly quipped, 'That one's for Albert', knowing full well that I would understand that King's own playing was the genesis for that solo."

Over and above its obvious disco-floor value, 'Let's Dance' maintains a gravity absent from the rest of the album by virtue of its surprising bleakness. It might be a party classic, but like '"Heroes"' its apparent optimism falls away on close inspection. In common with all Bowie's best lyrics nothing is made explicit, but a cryptic air of menace prevails. He isn't dancing beneath a lovers' moon, but "under the moonlight, this serious moonlight", and the future is a frightening blank: "Let's dance, for fear your grace should fall / Let's dance, for fear tonight is all." Nile Rodgers believes that the evocative "serious moonlight" is in part indebted to himself, telling Buckley that "I used to say 'serious' all the time. I would say, 'Man, that shit is serious!' meaning it's happening, it's great – it's a disco expression. In the disco *everything* is serious." However, the possibility of a more arcane inspiration can't be overlooked: among the erotic poetry of Bowie's long-time muse Aleister Crowley is a 1923 composition called 'Lyric Of Love To Leah', which includes the lines "Come, my darling, let us dance / To the moon that beckons us … Let us dance beneath the palm / Moving in the moonlight … Come my love, and let us dance / To the Moon and Sirius". So, is Bowie really singing about "the Sirius moonlight"? Well, possibly.

"It's ostensibly a dance song, but there's a particular type of desperation and poignancy about it," said Bowie. The poignancy was pressed home by the magnificent video, shot in Australia in February 1983 by Bowie and David Mallet; the principal locations were Sydney and the sheep-farming outpost of Carinda. By taking a lateral spin on the song's lyrics to espouse the cause of Aboriginal rights, the video offers the first substantial evidence of the hands-on sociopolitical role Bowie began carving for himself in the 1980s. "As much as I love this country," he told *Rolling Stone* during the shoot, "it's probably one of the most racially intolerant in the world, well in line with South Africa … There's a lot of injustice, so let's, you know, *say* something about it." But this is not the finger-wagging, just-say-no Bowie later to emerge on 'Crack City'; the 'Let's Dance' video remains oblique, relying on a series of powerful metaphors to dig deep into the Australian psyche. "One thing I'd been toying around with was the repellent and attractive qualities of the other side of the world, be it the Middle East or the Far East," Bowie said, "How we're both drawn and repulsed by what happens and who they are, and the fact that we're all one. That basic idea came through on 'Let's Dance' with the Aborigines and colonial English, and then in 'China Girl' and finally in 'Loving The Alien'."

Although not exactly linear, the 'Let's Dance' video portrays the seduction of a young Aboriginal couple by the commercialism of white urban Australia, a pair of expensive red shoes taking centre-stage as an icon of material status; in the city the boy and girl find themselves dehumanized by drudgery, and having finally earned the hard-won shoes they destroy them and return to the Outback. Along the way we have a vision of nuclear devastation, a parody of the then current American Express "That'll do nicely" commercials, and an unforgettable image of the couple painting Aboriginal designs on the wall of the Westerners' art gallery. Coming via Hans Christian Andersen and the 1948 Powell & Pressburger movie, the red shoes themselves have an aspirational symbolism already rooted in fairytale. "The red shoes are a found symbol," Bowie confirmed, "and it seemed *à propos* for this particular video. They are the simplicity of the capitalist society – luxury goods, red leather shoes. Also they're a sort of striving for success – black music is all about 'Put on your red shoes, baby'. Those two qualities were right for the song and the video." By choosing a symbol of capitalism which simultaneously references his beloved black music, Bowie confesses his own collusion in the process of cultural imperialism; at one point he appears in the video as an icy corporate manager, suggesting an implicit anxiety about his own role as a global rock star, the ultimate cultural colonist. Depressingly for a video so saturated in significances, the window-shopping sequence with the red shoes was later copied shot-for-shot by a 1990s advertising campaign for a "reassuringly expensive" lager.

The edited 'Let's Dance' single was released ahead of the album in March 1983. It entered the chart at number 5, and a fortnight later vanquished Duran Duran's 'Is There Something I Should Know?' to enjoy a three-week residency at number 1. The feat was repeated in America, ensuring that 'Let's Dance' became and remains the biggest international strike of Bowie's career (if not actually the biggest-selling single: that distinction belongs to the much-reissued 'Space Oddity'). It stayed in the UK chart for 14 weeks, relaunching the cult darling of the 1970s as a first-division superstar of the 1980s.

'Let's Dance' featured throughout the Serious Moonlight tour, which of course took its name from the lyric. On 23 March 1985 Bowie duetted on the number with Tina Turner at the Birmingham NEC, a performance later released on CD and video (see Chapter 3). The song was revived for the Glass Spider and Sound + Vision shows, but in the 1990s David dropped it from his repertoire, apparently regarding it as a threat to his creativity. In 1995 he spoke disparagingly of 'Let's Dance' as the epitome of what he would *not* be performing on the Outside tour. It came as a surprise, then, when it was revived for a one-off performance at the Bridge School benefit on 19 October 1996. "This started off as a joke for you all tonight, but we kind of got to like it," announced David. "In fact, we prefer this version to the original!" The barely recognizable stripped-down reworking that followed, with fabulous vocals from both David and Gail Ann Dorsey, won a standing ovation. Another radical makeover, for which the opening verse was performed in a dreamy acoustic style reminiscent of 'Wild Is The Wind' before pumping up to full speed on the first "tremble like a flower", was unveiled for the summer 2000 concerts and later reappeared on the Heathen and A Reality tours. A superb live recording of this version, from the BBC Radio Theatre concert on 27 June 2000, concludes the *Bowie At The Beeb* bonus disc.

Nile Rodgers included 'Let's Dance' in the reformed Chic's live repertoire in the early 1990s, while Smashing Pumpkins vocalist Billy Corgan has interpolated lines from the song into live performances of Joy Division's 'Transmission'. Bowie's original recording featured in the 1997 Howard Stern movie *Private Parts*, and was sampled in the same year by Puff Daddy & The Family for their top 20 hit 'Been Around The World'. The song has also been performed live by Beck and Aaron Carter, and in 2001 tribute artist Jean Meilleur performed a 58-piece classically orchestrated version on his Jeans'n'Classics tour.

A radical reworking of Bowie's original appeared in 2003 in the form of a major remix project, approved by David for release in South-East Asian territories and beyond. 'Let's Dance (Club Bolly Mix)' and 'China Girl (Club Mix)' were created under EMI's auspices by engineers and local musicians at Schtung Music, a production company based in Singapore, Hong Kong and Shanghai. Bolstered by the addition of sitars, tabla drums and Hindi backing vocals, 'Let's Dance (Club Bolly Mix)' even came with a new video produced by MTV Asia – effectively a remix itself, it laid elements of the original video into a kaleidoscopic montage of images, re-casting the narrative of the original video, red shoes and all, as a Bollywood-style romance. "Asian culture has had a fairly high profile within my work from the early 1970s," Bowie remarked in 2003. "It was not a difficult decision to give a green light to these remixes. I think they're pretty cool." An array of different versions of the two remixes appeared on a pair of extremely rare promo CDRs issued to radio stations in Singapore and Hong Kong in August 2003; the rest of the world was introduced to the Asian mixes later the same year via the *Club Bowie* album and the limited edition US reissue of *Best Of Bowie*, both of which also included the 'Club Bolly Mix' video. The results will not be to everyone's taste, but they're certainly among the most elaborate and interesting Bowie remixes ever released.

LET'S DANCE *(Lee)*
• Live Video: *Tina Live – Private Dancer Tour* *(Tina Turner)*

Not to be confused with the above, pop's first 'Let's Dance' took Chris Montez to number 2 in 1962. David sang the number live with the Kon-rads in the same year, and more than two decades later performed it as a medley with his own 'Let's Dance' during his guest appearance with Tina Turner at her Birmingham NEC concert on 23 March 1985.

LET'S SPEND THE NIGHT TOGETHER
(Jagger/Richards)
• Album: *Aladdin* • Live: *Motion* • Live Video: *Ziggy*

On an album as heavily influenced by The Rolling Stones as *Aladdin Sane*, this dazzling cover both acknowledges the debt and illustrates the extent to which Bowie takes his source material into new territory. The Spiders' electrically-charged rendition is faster and raunchier than the Stones' 1967 original, with Mike Garson's crazed piano once again adding depth to Ronson's fast-and-loose guitar, while the addition of some zappy synthesizer effects gives the whole a fresh, futuristic sheen.

In 1973 David's studied androgyny was still misunderstood by many (especially in the irony-free world of American rock journalism), and some reviewers commented on what they mysteriously believed to be a gay appropriation of a hetero-anthem. *Rolling Stone*'s Ben Gerson complained that "The rendition here is campy, butch, brittle and unsatisfying. Bowie is asking us to re-perceive 'Let's Spend the Night Together' as a gay song, possibly from its inception. Sexual ambiguity in rock has existed long before any audience was attuned to it. However, though Bowie's point is well taken, his methods are not."

The *Aladdin Sane* version, released as a single in America, Japan and various European countries, was recorded in December 1972. The song was added to The Spiders' stage show on 23 December and remained in the set until the end of the 1973 tour. During early performances Bowie would improvise an increasingly bizarre and vaguely suspect patter during the spoken section, usually revolving around the fantasy of picking up a schoolgirl and asking her to "educate" him – but in the version captured on *Ziggy Stardust: The Motion Picture*, he sticks to the original script.

LETTER TO HERMIONE
• Album: *Oddity*

Like 'An Occasional Dream' this is a painfully intimate song of lost love addressed to Hermione Farthingale, the lover and collaborator who left David in February 1969 after completing her part in *Love You Till Tuesday*. In November of the same year, Bowie told George Tremlett that *Space Oddity*'s two Hermione songs were "me in a maudlin or romantic mood. I'd written her a letter, and then decided not to post it. 'Letter To Hermione' is what I wished I'd said. I was in love with her, and it took me months to get over it. She walked out on me, and I suppose that was what hurt as much as anything else, that feeling of rejection."

The 2'43" demo recorded with John Hutchinson around April 1969 resembles the finished song in all but title: at this stage David was being more cryptic about the addressee and calling the song 'I'm Not Quite'.

For many years Bowie declined to speak further of Hermione, who has undoubtedly been over-hyped by some biographers as a vital key to understanding his music. In Radio 2's *Golden Years* documentary in 2000 he recalled that "as young love often does, it sort of, you know, went wrong after about a year," and at the same time he revealed that he had only recently made a startling discovery: "she had started writing to me again about two months, three months later, which was the most extraordinary thing. I'd sort of blanked it out of my mind, but obviously we could have got back together again, I realized, having read all these letters."

David has since revealed that he had nobody but himself to blame for the break-up with Hermione. "I was totally unfaithful and couldn't for the life of me keep it zipped," he admitted in 2002. "Bad move on my part, as I'm sure we would have lasted a good long time if I'd been a good boy. She, quite rightly, ran off with a dancer that she had met while filming. Then, I heard, she married an anthropologist and went to live in Borneo for a while, mapping out unknown rivers …

We met up again after I had become Ziggy, but it was gone. We spent a night or two together but the spark had been extinguished."

'Letter To Hermione' was covered by Human Drama on their 1993 album *Pin Ups*. Robert Smith, who duetted with David at the fiftieth birthday concert, has revealed that The Cure's 1992 hit 'A Letter to Elise' was named after the song.

LIEB' DICH BIS DIENSTAG (*Bowie/Busch*) : see LOVE YOU TILL TUESDAY

LIFE IS A CIRCUS (*Djin*)

This folksy number by obscure American group Djin, to whose work David had been introduced by Tony Visconti, was a staple of the Feathers repertoire. Around April 1969 Bowie recorded a 3'59" demo with John Hutchinson, which suggests that the song was being considered in the run-up to *Space Oddity*.

LIFE ON MARS?
• Album: *Hunky* • A-Side: 6/73 [3] • Live: *SM72* • Compilation: *The Best Of Bowie* • Bonus: *Aladdin* (2003) • Video: *Collection, Best Of Bowie* • Live Video: *Moonlight*

Bowie's 1971 masterpiece began as an attempt to construct a song around the chord sequence of 'My Way', the Frank Sinatra standard which already had a place in his history (see 'Even A Fool Learns To Love') – hence the words "Inspired by Frankie" on *Hunky Dory*'s handwritten liner notes. David's lyric, and indeed his performance of it, are among his finest ever, but it is Mick Ronson's operatic arrangement that elevates a great piece of songwriting to classic status, from the plaintive opening piano chord to the climactic *Also Sprach Zarathustra* timpani-roll at the beautiful false ending.

Many and ingenious have been the attempts of commentators to unravel the lyric of 'Life On Mars?'. After its elegiac introduction of "the girl with the mousy hair", seeking an escape from her quarrelsome parents in the fantasy world of the cinema, the song takes flight on wings of cryptic significances and surreal juxtapositions. "A sensitive young girl's reaction to the media" is how David described the song in

1971. After pausing for thought, he added 25 years later that "I think she finds herself let down. I think she finds herself disappointed by reality. I think she sees that although she's living in the doldrums of reality, she's being told that there's a far greater life somewhere, and she's bitterly disappointed that she doesn't have access to it … I guess I would feel sorry for her now. I think I had empathy with her at the time."

Some biographers, backing themselves up with the flimsiest of arguments, have suggested that "the girl with the mousy hair" is David's long-departed lover Hermione Farthingale, and that the song recounts her short-lived relationship with David. There is no evidence to substantiate this, and some to undermine it – Hermione's hair, for example, was red. But this is not a lyric to be decoded: the tumble of iconic images (John Lennon, Mickey Mouse, 'Rule Britannia', Ibiza, the Norfolk Broads, the snatches of scenes from the cinema) aren't in themselves significant. The point, surely, is their very proliferation, an explosion of chaotic glamour set against the drab isolation of the protagonist. Anyone tempted to apply too close an analysis to the song's evocative lyricism would do well to note that the line "Look at those cavemen go" comes straight from the chorus of the Hollywood Argyles' 1960 novelty hit 'Alley Oop', as covered in 1966 by the Bonzo Dog Doo-Dah Band.

'Life On Mars?' was belatedly released as a single at the height of Ziggymania in June 1973. Bowie mimed his way through a simple but impressive promo shot in a Ladbroke Grove studio on 12 May: resplendent in a turquoise Freddi Burretti suit and full Pierre Laroche make-up, he was almost whited-out against the stark backdrop. "It wasn't so much an idea as a moment in time," director Mick Rock later explained. "I wanted to do something that looked a little bit like a painting." Bowie later remarked that Rock "burnt the colours right out so that it had a strange, floaty pop-art effect." The single was a smash hit, holding fast at number 3 for three of its thirteen weeks on the chart; a combination of Slade, Gary Glitter and Peters & Lee prevented it from going higher. It has since featured on numerous compilations, appearing in a different edit on 1980's The Best Of Bowie, and in 2001 it was even reissued as a single in France, on a fresh wave of popularity generated by its use in a television commercial for the French Post Office.

In 1988 a cassette featuring a 1971 demo of 'Life On Mars?' was sold at Philips for £90, but this is not in circulation; neither is a rumoured second demo

featuring Ronson accompanying Bowie on the piano.

The song was added to The Spiders' repertoire for the Rainbow Theatre concerts in August 1972 and remained a feature of the Ziggy Stardust tour, becoming part of a medley with 'Quicksand' and 'Memory Of A Free Festival' during the final 1973 leg. A live performance recorded in Boston on 1 October 1972 was included on 2003's Aladdin Sane reissue. Apart from an excellent one-off performance on Johnny Carson's The Tonight Show on 5 September 1980, its next appearances were for the Serious Moonlight and Sound + Vision tours. Mike Garson later embellished the number with baroque piano frills for its superb revival on the 'hours…', 2000, Heathen and A Reality tours.

As great songs do, 'Life On Mars?' has attracted its fair share of interpreters: it has been recorded or played live by Eurythmics, Joe Jackson, The Divine Comedy, ABBA's Annifrid Lyngstad (whose Swedish version 'Liv På Mars?' appeared in 1975), The King's Singers, The Mike Flowers Pops, Marti Webb, All About Eve, The Flaming Lips, Frank Sidebottom (on his 1986 'Sci Fi EP'), Seal (in a 2003 BBC radio session), Jasper Steverlinck (whose excellent version topped the Belgian singles chart for several weeks in 2003) and, notoriously, Barbra Streisand on her album Butterfly. In 1976 Bowie described Streisand's version as "Bloody awful. Sorry, Barb, but it was atrocious." Over twenty years later he was still haunted by it, telling the audience at his 1999 VH1 Storytellers concert that Streisand "had her then husband-cum-hairdresser [Jon Peters] produce and arrange and probably blow-dry it!" Hunky Dory's Rick Wakeman has often reprised 'Life On Mars?' in concert, but the rumour that Mick Ronson cut a solo version is unfounded; the 'Life On Mars' he recorded in 1975 is his own composition and an entirely different song.

LIGHTNING FRIGHTENING
• Bonus: Man

Uncertainty surrounds the exact date of this early 1970s out-take, included as a bonus track on the 1990 reissue of The Man Who Sold The World, whose liner notes claim that it features John Cambridge on drums, Tim Renwick on guitar, and producer Tony Visconti on bass. This line-up would fix its date at some time during or immediately after the Space Oddity sessions, and certainly before Mick Ronson's arrival in February

1970. However, two factors cast doubt on this dating: firstly, the liner notes of this particular reissue are wholly inaccurate in at least one other instance ('Holy Holy'), and secondly, the remarkable similarity between 'Lightning Frightening' and Crazy Horse's 'Dirty, Dirty', which wasn't released until the beginning of 1971, is so absurdly close that it's unlikely to be a coincidence. Bowie's devotion to Neil Young during this period is well documented, and the presence of a chirpy sax solo also speaks more of his 1971 output than of his *Space Oddity* period, so perhaps a more likely hypothesis would be that 'Lightning Frightening' dates from the time of 'Rupert The Riley' and the various Arnold Corns demos of April 1971.

Referred to in some documentation as 'I've Got Lightning', it's a likeable slice of Neil Young-flavoured hippy rock, foot-tapping if not exactly ground-breaking, and is more remarkable for its raunchy harmonica line and jaunty sax than for its sub-'Maggie's Farm' protest lyric. Curiously, the official "bonus track" release fades into the song twenty seconds into the intro; a full-length 3'55" version has appeared on bootlegs.

LIKE A ROLLING STONE (Dylan)

Before his collaboration with Reeves Gabrels in early 1988, Bowie briefly hooked up with members of Bryan Adams's backing band and Bon Jovi producer Bruce Fairbairn to record some tracks in Los Angeles. The only results of this brief collaboration were the original demo of 'Pretty Pink Rose', an early version of 'Lucy Can't Dance', and a rock-heavy cover of Bob Dylan's 1965 hit 'Like A Rolling Stone', subsequently given to Mick Ronson and much enhanced by a guitar line of his own. The result appeared on Ronson's posthumous 1994 album *Heaven And Hull*, and reveals Bowie in competent but indifferent Tin Machine-era shape while his former guitarist immeasurably improves a dull rock-by-numbers backing. That David embellished his vocal becomes obvious when he ad-libs "Oh, rock 'em, Ronno, rock!" during Ronson's solo. The other musicians on the track are Keith Scott (guitar), Rene Wurst (bass), John Webster (keyboards) and Mark Curry (drums).

LITTLE BOMBARDIER
• Album: *Bowie*

Very few Bowie songs are in 3/4 time, and the nostalgic fairground waltz of 'Little Bombardier', recorded on 8 December 1966, sounds uncannily similar to the sorts of noises being cooked up by The Beatles just across town at the same time. Trombone, strings and bar-room piano provide a poignant backdrop to the lyric about an ageing war veteran who is rescued from loneliness and drink by the affection of two children, only to be hounded out of town as a suspected paedophile. Some biographers have attempted to link "Frankie" with Bowie's maternal grandfather on the flimsy basis that he served in the Great War, but this is mere conjecture. More noteworthy is the early appearance of one of Bowie's key motifs of fantasy and escape: Frankie "spent his time in a picture-house", seeking solace in the silver screen just like the disappointed heroine of 'Life On Mars?' and so many future Bowie characters. At the request of producer Bernie Andrews, David included 'Little Bombardier' in his first BBC session, recorded on 18 December 1967.

LITTLE DRUMMER BOY (Davis/Onorati/Simeone) : see PEACE ON EARTH

LITTLE EGYPT (Lieber/Stoller)

The Coasters' hit was among The Manish Boys' live repertoire.

LITTLE MISS EMPEROR (Pop/Bowie)

Co-written and co-produced by Bowie for Iggy Pop's *Blah-Blah-Blah*, 'Little Miss Emperor' appeared on the CD version and became the B-side of Iggy's hit 'Real Wild Child'.

LITTLE TOY SOLDIER

This obscure out-take, recorded with The Riot Squad at Decca Studios on 5 April 1967, is a truly remarkable curio. Like the contemporaneous 'Join The Gang' and 'We Are Hungry Men' it climaxes in an anarchic medley of comic sound effects (explosions, coughing, nose-blowing, smashing glass, car horns and even the speaking clock), but jettisons *David Bowie*'s serio-comic vignettes in favour of full-blown sexual fetishism. Bowie's manic vocal alternates between familiar Anthony Newley theatrics and a convincing attempt at Lou Reed's trademark snarl, as he tells the tale of a little girl who winds up her clockwork soldier every night so that he can whip her. Tellingly, the chorus lifts its melody and some of its lyrics ("Taste the whip, in love not given lightly / Taste the whip, now bleed for me") straight from The Velvet Underground's 'Venus In Furs'. Although the results are deliberately cartoonish the track is a turning-point of sorts, marking Bowie's first delve into a kinky netherworld that had been opened up to him by his recent discovery of bands like the Velvets. The 3'08" recording appears on some bootlegs under the alternative title 'Sadie'.

LITTLE WONDER (*Bowie/Gabrels/Plati*)
• A-Side: 1/97 [14] • Album: *Earthling* • Live: *Earthling In The City, liveandwell.com, Beeb* • Video: *Best Of Bowie*

Earthling's opening track shamelessly poaches its manic percussion and squalling power-chords from The Prodigy's 'Firestarter', a seminal UK number 1 in March 1996 which had been instrumental in bringing drum'n'bass rhythms to a mainstream audience. Nonetheless 'Little Wonder' subverts its own jungle pretensions by adopting a conventional rock sensibility for its "So far away" chorus, blessed with a soaring synthesizer line recalling the euphoria of '"Heroes"'. Reeves Gabrels revealed that the anarchic middle section was composited from "all sorts of shit. The bass track is Gail trying to get a sound from her pedalboard, not knowing it was being recorded. We constructed the track by grabbing bits of her bassline."

Bowie's vocals are all first-take recordings, and the utterly incomprehensible lyric, delivered in his finest bar-room cockney, is the result of another computer-enhanced cut-up session. On this occasion the starting-point is, of all things, *Snow White and the Seven Dwarfs*. "The key was to write one line about each dwarf, or using each dwarf's name," explained David, "but I ran out of dwarfs! I had Potty, Scrummy – all sorts of alternative names." He likened the track to 'Warszawa' in that "the sound of the words, the phonetics, against the musical context ... can give you quite strong, emotive feelings without having to have

a rational sense." Hence such magnificent nonsense as "Dopey morning, doc, grumpy nose" and "tits and explosions, sleepy time, bashful but nude." By the time he reaches "Sit on my karma, Dame Meditation", it's clear that we're facing an almost unprecedented degree of self-mockery; 'Little Wonder' needn't be taken too seriously.

Originally conceived as a nine-minute epic, 'Little Wonder' was whittled down to six minutes for *Earthling* and a further three were excised for the single release in January 1997, which reached number 14 in Britain and topped the chart in Japan. The extraordinary Brit-nominated video was directed by Floria Sigismondi, a Toronto-based Italian whose credits include the later (and very similar) videos for Marilyn Manson's 'The Beautiful People' and Tricky's 'Makes Me Wanna Die'. "I thought she just has a wonderful eye, great textures, fabulous cutting," said Bowie, "and also that she was really quite out on the proverbial limb in terms of subject matter; it was really quite odd." Set in a mutated dystopia somewhere between Fellini and *Eraserhead*, 'Little Wonder' depicts Bowie and a latter-day Ziggy clone prowling subway stations and New York streets against a relentless background of distorting images, shifting film speeds, and unearthly faces projected onto giant eyeballs and nightmarishly deformed animals. These are the work of sculptor Tony Oursler, whose video assemblages had been shown at the Pompidou Centre in Paris and at London's Saatchi Gallery; he later collaborated with Bowie on an exhibit for 1997's Florence Biennale. The projections of David's face onto the sculptures was achieved at Oursler's New York studio, where further examples were prepared for Bowie's fiftieth birthday concert and the subsequent tour.

'Little Wonder' was added to the live set for the East Coast Ballroom tour of September 1996. It was the opening number of the fiftieth birthday concert and featured throughout the 1997 and 2000 tours. A recording of the birthday performance appeared on the *GQ* magazine CD *Earthling In The City*, while the 'Danny Saber Dance Mix' appeared on the UK release of the movie soundtrack *The Saint*. 'Little Wonder' cropped up again in the soundtrack of *Hackers 2*, while another live version, recorded in New York on 15 October 1997, appeared on *liveandwell.com*. A third live recording, this time from the BBC Radio Theatre gig on 27 June 2000, was included on the *Bowie At The Beeb* bonus disc.

LIZA JANE *(Conn)*
• A-Side: 6/64 • A-Side: 9/78 • Compilation: *Early*

Although not quite where it all started, 'Liza Jane' is certainly among the most significant of David Bowie's early landmarks – released on 5 June 1964, it was his first ever record.

The single is credited to Davie Jones with The King Bees (see Chapter 3 for the band's history). Leslie Conn, who had negotiated a one-single deal with Decca and now effectively became Davie's manager, was controversially credited as songwriter. "It was an old Negro spiritual that we played around with," band member George Underwood later said. "I don't know how he came to put his name on it." Conn later admitted that "'Liza Jane' has my name on it, but I think it was a joint composition." What is certain is that The King Bees' adaptation bears only fleeting similarities to the original spiritual, which is transformed into a furious Rolling Stones-influenced R&B rave-up.

Both sides of the single were recorded in a seven-hour session at Decca Studios in West Hampstead, where David had had his ill-fated audition with The Kon-rads a few months earlier. Although producer Glyn Johns was in attendance, Conn took the credit for "Musical Director and Production". The single was released on Decca's subsidiary Vocalion Pop, which specialised in jazz and R&B releases.

On 6 June 1964, the day after its release, 'Liza Jane' was aired on BBC Television's *Juke Box Jury*. The panellists deciding the single's fate were Jessie Matthews (BBC radio's Mrs Dale), Bunny Lewis, Diana Dors and Charlie Drake, of whom only the last voted it a "hit". Making his very first television appearance, David was briefly seen reacting to the verdict. A fortnight later on 19 June he gave his first full-blown TV performance, as Davie Jones with The King Bees played 'Liza Jane' on ITV's *Ready, Steady, Go!* There was a further performance on 27 July for BBC2's *The Beat Room* – but live gigs, television exposure and the endorsement of Charlie Drake were all to no avail. The single flopped, and David's days with the King Bees were numbered. By August he was fronting his next outfit, The Manish Boys, who continued to play 'Liza Jane' live.

"When David and I parted company I went off to live and work in Majorca for a few years," Leslie Conn recalled in 1997. "One day I was on the phone to my mother and she said, 'What shall I do with those records I have in the garage?', which were a few hundred copies of 'Liza Jane'. So I replied, 'Throw them out,' and she did." Seldom can a nugget of filial advice have been so misguided, for original copies of the single now change hands for anything up to £900 apiece. Collectors are advised to beware of immaculate American counterfeits created in the 1970s (on the genuine article, the matrix number is machine-stamped on the vinyl; on the fake it is handwritten). In 1978 Decca reissued 'Liza Jane' to no avail, and it now appears on *Early On*. An unreleased acetate featuring a slightly longer fade-out is said to exist, but it has yet to appear on the collectors' circuit.

THE LONDON BOYS
• B-Side: 12/66 • A-Side: 5/75 • Compilation: *Deram*
• Download: 6/02

By the time 'The London Boys' appeared as the B-side of Bowie's first Deram single in December 1966, the song had been kicking around in one form or another for over a year. In an interview for *Melody Maker* in February 1966, ostensibly to publicise 'Can't Help Thinking About Me', Bowie had referred to the number by its original title: "It's called 'Now You've Met The London Boys', and mentions pills, and generally belittles the London night-life scene ... It goes down very well in the stage act and lots of fans said I should have released it – but Tony [Hatch, producer] and I thought the words were a bit strong." The first recording, now lost, was made with The Lower Third at Pye's Marble Arch studios in late 1965 but, with its unambiguous references to drug-taking, it was promptly rejected by the label. "I was choked, and David was as well," recalled drummer Phil Lancaster. Bowie later recalled that 'The London Boys' was also among the numbers played at The Lower Third's failed audition for the BBC on 2 November 1965.

The familiar studio version of 'The London Boys' was one of the tracks recorded on 18 October 1966 at R G Jones Studios in Surrey and used by Kenneth Pitt to secure David his Deram contract, going on to become the B-side of 'Rubber Band'. In America, Decca baulked at the drug references and chose to replace the B-side with 'There Is A Happy Land', but it appears that this scheduled June 1967 release never went ahead in any case.

"I thought it was a remarkable song," Pitt wrote in his memoir, "and in it David had brilliantly evoked the atmosphere of his generation and his London." Certainly 'The London Boys' is among Bowie's most sophisticated recordings of the period, demonstrating a mature grasp of pace and dynamics as his catatonic, drugged-out vocal gathers impetus over a swirling organ backing, anatomizing a teenager's initiation into swinging London ("You're gonna be sick, but you mustn't lose face – to let yourself down would be a big disgrace"), culminating in a bleak finale which prefigures his own downfall in the mid-1970s: "Now you wish you'd never left your home, you've got what you wanted but you're on your own."

Although for many years Bowie gave the impression of virtually disowning his Deram work, 'The London Boys' was something of an exception. During the *Pin Ups* sessions in 1973 he considered re-recording the song as a series of one-verse vignettes to alternate with the cover versions, creating a self-penned narrative bridging the sounds of his youth, but the idea was abandoned. Nearly a quarter of a century later, 'The London Boys' reappeared in the acoustic set David rehearsed for Radio 1's 1997 broadcast *ChangesNowBowie*, but was dropped at the rehearsal stage. The song finally received its long-awaited live resurrection in the summer 2000 concerts, and a new studio version was recorded later the same year for inclusion on *Toy*. In June 2002 a downloadable 1'26" excerpt from this recording was made available to BowieNet members via the enhanced CD of *Heathen*, followed by a further 1'30" snippet a couple of months later, but the full track has yet to be released.

LONDON BRIDGE IS FALLING DOWN
(*Traditional*) : see **FAME**

LONDON BYE TA TA
• Compilation: *S+V*, *S+V (2003)* • Live: *Beeb*

Hijacking the melody of Bowie's earlier composition 'Threepenny Pierrot', the swishing 'London Bye Ta Ta' is a vigorous step away from the whimsy of *David Bowie* and towards the proto-rock of *Space Oddity*. According to Kenneth Pitt the title and content derived from the West Indian patois David had overheard one day from a family saying their farewells at Victoria station, which explains the pseudo-Jamaican vocal affectation he adopts on both recorded versions. The rhythms and phrasing owe a firm debt to The Kinks' 1967 hit 'Waterloo Sunset', but the lyric is all Bowie's own. The line "Don't like your new face, that's

not nice" offers an early intimation of his identity-hopping, anticipating 'Sweet Thing' ("D'you think that your face looks the same?") by six years, while a distant ghost of the "red light, green light, make up your mind" bridge returns on 1980's 'Fashion'.

The first studio version was a proposed B-side recorded at Decca on 12 March 1968. With classic Tony Visconti strings, some superb percussion and an unusual outro of horses' hooves, this version fell by the wayside when 'In The Heat Of The Morning', recorded the same day, was rejected as a single. The master tape of this version went missing not long afterwards, explaining its absence from subsequent Deram repackages, although a 2'35" acetate copy has cropped up on bootlegs. Two months later a new rendition appeared in Bowie's BBC session recorded on 13 May, and this version now appears on *Bowie At The Beeb*.

'London Bye Ta Ta' was resurrected in 1970 as a side-effect of Kenneth Pitt's negotiations with Decca over their forthcoming repackage *The World Of David Bowie*. When it became apparent that the original master was lost, Bowie elected to re-record the song under his Philips contract. A new and superior take, with a shimmering guitar line and added backing vocals, was begun during the session for 'The Prettiest Star' on 8 January 1970 and completed on 13 and 15 January. This recording was initially earmarked as the follow-up single to 'Space Oddity' and was duly selected for performance on Grampian TV's *Cairngorm Ski Night* on 29 January, for which David played acoustic guitar to the accompaniment of a studio orchestra. The song reappeared in the BBC concert session on 5 February but not long afterwards, against Pitt's wishes, David chose 'The Prettiest Star' to replace it as the next single. 'London Bye Ta Ta' was denied an official release until the 1970 version appeared on *Sound + Vision*, the 2003 reissue of which featured a previously unreleased stereo mix.

THE LONELIEST GUY
• Album: *Reality* • Live Video: *Reality*

The fading chimes of 'Never Get Old' segue into *Reality*'s quietest, most contemplative track. Backed only by acoustic piano and ambient guitar textures, Bowie's vocal is at its most artfully fragile and naïve in this haunting meditation on memory, fortune and happiness. Vague, impressionistic images tumble together in the fractured lyric: "Streets damp and warm / Empty smell metal / Weeds between buildings / Pictures on my hard drive … Steam under floor / Shards by the mirror's frame". As ever the specific resonances are left to the listener, but the overall impression is of an isolated soul wallowing in the emptiness of his existence, repeatedly insisting "I'm the luckiest guy, not the loneliest guy", while the tone of his voice and the mournful music tell us otherwise. It's a bleak, morose reflection on a barren life: "All the pages that have turned / All the errors left unlearned".

"That song is a very despairing piece of work," David reflected in *Interview* magazine. "A guy qualifying his entirely hermetic, isolated existence by saying, 'Actually I'm a lucky guy. I'm not really alone – I just have myself to look after.' But in setting up the analogy of the city taken over by weeds, there is this notion that our ideas are inhabited by ghosts and that there's nothing in our philosophy – that all the big ideas are empty containers. I keep touching on something that I am awfully scared of: the prospect that there really is no meaning to anything. I was trying to avoid it like crazy on this album, but it did slip into that song."

The image of the entropic, weed-infested city was inspired by a genuine model, as Bowie revealed: "I had this image of Brasilia – it seemed to be the perfect standard for an empty, godless universe. I think it's the most extraordinary city: these huge public squares with these 1950s, 1960s kind of sci-fi buildings. The architect Oscar Niemeyer designed all these places thinking that they were going to be filled with millions of people, and now there are about 200,000 people living there, so the weeds and the grass are growing back up through the stones of this brilliantly modernistic city. It's a set of ideas – the city which is being taken back over again by the jungle."

Unusually, Mike Garson recorded his piano part for 'The Loneliest Guy' not at Looking Glass Studios, but at his home studio in Bell Canyon in the San Fernando Valley. "I recorded it on synthesizer originally," Garson explained, "and then took home the MIDI file and re-recorded it on my 9-foot Yamaha Disklavier, recording it as it played back."

The *Reality* promotional film included a performance clip of 'The Loneliest Guy', in which a dark-suited Bowie emoted into a studio microphone in a set-up reminiscent of the *Black Tie White Noise* promos. The song made regular appearances on A Reality Tour, captivating even the most boisterous of audiences with its dramatic tone and delicate acoustics. Bowie

squeezed out every ounce of its drama on stage and was often visibly touched by the vigorous applause. A performance on BBC1's *Parkinson* in November 2003 was of particular note, bringing this most delicate of the *Reality* songs to an even wider audience.

LOOK BACK IN ANGER *(Bowie/Eno)*
• Album: *Lodger* • Bonus: *Lodger* • Video: *Collection, Best Of Bowie* • Live Video: *Moonlight, Ricochet*

A magnificent symbiosis of frenetic percussion and guitar, including a joyous rhythm solo from Carlos Alomar, is punctuated by Brian Eno's unlikely interjections on "Horse trumpets" and "Eroica horn" to propel one of *Lodger*'s dramatic highlights. There's no apparent connection with John Osborne's 1956 kitchen-sink drama; instead the song concerns itself with sinister intimations of mortality as a fatalistic Bowie is visited by a down-at-heel angel of death who "coughed and shook his crumpled wings, closed his eyes and moved his lips" to declare "it's time we should be going."

David Mallet's superb video, inspired by *The Picture Of Dorian Gray*, casts Bowie as a Bohemian painter in an attic studio whose self-portrait has the reverse effect of Dorian's: Bowie finds the skin of his own face beginning to corrupt and melt. Despite the video 'Look Back In Anger' failed to make any chart impact in America, where it was released in preference to 'Boys Keep Swinging'. It was never a single in Britain.

'Look Back In Anger' was performed live throughout the Serious Moonlight, Outside, Earthling and Heathen tours, a fine version being included in the BBC radio session of 18 September 2002. Following Bowie's significant makeover of the song for his ICA benefit performance in July 1988, a new seven-minute studio version was recorded with lead guitar by Reeves Gabrels (his first recording with Bowie) and Erdal Kizilcay on drums and bass. This version later appeared as a bonus track on *Lodger*.

LOOKING FOR A FRIEND
• Live: *Beeb*

'Looking for a Friend' received its first public airing as part of Bowie's BBC session on 3 June 1971, at which David shared vocals with Mark Carr Pritchard. This version, which now appears on *Bowie At The Beeb*, is the only recording of the song to have received an official release. A superior 3'15" studio version was recorded at Trident on 17 June by the short-lived Arnold Corns (see *Hunky Dory* in Chapter 2). Intended as a single, this version remained unreleased until 1984 when the Scandinavian Krazy Kat label issued an unofficial 12" of all four Arnold Corns recordings. Lead vocal on the studio version is taken by Freddi Burretti, demonstrating a convincingly swishy relish as he tackles the song's less than subtle subtext: "Been trolling too long, been losing out strong for the strength of another man." With barrelling piano, mincing handclaps and a singalong chorus, the Lou Reed demi-monde of 'Waiting For The Man' (note the obvious titular similarity) crosses paths with the satin and tat of 'Queen Bitch' in one of Bowie's most overtly gay lyrics. The guitars of Trevor Bolder and Mick Ronson are unmistakable in the mix, but lead guitar is almost certainly played by Mark Carr Pritchard. The lyric of the Arnold Corns version differs slightly from the other recordings, substituting the line "I'm pretty as a picture, oh so nice, hoping that you might call" in place of "With a mirror on your backside face-to-face with the spaceman on the wall".

'Looking for a Friend' was still in Bowie's live repertoire at the Aylesbury gig of 25 September 1971, and at around the same time it was re-recorded during the early *Ziggy Stardust* sessions. However, unlike some of its Arnold Corns bedfellows the song was not destined for glory. The ragged and non-committal 2'12" *Ziggy* demo is wholly inferior to the Arnold Corns version, which is one of the most deliciously wonderful Bowie rarities to be found on the bootleg circuit.

LOOKING FOR LESTER
• Album: *Black* • B-Side: 10/93 [40]

The spunky jazz trumpet of Lester Bowie is the defining sound of *Black Tie White Noise* and this instrumental, in which the two Bowies chase each other's riffs on trumpet and saxophone, is at the album's musical heart. It's a sophisticated slice of techno-jazz whose title, Bowie admitted, is borrowed from John Coltrane's 'Chasing The Trane'. 'Looking For Lester' also marks the return of pianist Mike Garson, last heard on *Young Americans* and hereafter reinstated as an integral contributor to Bowie's sound. "He really

has a gift," David told *Record Collector* in 1993. "He kind of plops those jewels on the track and they're quite extraordinary, eccentric pieces of piano playing."

LOOKING FOR SATELLITES (*Bowie/Gabrels/Plati*)
• Album: *Earthling* • US Promo: 1997

In August 1996, shortly before the commencement of the *Earthling* sessions, the world's press erupted with reports that possible traces of life had been detected on Mars. As well as guaranteeing airplay for a certain track in Bowie's back catalogue, the news both enthralled and appalled David. "The idea that there's formed ice on the other side of the moon, and that there are water patterns on some of the planets, I think that's scintillating," he remarked later. "It absolutely, definitely points to life. Oh, what would we *do then*?" 'Looking For Satellites', the second *Earthling* track to be recorded, taps into a story which for a few weeks had held the world's collective breath, pondering not so much the nature of alien life as the human ramifications of discovering its existence: "Where do we go from here? / There's something in the sky … Who do we look to now?"

The shuffling backbeat recalls the ambient funk of the previous album's 'I Have Not Been To Oxford Town' but here, courtesy of one of Bowie's most beautiful chord progressions, the atmosphere is one of wistful uncertainty rather than chilly inevitability. The background textures are unified by a repetitive vocal cut-up which underscores the track like a mantra, creating a phonetic rather than a textual resonance. "I used words randomly," David explained, "'Shampoo', 'TV', 'Boy's Own', whatever I said first, stayed in." He described the song as "a straight, rational piece about where we find ourselves at this particular point in this era: somewhere between religion and technology, and not quite sure where to go next. It's kind of a poignant feeling, standing alone on a beach at night looking for a satellite … but what you're really looking for is an answer." In *Alien Encounters* magazine he added, "It's as near to a spiritual song as I've ever written: it's measuring the distance between the crucifixion and flying saucers."

'Looking For Satellites' features a remarkable contribution from Reeves Gabrels, whose intricate, fuzzy guitar solo builds to an extraordinary climax. "I didn't think the song should have a solo and David insisted," Gabrels later revealed, "So what you're hearing is me being pissed off that I had to put a guitar solo in a song that I thought shouldn't have one. After it I left the room, got a cup of coffee and thought that it might have been one of the best things I have ever done." David explained that "I told him I only wanted him to play on one string at a time. He had to stay on the low E string until the chord changed, then he could go up to the A. When it changed again he could go to the D. He was hemmed in by the chord until it changed, and that made his run-up most unorthodox. He just loved it." Gabrels continues: "When I got to the section where I was supposed to stop, I just thought, 'Fuck this!' and broke out of the rule, playing through the chorus ... Because of the restriction David put on me, it has a nice developmental curve, even though I'm overplaying. It has a nice orgasmic release."

A radio-friendly edit appeared as a promo in America, but plans to release the track as a single (with an unheard Mandarin vocal version as the B-side) were abandoned – to the disappointment of Mike Garson, who considered it the best track on the album. The song was performed at Bowie's fiftieth birthday concert and throughout the Earthling tour.

LOOKING FOR WATER
• Album: *Reality* • Live Video: *Reality*

'Looking For Water' appears initially to be one of *Reality*'s more straightforward rock numbers, laying Earl Slick's discordant guitar squeals over a repetitive descending bassline and a metronomic drum figure. Not for the first time on *Reality*, there are strong echoes of *Never Let Me Down*: the rhythmic and melodic phrasing, not to mention the hypnotic reiteration of the song's title, strongly recall the "Mummy come back cause the water's all gone" chorus of 'Glass Spider'.

However, the direct musical attack is offset by one of *Reality*'s most intriguing lyrics. The bleakness of 'The Loneliest Guy' appears to have transmuted into wholesale post-9/11 nihilism ("I lost God in a New York minute / Don't know about you but my heart's not in it"), but the underlying anger of the song is quite new. "I think probably it must have something to do with the Middle East," Bowie deadpanned disingenuously when asked about the lyric in 2003. "When I wrote it, I just had this image of somebody crawling through the desert looking for the water, which is the

most clichéd image that you can come up with. But then that made me think, well, the only thing he *would* be looking at would be the oil pumps. And the oil pumps seem to be working, but there is no water. This must be about a military, industrial situation – a complex of some kind. It must be about an administration that has a manifesto that was probably written in the late nineties that's being carried through now. That's kind of what was on my mind."

As if to seal the lyric's ironic broadside against American foreign policy, 'Looking For Water' also contains the first of two references on *Reality* to "the dawn's early light" which, as well as being a line from Mort Shuman's translation of 'Amsterdam', is of course a quotation from the opening line of 'The Star-Spangled Banner'.

'Looking For Water' initially made only rare appearances on A Reality Tour, becoming a more frequent fixture on the repertoire during 2004.

LOUIE, LOUIE GO HOME (*Revere/Lindsay*)
• B-Side: 6/64 • B-Side: 9/78 • Compilation: *Early*

The B-side of Bowie's first single, originally pencilled in as the A-side, is a cover version of an obscure track by Paul Revere & The Raiders, whose own 1960 debut had been a cover of Richard Berry's better-known 'Louie Louie'. The Raiders' 'Louie, Go Home' (as they called it) appeared in 1964 as a self-penned follow-up. To confuse matters further, 1964 was the year that The Kingsmen's hit version of the original 'Louie Louie' transformed the song from a mildly influential R&B standard into a notorious *succès de scandale* and the subject of a ludicrous FBI investigation. But that's another story.

'Louie, Louie Go Home' by Davie Jones with The King Bees, a blatant *faux*-Beatles makeover to complement the A-side's Rolling Stones pretensions, was added to the band's live repertoire and later performed by The Manish Boys.

LOVE ALADDIN VEIN : see ZION

LOVE IS ALWAYS (*Giroud/Albimoor/Bowie*) : see PANCHO

LOVE IS STRANGE *(Baker/Robinson)*:
see **HELLO STRANGER**

LOVE ME DO *(Lennon/McCartney)*:
see **THE JEAN GENIE**

LOVE MISSILE F1-11 *(Degville/Whitmore)*
• B-Side: 9/03

If *Heathen*'s 'I Took A Trip On A Gemini Spaceship' had seemed an unlikely choice of cover version, then Bowie's decision to revive Sigue Sigue Sputnik's much-derided 1986 hit during the *Reality* sessions surely takes the biscuit. In its day, the original's notoriety rested on the shameless fashion in which the band had ridden a wave of hype that allowed them to sign a reputed £4 million deal with EMI and propel the flimsy glam-punk nonsense of 'Love Missile F1-11' to number 3 in the UK chart. Debate raged over whether Sigue Sigue Sputnik's media-manipulation was part and parcel of their post-ironic art (they certainly antic-ipated the antics of artists like the KLF when they included genuine commercials between the tracks on their debut album), or whether they merely represent-ed a preposterous triumph of style over content.

Either way, 'Love Missile F1-11' is a tongue-in-cheek, unashamedly trashy and undeniably enjoyable excursion into the dumbness of rock and roll, setting a watered-down posture of post-Pistols anarchy against a glammed-up rendering of an archetypal Eddie Cochran-style riff – in fact, it's not a million miles removed from 'Round And Round', the Chuck Berry song played live by Bowie during his own break-through, so perhaps the connection was always there. Certainly Sigue Sigue Sputnik's methods in 1986 closely echoed Bowie's in 1972; the difference, one suspects, was one of talent.

Bowie's entertaining cover faithfully reproduces the tinny production, low-tech synthesizers, angry guitars and stereo pyrotechnics of the original. The track was included on the CD and DVD formats of the 'New Killer Star' single.

LOVE SONG *(Duncan)*

Lesley Duncan's song, later covered by Elton John on *Tumbleweed Connection*, featured in Feathers' folkish

repertoire. Bowie recorded a 3'30" acoustic demo around April 1969, providing harmonies to a lead vocal by John Hutchinson.

LOVE YOU TILL TUESDAY
• Album: *Bowie* • A-Side: 7/67 • B-Side: 5/75 •
Compilation: *Deram* • Video: *Tuesday*

This piece of worldly-wise cynicism masquerading as a paean to free love is one of Bowie's better-known Deram tracks and boasts one of his catchiest early melodies, later to be aped note-for-note by the theme tune of the BBC game show *Blankety Blank*.

The *David Bowie* version was recorded on 25 February 1967. A second take, featuring a new vocal, a vigorous string arrangement by Ivor Raymonde and a vaudeville play-out of 'Hearts And Flowers' from Czibulka's *Winter Marching*, was recorded at Decca on 3 June 1967, two days after the album's release. It was this second version that appeared as a single on 14 July, becoming the first Bowie release to receive sub-stantially favourable reviews. *Record Retailer* called it a "mature and stylish performance which could easily make it", while *Record Mirror* added that "This boy really is something different ... I reckon it's a stand-out single. Liked it; recommend it." In *Disc*, Penny Valentine declared that "This is a very funny rather bit-ter little love song about how he'll always love her – at least for four days. His incredible sense of timing and humour come over perfectly in this record. It would be nice if more people appreciated him." *Melody Maker*'s Chris Welch positively glowed, describing Bowie as "one of the few really original solo singers operating in the theatre of British pop ... Very funny, and deserves instant recognition."

In the same paper, no less a personage than Syd Barrett reviewed 'Love You Till Tuesday' during a monosyllabic overview of the week's new releases: "Yeah, it's a joke number. Jokes are good. Everybody likes jokes. The Pink Floyd like jokes. It's very casual. If you play it a second time, it might be even more of a joke. Jokes are good. The Pink Floyd like jokes. I think that was a funny joke. I think people will like the bit about it being Monday, when in fact it was Tuesday. Very chirpy, but I don't think my toes were tapping at all." Kenneth Pitt took great exception and later described Barrett's remarks as "moronic". Interestingly, Barrett's comments were made just as his own hit single 'See Emily Play', later covered by Bowie, was storming up the charts – and only a month before *Melody Maker* reported the first attack of "nervous exhaustion" that was soon to deprive British rock of one of its brightest talents.

Even in America, where the single appeared in September, 'Love You Till Tuesday' received critical plaudits. *Cash Box* announced that "orchestrations packed with zest, a delivery with all the punch of an on-stage pub performance, and some wild lyrics should put this power-house platter high in the running for a top chart spot." Despite the unprecedented notices, the single failed on both sides of the Atlantic.

Bowie included the song in his first BBC radio session on 18 December 1967, faithfully recreating the arrangement of the single version, and performed it for German TV's *4-3-2-1 Musik Für Junge Leute* on 27 February 1968; in August of the same year it was included in his ill-fated cabaret showcase. The song also featured over the opening credits of the 1969 film *Love You Till Tuesday*, for which David mimed to the single version (now minus the 'Hearts And Flowers' coda) against a white backdrop and sporting a groovy blue suit. At Trident on 29 January 1969 he recorded 'Lieb' Dich Bis Dienstag', a German language version set to the single arrangement with lyrics translated by Lisa Busch, intended for the proposed German cut of the film.

A 3'15" demo, recorded in 1966 with Bowie accompanying himself on guitar, has appeared on bootlegs. Of particular interest is a middle-eight cut from the later versions, in which David sings "I'm the coffee in your coffee [sic], the spoon in your tea / If you've got a problem then it's probably me / I'm hiding every place that you are."

LOVER TO THE DAWN

Bowie recorded this 4'48" acoustic demo with John Hutchinson around April 1969. Blessed with the duo's customary Simon and Garfunkel-influenced harmonies, it's of immense interest as the prototype for 'Cygnet Committee'. There's none of the later song's rhythmic intensity, musical complexity or anti-hippy sentiment, the familiar opening lyrics developing instead into a furious harangue aimed, one can only assume, at the recently-departed Hermione Farthingale: "Don't be so crazy, bitter girl ... we're not just sitting here digging you." A fascinating curio.

LOVING THE ALIEN
• Album: *Tonight* • A-Side: 5/85 [19] • A-Side: 4/02 [41] • Compilation: *Best Of Bowie, Club* • Video: *Collection, Best Of Bowie* • Live Video: *Glass*

The opening track of *Tonight* perfectly summarizes the album's malaise: it's a terrific piece of songwriting, but what should be a flight of operatic grandeur is dragged from the heights by insipid, over-elaborate production, spangly synth flourishes, uninspired and now dated echo-laden drumbeats and a ridiculously polite guitar break. Bowie later admitted apologetically that the demo was far superior. Still, 'Loving The Alien' is far from being a disaster. Arif Mardin's string arrangement is epic and the lilting marimba line is a pointer to *Tonight*'s tentative embracing of world music, recalling the sight of Bowie raptly listening to a Thai percussion band in *Ricochet* not long before the sessions. David later said that the breathy "ah-ah-ah" backing vocals, reminiscent of Laurie Anderson's 'O Superman', were borrowed from Philip Glass's *Einstein On The Beach*.

The mere sight of the word "alien" has prompted many to assume that the song restates the sci-fi themes of the Ziggy period, but a moment's attention to the lyric reveals otherwise. Beneath the mild-mannered production 'Loving The Alien' is a vehement diatribe against the blinkered sanctimony of organized religion: "If you pray all your sins are hooked upon the sky / Pray and the heathen lie will disappear / Prayers, they hide the saddest view." At the time Bowie described the song as "the most personalized bit of writing on the album for me; not to say that the others were written from a distance, but they're a lot lighter in tone. That one was me in there dwelling on the idea of the awful shit we've had to put up with because of the Church. That's how it started out: for some reason I was very angry." Using the bloodshed of the Crusades as its central image, 'Loving The Alien' makes a plea for inter-denominational harmony – particularly between Christianity and Islam – and questions the motives of religious leaders. "The crunching thing about the Church is that it has always had so much power," Bowie explained. "'Alien' came about because of the feeling that so much history is wrong – as is being rediscovered all the time – and that we base so much on the wrong knowledge that we've gleaned ... It's extraordinary considering all the mistranslations in the Bible that our lives are being navigated by this misinformation, and that so many people have died because of it."

In May 1985 'Loving The Alien' was remixed and released as a single, apparently after David had come across a review of the album that suggested the track could be a hit. It was only a moderate success, stalling at number 19 despite the twin attractions of lavish packaging (the 12" included a pull-out poster), and a stunningly grandiose video. Co-directing with David Mallet, Bowie performs the song on an angular, Escher-like set alongside two bizarrely decorated backing musicians, spliced with a jumble of impressionistic shots of him walking on water, finding blood in a font, as a burning Templar, an organist rising on a Wurlitzer in front of a *Raiders Of The Lost Ark*-style fountain, and a groom in morning suit and top hat whose bride, in full Islamic dress, angrily tears the dollar bills from her clothes and discards them in a devastated wasteland. As an assault on religion's materialist edifices, its commodification of women and its culturally divisive teachings, the video is intermittently successful, although its undisciplined sprawl of ideas falls short of Bowie's finest promos. The linking image of a blue-skinned David, derived from *Tonight*'s cover artwork, is presumably a symbolic attempt to cast himself as an outsider, neither white nor black, while the bizarre lightbulb-in-mouth image hails once again from Laurie Anderson's batty 'O Superman' video. Two different edits exist, one of which excises the shots of Bowie's nosebleed.

David's wife Iman would later cite the song as "one I'm particularly fond of. It seemed to anticipate our meeting," while David himself remarked in 1993 that "What I was trying to do was set up some line of thought that surrounded the possibility of harmony between Islam and Christian peoples. Little did I know that one day I'd marry a Muslim. This must have been prophetic!" Unsurprisingly then, 'Loving The Alien' was selected by the couple for inclusion on a five-track CD packaged with early editions of Iman's 2001 autobiography *I Am Iman*.

April 2002 saw the release of an excellent club remix by New York producer The Scumfrog, credited to "The Scumfrog vs Bowie". A minor UK hit (it did rather better in the dance chart, where it peaked at number 9), the remix was accompanied by a new video in which scenes from Bowie's original clip were projected onto the walls of animated skyscrapers in an ever-shifting urban jungle. This video appeared on the enchanced CD single, while the remix was later included on *Club Bowie* and The Scumfrog's 2003

album *Extended Engagement*.

'Loving The Alien' was performed throughout the Glass Spider tour. Sixteen years later, in a timely restatement of its central notion of "the possibility of harmony between Islam and Christian peoples", the song was revived in a beautiful new acoustic arrangement for the Tibet House Benefit concert on 28 February 2003. A variation of this version, for which David was accompanied by Gerry Leonard on guitar, reappeared throughout A Reality Tour.

LUCY CAN'T DANCE
• Bonus: *Black, Black (2003)*

Beginning life in early 1988 as a demo called 'Lucille Can't Dance' (see 'Like A Rolling Stone'), this composition was salvaged with splendid results during the *Black Tie White Noise* sessions. It's one of the album's strongest numbers and might have done well as a single; Nile Rodgers tells David Buckley that it was "a guaranteed number 1 record, and everyone around [Bowie] was totally perplexed when it only appeared as a bonus track on the CD. He was running from success and running from the word 'dance'."

Rodgers may be right; although a likely hit, 'Lucy Can't Dance' may have invited accusations that Bowie was once again pandering to the mainstream. The heavily treated vocal is laid over a pulsing beat filched straight from the mid-1980s "hi-energy" fad exemplified by Frankie Goes To Hollywood's 'Relax', and the sense of 1980s nostalgia is increased by a passing reference to Madonna's 'Material Girl'. It's good, catchy, sophisticated pop, and nobody but Bowie could get away with such a preposterous couplet as "So I spin while my lunatic lyric goes wrong / Guess I put all my eggs in a postmodern song". The melody bears strong similarities with 1992's 'Real Cool World' and, particularly, 1997's 'Dead Man Walking'.

LUST FOR LIFE *(Pop/Bowie)*

The title track of Iggy Pop's 1977 album has lyrics by Iggy and music by David who, as Pop later recalled, composed it on an unlikely instrument: "David Bowie wrote that in Berlin, in front of the TV, on a ukulele." David explained that the pair would often watch the American Forces Network news, "one of the few things that was in English on the telly, and it had this great pulsating riff at the beginning of the news." According to Iggy, the riff in question was "a guy tapping out that beat on a Morse code key. Ever the sharp mimic, David picked up the nearest available instrument and started strumming."

With co-production, keyboards and backing vocals also provided by Bowie, 'Lust For Life' is usually construed as a celebration of the pair's successful clean-up during their Berlin exile: "I'm through with sleeping on the sidewalk – no more beating my brains with the liquor and drugs". This doesn't quite tally with the reality of their recreational habits in 1977, but they'd certainly come a long way since the insanity of Los Angeles. The exuberant intro, borrowing freely not just from the AFN news but from The Supremes' 1966 hit 'You Can't Hurry Love', enjoyed extensive airplay in 1996 thanks to the track's prominent use in *Trainspotting*. Following this media saturation 'Lust For Life' was released as a single, reaching number 26 in November 1996. Nobody's fool, Bowie had already incorporated a splendid new arrangement into his live set for his Summer Festivals tour.

LUV

See Chapter 6 for details of Bowie's 1969 ice cream commercial.

M.O.R. *(Blur/Bowie/Eno)* :
see **BOYS KEEP SWINGING**

MADAME GEORGE *(Morrison)*

Van Morrison's number, from 1969's *Astral Weeks*, was performed live by Hype.

MADMAN *(Bowie/Bolan)*

This unfinished collaboration between Bowie and Marc Bolan is thought to date from September 1977, when David made his guest appearance on Granada TV's *Marc* (see 'Sleeping Next To You'), although it's possible that it dates from the previous March, when he stayed with Bolan in London for a few days during the Iggy Pop tour. The demo, featuring the pair sharing vocals and guitars, has appeared on bootlegs. In

1980 The Cuddly Toys recorded a cover version (likeable enough but clearly demonstrating the sketchiness of the almost nonexistent lyric), released as a single and on their album *Guillotine Theatre*.

Several other demo collaborations said to date from 1977 (with titles coined by bootleggers) are 'Casual Bop', 'Exalted Companions', 'Companies Of Cocaine Nights', 'Skunk City' and 'Walking Through That Door'. Only the last, a discoish number swathed in falsetto vocals, is unmistakably Bowie, and is believed by some to date from his earlier rumoured collaborations with Bolan in Los Angeles in 1975.

MAGGIE'S FARM *(Dylan)*
• A-Side: 9/89 [48]

Bob Dylan's 1965 single (from *Bringing It All Back Home*) was added to Tin Machine's repertoire during the 1989 tour, restructured around the riff from Marc Bolan's 'Jeepster'. For British audiences the refrain "I ain't gonna work on Maggie's farm no more" had acquired a satisfying new resonance in recession-hit, poll-tax-looming 1989. A version recorded at La Cigale in Paris on 25 June was released as a double A-side with 'Tin Machine'. The little-seen video, shot at the previous night's Amsterdam gig, was a useful commemoration of the tour but failed to push the single any higher than number 48.

MAGIC DANCE
• Soundtrack: *Labyrinth* • US A-Side: 1/87 •
Compilation: *Best Of Bowie (New Zealand)*, *Club* •
Promo: 12/03

Bowie's first on-screen number in *Labyrinth* is a surprisingly hard-rocking workout, constructed around traditional children's rhymes and much benefiting from funky rhythm guitars and a searing electric solo. An unusual problem occurred during recording when backing singer Diva Gray's baby refused to gurgle on cue: "It really buttoned its lip," recalled Bowie, "so I ended up doing the gurgles, so I'm the baby on that track as well!"

In the film, 'Magic Dance' (referred to in the closing credits, and by Bowie during filming, as 'Dance Magic') is the cue for a full-blown Muppet showstopper, in which David dances with 48 puppets and 12 costumed extras. The nursery-rhyme lyric ("slime and snails, puppy-dogs' tails") and chorus of comic goblin voices bring back distant memories of another notorious song, revealing a strand of continuity in Bowie's work that is seldom acknowledged. "I never thought in twenty years I'd come back to working with gnomes!" he laughed at the time. The "Power of voodoo / Who do? / You do" patter which underscores the song is an old playground nonsense-chant originally popularized by Cary Grant and Shirley Temple in the 1947 film *The Bachelor and the Bobbysoxer*; but intriguingly, the melodic "I saw my baby…" opening suggests a more sinister throwback to Iggy Pop's original version of 'Tonight'.

'Magic Dance' was remixed for a 12" release in America, Italy and Spain, making full use of Dan Huff's muscular middle-Eastern guitar break. A 4'09" single edit was prepared for radio play in various territories, but this got no further than the promo stage; oddly, this mix appeared on the New Zealand edition of 2002's *Best Of Bowie*, while the following year's *Club Bowie* featured a new 'Danny S Magic Party Mix', which also appeared on a 12" promo alongside the otherwise unavailable 'Magic Dust Dub'.

MAID OF BOND STREET
• Album: *Bowie*

Recorded on 8 December 1966, the quietly superb 'Maid Of Bond Street' features a vaudeville piano, acrobatically syncopated vocals and a typical Deram-era lyric of frustrated lives blighted by London's cruel underside, where celebrity and surface show are the only guarantors of success. Like 'Little Bombardier', the lyric contains one of Bowie's earliest references to the fantasy of cinematic glamour as a panacea for drab lives: "This girl, her world is made of flashlights and films / Her cares are scraps on the cutting-room floor". Perhaps because of its parochial references, the track was left off the American release of *David Bowie*.

MAKE UP *(Reed)*

Co-produced by Bowie for Lou Reed's *Transformer*, 'Make Up' publishes a virtual manifesto for the gay following that had gathered around the pair: "Gowns lovely made out of lace, and all the things that you do to your face … Now we're coming out, out of our closets, out on the streets." At the time, Reed explained

that "The gay life at the moment is not that great. I wanted to write a song which made it terrific, something that you'd enjoy. But I know if I do that, I'll be accused of being a fag; but that's all right; it doesn't matter. I like those people, and I don't like what's going down, and I wanted to make it happy."

MAN IN THE MIDDLE
• B-Side: 8/72

The most obscure of the Arnold Corns recordings (see *Hunky Dory* in Chapter 2) was cut at Trident on 17 June 1971. The backing is an indifferent slab of sub-*Man Who Sold the World* hippy rock not unlike the original take of 'Holy Holy', but Mick Ronson provides a superb solo while vocalist Freddi Burretti, clearly under Bowie's tutelage, attempts a pleasant enough impression of Lou Reed. Of greater interest is the lyric, a dummy-run for the androgynous alien superstar character towards whom David was rapidly groping his way: "He is a symbol of a new age, he glides above the realms of you and me … His gowns come from Paris, occasionally from Rome, he can go anywhere, except back to his home … He's the man in the middle, you can't tell which way he lays…" Speaks for itself, really. 'Man in the Middle' became the B-side of the group's second single in 1972. Bowie received the sole songwriting credit, although he has recently intimated that the song was in fact co-written with guitarist Mark Carr Pritchard.

THE MAN WHO SOLD THE WORLD
• Album: *Man* • B-Side: 6/73 [3] • A-Side: 11/95 [39]
• Live: *Beeb*

A top ten hit for Lulu in 1974, and memorably covered by Nirvana in their 1993 *Unplugged* set (during which Kurt Cobain spoke of "the debt we all owe David"), 'The Man Who Sold The World' has become a familiar title in the roll-call of Bowie classics – even if many people still seem unaware that he actually wrote it. "In America especially," David commented ruefully in 2000, "when I do 'The Man Who Sold The World', the amount of kids that come up afterwards and say, 'It's cool you're doing a Nirvana song.' And I think, 'Fuck you, you little tosser!'" Certainly the song's many high-profile cover versions have tended to obscure Bowie's original recording which, with its sinister percussion, circular guitar riff and ghostly vocal, achieves an unassuming air of pathos and menace far in advance of its subsequent imitations. Tony Visconti recalls that David's vocal was recorded at Advision on the very last day of mixing *The Man Who Sold The World*.

Like most of his work of the period Bowie has kept his counsel about the song, although he did once remark that it might have been unfair to unload it onto Lulu because it dealt with the "devils and angels" within himself (for her part Lulu later confessed she "didn't know what it meant"). In 1997's *Changes-NowBowie* documentary he revealed that "I guess I wrote it because there was a part of myself that I was looking for ... that song for me always exemplified kind of how you feel when you're young, when you know there's a piece of yourself that you haven't really put together yet – you have this great searching, this great need to find out who you really are."

This anxious grapple with the elusiveness of identity has led many to conjecture that the song was triggered by David's family troubles. The opening lines ("We passed upon the stair, we spoke of was and when / Although I wasn't there, he said I was his friend") evince a sinister echo of Hughes Mearns' famous nursery rhyme *The Psychoed*: "As I was going up the stair / I met a man who wasn't there / He wasn't there again today / I wish, I wish he'd stay away." Bowie compounds the identity crisis by claiming that he himself "wasn't there", while he thought his companion "died alone, a long, long time ago". The effacement of the individual and dread of mortality provide grim counterpoints to the immortal anguish of 'The Supermen' and the meditations on "impermanence" and "rebirth" in 'After All'. David only chose to name the album after this song at the very last minute, and it's been suggested that the title partly reflects an element of self-loathing over the question of "losing control" and "selling" his private life via such profoundly personal music.

In their biography, the Gillmans suggest another poetic model in Wilfred Owen's war poem 'Strange Meeting', whose narrator enters a mystical dreamscape to meet the enemy soldier he killed in battle. Certainly there's a persuasive correlation between "He said I was his friend ... I thought you died alone" and "I am the enemy you killed, my friend".

The album cut became a B-side in 1973 (for 'Life On Mars?' in Britain, and for 'Space Oddity' in America, Australia and Europe), but the song only really entered the public consciousness when Bowie produced Lulu's hit cover version. He had first encountered the singer at 1970's *Disc & Music Echo* Awards ceremony, and after meeting again during the final Ziggy tour David invited her to the "Last Supper" at the Café Royal. "We started talking about the possibility of working together," he explained later. "I was keen to get something fixed up, because I really have always thought that Lulu has incredible potential as a rock singer. I didn't think this potential had been fully realized ... we decided on 'The Man Who Sold The World' as being most suitable." Having laid down backing tracks and Lulu's vocals during the *Pin Ups* sessions at the Château d'Hérouville, Bowie added saxophone overdubs at Morgan Studios in Willesden, shortly before work commenced on *Diamond Dogs*. "I used the Pin Ups line-up to back her, including Ronson and drummer Aynsley Dunbar," Bowie recalled in 2002, "and played the sax section on overdubs. I still have a very soft spot for that version, though to have the same song covered by both Lulu and Nirvana still bemuses me to this day."

Boasting a prominent Bowie saxophone solo and backed by her cover of 'Watch That Man', Lulu's version was released in January 1974 and reached number 3 in the UK, where its substantial airplay included a television performance for which Lulu devised "an androgynous look" in charcoal suit, tie and gangster hat which bore a remarkable resemblance to the future Thin White Duke's wardrobe. "Bowie loved that look," said Lulu later. Rumours persist of a longer edit, possibly featuring a heavier vocal contribution from David. The pair would go on to record unreleased versions of 'Dodo' and 'Can You Hear Me'.

Lulu's version of 'The Man Who Sold The World' later appeared on her 1977 album *Heaven And Earth And The Stars*, and latterly on the 1994 compilation *From Crayons To Perfume – The Best Of Lulu*. Nirvana's cover appeared on their 1994 album *Unplugged In New York* and on 2002's *Best Of Nirvana*. The countless other covers include versions by Richard Barone (on 1987's *Cool Blue Halo*), No Man (on 1990's *Whamon Express*), Ed Kueffer (on 1995's *Exotic Mail Order Moods*), Simple Minds (on 2001's *Neon Lights*), and Midge Ure (on the 12" format of 1985's single 'If I Was', and later on a reissue of that year's album *The Gift* as well as on *David Bowie Songbook*).

Bowie himself has revived the song on a number of occasions, including the superb version in his *Saturday Night Live* set recorded in December 1979.

The Outside tour's radical trip-hop revamp was commemorated by an excellent studio recording, mixed by Brian Eno for release as a double A-side. "It sounds completely contemporary," Eno recorded in his diary on 30 October 1995, the day he mixed the track at Westside Studios: "I added some backing vocals and a sonar blip and sculpted the piece a little so that there was more contour to it." An acoustic rendition, closer to the original, appeared during Bowie's Bridge School benefit appearances in October 1996, and again for his BBC session for *ChangesNowBowie*. The live trip-hop version continued to crop up on the Earthling tour, while a superb recreation of the original arrangement, complete with phased vocal effects, was included on the summer 2000 tour, from which a live version recorded at the BBC Radio Theatre on 27 June 2000 was included on the *Bowie At The Beeb* bonus disc. A similarly faithful arrangement reappeared throughout A Reality Tour.

MAN WITHOUT A MOUTH
(Gutter/McNaboe/Zoidis/Albee/Roods/Ward)

Bowie sings backing vocals on this dark, edgy funk-rock number which closes the Rustic Overtones' *Viva Nueva*. His vocals were recorded in July 1999, on the same day as his more substantial contribution to 'Sector Z'. "He listened only once, then asked if I had three spare tracks left on the multitrack tape," explained Tony Visconti. "Within minutes he was in front of the microphone, and he started to sing a very haunting backing vocal. Afterwards he triple-tracked it. It was so perfect, that he could think of lines like that! He was finished in only twenty minutes." In February 2000, eighteen months before the album's delayed release, 'Man Without A Mouth' appeared on a limited-edition promo EP, and cropped up again a year later in the soundtrack of the film *Attraction*.

MARIA *(Bernstein/Sondheim)* :
see **THE JEAN GENIE**

MARS, THE BRINGER OF WAR *(Holst)*

The Lower Third's 1965 live shows usually culminated in a hard-rock rendition of 'Mars, The Bringer Of War' from Gustav Holst's *The Planets*, forever enshrined for

David's generation as the theme tune of *Quatermass*, Nigel Kneale's famous sequence of futuristic thriller serials screened by the BBC between 1953 and 1959. "David wanted to make it terrifically powerful, with World War Two sirens and explosions," recounted The Lower Third's drummer Phil Lancaster.

Many years later David would describe the original serial, 1953's *The Quatermass Experiment*, as "tremendous", recalling that he watched it "from behind the sofa when my parents thought I had gone to bed. After each episode I would tiptoe back to my bedroom rigid with fear, so powerful did the action seem to me. The title music was 'Mars, The Bringer Of War', so I already knew that classical music wasn't boring."

The popular impact of *Quatermass* in an age before *Star Trek* and *Doctor Who* is now difficult to recall. Kneale's postwar re-readings of HG Wells rooted the fantastic in 1950s suburbia, becoming a national talking-point and penetrating deep into the public consciousness. Their influence on Bowie's enduring sci-fi *shtick* cannot be underestimated; more than one childhood acquaintance has told biographers that *Quatermass* was second only to *The Flowerpot Men* as David's favourite television show. The *Quatermass* stories were founded on a compassionate juxtaposition of man's loneliness and spiritual hunger with his newly-acquired capacity to obliterate himself, apocalyptic themes which remained central to Bowie's lyrics throughout the 1970s. Elements of the mood and content of the serials trickle through his early work, from the Major Tom-like lost astronaut of *The Quatermass Experiment* to the portentous, *Quatermass II*-like advent of the 'Starman' and "the strange ones in the dome" who populate 'Drive In Saturday'. Bowie's dabblings in older mythologies during the *Station To Station* period echo the primeval rationale granted to the ascent of black magic, Kabbalistic symbols and racism in the third serial *Quatermass And The Pit*. For those willing to seek out the original serials (and for all their technical naivety, the television episodes are far superior to the subsequent cinema versions), the associations are legion.

MARY ANN *(Charles)*

Ray Charles's 1956 B-side was played live by The Manish Boys.

MASS PRODUCTION *(Pop/Bowie)*

Produced and co-written by Bowie for Iggy Pop's *The Idiot*, this is a frighteningly bleak slab of manic depression whose ambient atmospherics and woozy synthesizers prefigure Bowie's imminent *Low*. According to Iggy, the lyric was suggested by Bowie: "He just said, 'I want you to write a song about mass production,' because I would always talk to him about how much I admired the beauty of the American industrial culture that was rotting away where I grew up. Like the beautiful smoke-stacks and factories – whole cities devoted to factories."

MAYBE *(Barrett)*

The Chantels' 1957 US hit was included in David's medley with Cher on *The Cher Show* in November 1975...

MAYBE BABY *(Hardin/Petty)*

...as was The Crickets' 1958 hit.

MEMORY OF A FREE FESTIVAL
• Album: *Oddity* • A-Side: 6/70 • Live: *Beeb*

Bowie's valediction to his short-lived hippy summer initially looks like an unqualified eulogy for the Woodstock generation. The childlike melody and the album version's low-tech arrangement evoke a doped-out atmosphere reinforced by some open drug references – "someone passed some bliss among the crowd" is hardly ambiguous, while the opening reference to the children who "gathered in the dampened grass" is a neat prepositional pun allowing two distinct readings. The hallucinatory space-trips and references to the Buddhist ideal of satori (sudden enlightenment) are very much of a piece with David's 1969 worldview, and in selecting it as *Space Oddity*'s closing track, he told *Disc & Music Echo* that he intended to "...go out on an air of optimism, which I believe in. Things will get better. I wrote this after the Beckenham festival when I was very happy."

But the story behind 'Memory Of A Free Festival' is rather less straightforward. It commemorates the open-air event staged by the members of Growth,

Bowie's Beckenham Arts Laboratory, on 16 August 1969 (see Chapter 3), mid-way through the *Space Oddity* sessions and just a few days after the death of David's father. The twist, undoubtedly exaggerated in some quarters, is that sources have attested to the fact that David's disposition on the day couldn't have been further removed from the sentiments expressed in the song. Apparently he spent the festival quarrelling with his friend Calvin Mark Lee and future wife Angela, calling her and friend Mary Finnigan "materialistic arseholes" when he spotted them counting money they'd raised selling hamburgers and psychedelic posters. Later that year Bowie would tell journalist Kate Simpson that the attitudes of many of his contemporaries were "hypocritical ... They're striving like mad for some kind of commercial success ... I've never seen so many dishonest people in my life." Tune-in, turn-on hippies he dismissed as "so apathetic, so lethargic. The laziest people I've met in my life."

Thirty years later David admitted that "I think I stomped off in a temper tantrum at the end of the day, but I certainly turned it around by the time I came to write the song, because I felt, well, the idea of it was great, so I'll write about the idea more than anything else." While his low spirits at the festival might very understandably be put down to his father's funeral only five days earlier, there was a palpable reality in Bowie's sense of disillusion with what he considered the low ideals and flimsy convictions of the hippy movement. His anger would find a fuller expression in *Space Oddity*'s blistering 'Cygnet Committee', but on closer inspection the popular reading of 'Memory Of A Free Festival' as a hippy panegyric simply doesn't stand up. The lyric systematically undermines "the ecstasy that swept that afternoon" as a falsehood buoyed up by drugs and simplistic slogans, and his estimation of the festival as "ragged and naïve, it was heaven" is surely a deliberate exposure of the paradox rather than a celebration of it. Hence "We claimed the very source of joy ran through / It didn't, but it seemed that way", and hence the yearning "to capture just one drop" of the ideal in a real, grown-up world, rather than in a stew of dope. Like 'Cygnet Committee' it's an assertively retrospective song with past tenses in nearly every line; it's Bowie's end-of-project report on the failure of the Beckenham Arts Lab, a "Memory" about "the summer's end". Mary Finnegan's dismissal of the song as "sheer hypocrisy" reveals merely that she thinks it's about getting stoned and kissing people. It isn't; it's the close of a chapter and, in its evocation of spacecraft and "tall Venusians", a furtive taste of things to come.

The original album version was recorded at Trident not long after the event, David himself playing the shaky psychedelic intro on a Rosedale electric chord organ. He was joined by a motley crew of acquaintances to track and multi-track the hypnotic closing mantra of "The Sun Machine is coming down, and we're gonna have a party", a sequence echoing the singalong playout of The Beatles' 'Hey Jude' which Bowie had tacked onto his demo of 'Janine' a few months earlier. Among those lending their vocal talents to this section were The Rats' vocalist Benny Marshall, future Sony vice-president Tony Woollcott and, believe it or not, rising Radio 1 stalwart "Whispering" Bob Harris and his wife Sue, who had befriended David the previous year.

What Tony Visconti would later describe as a "terrible" version of 'Memory Of A Free Festival' was recorded during Bowie's BBC session on 5 February 1970; cut down from 6'40" to just over three minutes for the broadcast, this admittedly rather ropey version, in which David seems a little unsure of the lyrics, now appears on *Bowie At The Beeb*. Two months later, just before *The Man Who Sold The World* sessions, a tighter and more energetic re-recording was made at the express request of Mercury in America, who believed the song had stronger hit potential than the UK single 'The Prettiest Star'. In March Mercury's Robin McBride had written to Tony Visconti with detailed suggestions regarding the new version, asking him to "consider the possibility of picking up the tempo" and to "come to the *sun machine* take out lines at approximately two minutes and twenty seconds into the record … it is very important that we have a short mix in order to give us the maximum opportunity for radio exposure." Recording, produced by Visconti, took place at Advision on 3, 14 and 15 April. It was drummer John Cambridge's last Bowie engagement, marking the end of the Hype line-up. The timing problems that had concerned McBride were overcome by editing the track as a two-part single, the B-side consisting of the closing "Sun Machine" chant. Even so the A-side ran to four minutes, and like its predecessors on both sides of the Atlantic the single, released on 12 June, was a flop, selling no more than 240 copies across America by the end of its first month.

The single version, later included on 1990's *Space Oddity* reissue, is often held to be Mick Ronson's first appearance on a Bowie recording, but it appears this is not the case (see 'Wild Eyed Boy From Freecloud').

'Memory Of A Free Festival' was played live between 1969 and 1971, and was briefly revived as part of a medley with 'Quicksand' and 'Life on Mars?' for a few UK dates in May 1973. During the Philly Dogs tour a *Young Americans*-style gospel makeover became the standard closing number of the The Garson Band's support set.

In June 1990 E-Zee Possee scored a minor hit with 'The Sun Machine', an uninteresting dance-trance single on which the closing refrain of 'Memory Of A Free Festival' was sung over a house piano. The idea was repeated with greater success in 1998 by Dario G's top 20 hit 'Sunmachine', this time sampling Bowie from the original version and featuring a guest appearance by Tony Visconti on recorder. An eccentric folk/rap hybrid version of 'Memory Of A Free Festival' by 1 Giant Leap was premiered on the main stage on the closing night of 2002's Glastonbury Festival with an accompanying film; recorded and mixed over the preceding three days, it included live contributions from various acts at the festival, including Badly Drawn Boy and members of Faithless and Spearhead, and was intended as a tribute to the event's history.

MIRACLE GOODNIGHT
• Album: *Black* • A-Side: 10/93 [40] • Bonus: *Black (2003)* • Video: *Black, Best Of Bowie*

Constructed around an infectious five-note synthesizer bleep, which in Bowie's words "just keeps coming and coming", 'Miracle Goodnight' is a breathless vow of love which, as a mark of its romanticism, breaks at one point into a full-blown rearrangement of Handel's *The Arrival of the Queen of Sheba*. It's perhaps the most unabashed love song Bowie has ever produced: "I love you in the morning sun, I love you in my dreams, I love the sound of making love, the feeling of your skin, the corner of your eyes…" David Buckley reports that the insistent riff is identical to the night chorus of Balinese frogs, and although this might seem a ludicrous proposition, we know that David has holidayed on Bali several times, notably during his honeymoon with Iman immediately prior to the *Black Tie White Noise* sessions – so it's not impossible.

'Miracle Goodnight' performed disappointingly as the third *Black Tie White Noise* single – released ahead of the album, it could well have been a major hit. Matthew Rolston's quite brilliant video shuffles images of Bowie in a Harlequin costume (shades of 'Ashes To Ashes') and playing the fool as a latter-day Buster Keaton (to whose physical characterizations David had expressed a debt as long ago as the 1970s), against shots of him suavely unaffected by a bevy of busty women. There are playful mirror-images and split-screens, and even an image of David as Eros. The effect is of a little boy bashfully declaring his love; it's very endearing and certainly among Bowie's most undervalued videos. A selection of out-takes and mishaps from the shoot appear at the end of the *Black Tie White Noise* documentary, which also features a superfluous second video directed by David Mallet.

THE MIRROR

Written and performed by David during the 1967 production *Pierrot In Turquoise*, 'The Mirror' survives as a 1'26" demo made for the 1970 TV adaptation *The Looking Glass Murders*. The opening lyric, "Wash your face before the faded make-up makes a mark", sounds like an uncannily prescient mission statement for Bowie's future career.

MISS AMERICAN HIGH

This unreleased track was apparently recorded during the *Toy* sessions in 2000.

MISS PECULIAR : see HOW LUCKY YOU ARE

MIT MIR IN DEINEM TRAUM *(Bowie/Busch)* : see WHEN I LIVE MY DREAM

MODERN LOVE

• Album: *Dance* • A-Side/B-Side: 9/83 [2] • Compilation: *S+V (2003)* • Video: *Collection, Best Of Bowie* • Live Video: *Glass*

The opening track of *Let's Dance* epitomizes the album: bursting with energy, brilliantly performed and undeniably catchy, but depressingly superficial by comparison with practically anything Bowie had

recorded before. Lyrically it establishes the album's recurring theme of conflict between "God and Man" in a secular world, but the attempts of some to interpret the title (and the opening line "I catch a paper boy") as a restatement of sexual ambiguity fail to convince.

Tony Visconti considered 'Modern Love' one of the best tracks on *Let's Dance*, but despite its gleaming production it's a number that has not worn well. Almost buried in the mix, Rob Sabino's boogie-woogie piano gives the song its best moments, but it's the wall of cacophonous drums and honking saxophones which sets the template for the mid-1980s. David later revealed that the song's ancestry lay in his earliest rock hero: "When I do my little call-and-response things on songs like 'Modern Love', it all comes from Little Richard." The track was a favourite of the album's producer Nile Rodgers, who described it in 1983 as "an old barrelhouse rocker with a real pounding Little Richard-type piano, while on top it has a very sophisticated jazz horn sound."

An edited version became the third *Let's Dance* single, successfully following 'China Girl' to number 2 in Britain (it was held off the top by Culture Club's million-seller 'Karma Chameleon'), while in America it made number 14. The B-side was a live version recorded in Montreal on 13 July 1983, which made its CD debut 20 years later on 2003's *Sound + Vision* reissue. The video, directed by Jim Yukich, was a composite of performance shots filmed on 20 July in Philadelphia. By the time of the single release Elton John's astonishingly similar-sounding 'I'm Still Standing' was already riding high in the chart, although both tracks were recorded around the same time and any malice aforethought seems unlikely.

'Modern Love' became a staple final encore (rather cheesily allowing David to "wave bye-bye" to the crowd as per the lyric) for the Serious Moonlight, Glass Spider and Sound + Vision tours, later making the occasional appearance on A Reality Tour. It also featured in Bowie's Live Aid set in 1985, while in 1987 a new duet version with Tina Turner was used as the soundtrack of the pair's little-seen Pepsi commercial (see Chapter 6). In 2001 tribute artist Jean Meilleur performed a classically orchestrated version on his Jeans'n'Classics tour, while teen idol Aaron Carter performed 'Modern Love' back-to-back with 'Let's Dance' on his 2003 Jukebox tour.

MOMMA'S LITTLE JEWEL *(Hunter/Watts)*

Produced by David for Mott The Hoople's *All The Young Dudes*. Listen carefully and you can hear Bowie overriding a mishap with the words, "No, don't stop – carry on!"

MOON OF ALABAMA *(Brecht/Weill)*:
see **ALABAMA SONG**

MOONAGE DAYDREAM
• A-Side: 5/71 • Album: *Ziggy* • Live: *David, Motion, SM72, Beeb* • Bonus: *Man, Ziggy (2002)* • B-Side: 2/96 [12] • Live Video: *Ziggy*

If the opening and closing tracks of *Ziggy Stardust* are the album's framework, then 'Moonage Daydream' is surely its keystone. The opening thunderbolt of guitar cuts rudely across the fade-out of 'Soul Love' (and yet, brilliantly, maintains its tempo), plunging the listener headlong into the morass of sleazy sex and surreal science fiction that occupies the album's heart. Three tracks in, and here at last is Ziggy Stardust, proclaiming himself an exotic hybrid of rock's past and mankind's future: "an alligator", "the space invader", "a mama-papa" and "a rock'n'rollin' bitch". Occasionally during the Ziggy Stardust tour (as captured on *Santa Monica '72*), Bowie introduced 'Moonage Daydream' as "a song written by Ziggy", and at various times it's been cited as the album's best track by Trevor Bolder, Woody Woodmansey and producer Ken Scott.

Although irrevocably linked to Ziggy, 'Moonage Daydream' began life several months earlier. Bowie recalls having already written the song by February 1971, but the earliest extant version is a recording by the short-lived Arnold Corns (see *Hunky Dory* in Chapter 2). This cut, taped at London's Radio Luxembourg Studios in April 1971, became the group's first single the following month and later appeared (without the spoken "Whenever you're ready" intro) as a bonus track on *The Man Who Sold the World* and on the 2002 *Ziggy Stardust* reissue. It sorely lacks the *Ziggy* version's lightness of touch, suffering from a ponderous arrangement and David's strained attempt at an American rock'n'roll vocal, complete with a gauche whoop of "Come on, you mothers!" Although both lyrics and delivery would be

massively improved, the essential Americanism remains in the definitive *Ziggy* version, recorded at Trident on 12 November 1971. 'Moonage Daydream' continues the album's systematic plundering of the American rock idiom, replete with abbreviations ("comin'", "'lectric", "rock'n'rollin'") and phrases like "busting up my brains", "freak out", "far out" and "lay the real thing on me". What to Bowie was still the distant glamour of America is here invested with a literal sense of alienness. Consciously or not, the hotchpotch of opening images recalls some of rock's American antecedents: Bill Haley's 'See You Later, Alligator', The Mamas And The Papas, the "rock-'n'rollin' bitch" Little Richard, perhaps even the 1958 Sheb Wooley/Jackie Dennis hit 'Purple People Eater', which David once recalled "was big on my agenda" when, as an 11-year-old, he had first discovered American music. Only one album later, his long-awaited fulfilment of the American Dream would alter the frame of his songwriting forever.

According to Ken Scott the unison playing of baritone sax and piccolo in the song's instrumental break also derived from Bowie's youth: "He'd heard it on an old Coasters record, loved the sound, and made it clear that was what he wanted." David has said the inspiration was actually The Hollywood Argyles' 'Sure Know A Lot About Love', the B-side of their hit 'Alley Oop'. The strings over the final fade were orchestrated by Mick Ronson, but the swirling phased effect was Scott's idea during the mixing stage.

Another vital ingredient is Mick Ronson's spectacular guitar solo, arguably his finest on a Bowie recording and long renowned among guitarists as an all-time classic. Like many of Ronson's moments of genius, it was improvised after Bowie had conveyed the mood he wanted by the most unconventional of means: David explained in 2002's *Moonage Daydream* book that he would "literally draw out on paper with a crayon or felt-tip pen the shape of a solo. The one in 'Moonage Daydream', for instance, started as a flat line that became a fat megaphone type shape, and ended as sprays of disassociated and broken lines. I'd read somewhere that Frank Zappa used a series of drawn symbols to explain to his musicians how he wanted the shape of a composition to sound. Mick could take something like that and actually bloody play it, bring it to life. Very impressive."

'Moonage Daydream' was included in the BBC radio session recorded on 16 May 1972 (a superb version which later appeared on *Bowie At The Beeb*), and featured throughout the Ziggy Stardust tour. Early on the first UK leg an accompanying video was shot by Mick Rock: "That was the first video I ever did with David," he recalled in 1998. "It was shot on a Bowlex 16mm camera in April of 1972. It was a collage of live footage. I can't remember if it's ever been publicly shown, but I'm sure that at some point in the not-too-distant future it will get seen." 'Moonage Daydream' reappeared on the Diamond Dogs tour, and latterly on the Outside, Earthling and Heathen tours. A live version recorded on 13 December 1995 appeared on the 'Hallo Spaceboy' single, while a previously unreleased remix by Alan Moulder, originally heard in a 1998 commercial for Dunlop tyres, was included on the 2002 reissue of the *Ziggy Stardust* album.

Cover versions have been released by numerous artists including Terrorvision, Racer X, Patti Rothberg (on her 2001 album *Candelabra Cadabra*) and 10,000 Maniacs (as a medley with 'Starman'). Mick Ronson retained it in his solo repertoire during the 1970s, and a live tribute version by The Spiders From Mars, fronted by Joe Elliott, appears on the album of 1994's *Mick Ronson Memorial Concert*.

MOSS GARDEN (Bowie/Eno)
• Album: *"Heroes"*

Elsewhere on *"Heroes"* Bowie sings about being "under Japanese influence", and 'Moss Garden' consolidates his long-time fascination with a country he had first visited as Ziggy Stardust. Here he plucks an evocative koto over a soft backing of synthesizer atmospherics that phase from speaker to speaker, suggesting the sound of distant aeroplanes. In the 1980s Bowie's taste for Japanese gardens would extend as far as creating one at his Mustique hideaway. The love affair would continue with 'Crystal Japan', and the gentle ambient textures of 'Moss Garden' itself would be recalled on 1993's *The Buddha Of Suburbia* and 1999's 'Brilliant Adventure'.

THE MOTEL
• Album: *1.Outside* • Live: *liveandwell.com*

With a title redolent of Hitchcock's *Psycho* (presumably intentionally, given *1.Outside*'s subject matter), this long and complex track lurks unobtrusively at the album's heart and repays attention as arguably its finest moment. It's a favourite of pianist Mike Garson, who tells David Buckley that "It's probably in [Bowie's] top ten songs ever." Bowie's funeral vocal is mournfully tugged along by weeping guitars, Garson's melancholic piano and a shuffling drumbeat reminiscent of 'Five Years', burning a slow fuse towards a final orgiastic explosion of feedback. It invites comparison with the *Diamond Dogs* classic 'Sweet Thing', and the lyrics, with a similar refrain of "boys", are about as cheerful: "Explosion falls upon deaf ears, while we're swimming in the sea of shame / Living in the shadow of vanity, a complex passion for a simple man / There is no hell like an old hell…" The last line, repeated throughout the song, is a lift from The Walker Brothers' 'The Electrician' (from 1978's *Nite Flights*, whose title track Bowie had already covered), and may also refer to David's 1994 visit to the Guggin psychiatric hospital in Austria, where he later explained that in the wing "where all the psychos and murderers live … the only thing written on the wall is 'THIS IS HELL'." According to *1.Outside*'s sleeve notes, 'The Motel' is "To be sung by Leon Blank", the young murder suspect in the narrative's art-crime investigation.

'The Motel' was performed live during the European legs of the Outside and Earthling tours, and reappeared throughout A Reality Tour. A version recorded in Amsterdam on 10 June 1997 appeared on *liveandwell.com*, introduced by David as "a love song to desperation." The original version reappeared on the soundtrack album of the 2001 film *Intimacy*.

MOTHER (Lennon)

In 1973 *Rock* magazine recorded the spectacle of Bowie sitting by an open fire at the Château d'Hérouville, listening intently to John Lennon's anguished 1970 single during a break in the *Pin Ups* sessions. Twenty-five years later, in August 1998, Bowie recorded a cover of 'Mother' for a tribute album being assembled by Yoko Ono. Following the abandoned 'Safe', 'Mother' saw the continuation of Bowie's long-awaited reunion with producer Tony Visconti. "It was a good excuse for us to get back into the studio," said David. "In fact we were looking for a project to do together, and this song, completely autonomously, seemed to fit. We didn't want to run the risk of doing a whole album and then discovering after three songs that there was no more current between us. And it worked very well, to the point that we are going to work together again in the near future." Another reunion for the 'Mother' session was with drummer Andy Newmark, whose last Bowie credit had been 1974's Philly Dogs tour, and the recording also featured backing vocalist Richard Barone and keyboard player Jordan Ruddess. Ono's tribute album was originally intended for release in October 2000 to mark Lennon's sixtieth birthday, but at the time of writing it remains unreleased.

MOTHER, DON'T BE FRIGHTENED (Gillespie)

Co-produced and arranged by David for Dana Gillespie's *Weren't Born A Man*.

MOTHER GREY

Abandoned at the demo stage in early 1968, this little-known song later became the subject of a copyright dispute with Essex Music (see 'April's Tooth Of Gold').

MOVE ON
• Album: *Lodger* • B-Side: 8/80 [1]

'Move On' consolidates the theme of wanderlust spread across the first side of *Lodger*. Its reputed working title 'Someone's Calling Me' discloses a special poignancy, for here Bowie contemplates his own restless shifting from country to country and, in the process, creates a metaphor for his musical backpacking. He considers many of the environments that have informed his work throughout the 1970s – including Cyprus, the former home of Angela Barnett which he had visited at the beginning of the decade – but particularly prominent are the scenes of his Kenyan safari and Kyoto Christmas of 1978: "Africa is sleepy people, Russia has its horsemen / Spent some nights in old Kyoto, sleeping on the matted ground." Here, at the height of Bowie's new Europeanism, America is noticeable by its absence – except, perhaps, in his recently perfected pseudo-Elvis baritone, which suits the song perfectly.

In 1979 Bowie described 'Move On' as "blatantly romantic", and revealed that the backing track was another reminder of his own musical heritage. Evidently he had been playing some of his old tapes on the studio Revox: "I accidentally played one back-

wards and thought it was beautiful. Without listening to what it was originally, we recorded the whole thing note-for-note backwards, then I added vocal harmonies with Tony Visconti. If you play it backwards, you'll find that it's 'All The Young Dudes'."

MOVING ON

Little is known about this track except that it was recorded in Los Angeles in May 1975 at the tail-end of an abortive session with Iggy Pop, who had been attempting to assemble a solo album with the assistance of ex-Stooges James Williamson and Scott Thurston. Bowie hired the four-track Oz Studio, where early versions of 'Sell Your Love' (later featured on Iggy's *Kill City*) and two new songs, 'Drink To Me' and 'Turn Blue' (later revamped on *Lust For Life*) were attempted, but neither David nor Iggy was in the best of conditions in mid-1975 and the sessions were unproductive. Williamson later recalled Bowie being at the height of his "stick insect paranoia", while Iggy was permanently the worse for drink and drugs. After the session collapsed, Bowie remained in the studio and improvised 'Moving On' on acoustic guitar. On finishing it, he is said to have complained, "Another song; that's the last thing I need." Any connection with the *Lodger* track 'Move On' is pure supposition.

MUSIC IS LETHAL (Battisti/Bowie)

Bowie's English lyrics for this cover on Mick Ronson's *Slaughter On 10th Avenue* tellingly bridge the gap between Jacques Brel's 'Amsterdam' and his own 'Rock'n'Roll Suicide', a connection which Ronson seems implicitly to acknowledge in his instrumental arrangement and vocal delivery. Bowie pens a melodrama of drunken bar-fights, "mulatto hookers, cocaine bookers, troubled husbands, stolen freedoms" and sexual redemption, themes common in his work as *Diamond Dogs* loomed large.

MY DEATH (Brel/Shuman/Blau)
• Live: *Motion*, *SM72*, *Rarest* • Live Video: *Ziggy*

With 'Amsterdam' already established as a popular number during the early Ziggy concerts, Bowie struck gold when he elected to co-opt a second Jacques Brel composition, the doom-laden melodrama 'My Death', into The Spiders' repertoire. Blessed with a poetic but free English translation by Mort Shuman and Eric Blau, Bowie's version was unveiled for the Rainbow Theatre shows in August 1972 and thereafter became an eagerly anticipated live highlight. Versions of the early acoustic guitar rendition, recorded in September and October of 1972 respectively, appear on *RarestOneBowie* and *Santa Monica '72*.

On 17 January 1973 Bowie performed 'My Death' alongside 'Drive In Saturday' on LWT's *Russell Harty Plus*. Legend has it that a guitar string broke during the actual performance, but in fact this mishap occurred during camera rehearsals. For the 1973 tour, the addition of a romantic Mike Garson piano arrangement transformed 'My Death' from a softly-strummed acoustic number into a full-blown torch song, as recorded on *Ziggy Stardust: The Motion Picture*. The torrid romanticism, existential bleakness and high dramatics of 'My Death' perfectly suited the style and subject matter of the *Ziggy Stardust* and *Aladdin Sane* compositions, eloquently underlining their debt to Brel's chanson tradition. As recently as 2003, Bowie described 'My Death' as "very important to me as a song."

'My Death' was revived for the Outside tour in a magnificent full-blooded orchestration, although one of the finest performances was a stripped-down version accompanied only by Mike Garson on piano, which Bowie performed at a private charity function on New York on 18 September 1995. The song reappeared occasionally on the Earthling tour's American leg.

MY WAY (François/Thibault/Revaux/Anka) :
see EVEN A FOOL LEARNS TO LOVE

THE MYSTERIES
• Album: *Buddha*

The longest track on *The Buddha Of Suburbia* is also the most reminiscent of Bowie's Berlin period: a long, ambient instrumental, devoid of percussion and relying instead on a droning glissando of synthesizer sound overlaid with plaintive hints of acoustic guitar and Erdal Kizilcay's reverse-tracked keyboard. Bowie explained that "the original tape was slowed down, opening up the thick texture dramatically and then Erdal would play the thematic information against it."

The minimal, magnificent result is a staggering artistic *volte face* from a man who was still performing with Tin Machine only eighteen months previously.

THE MYTH (Bowie/Moroder) :
see CAT PEOPLE (PUTTING OUT FIRE)

NA NA HEY HEY (KISS HIM GOODBYE)
(Carlo/Frashuer/Leka) : see HEAVEN'S IN HERE

NATURE BOY (Ahbez)
• Soundtrack: *Moulin Rouge*

Bowie recorded two versions of Eden Ahbez's haunting classic (originally a US hit for Nat King Cole in 1948, and subsequently covered by the likes of Frank Sinatra, Sarah Vaughan, Dinah Shore, John Coltrane and Bobby Darin) for use in Baz Luhrmann's 2001 film *Moulin Rouge*, which adopts as its central motif the song's final line: "The greatest thing you'll ever learn is just to love and be loved in return". Although both of Bowie's recordings appear on the soundtrack album, only the first version features in the film itself, and very fleetingly at that: it's heard in the background in a couple of scenes while Ewan McGregor's character sits at his typewriter. 'Nature Boy' is sung more prominently in the film by John Leguizamo and, later, by McGregor himself. The picture's composer Craig Armstrong explained that "It's a very interesting, opaque piece of music, and the more we worked on it, the more that song became Ewan's theme."

With its spine-tingling Bowie vocal (recorded in New York by Tony Visconti) and a lavish orchestral arrangement by Craig Armstrong, the solo version which opens the soundtrack album is the more conventional of the two recordings. The second version, credited to David Bowie and Massive Attack, closes the album and substitutes a more laid-back vocal over a sophisticated dub backing. Bowie recorded the second vocal in New York in February 2001, and the mix was completed in London by Massive Attack's Robert "3D" Del Naja. "It's slinky and really mysterious," David later commented. "3D has put together a riveting piece of work."

NEEDLES ON THE BEACH
(Bowie/Gabrels/H.Sales/T.Sales)
• Compilation: *Beyond The Beach*

This instrumental out-take from the Australian *Tin Machine II* sessions, distinguished by twanging Shadows-style guitar work of the kind previously heard on 'Prisoner Of Love', remained unreleased until 1994's Various Artists compilation *Beyond The Beach*. According to Reeves Gabrels, "The title came as a reference to surf music combined with the fact that we kept finding used needles on the beaches. Simple explanation really. Plus, two of the chord changes come from Hendrix's 'Third Stone From The Sun' where he says, 'We'll never listen to surf music again.'"

NEIGHBORHOOD THREAT *(Pop/Bowie/Gardiner)*
• Album: *Tonight*

Originally on Iggy Pop's *Lust For Life*, with co-production, piano and backing vocals from Bowie, 'Neighborhood Threat' was re-recorded for *Tonight* in 1984. This is a rare instance of Bowie's version actually boasting a heavier, rockier guitar line than Iggy's, although it lacks the original's doom-laden percussion and wall-of-sound atmospherics. Even so, 'Neighborhood Threat' kicks like nothing else on *Tonight* and provokes a surprisingly fierce vocal out of David, who was nonetheless displeased, describing it as "a disastrous recording" as early as 1987. "That's one I wish I'd never touched, or at least touched differently," he told *Musician* magazine. "It went totally wrong. It sounded so tight and compromised, and it was such a gas doing it. It was the wrong band to do it with – wonderful band, but it wasn't right for that song. I had this huge bunch of people and it just made the whole thing claustrophobic, tightened the whole thing up and it sounds squeaky."

NEUKÖLN *(Bowie/Eno)*
• Album: *"Heroes"*

One of the bleaker instrumental soundscapes on *"Heroes"* is this chilly lament for a displaced people. "Neuköln is an area of Berlin which is primarily Turkish and I had to work out a way of putting a Turkish modal thing into it," explained Bowie in 1983 – hence his plaintive squalls of saxophone, picking out evocative Middle Eastern figures against oppressive European blasts of bass and synthesizer. The impression is of a culture struggling to retain its identity in a cold land far from home, and the morose conclusion reduces the saxophone to a succession of futile blasts and a final, dying fall. 'Neuköln' later formed the basis for the fifth movement of Philip Glass's *"Heroes" Symphony*.

NEVER GET OLD
• Album: *Reality* • Download: 11/03 • Japanese A-Side: 3/04 • Live Video: *Reality*

From low-key opening bars to resounding operatic finish, 'Never Get Old' is a classic Bowie song in the finest tradition, beginning with an echoing drumbeat and a wonderfully catchy rhythm guitar hook, building with the arrival of Mark Plati's slinky bassline, and then piling on the multi-layered "Better take care" backing vocals and an infectious synth riff before Bowie's lead vocal arrives, deploying his most appealing style in a fragile lyric that recalls the world-weary themes of *Heathen* and the depressive withdrawal of *Low* and *"Heroes"*: "I think I better go, better get a room, better take care of me", and – a key line for the *Reality* album – "I think about this and I think about personal history".

'Never Get Old' isn't quite like any previous Bowie number, but it positively bristles with echoes and inversions of the past. The "countdown, 3, 2, 1" in the first verse inevitably recollects 'Space Oddity', and the moment when "the movie gets real when the star turns round" draws us once again into Bowie's long-held fascination with the blurring of fact, fiction and glamour that informs our relationship with the silver screen. The bridge of textured synthesizers and backing vocals leading into the second verse suggests something of the Berlin albums and also of *Heathen*'s quieter moments, while "The sky splits open to a dull red skull, my head hangs low cause it's all over now" conflates the depression of *Low* with *Hunky Dory*'s sinister "crack in the sky". Best of all is the triumphant, pile-driving chorus in the full-blown '"Heroes"' tradition, with a little of the melody of 'Crack City' even making a return visit. Here, as in 'New Killer Star', the anxiety of the verse appears to be blown away by a blast of optimism, but this time it's an optimism that is at best ironic and at worst deluded. The repeated insistence that "I'm never ever gonna get old" runs counter to the dignified acknowledgements of age found elsewhere on *Reality* and *Heathen* – and, of course, it runs counter to reality itself. "I feel bitterly angry that I won't be doing all this for the rest of eternity," David remarked in 2003. "Rage, that's what you get more than anything else. You get a bit angry, because it's good down here. On one of my new songs, 'Never Get Old' – the song's ironic – there is the image of a petulant rock singer sitting in a half-darkened room saying, 'I'm not gonna get old.' I thought it was a funny image." In another interview he remarked that "It just brought a grin to my face singing it. I grow old hourly, but it was a line too good not to sing. One of my generation was going to sing it at some point, so I thought I'd do it."

Television viewers in France were among the first to receive a sneak preview of *Reality* when, as early as June 2003, 'Never Get Old' appeared as the backing music in a TV commercial for Vittel mineral water. Bowie appeared in the commercial himself, which was filmed in his friend Julian Schnabel's New York apartment. As David moves from room to room he encounters various *alter egos* played by Bowie tribute act David Brighton: Ziggy Stardust, the 'Ashes To Ashes' pierrot, the Thin White Duke, the 'Rebel Rebel' pirate, the long-haired 'Man Who Sold The World', and even a CGI animated rendering of the *Diamond Dogs* sleeve image. The inherent irony of the lyric was apparently lost on the makers of the commercial, who understandably chose to accentuate the optimistic angle: taking his trusty bottle of Vittel from the fridge, Bowie runs down the stairs and steps out into the street, as if symbolically leaving his past behind him, while the voiceover adds the appropriate slogan: "Vittel – chaque jour une vie nouvelle."

Bowie later admitted that he had consented to the Vittel commercial purely to win some airplay for 'Never Get Old' on French television: "They said, 'We want you to do zis thing wiz ze Ziggy', and I said, 'Oh yeah, all right then, what do I get out of it?' 'What do you want to put in ze advert?' I said, 'Play a new song!' ... So I've got all this fantastic play over this bottle of water – it's really good!" An adulterated version of the Vittel commercial was later used in various countries to advertise *Reality* itself, while a separate mimed performance of 'Never Get Old' appeared in the *Reality* promotional film. In 2004 the song was again used for commercial purposes, this time in the form of a "mash-up" with 'Rebel Rebel' which appeared in an advert for Audi cars (see 'Rebel Never Gets Old').

'Never Get Old' was scheduled as *Reality*'s second single to coincide with Bowie's UK tour dates in November 2003, but in a repeat of the previous year's 'Slow Burn' saga, the European release was shelved at the last minute. Promo CDs of the 3'40" single edit backed by 'Waterloo Sunset' immediately rose in value, while in Britain the proposed release was replaced by a downloadable "cyber-single" of the two tracks, available from the Sony Music UK site. As an added incentive to purchase the download, buyers were entered into a draw to win a framed gold *Reality* presentation disc, engraved to the winner and signed by David. A conventional CD single was released the following year in Japan.

'Never Get Old' established itself as a reliable mainstay of A Reality Tour, usually receiving a rapturous response from the crowd. And quite right too: it's not only one of the best songs on *Reality*, but one of the best songs Bowie has ever written.

NEVER LET ME DOWN (Bowie/Alomar)
• Album: *Never* • A-Side: 8/87 [34] • Video: *Collection, Best Of Bowie* • Live Video: *Glass*

By virtue of its unaffected simplicity, 'Never Let Me Down' is among the strongest material on this over-wrought album. Although heralded by the familiar machine-gun percussion, it settles down via Bowie's impressive harmonica solo into a softer, rhythm guitar-led style reminiscent of Bowie's erstwhile muse John Lennon: "That owes an awful lot to John," he admitted at the time. The obvious model is 'Jealous Guy', whose plaintive whistling solo Bowie replicates in a self-portrait of an emotionally battered loner sustained by the "soul revival" of his supportive companion – a more substantial development of the earlier 'Without You'. "'Never Let Me Down' is a pivotal track for me," David said in 1987. "I don't know if I've written anything quite that emotive of how I feel about somebody." He dedicated the song to his long-time personal assistant Coco Schwab, fuelling the rumours already flying that the pair were about to marry. They weren't, David calmly denying that it was that sort of relationship, but the song bears touching witness to Ms Schwab's role in saving him from "falling to pieces" during darker times.

That the album was promptly named after this last-minute addition suggests that its refreshing spontaneity was more to Bowie's taste than the prevailing overproduction. The song was conceived in the last days of the sessions, as David Richards and Bob Clearmountain were mixing at New York's Power Station. "David came in one day and said he had a great idea for a new song," Richards explained. "Studio A just happened to be free. So we flew down in the elevator to start recording in the other room, leaving Bob on the third floor to mix 'Zeroes'. We already had a drum track from a song that had been abandoned in Montreux, and after David had sung over this, it already sounded fantastic. By eleven o'clock that night, Carlos [Alomar] had been in to add some guitars and Crusher [Bennett] some percussion." Bowie later credited Alomar with overlaying the chord sequence: "I had a basic chord change I wanted to use, but it sounded ponderous and funereal. I gave it to Carlos, and he did something with it." Alomar later revealed that the chords originated from an abandoned song of his own called 'I'm Tired' – hence his co-writing credit. Of the finished track, Bowie admitted to being "…very pleased with it. It was literally written and recorded overnight, whereas most of the others took a few weeks to put together and arrange. It was completely finished in twenty-four hours from the beginning of the writing to the end of the arranging."

As the album's third single 'Never Let Me Down' peaked at 34 in the UK, faring better in America, where it reached number 27. The video was directed by Jean-Baptiste Mondino, who had made his name in 1985 with Don Henley's 'The Boys Of Summer' and Sting's 'Russians', and would later direct Madonna's controversial 'Justify My Love'. "That's an experiment," declared Bowie prior to filming. "I'm really putting myself in his hands … I think if I did it, it would be very abrasive, and I'm not quite sure if that's how I want the song to come off visually." Years ahead of its time (indeed Bowie later noted that "it has a very sort of nineties look to it"), Mondino's video beautifully captures the song's dreamlike quality, with sepia-tinted shots of sleepy couples at an American "dance marathon" straight from Sydney Pollack's 1969 melodrama *They Shoot Horses, Don't They?*. The spoken preamble ("Put on your red shoes and dance to your heartbeat!") harks back to an earlier hit.

The song was performed on the Glass Spider tour.

NEW ANGELS OF PROMISE *(Bowie/Gabrels)*
• Album: *'hours…'*

This dissonant, stately track revisits Bowie's Berlin period, its oblique lyric resurrecting the visions of alien supermen who people his earlier work. Lyrically it recalls 'Sons Of The Silent Age' ("we are the silent ones … take me to the edge of time"), even borrowing a snatch of the melody for "I am a blind man, she is my eyes". With some late-Beatles vocal harmonies and a lyrical nod to Presley's 'Suspicious Minds', there are time-travelling echoes of earlier musical trends. As suggested by the variant lyrics in the CD inlay, the song (originally called 'Omikron') features heavily in the *Omikron* computer game, for which a shorter 2'23" edit forms the introductory music.

A NEW CAREER IN A NEW TOWN
• Album: *Low* • B-Side: 2/77 [3]

The title of this beautiful instrumental suggests a statement about Bowie's creative resettlement in Berlin; in fact 'A New Career In A New Town' was recorded in France during the early stages of the *Low* sessions, but what seems important is the transitional nature of the music. There's an engaging friction between, on the one hand, everything David's harmonica solo suggests about Stateside authenticity and R&B roots, and on the other, the shiny, robotic pulse of a particularly Kraftwerk-esque synthesizer backing: the opening electronic percussion is a straight lift from the title track of 1975's *Radio-Activity*. Over 25 years after the release of *Low*, 'A New Career In A New Town' made its live debut on the Heathen tour, subsequently reappearing on A Reality Tour.

NEW KILLER STAR
• Album: *Reality* • DVD A-Side: 9/03 •
Italian/Canadian A-Side: 9/03 • Live Video: *Reality*

The opening track of *Reality* kicks off the album in style, its initial bars of woozy treated guitar fleetingly recalling the gentle beginnings of *Heathen* before Earl Slick's crackling riff blasts into life. 'New Killer Star' reclaims the swaggering guitar style beloved of classic mid-1970s albums like *Diamond Dogs* (texturally its closest relative in the Bowie canon is perhaps the guitar jam that bridges 'Sweet Thing' and 'Rebel Rebel' on that album), while also recalling some of the 1990s work of Blur, whose album *Think Tank* was championed by David at the time of the *Reality* sessions and whose 1999 single 'Coffee + TV' is readily recalled in the lolloping riff. An influence rather closer to home, although it's one that many Bowie fans will prefer to overlook, is 1987's much-pilloried *Never Let Me Down*. The production of *Reality* is far superior and the execution more heartfelt and successful, but in terms of melody and style there's no denying the close similarity with, in particular, "87 And Cry' (the line "A new killer star" revisits the melody of "It couldn't be done without dogs", while the "ready, set, go!" section recalls the yell of "'87 and cry!" in the earlier song).

Lyrically 'New Killer Star' sets out *Reality*'s stall as an album of modern, urban angst: if *Heathen*'s apparent echoes of 9/11 were coincidental, here they assuredly are not. The album's opening line – "See the great white scar over Battery Park" – cannot help but conjure up memories of the pall of smoke that hung over Ground Zero after the terrorist attacks. "The ghost of the tragedy that happened there is reflected in the song," David told *Performing Songwriter*, "but I'm trying to make something more positive out of it. The birth of a new star." In another interview he explained that "The lyrics weren't really reflections of 9/11 itself, but on the state of New York as it is at the moment, the scattered pieces, the idea of collecting things back together, and is it worth trying to keep a community going, or do we kind of disperse at this point in time?" Hence the first verse's advancement of a dogged optimism, of accentuating the positive in the face of adversity, as Bowie sings "But I won't look at that scar" and instead suggests, in Irving Berlin's time-honoured response to trouble ahead, "Let's face the music and dance". "I use it as the cliché it is," David said of the quotation, "from those old Fred Astaire movies or whatever – 'Well, times can be real bad, but we'll work our way through this.' Because it brings all that luggage with it."

As if to lend these optimistic sentiments an up-to-the-minute validation, a month before the release of *Reality* Bowie witnessed something of New York's social cohesiveness during the devastating power blackout, reckoned to be the biggest in history, that crippled a large area of America's Eastern seaboard in August 2003. "A hard black line was scored through the history of New York on 9/11," Bowie said. "It really has changed everything in this culture. Even in the most subtle ways. I was amazed at the way New Yorkers came together during the blackout. That was absolutely unprecedented. I think the last time was in about 1977 and I wrote a song called 'Blackout' because I was there then as well. I remember burnings, looting, it got very nasty. But this time around everybody was looking out for everybody else. It was extraordinary. There was no looting. Normally it's rule number one, there's a blackout, all the alarms are off, loot. But this time was extraordinary. There is definitely a sense of community here that there wasn't before."

The second verse touches on another familiar Bowie theme: pop culture's trivialization of the search for profundity and meaning. The absurdity of "seeing Jesus on *Dateline*" recalls some of the bleaker images in 'I Can't Read' and 'Goodbye Mr. Ed', while the opening lines of the verse establish the argument at the heart of the *Reality* album: "See my life in a comic / Like the way they did the Bible / With the bubbles and action / The little details in colour". This usurpation of the "real" by the counterfeit, the dumbing-down of experience into the banality of a comic strip, opens the door onto many of the album's later lyrics – and also expresses very neatly what the cover artwork is all about.

But the radical shift is withheld until the chorus, as the song itself undergoes a change from minor to major key and the lyrics grasp at a sudden optimism: "I got a better way – I discovered a star!" This, as Bowie explained to *Interview* magazine, is the key to the song and to its position on *Reality*: "I led off the album with that song because I realized that if I opened with the wrong track, it would set the album up as being negative, which it is not. The one thing I tried to muster all the way through was a sense of positivism. 'New Killer Star' is built around a rather corny idea – that in all our troubles, there are things that are clear and bright and beautiful. It's a very simplistic thought, decorative in a way because there's a bit of wordplay in there." Nowhere is this wordplay clearer than in the song's punning title: the multiple meanings of the word 'star' have provided the mainspring for numerous other Bowie songs (this is indeed the seventh Bowie composition to feature the word in its title), but when David sings "new killer", he's also replicating the increasingly prevalent dumbed-down mispronunciation of "nuclear" whose most celebrated exponent is George W Bush.

'New Killer Star' was accompanied by Bowie's first full-blown video since 1999's 'Survive'. Directed by the Los Angeles-based filmmaker and animator Brumby Boylston, erstwhile creative director of the cutting-edge animation company Humunculus, the 'New Killer Star' clip is notable for several unusual features, not least the absence of David Bowie himself. Presented in a lenticular style akin to the original sleeve of the *'hours...'* album, the video consists of a succession of still images which simulate movement as each frame "rotates" through different angles. This initially jarring effect gradually builds into a curious impression of narrative coherency as the images flit from one wobbly snapshot to another: a shoeshine boy, a call girl, a factory foreman, railroad construction workers, gardeners and airline stewards go about their business as the sun rises over the patchwork fields, white picket fences and power-stations of a kitsch, idealized 1950s America; eyes gradually turn skyward as an astronaut's space capsule narrowly avoids crashing to earth; disaster is averted, and all returns to normal. Without a doubt one of the oddest pop videos ever made, it left many fans bemused – but it provides a striking demonstration of Bowie's commitment to the new, even at a time when his enthusiasm for singles in general and videos in particular appeared to be on the wane.

The 3'42" 'New Killer Star' video was released as a DVD single in the UK, US and various other territories on 29 September 2003, its DVD-only status disqualifying it from the singles chart. Meanwhile in Canada and Italy the album version of 'New Killer Star' was released as a conventional CD single. Both formats were backed by the cover of Sigue Sigue Sputnik's 'Love Missile F1-11' recorded during the *Reality* sessions, while the DVD single also included the four-minute *Reality* EPK featuring interview footage and performance clips from the *Reality* promotional film. The sleeve photo was a close-up from a Frank Ockenfels photo of David playing his 1956 Supro guitar. The top half of the same photo would later form the CD sleeve of the 'Never Get Old' promo single, allowing the two to fit seamlessly together.

As *Reality*'s debut single, 'New Killer Star' received extensive airplay during the round of TV appearances to promote the album and tour, including performances on, among others, *Friday Night With Jonathan Ross* and *The Late Show With David Letterman*. For the first seven nights of A Reality Tour 'New Killer Star' was the opening number, before being relegated to second place for many of the subsequent shows.

NEW YORK TELEPHONE CONVERSATION
(Reed)

Co-produced by Bowie for Lou Reed's *Transformer*, this black comedy was salvaged from an abandoned 1968 Broadway musical planned by Andy Warhol. Bowie can be heard in the background, ghosting Reed's vocal an octave higher.

NEW YORK'S IN LOVE
• Album: *Never*

This strong contender for the *Never Let Me Down* wooden spoon is a duff space-filler which makes a half-hearted stab at a prosopopoeic rendering of New York City as a living character, observing the comings and goings in her own streets. David called it "a rather sarcastic song about New York, that real vain aspect of big cities. They're so pompous and big and in love with themselves." Instrumentally it veers between poppy synthesizers and tough guitar breaks, offering a foretaste of the impending sound of Tin Machine, and there's an unsuccessful attempt to recapture the racketing work-out funk of 'Red Sails' or 'It's Hard To Be A Saint In The City' towards the end. The song was performed on the first seven shows of the Glass Spider tour.

NEXT *(Brel/Schuman)*

Jacques Brel's classic, later famously covered by Alex Harvey, was performed by Feathers.

NIGHT TRAIN *(Washington/Simpkins/Forrest)*

This blues classic was played live by The Manish Boys; a version appears on James Brown's 1962 LP *Live at the Apollo*, much admired by David at the time. On 1997's Earthling tour Bowie would occasionally call "All aboard the Night Train!" during 'Little Wonder'.

NIGHTCLUBBING *(Pop/Bowie)*

Produced and co-written by Bowie for Iggy Pop's *The Idiot*, this composition is decidedly more David than Iggy, wallowing in the metronomic *motorik* rhythms and menacing synthesizers soon to spill forth on *Low*. Iggy Pop later remarked that "Bowie and I really just brought out the best in each other. 'Nightclubbing' was my comment on what it was like hanging out with him every night." Only Iggy could deliver quite such a superbly sleazy lead vocal, but David can clearly be heard singing along in the background.

"We had the idea on the last day of recording," Iggy Pop recalled many years later. "The musicians had all packed everything away, some of them had already left on the plane. Coco Schwab came in armed with two ugly plastic masks. Bowie put one on for a laugh and sat down at the piano and played some old Hoagy Carmichael stuff. I went in and told him, 'That's it, that's exactly what I want.' I wrote the lyric in ten minutes and we recorded the song with a lousy drum machine. Bowie kept on saying. 'But we gotta call back the drummer, you're not gonna have that freaky sound on the tape!' And I replied 'Hey, no way, it kicks ass, it's better than a drummer.' I always encouraged him to express the darkest and most deranged part of his art. Bowie helped me with some of the lyrics and said, 'Why don't you write a description of walking through the night like ghosts?'"

Among several well-known cover versions of 'Nightclubbing' are those by Grace Jones (who named an album after it), The Creatures and The Human League, while Iggy's original enjoyed a revival in 1996 after its appearance in *Trainspotting*.

1984

• Album: *Dogs* • Live: *David* • Compilation: *S+V* • Bonus: *Dogs (2004)*

One of Bowie's favourite tracks from *Diamond Dogs* and the song that was to herald his next change of musical direction, '1984' began life as the signature number of his planned adaptation of George Orwell's novel. The song received its first performance at the Marquee on 19 October 1973 when, in a medley with the soon-to-be-abandoned 'Dodo', it became the opening number of NBC's *The 1980 Floor Show*. The same month saw the recording of a studio version of the medley, marking David's last session at Trident, his last with producer Ken Scott, and for nearly twenty years his last with Mick Ronson. Although slower in pace and less disco-flavoured than the later version (and with marginally different lyrics), '1984/Dodo' tentatively signals David's flirtation with the soul and

funk of Gamble and Huff's "Philly" sound. The track later appeared on *Sound + Vision* and the 2004 reissue of *Diamond Dogs*.

Not long afterwards '1984' was radically re-recorded for *Diamond Dogs*. Taken at a faster tempo, and awash with Alan Parker's crackling wah-wah guitar and a cascading Tony Visconti string arrangement, the album version betrays a heavy debt to Isaac Hayes's 1971 'Theme From *Shaft*', arguably the precursor of the entire disco movement. Despite being an obvious single if ever there was one, and released as such in America and Japan, '1984' remained an album track in Britain.

Although the uptempo arrangement and instrumental fireworks suggest a less doom-laden atmosphere, '1984' maintains the dark foreboding that dominates *Diamond Dogs*, and its succession of violent vignettes recall the psychological horror of compositions like 'All The Madmen': "they'll split your pretty cranium and fill it full of air" is a virtual rewrite of "day after day, they take some brain away". There's also a direct reference to Dylan's 'The Times They Are A-Changing' (even more explicit in the *1980 Floor Show* version, which quotes the title verbatim), while Bowie's "all-night movie role" and the portents of doom ("you've read it in the tea-leaves") recall the Armageddon foreshadowed in 'Five Years'. In keeping with the bleak *Diamond Dogs* philosophy, the only escape is to blank out "tomorrow" by "shooting up on anything".

'1984' became the opening number of the Diamond Dogs show; as the cheers on *David Live* bear witness, Bowie remained invisible until revealed in a spotlight at the end of the first verse. It remained in the Philly Dogs set, but has not been performed since. Tina Turner later covered the song on her 1984 (geddit?) album *Private Dancer*. In 2003 Bowie's original recording was included on a charity CD called *Songs Inspired By Literature: Chapter 2*, an educational fund-raiser produced by Artists For Literacy.

1917 *(Bowie/Gabrels)*
• B-Side: 9/99 [16]

Enigmatic of title, this *'hours…'* B-side builds guitars and synthesized strings over a programmed rhythm track borrowed from Led Zeppelin's 1975 classic 'Kashmir' (it's probably coincidence, but 1917 was the year in which Count von Zeppelin died!). With vocals treated to the point that they blend unintelligibly with the organic whole, '1917' boasts the steely art-rock attack of *Scary Monsters* and, moreover, successfully regains its air of mystery.

1969 *(The Stooges)*

This song from The Stooges' self-titled debut album was performed on the 1977 Iggy Pop tour. A version featuring Bowie apears on *Suck On This!*.

96 TEARS *(Martinez)*

This 1966 hit for the unusually named ? And The Mysterians was performed on the 1977 Iggy Pop tour.

NITE FLIGHTS *(Engels)*
• Album: *Black* • Promo: 1993 • Bonus: *Black (2003)*
• Compilation: *S+V (2003)* • Video: *Black*

Scott Walker remains one of Bowie's unsung heroes, rarely discussed by commentators but often cited by David with such emphasis as to leave little doubt of his abiding influence. When Radio 1's fiftieth birthday tribute *ChangesNowBowie* secured a rare message from the reclusive Walker, in which he told how David had "freed so many artists" and thanked him "for all the years, and especially for your generosity of spirit," Bowie was more audibly choked than he has ever been in a mainstream interview. After a long pause he almost sobbed: "You've really got to me there, I'm afraid. I think he's probably been my idol since I was a kid. That's very moving … that's really thrown me. Thank you very much."

In 1993 David explained that "in the late seventies Scott Walker brought out the most extraordinary album of his own songwriting – quite the most lovely songs that I'd heard in years." The album in question was The Walker Brothers' *Nite Flights*, released in July 1978 only a few weeks in advance of Bowie's *Lodger* sessions. The title track seems more than likely to have influenced that album's 'African Night Flight', but it would be another fifteen years before David covered the song itself.

Bowie's re-reading of 'Nite Flights' proved to be one of the dramatic highlights of *Black Tie White Noise*, whose Euro-disco and jazz-funk fusions are here twisted into a darker soundscape, the most evocative of the album's many echoes of Bowie's Berlin period. Lyrically 'Nite Flights' prompts Bowie towards the macabre surrealism of *1.Outside*: "The dark dug up by dogs, the stitches torn and broke, the raw meat fist you choke has hit the bloodlight…"

A mimed studio performance appears in David Mallet's *Black Tie White Noise* documentary. A week after the filming, on 13 May 1993, Bowie gave a studio performance on NBC's *The Tonight Show With Jay Leno*. 'Nite Flights' was slated as a possible fourth single from *Black Tie* but shelved after the unspectacular sales of 'Miracle Goodnight'. A 12" club promo released in 1993 contained the 'Moodswings Remix' which reappeared as a bonus track on 2003's *Black Tie White Noise* reissue and, in 'Radio Edit' form, on the same year's *Sound + Vision* repackage. The song was performed on the Outside tour.

NO CONTROL *(Bowie/Eno)*
• Album: *1.Outside*

'No Control' darkens the tone of *1.Outside* with a hard-edged synth bassline pitched somewhere between the Pet Shop Boys' bleaker moments and, of all things, Paul Hardcastle's 1985 hit 'Nineteen'. Bowie's menacing, nursery-rhyme vocal ("To be sung by Nathan Adler," according to the Outside tour brochure) conjures up memories of ancient tracks like 'After All' and 'The Man Who Sold The World', alluding to the latter's perennial Bowie anxiety about losing "control": "Stay away from the future, back away from the light / It's all deranged, no control / Sit tight in your corner, don't tell God your plans…" Middle Eastern wails of synthesizer build the atmosphere as Bowie dives into *1.Outside*'s abyss of paranoia, intellectual chaos and neo-spirituality.

'No Control' was recorded on 20 January 1995 and, according to Brian Eno's diary, was "effectively finished in the hour". Eno considered Bowie's vocal "gorgeous, mature. There's a stunning section in it where he alludes to that style of singing you get in Broadway musicals, when the hero looks up into the sun, one arm extended to the future, and sings in this gloriously open-throated, honest, touchingly trusting way … Watching him tune it to just the right pitch of sincerity and parody was one of the most fascinating things I've ever seen in a studio … It's funny that the song is called 'No Control', because this performance by him is a paradigm of control."

'No Control', which might have made a fine single, remains one of the few 1.*Outside* tracks yet to be performed live. In 1998 a rare Dutch radio promo CD featured an instrumental version backing Bowie's spoken appeal on behalf of the War Child charity.

NO FUN (*The Stooges*)

The 1969 Stooges number, later covered by The Sex Pistols, was performed on the 1977 Iggy Pop tour. A version featuring Bowie appears on *Suck On This!*.

NO ONE CALLS (*Bowie/Gabrels*)
• B-Side: 9/99 [16]

With walls of queasy synthesizer and a Kraftwerk-style robotic rhythm, this cold and disturbing B-side surprisingly resurrects a sound Bowie had embraced on mid-1980s tracks like *Labyrinth*'s 'Within You'; in fact, the resemblance to Trevor Jones's incidental *Labyrinth* track 'Thirteen O'Clock' is positively uncanny. Repetitive lyrical fragments suggest a return to the frozen, psychotic withdrawals of *Low* and 1.*Outside* ("Nobody calls, falling to pieces … nobody phones, anyone at all").

NOON-LUNCHTIME : see ERNIE JOHNSON

NOTHING TO BE DESIRED (*Bowie/Eno*)
• US B-Side: 9/95

This 1.*Outside* out-take, a B-side in America and Canada only, reprises the relentless tumbling rhythm of 'A Small Plot Of Land' and adds swathes of guitar, 'Hearts Filthy Lesson'-style backing vocals and tinkling Garson piano. Bowie repeats an endless chant of the title and the phrase "mind-changing" until, just as the track fades away, he starts quoting the German lyric of '"Helden"'. Mad, but strangely marvellous.

NOW (*Bowie/Armstrong*)

Some audiences on the 1989 Tin Machine tour were treated to this work-in-progress composition which,

although a typical Tin Machine thrash-up, would prove of no little significance five years later as the basis for 'Outside'. 'Now' was at best half-formed, beginning with a recreation of the power-chords and backbeats of the 1988 version of 'Look Back In Anger' before slipping rather clumsily into the familiar opening chords of 'Outside'. The lyrics, although sketchy, were similar to those of the later track.

O SUPERMAN (*Anderson*)

An interesting addition to the Earthling tour was a brilliant, hypnotic cover of Laurie Anderson's avant-garde classic, a UK number 2 in 1981 which appeared on her debut album *Big Science*. Lead vocal was taken by Gail Ann Dorsey, while Bowie contributed harmonies and baritone sax. "I'm doing it for Gail because I thought it would suit her," David explained. Indirectly, the idea evolved from David's stage reunion with Lou Reed in January 1997. Reed had not long embarked on his relationship with Laurie Anderson, the two appearing on each other's albums as of Anderson's Eno-produced *Bright Red* in 1994. "We knock around a lot, actually," revealed Bowie. "Laurie and my wife, Lou and myself go to the theatre and all that bourgeois stuff." In 1998 David collaborated with Laurie Anderson on *Line*, an art exhibit for the Museum Ludwig in Cologne.

AN OCCASIONAL DREAM
• Album: *Oddity*

"This is another reflection of Hermione who I was very hung up about," Bowie said in 1969, and indeed 'An Occasional Dream' covers much the same territory as 'Letter To Hermione', lamenting the march of time and recalling the "madness" of frittering away "one hundred days" until "the days of fate" caught up – now a photograph of happier hours "burns my wall with time". Bowie's obsessive fascination with the destructiveness of nostalgia and the relentless movement of time would continue to be a lynchpin of his 1970s work, perhaps most obviously in a clutch of songs on *Aladdin Sane*.

The 2'34" demo, recorded with John Hutchinson around April 1969, closely resembles the finished track save for an extra lyric sung by Hutch beneath David's lead vocal. The song was included in the BBC session recorded on 5 February 1970.

OH DARLING : see DON'T BE AFRAID

OH! YOU PRETTY THINGS
• Album: *Hunky* • Live: *Motion, Beeb* • Live Video: *Ziggy, Best Of Bowie*

Probably the earliest *Hunky Dory* track to be composed, 'Oh! You Pretty Things' was demoed at Radio Luxembourg's studios as early as December 1970. "I couldn't sleep," Bowie later said. "It was about four o'clock in the morning. I woke up and this song was going round in my head. I had to get out of bed and just play it to get it out of me so that I could get back to sleep again."

Before the song was recorded for *Hunky Dory*, a cover version was cut by former Herman's Hermits vocalist Peter Noone. Produced by Mickie Most and released in April 1971, Noone's solo debut was a number 12 hit, making it Bowie's most significant success since 'Space Oddity'. David provided backing vocals and played piano on the Noone single, which avoided potential airplay bans by changing "The earth is a bitch" to "The earth is a beast". Noone declared that "David Bowie is the best songwriter in Britain at this time … certainly the best since Lennon and McCartney, and in fairness, you don't hear so much of them nowadays … David Bowie has more than enough talent to write hit songs, automatic hit songs, for just about any kind of singer." Bowie, who played piano for Noone's performance on a long-lost edition of *Top Of The Pops*, commented: "I don't know if Peter knows what it means. It's all about Homo Superior. Herman goes heavy."

Indeed, 'Oh! You Pretty Things' belies its jaunty, stomping piano arrangement, teetering on the sinister Nietzschean brink occupied by much of *Hunky Dory*. Bowie's version is notably darker in tone than Noone's chart-friendly recording: there's a sinister element to "the Homo Superior" who drive their "Mamas and Papas insane", while "the golden ones" and the suggestion that "Homo Sapiens have outgrown their use" sound like pronouncements from the occult writings of Aleister Crowley. There's also a strong hint of Arthur C Clarke's 1953 science-fiction novel *Childhood's End*, in which an alien influence causes mankind's children to evolve into something

incomprehensible to their parents. The song's key reference, however, is to an earlier science-fiction fantasy: Edward Bulwer-Lytton's 1871 novel *The Coming Race*, in which the narrator discovers a super-advanced species of quasi-humans living in the depths of the earth. Aided by a mystical energy force called the Vril, their superior civilization has banished war, crime and inequality, and women are the victors in the battle of the sexes. At the end of the novel the narrator predicts the death of the human race at the hands of "our inevitable destroyers".

"I think," Bowie told Michael Watts in his famous coming-out interview for *Melody Maker* in January 1972, "that we have created a new kind of person in a way. We have created a child who will be so exposed to the media that he will be lost to his parents by the time he is 12." Bowie insisted that his imminent race of supermen constituted an optimistic vision: "all the things that we can't do they will." Bearing in mind his endearing fixation with bargain-basement sci-fi, it's amusing to note that "the Homo Superior" was later appropriated as the name of the young generation of telepaths in *The Tomorrow People*, Thames Television's chronically low-budget answer to *Doctor Who*, which began screening in 1973. The show's creator, Roger Price, was a fan of Bowie who had interviewed him at around the time of *Hunky Dory*, so his adoption of the term was certainly no coincidence.

"The reaction of me to my wife being pregnant was archetypal daddy – oh, he's gonna be another Elvis," David said during pre-publicity for *Hunky Dory*. "This song is all that plus a dash of sci-fi." In 1976, during a less coherent but intermittently revealing interview, he hinted at the song's darker side: "a lot of the songs in fact do deal with some kind of schizophrenia, or alternating id problems, and 'Pretty Things' was one of them," he explained. "According to Jung, to see cracks in the sky is not, is not really quite *on* … I hadn't been to an analyst, no, my parents went, my brothers and sisters and my aunts and uncles and cousins, they did that, they ended up in a much worse state, so I stayed away. I thought I'd write my problems out."

'Oh! You Pretty Things' was re-recorded for three BBC radio sessions, on 3 June and 21 September 1971 and 22 May 1972. The first of these recordings was cut from the show prior to broadcast and is now sadly lost, while the last of the three appears on *Bowie At The Beeb*. The second, from the acoustic Bowie/ Ronson session, was included as an extra track on the Japanese release of *Bowie At The Beeb*. The song also featured in Bowie's 8 February 1972 appearance on *The Old Grey Whistle Test*, offering the rare spectacle of David singing one of his songs at the piano, albeit miming to the keyboard track from *Hunky Dory*. Two takes from the *Whistle Test* session appear on the *Best Of Bowie* DVD, while a fluffed first take surfaced on BBC2's *John Peel Night* in 1999. The song featured in a few Ziggy concerts from May 1973 onwards, in a medley incorporating 'Wild Eyed Boy From Freecloud' and 'All the Young Dudes'.

ON BROADWAY (*Mann/Weill/Lieber/Stoller*)

A snatch of the Lieber & Stoller standard, a US hit for the Drifters in 1963 and covered by a host of other artists, appears in 'Aladdin Sane'.

ONE (*Nilsson*)

Harry Nilsson's 'One', a US hit for Three Dog Night in 1969, was included in David's medley with Cher on *The Cher Show* in November 1975.

ONE HUNDRED YEARS FROM TODAY
(*Young/Washington*)

As recorded by Frank Sinatra and Doris Day, this standard appeared in the 1968 Feathers repertoire.

ONE LOVE (*Marley*) :
see **DANCING IN THE STREET**

ONE MORE HEARTACHE
(*Robinson/White/Moore/Rogers*)

Marvin Gaye's 1966 single was covered live by The Buzz.

ONE NIGHT (*Bartholomew/King*)

On 16 August 2002, the final date of the Area: 2 tour, Bowie marked the 25th anniversary of Elvis Presley's death by opening his encores with a one-off performance of the Presley hits 'I Feel So Bad' and 'One Night'.

The latter, written by Dave Bartholomew and Pearl King, was first recorded in 1956 by Smiley Lewis under its original title 'One Night Of Sin (Is What I'm Praying For)'. When Elvis Presley recorded the number in 1958 his management elected to bowdlerize this unwholesome sentiment, and thus the lyric's desire became "One night with you" instead. In this form the song was a worldwide smash for Presley, topping the UK chart in 1959 and reaching number 4 in America. The famously raunchy number would later be covered by artists as diverse as Fats Domino and Mud (who stuck to the cleaned-up Presley lyrics), and Joe Cocker and Marc Almond (who didn't). Despite following the Presley version, Bowie's live rendition succeeded in sounding as suggestive as any of them.

ONE OF THE BOYS (*Ralphs/Hunter*)

Produced by David for Mott The Hoople's *All The Young Dudes*, this B-side was recorded on 14 May 1972.

ONE SHOT (*Bowie/Gabrels/H.Sales/T.Sales*)
• Album: *TM2* • European A-side: 1991 •
Live Video: *Oy*

After the early promise of 'Baby Universal' *Tin Machine II* returns to its predecessor's unlovely cock-rock instincts with this unspectacular grunge-up, outstaying its welcome with an excessively tiresome guitar break while the lyric's bitter account of a loveless liaison veers uncomfortably towards misogyny. Still, the melody is decent, Bowie's split-octave vocal continues the album's revival of his 1970s techniques, and the dynamics and mixing are a general improvement on *Tin Machine*. Although recorded separately in Los Angeles in March 1991, with engineering and production by *Tonight*'s Hugh Padgham, the track doesn't sound significantly different from the rest of *Tin Machine II*.

A remixed edit of 'One Shot' was released as a single in some mainland European territories, and was performed during the It's My Life tour.

ONLY ME

Produced by Bowie for the ill-fated Astronettes album

and eventually released on 1995's *People From Bad Homes*, this song's authorship remains in doubt.

ONLY ONE PAPER LEFT

Nothing is known about this unfinished track except that it was demoed during the *Ziggy Stardust* sessions, probably around September 1971.

ONLY YOU *(Ram/Rand)*

Originally a 1956 hit for both the Hilltoppers and the Platters, 'Only You' was included in David's medley with Cher on *The Cher Show* in November 1975.

OPENING TITLES INCLUDING UNDERGROUND : see UNDERGROUND

OUTSIDE *(Bowie/Armstrong)*
• Album: *1.Outside*

The title track of *1.Outside* triumphantly plunges Bowie back into the realm of stately, narcissistic, grandiloquent rock from which he had for so long absconded. Despite being a revamp of a Tin Machine composition (see 'Now'), and despite being recorded in early 1995 as a late addition to the album, it makes a magnificent opener. Subtitled 'Prologue' in the Outside tour booklet, the song expands the chord sequence previously used for the 1988 re-recording of 'Look Back In Anger', embellishing it with weird, Eno-inspired electronic warbles as the unhinged lyric opens up the cyclical timelessness of the album's *fin de siècle* setting and offers a taste of its brutalist vocabulary: "the crazed in the hot-zone, the mental and diva's hands, the fisting of life to the music outside…" 'Outside' was performed live on the Outside and Earthling tours, Gail Ann Dorsey often taking lead vocal on the latter.

OVER THE WALL WE GO

Those acquainted with the obscure backwaters of Bowie's work are aware that there are some songs which leave 'The Laughing Gnome' standing. 'Over The Wall We Go' is one such, and even your present guide, who can find it in his heart to praise elements of *Never Let Me Down*, has his limits.

The song was demoed in 1966, although confusion reigns over the exact date. It has been claimed that Bowie's version was broadcast on Radio London in the summer of 1966 alongside an early interview conducted at one of the Marquee's "Bowie Showboat" concerts, but this is almost certainly a misconception perpetrated by a ham-fisted bootleg which blatantly inserts Bowie's 2'44" studio demo into the authentic interview. The evidence points strongly to the demo being recorded later in the year, probably in December at the time of the *David Bowie* sessions.

As revealed by the demo, 'Over The Wall We Go' is a comic *Carry On* burlesque, reputedly inspired by a recent spate of prison break-outs. The repetitive battle-cry of "All coppers are nanas!" is set to the melody of 'Pop Goes The Weasel', while the verses hang on the tune of the traditional nursery song 'Widecombe Fair', which should give some indication of the overall tone. David affects a string of comedy voices of the kind found on the contemporaneous 'We Are Hungry Men', pulling off a startlingly accurate Bernard Bresslaw ("My name is 'Enery, some say I'm fick / I've spent 'arf me life in and out of nick") and even attempting John Lennon's Scouse drawl ("We crawled back to safety, our hearts filled with gloom / Cos we'd dug ourselves through to the smallest room"). Bowie's demo is a rough-and-ready affair on acoustic guitar and bass, peppered with references to the Christmas season which suggest he may have considered the song little more than a seasonal *jeu d'esprit*.

On 3 January 1967 Kenneth Pitt took the demo to the agent Robert Stigwood, who rejected the suggestion that it would suit novelty singer Mike Sarne (best known for 'Come Outside', his chart-topping 1962 duet with Wendy Richard), but passed it instead to a new client: Oscar Beuselinck, later to find fame as Paul Nicholas.

For the resulting single, credited simply to Oscar and released in 1967 on Stigwood's Reaction label, Bowie excised the Christmas references and replaced the Liverpudlian character with a verse which, for better or worse, stands as his first explicitly homosexual lyric. Here, however, the aim is not the mercurial gender-blurring of the Ziggy years, but pure limp-wristed innuendo direct from *Round The Horne*. Oscar rises to the occasion with a creditable impersonation of Julian and Sandy's strangulated vowels: "I'm a privileged con, so my uniform's blue / The new lads will ask me if I am a screw / I'll tell them, 'Ooh, cheeky, not even for you!'" Bowie is on hand to provide backing vocals and the voice of the prison warder.

Mercifully for all concerned, and despite a performance on Ken Dodd's ITV show *Doddy's Music Box*, the Oscar single was a flop. A 1978 re-release, this time under the pseudonym Ivor Bird, was no more successful. Oscar's version later appeared on *David Bowie Songbook*, where it should be hunted down and heard by everyone. But probably just the once.

PABLO PICASSO *(Richman)*
• Album: *Reality* • Live Video: *Reality*

Heathen's second track is a cover version of an influential number by an eccentric Boston band, and *Reality* follows suit, devoting track two to an exuberant reading of the Jonathan Richman classic 'Pablo Picasso'. Richman's original version was recorded in 1972, but shelved along with the rest of his early recordings until the release of his band's debut album *The Modern Lovers* in 1976 (by which time John Cale, who produced Richman's recording, had already included his own cover on his 1975 album *Helen of Troy*). "There was something so light and dotty about his lyrics," recalled Bowie. "The stuff he used to write was insanely comical. I just salvaged this one from the past because I always thought it was a fantastically funny lyric." In another interview he confessed that "I've always wanted to do it. It's just a treat. On *Heathen* I did a piece by the Pixies, called 'Cactus'. 'Pablo Picasso', at least the way we've done it, occupies a similar place on the album."

Showcasing Tony Visconti's virtuoso production, with a wall of squealing synthesizers underscoring slabs of guitar and wildly energetic percussion, Bowie's version supplants the minimalist deadpan of Richman's original with a faster, rockier interpretation which loses none of the original's tongue-in-cheek absurdity. Alongside some lyrical embellishments (the "Swinging on the back porch, jumping off a big log, Pablo's feeling better now, hanging by his fingernails" sequence is pure Bowie), perhaps the most flagrant addition is Gerry Leonard's stuttering Spanish guitar, a wilfully corny reminder of Picasso's nationality which serves the same tongue-in-cheek purpose as the oriental riff imposed on 'China Girl' by Nile Rodgers twenty years earlier. "Apologies now to

Jonathan Richman," laughed Bowie in 2003, "but I took the lyrics and made a song that is completely different. The original is a little dirge-like, and it's all on one note. It doesn't move much, which gives it a power, but it gives it the power of another era. I wanted to change the era and give it a more contemporary feel."

'Pablo Picasso' was performed throughout A Reality Tour.

PALLAS ATHENA
• Album: *Black* • B-Side: 3/93 [9] • A-Side: 8/97 • B-Side: 8/97 [61] • Bonus: *Black (2003)* • Compilation: *S+V (2003)*

Demonstrating that it was Bowie's unfashionable image and not his music that unfairly mitigated against him in the 1990s, when club promos of 'Pallas Athena' were released anonymously ahead of *Black Tie White Noise* the track became a hit on American dance floors. It's the first of several ambient dance instrumentals Bowie recorded in the 1990s, its fashionable club beats overlaid with a distorted vocal sample proclaiming "God is on top of it all – that's all!" Although Bowie claimed to the *NME* in 1993 that "I don't know what the fuck it's about," he is unlikely to have forgotten that Pallas Athena, who sprang from the brow of Zeus, was "the same old painted lady from the brow of the superbrain" he had evoked over 20 years earlier in 'Song For Bob Dylan'. But if the music bears any relation to Bowie's previous output, it's the second side of *Low* with an added disco beat, and in many ways this anticipates much of his remaining work of the decade. In *Arena* magazine in 1993, David's personal assistant Coco Schwab described him "grinning happily, dancing wildly all over the studio, listening to the first mix of 'Pallas Athena' – still excited after all these years..."

Bowie gave a playback performance of 'Pallas Athena' on *The Arsenio Hall Show* on 6 May 1993, and went on to perform the number on the Earthling tour, from which a live version recorded in Amsterdam was released on the *Tao Jones Index* 12" and the 'Seven Years In Tibet' CD. Various other remixes have appeared as B-sides and on 2003's reissues of *Black Tie White Noise* and *Sound + Vision*.

PANCHO *(Giroud/Albimoor/Bowie)*

Two songs, composed by Andrée Giroud and Willy Albimoor for the Belgian singer Dee Dee, were farmed out to Bowie by Essex Music in mid-1967 for English lyrics. David titled his versions 'Love Is Always' and 'Pancho', and Dee Dee's recordings duly appeared as a single in Belgium (Palette PB 25.579) on 10 June 1967, a few days after the release of *David Bowie*. David's demos of both songs, prepared to demonstrate the pronunciation of the English lyrics, still exist on tape. In 1997 a cover of 'Pancho' (about a Latin ladykiller from the wrong side of the tracks) appeared on RCA's easy-listening compilation *Another Crazy Cocktail Party*.

PANIC IN DETROIT
• Album: *Aladdin* • B-Side: 9/74 [10] • Live: *Rare* • Bonus: *Scary, Heathen*

Like most of *Aladdin Sane*, 'Panic In Detroit' was written in America during the autumn of 1972. Iggy Pop, who flew from Los Angeles to be at Bowie's Carnegie Hall concert on 28 September, apparently spent the night telling David colourful tales of the Detroit revolutionaries he had known during his youth in Michigan. Thus emerged the gun-toting Che Guevara lookalike at the centre of the lawless urban meltdown of 'Panic In Detroit'. David later cited another source, claiming that after the same gig he was astounded to meet a former classmate from Bromley Tech who had come to pay his respects: "It was somebody who I used to go to school with who ended up as a very big drugs dealer in South America. And he flew in to see one of the shows and reintroduced himself. 'I don't believe it,' I said, 'Is this what you are now?' He was the full bit, with the clothes and the piece and everything, and I thought, my God – him?"

The song was written the following month – allegedly in Detroit itself, where The Spiders played on 8 October – but the studio version was not completed until 24 January 1973, when David's vocal was laid down at the end of the *Aladdin Sane* sessions at Trident. The lyric pursues the album's brutal visions of urban America, riddled with images of violence juxtaposed with celebrity ("I asked for an autograph"), drugs ("scored", "made a run"), emotional isolation ("I wish someone would phone") and suicide ("found him slumped across the table, a gun and me

alone"). Musically, the track is a taste of things to come the following year: building on one of David's customary Bo Diddley riffs, Mick Ronson's guitar is never more bluesy than here, and there are some full-throated soul backings from Linda Lewis and Juanita Franklin.

'Panic In Detroit' was added to the live set for the 1973 US tour, although it remained a rarity in The Spiders' repertoire. It returned more prominently for the Diamond Dogs show, from which a splendid live version appeared as the 'Knock On Wood' B-side and later on *Bowie Rare*. The song reappeared on the Station To Station, Sound + Vision, Earthling and A Reality tours.

A new studio version was cut in December 1979, originally intended for broadcast on ITV's *Kenny Everett's New Year's Eve Show*. In addition to Bowie on guitar and vocals, the musicians on this recording were Zaine Griff on bass, Andy Duncan on drums and Tony Visconti (who also produced the track) on guitar and backing vocals. In the end the 1979 version of 'Panic In Detroit' was dropped in favour of the same session's acoustic re-recording of 'Space Oddity', and it eventually appeared as a bonus track on *Scary Monsters* and on the bonus disc included with initial pressings of *Heathen*. Although inferior to the original it's an interesting curio, incorporating the "Speak and Spell" toy a good three years before OMD's 'Genetic Engineering'.

Finally, an honourable mention for the theme tune of the seminal BBC kids' show *Cheggers Plays Pop*, which fused the 'Panic In Detroit' riff to Led Zeppelin's 'Whole Lotta Love' with immortal results.

THE PASSENGER *(Pop/Gardiner)*

This classic track on Iggy Pop's *Lust For Life* was co-produced by Bowie, who also plays piano and provides some unmistakable backing vocals. David had no hand in writing the song which, as Iggy later explained, was based on a Jim Morrison poem "about modern life as a journey by car." Some have seen Iggy's lyrics as a portrait of Bowie himself as the ever-observant traveller, cultural sponge and style-collector. 'The Passenger' became the B-side to the flop 'Success' single in October 1977, but became a hit in its own right after featuring in a car commercial twenty years later. Siouxsie And The Banshees' cover was a minor UK hit in 1987.

PEACE ON EARTH/LITTLE DRUMMER BOY

(Grossman/Fraser/Kohan; Davis/Onorati/Simeone)
• A-Side: 10/82 [3] • Bonus: *SinglesUS* • Live Video:
Bing Crosby's Merrie Olde Christmas

Bowie's duet with Bing Crosby was recorded at ATV's
Elstree Studios on 11 September 1977 for the fifty-
minute television special *Bing Crosby's Merrie Olde
Christmas*. Only two days earlier, David had taped his
appearance with Marc Bolan on Granada's *Marc*.
"Poor old Bing copped it as well just after I'd done this
with him," David later recalled. "I was getting seriously worried about whether I should appear on TV
because everyone I was going on with was kicking it
the following week." Crosby collapsed and died in
Madrid on 14 October.

Like the *Marc* show, *Bing Crosby's Merrie Olde
Christmas* allowed David to perform '"Heroes"' (featuring a superb new vocal and a shock reprise of
Ziggy's invisible-wall mime), but the main attraction
was his duet with the great man. Conforming to the
old-fashioned variety style so mercilessly satirized by
Steve Coogan's *Knowing Me, Knowing Yule*, the show
had Bing answering the doorbell to welcome various
celebrity visitors to his festive home. After a cosy chit-
chat about what went on in "the Bowie household at
Christmas time" (ironically, Angela Bowie's conduct
was to make Christmas 1977 one of the more turbu-
lent times in that particular residence), David invited
Bing to join him in a seasonal duet which he
described as "my son's favourite". 'Peace On Earth/
Little Drummer Boy' was every bit as saccharine as the
occasion demanded, and although it's certainly one of
the more surreal moments in Bowie's career, only the
most hard-hearted could fail to agree that it achieves
its aims with considerable charm.

"He was not there at all," Bowie told *Q* in 1999.
"He had the words in front of him. 'Hi Dave, nice to
see ya here…' And he looked like a little old orange
sitting on a stool. He'd been made up very heavily and
his skin was a bit pitted, and there was just nobody
home at all, you know? It was the most bizarre experience. I didn't know anything about him. I just knew
my mother liked him."

The show was broadcast on Christmas Eve 1977.
Five years later 'Peace On Earth/Little Drummer Boy'
was released as a Christmas single by RCA, a piece of
opportunism which did little to improve Bowie's relationship with his soon-to-be-former label. The single,
which peaked at number 3, has since appeared on

numerous Christmas compilations, although its only
official release on a Bowie collection was as a limited-
edition bonus disc with the American compilation
The Singles 1969 To 1993. An enhanced CD single featuring the video clip, released on the American label
Oglio in 1999, has been heavily imported into
Britain.

PENETRATION *(Pop/Williamson)*

Mixed by Bowie for Iggy And The Stooges' 1973
album *Raw Power*.

PEOPLE ARE TURNING TO GOLD :
see **ASHES TO ASHES**

PEOPLE FROM BAD HOMES

This obscure Bowie composition was recorded by the
Astronettes in late 1973 and eventually released on
1995's *People From Bad Homes*. It's a somewhat meandering soul-pop number propelled by electric keyboard and boasting a jaunty sax solo from David. The
lyric is less than inspiring, although the exhortation to
face down detractors ("Just stand on your own line,
stand high above") echoes 'I Am Divine' ("I walk a
fine line") and prefigures 'Golden Years' with its
injunction to "walk tall, act fine". The title was later
recycled in the lyric of 'Fashion'.

PEOPLE HAVE THE POWER *(Smith/Smith)*

Bowie provided backing vocals during Patti Smith's
rousing performances of her 1988 single (from the
same year's album *Dream Of Life*) which concluded
each of the Tibet House Benefit concerts on 26
February 2001 and 22 February 2002.

PERFECT DAY *(Reed)*

Co-produced by Bowie for Lou Reed's *Transformer*,
'Perfect Day' has taken its place in the pantheon of
classic rock ballads. Even to the uninitiated it's familiar from a dozen films and commercials, perhaps
most famously 1996's *Trainspotting* (although the

notion that the lyric might be addressed to heroin rather than to a lover predates that film by many years). Countless covers include a 1995 version by Kirsty MacColl and Evan Dando, and another – produced by Ken Scott – on Duran Duran's 1995 album *Thank You*.

In September 1997 both Bowie and Reed featured in the BBC's new recording of 'Perfect Day', for which individual lines were taped by a plethora of celebrity artists across the spectrum of musical styles as an extended advertisement for the Corporation's public service remit. A more bizarre choice of song as the vessel for an exercise in corporate branding would be difficult to imagine, but somehow it worked. Among those also taking part were Bono, Suzanne Vega, Elton John, Boyzone, the Brodsky Quartet, Lesley Garrett, Tammy Wynette, Dr John, Burning Spear, Shane McGowan, Courtney Pine, the BBC Symphony Orchestra, Laurie Anderson, Tom Jones and Joan Armatrading. "It's a way of saying thank you for *The Flowerpot Men*," said Bowie, who appeared in the accompanying video in a loose-fitting Asian suit and enormous earring of the kind he had taken to wearing on the Earthling tour. 'Perfect Day '97' attracted enormous interest and in November it was released as a single in aid of the BBC's Children In Need charity, going straight to number 1 in the UK. The 'Male Version' B-side reused Bowie's vocal contribution, while a new CD released in June 2000 featured the 1997 tracks and video, plus a new performance (featuring Reed but not Bowie) from the BBC's Music Live event.

PIANOLA *(Bowie/Cale)*

Also documented as 'Piano-La', this is one of two demos in collaboration with former Velvet Underground maestro John Cale. The recordings took place at New York's Ciarbis Studios on 15 October 1979 (not May 1979 as some accounts have claimed). The two-minute 'Pianola' reveals little of Bowie, who merely provides some "la la la" vocals to Cale's Chopinesque piano backing. "Yeah, that's Bowie wailing away in the background," Cale confirmed several years later, while in 2000 David recalled the songs in an online chat: "As far as I know, these have always just been bootleg songs. Unfortunately, there is nothing at a higher quality to release. I would grab those bootlegs when you see them. Don't say you heard it

from me."

The second number, 'Velvet Couch', is a little longer and more melodically finished but is likewise no more than a rough piano demo, featuring an ad-libbed and almost inaudible vocal in which David sings about "a red velvet couch with no guitar". In the same year Bowie appeared on stage with Cale and Philip Glass in New York (see 'Sabotage'), but despite claims to the contrary he is unlikely to have played on a series of further Cale demos, dated May 1979, which have appeared on bootlegs.

PICTURE MORE

The performing rights organization BMI lists this mysterious title as a Bowie composition, published by his company Tintoretto Music.

PICTURES OF LILY *(Townshend)*
• Compilation: *Substitute: The Songs Of The Who*

In October 2000, towards the end of the *Toy* sessions at Looking Glass Studios, Bowie recorded a cover version of The Who's 1967 hit 'Pictures Of Lily' for inclusion on the 2001 tribute album *Substitute: The Songs Of The Who*. Masterminded by Cast producer Bob Pridden, the album included covers by Pearl Jam, Sheryl Crow, Paul Weller and Stereophonics but, as Pridden later remarked, "things really began to take off when David Bowie agreed to record 'Pictures Of Lily'."

David, who apparently joined the project at the request of Pete Townshend, described his version as "Rather glam, actually. We slowed it down quite a lot. I'm pleased to say that Pete liked it, so that makes me pretty happy." Accompanied by Sterling Campbell on drums and Mark Plati on guitar and bass, David himself plays the Stylophone, an instrument already revived for some of the *Toy* tracks. All three provide backing vocals in a lush, multi-tracked and guitar-heavy arrangement which, as Bowie pointed out, is considerably slower than the original and succeeds in emphasizing the lyric's wistful subject matter. Popularly assumed to be a paean to teenage masturbation, 'Pictures Of Lily' was described by Townshend in 1967 as "a look back to that period in every boy's life when he has pin-ups. The idea was inspired by a picture my girlfriend had on her wall of an old vaudeville star – Lily Baylis. It was an old 1920s postcard and someone had written on it, 'Here's another picture of Lily'. It made me think that everyone has a pin-up period." It seems likely that Townshend was in fact thinking of Lillie Langtry, who did indeed die in 1929 as in his lyric; Lilian Baylis (1874-1937) was a noted theatre manager.

Prior to the album's release, Bowie's 'Pictures Of Lily' was also included on a three-track sampler CD made available via an exclusive offer to purchasers of the *Daily Telegraph*.

PLANET OF DREAMS *(Bowie/Dorsey)*
• Compilation: *Long Live Tibet*

This exclusive track on the 1997 charity album *Long Live Tibet*, credited to David Bowie and Gail Ann Dorsey, is a rather old-fashioned affair propelled by a grandiose piano somewhere between late-1970s Elton John and Talk Talk's 'Life's What You Make It'. The slight lyric has a vague echo of Lou Reed (David sings of "the poor huddled on the kerb" and "pain that comes and goes"), an impression pushed home when Gail launches into a "do-do-do" backing vocal straight from 'Walk On The Wild Side'.

PLAY IT SAFE *(Pop/Bowie)*

Bowie's only collaboration on Iggy Pop's 1980 album *Soldier* was recorded in May 1979 at Rockfield Studios in Monmouthshire, during a break from promoting *Lodger*. As well as co-writing the song Bowie sang backing vocals with various members of Simple Minds, who were recording *Empires And Dance* in the neighbouring studio. Simple Minds had initially asked Bowie to play saxophone on one of their tracks, but David declined and roped them into the Iggy session instead.

PLEASE DON'T TOUCH : see SWEET JANE

PLEASE MR GRAVEDIGGER
• Album: *Bowie*

Bowie's first recording of this number, made on 18 October 1966 at R G Jones Studios, has long since dis-

appeared, either junked or snapped up by a private collector. It was part of the three-song package with which Ken Pitt sold Bowie to the Deram label, and was promptly re-recorded on 13 December for inclusion on *David Bowie*. More a tone-poem than a song, this bizarre experiment features no instruments: instead atmospheric sound effects underscore David's *a cappella* vocal, delivered in a congested whine and punctuated by sniffs and sneezes, as he enacts the role of a grumbling child-murderer contemplating his next victim in the pouring rain of a Lambeth graveyard. It's hardly Anthony Newley, but it's certainly a black joke at the expense of music-hall numbers like 'Oh Mr Porter' and perhaps, some have suggested, a macabre response to the mid-1960s vogue for bubblegum "death-discs" like 'Leader Of The Pack'.

Engineer Gus Dudgeon painted a vivid picture of the recording session for David Buckley, indicating that even at this stage in his career Bowie was adopting unorthodox studio methods in order to get into a role: "What I remember is Bowie standing there wearing a pair of cans with his collar turned up as if he was in the rain, hunched over, shuffling about in a box of gravel. And you thought Brian Wilson had lost it!" Dudgeon also revealed that he had mixed feelings about Bowie's comic contraction of the doomed "Mr Gravedigger" to "Mr G D": "They're my initials and it bugs me!"

Unlikely as it may seem, Bowie performed 'Please Mr Gravedigger' on German TV's *4-3-2-1 Musik Für Junge Leute* on 27 February 1968.

PLEASE PLEASE PLEASE *(Brown/Terry)* : see YOUNG AMERICANS

PORT OF AMSTERDAM : see AMSTERDAM

THE PRETTIEST STAR
• A-Side: 3/70 • Album: *Aladdin* • Compilation: *S+V*, 69/74

Reputedly played down the telephone in December 1969 as part of David's marriage proposal to Angela Barnett (she was spending Christmas in Cyprus while waiting for her British visa to be reinstated), 'The Prettiest Star' is unlikely ever to be hailed as one of Bowie's key songs – but his vow that "One day ... you and I will rise up all the way" is a rousing mission-statement on the eve of the decade he and Angie were to conquer.

The original version was begun at Trident on 8 January 1970, Bowie's twenty-third birthday, and completed on 13 and 15 January. Not long afterwards the song received its first public airing in the live BBC session recorded on 5 February. The single appeared a month later on 6 March, a fortnight ahead of the Bowies' wedding. As the follow-up to 'Space Oddity' it received considerable coverage in the music press, garnering positive reviews in the NME ("a thoroughly charming and wholly fascinating little song … the self-penned lyric is enchanting, if somewhat enigmatic – and the melody is haunting and hummable … I like it immensely"), Music Business Weekly ("an immediately infectious number and a very strong follow-up"), Record Mirror ("a melodic and interesting production … chart cert") and Disc & Music Echo ("a lovely, gentle, gossamer piece … the most compact, catchy melody I've ever heard. A hit indeed"). Such predictions were quickly dashed, however: the single sold fewer than 800 copies and failed to chart.

The 1970 mono single was later included on Sound + Vision, while a previously unavailable stereo version appeared on The Best Of David Bowie 1969/1974 and 2003's reissued Sound + Vision. Although it's one of Bowie's more pedestrian recordings of the period, sounding positively turgid by comparison with the sparkly Aladdin Sane version, it's assured a place in the history books by virtue of its lead guitarist being one Marc Bolan. The two future stars had known each other since 1964, and the ties had been reinforced by Tony Visconti's production work with both. In 1969 Bowie had supported Bolan on tour, and mutual jam sessions at Visconti's flat were commonplace. "That was the only time when they could have worked together," Visconti later said of the 'Prettiest Star' session, "the only time their egos would have allowed it. But you could tell the rivalry between them was there. Marc was OK about it. He loved the fact he'd been asked to play electric guitar on that record because he'd only just got out of his acoustic days on his own releases. But June, Marc's wife, sat through the playback, announced that the best thing about the record was Marc's playing, and walked out of the room." Many years later, Bowie recalled that "I don't think we were talking to each other that day. I can't remember why, but I remember a very strange atmosphere in the studio. We were never in the same room at the same

time. You could have cut the atmosphere with a knife."

Later in 1970 Bolan's chart career took off, depriving Bowie of Tony Visconti but, it has often been suggested, offering the essential competition that would galvanize him into action. Once Ziggy Stardust had assured Bowie's place in the rock firmament two years later, his old friend's jealousy was never far from the surface: at the end of 1972 Bolan told the press that "With no disrespect to David, it's much too soon to put him in the same class as me," and that Bowie was "very much a one-hit wonder, I'm afraid." The pair's much-vaunted rivalry has since been the subject of many a second-hand anecdote, but Visconti, who is uniquely qualified to discuss the subject, told Dave Thompson in his book Moonage Daydream that the relationship was a complex one: "Marc was in rivalry with everybody. He simply couldn't stand attention going in anyone else's direction. He was a total megalomaniac, God bless him. David, on the other hand, is very gregarious, a very open-minded person, and apart from a normal, healthy type of rivalry he was never obsessed with Bolan … David always loved Marc, he loved to be with him, he would come home after a social session with Marc feeling quite hurt after Marc had taken too many digs at him … But there was a lot of love between them … Bowie never had anything but kind words to say about him." Despite a few mid-1970s jams in Los Angeles, the two only worked together in public once more (see 'Sleeping Next To You').

In addition to its appearances on various Bowie compilations, the 1970 recording of 'The Prettiest Star' was later included on the 2002 Marc Bolan box set 20th Century Superstar. Meanwhile, in 1973 'The Prettiest Star' was re-recorded in its more familiar Aladdin Sane version, complete with 1950s doo-wop backings and a meaty guitar solo from Mick Ronson. The lyrical references to screen starlets and "the movies in the past" fit snugly with the nostalgic Hollywood themes found elsewhere on Aladdin Sane. This version provided inspiration for one of the most underrated British guitar talents: Marco Pirroni, best known for his work with Adam Ant and Sinead O'Connor, said in 1999 that "Mick Ronson was a huge influence on The Ants," and described the Aladdin Sane take of 'The Prettiest Star' as "the best guitar sound ever … Ronson has got this brilliant, overdriven, mad guitar sound. I'm still trying to get that sound today." Ian McCulloch pulled off an excellent impersonation of it on his 2003 cover version, recorded for *Uncut* magazine's *Starman* CD and released as a B-side on the same year's single 'Love In Veins'.

PRETTY PINK ROSE
• A-Side: 5/90

Originally demoed in early 1988 (see 'Like A Rolling Stone') before becoming a *Tin Machine* reject, 'Pretty Pink Rose' was brought to fruition in January 1990 when it was re-recorded for inclusion on *Young Lions*, the forthcoming solo album by Sound + Vision tour guitarist Adrian Belew. "I sent him five tracks that didn't have any vocals," said Belew later, "and he sent me back a song called 'Pretty Pink Rose' that he hadn't used but thought it might fit in with my album. We went to record that in New York and because we'd been rehearsing for the tour, his voice was shot. He said, 'I'm sorry, but I can't sing it today.' I said okay, I'd work on another song that hadn't got vocals and he could go home and rest. But he said, 'Let me hear that.' He began writing lyrics and about half an hour later, he'd finished a song called 'Gunman'. I was amazed. He then went in and sang it two or three times and that was it."

Both 'Gunman' and 'Pretty Pink Rose' subsequently appeared on *Young Lions* in May 1990 while the latter, in slightly edited form, was also released as a single. Although credited to "Adrian Belew featuring David Bowie", 'Pretty Pink Rose' is dominated by David's vocal performance and is a Bowie single in all but name. It's a great song, too, powered along by searing guitar and featuring some fabulously barmy lyrics ("She's a poor man's goal, she's the anarchist crucible, flying in the face of the despot cannibal…"). The video, directed by 'Time Will Crawl' veteran Tim Pope, featured Bowie and Belew in their Sound + Vision regalia, succumbing to the charms of Julie T Wallace (then familiar as the star of the BBC's sexual melodrama *The Life And Loves Of A She-Devil*) resplendent in traditional Russian dress. The single didn't chart, which is a pity as it might have been a hit if released under Bowie's name. 'Pretty Pink Rose' was performed throughout the Sound + Vision tour.

PRETTY THING
• Album: *TM*

Although the title unavoidably conjures up memories of past glories (and in case of doubt, the chorus goes "Oh, you pretty thing!"), this is sadly one of the least engaging tracks on *Tin Machine*. The initial stop-start dynamics are fun, owing an obvious debt to 'Don't Bring Me Down', one of the *Pin Ups* covers originally recorded by (who else?) The Pretty Things, but the track degenerates into one of Tin Machine's blustering rock-outs – and the laddish, sexist lyrics are beyond the pale. When *Q* asked him about the line "Tie you down, pretend you're Madonna," Bowie slipped into the least appealing side of his 1989 idiom ("Hey, we were hanging out with Sean and he told us a few things! You know what I mean?") before back-pedalling rapidly ("Nah, it's a throwaway. I was just trying to think of a – it's such a silly song anyway.").

A performance-style excerpt of 'Pretty Thing', featuring Bowie gliding above the crowd on a hydraulic arm, was included in Julien Temple's 1989 Tin Machine video. The song was played on both Tin Machine tours.

THE PRETTY THINGS ARE GOING TO HELL
(Bowie/Gabrels)
• Soundtrack: *Stigmata* • Album: *'hours…'* • Australian A-Side: 9/99 • B-Side: 1/00 [28] • B-Side: 7/00 [32]

Starting life as an instrumental track originally intended for Reeves Gabrels's solo album *Ulysses (della notte)*, 'The Pretty Things Are Going To Hell' was furnished with lyrics by Bowie, whose hugely self-referential title simultaneously recalls 'Oh! You Pretty Things', 'Pretty Thing', 1960s beat group The Pretty Things (as covered on *Pin Ups*), and Iggy And The Stooges' *Raw Power* track 'Your Pretty Face Is Going To Hell'. According to Gabrels, the track was "one of the first songs we recorded, but one of the last to get completed vocals. The main guitars took me about 20 minutes to do in London, February 1999, and the vocals are largely from a rough vocal demo done in May 1999. I thought that it was going to remain unfinished but it lived through David's period of dislike for it to become a fan favourite."

The result is the rockiest piece on *'hours…'*, fusing a chugging glam-punk bassline with 'Little Wonder'-style blasts of guitar and some manic 'Diamond Dogs' cowbell percussion. The nervy references to "reaching the very edge" and "going to the other side" restate Bowie's efforts to position himself outside the mainstream, but he explained that the lyric was chiefly inspired by the same source as 1973's 'Aladdin Sane': "I think these are tough times," he told *Uncut*. "It's a tough period to live in. And I was thinking of that Evelyn Waugh idea of the bright young things, the pretty things ... I think their day is numbered. So I thought, well, let's close them off. They wore it well but they did wear themselves out, y'know, there's not much room for that now. It's a very serious little world."

The darkly funny observation that "they wore it out but they wore it well", with its promise of a damnation that is at least stylish, recollects the cultural critiques of 'Teenage Wildlife' and 'Fashion', as does the quasi-Biblical enquiry "What is eternal, what is damned? / What is clay and what is sand?" This is Bowie at his most mischievous, turning the tables on his own premonition in 'Changes' that "pretty soon now you're gonna get older" when he crows, "I found the secrets, I found gold / I find you out before you grow old".

A remixed version featured in the film *Stigmata*, whose soundtrack album was released two months ahead of 'hours...'. The *Stigmata* album mix differs from the minute-long snippet heard in the film itself, and yet another variant *Stigmata* version appeared on the 'Survive' CD single. The *Stigmata* version also features in *Omikron: The Nomad Soul*, while the original recording was later used in the soundtrack of the 2001 film *Fat Girl*.

A further edit replaced the 'Thursday's Child' single in Australia and some other territories. The little-known video, directed by Dom and Nic of 'I'm Afraid Of Americans' fame, was shot at New York's Kit Kat Club on 7 September 1999. In keeping with the retrospective mood of the album, the video features David being attacked by life-size puppets of four of his past incarnations: Ziggy Stardust, the dress-wearing Man Who Sold The World, the Thin White Duke and the 'Ashes To Ashes' Pierrot. The puppets, constructed by Jim Henson's Creature Shop at a reported £7000 each, appear to represent one of Bowie's most pressing concerns as an artist: the constant struggle to avoid being overwhelmed by his own past. Canadian actor Chad Richardson secured the supporting role of Bowie's young *alter ego* after imitating his Ziggy-era mannerisms at an audition. Richardson told reporters that "at

the very end of the video, where I'm the new Bowie reborn, it was very cool because Bowie was watching ... and he said, 'Oh my God, it's unbelievable. You've got all my moves down proper. I can't believe it.'" Sadly the video was never released. "It was abandoned after we found that the puppets ended up looking like puppets," David explained a year later. "What I mean is it didn't have the East European darkness that Dom and Nic had wanted to achieve. Some of it is downright funny and I'm sure it will make its way onto a video compilation one of these days – to be a source of endless amusement to you all and another form of Chinese torture for myself."

'The Pretty Things Are Going To Hell' was played live on the 1999-2000 dates; a live version recorded in New York on 19 November 1999 appeared on some formats of the 'Seven' single.

PRISONER OF LOVE
(Bowie/T.Sales/H.Sales/Gabrels)
• Album: *TM* • A-Side: 10/89

This is one of *Tin Machine*'s more conventional offerings, an uncomplicated blues-rocker constructed around a twanging, Hank Marvin-style riff strangely reminiscent of Blondie's 'Atomic'. Despite featuring the catastrophic line "Like a sermon on blues guitar, love walked into town," it's actually quite an affecting lyric, a combination of lover's vows and worldly advice ("just stay square," exhorts the new, socially conscious Bowie) addressed in part, he explained at the time, to his then partner Melissa Hurley. "The fact that my girlfriend is young, very naïve and kind of straight is, for me, something I just would like her to retain for as long as she can," he said in 1989. "'Cause there is so much crap out there, you know, and there's nothing wrong with being like that. That's why it's got a very kind of corny 'Just stay square' line in it."

The fade-out features a paraphrase of Allen Ginsberg's 1955 poem *Howl* ("I've seen the best minds of my generation laid down in cemeteries..."), previously quoted on Iggy Pop's Bowie-produced track 'Little Miss Emperor'. The line may originally have reached Bowie via The Fugs, whose 1965 debut album *The Virgin Fugs* includes the track 'I Saw The Best Of My Generation Rot'. It's also worth noting that *Prisoner Of Love* is the title of Jean Genet's final work, an exploration of the Palestinian conflict completed just before his death in 1986.

'Prisoner Of Love' failed to chart as Tin Machine's third single, despite the added incentive of live tracks recorded in Paris during the 1989 tour, on which the song was also performed. The so-called 'LP Version' on the extended formats was in fact a marginally longer version of the single edit. Julien Temple's 1989 Tin Machine video featured a staged performance of 'Prisoner Of Love' in blue-tinted slow-motion.

PURPLE HAZE (*Hendrix*) : see **THE JEAN GENIE**

PUSSY CAT : see **BUNNY THING**

QUALISAR (*Bowie/Gabrels*)

An instrumental track recorded by Bowie with Reeves Gabrels in 1999 for exclusive use in the *Omikron* computer game.

QUEEN BITCH
• Album: *Hunky* • B-side: 2/74 [5] • Live: *SM72, Rarest, Beeb* • Live Video: *Best Of Bowie*

This is *Hunky Dory*'s least representative track – the only one devoid of Rick Wakeman's piano, and the only one on which Mick Ronson's guitar dominates – and notwithstanding the excellence of the numbers surrounding it, it's 'Queen Bitch' that reveals the shape of things to come. The last of the album's cycle of tribute numbers, it's an energetic pastiche of the Velvet Underground, and specifically the hardcore guitar and half-spoken delivery of Lou Reed. The scrawled sleeve-notes for the track read "Some V.U. White Light returned with thanks", referring to the seismic influence of Reed's 'Waiting for the Man' and 'White Light/White Heat' on Bowie's own songwriting. The lyric, too, is indebted to Reed's urban poetry, a coded portrait of seduction and betrayal larded with the sassy gay street argot of Greenwich Village. There are sly references to other icons, too: the narrator's friend is "trying hard to pull sister Flo", which is not just a nod to Reed's 'Sister Ray' but surely an allusion, more immediate then than now, to the excessively camp backing singers Flo and Eddie who regularly whooped along to T Rex's breakthrough hits on *Top Of The Pops* at the time. The chorus finds Bowie doffing

his hat to another influence: "satin and tat" had long been one of Lindsay Kemp's favourite throwaway phrases when describing his taste in theatricality. Part of the genius of 'Queen Bitch' is that it filters the archness of Bolan and Kemp through the streetwise attitude of Reed: this is a song that succeeds in making the phrase "bipperty-bopperty hat" sound raunchy and cool.

The song was a favourite during Bowie's BBC sessions, and was first aired ahead of *Hunky Dory* in the concert set recorded on 3 June 1971, in a quieter and less raucous rendition than later versions. Further BBC recordings were taped on 11 and 18 January 1972 (the second of these can be heard on *Bowie At The Beeb*), and yet another featured on Bowie's *Old Grey Whistle Test* appearance on 8 February. Two fluffed takes of this performance, both of which peter out in the opening seconds, have been aired on various out-take shows over the years, notably ITV's *Changes: Bowie at 50* documentary. The successful full-length take appears on the *Best Of Bowie* DVD.

'Queen Bitch' featured on the 1972 Ziggy tour, the Station To Station tour (from which a spunky live version recorded on 23 March 1976 appears on *RarestOneBowie*), and latterly the Sound + Vision and Earthling tours. At his fiftieth birthday concert Bowie performed the song as a duet with Lou Reed himself.

QUEEN OF ALL THE TARTS (OVERTURE)
• Bonus: *Reality*

Piped into the auditoria immediately before curtain-up on each show of A Reality Tour (hence, presumably, its subtitle), 'Queen Of All The Tarts' was included on the bonus disc that came with initial pressings of *Reality*. It's a likeable piece, consisting of a splendidly dramatic series of instrumental swoops punctuated by multi-tracked vocals intoning the track's curious sub-Lewis Carroll title. The vocal quality is reminiscent of some of the *'hours...'* B-sides, although the dynamics and synth-heavy arrangements are firmly in the *Heathen* and *Reality* mould, and there's some very 'Pablo Picasso'-style guitar work towards the end.

QUICKSAND
• Album: *Hunky* • B-Side: 4/74 [22] • Bonus: *Hunky*

At the time of *Hunky Dory*'s release in December 1971,

Bowie revealed that 'Quicksand' had been inspired by his first trip to America the previous February. "The chain reaction of moving around throughout the bliss and then the calamity of America produced this epic of confusion," he declared. "Anyway, with my esoteric problems I could have written it in Plainview or Dulwich." Several years later he would describe 'Quicksand' as a mixture of "narrative and surrealism", and a precursor to the compositions on *Low*.

Like all the best tracks on *Hunky Dory*, 'Quicksand' combines a deceptively simple melody with a sumptuous arrangement and an almost impenetrable lyric. This is Bowie bewildered, disempowered and intimidated by politics and religion, "sinking in the quicksand of my thought", hemmed in by "logic" and "bullshit faith", rejecting "belief" and foreseeing "the death of Man". The song's "dream-reality" reprises the cinematic role-playing found throughout the album ("I'm living in a silent film … I'm the twisted name on Garbo's eyes"), as Bowie, "caught between the light and dark", ponders his "potential" in an increasingly sinister whirl of references to Churchill, Himmler, Aleister Crowley's "Golden Dawn" and, once again, Nietzsche's supermen. It's a listless, withdrawn lyric apparently wallowing in depression, but for all its dark foreboding it's a strangely lovely song and a confirmed favourite among Bowie aficionados.

A 1971 acoustic demo appeared on Rykodisc's *Hunky Dory* reissue, while a further, purely instrumental demo is said to exist on acetate. 'Quicksand' was performed during the final 1973 leg of the Ziggy Stardust tour, in a medley with 'Life On Mars?' and 'Memory of a Free Festival'. Thereafter the song was laid to rest until 1997, when Bowie recorded a new version for Radio 1's *ChangesNowBowie*. "It was somebody in the band that said I should do it," he explained in the broadcast. "I'd forgotten all about it, and since I've done it for you guys I've started using it on stage. I'd forgotten – it's a really lovely song." At his fiftieth birthday concert a few days later, Bowie performed 'Quicksand' as a splendid duet with Robert Smith of The Cure, who later revealed to the *NME* that "You didn't get a choice of duet, which was annoying. David rang up and said, 'What song would you like to do?' so I started reeling off all these songs like 'Drive In Saturday', 'Young Americans'. Then he said, 'How about 'Quicksand'?' and I thought, 'You bastard!'" Following the superb Bowie/Smith duet, 'Quicksand' became the Earthling tour's regular curtain-raiser, with a revamped guitar intro borrowed from 'The Bewlay

Brothers'. The song resurfaced on the 2004 leg of A Reality Tour.

A notable cover version was performed by Seal during his MTV *Unplugged* appearance in 1996, while Dinosaur Jr. included a version on their 1991 album *Whatever's Cool With Me*.

RADIOACTIVITY *(Hütter/Schneider/Schult)*

The title track of Kraftwerk's 1975 album was played as pre-show music on the Station To Station tour. During Tin Machine's It's My Life tour, David occasionally sang a few lines from the number during the extended rendition of 'Heaven's In Here'.

RAGAZZO SOLO, RAGAZZA SOLA
(Bowie/Mogol) : see **SPACE ODDITY**

RAW POWER *(Pop/Williamson)*

Mixed by Bowie for Iggy And The Stooges' *Raw Power*, the title track was later performed on Iggy's 1977 tour. A version featuring Bowie appears on *Suck On This!*.

READY FOR LOVE/AFTER LIGHTS *(Ralphs)*

Produced by David for Mott The Hoople's *All The Young Dudes*.

REAL COOL WORLD
• A-Side: 8/92 [53] • Bonus: *Black (2003)*

Bowie's first post-Tin Machine single secured only one week in the lower reaches of the UK chart, but provided the faithful with a significant foretaste of things to come. The theme song for the little-seen movie comedy *Cool World* was the first fruit of Bowie's rekindled relationship with producer Nile Rodgers in the run-up to *Black Tie White Noise*, foreshadowing that album's fusion of 1990s dance beats with European electro-funk and Middle Eastern saxophone breaks. There are hints, too, of abiding Bowie mythologies in the sketchy lyric, as he sings of "saint-like and fantastic heroes feeling like lost little children in fabled lands."

Although released in half a dozen remixed forms

aimed at club and radio airplay, and supported by a video of scenes from the movie, 'Real Cool World' sank without trace. Excepting the soundtrack album *Songs From The Cool World*, its sole compilation appearance is the previously unreleased edit that appears as a bonus track on the 2003 reissue of *Black Tie White Noise*.

REAL WILD CHILD (WILD ONE)
(O'Keefe/Greenan/Owens)

Co-produced by Bowie for Iggy Pop's *Blah-Blah-Blah*, 'Real Wild Child' took Iggy to number 10 with the first and still biggest hit of his career.

REALITY
• Album: *Reality* • Live Video: *Reality*

The first track to be recorded during the *Reality* sessions is also the album's loudest, rockiest moment, its thrashing drums and squalling guitar riffs recalling the sensory assault of 'Hallo Spaceboy' and some of the more artful Tin Machine pieces. However, underpinning the wall of noise is the classic simplicity of an instantly recognizable acoustic strum that goes right back to Bowie's 1960s recordings: at one point the layers of electric sound even break down, 'Space Oddity'-style, to leave only the acoustic guitar as Bowie sings, "I've been right and I've been wrong / Now I'm back where I started from", as if purposely exposing the songwriter behind the rock'n'roller. This is an entirely appropriate sentiment, because the quasi-autobiographical shorthand of 'Reality' lies at the heart of the album's loosely managed theme. As Bowie himself said, "The basis is more an all-pervasive influence of contingency than a defined structure of absolutes": in other words, the quest for structure and meaning in life is doomed to failure, because however hard one searches, no pattern will ever emerge – and so, as this song pointedly concludes, "I look for sense but I get next to nothing / Hoo boy, welcome to reality".

"The thing, probably, that keeps me writing is this awful gnawing feeling that there are no absolutes," Bowie told *Los Angeles City Beat*. "That there is no truth. That we are, as I've been thinking for so many years now, fully in the swirl of chaos theory." In *Interview* magazine he elaborated on the same idea: "We set up these plays for ourselves because if we were

to open ourselves up to the idea that there is no plan, no evolution, no point in our being here, we could not struggle through to the next day. The days work for us. A stage play will set up certain laws within itself – it doesn't mean they're real laws, they just work for the play which in itself is only a metaphysical arena. You know that line from *As You Like It*: 'All the world's a stage / And all the men and women merely players'? What truth there is in that cliché!"

Thus, appropriately enough, *Reality*'s title track adopts the form of an artificial narrative, the better to convey the notion that a real life *has* no formal narrative. Looking back on earlier times, Bowie confesses that he "built a wall of sound to separate us" and "hid among the junk of wretched highs". The second verse turns, as do so many later Bowie songs, to intimations of mortality: the line "Now my sight is fading in this twilight" recalls the approaching dissolution of 'Heathen (The Rays)', while "Now my death is more than just a sad song" offers an elegant and self-lacerating pun with its pointed recollection of the Jacques Brel number so beloved of his younger self, in the days when the reality of death lay too far in the future to warrant any contemplation beyond the purely dramatic. "I still don't remember how this happened" sounds like Bowie's variation on John Lennon's famous observation that "Life is what happens to you while you're busy making other plans", while the couplet "I've been right and I've been wrong / Now I'm back where I started from" pertinently recalls the celebrated "I've never done good things / I've never done bad things" line in 'Ashes To Ashes'. It's a dense, clever, end-of-term report of a song, replete with evocative echoes. Like all of its parent album, the song was performed live throughout A Reality Tour.

REBEL NEVER GETS OLD

In March 2004, a "mash-up" remix of 'Rebel Rebel' and 'Never Get Old' created by Endless Noise appeared in a TV advertising campaign for Audi of America, who sponsored the North American leg of A Reality Tour. Over the previous couple of years Bowie had made no secret of his fondness for mash-ups, which combine unlikely bedfellows to create new pieces of music. In 2003 EMI/Virgin had invited Mark Vidler of Go Home Productions to create two Bowie mash-ups; Vidler produced 'I'm Afraid Of Making Plans For Americans' (which combined 'I'm Afraid Of

Americans' with XTC's 'Making Plans For Nigel') and 'Jacko Under Pressure' (an ironic pairing of 'Under Pressure' with Michael Jackson's 'Rock With You'). Towards the end of the year Vidler was contracted by Bowie's organization to create a further mash-up, and this time the result was 'Rebel Never Gets Old', a development of the idea suggested by the Audi commercial. Vidler produced three versions: a 3'25" 'Single Mix', a 7'22" 'Seventh Heaven Mix', and a 4'17" edit of the latter.

In April 2004, Audi and Sony launched an online remix competition which invited contestants to create their own "mash-ups" from pre-selected Bowie clips using downloadable software. At the time of writing, 'Rebel Never Gets Old' was scheduled for release in May 2004 as a download via the iTunes Music Store, with a 12" vinyl picture disc containing all three mixes due to follow in European territories.

REBEL REBEL

• A-Side: 2/74 [5] • US A-Side: 5/74 • Album: *Dogs* •
Live: *David* • Compilation: *S+V* • Soundtrack: *Charlie's Angels: Full Throttle* • Bonus: *Reality, Dogs (2004)* •
Video: *Best Of Bowie* • Live Video: *Moonlight, Glass*

Released two months ahead of its parent album, 'Rebel Rebel' gave little indication of the dark intensity of Bowie's new work. If, as is believed, it was originally written for the aborted Ziggy Stardust musical David was planning in late 1973, its incongruity amid the apocalyptic prog-rock nightmare of *Diamond Dogs* becomes a little more understandable. Arguably the flimsiest and most disposable product of the album sessions, for all its iconic status 'Rebel Rebel' is little more than a bankable retread of previous gender-bending stompers like 'The Jean Genie' and 'Suffragette City', representing a rare instance of Bowie treading water and playing safe at the height of his 1970s creativity. This is not to suggest it isn't a fine pop song, and moreover one that offers evidence that David can handle lead guitar with great proficiency. Bowie plays the lion's share of the lead guitar on 'Rebel Rebel', with an additional contribution from '1984' guest guitarist Alan Parker, who added the three descending notes at the end of each loop of the riff.

Keith Richards, who socialized with Bowie during the *Diamond Dogs* sessions, is also reputed to play on 'Rebel Rebel', and although this rumour is highly unlikely the song's antecedents are obvious. The riff is

pure 'Satisfaction'-era Rolling Stones – "It's a fabulous riff!" Bowie later recalled, "Just fabulous! When I stumbled onto it, it was 'Oh, thank you!'" – while his pouty-shouty vocal is unadulterated Mick Jagger. Another likely influence is the New York transsexual Wayne (later Jayne) County, a member of the cast of *Pork* who had been among the Bowie entourage since the time of *Ziggy Stardust*, and whose 1973 composition 'Queenage Baby' included the line "Can't tell whether she's a boy or a girl".

Viewed historically, 'Rebel Rebel' stands as Bowie's valediction to a musical movement that was already heavily in decline. By the beginning of 1974 the trappings and sounds of glam had been annexed by pop's establishment and the charts coarsened by a host of second-generation imitators. In the week that 'Rebel Rebel' peaked at number 5 in the UK chart, Suzi Quatro's 'Devil Gate Drive' was at number 1 and the top ten also included Alvin Stardust's 'Jealous Mind', Mud's 'Tiger Feet' and the Bay City Rollers' 'Remember'. Bowie was by no means the only glam architect peppering his songs with farewell gestures. Roxy Music's November 1973 album *Stranded*, the first without Brian Eno, signalled a retreat from their glam sound. Alice Cooper released 'Teenage Lament '74' ("what a drag it is in these gold lamé jeans"), and later in the year Mott The Hoople (now including Mick Ronson, fresh from recording the revealingly titled 'Growing Up And I'm Fine') would be asking "Did you see the suits and the platform boots?" in their final hit 'Saturday Gigs'. Most telling of all was Marc Bolan's February 1974 single, the poignantly titled '(Whatever Happened To The) Teenage Dream?' It was time to move on, and 'Rebel Rebel' drew a line beneath Bowie's glam rock career.

According to David's ghostwritten diary in *Mirabelle* – not the most reliable of sources – the recording of 'Rebel Rebel' was "all completed in three days." An alternative take was cut in New York in April 1974 and released briefly as an American single in May, thereafter disappearing until it inclusion on *Sound + Vision* and 2004's *Diamond Dogs* reissue. The rough-cut garage sound of the more familiar version is abandoned on the alternative take, which is awash with phased echo effects and rattling percussion, while Geoff MacCormack's congas and the syncopated backing vocals push the song, tellingly enough, in a quasi-soul direction. Interestingly it's this version that would be used as the blueprint for nearly every subsequent live rendition until the end of the 1990s.

On 13 February 1974 a mimed performance of 'Rebel Rebel' was recorded at Hilversum's Avro Studio 2 for the Dutch television show *Top Pop*. Broadcast two days later, it featured David superimposed over flashing disco lights by the miracle of chromakey. This clip, which became the song's semi-official video, premiered Bowie's short-lived pirate image – a spotted neckerchief and black eyepatch which, as he later recalled, made a virtue of necessity: "I had conjunctivitis, so I made the most of it and dressed like a pirate. Just stopped short of the parrot! I had this most incredible jacket that I was wearing that night. It was a bottle-green bolero jacket that Freddi [Burretti] made for me and he got an artist to paint, using the appliqué technique, this supergirl from a Russian comic on the back. Anyway, I did a press conference and performed 'Rebel Rebel' on Dutch television with a bright red Fender Stratocaster. But I took the jacket off during the press conference and somebody stole it. I was really pissed off." The pirate look, along with the Ziggy hairstyle, was soon ditched in favour of the swept-back parting and double-breasted suits of the Diamond Dogs tour.

A pre-recorded performance of 'Rebel Rebel' was scheduled to appear on *Top Of The Pops* on 21 February 1974, but the promo film failed to arrive at the studio on time and the item was dropped. The cancellation led to rising hopefuls Queen being granted their first *Top Of The Pops* appearance, in a hastily arranged performance of what would soon become their first hit, 'Seven Seas Of Rhye'.

For many years 'Rebel Rebel' remained a live standard in Bowie concerts, featuring on every solo tour from Diamond Dogs to Sound + Vision, while an unusual, sax-heavy version appeared in his Live Aid set. By 1990, however, the song had become symbolic of David's fear of entrapment on the greatest hits circuit: "I haven't done 'Rebel Rebel' since the Glass Spider thing," he said at the outset of the Sound + Vision tour. "It felt odd then and it feels odder now … the ones that are generationally message-oriented like 'Rebel Rebel' I feel very uncomfortable with, and I find I'm throwing them away a bit. I hope it won't show." After 1990 it seemed unlikely that Bowie would revive 'Rebel Rebel' again, and it came as some surprise when a rock-heavy, back-to-basics version was included on the 1999-2000 dates.

For the latter dates of the Heathen tour in the autumn of 2002, Bowie unveiled a new and heavily reworked interpretation which, not unlike the 1974 live version of 'The Jean Genie', began with a quiet, minimalist opening verse picked out on rhythm guitar, before plunging into the familiar riff for the choruses. "I hadn't done it in quite a few years," said Bowie, not entirely accurately, "so we restructured it and made it more minimal, and it works really well." This excellent new interpretation was premiered at the live BBC radio session of 18 September 2002, and reappeared throughout A Reality Tour, usually as the opening number. A studio version of the new arrangement, produced by Tony Visconti, was recorded in the initial stages of the *Reality* sessions and appeared on the June 2003 soundtrack of *Charlie's Angels: Full Throttle* (in the film it accompanies the vision of Drew Barrymore resplendent in Aladdin Sane wig and make-up), and later as a bonus track on the two-disc version of *Reality* and the 2004 reissue of *Diamond Dogs*.

Unsurprisingly considering its anthemic status, 'Rebel Rebel' has been performed by a vast number of other artists, and is almost certainly the most frequently covered title in the Bowie songbook. Among its many interpreters are The Bay City Rollers, Joan Jett, Bryan Adams, Duran Duran, Rick Derringer, Def Leppard, Smashing Pumpkins, Dead Or Alive, The Mike Flowers Pops, Shaun Cassidy, Bruce Lash, Lyn Todd, Rickie Lee Jones, Adamski (under his early moniker The Legion of Dynamic Discord), Jean Meilleur and Sigue Sigue Sputnik, whose horrid live recording can be heard on *David Bowie Songbook*. Iggy Pop and Lenny Kravitz joined forces on a live version at 1998's VH1 Fashion Awards. Bowie's original recording appeared in the soundtrack of the 1999 comedy *Detroit Rock City*. 'Rebel Rebel' also has the dubious honour of being one of the earliest Bowie songs to feature in a commercial: it was used to advertise "Rebel" perfume in the mid-1970s. In 2004 the song was subjected to a number of "mash-up" remixes with 'Never Get Old' and used in an advertising campaign for Audi cars (see 'Rebel Never Gets Old').

RED MONEY *(Bowie/Alomar)*
• Album: *Lodger*

Musically *Lodger*'s closing track is a straight retread of Bowie's 1976 Iggy Pop collaboration 'Sister Midnight', and has been widely dismissed as an inferior remake. This is unfortunate because, with its brand-new set of lyrics, 'Red Money' has an intrigue all its own. Bowie explained in 1979 that the "small red box" was a reference to a recurring image he used in his paintings: "This song, I think, is about responsibility. Red boxes keep cropping up in my paintings and they represent responsibility." Accordingly, 'Red Money' ends with the proposition: "Such responsibility, it's up to you and me."

A constant in Bowie's career is the impulse to smash each edifice he constructs, to "break up the band", to "pack a bag and move on" before stagnation sets in. If the red box is a symbol of responsibility, then the sheer weight of oppression it brings in 'Red Money' is hugely revealing: "I could not give it away, and I knew I must not drop it, stop it, take it away!" It's tempting to read 'Red Money' as pure metaphor, an artful statement of deconstruction, dismantling the European phase that had begun in 1976 with the recording of the original 'Sister Midnight'. It is, after all, the last track on *Lodger*, Eno is gone, and the repeated refrain is "Project cancelled." It may not be deliberate, but it's jolly neat.

RED SAILS *(Bowie/Eno)*
• Album: *Lodger*

The last of *Lodger*'s opening salvo of exotic, continent-hopping tracks is this madly exuberant piece of nonsense, an upbeat slab of new wave pop that would have made an infinitely better second single than 'D.J.'. An obvious keynote is Düsseldorf band Neu!, whose influence on Bowie's music is seldom as widely acknowledged as that of their compatriots Kraftwerk. According to David "That drum and guitar sound, that especially" derived from Neu!, but "The moments of difference … came from Adrian [Belew] not being played Neu!; he'd never heard of them. So I told him the atmosphere I wanted and he came up with the same conclusions that Neu! came up with, which was fine by me. That Neu! sound is fantastic."

Against a backdrop of German and Far Eastern motifs, with bellowing back-up vocals from Brian Eno, Tony Visconti and himself, Bowie unleashes one of his most devil-may-care vocal performances, and although recorded several months earlier the result sounds remarkably like Lene Lovich's loopy 1979 hit 'Lucky Number'. Speaking in the same year, Bowie explained: "Here we took a new German music feel and put it against the idea of a contemporary English mercenary-cum-swashbuckling Errol Flynn, and put

him in the China Sea. We have a lovely cross-reference of cultures. I honestly don't know what it's about." Maybe, but there are obvious thematic comparisons with the nomadic self-portrait found throughout the album: "Wake up in the wrong town, boy I really get around."

'Red Sails' was performed during the early leg of the Serious Moonlight tour.

REMEMBERING MARIE A.
(Traditional, adapted Brecht/Muldowney)
• B-Side: 2/82 [29]

The second track on the *Baal* EP is a typically Brechtian collision of bitterness and sentimentality: Baal finds it easier to recall the cloud drifting overhead during a long-ago liaison than the face of the girl herself. Brecht's ironic working title was 'Sentimental Song no. 1004', and he adapted the music from a traditional nineteenth-century melody called 'Lost Happiness' which he had heard sung by factory girls. He described it as "a hymn to summer … a song of the countryside, its swansong."

REPETITION
• Album: *Lodger* • B-Side: 6/79 [29]

Lodger's vignettes of Western civilization continue with this sombre excursion into the unusually direct topic of wife-beating. Over a hypnotic pulse of drunken bass, wavering synthesizers and discordant guitars Bowie's numbed vocal sketches the portrait of a frustrated, mediocre husband who "could have had a Cadillac if the school had taught him right, and he could have married Anne with the blue silk blouse", and so vents his impotent anger on his wife: "I guess the bruises won't show if she wears long sleeves". Inevitably reminiscent of Lou Reed's similarly-themed 'Caroline Says', it's probably Bowie's most unambiguous attack on a specific social ill until the days of Tin Machine – but its subtle power is something they would seldom achieve.

After languishing in relative obscurity for nearly twenty years, 'Repetition' was unexpectedly reworked in 1997 for Radio 1's *ChangesNowBowie*. "I wanted to try it acoustically because it was so much an electronic piece of work on the album," Bowie explained. "I wanted to see what it was made of just as a song, when it was really stripped down, and it's interesting to see how something that's really so minimal works quite well as a straightforward rendition." On 9 January 1997 a performance was recorded backstage at Madison Square Garden for inclusion in the pay-per-view broadcast of Bowie's fiftieth birthday concert. Thereafter the song was revived for the *'hours…'* tour, during which another BBC version surfaced in the live set recorded on 25 October 1999.

REPRISE : see EVEN A FOOL LEARNS TO LOVE

REPTILE *(Reznor)*

Bowie joined Nine Inch Nails to perform this song from *The Downward Spiral* during the Outside tour's US leg.

THE REVEREND RAYMOND BROWN

Kenneth Pitt cites this as a discarded 1968 Bowie composition. No other sources mention the number; it's possibly an alternative title for one of the 'Ernie Johnson' songs.

REVOLUTIONARY SONG *(Bowie/Fishman)*
• Japanese A-Side: 6/79 • Soundtrack: *Just A Gigolo*

Bowie's sole contribution to the *Just A Gigolo* soundtrack remains an overlooked rarity. Credited to "David Bowie and the Rebels", it appears on the film's long-deleted soundtrack album and was released in edited form as a Japanese single in 1979. Both flopped, and copies of the single now command surprisingly large sums. The track is sometimes listed as 'David Bowie's Revolutionary Song', as billed on the album sleeve, but not on its label or on the single.

According to the co-writer and soundtrack supervisor Jack Fishman, the number was composed by David "on the set between scenes. He recorded the accompaniment for his 'Revolutionary Song' himself. The track opens with David playing and 'la-la-ing', then combines with an instrumental and full chorus version, finally returning to David departing, accompanied by the chorus." Frankly, like much else about *Just A Gigolo*, this account smacks of a certain desper-ation; it seems probable that Fishman was simply permitted to expand on what was no more than a doodle in order that he might boast a David Bowie song on his soundtrack album. Bowie's vocal contribution consists only of "la-las", while the backing singers' painfully forced lyrics ("It isn't wrong to be prepared to fight … it shouldn't matter if we're brown or white") were quite obviously written and added later. But the overall result is decent enough, evoking the same German pit-band atmosphere as Bowie's later *Baal* recordings. The instrumental B-side was performed by The Pasadena Roof Orchestra, who feature on the soundtrack album alongside Marlene Dietrich and, bizarrely, The Village People.

RICOCHET
• Album: *Dance*

Quite the oddest thing on *Let's Dance*, 'Ricochet' avoids the bathos of some of its bedfellows and, if nothing else, deserves credit as the album's only excursion into the experimental realms we had hitherto come to expect on a Bowie record. With no readily discernible melody it relies on a repetitive R&B/swing backing, anticipating the Creole structures of *Tonight* tracks like 'Tumble And Twirl', while Bowie intones bleak images of industrialized communities in a world devoid of spirituality. Stranger still are the dead-pan spoken interjections treated with a loud-hailer effect: "Men wait for news while thousands are still asleep, dreaming of tramlines, factories, pieces of machinery, mine-shafts, things like that…" Despite its avant-garde pretensions and enticing reminders of Bowie's earlier *Metropolis*-inspired dystopias, the resultant whole is distinctly less than the sum of its parts.

In 1987 Bowie revealed that he "adored" the composition, but "the beat wasn't quite right. It didn't roll the way it should have, the syncopation was wrong. It had an ungainly gait; it should have flowed … Nile [Rodgers] did his own thing on it, but it wasn't quite what I'd had in mind when I wrote the thing." Tony Visconti, meanwhile, singled out 'Ricochet' as one of his favourite *Let's Dance* tracks. It was the only one on the album not to be released as a single or B-side in any territory.

RIGHT

• Album: *Americans* • B-Side: 8/75 [17]

This great track is the funkiest thing on *Young Americans* and cuts to the heart of the album's James Brown/Stax aspirations. The laid-back bass and the complex syncopation of call-and-response vocals between David and the backing singers (a sequence captured in rehearsal for Alan Yentob's *Cracked Actor*) lends an air of immaculate sophistication to the lyric's paean to positive thinking. In 1975 Bowie described the song as "putting a positive drone over. People forget what the sound of Man's instinct is – it's a drone, a mantra. And people say, 'Why are so many things popular that just drone on and on?' But that's the point really. It reaches a particular vibration, not necessarily a musical level."

A 4'46" demo has appeared on bootlegs, revealing the song at an earlier but already intricate stage with David trying his vocal an octave higher. Perhaps because of its vocal complexity, 'Right' has never been performed live.

RIGHT ON MOTHER

Bowie's 2'39" demo of this *Hunky Dory*-flavoured 1971 composition has appeared on bootlegs. Apparently celebrating an improved relationship with his mother, who according to the lyric has come to terms with David's marriage and lifestyle, the song features a thumping piano very much in the style of 'Oh! You Pretty Things'. Also in common with that song, it was subsequently recorded by Peter Noone and released in October 1971 as the B-side of his single 'Walnut Whirl', with Bowie providing piano and backing vocals.

ROCK'N'ROLL SUICIDE

• Album: *Ziggy* • Live: *David, Motion, SM72, Beeb* • A-Side: 4/74 [22] • Live Video: *Ziggy*

The final track on *Ziggy Stardust* is Bowie's own 'A Day in the Life', lowering the curtain on a classic album with a majestic arrangement and a closing chord that has become one of rock's magic moments. Like so many great album-closers (Suede plainly had an eye on this song when constructing their 1994 epic 'Still Life'), it's a theatrical number that builds from a quiet,

acoustic strum to a lush arrangement of strings, guitars and operatic vocals. Lyrically it spells the dissolution of Ziggy himself, now a hollow figure caught in the headlights of braking cars as he stumbles across the road. The intimation of mortality which opens the song is a deliberate paraphrase of a poem – "something to the effect of life is a cigarette, smoke it in a hurry or savour it," Bowie explained. He claimed the source was Baudelaire, but in fact it comes from the Spanish poet Manuel Machado's *Chants Andalous*: "Life is a cigarette, / Cinder, ash, and fire / Some smoke it in a hurry, / Others savour it." In Bowie's own lyrical landscape the image reiterates the dread inhabiting many of the pivotal songs of the Ziggy period, notably 'Five Years', 'My Death' and 'Time'.

Compositionally, 'Rock'n'Roll Suicide' owes less to the conventional tenets of rock music than to the European chanson tradition. "To go from a fifties rock-flavoured thing with an Edith Piaf nuance on it produced that," Bowie remarked in 2003. "There was a sense of French chanson in there. It wasn't obviously a fifties pastiche, even though it had that rhythm that said total fifties. But it actually ends up being a French chanson. That was purposeful. I wanted that blend, to see if that would be interesting. And it was interesting. Nobody was doing that, at least not in the same way."

A more specific inspiration, albeit one that Bowie has never explicitly acknowledged, is Jacques Brel's 1964 chanson 'Jef' which, courtesy of translator Mort Shuman, appeared in the 1966 stage revue *Jacques Brel Is Alive And Well And Living In Paris* under the giveaway title 'You're Not Alone'. As if to stress the obvious, the song's repeated refrain of "Non, Jef, t'es pas tout seul" appears in Shuman's translation as "No love, you're not alone". Bowie has often cited the show's original cast recording (which also features the Shuman translations of 'Amsterdam' and 'My Death' that were to become significant items in his own repertoire) as one of his favourite records, and the lyrical, melodic and dynamic similarities between 'You're Not Alone' and 'Rock'n'Roll Suicide' are quite unmistakable.

Another source was one of the most prized albums of David's teenage years, James Brown's 1962 release *Live At The Apollo* (also known by the ungainly title *The Apollo Theatre Presents: In Person! The James Brown Show*). "Two of the songs on this album, 'Try Me' and 'Lost Someone', became loose inspirations for 'Rock'n'Roll Suicide'," David confirmed many years later. "Brown's Apollo performance still stands for me as one of the most exciting live albums ever."

When planning his aborted stage production of *Ziggy Stardust* in late 1973 Bowie extrapolated on the song's storyline, telling *Rolling Stone* that the alien "infinites" would "tear [Ziggy] to pieces on stage during the song 'Rock'n'Roll Suicide'. As soon as Ziggy dies on stage the infinites take his elements and make themselves visible." This explicit sci-fi reading seems less satisfactory than the more universal implications of the track itself which, like so much on *Ziggy Stardust*, seems almost prophetic with regard to its creator's immediate future: "You got your head all tangled up ... I've had my share, so I'll help you with the pain" might be Ziggy addressing David's future self as he heads for the abyss.

"At this point I had a passion for the idea of the rock star as meteor," said Bowie later. "And the whole idea of The Who's line: 'Hope I die before I get old.' At that youthful age you cannot believe that you'll lose the ability to be this enthusiastic and all-knowing about the world, life and experience. You think you've probably discovered all the secrets to life. 'Rock'n'Roll Suicide' was a declaration of the end of the effect of being young." Hence the cruel irony of Ziggy, who had once declared "let the children lose it", now finding himself "too old to lose it".

The song concludes on a cautious promise of redemption, although David's cry of "You're not alone, gimme your hands, 'cos you're wonderful!" is a savagely ironic take on the Las Vegas schmaltz that is the last resort of the fallen superstar. It became the most theatrical of Ziggy's stage enactments, as Bowie reached out imploringly to the front row of the audience to touch their outstretched fingertips, whipping them into a frenzy at the end of each concert. Initially, however, audiences took a while to catch on to the idea. "I remember him doing 'Rock'n'Roll Suicide', maybe for the first time," recalls David Stopps, who managed the Friars club in Aylesbury where The Spiders played their debut gig on 29 January 1972 – some six days before the studio version of 'Rock'n'Roll Suicide' was completed at Trident. "He shouted at the audience, 'Gimme your hands, 'cos you're wonderful!', and nobody got up. In those days they used to sit on the floor, and the stage was reasonably high and somebody got up to give him their hands, but only half-heartedly ... I remember thinking, 'Oh, that's a strong song,' but nobody knew it."

Such apathy was not to last, however: as the Ziggy juggernaut gathered speed over the following months

Bowie's final moment of interplay with the audience became the show's cathartic highlight. The hysteria is brilliantly captured in the film of the final Ziggy concert, first as a huge security guard drags David's vulnerable figure back from the grasping sea of hands (all for theatrical effect, one suspects), and again, seconds later, when an ecstatic young fan makes it onto the stage and hugs David for a split second before being whisked away by the bouncers. The notion of writing a song with an eye specifically on its staging potential was new to David, but would hereafter remain a vital element of his craft. Angela Bowie has claimed that she conceived this consummate fusion of music and theatre, urging David to write a song "...where you can go to the front of the stage, and he wrote 'give me your hands' ... it looked good when he did that whole sort of Messiah thing."

'Rock'n'Roll Suicide' closed nearly every concert on the Ziggy Stardust tour, from which Mick Rock compiled what he later called a "wonderful" video. The song also closed the Diamond Dogs shows and returned for a few early gigs on the Stage and Sound + Vision tours. A second studio version was recorded at David's BBC session on 23 May 1972, and can now be heard on *Bowie At The Beeb*. A superfluous 7" release of the original album track reached number 22 in 1974, a testament to Bowie's commercial stock at the time which unfortunately gave the green light to RCA's money-for-old-rope approach to his back catalogue for the remainder of the decade.

Foremost among the many cover versions of 'Rock'n'Roll Suicide' are a gruesome 1993 recording by Tony Hadley, latterly included on *David Bowie Songbook*; an extraordinary acoustic version by Hazel O'Connor, now available on 2001's *Diamond Gods*; and an excellent interpretation by Black Box Recorder, taped for a BBC radio session in 2000 and later included on *Uncut* magazine's *Starman* CD.

ROCK'N ROLL WITH ME *(Bowie/Peace)*
• Album: *Dogs* • Live: *David*

Cover versions and lyric translations aside, the earliest song for which Bowie took a co-writing credit was Mick Ronson's 1974 number 'Hey Ma Get Papa'. Following swiftly in its wake came the first co-writing credit on one of Bowie's own albums: the *Diamond Dogs* track 'Rock'n Roll With Me' is co-credited to David's schoolfriend, backing singer and sometime

Astronette Geoffrey MacCormack, now re-styling himself "Warren Peace". The song emerged one day at Bowie's Oakley Street house when MacCormack played some chord sequences on the piano; these became the basis of the verse melody, to which David added the chorus and the lyric. Co-writing credits were to become relatively common in the Bowie songbook hereafter.

Rumoured in some quarters to have been composed originally for the scrapped *Ziggy Stardust* stage musical, 'Rock'n Roll With Me' was cited by David in 1975 as one of his favourite *Diamond Dogs* tracks. With *Young Americans* already under his belt this was a revealing comment: the track betrays definite leanings towards his soul-singer phase, with a piano intro blatantly evoking Bill Withers's much-covered 1972 hit 'Lean On Me'. Few others have singled out 'Rock'n Roll With Me' as a true highlight of *Diamond Dogs*, but it's nevertheless a charmingly performed ballad with lyrical hints at the meditation on rootlessness ("I always wanted new surroundings") that would become a staple of later recordings like 'Be My Wife' and 'Move On'. After the apocalyptic 'Sweet Thing', the impression is of a calmer effort to confront the same feelings of entrapment in the gilded cage of celebrity: "I would take a foxy kind of stand while tens of thousands found me in demand … I've found the door which lets me out". Halfway through performing the song at a Philly Dogs concert in Boston, David suddenly broke off and launched into a barely coherent explanation for the audience's benefit, which would seem to suggest that the lyric is a celebration of the artist's relationship with his public: "it's about me, and singing, and why people would do – getting on stage and singing. I wouldn't be able to – you start off thinking one thing, and you would end up thinking another – the music sings for you, and kind of makes it work that way. I suppose that's what it's about."

'Rock'n Roll With Me' was performed throughout 1974, the *David Live* cut appearing as a US single in September to capitalize on the interest caused by Donovan's quick-off-the-mark cover version, released the same month.

ROSALYN *(Duncan/Farley)*
• Album: *Pin*

The first of two *Pin Ups* numbers originally recorded by The Pretty Things, 'Rosalyn' was the group's first hit

in 1964. Bowie's version is both energetic and faithful: "Dave even screamed in the same places I did," Pretty Things vocalist Phil May told Christopher Sandford.

ROSIE GIRL : see CHINA GIRL

ROUND AND ROUND *(Berry)*
• B-Side: 4/73 [3] • Compilation: S+V, Ziggy (2002), S+V (2003)

The Spiders' lively cover of Chuck Berry's classic (originally backing his 1958 single 'Johnny B. Goode') was recorded during the *Ziggy Stardust* sessions in late 1971, originally for inclusion on the album. As late as 9 February 1972 a master tape notes the latecomer 'Starman' ousting 'Round And Round' as track 4 of *Ziggy Stardust*. "It would have been the kind of number that Ziggy would have done onstage," explained Bowie in January 1972 during his earliest interview about the album and its title character. "He jammed it for old times' sake in the studio, and our enthusiasm for it probably waned after we heard it a few times. We replaced it with a thing called 'Starman'. I don't think it's any great loss, really."

'Round And Round' (re-titled, incidentally, from Berry's 'Around And Around', although some Bowie sources persist with the original) was eventually released in 1973 as the B-side of 'Drive In Saturday', appropriately stressing that single's implicit 1950s nostalgia. The recording resurfaced on *Bowie Rare*, *Sound + Vision* (from which Rykodisc also released it as a one-track promo CD), and 2002's *Ziggy Stardust* reissue. Meanwhile the 2003 repackage of *Sound + Vision* included a previously unreleased version featuring an alternative and joyously unrestrained 1971 vocal. Bowie played 'Round And Round' at the Aylesbury gig on 25 September 1971 and at a few Ziggy Stardust concerts, most memorably with guest guitarist Jeff Beck during the final Hammersmith Odeon encores on 3 July 1973.

RUBBER BAND
• A-Side: 12/66 • Album: *Bowie* • Compilation: *Deram*
• Video: *Tuesday*

Bowie's first version of 'Rubber Band' was recorded at R G Jones Studios on 18 October 1966, as part of the three-song package with which Kenneth Pitt secured his Deram contract. It's the earliest recording to showcase the infamous Anthony Newley fixation which, depending on taste, either graced or bedevilled Bowie's output during the Deram period. Although firmly rooted in vaudeville, it's a melancholy number about a war veteran whose lady-friend has been poached by a brass band conductor. The lyric's "Library Gardens" are to be found in David's native Bromley (indeed, he would perform there in 1969), but attempts to identify the narrator as his maternal grandfather Jimmy Burns are too ludicrous for words. Regardless of its actual merit, 'Rubber Band' reveals enormous leaps in the sophistication of David's songwriting and arrangements by comparison with his earlier 1966 material. There's a dramatic drive in the melodic as well as the lyrical narrative, and in many ways the song represents a creative breakthrough.

The original recording was released as a single on 2 December 1966, heralded by a Decca press release which informed the industry that the number was "a love story without a happy ending, it is pathos set to tubas … There's a neat off-beat approach to the lyrics that touch on such topics as garden tea parties, waxed moustaches and the First World War. Yet the underlying sentiment reflects the ideals and humour of this London-born singer." Despite this rather leaden publicity, 'Rubber Band' succeeded in garnering some of David's first significant reviews. *Disc* declared: "I do not think 'Rubber Band' is a hit. What it is is an example of how David Bowie has progressed himself into being a name to reckon with, certainly as far as songwriting is concerned. He is not the David Bowie we once knew. Even a different voice – distinctly reminiscent of a young Tony Newley – has emerged. Listen to this record then turn it over and listen to 'The London Boys', which actually I think would have been a much more impressive topside. But both are worth thinking about."

As *Disc* predicted the single was another flop, but nevertheless 'Rubber Band' was re-recorded on 25 February 1967 for inclusion on *David Bowie*. Although the arrangements are very similar, the superior album version is easily differentiated by Bowie's more animated vocal and by the change of date from "1912" to "1910". The second version was intended for single release in America, where Decca had been slower to market their new discovery, but it appears the US release never went beyond the promo stage. The album version later featured in 1969's *Love You Till*

Tuesday film, accompanied by a suitably whimsical sequence showing a moustachioed David, in blazer and boater, watching an imaginary bandstand concert.

RUMBLE *(Grant/Wray)*

During A Reality Tour, David and the band would occasionally play a short snippet of Link Wray's 1958 rockabilly guitar classic between numbers.

RUN *(Bowie/Armstrong)*
• Album: *TM*

This CD-only *Tin Machine* track is co-written by Kevin Armstrong, the band's unsung fifth member, and draws some obvious inspiration from The Velvet Underground's 1966 track 'Run Run Run'. Nevertheless it's one of the weakest in the set, its melody simply too slight to withstand the inevitable barrage of percussion unleashed during the choruses. The quieter, well-played verses, which fleetingly recall the "kiss you in the rain" passage of 1977's 'Blackout', feature some of Tin Machine's best guitar work and offer a glimpse of how much better the whole album might have been if liberated from the apparently obligatory bursts of destructive noise. 'Run' was performed live on the 1989 tour.

RUNNING GUN BLUES
• Album: *Man*

This is *The Man Who Sold The World*'s most obvious hangover from the style of Bowie's previous album, reviving *Space Oddity*'s penchant for the topical protest number. Taking an unusually direct lyrical line, Bowie assumes the persona of a deranged Vietnam veteran who indulges in killing sprees at home. There had been several horrific gun massacres in America during late 1969 and early 1970, but perhaps a specific source was the high-profile 1969 court martial of Lieutenant William Calley, who had answered charges of killing 300 Vietnamese villagers by claiming that he believed the mass murder of civilians was US government policy. It seems that newsmen were very much in evidence when the lyric was written: Angela Bowie recalls that David composed the number during an afternoon when he and Tony Visconti were continual-ly interrupted from their work to give interviews.

Although the lyrics may be a throwback to *Space Oddity*, in performance and production 'Running Gun Blues' provides a taste of things to come. Vocally Bowie throws caution to the wind with an exaggerat-ed prototype of the demented falsetto much loved of *Hunky Dory* and *Ziggy Stardust*, while the tight rela-tionship between guitar, bass and vocal prefigures the sound of the future Spiders From Mars.

RUPERT THE RILEY

Recorded at Trident on 23 April 1971 under the name Nick King All Stars, this polished three-minute out-take has been ridiculed in some quarters for being a tongue-in-cheek paean to David's car – as though his songs are usually about something more sensible. Featuring tight proto-*Ziggy* production, a bluesy piano riff lifted from the Stones' 'Let's Spend The Night Together' (a good eighteen months before Bowie's own version), a sinewy sax line prefiguring *Diamond Dogs*, and even a "beep-beep" motif lifted a decade later for 'Fashion', 'Rupert The Riley' is a veritable ground-zero of Bowie influences.

Two versions were recorded, one with David on lead vocal and the other, more commonly found on bootlegs, relegating David to backing vocals while the lead is taken by Mickey King, also known as both Sparky and Nick (hence "Nick King All Stars"). Angela Bowie's memoir *Backstage Passes* devotes a page to Mickey King, whose minor contribution to David's recording career passes without mention but whose talent in other departments is discussed at some length. One of the circle of exotic characters intro-duced to the Bowies by Freddi Burretti, King was mur-dered not long afterwards (in 1974, according to David), apparently on the orders of a colonel whom King had been blackmailing over their gay relation-ship.

The Riley Gamecock of the song's title was David's mode of transport during his time at Haddon Hall, but was not always the source of untrammelled joy commemorated in the song. On one occasion David stalled outside Lewisham police station and acciden-tally left the car in gear while cranking the engine, causing Rupert to lurch forward and put his owner in Lewisham Hospital. "I had really long hair in those days," David recalled in 2003. "I was standing round

the front of the car, trying to pump it back into life again, and all the cops were at the windows laughing at me. And the bloody thing started up, and I'd left it in first gear and it came at me. The crankshaft went through my leg and I was pumping blood like a foun-tain. I cracked both my knees as the bumper had kind of got me pinned to another car that was just behind it."

SABOTAGE *(Cale)*

In March 1979 Bowie joined Philip Glass, Steve Reich and John Cale on stage at New York's Carnegie Hall, in an event billed as "The First Concert Of The Eighties". In an unusual instrumental departure David played viola on Cale's 'Sabotage' (interestingly he mimed with a violin on *The Kenny Everett Video Show* only a month later). This rare performance does not, however, feature on Cale's 1979 live LP *Sabotage*.

SACRIFICE YOURSELF *(Bowie/T.Sales/H.Sales)*
• Album: *TM* • B-Side: 6/89 [51] • Live Video: *Oy*

There are enticing hints here that Bowie is indulging in some cathartic career-analysis ("twenty-five years pass him like an evening at the circus", and later "Wham bam, thank you Charlie!"), but there's little else of interest in this messy thrash, during which even the most dedicated listener begins to feel that *Tin Machine* is outstaying its welcome. Included only on the CD version of the album but also released as a B-side, 'Sacrifice Yourself' was performed live on both Tin Machine tours. Amusingly, the lyric includes the very nearly prophetic line "married to a Klingon": it would be another eighteen months before David met his future wife Iman, later a shape-shifting alien in *Star Trek VI*.

SADIE : see LITTLE TOY SOLDIER

SAFE *(Bowie/Gabrels)*
• B-Side: 9/02 [20] • Bonus: *Heathen (SACD)*

Originally recorded under the title '(Safe In This) Sky Life', this little-known recording is of immense his-toric interest in the Bowie canon. Written in early 1998, '(Safe In This) Sky Life' was originally destined for inclusion in the soundtrack of the *Rugrats* movie. Having recorded an initial version with Reeves Gabrels, Bowie decided that a second attempt would benefit from the expertise of Tony Visconti, with whom he hadn't shared a studio since the *Baal* sessions in 1981. According to Visconti the film's producers had requested a classic Bowie sound, "a little bit of 'Space Oddity', '"Heroes"' and 'Absolute Beginners' all rolled into one. I don't know whose idea it was to get me, but I got the phone call from David." On Radio 2's *Golden Years* documentary in 2000, Visconti revealed that the reunion was a success on every level: "We still have a great affection for each other. That's become obvious lately. He really did make amends, and he sought me out … we're back together again as friends."

In August 1998 the long-awaited reunion spawned a new version of 'Safe'. Backing vocals were provided by Richard Barone of The Bongos (who had covered 'The Man Who Sold The World' on their 1987 album *Cool Blue Halo*). Barone later revealed that he sang multi-tracked harmonies on 'Safe', which also featured the talents of Blondie drummer Clem Burke, sometime Prefab Sprout keyboardist Jordan Ruddess and, in classic Tony Visconti tradition, a 24-piece string section.

Bowie and Visconti immediately went on to collaborate on David's cover of John Lennon's 'Mother', but sadly 'Safe' disappeared from the *Rugrats* project when the scene containing it was cut altogether. "I have always wanted to work with David Bowie and I finally had my chance," the film's music coordinator Karyn Rachtman said afterwards. "He delivered a song far beyond my wildest dreams and now I can't even use it! The song is beautiful." For his part, Bowie indicated in 1999 that a release was now unlikely: "Unfortunately, it doesn't really fit in with what I'm doing at the moment. A shame really, as it was quite sweet for what it was."

In June 2002 the track was made available online to purchasers of the enhanced *Heathen* CD, reappearing in more conventional form three months later as one of the 'Everyone Says 'Hi'' B-sides, while the subsequent SACD release of *Heathen* carried a 5.1 remix which is over a minute longer than the B-side version. Powered throughout by an acoustic strum familiar from much of the *'hours…'* material, 'Safe' is a soaring Eastern-tinged rock ballad dripping with strings and keyboards, with trademark Gabrels-style guitar squeals during the final fade. The lyric covers the same themes of spiritual uncertainty found throughout *'hours…'* and, more particularly, *Heathen* ("Tomorrow's really on my mind / Sure to pick up from now on / Things will move more slowly / But the air is thin and chance is slim / Sometimes we all have these dreams … Are things getting better now? / Are things getting worse?"). In 2001 Bowie had intimated that he might rework the song with "a lyric change", so it remains uncertain whether the released version boasts the original vocal or a new one recorded during the *Heathen* sessions.

(SAFE IN THIS) SKY LIFE *(Bowie/Gabrels)* : see SAFE

SATELLITE OF LOVE *(Reed)*

Originally demoed for The Velvet Underground's 1970 album *Loaded*, one of Lou Reed's loveliest compositions was reinvented for *Transformer* with co-production by Bowie and a superb Mick Ronson arrangement, matching the melody to a dainty piano line and snappy finger-clicks of the kind familiar from Bowie's recordings of the time. David's backing vocals are unmistakable, particularly in the 'Memory Of A Free Festival'-style playout. "David Bowie's background vocals," wrote Lou Reed in the liner notes of his 2003 compilation album *NYC Man*, "I love them on his records, I love them when he did them on my record. It's not the kind of part I would have ever come up with if you left me alone with a computer program for a year. But David hears those parts. Plus he's got a freaky voice and he can go up that high and do that. It's very, very beautiful. And he's a great singer."

'Satellite Of Love' is the only directly Bowie-related track to feature in Todd Haynes's film *Velvet Goldmine*.

SATISFACTION *(Jagger/Richards)* : see THE JEAN GENIE

SAVIOUR *(Young)*

St Louis-born singer-songwriter Kristeen Young's 2000 album *Enemy* brought her to the attention of Tony Visconti, who introduced her to David Bowie, who in turn invited her to record some vocal and piano overdubs for *Heathen*. Not long afterwards, Bowie duetted with Young on 'Saviour', one of the Visconti-produced solo tracks recorded in 2002 which were eventually released the following year on her splendidly titled album *Breasticles*.

Kristeen Young was evidently delighted to be working with Bowie, and promptly incorporated several of his songs, including 'Boys Keep Swinging', 'Conversation Piece' and 'The Man Who Sold The World', into her live repertoire. At a gig in London in 2003, she explained that 'Saviour' was inspired by her friendship with Tony Visconti, its lyric celebrating the redemptive qualities of a relationship that had helped them both to overcome hard times: "We could rise up from this grave / We could prepare to ascend / We could walk on water / Be my reciprocal saviour." Both instrumentally and vocally, Kristeen Young's work bears a striking resemblance to the mighty Kate Bush at her most uncompromisingly intense, and nowhere more so than on this track, which recalls some of the more left-field offerings on *The Dreaming*. Bowie rises to the occasion with a committed, anguished vocal performance on a song which, like the rest of the album, is original, unapologetically avant-garde, and absolutely superb.

A promo CDR of *Breasticles*, privately distributed by Young prior to the official release of the album, features a different track-listing and an alternative version of 'Saviour' known as the 'Bowie Mix'. This is more or less identical to the track that eventually appeared on the album with the exception of David's vocal itself, which is a different recording. The vocals for the released version were added in February 2003: "We re-did some things to it," explained Young, "which included David re-singing some of his parts."

SAVIOUR MACHINE
• Album: *Man*

With its lush, almost big-band arrangement and cinematic fade-in opening, 'Saviour Machine' is poised somewhere between the protest-song sensibilities of *Space Oddity* and the totalitarian sci-fi of *Diamond Dogs*. In an interview for *Music Now!* at the end of 1969 Bowie had voiced his distaste for the dangerous gullibility of those who are "happy to be able to follow other people", and here he spins a parablaic yarn about "President Joe" who sweeps to power ("the world held his hand") but abdicates responsibility to

a utopian super-computer which turns on its human creators: "A plague seems quite feasible … or maybe a war, or I may kill you all!" The inspiration is likely to be Joseph Sargent's 1969 film thriller *The Forbin Project* (publicity tag line: "We built a super computer with a mind of its own and now we must fight it for the world!"), which opened in the UK in early 1970. Once again Bowie is dabbling in his pet themes of leadership's dangerous glamour, and the secular's usurpation of the spiritual (the computer is called "The Prayer") – themes which would go on to fashion much of his most successful and controversial 1970s work. It's all the more surprising, then, that the lyric of 'Saviour Machine' was hastily written at the last minute after repeated prompting from Tony Visconti (Angela Bowie records David staying up into the early hours to complete it), while the guitar break is taken straight from the chorus of the whimsical folk number 'Ching-a-Ling', discarded only a year earlier but already light years away musically.

The rare original German release of *The Man Who Sold The World* featured a reprise of the 'Saviour Machine' intro at the end of the album, cross-faded with the end of 'The Supermen'.

SCARY MONSTERS (AND SUPER CREEPS)
• Album: *Scary* • A-Side: 1/81 [20] • Live: *SNL 25* • Compilation: *Best Of Bowie* • Live Video: *Moonlight*

The title track and third single from *Scary Monsters* is an aggressive, guitar-driven piece in which Bowie, in a heavily distorted rendering of his fruitiest Cockney whine, revisits the brutalized inner world of claustrophobic romance etched out to such memorable effect on Iggy Pop's two Berlin albums. This time David's girlfriend has "a horror of rooms" and is "stupid in the street and she can't socialize"; and not unlike Iggy's China Girl, "she asked for my love and I gave her a dangerous mind". It's a cryptic and disturbing return to the "monster" who had plagued David in 'The Width Of A Circle' a decade earlier, and just like Mick Ronson on that classic track, Robert Fripp delivers a frenzied masterclass in how to go heroically over the top without a shred of hard-rock machismo.

'Scary Monsters' was performed live on the Serious Moonlight, Glass Spider, Outside and Earthling tours, while Frank Black duetted on the number at the fiftieth birthday concert. The song made regular appearances on television and radio spots during 1997, including *Saturday Night Live* on 8 February (later released on the show's 1999 compilation *SNL25 – Volume 1*), and *The Jack Docherty Show* on 18 April. An unlikely Johnny Cash-style "Country" version was included in several of the two-man acoustic sessions Bowie recorded with Reeves Gabrels for American and Canadian radio stations at around the same time. In 1998 a remastered version of the original album cut appeared in the PlayStation game *Gran Turismo* and its accompanying "soundtrack" CD, while the original 7" edit made its CD debut on the UK, US/Canada and Greek formats of 2002's *Best Of Bowie*.

SCREAM LIKE A BABY
• Album: *Scary* • B-Side: 10/80 [5]

Once again Bowie recycles obscure early 1970s material for inclusion on *Scary Monsters*, in this case the basic melody of 'I Am A Laser', written for The Astronettes and recorded at Olympic in 1973. In all other respects 'Scream Like A Baby' is every bit a *Scary Monsters* track, its ultra-modern new wave guitar/synth sound instantly identifiable with contemporaneous autumn 1980 releases like Hazel O'Connor's 'Eighth Day' and OMD's 'Enola Gay'. Bowie's fantastically accomplished vocal bristles with bizarre techniques, notably the extraordinary vari-speed segment in which two parallel vocal lines are simultaneously raised and lowered in pitch while maintaining the same tempo, raising the ghost of the split-personality themes prevalent on *The Man Who Sold The World* and *Hunky Dory*. The lyric bears out such comparisons, offering a brutal story of mental instability and *Clockwork Orange*-style totalitarianism. In a direct echo of his 1973 description of 'The Supermen', Bowie described the setting as "future nostalgia … a past look at something that hasn't happened yet."

A 3'17" demo has appeared on bootlegs, featuring an inferior, synthesizer-free arrangement, slightly different lyrics and a more cautious vocal performance: notably, Bowie sings "I'm learning to be an *integrated* part of society", and doesn't stammer the final word as he does to such memorable effect on the album. 'Scream Like A Baby' was rehearsed for the Glass Spider tour, but was dropped before the show opened and has yet to be performed live.

SEA DIVER *(Hunter)*

Produced by David for Mott The Hoople's *All The Young Dudes*.

SEARCH AND DESTROY *(Pop/Williamson)*

Mixed by Bowie for Iggy And The Stooges' *Raw Power*, 'Search And Destroy' was performed during Iggy's 1977 tour; a version featuring David appears on *Suck On This!*.

SEASON FOLK : see ERNIE JOHNSON

THE SECRET LIFE OF ARABIA *(Bowie/Eno/Alomar)*
• Album: *"Heroes"*

The unjustly overlooked final track of *"Heroes"* is probably the most conventional song in the entire "Berlin" trilogy. A complex multi-tracked vocal counterpoints David's baritone with outrageous extremes of bass and falsetto, while his saxophone, Dennis Davis's brilliant drumming and Carlos Alomar's funk guitar conspire to create a commercial, almost disco-rap sound. The lyric returns once again to Bowie's predilection for casting himself as an actor trapped in a film: this time he becomes a torrid Rudolph Valentino in *The Sheik* or perhaps John Boles in *Desert Song* ("You must see the movie, the sand in my eyes / I walk through a desert song when the heroine dies").

The superb 1981 cover version by Heaven 17 spin-off The British Electric Foundation, with Billy MacKenzie of The Associates on lead vocal, was included on *David Bowie Songbook*.

SECTOR Z
(Gutter/McNaboe/Zoidis/Albee/Roods/Ward)

Bowie provides guest vocals on this brilliant track from the Rustic Overtones' *Viva Nueva*, an archly spacey soul-pop confection with DJ-meets-sci-fi lyrics reminiscent of 'Starman' and 'Lady Stardust', described by Tony Visconti as "a humorous song about making contact with aliens". Bowie initially appears as a disc-jockey interrupting lead singer Dave Gutter's verses with the repeated enquiry "Are you listening?", before taking over the lead vocal to create a call-and-response with himself (much in the style of 'Ashes To Ashes') for the 'Starman'-esque chorus line ("Is your volume up, is your power on? / To your solar system at the speed of sound / Are you listening? Which way does your antenna go? / On your radio, this is rock'n'roll!"). Bowie's wildly exuberant, high-pitched vocal was described by a delighted Visconti as "nothing less than his Ziggy voice! I was thrilled to hear that tone and style again. Afterwards I said, 'You haven't used that voice for a while!' David waved a cigarette and said, 'There's a very good reason for that!'"

SEE EMILY PLAY (Barrett)
• Album: Pin

"I only met him on a couple of occasions," said David in 1973 of Syd Barrett, who had rather cruelly reviewed 'Love You Till Tuesday' for Melody Maker back in 1967, "and then we didn't get on all that well. But I'm a great fan of his." Years later he went further, describing Barrett's as "probably one of the most languid, poignant voices in English popular music. I thought he was an absolutely superb poet and a stunning performer, which has not really been said about him, but he had a hypnotic, charismatic effect on stage. Also the first bloke I'd seen wearing make-up in a rock band to great effect. Me and Marc Bolan both noted that!"

Bowie's radical reworking of Pink Floyd's 1967 hit is one of the highlights of Pin Ups. From the opening tick-tock of guitar to the elaborate violin fade-out, the psychedelic Sgt Pepper production is marvellous, displaying a lightness of touch unique on the album. Subtle lines on piano and synthesizer counterpoint the emotive guitar work, and there's a devastatingly effective use of Bowie's favourite trick of adding backing voices an octave lower than the lead vocal, lending the whole a Hunky Dory-ish feel.

SEE-SAW (Cropper/Covay)

Don Covay's 1965 single was played live by The Buzz.

SEGUE – ALGERIA TOUCHSHRIEK
(Bowie/Eno/Gabrels/Garson/Kizilcay/Campbell)
• Album: 1.Outside

For the longest and best of 1.Outside's "segues" Bowie plays a 78-year-old dealer in "art-drugs and DNA prints". The unsettling Mr Touchshriek, who speaks in David's finest Cockney, is considering renting a room to a fellow "broken man", because "We could have great conversations, looking through windows for demons and watching the young advancing all electric." The backing is a curious piece of cod-reggae lift music, midway between Tonight's version of 'Don't Look Down' and Brian Eno's full-blown excursions into the weird.

SEGUE – BABY GRACE (A HORRID CASSETTE)
(Bowie/Eno/Gabrels/Garson/Kizilcay/ Campbell)
• Album: 1.Outside

The first of the spoken "segues" on 1.Outside is supposedly a cassette-recording of the 14-year-old murder victim's last words, spoken as she slips from consciousness. Like much of the album, it treads a fine line between absurdity (Bowie's high-pitched vocal treatment wittering about "popular musics and aftershocks") and horror (the obvious echo of the Moors Murderers' tape-recordings). Backed by a slow, hallucinatory wall of guitar feedback and piano, Baby Grace reveals that "Ramona put me on these interest-drugs, so I'm thinking very, too, bit too fast, like a brain-patch," and concludes: "Now they just want me to be quiet, and I think something is going to be horrid." Bowie later joked that "I've gone from wearing dresses to being a 14-year-old girl," and described the "rather sad, poignant little cassette" as "delightful stuff."

SEGUE – NATHAN ADLER
(Bowie/Eno/Gabrels/Garson/Kizilcay/Campbell)
• Album: 1.Outside

Detective Professor Nathan Adler of Art-Crime Inc is granted two spoken interludes on 1.Outside, the first of which is credited to the album's six-man core band and the second to Bowie and Eno only. Both allow David to indulge in some cod private-eye narration straight out of a 1940s dime novel: against a funky rhythm guitar backdrop, Bowie affects a creditable Bogart to discuss the suspects in the case, describing his ex-girlfriend Ramona as "an update demon" and recounting how Leon Blank cut "a zero in the fabric of time itself."

SEGUE – RAMONA A. STONE
(Bowie/Eno/Gabrels/Garson/Kizilcay/Campbell)
• Album: *1.Outside*

For the silliest of his *1.Outside* segues, Bowie adopts a vocoder-treated alien voice for the character of body-parts jeweller Ramona, whose experiences sound amusingly (and surely intentionally) similar to those of her creator: "I was an artiste in a tunnel, and I've been having a mid-life crisis," she waspishly informs us, as the atmospheric textures of the next track, 'I Am With Name', gather momentum in the background.

SELL ME A COAT
• Album: *Bowie* • Compilation: *Deram* • Video: *Tuesday*

This melancholy ballad employs standard Freudian imagery (summer as love and happiness, winter as loss and frigidity) in a tale of poisoned love. The Gillmans propose in their biography that Bowie's fairytale metaphors ("Jack Frost ain't so cool … see my eyes, my window pane") bear striking similarities to a poem written a generation earlier by his grandmother ("Old Jack Frost has come again / He's busy on the window pane"). The track was recorded on 8 December 1966, and David later performed it during the Lindsay Kemp show *Pierrot In Turquoise*. In 1968 it was offered without success to both Judy Collins and Peter, Paul and Mary.

'Sell Me A Coat' was dusted down in 1969 for inclusion in the *Love You Till Tuesday* film. Some additional instrumentation and rather overpowering backing vocals from Hermione Farthingale and John Hutchinson were added to the original recording, but the poorly mixed result is by no means an improvement, swamping the delicacy of the arrangement and muffling David's lead vocal. The film sequence is worthier of attention as it includes a shot of Mr Fish, the London boutique that would later supply David with his *Man Who Sold The World* dresses. Like the film's rendition of 'When I Live My Dream', the lyric's

poignancy is given a twist by the knowledge that David and Hermione were parting company during the shoot.

SELL YOUR LOVE *(Pop/Williamson)* :
see **MOVING ON**

SENSE OF DOUBT
• Album: *"Heroes"* • B-Side: 1/78 [39] • Live: *Stage*

Created almost entirely by the "Oblique Strategies" cards used to generate random effects during the *"Heroes"* sessions, this doomy, minimalist instrumental is constructed around a simple four-note piano line and a bank of piping synthesizers of the kind familiar from Walter Carlos's *A Clockwork Orange* theme. "It was an organic sound set against a synthesized horn section, a trumpet fanfare," said Bowie in 1978. "It retains a human quality. [If] it becomes completely electronic, I think it misses the point … my wish is to encapsulate what I see around me, the environment and the time … so I can look back and see the seventies through my eyes like a series of paintings."

'Sense Of Doubt' was one of the more high-profile *"Heroes"* tracks in its day, being performed on Italian television's *L'Altra Domenica* in 1977 and featuring throughout the Stage tour. Gerry Troyna's 1984 film *Ricochet* includes what is effectively a full-length video for 'Sense Of Doubt', a sequence showing Bowie exploring a deserted shopping mall in Singapore, gliding up and down escalators and past fountains and Christmas trees.

Philip Glass used 'Sense Of Doubt' as the basis for the third movement of his 1997 *"Heroes"* Symphony.

SEVEN *(Bowie/Gabrels)*
• Album: *'hours…'* • B-Side: 1/00 [28] • A-Side: 7/00 [32] • Live: *Beeb*

The second great throwback number on *'hours…'* is delivered in the fragile acoustic style of Bowie's softer *Hunky Dory* recordings, blessed with a gorgeous melody and a weeping slide guitar of perfect, unadorned simplicity. "My God, it's like right out of the sixties, real hippy-dippy!" was David's observation. The appearance in the lyric of a mother, father and brother, the latter pictured weeping with the narrator "on a bridge of violent people", led to inevitable conclusions which Bowie was quick to play down: "They're not necessarily my mother, father and brother," he told Q, "it was the nuclear unit thing."

'Seven' is clearly not concerned with specific remembrances: quite the contrary, in fact. Like many tracks on the album it addresses the poignant inconstancy of memory and concludes that the present is what matters. "Seven days to live, seven ways to die … I'd actually reduce that further to twenty-four hours to live," David told Q. "I'm very happy to deal and only deal with the existing twenty-four hours I'm going through. I'm not inclined to even think too heavily about the end of the week or the week I've just come through. The present is really the place to be." For VH1's Storytellers he introduced 'Seven' as a "song of nowness", reflecting that "tomorrow isn't promised."

Like 'Thursday's Child', 'Seven' uses the days of the week as an index of time, and it's worth considering that the medieval Book of Hours typically includes seven penitential psalms. But here the album's devotional imagery recedes into the Nietzschean probings of Bowie's early 1970s songs, realigning the famous proposition in Die Fröhliche Wissenschaft that "God is dead": "The gods forgot they made me, so I forgot them too / I listen to their shadows, I play among their graves."

'Seven' featured on most of the 1999-2000 dates; a live version recorded in Paris on 14 October 1999 was included on single formats of 'Survive', while a recording from the BBC Radio Theatre concert on 27 June 2000 appears on the Bowie At The Beeb bonus disc. The July 2000 A-side release included Bowie's original demo, together with remixes by Beck and Marius de Vries, and another live version taped in New York on 19 November 1999. Yet another live version, recorded on 22 November 1999 for Canada's Musique Plus channel, was later included as a QuickTime video on a CD cover-mounted on the August 2000 issue of Yahoo! Internet Life magazine, tying in with Bowie's appearance at the Yahoo! awards. Another version, similar to the demo, appeared in the Omikron computer game.

SEVEN DAYS (Peacock)

Annette Peacock's ballad was produced by Bowie for The Astronettes in 1973, and eventually released on 1995's People From Bad Homes.

SEVEN YEARS IN TIBET (Bowie/Gabrels)
• Album: Earthling • A-Side: 8/97 [61] • Live: liveandwell.com • Video: Best Of Bowie

Inspired by Heinrich Harrer's autobiography of the same name, the gorgeously atmospheric 'Seven Years In Tibet' was added to Bowie's live repertoire in September 1996 while the Earthling sessions were still in progress. "One thing I've learned about my writing is that I'm not a didactic writer," explained David, who had presumably learned a thing or two from 'Crack City'. "When I try and make a very strong point simply, I fall on my ass. I'm really bad at it so I stay away from that, but I wanted to say something about the Tibetan situation. When I was about nineteen … a very influential book for me was Seven Years In Tibet … and that book kind of stayed with me over the years. I wanted to relay what had been happening politically with Tibet through that book. And the subtext of the song is really some of the desperation and agony felt by young Tibetans who have had their families killed and themselves have been reduced to mere ciphers in their own country. I wouldn't explore it too thoroughly because it really works in more of an expressionistic level. It's a feeling that comes over in the song."

The track was nearly abandoned during recording; beginning as a Reeves Gabrels composition called 'Brussels' it was, Bowie recalled, "something we started that seemed incredibly hack, with a very predictable, self-serious quality. I said, 'Dump this one, Reeves,' but he worked on it during my absence and turned it into something absolutely magical. It went from being something I wanted off the album to almost my favourite song on the album."

It was a narrow escape, for 'Seven Years In Tibet' is unquestionably one of Bowie's finest tracks of the 1990s, harnessing a slinky saxophone riff and the distant squeals of Reeves Gabrels's guitar to a superbly dark, lolloping rhythm for the softly sinister verses, before sledgehammering the listener into submission with a tidal wave of guitar for the shrieking chorus. Best of all are David's treated vocals and Mike Garson's dementedly wonky synthesizer line. Bowie described the backing as "the juxtaposition of a Stax influence with a late eighties Pixies style", while Gabrels claimed that for the verses "I deliberately evoked a Fleetwood Mac 'Albatross' feeling, but mainly so I could oppose it to the ton-of-bricks chorus."

The revival of Bowie's fascination with all things Tibetan coincided with a wave of high-profile American support for the country's plight during the mid-1990s. Major motion pictures like *Kundun* and *Seven Years In Tibet* (a 1997 dramatization of Harrer's memoir which had no direct connection with the Bowie track) enshrined the subject as Hollywood's *cause du jour*. In the same year, Bowie contributed 'Planet Of Dreams' exclusively to the Tibet House Trust's charity album *Long Live Tibet*, while in 2001, 2002 and 2003 he performed short but memorable sets at the Trust's benefit concerts at Carnegie Hall.

Bowie's Mandarin vocal version of 'Seven Years In Tibet' sat at number 1 in the Hong Kong chart at the time of the Chinese takeover in June 1997. "I thought what a perfect time to release a single in Hong Kong, just as the Chinese take over," he said later. "It got super-popular but I'm not sure we'll be able to tour there now of course … I've probably fallen out with the Chinese now." (Some years later he would in fact play Hong Kong without incident on A Reality Tour.) With lyrics translated by Lin Xi, the Mandarin version was released in some territories under the title 'A Fleeting Moment', and appeared on the B-side of the UK single.

'Seven Years In Tibet' was performed with Dave Grohl at Bowie's fiftieth birthday concert, and featured throughout the Earthling tour. Released in August 1997, the edited single did little chart business, and the video was seldom seen until its inclusion (in both English and Mandarin forms) on 2002's *Best Of Bowie* DVD. Directed by the "Torpedo Twins" of *Tin Machine Live At The Docks* fame, it interspersed live footage with images of Tibetan lamas, religious icons and our old friend the dancing Minotaur, the studio sequences being shot in Italy on 9 July. A live version recorded in New York on 15 October 1997 later appeared on *liveandwell.com*.

SEX AND THE CHURCH
• Album: *Buddha*

Sexuality and spirituality are key elements in Hanif Kureishi's *The Buddha Of Suburbia*, and 'Sex And The Church' is Bowie's fugue on the confluence of the two themes. Against a club-friendly 'Pallas Athena' beat, David mutters disjointed thoughts through a vocoder, demanding "Give me the freedom of the spirit and the

joys of the flesh," and returning to a cyclical refrain of the track's title. After six surprisingly hypnotic minutes it comes to a sudden end with an insistent rhythmic build-up borrowed from 'The Jean Genie'.

SHADES *(Pop/Bowie)*

Co-written and co-produced by Bowie for Iggy Pop's *Blah-Blah-Blah*, the excellent 'Shades' was remixed and released as a single without success in 1987.

SHADOW MAN
• European B-Side: 6/02 • B-Side: 9/02 [20]

Existing only as a rough 3'45" demo on guitar, drums and vocal, the original unfinished 'Shadow Man' (also documented variously as 'The Man' and 'Shadow-man') was recorded at Trident on 14 September 1971 in the early stages of the *Ziggy Stardust* sessions. There is some evidence to suggest that an earlier version was taped on 23 April along with 'Rupert The Riley', although an unlikelier pairing is hard to imagine. The lyric is a meditation on the future impact of our present lives, as disclosed by the mysterious Shadow Man himself: "He'll show you tomorrow / He'll show you the sorrows / Of what you did today." Ultimately it seems that he is a projection of the future self: "Look in his eyes and see your reflection … the Shadow Man is really you … He knows your eyes are drawn to the road ahead / And the Shadow Man is waiting round the bend."

Clearly evoking earlier *doppelgänger* lyrics like 'The Man Who Sold The World' and, in particular, 'Wild Eyed Boy From Freecloud' ("really you and really me…"), 'Shadow Man' is often cited as one of the finest Bowie rarities. Certainly it's a fascinating curiosity and a wonderful song – but, as a melancholy folk-ballad imbued with the introspective isolation of *Space Oddity*-era compositions like 'Conversation Piece', it's hard to imagine how it might have fitted into the *Ziggy Stardust* concept.

In 2000 'Shadow Man' became one of the more surprising titles selected for re-recording during the *Toy* sessions, although it's uncertain whether this new version was originally intended for inclusion on *Toy* or as part of the mooted thirtieth anniversary *Ziggy Stardust* project. It eventually appeared on some formats of 2002's 'Slow Burn' single, and later as a B-Side of 'Everyone Says 'Hi''. Bowie gives a magnificent vocal performance over a gorgeously evocative arrangement for piano and strings, and the result is outstanding: this is without question one of the most beautiful recordings of his career.

SHAKE (Cooke)

Sam Cooke's posthumous 1965 hit was played live by The Buzz.

SHAKE APPEAL (Pop/Williamson)

Mixed by Bowie for Iggy And The Stooges' *Raw Power*.

SHAKE IT
• Album: *Dance* • B-Side: 5/83 [2]

Let's Dance concludes with this likeable enough piece of fluff, topping a bassline almost identical to that of the title track with a dated synthesizer vibro-twang familiar from countless early 1980s hits like Chaka Khan's 'I Feel For You' and Nik Kershaw's 'I Won't Let The Sun Go Down On Me'. Lyrically 'Shake It' neatly wraps up the *Let's Dance* motif of partying as a bulwark against spiritual despair ("We're the kind of people who can shake it if we're feeling blue"), and draws on the images of moonlight and boxing which pervade the album's lyrics and sleeve artwork ("I duck and I sway, I shoot at a full moon"), but it's unlikely to be hailed as one of Bowie's most substantial achievements.

SHAKIN' ALL OVER (Kidd)
• B-Side: 8/91 [33]

Johnny Kidd and the Pirates, later supported live by The Lower Third, enjoyed a number 1 hit in 1960 with 'Shakin' All Over'. Many years later 'Shakin' All Over' was revived for the two Tin Machine tours, a live 1989 recording appearing as a B-side. At the Bradford concert on 2 July 1989, Bowie dedicated 'Shakin' All Over' to his former drummer John Cambridge, who had appeared out of the woodwork to attend the gig. Incidentally, the fact that Bowie occasionally announced the number by yelling "There's a whole

lotta shakin' goin' on!" has given rise to an erroneous belief that Tin Machine also played Jerry Lee Lewis's 1957 hit of that name. They didn't. Another unreliable rumour has Bowie jamming on the number with Mott The Hoople in 1972: see 'Sweet Jane'.

SHAPES OF THINGS (Samwell-Smith/McCarty/Relf)
• Album: *Pin*

The second Yardbirds cover on *Pin Ups* was originally a number 3 hit in 1966. Bowie here gives a more convincing account of himself than on 'I Wish You Would', with a declamatory vocal complemented by swaggering percussion and some pleasingly intricate production. Even so, in songs like 'Five Years' and 'Drive In Saturday' David had already explored similar territory, arguably to far greater effect.

SHE BELONGS TO ME (Dylan)

Bob Dylan's song (from 1965's *Bringing It All Back Home*) was among Bowie's live repertoire in 1969.

SHE SHOOK ME COLD
• Album: *Man*

Tony Visconti has cited this track as one of *The Man Who Sold The World*'s "classic moments", confessing that parts of it still leave him "smiling from ear to ear", but his opinion is not universally shared. Given the well-documented apathy with which Bowie is said to have approached the sessions, it's tempting to conclude that this was a track on which he bestowed particular indifference. The lyric is little more than a swaggering rock'n'roll boast about a sexual conquest with a dash of occult nastiness thrown in (the line "she sucked my dormant will", together with the callous confession about "many young virgins", hint at the Crowley-inflected "Sexmagickal" overtones of 'Holy Holy'), while the Cream-indebted prog-rock arrangement is undiluted Mick Ronson. Untempered by Bowie's more delicate touch – a combination that made classics out of the album's other rock numbers – Ronson's Jeff Beck/Jimmy Page impersonation falls a long way short of his brilliant arrangements on later albums. It's perfectly competent early 1970s rock, but it's hardly a David Bowie song at all. "I had to peel them apart to get David to listen to what the band had just done," Visconti later said of David and Angie's behaviour during the sessions. Here, it shows.

SHE'LL DRIVE THE BIG CAR
• Album: *Reality* • Live Video: *Reality*

Introducing 'She'll Drive The Big Car' at the Riverside Studios concert in September 2003, Bowie explained that it is "a tragic little story about a lady and her family. And she lives in the wrong part of town, but she wants to live in an even badder, wronger part of town – but her would-be affair, her boyfriend, doesn't turn up."

The resulting excursion into shattered illusions and thwarted fantasies must rank among the most affecting lyrics on *Reality*, and like many of them it is steeped in the mood and environs of downtown New York. The opening lines relate the protagonist's failed attempt to run away ("She waited by the moon / She was sick with fear and cold / She felt too old for all of this / Of course he never showed"), and thence her return to a disappointing marriage, where "love lies like a dead cloud on a shabby yellow lawn". The sense of dashed expectations is pressed home in the second verse: the line "Way back when 'millennium' meant racing to the light" reflects Bowie's oft-repeated comments at the time of *Heathen* regarding his sense of disappointment that the optimism with which the world ushered in the year 2000 had melted away within months. The only respite for the heroine in this song, not unlike the protagonist in 'Fly', is to get into her car "and talk herself insane" as she drives "south along the Hudson" listening to "sad sad soul" on the radio. Like several of the *Reality* tracks, it's a mournful, disturbing window onto a wretchedly disappointed life.

"All her plans have been disassembled by her thoughtless boyfriend who didn't show up to take her back to the old bohemian life," David explained to *Interview* magazine, "so she's stuck with this middle-class family and absolutely, desperately unhappy as she's peeling along Riverside Drive. In my mind, she just swings it off to the left and takes the whole lot down. You know what I mean? I see it as a sad song, but I kind of left it open. She's turning the radio up high so she doesn't have to think any more when she makes her decision to go over the edge."

Despite this overwhelming tone of suicidal melan-

choly, 'She'll Drive The Big Car' is also one of the most infectious numbers on *Reality*, combining a funky backbeat with sophisticated, soulful backing vocals and a series of irresistibly catchy motifs, from Mike Garson's repetitive four-note piano figure to the appealing flourishes of Bowie's harmonica, and a series of rhythm guitar hooks, percussion trick-shots and handclaps in the choruses that recall that milestone of Bowie funk 'Golden Years'. David's lead vocal is masterful, moving from a bleak, emotionally burned-out and heavily distorted drone in the verses to a soulful, heartfelt croon in the choruses, even treating us to an exhilarating snatch of his *Young Americans* falsetto when he unexpectedly leaps an octave on the second "sad sad soul". That phrase admirably describes 'She'll Drive The Big Car', which was performed live throughout A Reality Tour.

SHE'S GOT MEDALS
• Album: *Bowie*

Recorded on 14 November 1966, this knockabout novelty number has received some attention as the earliest lyrical evidence of Bowie's dalliance with gender-bending and cross-dressing. Concerning a tomboy who joins the army in the guise of a man, only to cheat death in a bombing raid by returning home as a woman, it enjoys the same cheeky-chappie delivery as 'Love You Till Tuesday': Bowie delivers another of his Tony Hancock impressions on "She went and joined the army, passed the medical – don't ask me how it's done!" In the mid-1960s, incidentally, "medals" was still a slang term for "balls", originally derived from the Bengal Medal's reputation for being so commonplace that soldiers would use them as fly-buttons.

In 1967 'She's Got Medals' was offered by Bowie's American publisher to Big Brother & The Holding Company and to Jefferson Airplane; both turned it down.

SHILLING THE RUBES :
see **ARE YOU COMING ARE YOU COMING**

SHINING STAR (MAKIN' MY LOVE)
• Album: *Never*

After the flawed excellence of 'Glass Spider', *Never Let*

Me Down gets into trouble with this, the first in a series of insipid and featureless tracks which drag the album through its protracted demise. The arrangement is a flimsy, negligible combination of rhythm guitar and synthesized handclaps, but the real problem is the lyric. Bowie described it as "a strange little piece" which "reflects back-to-street situations, and how people are trying to get together in the face of so many disasters and catastrophes socially around them, never knowing if they're going to survive it themselves. The one thing they have got to cling on to is each other … It's just a little love song coming out of that environment." But whereas 'Time Will Crawl' capitalizes on Bowie's cut-up style to create some sinister images, and even 'Day-In Day-Out' gets by on a bit of righteous anger, here the attempt to muster some kind of eschatological relevance smacks of desperation. Topical references to a "crack-house", "Sinn Fein" and "Chernobyl" were embarrassing even in 1987, particularly as Prince had only just ploughed the same furrow far more effectively with the laid-back rage of 'Sign "O" The Times', a top ten single immediately prior to the release of *Never Let Me Down*.

David's high-register delivery is indebted to Smokey Robinson, one of several obvious vocal influences on the album. "I tried 'Shining Star (Makin' My Love)' with another voice, and it just sounded wrong," he explained. "It needed a high, little voice, a bit Smokey Robinson. That never bothered me, changing voices to suit a song." The final nail in the coffin is the incongruous arrival of guest vocalist Mickey Rourke, who joins Bowie on what the credits refer to as a "mid-song rap".

The song was rehearsed for the Glass Spider tour, but dropped before the opening date.

SHOPPING FOR GIRLS (*Bowie/Gabrels*)
• Album: *TM2*

Hard on the heels of the horror that is 'Stateside' comes one of the most undervalued Tin Machine songs, based on a subject brought to Bowie's attention by Reeves Gabrels's wife Sarah. An investigative journalist by trade, she had spent the six months immediately prior to her press engagement on the Glass Spider tour working on a news project called *Children Of Darkness*, during which she had investigated such scandals as child slavery in South American silver

mines, child soldiers in Uganda, and child prostitution in Thailand and the Philippines.

By contrast with the unattractive stridency of the political lyrics on the first Tin Machine album, Bowie displays an admirable lightness of touch in 'Shopping For Girls', a quietly furious song about underage sex tourism in the Far East. The lyric is one of his best, evoking a culture of emotional and educational deprivation by dint of some hard-edged wordplay (the familiar acrostic becomes "A small black someone jumps over the crazy god," while "That's a mighty big word for a nine-year-old" deftly exposes the premature worldliness of a ruined childhood). There are echoes of the brutal assignations of 'Cracked Actor' and 'Time', but here there's no shred of residual glamour to counterbalance the sordid reality: "These are children riding naked on their tourist pals, while the hollows that pass for eyes swell from withdrawal … You gaze down into her eyes for a million miles, you wanna give her a name and a clean rag doll."

'Shopping For Girls' was performed during the It's My Life tour, and later unexpectedly revived in Bowie's BBC session for *ChangesNowBowie*. This slower, acoustic version was a vast improvement on the original, allowing a wordy song the necessary breathing space denied by its stodgy *Tin Machine II* arrangement.

SHOUT : see **FASHION**

SILLY BOY BLUE
• Album: *Bowie* • Live: *Beeb*

This is one of Bowie's outstanding Deram tracks and, recorded on 8 December 1966, it's also among the earliest evidence of his emerging Buddhist phase. He had told *Melody Maker* the previous February that "I want to go to Tibet. It's a fascinating place, you know … The Tibetan monks, lamas, bury themselves inside mountains for weeks and only eat every three days. They're ridiculous – and it's said they live for centuries." David's dabblings in Buddhism would inform several other tracks of the period, but 'Silly Boy Blue' is the first and the most obvious: the surreal lyric addresses a "Child of Tibet" and evokes "Mountains of Lhasa", "reincarnation" and even "Yak-butter statues". In 1968-1969 it would provide the backing for David's Tibetan mime sequence *Yet-San And The Eagle* (see Chapter 3).

New recordings featured in David's first two BBC radio sessions, taped on 18 December 1967 and 13 May 1968. The first of these remains close in style to the album version, while the second, now available on *Bowie At The Beeb*, showcases an expansive and intricate Tony Visconti arrangement for strings, keyboards and percussion which really opens up and enriches the song's potential: as Tibetan cymbals and gongs echo around him, Bowie chants "Chimi Chimi Chimi" during the instrumental section in tribute to his Buddhist teacher and friend Chimi Youngdong Rimpoche.

Like many of David's Deram songs 'Silly Boy Blue' was pitched to other recording artists, and although rejected by Judy Collins, Jefferson Airplane and Big Brother & The Holding Company, it was taken up by Billy Fury, whose unsuccessful cover was released by Parlophone in March 1968. In America the song was apparently recorded by the obscure Elephant's Memory, who later went on to work with John Lennon.

Meanwhile, the melody of 'Silly Boy Blue' reappeared almost note-for-note in the chorus of Right Said Fred's 1991 top three hit 'Don't Talk Just Kiss' – conscious or not, it certainly wouldn't be the band's first connection with Bowie (see *Jazzin' For Blue Jean* in Chapter 5).

The 2'56" demo which has appeared on bootlegs was recorded with The Lower Third at R G Jones Studios as early as October 1965. Its entirely different lyric has more to do with suburban London than distant Tibet, while the bass guitar and handclap interjections will be instantly recognizable to fans of The Beatles' 'I Want To Hold Your Hand'.

A new studio version of 'Silly Boy Blue' was among the songs recorded during 2000's prolific *Toy* sessions. On 26 February 2001, David performed a spectacular live version (which retained the "Chimi" chant) at the Tibet House Benefit concert at Carnegie Hall, backed by the Scorchio Quartet and a troupe of monks from the Drepung Gomang Buddhist Monastic University.

SILVER TREETOP SCHOOL FOR BOYS

This little-known Bowie composition, reprising the *David Bowie* album's atmosphere of nostalgic whimsy with a dash of obscure menace, was inspired by a newspaper report David had seen about a pot-smok-

ing scandal among the boys of Lancing College. On 22 May 1967 Kenneth Pitt sent Bowie's demo (now believed lost) to producer Steve Rowland. Nothing came of this, but later the same year the song was recorded and released by two different groups. Slender Plenty's version was first off the mark, released as a single on Polydor in September. The better-known version by The Beatstalkers, a Scottish band managed by Kenneth Pitt, appeared in December as the B-side of their CBS single 'Sugar Chocolate Machine'; it later surfaced on *David Bowie Songbook*. Unlike The Beatstalkers' subsequent Bowie cover 'Everything Is You', David made no contribution to the recording.

SISTER MIDNIGHT *(Pop/Bowie/Alomar)*

Written in January 1976 during rehearsals for the Station To Station tour and performed at several early US dates, 'Sister Midnight' was a collaborative effort: Carlos Alomar devised the guitar riff, Bowie wrote the first verse, and Iggy Pop completed the lyrics. Rehearsal recordings for the 1976 tour reveal the song's origins in the Carlos Alomar-driven funk groove that had shaped earlier compositions like 'Fame' and 'Stay', an element largely eliminated from subsequent renditions as the song's colder, spikier characteristics began to emerge. Iggy's stark and definitive studio version, produced by David and featuring a revised lyric, was recorded at the Château d'Hérouville in late June at the commencement of sessions for *The Idiot*, which takes its title from the song. It was released as a single in America, but failed to chart.

'Sister Midnight' appeared throughout the 1977 Iggy Pop tour (a version appears on *Suck On This!*), and was performed by Iggy and David on CBS's *The Dinah Shore Show* on 13 April. Although David never recorded his own studio version, the melody was later revamped with another new lyric (only "can you hear it at all?" survived from the original) as 'Red Money', the closing track on *Lodger*. Bowie introduced snatches of the original 'Sister Midnight' into 'Young Americans' on some dates of the Sound + Vision tour, and later revived the number in full for A Reality Tour.

SIXTEEN *(Pop)*

Bowie co-produced and played piano on this track

from Iggy Pop's *Lust For Life*.

SKUNK CITY (*Bowie/Bolan*) : see **MADMAN**

SKY LIFE : see **SAFE**

SLEEPING NEXT TO YOU (*Bowie/Bolan*)

Although Marc Bolan's career took off ahead of Bowie's, with an uninterrupted run of 11 top ten singles which firmly established him as glam's first superstar, he failed to maintain his early momentum. Unlike Bowie, Bolan was unable or unwilling to present a moving target, and with glam on the wane his music deteriorated catastrophically. "Sadly, Marc would never develop further than the three-minute single," Tony Visconti later told Barney Hoskyns. After spending the mid-1970s languishing in Los Angeles and Monte Carlo in much the same cocaine blizzard as Bowie (but, unlike Bowie, with no classic albums to show for it), Bolan began a cautious recovery in 1976 with his hit 'I Love To Boogie', followed in March 1977 by his best album for some time, *Dandy In The Underworld*. Later the same year Bolan was thrown an unlikely lifeline as the presenter of a teenage pop show for Granada Television, and it was on the set of *Marc* that the two old sparring partners met once again.

Bowie was in the midst of his publicity push for *"Heroes"*, and it was primarily in order to showcase the title track that he agreed to appear. Recording took place on 9 September 1977 at Granada's Manchester studios where, despite all manner of provocative circumstances, spirits were high. Bowie was apparently untroubled by the discovery that Bolan's studio band included Herbie Flowers and Tony Newman, two members of the infamous *David Live* pay revolt of 1974, and despite some biographers' attempts to portray the occasion as a bitter battle of egos, the only major mishap was the late arrival of guest band Generation X. For the climax of the show, David was to join Marc on a brand new number called 'Sleeping Next to You' which the pair had co-written for the occasion. The studio schedule had over-run and there was only time for one messy and abortive take, which degenerated into chaos when Bolan fell off the stage a few seconds into the guitar intro. The electricians

pulled the plugs and apparently Bolan ran to his dressing room in tears, only emerging when Bowie suggested they try to salvage something from the footage. Everyone, Bolan included, saw the funny side as the tape was replayed. "Oh, that's really Polaroid!" David is said to have remarked, "You've got to keep that ending!" They did, but Bolan would not live to see it aired. Seven days later, in the small hours of 16 September, he was killed in a car crash just off Roehampton Lane in Barnes. Accompanied by Tony Visconti, Bowie attended the funeral at Golders Green on 20 September, and subsequently established a trust fund for Bolan's son.

In addition to the brief televised snatch of 'Sleeping Next To You' – little more than a 'Jeepster'-style guitar intro – around twenty minutes of audiotape exists of Bowie and Bolan rehearsing the song. It's also referred to as 'Standing Next To You' in some documents, but Bolan clearly sings "sleeping" on the tape. This version, however, is neither as complete nor as satisfying as 'Madman', 1977's other Bowie/Bolan composition.

SLIP AWAY
• Album: *Heathen*

One of the undoubted highlights of *Heathen*, the majestic 'Slip Away' is a sweeping ballad whose wistful piano, soaring strings and heartfelt chorus immediately evoke classics like 'Space Oddity' and 'Life On Mars?'. The lyric is a melancholy meditation on lost happiness and faded glory, in this case somewhat cryptically expressed through the perspectives of two puppets from the obscure low-budget children's television series *The Uncle Floyd Show*. Fronted by pianist and entertainer Floyd Vivino, the show began airing on New Jersey networks in January 1974 and continued on and off, amid fluctuating fortunes and ever-changing TV channels, until 1999, when the Cablevision network finally sounded its death-knell. An anarchic and irreverent early evening children's variety show pitched somewhere between *Banana Splits* and *The Muppet Show*, *Uncle Floyd* enjoyed its first flush of success on the WTVG channel in the late 1970s, when it began to attract wider media attention and enticed guest bands like Squeeze and The Ramones to perform in the studio. During one recording in 1980 the show's performers were astonished to see David Bowie in the studio audience, singing and clapping along to the signature song 'Deep In The Heart Of Jersey'. David went backstage afterwards to tell the cast how much he loved the show, revealing that he watched it every night during his make-up sessions for *The Elephant Man*. When the flabbergasted performers enquired how he had first come across the show, he told them that he had been introduced to it by another fan, John Lennon.

"Back in the late seventies, everyone that I knew would rush home at a certain point in the afternoon to catch *The Uncle Floyd Show*," David recalled in 2002. "He was on UHF Channel 68 and the show looked like it was done out of his living room in New Jersey. All his pals were involved and it was a hoot. It had that Soupy Sales kind of appeal, and though ostensibly aimed at kids, I knew so many people of my age who just wouldn't miss it. We would be on the floor, it was so funny."

Although Uncle Floyd was joined by a supporting cast of human entertainers, the show's central appeal was his interaction with the many and varied puppet characters, foremost among whom was Oogie, a clown-faced wooden *alter ego* voiced and operated by Floyd himself in the manner of a ventriloquist's doll (no ventriloquist himself, Floyd would wait for the camera to cut to a close-up of Oogie's face during their conversations). Another favourite puppet was Bones Boy, a cynical wisecracking skeleton doll whose catchphrase "Snap it, pal!" became one of the show's trademarks.

The Uncle Floyd Show inspired fierce devotion among its homegrown New Jersey audience, but never achieved the hoped-for transition to nationwide success. The nearest it came was in 1982, when the series enjoyed a brief period of national syndication by the broadcasting giant NBC, but it was soon pulled after the customary complaints (one station denounced it as "garbage", and many others objected to the perceived religious irreverence of a character called Brother Billy Bobby Booper). By 1983 the show was once again relegated to the New Jersey cable circuit.

Hence, in Bowie's 'Slip Away' lyric, the wistful image of the abandoned puppets recalling how fame was once within their grasp ("Once a time they nearly might have been / Bones and Oogie on a silver screen"), and the knowledge that their brief moment of glory is now no more than a series of radio waves travelling ever deeper into space ("Oogie knew there's never ever time / Some of us will always stay behind / Down in space it's always 1982"), and that the show,

as it recedes into history, will be known only by the few who saw it ("No-one knew what they could do / Except for me and you / They slip away…"). But the greatness of 'Slip Away' lies in the fact that its meditative beauty effortlessly transcends the specific and eccentric lyrical references: as a song of loss and yearning, its themes are universal.

Originally recorded under the title 'Uncle Floyd' during the *Toy* sessions in 2000, the track was revamped from scratch for *Heathen*, as evidenced by its stately and grandiose Tony Visconti production. In addition to the majestic washes of synthesized strings, plaintive bar-room piano and fluid bass, 'Slip Away' is notable for once again featuring the Stylophone, the electronic toy famously employed on 'Space Oddity' and brought out of retirement in 2000 for use on a number of tracks including David's cover of 'Pictures Of Lily'. "Somebody from England had sent me one with the original Rolf Harris boxing on it, and I was absolutely delighted," he said in 2002. "I hadn't seen the thing since '69, '70, whenever it was. So I used it as the solo instrument for 'Pictures Of Lily' with, I thought, great results … I said, I really should start using this again on something. So I put it with my collection of old synthesizers. I've got a lot of old stuff that I've kept over the years, that I really dragged out for this album." The pulse of low-tech synthesizers and reversed-tape trickery that opens and closes the track recalls the experimental textures of Bowie's Berlin albums, in particular 'Subterraneans'. "You hear [the Stylophone] really well at the end of 'Slip Away'," David pointed out. "Tony suggested that I cover the top note of some of his string parts with it, and it gives them a kind of lift."

The 5.1 remix of the track on the *Heathen* SACD is marginally longer than the CD version. David's Stylophone made regular live appearances on the Heathen and A Reality tours, during which the magnificent live performance of 'Slip Away' (accompanied on the latter tour by the screening of a clip from *The Uncle Floyd Show*) was a regular highlight.

SLOW BURN
• Album: *Heathen* • European A-Side: 6/02 •
Compilation: *Best Of Bowie*

If 'Slip Away' harks back to some of Bowie's classic ballads, then the next track on *Heathen* revisits another vintage Bowie sound: the futuristic revamping of the old-fashioned R&B style epitomized by tracks like '"Heroes"' and 'Teenage Wildlife'. Both songs are instantly recalled in the rolling bassline and soaring lead guitar of 'Slow Burn', although the shifting chords, doom-laden lyrics and soulful saxophone harmonics offer something entirely new.

As most reviewers noted at the time, 'Slow Burn' is distinguished by an excellent lead guitar performance by The Who's Pete Townshend, returning to the Bowie stable 22 years after his contribution to 'Because You're Young'. Bowie described Townshend's performance on 'Slow Burn' as "the most eccentric and aggressive guitar I've heard Pete play, quite unlike anything else he's done recently." The collaboration came about after a meeting in October 2001, by which time the main *Heathen* sessions had already been completed. "He came over to New York to do the Concert For New York," explained Bowie, "and I was on that too. But rehearsals kind of took everything over and we got no time to do any recording, so he had to go back to England. I sent him an MP3 of it, and then he sent his parts back on Pro-tools, so we just transferred it in the studio. So it was kind of done by mail, the entire thing."

Three months later, on 29 January 2002, further overdubs were added by The Borneo Horns, the three-man sax section last heard on *Never Let Me Down*. At the time Bowie cited 'Slow Burn' as "probably my favourite track on the album so far," describing it as "moody and sad, with a strong R&B feel."

'Slow Burn' continues *Heathen*'s preoccupation with what David referred to as "a low-level anxiety", and, like the album's opener 'Sunday', it was popularly but inaccurately suggested by reviewers that the lyric referred in some way to the events of 11 September 2001. In fact, as Bowie explained, the anxious intimations of "fear overhead" in "this terrible town" were grounded in feelings he had been nurturing long before the terrorist attacks. Indeed, many of the same concerns can be traced to earlier Bowie compositions. The sense of urban paranoia ("The walls shall have eyes and the doors shall have ears / But we'll dance in the dark and they'll play with our lives") echoes dozens of lyrics on albums like *Scary Monsters* and *Diamond Dogs*, while the portentous menace of the line "These are the days" had already been put to good use in both 'Under Pressure' and 'The Dreamers'. But this is not to say that 'Slow Burn' lacks individuality; on the contrary, it's one of the strongest compositions on *Heathen*. Tony Visconti's

razor-sharp production abounds with splendid touches such as the tight saxophone blasts that punctuate the second verse, while his recording of David's voice is strongly reminiscent of its treatment on '"Heroes"'.

The 5.1 remix of 'Slow Burn' on the *Heathen* SACD is marginally longer than the CD version. As the debut single from *Heathen*, 'Slow Burn' made several appearances during live television spots in the summer of 2002, including a *Top Of The Pops* performance pre-recorded in New York on 2 June. However, owing to changes in plan by the record company the release of the single was sporadic. In most of mainland Europe it appeared on 3 June 2002 on two separate discs: a card-case CD backed by 'Wood Jackson' and 'Shadow Man', and a maxi CD featuring the same tracks plus 'When The Boys Come Marching Home' and 'You've Got A Habit Of Leaving'. Both formats featured the full-length album version of 'Slow Burn', while a 3'55" radio edit appeared on a promo CD and later on *Best Of Bowie*. Small quantities of the European single were imported to Britain but the official UK release, originally scheduled for July 2002, was cancelled; no *Heathen* single would be forthcoming in Britain until 'Everyone Says 'Hi'' two months later. Unexpectedly for a number that had initially been marketed as the album's flagship song, 'Slow Burn' disappeared from the Heathen tour repertoire after just two concerts, making its second and last stage appearance at Meltdown on 29 June.

A SMALL PLOT OF LAND
(Bowie/Eno/Gabrels/Garson/Kizilcay/Campbell)
• Album: *1.Outside* • Soundtrack: *Basquiat*

Falling somewhere between the accumulative symphonic sound of Philip Glass and the avant-garde jazz of pianist Mike Garson, 'A Small Plot Of Land' is one of *1.Outside*'s more challenging tracks, a cold, pared-down arrangement for drums and piano over which atonal howls of guitar, bass and ghostly voices build into a pandemonium of sound. According to the Outside tour brochure, the song is "To be sung by the residents of Oxford Town, New Jersey," and Bowie's lyric seems to be an almost Biblical lament. The doomed plight of the "poor dunce" who "pushed back the pigmen" and "never knew what hit him" recalls Bowie's early classic 'Wild Eyed Boy From Freecloud', and the observation that "prayer can't travel so far these days" taps into *1.Outside*'s theme of pre-millennial paganism. The line "swings through the tunnels and claws his way" is plainly indebted to Scott Walker's 'Nite Flights' ("turns its face into the heat and runs the tunnels"), covered by Bowie only a year earlier. Indeed, the entire recording is without doubt influenced by Walker, whose superb 1995 album *Tilt*, although released after the *1.Outside* sessions, bears uncanny similarities with this track in particular.

In October 1994 Bowie discussed the as-yet unheard 'A Small Plot Of Land' in an Internet conversation with Brian Eno published in Q magazine. Eno revealed that he was working on "a new beginning to that song which I like very much. It's an atmospheric piece about 90 seconds long using your 'poor soul' phrase played very slowly and forming long drifting overlays. In the background is a sound like motors or machines or transmissions of some kind. I think it's lovely…" This certainly isn't the finished album track, although it might be the early, percussion-free Eno mix used in Julian Schnabel's 1996 film *Basquiat* to underscore the emotional aftermath of Andy Warhol's death. Eno later recorded in his diary that Schnabel considered this mix "Much better than what went on the record".

Bowie gave a magnificent unadorned live performance of 'A Small Plot Of Land', taken at a languid tempo and accompanied only by Mike Garson on piano, at a charity function in New York on 18 September 1995. In its more familiar album arrangement, the song was played throughout the Outside tour, and in 1996 a further instrumental remix was used as the theme music for Andrew Graham-Dixon's excellent revisionist BBC series *A History Of British Art*.

SO NEAR TO LOVING YOU

An unrealized Davie Jones composition rehearsed with The Manish Boys in 1965.

SO SAD : see SWEET JANE

SOCIAL KIND OF GIRL

An acetate of this mysterious Bowie demo, coupled with 'Everything Is You' and thus probably dating from around May 1967, was privately sold in 1996.

SOFT GROUND *(Allen)*

Produced by Bowie for Mott The Hoople's *All The Young Dudes*.

SOME ARE *(Bowie/Eno)*
• Bonus: *Low*

This out-take from the *Low* sessions was mixed in 1991 for release as a bonus track. Although co-credited to Brian Eno, the original composition is said to predate *Low*: according to some sources it was written in Los Angeles in 1975 as part of Bowie's abandoned soundtrack for *The Man Who Fell To Earth*, and was intended to underscore the scene near the end of the film in which Mary-Lou sees Santa Claus driving his sleigh down the street, although Bowie himself has denied this. It's a soft, emotive track over which David's breathy and indistinct vocal captures fleeting images of "sleigh-bells in snow". The version re-orchestrated by Philip Glass for the second movement of his 1993 *Low Symphony* was played as pre-show music on the Outside tour, and later appeared on the 2001 compilation *All Saints*.

SOME WEIRD SIN *(Pop/Bowie)*

Bowie co-wrote and co-produced this track on Iggy Pop's *Lust For Life*, also providing keyboards and backing vocals. It was performed on Iggy's 1977 tour.

SOMEBODY UP THERE LIKES ME
• Album: *Americans*

Developed from Bowie's earlier composition 'I Am Divine' and briefly considered as the title for *Young Americans*, 'Somebody Up There Likes Me' was recorded at Sigma Sound in August 1974. The title derives from the 1956 biopic starring Paul Newman as the boxer Rocky Graziano, but the lyric addresses a wider cult of celebrity. David described it as a "Watch out mate, Hitler's on his way back" warning, and his portrait of the charismatic, media-obsessed politician "on everybody's wall, blessing all the papers, thanking one and all, hugging all the babies, kissing all the ladies" is all too clear. Significantly, the lyric could just as well describe any celebrity (even a rock star – David added that the song was "your rock and roll sociological bit"), and exposes the implicit fiction of image-construction and the hollowness of fame and adulation: "Worlds away when we were young, any man was judged by what he'd done / But now you pick them off the screen, what they look like, where they've been." Yet again, Bowie warns us to choose our leaders carefully – a theme he would soon pursue to dangerous extremes – but 'Somebody Up There Likes Me' muffles its ominous tone behind a slick, shimmering wall of saxophone and synthesizer, and you have to listen quite carefully to deduce that it's not just another smoochy soul number.

A 6'39" demo, similar to the finished version but for a different keyboard arrangement, has appeared on bootlegs. The song was performed occasionally during the Philly Dogs tour, receiving its live premiere on 10 October 1974.

SOMETHING HAPPENS

This unfinished track (also referred to as 'Something') was demoed in the late summer of 1971. In a contemporary radio interview, Bowie named the song as one that would appear on his next (i.e. post-*Hunky Dory*) album. In the event it never got beyond the demo, of which an almost inaudible 2'11" copy has surfaced on bootlegs.

SOMETHING I WOULD LIKE TO BE

Kenneth Pitt claims that this otherwise unknown track was recorded at Bowie's BBC session on 18 December 1967, but it seems likely that this is incorrect (see Chapter 4).

SOMETHING IN THE AIR *(Bowie/Gabrels)*
• Album: *'hours…'* • Soundtrack: *American Psycho* • B-Side: 7/00 [32]

There are countless evocative echoes of Bowie's past in the building intensity of 'Something In The Air', whose chorus chords reprise 'All The Young Dudes' while the hushed verses, with their ambient 'Albatross'-style guitars and fragmented vocoder vocals, recall 'Seven Years In Tibet'. A snatch of the melody (on the lines "nothing left to save" and "place

of no return") comes straight from 'The Motel', while lyrics like "We lay in each other's arms but the room is just an empty space / I guess we've lived it out" recollect older regrets like 'An Occasional Dream'. The repeated cry of "I've danced with you too long" resurrects the "last dance" of 'Under Pressure' and, as Bowie himself has pointed out, the song's coda includes an obvious homage to 'I'm The One', a 1972 recording by Annette Peacock, whom David had approached that same year with a view to performing on *Aladdin Sane*.

Even the title hints at a tantalizing relevance to Bowie history: Thunderclap Newman's unrelated one-hit wonder 'Something In The Air' topped the UK chart during the *Space Oddity* sessions in July 1969, which tempts one to read suggestive David/Angie resonances into lines like "We used what we could to get the things that we want / But we lost each other on the way". Ultimately, though, 'Something In The Air' is a bigger song than that; it's a study in regret which portrays, in David's words, "somebody who really can't stand the relationship he's in, so he's kicking out his partner." Like all his best compositions it operates in an elliptical, elusive territory, addressing universal truths and specific moments simultaneously. It's a grandiose, heartbreaking song, and one of the highlights of Bowie's 1990s output. It was played on the *'hours…'* tour (fine versions were recorded at the BBC session on 25 October 1999 and for *Later… With Jools Holland* on 29 November), and a live version recorded in New York on 19 November 1999 appeared on some formats of the 'Seven' single. An edited version of the album cut appears in the *Omikron* computer game. In 2000 a Mark Plati remix appeared over the end credits of the film *American Psycho* (later appearing as a bonus track on the 2004 US reissue of *'hours…'*), while the original version was used in the soundtrack of the 2001 film *Memento*.

SOMEWHERE *(Bernstein/Sondheim)* :
see **HEAVEN'S IN HERE**

SONG FOR BOB DYLAN
• Album: *Hunky*

"This is how some see BD," was David's summary of this little-regarded track at the time of *Hunky Dory*'s release. The title parodies 'Song To Woody', Bob

Dylan's 1962 paean to his idol Woody Guthrie, but Bowie's tribute becomes a harangue rather than a eulogy. Addressed directly to "Robert Zimmerman" (highlighting David's growing preoccupation with layers of identity), the lyric suggests that the radical folk-rocker of old should implore his "good friend Dylan" to return to his songwriting roots ("gaze a while down the old street") and come to the rescue of those who have lost faith ("Tell him they've lost his poems … Give us back our unity"). There's a sense, too, in which Bowie is staking a claim on Dylan's territory: in 1976 he told *Melody Maker* that the song "laid out what I wanted to do in rock. It was at that period that I said, OK, if you don't want to do it, I will. I saw the leadership void."

The full-scale glam chorus pilfers incongruously from The Velvet Underground (the titles of 'Here She Comes Now' and 'There She Goes Again' effectively provide the hook), while celebrating the power of Dylan's "old scrapbook" to rout the world's corruption. In his evocation of the goddess Athene, Bowie renews *Hunky Dory*'s plea for the artist to be visited by inspiration. 'Song For Bob Dylan' thus seems to be both tribute and reprimand, and a reminder amid the album's cryptic amoralities that, two years on from the protest numbers on *Space Oddity*, Bowie still identifies himself at least in spirit with a more polemic school of songwriting.

'Song For Bob Dylan' was premiered at Bowie's BBC concert session recorded on 3 June 1971, with lead vocals by schoolfriend and erstwhile King Bee George Underwood. As David's rambling introduction made (un)clear, at this early stage it was called 'Song For Bob Dylan – Here She Comes'. The number featured frequently during the early Ziggy concerts, before disappearing altogether in mid-1972.

SONG SUNG BLUE *(Diamond)*

Neil Diamond's 1972 hit was included in David's medley with Cher on *The Cher Show* in November 1975.

SONG 2 *(Albarn/Coxon/James/Rowntree)*

During tour rehearsals in July 2003, David and several of his band saw Blur in concert at New York's Hammerstein Ballroom. Bowie sang the band's prais-

es for months thereafter, and during A Reality Tour would often launch into a short burst of their 1997 hit between numbers.

SONS OF THE SILENT AGE
• Album: *"Heroes"* • Live Video: *Glass*

This is one of the outstanding tracks on *"Heroes"* and also among the most unsettling. The cloud of depression and retreat that hangs over so much of Bowie's Berlin work is here manifested in a cryptic portrait of shadowy characters who, perhaps like Hitler's Nazis, "stand on platforms, blank looks and no books" and "rise for a year or two then make war". Like the cursed immortals of 'The Supermen', the sons of the silent age "don't walk, they just glide in and out of life" and "they never die, they just go to sleep one day". Interspersed between these mystic, almost catatonically droned verses – also showcasing one of Bowie's finest saxophone performances – we get triumphant bursts of "Bowie histrionics" as David howls pledges of eternal love.

'Sons Of The Silent Age' was performed on the Glass Spider tour, during which guitarist Peter Frampton took over vocal duties for the choruses while Bowie concentrated on a piece of gymnastic choreography with dancer Constance Marie. The song was later reworked by Philip Glass as the fourth movement of his 1997 *"Heroes" Symphony*.

SORROW *(Feldman/Goldstein/Gottehrer)*
• A-Side: 9/73 [3] • Album: *Pin* • Live Video: *Moonlight*

Originally a one-hit wonder for The Merseys in 1966, 'Sorrow' is one of the highlights of *Pin Ups* and an obvious choice of single. Entering the chart just as Deram's reissue of 'The Laughing Gnome' peaked at number 6 (rumour has it that RCA delayed 'Sorrow' for this very reason), it pulled focus onto David's new work and spent a healthy five weeks in the top ten. Bowie turns in a convincing forgery of Bryan Ferry's affected consonant-dropping baritone, lending credence to the rumour that he was stealing the march on Ferry's own covers project *These Foolish Things*. Melodically 'Sorrow' ploughs the same commercial sax-and-strings furrow as Bowie's contemporaneous Lulu recordings, and like them it belongs to that short-lived moment when the Ziggy hairstyle was still in place but the leotards had given way to double-breasted jackets and ties.

As the current single, 'Sorrow' was included in NBC's *The 1980 Floor Show* in October 1973, with Bowie singing a new vocal over the *Pin Ups* backing track. 'Sorrow' subsequently featured in the Philly Dogs and Serious Moonlight tours.

SORRY (H.Sales)
• Album: *TM2*

The 1989 Tin Machine gigs occasionally featured a raucous hard-rock version of this Hunt Sales composition, reworked for *Tin Machine II* as a slushy ballad. Although marginally less hideous than 'Stateside', Hunt's second stint as lead vocalist is another unwelcome intrusion, dragging the album in the direction of Bryan Adams at his most schmaltzy or Roger Waters at his most self-indulgent. Ironically Hunt's drums, often such an intrusive presence, are here at their most restrained. The acoustic guitar intro and Bowie's soft saxophone breaks promise more than the song, an uninteresting "didn't mean to hurt you" ramble, ever manages to deliver. 'Sorry' was again performed on the It's My Life tour.

SOUL LOVE
• Album: *Ziggy* • Live: *Stage*

Only the most overworked imagination could slot this song directly into a *Ziggy Stardust* narrative, but the sublimely melodic 'Soul Love', with its tight guitar work and charming sax solo, provides a perfect bridge between the apocalyptic foreboding of 'Five Years' and the glam meltdown of 'Moonage Daydream'. Compared with the rest of the album it initially seems an unusually compassionate song, a series of wistful moments in love: a mother grieving at her son's grave, the son's love of the ideal for which he died (and thus the further resonance of Mary grieving at Christ's tomb), a pair of young lovers believing in their "new words", and the love of "God on high". But on closer inspection there's a nihilistic undercurrent and a cynical re-reading of love that stands in sharp contrast with Bowie's earlier songwriting: he rails against "idiot love" which "descends on those defenceless" and bleakly concludes that "love is not loving". These are

sentiments reflected in a comment he made in 1976 regarding his short but passionate relationship with Hermione Farthingale: love, he said bleakly, "was an awful experience. It rotted me, drained me, and it was a disease."

Other vignettes revive Bowie's scorn for institutions and causes: the dead son/Christ "gave his life to save the slogan", reprising the futility of 'Cygnet Committee' and prefiguring "Tony went to fight in Belfast" later on the album. "The priest", already a character in 'Five Years', here "tastes the word" amid "the blindness that surrounds him", recollecting the "bullshit faith" of 'Quicksand' and clearing the way for a secularized "church of man, love" (or, in a more provocative reading, the "church of man-love") in the following song.

'Soul Love' was recorded at Trident on 12 November 1971. The song made a couple of appearances on the 1973 American tour, and again for the first two Serious Moonlight shows, but its only stint as a regular live fixture was on 1978's Stage tour. The excellent *Stage* version was released as a single in Japan.

Mick Ronson recorded an unlikely Country & Western solo version in 1975. Inelegantly retitled 'Stone Love (Soul Love)', it remained in the vaults until appearing as a bonus track on various 1990s Ronson re-releases. On 22 February 2002 Chocolate Genius opened the Tibet House Benefit concert – at which Bowie was also performing – with an acoustic version of 'Soul Love'.

SOUND AND VISION
• Album: *Low* • A-Side: 2/77 [3] • Bonus: *Low* • Live: *Rarest* • US A-Side: 12/91

RCA officials who had thrown up their hands in horror at *Low* were placated by the meteoric success of its first single, which hit the top 3 in Britain to become Bowie's biggest hit, reissues excepted, since 'Sorrow' in 1973. Dennis Davis's distorted snare-drum, the insistent *plish* of cymbals, the emotive backing vocals of Tony Visconti's wife Mary (formerly Mary Hopkin of 'Those Were The Days' renown), and the layered washes of synthetic strings played by Bowie himself, contribute to one of his most iconic and brilliant recordings. The infectious rhythm and catchy melody seem strangely at odds with the fragmentary lyric, a depressive meditation on retreat and creative bankruptcy characteristic of *Low*'s sombre introspection: "Pale blinds drawn on day, nothing to do, nothing to say," muses Bowie dismally as, recalling 'Quicksand', he finds himself anxiously "waiting for the gift of sound and vision".

In 2003 Bowie described 'Sound And Vision' as "a very sad song for me … I was trying very hard to drag myself out of an awful period of my life. I was locked in a room in Berlin telling myself I was going to straighten up and not do drugs anymore. I was never going to drink again. Only some of it proved to be the case. It was the first time I knew I was killing myself and time to do something about my physical condition."

In common with the rest of *Low*, Bowie's vocals were added after the studio band had packed up and left; Tony Visconti recalls that even his wife's backing vocals were "recorded before there was a lyric, title or melody." Intriguingly, he tells David Buckley that originally "there were more verses, but we honed it down during the mix to what you've heard."

Released in February 1977, 'Sound And Vision' was an instant turntable favourite and its lengthy intro was co-opted by BBC television to back its programme trailers. It was this exposure that helped boost sales of the single, which Bowie himself did nothing to promote. Despite no video, *Top Of The Pops* appearance or even so much as an interview, 'Sound And Vision' became a huge hit – at least in Britain. It proved too much for the American singles market, only managing number 69 and signalling the end of Bowie's short commercial honeymoon in the US until 1983.

Low's 1991 reissue came with a bonus remix by David Richards which allows an unpleasant honking saxophone to disrupt the original's textured atmospherics. In the same year this version and two further remixes appeared on an American single by 808 State. Despite being the Berlin albums' biggest commercial hit, 'Sound And Vision' received only one performance on the Stage tour, at Earls Court on 1 July 1978; this one-off rendition later appeared on *RarestOneBowie*. The song was later revived for the Sound + Vision, Heathen and A Reality tours.

SOUTH HORIZON
• Album: *Buddha* • B-Side: 11/93 [35]

Bowie's favourite track on *The Buddha Of Suburbia* anticipates the more experimental tracks on *1.Outside*, notably 'A Small Plot Of Land'. Mike Garson's piano improvisation is here at its wildest, prompted by a constantly shifting background of rhythms and atmospheric effects peppered with Bowie's saxophone and Erdal Kizilcay's plaintive trumpet. As Bowie explained, "all elements, from lead instrumentation to texture, were played both forwards and backwards. The resulting extracts were then intercut arbitrarily giving Mike Garson a splendidly eccentric backdrop upon which to improvise. I personally think Mike gives one of his best ever performances on this piece and it thrills on every listening."

SPACE ODDITY
• A-Side: 7/69 [5] • US A-Side: 7/69 • Italian A-Side: 1/70 • Album: *Oddity* • A-Side: 9/75 [1] • B-Side: 2/80 [23] • Live: *Motion, SM72, BBC, Beeb* • Compilation: *Rare, Tuesday, S+V, Deram* • Bonus: *Scary* • Video: *Tuesday, Collection, Best Of Bowie* • Live Video: *Ziggy, Moonlight*

Even after all these years 'Space Oddity' remains Bowie's best-known, most influential and perhaps most remarkable song. Having been a hit twice over, it also enjoys the distinction of being his biggest-selling single in the UK, knocking 'Let's Dance' and 'Dancing In The Street' into second and third place.

The story of Major Tom's fateful trip into space has become part of pop mythology, and Bowie has wisely preserved the song's mystique by declining to discuss it at length. "It was about alienation," he once said, adding that he had "a lot of empathy" with Major Tom. Certainly the sudden and painful end of his relationship with Hermione Farthingale is part of the story: the quarrel that attended Hermione's final contribution to the *Love You Till Tuesday* film, which Kenneth Pitt believes was probably the couple's last gasp, occurred the day before David recorded his first studio version of the song. The melancholic subtext ("planet earth is blue and there's nothing I can do") and the submission to a pre-ordained fate ("I think my spaceship knows which way to go") bolster the sense of 'Space Oddity' as a song of withdrawal and resignation. The tantalizing uncertainty about whether Major Tom's fate is of his own making (is his circuit really dead, or is he simply ignoring Ground Control's pleas at the end?) adds a further dimension to an almost Hamlet-like meditation on the consequences of inaction. Bowie's anxiety about the loss of "control" (a word to which he repeatedly returns in songs like 'The Man Who Sold The World', 'I Am Divine' and 'No Control'), sponsors the notion that Ground Control itself is a metaphor for motherhood, a nurturing environment of spiritual comfort and moral certainty, an environment lost to the individual as he lifts off into life. Some have found a drug-fixated subtext in Major Tom's "trip", suggesting that the countdown, "lift-off" and "floating in a most peculiar way" reflect the process of injecting heroin and waiting for the hit. David later claimed to have had "a silly flirtation with smack" in 1968, "but it was only for the mystery and enigma of trying it. I never really enjoyed it at all."

One undisputed source is Stanley Kubrick's epoch-making 1968 movie *2001: A Space Odyssey*, which furnishes Bowie's "odd ditty" with its punning title. An anonymous friend records in Christopher Sandford's biography that *2001* had a "seismic impact" on Bowie at the time of its release. "It was the sense of isolation that I related to," David later explained. "I was out of my gourd anyway, I was very stoned when I went to see it, several times, and it was really a revelation to me. It got the song flowing."

And, of course, July 1969 was also the month that Neil Armstrong set foot on the moon. It's nigh on impossible for us to recall the extent to which spacemen had suddenly become the darlings of the media, but in 1969 the *Observer*'s Tony Palmer considered 'Space Oddity' a welcome breath of cynicism "at a time when we cling pathetically to every moonman's dribbling joke, when we admire unquestioningly the so-called achievement of our helmeted heroes without wondering why they are there at all." Certainly 'Space Oddity', with its pressmen who "want to know whose shirts you wear", is one of Bowie's key meditations on the vanity and transience of fame, prefiguring Ziggy Stardust's conflation of the different meanings of "star" and questioning the criteria of celebrity like many other lyrics ('Fame', 'It's No Game', 'Somebody Up There Likes Me'). But the most ingenious and delightful theory of all regarding the song's provenance is that Bowie might have called his astronaut after a name he saw as a boy on a variety bill posted in Brixton: Tom Major, father of the future Prime Minister.

Musically, 'Space Oddity' demonstrates the new acoustic bent David's compositions had taken since the formation of his multimedia trio Feathers in 1968. The style, arrangement and indeed lyrics owe a debt to the transatlantic folk-rock sounds of the late 1960s, in particular the Bee Gees' 1967 debut hit 'New York Mining Disaster 1941', whose chorus ("Have you seen my wife, Mr Jones?") is almost too close for words. "'Space Oddity' was a Bee Gees type song," Bowie's colleague John "Hutch" Hutchinson told the Gillmans. "David knew it, and he said so at the time … the way he sang it, it's a Bee Gees thing."

There exists a bewildering array of versions, edits and re-recordings of 'Space Oddity'. A very short and poor quality snippet from an early demo, which fizzles out after the "lift-off" sequence, has appeared on bootlegs and is difficult to date. On 2 February 1969, the day after Hermione's departure, the earliest full version was recorded at Morgan Studios, Willesden, for inclusion in the *Love You Till Tuesday* film. For this one-off session, produced by Jonathan Weston, David and Hutch were joined by Dave Clegg (bass), Tat Meager (drums) and Colin Wood (Hammond organ and Mellotron). Taken at a rattling pace and with a curiously jaunty and dated arrangement, this recording is markedly inferior to the later, more famous version. It's also notable for the fact that Hutch sings lead vocal for the "Ground Control" sections while David plays Major Tom, their close vocal harmonies emphasizing the Bee Gees connection. It was later released on the *Love You Till Tuesday* album, while the shorter edit used in the film appears on *The Deram Anthology 1966-1968*. "Quaint" is probably the kindest description of the accompanying film clip, which features the young David heading for the stars in what looks like a moped helmet, to be accosted and undressed by a dodgy pair of proto-*Blake's 7* space sirens.

The acoustic demo recorded with Hutch not long afterwards (and later released on *Sound + Vision*) secured Bowie his contract with Mercury Records, and the song's most famous version was recorded on 20 June 1969 (see *Space Oddity* in Chapter 2). Tony Visconti, who produced the remainder of the album, hated the song, regarding it as "a cheap shot – a gimmick to cash in on the moon landing". It was he who delegated the track to his colleague Gus Dudgeon, later explaining that "David was writing such beautiful songs then, and suddenly he comes up with 'Space Oddity' which was just so *topical*. Men were going to be walking on the moon within weeks, and he comes up with something like that. I told him he would probably have a hit with it, but I didn't want anything to do with it." More recently Visconti has relented, saying "when I saw the way this song fitted into the scheme of things, I wished I'd dropped my peacenik hippie ideals and recorded this classic track." The chance to produce 'Space Oddity' represented a considerable feather in Gus Dudgeon's cap, although many years later he would claim that he had received only his recording fee and was never paid an agreed 2 per cent of royalties on the track. (In June 2002 reports circulated that Gus Dudgeon was intending to sue the relevant record companies for a one-off settlement of £1 million, but the story was swept away a month later by the tragic news that he and his wife Sheila had died in a car accident on the M4 motorway.)

The album version of 'Space Oddity' was considerably longer than the single edit, but contrary to some reports it's not a re-recording. Among the track's gimmickry was its use of a new musical toy, the Stylophone, whose manufacturers roped Bowie into an advertising campaign that ran "David Bowie plays Stylophone in his greatest hit!" Bowie later revealed that it was Marc Bolan who had introduced him to the Stylophone's electronic warble: "He said, you like this kind of stuff, do something with it. And I put it on 'Space Oddity', so it served me well. It was just a little signal responding to electrodes. Sounded atrocious." The Stylophone reappeared on *The Man Who Sold The World* (most notably on 'After All'), and three decades later Bowie would bring it out of retirement to great effect on *Heathen* and *Reality*.

The topicality of 'Space Oddity' was lost on neither Mercury nor the many broadcasters they lobbied, several of whom adopted the song as an unofficial accompaniment to the momentous events of 20 July 1969. The single was rush-released on both sides of the Atlantic, appearing on 11 July – only three weeks after recording – to catch the Apollo 11 landing. BBC television played 'Space Oddity' during its coverage of the event, and the song has popped up in documentaries about space exploration ever since. "I'm sure they really weren't listening to the lyric at all," laughed Bowie in 2003. "It wasn't a pleasant thing to juxtapose against a moon landing. Of course, I was overjoyed that they did. Obviously some BBC official said, 'Oh, right then, that space song, Major Tom, blah blah blah, that'll be great.' 'Um, but he gets stranded in space, sir.' Nobody had the heart to tell the producer that!"

Released in different edits in Britain and America, the single turned out to be a slow burner despite some excellent reviews. "I have a bet on in the office that this is going to be a huge hit," wrote Penny Valentine in *Disc & Music Echo*, adding that she "listened spellbound throughout ... the sound is amazing ... It's obviously going to do well in America, which is nice."

Although Ms Valentine won her bet – eventually – her final prediction was wide of the mark. Six weeks after release the single still hadn't charted, and Kenneth Pitt's half-hearted attempt at chart-rigging ("I don't defend my conduct," he later wrote, "I explain it") was a failure. He had paid £140 to a shady figure called Tony Martin, who promised to get the single into various music weeklies' charts but instead vanished with the money. However, in Britain at least, 'Space Oddity' prospered without such assistance. The single finally charted in September, slowly rising to number 5 by early November. In America it flopped completely, despite a brazen letter sent to thousands of American journalists by Mercury's publicity director Ron Oberman, describing it as "one of the greatest recordings I've ever heard. If this already controversial single gets the airplay, it's going to be a huge hit." It didn't, it wasn't, and not even a relaunch in November succeeded in getting the single into the US chart. Kenneth Pitt has raised the intriguing possibility – hinted at by Oberman's mysterious use of the word "controversial" – that the single was clandestinely banned by radio stations and other outlets across the States because of its un-American attitude to the space programme. There are certainly reports of radio stations ignoring repeated requests to play the single, and even one account of an American schoolteacher who stopped pupils listening to it because of the lyrics.

The number of different versions continued to grow with the release of the British single in both mono and stereo. The latter was still a comparative novelty in the singles market, and Rick Wakeman later recalled that it was Bowie's own persistence that led to the innovation: "To the best of my knowledge nobody released stereo singles at that time, and they pointed that out to David ... and I can remember David saying, 'That's why this one will be stereo!' And he just stood his ground ... he wasn't being awkward, but he had a vision of how things should be."

The UK single saw yet another innovation. Although 7" picture sleeves were common in America and mainland Europe, they were practically unheard of in Britain. As recently as 1996 collectors discovered two previously unsuspected UK 'Space Oddity' picture sleeves, showing David strumming his acoustic guitar – the image used in most other territories. Initially dismissed as fakes, they were authenticated by Bowie discographer Marshall Jarman, who traced a third copy in the hands of a former Philips employee. Only these three copies are known to exist, prompting *Record Collector* to nominate the UK picture-sleeve 7" of 'Space Oddity' not only as the rarest single item of Bowie merchandise, but also the fourth rarest record in existence, valued at around £3000.

Still the alternative versions came. With an eye on European markets, Bowie recorded an Italian vocal with lyrics by Ivan Mogol. 'Ragazzo Solo, Ragazza Sola' means 'Lonely Boy, Lonely Girl', and the rest of the words are equally at variance with the original. "I thought it ridiculous that David should be recording this lyric," recalls Kenneth Pitt, "but it was explained to us that 'Space Oddity' could not be translated into Italian in a way that the Italians would understand." This version was recorded at Morgan Studios on 20 December 1969, with production and accent coaching by Claudio Fabi. Released in Italy in 1970, it later appeared on *Bowie Rare*. Covers of the Italian version by Equipe 84 and The Computers were released in Italy before David's own recording – indeed, according to Gus Dudgeon, Bowie's version was only recorded at all because his publisher wanted to eclipse the Italian releases. A French translation was also made by Boris Bergman, entitled 'Un Homme A Disparu Dans Le Ciel' ('A Man Has Disappeared In The Sky'), although opinions differ about whether Bowie ever recorded a version of this.

Unsurprisingly the success of the 'Space Oddity' single led to a rash of public appearances, beginning with a performance on Dutch TV's *Doebidoe* recorded on 25 August 1969 and shown five days later. On 2 October Bowie made his first ever appearance on *Top Of The Pops*, playing his Stylophone against a black background at the express request of Kenneth Pitt, who dreaded David being upstaged by a studio audience "less interested in seeing the artist than itself on the monitor sets." The performance was transmitted on 9 October and repeated the following week, propelling the single to its number 5 peak. Further performances came on Germany's *4-3-2-1 Musik Für Junge Leute* (recorded 29 October, shown 22 November) and Switzerland's *Hits A-Go-Go* (2 November). On 10 May 1970 David performed 'Space Oddity' at the Ivor Novello Awards, receiving a Songwriters' Guild award for the composition. It's perhaps not surprising that as early as December 1969 David responded to an interviewer's question, "'Space

Oddity – are you bored with it?", with the frank reply, "Oh yes. It's only a pop song after all."

'Space Oddity' was to be Bowie's only taste of chart success until 'Starman' three years later. While it was a useful dry run for the fame and fortune that would one day be his, in its day 'Space Oddity' was destined to be nothing more than an example of that most despised of phenomena, the novelty hit. 1969, which began with the Scaffold's 'Lily The Pink' and ended with Rolf Harris's 'Two Little Boys' in the number 1 spot, was a year curiously dominated by such confections, and it's worth noting that Zager And Evans's sci-fi hit 'In The Year 2525' sat atop the singles chart for the three weeks immediately preceding 'Space Oddity''s top 40 entry. To an extent Tony Visconti's misgivings were justified – 'Space Oddity' emerged into a world already tiring of space-age novelties, and only retrospectively did it transcend such associations to become a genuine classic. In 1983 Bowie opined that "it was, unfortunately, a very good song that possibly I wrote a bit too early, because I hadn't anything else substantial at the time."

'Space Oddity' was included in a BBC radio session recorded on 22 May 1972, later appearing on the *BBC Sessions 1969-1972* sampler and on *Bowie At The Beeb*. In a sideswipe at Elton John's then number 5 hit, Bowie cheekily interjected "I'm just a rocket man!" between verses. In *Backstage Passes* Angela Bowie claims David was piqued by the Gus Dudgeon-produced 'Rocket Man', considering it an opportunistic rip-off of 'Space Oddity' at a time when 'Starman' had yet to enter the chart. Intentionally or otherwise, the similarities in Bernie Taupin's lyric certainly extend beyond the basic spaceman theme – there has never been much doubt that 'Rocket Man' is a metaphor for drug-taking, and the line "I miss the earth so much, I miss my wife" is remarkably familiar.

At the end of David's American sojourn in December 1972, on the very day that he sailed for Britain on the *QEII*, a new video was shot by Mick Rock featuring a guitar-strumming Bowie amid the pseudo-space-age paraphernalia of RCA's New York Studios. "I really hadn't much clue why we were doing this, as I had moved on in my mind from the song," David later recalled, "but I suppose the record company were re-releasing it again or something like that. Anyway, I know I was disinterested in the proceedings and it shows in my performance. Mick's video is good, though." The clip did indeed support RCA's American reissue in January 1973 (which reached number 15 in the *Billboard* chart, becoming Bowie's first US hit) and was later used to promote the British re-release in September 1975, which pushed Art Garfunkel's 'I Only Have Eyes For You' from pole position in November to give David his first British number 1. With Bowie firmly ensconced in Los Angeles recording *Station To Station* at the time, the BBC's legendary dance troupe Pan's People were pressed into service for a *Top Of The Pops* performance.

In 1980 yet another new version, recorded for *Kenny Everett's New Year's Eve Show* the previous December, was released as the B-side of the 'Alabama Song' single (and latterly on 1992's *Scary Monsters* reissue). The lush arrangements of the Gus Dudgeon-produced original were stripped down to the bare essentials of acoustic guitar, drums and piano, and accordingly the message 'Sorry Gus' could be found scratched into the run-out vinyl. The idea for the re-recording had come from the Everett show's director David Mallet. "I agreed as long as I could do it again without all its trappings and do it strictly with three instruments," David explained. "Having played it with just an acoustic guitar on stage early on, I was always surprised at how powerful it was just as a song, without all the strings and synthesizers." Tony Visconti, who produced this version, later added that the recording "was never meant to be a single. Andy Duncan is on drums and a Bowie lookalike, Zaine Griff, is on bass. I temporarily forget the pianist. David, again, played twelve-string."

Later in 1980 came Bowie's disinterring of Major Tom in 'Ashes to Ashes', which appropriately enough became his second British number 1, and whose famous video revisited visual elements from the Kenny Everett performance of 'Space Oddity'. Nor was this the only Major Tom revival: 'Space Oddity' itself has been subjected to a vast number of live and studio covers by artists including Rick Wakeman, Pentangle (whose drummer Terry Cox had, like Wakeman, contributed to the original single), The Flying Pickets (whose extraordinary 1983 *a cappella* version was later compiled on *David Bowie Songbook*), Hank Marvin, Jonathan King, The Barron Knights, Rudy Grant, Cut, Saigon Kick, Steel Train and Natalie Merchant. The recording by the Langley Schools Music Project, a 60-voice choir of Canadian children recorded in the late 1970s and reissued on CD in 2002, is one of Bowie's favourite versions: "The backing arrangement is astounding. Coupled with the earnest if lugubrious vocal performance, you have a piece of art that I

couldn't have conceived of, even with half of Colombia's finest export products in me." The revived Langley Schools Music Project formed part of Bowie's 2002 Meltdown programme.

In 1984 the German vocalist Peter Schilling had a one-hit wonder with his 'Space Oddity' sequel 'Major Tom (Coming Home)', also included on his album *The Different Story (World Of Lust And Crime)*. The little-known Panic On The Titanic produced a song called 'Major Tom', while Def Leppard's 'Rocket' (from their 1987 album *Hysteria*) also resurrected the character. "Ground Control to Major Tom" is among the many pop quotations hilariously shoe-horned into Ben Elton's dialogue in the 2002 Queen stage musical *We Will Rock You*, while two decades earlier the BBC's comedy classic *The Young Ones* had featured Neil complaining that "planet Earth is blue and there's nothing I can do!" as he floated in space. 'Space Oddity' has been sung by both Chandler and Joey in the US sitcom *Friends*, by Phil Mitchell in *EastEnders*, by comedian Vic Reeves on *Shooting Stars*, and even by the BBC's intrepid journalist Louis Theroux during his 1998 *Weird Weekend* in the company of UFO-spotters in the American west.

'Space Oddity' has remained a live favourite throughout Bowie's career, featuring in his 1969-1971 sets and on the Ziggy Stardust, Diamond Dogs, Serious Moonlight and Sound + Vision tours. On 19 October 1973 a fine *Pin Ups*-era version, leaning heavily on piano and saxophone, was shot for *The 1980 Floor Show*, accompanied by NASA footage of rockets taking off. In 1997 Bowie closed his fiftieth birthday concert with an acoustic rendition of 'Space Oddity', later included on a limited-edition CD-ROM issued with *Variety* magazine in March 1999. A sumptuous new version orchestrated by Tony Visconti, with string accompaniment by the Scorchio and Kronos Quartets, was the highlight of Bowie's set at the Tibet House Benefit concert at Carnegie Hall in February 2002. A more conventional rendition made a one-off appearance at Denmark's Horsens Festival on the same year's Heathen tour.

SPEED OF LIFE
• Album: *Low* • B-Side: 6/77 • Live: *Stage*

Low opens with this superb, spirited instrumental, faintly recalling the chorus melody of 'The Jean Genie' and firmly establishing the album's sonic manifesto of distorted snare-drums and buzzing synthesizers, including a descending synth line reused on several later recordings including 'Scary Monsters'. The rapid fade-up at the beginning makes for a bizarre album-opener, as though the listener has just arrived within earshot of something that's already started. 'Speed Of Life' featured on the Stage and Heathen tours.

SPIRITS IN THE NIGHT *(Springsteen)*

For the ill-fated Astronettes project in 1973 Bowie produced a lively cover of this number from Bruce Springsteen's debut album, *Greetings From Asbury Park, N.J.* Shelved until 1995's *People From Bad Homes*, it's one of the best of the Astronettes' recordings, boasting a fine Mike Garson piano performance and a confident groove noticeably lacking elsewhere on the album. During the quiet middle section, Bowie can be heard in the background offering a spot of technical advice to singer Geoffrey MacCormack. One can't help but wonder whether Springsteen's lyric "Now Wild Billy was a crazy cat" might have directly influenced an almost identical line in Bowie's contemporaneous composition 'Diamond Dogs'.

STANDING NEXT TO YOU :
see **SLEEPING NEXT TO YOU**

STAR

• Album: *Ziggy* • Live: *Stage*

For those who buy into the theory that *Ziggy Stardust* has a narrative concept, the fast and furious 'Star' eavesdrops on a fatal moment of hubris as Ziggy ponders how he "could make it all worthwhile as a rock-'n'roll star" while scorning those who have sacrificed their lives to loftier ideals – fighting in Belfast or, in the case of (presumably Nye) Bevan, trying "to change the nation". There's even a mention of "Rudi" who "stayed at home to starve" – could this be Freddi Burretti's *alter ego* "Rudi Valentino", fashioned into star material by Bowie only months earlier and then discarded during the run-up to the realization of his own ambitions? In this reading 'Star' provides a vital narrative bridge between the "awful nice" singer wistfully captured in 'Lady Stardust' and the self-regarding megalomania of 'Hang On To Yourself', a movement

conveyed with a Bolanesque yell of "get it on!" in the instrumental bridge between verse and chorus.

Beyond the *Ziggy* concept 'Star' operates on a wider scale, encapsulating the fantasies of every adolescent dreamer miming into a hairbrush in a suburban bedroom, and voicing Bowie's own frustration at not having fulfilled his potential: "I could fall asleep at night as a rock'n'roll star / I could fall in love all right as a rock'n'roll star." Set against the romance is the cynical reality: he proposes merely "to play the part" because he "could do with the money". It's a pleasing paradox that in the very act of producing such an ironic twist on every teenager's fantasy – for Ziggy will pay for his stardom – Bowie himself achieves it.

David Stopps, manager of the Friars club in Aylesbury where Bowie played some of his key early Ziggy dates, recalls that Bowie had offered 'Star' to a little-known Princes Risborough band called Chameleon in early 1971, and it was only after being reminded of the number at his Aylesbury gig on 25 September that Bowie said, "Ooh, I must dig that one out." Sure enough, in September 2000 a previously unknown demo of the song, given to Chameleon's singer Les Payne in early 1971, fetched £1527 at Christie's. Recorded by Bowie at the Radio Luxembourg studios where much of *Hunky Dory* was demoed, this early version features a few lyrical variations: the opening line is "If someone had the sense to hear me / If someone had the time to see", while later David sings "I could make a big-time noise as a rock-'n'roll star". Although Chameleon apparently recorded a version later the same year, it was never released.

Meanwhile, the *Ziggy Stardust* version was completed on 11 November 1971 under the working title 'Rock'n'Roll Star', its manic backing vocals copied, by David's own admission, from The Beatles' 'Lovely Rita'.

Although Bowie transplanted the parting shot "Just watch me now!" into live performances of 'Queen Bitch' in 1976, 'Star' itself was not performed until 1978, when the live *Stage* version was released as a 12" promo in the US. 'Star' was resurrected for the Serious Moonlight tour, initially as the opening number after a brief intro from 'The Jean Genie'. The song has been covered live by several artists, notably Billy Bragg.

STARMAN

• A-Side: 4/72 [10] • Album: *Ziggy* • Live: *Beeb* • Live Video: *Best Of Bowie*

On 5 July 1972 David Bowie and The Spiders From Mars appeared on *Top Of The Pops* to perform 'Starman', released ahead of the *Ziggy Stardust* album from which it came. More than any other individual performance it was this one iconic television spot, transmitted the following day, which catapulted Bowie to stardom. It's deceptively easy to forget that in the summer of 1972 David Bowie was still yesterday's news to the average *Top Of The Pops* viewer, a one-hit wonder who'd had a novelty single about an astronaut at the end of the previous decade. Three minutes on *Top Of The Pops* in a rainbow jumpsuit and shocking red hair put paid to that forever. Having made no commercial impact in the two months since its release, 'Starman' stormed up the chart, going top ten a fortnight later and spawning everything that was to follow.

The famous *Top Of The Pops* performance, which was later included on the *Best Of Bowie* DVD, was not in fact the song's first television spot; that honour goes to Granada's *Lift-Off With Ayshea*, for which The Spiders had recorded a performance on 15 June against a backdrop of coloured stars, its earlier date betrayed by Woody Woodmansey's not-yet-peroxided hair. The show was transmitted six days later on 21 June. For both performances The Spiders were joined by tour pianist Robin Lumley, and David's newly-recorded vocal for *Top Of The Pops* interpolated a cheeky reference to Marc Bolan's trail-blazing hit of the previous year: "Some cat was laying down some *get-it-on* rock'n'roll".

'Starman' boasts one of Bowie's most infectious melodies, much enhanced by a cunning Mick Ronson arrangement for violins and guitar which is more in keeping with the gentler sounds of *Hunky Dory* than the rock attack of its successor. To those familiar only with 'Space Oddity', the title and acoustic intro must have initially suggested that this man had only one song in his playbook, but within moments it's the lyric that catches the attention. In the years since Major Tom left the chart, hippy whimsy has given way to "hazy cosmic jive" as a radio show is interrupted by a message from space. But, like 'Space Oddity', the subtext is all: this is less a science-fiction story than a self-aggrandizing announcement that there's a new star in town. Bowie exploits 'Starman' not just as a comeback hit, but as the vessel by which he reveals himself as a reconstructed icon. The chorus is at once Messianic and arrogant: "Let all the children boogie" conflates Christ's "Suffer little children to come unto me" with Marie Antoinette's "Let them eat cake". As in 'Moonage Daydream', Bowie saturates the lyric with slangy Americanisms ("boogie", "Hey, that's far out", "Don't tell your poppa", "Some cat was layin' down some rock'n'roll"), which vie with an intensely British sensibility to create a bizarre and beautiful hybrid.

According to Bowie, 'Starman' could be interpreted "at the immediate level of 'There's a Starman in the Sky saying Boogie Children', but the theme is that the idea of things in the sky is really quite human and real, and we should be a bit happier about the prospect of meeting people." This reading closely aligns the song with the much later 'Looking For Satellites'.

As the final *Ziggy Stardust* track to be written and recorded (it was completed on 4 February 1972), 'Starman' was immediately championed by RCA's Dennis Katz, who insisted it be released as a single and added to the album at the eleventh hour. A master tape dated 9 February duly notes the substitution of 'Starman' in place of 'Round And Round'. It's extraordinary to consider that one of Bowie's definitive songs replaced a Chuck Berry cover almost as an afterthought.

During an interview for *Rolling Stone* in November 1973, Bowie launched into a disquisition on the song's place in his planned *Ziggy Stardust* stage production: "The end comes when the infinites arrive. They really are a black hole, but I've made them people because it would be very hard to explain a black hole on stage … Ziggy is advised in a dream by the infinites to write the coming of a starman, so he writes 'Starman', which is the first news of hope that the people have heard. So they latch onto it immediately. The starmen that he is talking about are called the infinites, and they are black-hole jumpers. Ziggy has been talking about this amazing spaceman who will be coming down to save the earth. They arrive somewhere in Greenwich Village." Bowie's affinity with home-grown science-fiction permeates much of his work, and he has always enjoyed this *Quatermass*-style juxtaposition of the fantastic with the banal, of the mystical with the homely, of black holes with Greenwich Village. Remarkably, this account of "black-hole jumping" and of Ziggy's ultimate fate ("When the infinites arrive, they take bits of Ziggy to make themselves real because in their original state they are anti-matter and cannot exist in our world") is identical to the storyline of the BBC's tenth anniversary *Doctor Who* special *The Three Doctors*, a high-profile reunion of the show's lead actors which had been broadcast a few months earlier, while Bowie was in London recording *Aladdin Sane*.

Part of the song's innocent appeal – not to mention its commercial success – lies in the blatancy of its sources. It's within a whisker of being a cross-breed of T Rex's 'Hot Love' and 'Telegram Sam', the latter released in the month 'Starman' was recorded. The "la la la" chorus is straight out of 'Hot Love' and the cry of "let all the children boogie" is pure Bolan. The Morse-code tattoo on piano and guitar before each chorus is lifted from The Supremes' 'You Keep Me Hangin' On' via Blue Mink's 'Melting Pot', while the chorus melody itself is swiped from Judy Garland's signature tune 'Over the Rainbow', tapping into a ready-made signifier of yearning and stardom with built-in gay undertones. During his Rainbow Theatre shows in August 1972 Bowie explicitly acknowledged the link, altering the melody to sing "There's a Starman, over the rainbow, where I fly." And as he knows better than most, you can't keep a good tune down: twenty years later the same melody was rifled by Suede for the chorus of their Bowie-worshipping debut hit 'The Drowners'. Suede also made capital use of Bowie's favoured "la la la" play-out, typified by 'Starman' and 'Time', in numbers like 'The Power' and 'Beautiful Ones'.

The US single featured a slightly different edit, with some ten seconds shaved from the fade-out, while the Spanish release was entitled 'El Hombre Estrella'. A lively new recording, again interpolating the 'Get It On' reference, was included in a BBC session recorded on 22 May 1972 and can now be heard on *Bowie At The Beeb*. An instrumental mix of the studio backing, possibly prepared for one of the television appearances, was auctioned at Sotheby's in 1990 and now appears on bootlegs.

'Starman' was occasionally played on the Ziggy Stardust tour but was never a great live success for The Spiders; it reappeared for a few Sound + Vision dates before being put on ice until 2000, when its triumphant concert revival included a performance on Channel 4's *TFI Friday* on 23 June. It later made the occasional appearance on the Heathen and A Reality tours. Despite a comparatively low profile since 1972, Bowie's second hit has been covered by numerous artists including 10,000 Maniacs, Dar Williams, The

Cybernauts and notably Culture Club: a live favourite of the band during the early 1980s, the song was recorded in the studio for their 1999 comeback album *Don't Mind If I Do*. In October 2001, Boy George even dressed as Bowie to perform 'Starman' on the ITV celebrity special *Popstars In Their Eyes*. And who can forget the late Dustin Gee singing 'Starman' in full Ziggy regalia on the pisspoor early 1980s ITV impressions show *Go For It*? Not me, try as I might. More recently 'Starman' featured in Kevin Elyot's 1995 Olivier Award-winning play *My Night With Reg*, and to confirm its absorption into the end-of-millennium zeitgeist, it was given a plaintive rendition by Brian Murphy in 1999's brilliantly Beckettian BBC sitcom *Mrs Merton and Malcolm*.

STATESIDE (H.Sales/Bowie)
• Album: *TM2* • B-Side: 8/91 [33] • B-Side: 10/91 [48]
• Live: *Oy* • Live Video: *Oy*

The ominous opening drum-roll of 'Stateside' heralds Tin Machine's darkest hour. Although the blues had occupied a crucial place in Bowie's musical palette since his earliest days as a performer, he had never been so crass as to attempt a full-blown "I woke up this morning" job. Never, that is, until this, and there has seldom been a more incongruous or less welcome intrusion onto a Bowie album.

The lion's share of the responsibility – but by no means all – can be placed at the door of drummer Hunt Sales, who unusually precedes Bowie in the songwriting credit and howls on about "going Stateside with my convictions" for a few hours until David wrests control of the lyric, apparently attempting to redress the balance with some clunking anti-American irony ("Marilyn inflatables, home on the range, where the livin' is easy on a horse with no name / Kennedy convertibles, home on the range, where the sufferin' comes easy on a blond with no brain"). Lennon and McCartney's pass-the-parcel approach might have made a classic out of 'A Day In The Life', but the same cannot be said of 'Stateside'. Having taken one look at this undignified monstrosity, Bowie should have elected to stuff democracy. Instead, he capitulated to Mr Sales and in doing so compromised the album. It's not as if 'Stateside' is particularly badly performed, but the superannuated blues setting and crass apple-pie sentiment (even allowing for the attempted irony injection, with its reference to America's 1971 hit 'A Horse With No Name') represent an abdication of everything Bowie's music has ever achieved.

After the album take had already appeared on single formats of 'You Belong In Rock N'Roll', Tin Machine's BBC version, recorded on 13 August 1991, surfaced as a B-side on the 'Baby Universal' CD. The album cut later featured in the soundtrack of the 1992 film *Dr Giggles*. 'Stateside' was performed on the It's My Life tour (veterans will recall the spectacle of Mr Sales climbing down from his drumkit and attempting to whip the crowd into a pre-song frenzy by waving his drumsticks at them and repeatedly yelling "Y'all ready to go stateside?"), from which an alarming eight-minute live version found its way onto *Oy Vey, Baby*. Jointly, they're a close contender with *Tonight*'s 'God Only Knows' as the very worst items in Bowie's recorded legacy.

STATION TO STATION

• Album: *Station* • Live: *Stage* • Live Video: *Moonlight*

As well as unveiling the sinister figure of the Thin White Duke, the album cut of 'Station To Station' has the distinction of being the longest studio track Bowie has ever released. Scintillatingly performed and gorgeously produced, it represents one of the high watermarks in his studio work. David is in superb voice and Earl Slick's lead guitar is never finer, wailing across a relentless plod of piano, drums and rhythm guitar in the measured Germanic *motorik* of the first half, before igniting over the first flowering of the classic Murray/Davis/Alomar rhythm section in the galloping climax.

The opening sound effect of a rampaging steam-train acknowledges the influence of Kraftwerk's 1974 album *Autobahn*, which begins with the sound of a car revving up and driving across the stereo speakers. Kraftwerk later returned the compliment on 1977's *Trans-Europe Express*, whose title track includes the lyric "From Station to Station back to Düsseldorf city, meet Iggy Pop and David Bowie" over the synthesized sound of a speeding train (the line commemorates an actual meeting in mid-1976, a photo of which appeared in Kraftwerk's video at the appropriate moment).

However, the railway motif of 'Station To Station' is something of a red herring. Certainly it expresses what David later called the album's "wayward spiritu-

al search", restating the travelling metaphor familiar from earlier compositions: the stations recall the "new surroundings" of 'Rock'n Roll With Me', and the "mountains on mountains" reprise the questing motifs of 'Wild Eyed Boy From Freecloud' and *The Man Who Sold The World*. But, as Bowie has confirmed, the title actually alludes to the Stations of the Cross, the sequence of fourteen landmarks on Christ's path to the crucifixion, each a symbolic stopping-place for prayer in the carvings of medieval churches. What is less widely understood is that, in the maelstrom of spiritual confusion and occultism which infused his 1975 worldview, Bowie conflates the Stations of the Cross with the Sephiroth, the ten spheres of creation which form the basis of the thirteenth-century Jewish mystical system known as the Kabbalah.

Foremost among Bowie's reading in the summer of 1975 was *The Kabbalah Unveiled* by S L MacGregor Mathers, chief of the Hermetic Order of the Golden Dawn and life-long adversary of Aleister Crowley (he was responsible for Crowley's expulsion from the Order). According to the Kabbalah the divine sphere of the Godhead, or Crown of Creation, is called Kether, while the sphere of the physical Kingdom is known as Malkuth. For Bowie, whose work since the late 1960s had systematically pondered transmutations between divine and mortal states of being, the mythology of fall and redemption was now expressed as "one magical movement from Kether to Malkuth". The spheres exist at opposite ends of the Tree of Life, a Kabbalistic pattern which Bowie had adopted as a talismanic protection at the time (he can be seen drawing it on the floor in the contemporary photograph reproduced in subsequent reissues of *Station To Station*).

Alongside the Kabbalistic coding are further references to Aleister Crowley, previously mentioned in Bowie's man-and-superman song 'Quicksand'. The Thin White Duke's propensity for "making sure white stains" refers to Crowley's first book, the obscure *White Stains*, another treatment of the Gnostic myth of the Fall; the combined sexual, racial, occult and drug-related significances of the title would rebound on Bowie in 1976. Given that this album follows hard on the heels of the making of *The Man Who Fell To Earth* (and uses a monochrome still from the film on its front cover), it can be no coincidence that Bowie is here "flashing no colour": in his distressed mental state, he presumably wishes to fall to earth himself, rejecting his experimentation with the Tattva system which advocates "colour-flashing", a process of combining complementary colours to heighten consciousness and transport magicians to the astral plane.

But 'Station To Station', endlessly fascinating and allusive as it is, casts Bowie as yet another, more classical model of both magician and Duke. Standing "tall in this room overlooking the ocean", he is not just David Bowie in his secluded Los Angeles villa, but a timeless Prospero, "lost in my circle", preparing to break his wand and abjure his magic. Hence the misquotation from *The Tempest* ("Such is the stuff from where dreams are woven") giving way in the torrid finale to an altogether more optimistic paraphrase of Cole Porter's 'I Get A Kick Out Of You' ("It's not the side-effects of the cocaine / I'm thinking that it must be love"). Casting out the supernatural and the angelic ("does my face show some kind of glow? / It's too late"), Bowie appears to be throwing himself on the mercy of temporal power, cushioning himself with drink and toasting "the men who protect you and I". In conceding that "the European canon is here", 'Station To Station' draws the blinds on the coke-fuelled horror of his Los Angeles interlude and paves the way for a long, slow recovery.

It is, then, entirely appropriate that the sound of 'Station To Station', more than any other track on the album, should point the way towards Bowie's next musical phase, just as 'Rock'n Roll With Me' had presaged his soul-singer period two years earlier. "As far as the music goes, *Low* and its siblings were a direct follow-on from the title track," David remarked in 2001. "It's often struck me that there will usually be one track on any given album of mine, which will be a fair indicator of the intent of the following album."

'Station To Station' provided the opening number throughout the 1976 tour, and subsequently featured in the Stage, Serious Moonlight, Sound + Vision and summer 2000 shows. It made a memorable contribution to Ulrich Edel's 1981 film *Christiane F. Wir Kinder Vom Bahnhof Zoo*, in which Bowie lip-synched to the *Stage* version in a concert scene filmed in Manhattan in October 1980.

STAY

• Album: *Station* • B-Side: 7/76 • Bonus: *Station* • Live: *Beeb*

One of Bowie's classic hybrids, 'Stay' manages to be

funk, soul and hard rock all at the same time, showcasing Earl Slick's lead guitar to fine effect against *Station To Station*'s superb rhythm section. The rhythm guitar riff, among the best on any Bowie recording, was created by Carlos Alomar who tells David Buckley that the track was recorded "very much in our cocaine frenzy". It's an anxious confessional about the inscrutability of ships that pass in the night ("You can never really tell when somebody wants something you want too"), epitomizing the combination of racking self-doubt and confidently stylish production found throughout the album.

A heavily edited 3'21" version became the B-side of RCA's superfluous 'Suffragette City' single in the summer of 1976; in America and other territories it was released as an A-side backed by an edited 'Word On A Wing'. The 7" edit subsequently turned up on the soundtrack album *Christiane F. Wir Kinder Vom Bahnhof Zoo*.

Before the release of *Station To Station* 'Stay' was previewed in an excellent live performance for CBS's *The Dinah Shore Show* on 3 January 1976, and went on to become a staple of Bowie's concert repertoire over two decades, featuring in the Stage, Serious Moonlight, Sound + Vision, Earthling, 1999-2000 and Heathen tours. A superb live version recorded at Nassau Coliseum on 23 March 1976 appeared on *Station To Station*'s 1991 reissue, while another fine recording, this time from the BBC Radio Theatre concert on 27 June 2000, was included on the *Bowie At The Beeb* bonus disc.

STAY (Williams)

Not to be confused with the above, Maurice Williams and the Zodiacs' 1961 hit was played live by The Buzz.

STRANGERS WHEN WE MEET

• Album: *Buddha* • Album: *1.Outside* • A-Side: 11/95 [39] • Video: *Best Of Bowie*

This is one of *The Buddha Of Suburbia*'s more conventional tracks, dropping a riff borrowed from the Spencer Davis Group's 1966 hit 'Gimme Some Loving' into a setting that is pure late-1970s Roxy Music to forge a compassionate, melodic pop song for grown-ups. It seems to concern the give and take of a mature relationship, but it's just possible that the lyric also confronts the latest round of kiss-and-tell revelations made by Angela Bowie on chat-shows and in print when the so-called gagging order of her divorce settlement had expired in early 1993 ("Slinky secrets hotter than the sun … Cold tired fingers tapping out your memories … All your regrets ride roughshod over me / I'm so glad that we're strangers when we meet"). If this is an accurate reading – and it probably isn't – light-hearted lines like the "I'm in clover / Heel-head-over" couplet suggest that any bitterness is well reined in.

In most estimations 'Strangers When We Meet' was one of the less thrilling tracks on the otherwise radical *Buddha Of Suburbia*, and it came as something of a surprise when Bowie elected to re-record it in 1995 as a last-minute addition to *1.Outside*. This version abandons the spacey synth effects in favour of a lusher, more rounded arrangement augmented by Mike Garson's piano and Reeves Gabrels's guitar, holding long, sustained notes *à la* '"Heroes"'. Arriving at the end of *1.Outside*'s art-rock insanity 'Strangers When We Meet' seems even more incongruous, resolving all the album's angst and black comedy in a soothing slice of conventional pop. Still, released as a double A-side with the re-recorded 'The Man Who Sold The World' it made for a fine single which deserved better than its feeble number 39 peak. An American promo CD added a further single edit of the *Buddha Of Suburbia* version.

The single was accompanied by a handsome Sam Bayer video which lacked the bite of his promo for 'The Hearts Filthy Lesson' – again sepia-tinted and set in a dusty artist's studio, it consists of Bowie flirting with a rag-doll ballerina and vamping to camera. Equally lacklustre, unfortunately, was a live performance for *Top Of The Pops* on 10 November 1995 during rehearsals for the UK leg of the Outside tour, but matters were redressed by an excellent rendition on BBC2's *Later… With Jools Holland* on 2 December, and another for French TV's *Taratata* on 26 January. The song featured throughout the Outside and Earthling tours.

STUPIDITY *(Burke)*

A Solomon Burke number performed live by The Manish Boys.

SUBTERRANEANS
• Album: *Low*

Although originally written and, in some form or another, recorded for Bowie's abandoned soundtrack of *The Man Who Fell To Earth*, 'Subterraneans' was reinvented during the *Low* sessions as a portrait of Bowie's new surroundings: "'Subterraneans' is about the people who got caught in East Berlin after the separation," he said in 1977, "hence the faint jazz saxophones representing the memory of what it was." The result is one of the most melancholy tracks Bowie has committed to disc, taking as its cue the reversed-tape trick he had previously used at the beginning of 'Sweet Thing', and building the resulting blurts of sound into a bleak ambient edifice over which he wails semi-comprehensible vocals after the fashion of 'Warszawa'.

'Subterraneans' was reworked as the first movement of Philip Glass's 1993 *Low Symphony*, and was performed live with Nine Inch Nails during the US leg of the Outside tour, augmented by lyrics from 'Scary Monsters'. It was later revived in more conventional form for 2002's Heathen tour.

SUCCESS *(Pop/Bowie/Gardiner)*

Bowie co-wrote and co-produced this track on Iggy Pop's *Lust For Life*, also contributing piano and backing vocals, for which he is joined by the instantly recognizable Sales brothers. Three-quarters of the future Tin Machine gamely join a Simon-Says singalong, dutifully repeating the increasingly daft lines Iggy throws at them during the play-out ("I'm gonna do the twist … I'm gonna hop like a frog … I'm gonna go out on the street and do anything I want … Oh shit!").

Bowie's original ideas for the recording did not meet with his friend's approval. "He wanted me to sing like a crooner," Iggy Pop later revealed, "and I thought it was completely horrible. So I waited until he walked out of the studio and I changed everything. When he came back, he found it very good."

'Success' was released as a single – without success – in October 1977, and was covered by Duran Duran on 1995's *Thank You*.

SUCKER *(Hunter/Ralphs/Watts)*

Produced by Bowie for Mott The Hoople's *All The Young Dudes*.

SUFFRAGETTE CITY

• Album: *Ziggy* • Live: *David, Motion, SM72, Beeb* • B-Side: 4/72 [10] • A-Side: 7/76 • Live Video: *Ziggy*

Originally rejected by Mott the Hoople in January 1972, 'Suffragette City' was repossessed to become one of the last tracks recorded for *Ziggy Stardust*, completed at Trident on 4 February. With its stomping Little Richard piano, driving guitars and celebrated casual-sex whoop of "Wham bam, thank you ma'am!" (filched, as Bowie later confessed, from the title of a track on Charles Mingus's 1961 album *Oh Yeah*), the song quickly established itself as one of the pivotal Ziggy numbers. Depending on how much gender-bending one wishes to read into the lyric, it's either a laddish request to be left alone with a girlfriend ("don't crash here, there's only room for one and here she comes!") or else, in the same vein as 'John, I'm Only Dancing', it's an AC/DC switch from boyfriend to girlfriend ("I gotta straighten my face … I can't take you this time"). Notably Bowie addresses his male friend as "droogie", a direct reference to *A Clockwork Orange*: Stanley Kubrick's 1971 film adaptation was a major influence on Ziggy's cultural grab-bag, dictating both costumes and pre-show music on tour (see Chapter 3).

'Suffragette City' sees one of Bowie's earliest uses of the ARP synthesizer, an instrument that would later form the backbone of his Berlin albums. Here it's pressed into service to provide the ersatz saxophone blasts underscoring the guitar. "David had this idea for a big sax sound, bigger than anything he could play," Ken Scott told Mark Paytress, "so we hooked up this huge synth, fiddled around until we got the closest sound to a sax as possible, and left Mick Ronson to play the right notes."

A new version was included in Bowie's BBC session recorded on 16 May 1972, and this excellent cut, distinguished by some sharp guitar work from Mick Ronson and boogie-woogie piano from Nicky Graham, now appears on *Bowie At The Beeb*. Despite already having appeared as the B-side of 'Starman', the album original was reissued as an A-side in 1976 to promote *ChangesOneBowie*. Not surprisingly, it failed to chart.

'Suffragette City' featured throughout the Ziggy Stardust, Diamond Dogs, Station To Station, Stage, Sound + Vision and A Reality tours. As something of a primal rock classic it's been covered by countless artists in the studio or on stage, including U2, Alice In Chains, Duran Duran, Red Hot Chili Peppers, Big Audio Dynamite, Andy Taylor, LA Guns, Boy George (on his 1999 rarities compilation *The Unrecoupable One Man Biscuit*), Frankie Goes To Hollywood (on extended formats of their 1986 single 'Rage Hard'), Steve Jones (on 1989's *Fire And Gasoline*), and even sometime Bowie choreographer Toni Basil. A version by The Spiders From Mars, fronted by Joe Elliott, appears on the 1997 live album of *The Mick Ronson Memorial Concert*. Carter The Unstoppable Sex Machine used a sample of Bowie's original on their 1991 track 'Surfin' USM', and in 1999 *Suffragette City* was even used as the title of a novel by Kate Muir.

SUMMER KIND OF LOVE : see GOING DOWN

SUNDAY

• Album: *Heathen* • Bonus: *Heathen* • French/Canadian B-Side: 9/02

The dark sonic textures and bleak lyrics of *Heathen*'s sinister opening track led many reviewers to suggest that the song may have been inspired by the events of 11 September 2001. Certainly it's easy to see how such a conclusion might have been reached: the opening lines ("Nothing remains / We could run when the rain slows / Look for the cars or signs of life") are delivered with burned-out emotion against a backdrop of layered backing vocals and a repetitive bleeping guitar loop which seems to recall the tales told by New York firefighters of mobile phones ringing plaintively in the silent wreckage.

However, any such resonances are entirely coincidental, because 'Sunday' was in fact among the first songs to be written for *Heathen* and predates the September 11 attacks by several weeks. "It was quite spine-tingling to realize how close those lyrics came," Bowie later remarked. "There are some key words in there that really just freak me out." Far from being a blighted cityscape, the inspiration for 'Sunday' was in fact the barren beauty of the mountainous countryside surrounding Allaire Studios. "Strangely enough, you don't always write what you want to write," David told *Interview* magazine the following year. "'Sunday' and 'Heathen' were two pieces I didn't want to write, but this place was just dragging the lyrics out of me. I would get up very early in the morning, about six, and work in the studio before anybody else got there, assembling what I wanted to do as that day's work. And often the lyrics would come as I was sort of putting the music together. It was absolutely terrific. And the words to 'Sunday' were tumbling out, the song came out almost written as I was playing it through, and there were two deer grazing down in the grounds below and there was a car passing very slowly on the other side of the reservoir. This was very early in the morning, and there was something so still and primal about what I was looking at outside that there were tears just running down my face as I was writing this thing. It was just extraordinary."

The result is a superbly atmospheric album opener which establishes *Heathen*'s core themes of spiritual uncertainty and existential fear. Both melodically and lyrically, 'Sunday' is descended from a long line of compositions such as 'The Motel' and 'The Dreamers', and perhaps in particular the spiritual quest lyrics of *Station To Station* and *Low* (the line "All my trials, Lord, will be remembered" is strongly reminiscent of 'Word On A Wing'). The quasi-monastic chanting style of Tony Visconti's backing vocals ("It sounds like a synth," the producer later revealed, "but I taught myself how to sing two notes at once after studying Tuvan and Mongolian music for years") not only recalls some of the *Low* tracks but also reinforces the song's devotional atmosphere, paving the way for a beautiful, aspirational series of chord changes as the lyric strives to resolve its spiritual search and emerge onto a better, angelic plane: "Now we must burn all that we are / Rise together through these clouds / As on wings". But, as suggested by the sudden explosion of percussion and volume on Bowie's final swooping cry of "Everything has changed", it's at best an uncertain state of transcendence.

The song's title neatly encapsulates the album's sense of an uneasy balance between the spiritual and the secular: it might be no more than a bland diary entry, or it might just as conceivably carry the religious connotations obviously associated with Sunday (a day, incidentally, which features in a surprisingly large number of David's lyrics from 'The Pretty Things Are Going To Hell' to 'Julie', and from the reminiscences about "church on Sunday" in 'Can't Help Thinking

About Me' to the Sunday meetings of lovers in 'Rubber Band' and 'Love You Till Tuesday').

A remix by Moby, adding an upbeat rhythmic backing which lends the song a commercial sheen but perhaps robs the track of some of its original texture, was included on the bonus disc issued with initial pressings of *Heathen*. The rarer 'Tony Visconti Mix', which sets a more recognizable variation of the album version against a beat-box percussion loop, ominous rumbles of thunder and a closing string solo, appeared on some European formats of the 'Everyone Says 'Hi'' single and on the Canadian release of 'I've Been Waiting For You'. 'Sunday' was performed on the Heathen and A Reality tours, an excellent live version appearing in the BBC radio session of 18 September 2002.

THE SUPERMEN
• Album: *Man* • Compilation: *Glastonbury Fayre* • Live: *S+V, SM72, Beeb* • Bonus: *Hunky, Ziggy (2002), Aladdin (2003)*

The first studio version of 'The Supermen' was recorded at London's Playhouse Theatre on 25 March 1970, as part of a BBC radio session in advance of the *Man Who Sold the World* sessions. It was to prove the end of the road for drummer John Cambridge, who had been with Bowie since the *Space Oddity* album. Unable to handle a "tricky little bit" in the complex time signature, Cambridge was unceremoniously sacked the following month. "I just couldn't get it right and even Mick was saying, 'Come on, it's easy,' which makes you feel worse," Cambridge later recalled. According to Tony Visconti the removal of Cambridge was principally Ronson's doing. The BBC version (often wrongly labelled by bootleggers as a demo from the album sessions) does indeed feature some dodgy drumming, together with a fine vocal performance from Bowie and some marginally different lyrics.

The successful album take of 'The Supermen', featuring apocalyptic echo-tracked drumming from Cambridge's successor Woody Woodmansey, is a melodramatic helping of Teutonic fantasy, dabbling again in the Nietzschean overtones prevalent throughout the album. The barrelling timpani-rolls recall Richard Strauss's most celebrated composition *Also Sprach Zarathustra*, a Nietzschean fanfare famously used as the theme music for another Bowie source, *2001: A Space Odyssey*. David had been reading *Jenseits von Gut und Böse* and *Also Sprach Zarathustra* during the early part of 1970, and chilly observations derived from both can be found throughout *The Man Who Sold The World* and *Hunky Dory*. Here, as in 'Saviour Machine', the theme arises from Nietzsche's proposition of the superman's rejection of temporal morality, but Bowie has superimposed a nightmarish fairytale of the "tragic endless lives" of immortal beings "chained to life", while "sad-eyed mermen" suffer "nightmare dreams no mortal mind could hold". Within this mythic Wagnerian landscape (whose "mountain magic" recalls the fairytale setting of 'Wild Eyed Boy From Freecloud'), "man would tear his brother's flesh" in the desperate quest for "a chance to die".

"I set 'The Supermen' as a period piece," Bowie said in 1973, "but I think it was a forward rather than a backward thing." Three years later he told another interviewer that the song was "pre-Fascist", explaining that in 1970 he was "still going through the thing when I was pretending I understood Nietzsche … and I had tried to translate it into my own terms to understand it, so 'Supermen' came out of that."

On 12 November 1971 a radically rearranged version was recorded during the *Ziggy Stardust* sessions at Trident, alternating soft, acoustic verses with explosive, Ronson-led choruses. It was originally donated to the 1972 *Glastonbury Fayre* compilation, later appearing on 1990's *Hunky Dory* reissue and 2002's *Ziggy Stardust* repackage. It was this version that Bowie chose to emulate in live performances during the Ziggy Stardust tour, and although it's more of a piece with the classic Ziggy sound, my money's still on the drum-banging rollercoaster of the original album recording. In *Strange Fascination* Tony Visconti describes the first version as one of *The Man Who Sold The World*'s "outrageous sonic landscapes … kind of prescient for the sound that Queen eventually came up with – not only the vocal style, but the high-pitched backing vocals and the guitar solo, too."

In its "alternate" form 'The Supermen' was taped for two further BBC sessions on 3 June and 21 September 1971 (the second of these, a superb recording, now appears on *Bowie At The Beeb*), while a live version from Boston on 1 October 1972 later appeared on the *Sound + Vision Plus* CD and on 2003's *Aladdin Sane* reissue. An acoustic revival, with tempo and phrasing more faithful to the original version, was included in the 1997 *ChangesNowBowie* session. "The riff that I used on that I actually revived on

Earthling," David confessed in the accompanying interview. "You've got to spot it!" The riff in question, recycled for 'Dead Man Walking', was apparently given to David by Jimmy Page back in 1965 during the session for 'I Pity The Fool'. "He was quite generous that day," said David, "and he said 'Look, I've got this riff but I'm not using it for anything, so why don't you learn it and see if you can do anything with it?' So I had this riff, and I've used it ever since!" 'The Supermen' subsequently appeared on the Earthling and A Reality tours.

SURVIVE *(Bowie/Gabrels)*
• Album: *'hours…'* • A-Side: 1/00 [28] • Live: *Beeb* • Video: *Best Of Bowie* • Live Video: *Best Of Bowie*

"There's something I find really authentically early seventies about the writing structure of 'Survive'," Bowie declared of one of his favourite *'hours…'* tracks. Although a prime exhibit of the alleged *Hunky Dory* style which pre-release hype suggested was to be the album's keynote, in fact 'Survive' offers a deft blend of old and new, locking a classic twelve-string Bowie intro with a gradual build into a soaring Reeves Gabrels guitar break, but discreetly subjugating both to one of the most beautiful melodies Bowie has ever created. There are definite reminders of *Hunky Dory*'s slow ballads but perhaps the closest ancestor is 'Starman', whose luxuriant lead guitar sound and Supremes-influenced Morse Code guitar bleeps are resurrected to great effect. The shuffling drumbeat and stop-start verse melodies, meanwhile, are vaguely reminiscent of 'Five Years'.

Like 'Something In The Air' the song reviews an extinct relationship, although once again Bowie was keen to explain that it referred to nothing specific. "There was a time in my life where I was desperately in love with a girl," he told *Uncut*, "and I met her, as it happens, quite a number of years later. And boy, was the flame dead! So in this case on the album the guy's thinking about a girl he knew many years ago, and she was 'the great mistake he never made'. See, I know how it feels, but it's not part of my current situation. I'm much too jolly."

There are references to Bowie's age-old fantasies of escape and identity ("Give me wings, give me space / Give me money for a change of face") and, as elsewhere on *'hours…'*, an awareness of encroaching age ("Who said time is on our side?"), resolving into a determination to survive the mistakes of the past and forge ahead. 'Survive' is a complex, compassionate achievement and undoubtedly one of Bowie's finest songs of the 1990s. It was a regular highlight of the 1999-2000 tours, and among numerous television performances were fine renditions on Channel 4's *TFI Friday* on 8 October 1999 and, as a pre-recorded insert, BBC2's *TOTP2* special on 3 November. Three further versions were taped at the BBC's Maida Vale studios on 25 October for broadcast on various radio stations, and another live recording, this time from the BBC Radio Theatre concert on 27 June 2000, later appeared on the *Bowie At The Beeb* bonus disc. The song resurfaced on the Heathen tour, featuring in yet another BBC session on 18 September 2002.

In January 2000 'Survive' was released as a single, remixed by UK producer Marius de Vries with additional guitar by Karma County's Brendan Gallagher, who later revealed that de Vries "had a great idea of reintroducing several of David Bowie's music periods into his production of 'Survive' – a bit of 'Space Oddity' acoustic guitar, some Mick Ronson electric circa 'Jean Genie', and a bit of angular Adrian Belew kind of stuff as well." The video, shot in London by Walter Stern, depicts Bowie sitting alone in a dingy kitchen, gazing blankly ahead in deep thought as he waits for an egg to boil. As the song begins to take flight so does Bowie's egg, quickly followed by his table, his chair and himself, until he is floating in mid-air and clutching at the cooker for support. By the end all has returned to normal. It's a hallucinatory, curiously moving little drama that perfectly echoes the song's reflective, daydream quality, and once again hints obliquely at Bowie's past work – in this case the trippy anti-gravity and kitchen scenes in the classic 'Ashes To Ashes' video.

The first CD single included a PC-playable version of the video, while the second featured a live version recorded at the Elysée Montmartre, Paris, on 14 October 1999, plus a video of the same performance. Both these videos reappeared on the *Best Of Bowie* DVD, while the single edit also appeared in the soundtrack of the *Omikron* computer game.

SWEET HEAD

• Bonus: *Ziggy, Ziggy* (2002)

In 1990 'Sweet Head' took Bowie fans entirely by surprise: until its appearance on Rykodisc's *Ziggy Stardust* reissue, even the best-informed aficionados knew nothing of its existence. Even then they nearly didn't get to hear it – Rykodisc's Jeff Rougvie later revealed that Bowie initially barred its release, "and then two months later he changed his mind and said we could put it out." The edit later included on the 2002 reissue of *Ziggy Stardust* goes a step further, opening with some additional studio banter between David and the band, and in the same year the song won a little extra familiarity with its inclusion on the soundtrack of the film *Moonlight Mile*.

No timorous demo but a fully polished recording from the *Ziggy Stardust* sessions, 'Sweet Head' casts an intriguing light on the album's development. Completed on 11 November 1971, it boasts a hard-edged guitar sound, a driving tempo and a furiously quickfire vocal line, which interestingly makes direct lyrical reference to Ziggy himself – something otherwise found only on the title track. This has led to speculation that 'Sweet Head' was dropped because Bowie was reluctant to put all his eggs in one basket by overloading the album with "concept".

The riff's similarity to that of 'Hang On To Yourself' might also account for the song's drop into obscurity, but equally noteworthy is the fact that the lyrics are particularly strong for their time and would doubtless have courted controversy. Like a nastier version of 'Five Years', there are references to *Clockwork Orange*-style "mugging gangs", "spicks and blacks" and "burnt-out vans", together with a swaggering Messianic self-image that pushes the album's religious imagery to the borders of blasphemy ("Till there was rock you only had God"). As if that weren't enough there's a running streak of innuendo about the act suggested by the song's title, culminating in a cheeky "While you're down there" which anticipates Bowie's famous guitar-fellatio act on the 1972 tour. This is Ziggy as sexed-up godhead, a preening and phallic "rubber peacock" dispensing rock gratification ("Ziggy's gonna play, and I'm just about the best you can hear!") in return for sexual favours and mindless worship. Sinister, exhilarating, dumb and magnificent, it's quite beyond belief that 'Sweet Head' was dropped from the album and lost for nearly twenty years.

SWEET JANE (Reed)

Lou Reed joined Bowie on stage at the Royal Festival

Hall on 8 July 1972 to duet on The Velvet Underground's 'Sweet Jane' (from 1971's *Loaded*). In the same month Bowie produced Mott The Hoople's cover version for *All The Young Dudes*. Reed's guide vocal for Mott, recorded at Trident with Bowie on backing vocals, has appeared on bootlegs. Five other heavily bootlegged demos from the *All The Young Dudes* sessions ('It's Alright', 'Henry And The H-Bomb', 'Shakin' All Over', 'Please Don't Touch' and 'So Sad') also purport to feature Bowie, but his presence on the tracks is doubtful: he is unlikely to have played guitar with Mott and his voice is nowhere to be heard.

SWEET THING

• Album: *Dogs* • Live: *David* • Bonus: *Dogs (2004)*

Although 'Sweet Thing', 'Candidate' and 'Sweet Thing (reprise)' are listed as three distinct tracks on *Diamond Dogs*, they segue seamlessly and are musically inseparable, so we'll discuss them together.

The sequence enjoyed a gradual gestation, as evidenced by the entirely different version of 'Candidate' included on 1990's *Diamond Dogs* reissue and by the lesser-known 1973 demo 'Zion', which provided a prototype for elements of the 'Sweet Thing' melody. However, neither of these early tracks remotely hints at the quality of the nine-minute sequence which dominates the first side of *Diamond Dogs*.

'Sweet Thing/Candidate' not only offers the strongest evidence of the album's "concept" pretensions, but is also the arguable highlight of *Diamond Dogs* and one of the great Bowie recordings. Beginning with a slow fade-in of reversed instrumentation resolving into a sublime piano line from Mike Garson, 'Sweet Thing' drips with decadence and decay as Bowie paints "a portrait in flesh" of sex as a drug-like commodity ("if you want it, boys, get it here"), and of love reduced to a series of hasty assignations in the ruined doorways of Hunger City, where physical intimacy means "putting pain in a stranger".

Bowie's vocal performance is among his finest ever, achieving spectacularly dextrous swoops between sepulchral bass and full-throated falsetto howls. Then, from the low-key intensity of its opening, the song shifts gear into 'Candidate', where densely written cut-ups tumble relentlessly across the rising noise of fuzzy, demented guitars. There are disquieting images of violence in the references to

Charles Manson, Cassius Clay and *"les tricoteuses"*, the women who knitted at the foot of Madame Guillotine, while Bowie himself seems half destroyed by "rumours and lies and stories they made up", consumed by the fakery of his own stage creations ("My set is amazing, it even smells like a street, there's a bar at the end where I can meet you and your friend"), and driven to distraction by his own promiscuity ("I put all I had in another bed, on another floor, in the back of a car, in a cellar like a church with the door ajar"). As the melody self-destructs beneath the accelerating chant of the lyric, 'Candidate' expires in a final image of flailing despair: "We'll buy some drugs and watch a band, and jump in a river holding hands." Thereafter the melody resolves, via a desperate squall on the saxophone, into a resigned reprise of 'Sweet Thing' in which David grimly concludes that he might as well "let it be" because "a street with a deal" is "all I ever wanted"; but then the accelerating bad trip returns with a nightmare excursion into rumbling rock guitars and squeals of feedback, finally fizzling out on the threshold of 'Rebel Rebel'.

The 'Sweet Thing/Candidate' suite demonstrates Bowie's commitment to experimental methods during the *Diamond Dogs* sessions. The lyrics are among the most clearly indebted to the Burroughsian cut-up method, and Bowie is known to have asked his musicians to play "in character" during recording: percussionist Tony Newman recalls David asking him to imagine himself as a French drummer-boy watching his first guillotine execution during the *"tricoteuses"* section.

There are inevitable parallels between 'Sweet Thing' and Bowie's own increasingly high-octane lifestyle at the time of the *Diamond Dogs* album, suggesting that the lyric is a desperate confessional, offering no resolution beyond self-lacerating despair. "When it's good it's really good, and when it's bad I go to pieces" might be Bowie's watchword for the mid-1970s. It's a stunningly bleak glimpse into the abyss and remains one of the most comprehensively imagined and dramatically performed of all Bowie's recordings.

The 'Sweet Thing/Candidate' sequence was performed throughout the Diamond Dogs tour, but was dropped from the Philly Dogs show and has never been performed since. In the same week that Bowie's Philadelphia concerts were being taped for *David Live* (which features a tense rendering of the sequence) in July 1974, Ava Cherry is understood to have recorded a souled-up version of 'Sweet Thing' with Michael Kamen at Sigma Sound studios, but this recording has never been released. A 2'57" mix of the 'Candidate' section from *Diamond Dogs*, which fades up after 'Sweet Thing' and down before 'Sweet Thing (reprise)', appeared on the soundtrack album of the 2001 film *Intimacy* and on 2004's reissue of *Diamond Dogs*.

TAKE IT WITH SOUL

Nothing is known of this Bowie composition, included in The Buzz's repertoire in late 1966.

TAKE MY TIP

• B-Side: 3/65 • Compilation: *Manish, Early*

The B-side of The Manish Boys' only single has the distinction of being the first self-penned Bowie composition to be released. It has a more rootsy R&B feel than the A-side, with guest guitarist Jimmy Page providing a nifty rhythm guitar, while the fast-talking streetwise lyric and some of the melodic phrases strongly anticipate the 1971 out-take 'Sweet Head'. 'Take My Tip' was also the earliest Bowie song to be covered: by the time The Manish Boys' single was released a version had already been recorded by Kenny Miller and released on the Stateside label.

As with 'I Pity The Fool', two different versions of 'Take My Tip' were recorded by The Manish Boys on 8 February 1965. Organist Bob Solly told *Record Collector* in 2000 that "Davie fluffs his own line on that song. What should have been 'spider who possesses the sky' came out as '*bider* who possesses the sky'! It didn't really matter; the lyrics were secondary in those days." The released (and fluffed) version later appeared on *The Manish Boys/Davy Jones And The Lower Third*, while the previously unreleased take appears on *Early On*.

TEENAGE WILDLIFE

• Album: *Scary*

The sublime opening track on the less familiar second side of *Scary Monsters* was originally entitled 'It Happens Every Day'. Robert Fripp's serene guitar line is reminiscent of his work on '"Heroes"' – a song with which 'Teenage Wildlife' is often compared – but the

dramatic progression here is something quite new. On one level it's a critique of slavish fashion victims, a long-time preoccupation particularly prevalent on *Scary Monsters*, and the lyric is often glossed as an attack on the herd of Bowie imitators who rose to prominence at the end of the 1970s: Gary Numan believes he is one of the song's subjects, telling David Buckley that he was "quite proud about it at the time". As it unwinds, the long and complex lyric becomes increasingly introspective, ruthlessly picking apart Bowie's own status as a trend-setting benchmark of style. "I feel like a group of one," he complains, archly dismissing "the new wave boys" as the "same old thing in brand new drag", and renouncing the unwanted status of role model for a new generation: "You'll take me aside and say, 'David, what shall I do, they wait for me in the hallway?', and I'll say, 'Don't ask me, I don't know any hallways'".

There is, however, more to 'Teenage Wildlife' than taking pot-shots at Gary Numan; Bowie has bigger fish to fry. The song confronts those who, throughout the 1970s, had wanted him to stand still and repeat his last success. In 1980 he explained that "if I had my kind of mythical younger brother, I think it might have been addressed to him. It's for somebody who's not mentally armed [for] the shell-shock of actually trying to assert yourself in society and your newly found values. I guess the younger brother is my adolescent self." Of the lyric's ominous "midwives to history" who "put on their bloody robes", he added: "I have my own personal bloody midwives. We all have them. Mine shall remain nameless. For the sake of the song they're symbolic; they're the ones who would not have you be fulfilled."

The phrase "bloody robes" would crop up again in the lyric of 1995's 'No Control'. Interestingly, after fifteen years of comparative obscurity 'Teenage Wildlife' received its live debut on the same year's Outside tour, an excellent and entirely appropriate addition to a show that wilfully challenged the audience's traditional appetite for the over-familiar.

TELLING LIES

• Download: 9/96 • A-Side: 11/96 • B-Side: 1/97 [14] • Album: *Earthling* • B-Side: 4/97 [32] • Live: *liveandwell.com*

The first *Earthling* track to be written was added to Bowie's live set for the 1996 Summer Festivals tour, making its debut in Nagoya on 7 June. "I put together this track on my own in Switzerland," he later told *Mojo*, "and used it as a blueprint of where I wanted the *Earthling* album to go … We just kept re-moulding it throughout the tour." He later explained that 'Telling Lies' had begun life during the *1.Outside* sessions, during which he had "changed the arrangement all the time; we must have tried out 20 different approaches for that song. Ultimately I found that hybridising a very aggressive rock sound with drum'n'bass worked best."

'Telling Lies' offers an interesting bridge between the sonic landscapes of *1.Outside* and *Earthling*, retaining some of the former's studio artifice and lacking some of the latter's spontaneity, setting atonal wheezes of guitar and synthesizer over a backing that revisits the rhythm track of 'We Prick You'. The cut-up lyric similarly stands at a crossroads between the two, fuelled by *1.Outside*'s pre-millennial Messianism ("gasping for my resurrection … I'm your future, I'm tomorrow, I'm the end"), and *Earthling*'s hesitant grasp at a new spirituality ("through the chromosomes of space and time … feels like something's going to happen this year"). Throughout the chorus Bowie juxtaposes "telling lies" with "starting fires," a tongue-in-cheek revision of the playground chant "Liar, liar, pants on fire", and also surely a flagrant reference to The Prodigy's March 1996 chartbuster which furnished 'Little Wonder' with its backbeat and *Earthling* with much of its inspiration.

Just as Bowie had been among the first musicians to appreciate the potential of rock video and CD-ROM, so on 11 September 1996 he became the first major artist to release a track on the Internet when Mark Plati's 'Feelgood Mix' began clocking up a reported 250,000 hits. The conventional release came on 4 November, although its distribution was limited to 3500 copies available through a select list of small independent record shops. It's difficult to imagine any other mainstream artist coming up with a publicity stunt that involves ensuring that their latest single is almost impossible to find.

Two of the three single mixes were included on subsequent releases, where the variant titles caused some confusion: completists should note that the 'Paradox Mix' is in fact the same as the 'A Guy Called Gerald Mix', while the 'Bowie Mix' is the 'Feelgood Mix'. The *Earthling* version is a different mix altogether, and was David's personal favourite: "It's not so dance-oriented," he said at the time. "It has a very dark atmosphere to it. It's actually, I think, one of the strongest pieces on the album." 'Telling Lies' was performed at the fiftieth birthday concert and throughout the Earthling tour, from which a version recorded in Amsterdam on 10 June 1997 later appeared on *live-andwell.com*.

TEMPTATION *(Freed/Broan)*

Included in David's medley with Cher on *The Cher Show* in November 1975.

THAT'S A PROMISE

Also referred to as 'Baby', this Bowie composition was demoed with The Lower Third at R G Jones Studios in October 1965, and a scratchy copy of the 2'19" recording has appeared on bootlegs. An inessential sample of Kinks-flavoured R&B, its most notable feature is a brief and unexpected preview of David's full-blown *Young Americans* falsetto.

THAT'S MOTIVATION
• Soundtrack: *Absolute Beginners*

With a backing track based on the opening bars of the title song, Bowie's second major contribution to *Absolute Beginners* is nowhere near as successful. The melody is nonexistent and the result is a meandering anti-climax. It works better with the visuals: 'That's Motivation' is Bowie's big number in the film, allowing him to tap-dance on the keys of a giant typewriter as his repulsive ad-man introduces the hero to "the world of your dreams … where you can commit horrible sins and get away with it," and urges him to "learn to fall in love with yourself".

THAT'S WHERE MY HEART IS
• Compilation: *Early*

In all its crackling acoustic frailty, this mid-1965 demo of an unremarkable love lyric speaks volumes about the developing vocal style of the young Davy Jones. Interspersed with elements of Gene Pitney there are tentative inroads into the crooning baritone and the aggressive mock-Cockney that would later become Bowie staples.

THERE IS A HAPPY LAND

• Album: *Bowie*

Recorded on 24 November 1966, this sentimental number locates childhood innocence in a magical, Blakeian paradise symbolically removed from the impending darkness of adulthood. It was pencilled in as the B-side of the unreleased American 'Rubber Band' single after Deram's US division rejected 'The London Boys', and in 1967 the song was unsuccessfully offered to Judy Collins and to Peter, Paul and Mary, whose famous flower-power rendering of 'Puff The Magic Dragon' covers very similar territory.

THINGS TO DO

This Bowie composition was recorded by the Astronettes in 1973 and eventually released on 1995's *People From Bad Homes*, on which a brief snippet of David speaking can be heard at the beginning of the track. The arrangement is akin to the more uptempo soul recordings from the *Young Americans* sessions, notably prefiguring the rhythmic pattern of the outtake 'After Today'. The love-song lyric is undemanding, the only point of note being a proliferation of soul-by-numbers religious references, including a line from the 23rd Psalm ("the Lord is my shepherd"). It would be another couple of years before Bowie began peppering his own recordings with overt Biblical motifs on *Station To Station*.

THIS BOY *(Lennon/McCartney)*

The Beatles classic, originally a 1963 B-side, was an occasional addition to the Ziggy Stardust repertoire in the summer and autumn of 1972, including shows in Bristol on 27 August, Stoke on 7 September, and a couple of the subsequent US concerts. The most commonly available recording of 'This Boy' has appeared on numerous bootlegs, but in the absence of reliable confirmation its exact provenance remains uncertain. It is often said to hail from the Friars, Aylesbury on 15 July, but the evidence points more compellingly to the Bristol gig of 27 August.

THIS IS MY DAY : see **ERNIE JOHNSON**

THIS IS NOT AMERICA *(Metheny/Bowie/Mays)*

• A-Side: 2/85 [14] • Compilation: *SinglesUK, Best Of Bowie, Club* • Bonus: *Tonight* • Live: *Beeb* • Soundtrack: *Training Day*

Recorded in late 1984, the theme song for John Schlesinger's *The Falcon And The Snowman* is sleek, smooth and ever so slightly dull, adopting the smoochy jazz-fusion style then being popularized by acts like Sade and Shakatak. It's hardly Bowie's finest lyric ("Snowman melting from the inside, Falcon spirals to the ground", ahem), but 'This Is Not America' did reasonable business in Britain and America (where it made number 32), and in common with many of Bowie's 1980s film themes it became a huge hit in Germany. As early as September 1984 David spoke enthusiastically of the movie: "It's the story of two young American guys who sell secrets to the Russians. It's Tim Hutton and Sean Penn giving the performances of their lives, but I don't know how it will be received in the States given the current political climate. It's very objective, though one feels great sympathy for the two boys. It's a magnificent piece of filmmaking, the best Schlesinger movie I've seen in years." Bowie does not feature in the accompanying video, which was constructed from clips of the movie.

Fifteen years on, 'This Is Not America' received its live premiere on the summer 2000 dates, with a fine version recorded on 27 June appearing on the *Bowie At The Beeb* live bonus disc. July 2001 found Bowie collaborating with rapper P Diddy on a radical hip-hop re-recording at Daddy's House Studio in New York, for use in the soundtrack of the film *Training Day*. The result was retitled 'American Dream' and credited to P Diddy and The Bad Boy Family featuring David Bowie. "I'm in the studio recording with Sean," explained Bowie at the time. "We're doing live vocals. It's not really so much like a sampling kind of affair. The first time we did it [i.e. Puff Daddy's 'Let's Dance'-sampling 1997 hit 'Been Around The World'] we had a lot fun, it was kind of cool, but we might as well have phoned in our performances, because it was done 2000, 3000 miles apart. This time, really, it's like a nice thing … This version's definitely got a menace. The beats will be very interesting because it's definitely moved on from what you'd expect. There's a fast techno flavour to it. It's got an aggression to it that really reflects the movie."

A remix of the original 'This Is Not America' by The Scumfrog later appeared on *Club Bowie*, while the Ahn Trio included a "classical" cover version, played on violin, piano and cello, on their 2001 album *Ahn-Plugged*.

THREEPENNY JOE

Kenneth Pitt cites this as a discarded 1968 Bowie composition; a connection with 'Threepenny Pierrot' seems more than likely.

THREEPENNY PIERROT

This Bowie song from 1967's Lindsay Kemp production *Pierrot In Turquoise* survives as an unreleased 1'56" demo made for the 1970 adaptation *The Looking Glass Murders*. It's an introduction to the "comical hero" and his relationship with the *commedia dell'arte* archetypes Harlequin and Columbine. By the time of *The Looking Glass Murders* the melody, here bashed out on a tinkling vaudeville piano, had already been reused for 'London Bye Ta Ta'.

THRU' THESE ARCHITECTS EYES *(Bowie/Gabrels)*
• Album: *1.Outside*

This splendid, grandiose number in the *Lodger/Scary Monsters* vein was cut in New York in 1995 as a late addition to *1.Outside*, and despite being ascribed to the Leon Blank character it seems to bear little relation to the linking narrative. It's blessed with a superb Mike Garson solo and a chugging backbeat of guitars and drums, but the real treasure is the absurdly bombastic lyric. Only Bowie could namecheck Phillip Johnson and Richard Rogers and still make it sound thrilling, and who else would have the gall to attempt a metaphor built around the word "concrete"?: "All the majesty of a city landscape / All the soaring days of our lives / All the concrete dreams in my mind's eye..." The song occasionally appeared on the US leg of the Outside tour.

THRUST *(Bowie/Gabrels)*

An instrumental track recorded by Bowie with Reeves Gabrels in 1999 for exclusive use in the *Omikron* computer game.

THURSDAY'S CHILD *(Bowie/Gabrels)*
• A-Side: 9/99 [16] • Album: *'hours...'* • B-Side: 1/00 [28] • Video: *Best Of Bowie*

With its acoustic guitars, synth backings and fragile vocal, 'Thursday's Child' revives a wistful ballad style seldom heard in Bowie's work since the 1980s; in fact, the chords and arrangement are curiously reminiscent of The Cars' global 1984 hit 'Drive'. The song's nearest relatives in the Bowie canon are perhaps 'Buddha Of Suburbia' and the undervalued 'As The World Falls Down', although the addition of some fashionable soul-diva backing vocals brings the track firmly into 1999. According to Reeves Gabrels, "David originally wanted TLC to sing on 'Thursday's Child', which I wasn't really into at all. Through a stroke of good fortune I managed to get Holly Palmer, who is a friend I used to write songs with in Boston." Holly Palmer would go on to become one of Bowie's regular backing vocalists.

"It's a title not imbued with arcane knowledge, as you might think," David explained during his VH1 *Storytellers* concert in 1999. "It was prompted by the memory of the autobiography of Eartha Kitt ... it was called *Thursday's Child*, and that stayed with me since I was fourteen, I don't know why – but it just kind of bubbled up the other month when we wrote this. This song, I might point out, is not actually about Eartha Kitt!" Interestingly, what Bowie didn't mention was that 'Thursday's Child' was also the title of a ballad written by Elisse Boyd and Murray Grand, recorded by Eartha Kitt in 1956 and performed live on countless occasions, with a dolorous tempo and a strikingly similar lyric of melancholic retrospection ("I never know which way I'm bound / Heartbreak hangs round for Thursday's child / I'll always be blamed for what I was named / But still I'm not ashamed I'm Thursday's child"). It's possible that Bowie was unaware of the song, but this seems highly unlikely given his familiarity with other Eartha Kitt recordings like 'The Day The Circus Left Town' and 'Just An Old Fashioned Girl'.

Speculation inevitably arose that the song's title

might also refer to David's own birthday, but 8 January 1947 was in fact a Wednesday. According to the nineteenth-century nursery rhyme, which Bowie often recited on stage during the 1999 tour, "Wednesday's child is full of woe", while "Thursday's child has far to go." Another probable spark is a line from The Velvet Underground's classic 'All Tomorrow's Parties': "Thursday's child is Sunday's clown." And, as David confirmed, the arrangement recalls yet another nursery rhyme – the "Monday, Tuesday, Wednesday" underscore closely echoes the "two and two are four" backdrop of 'Inchworm', Danny Kaye's song from the 1952 film musical *Hans Christian Andersen*, which Bowie has often cited as a childhood influence: "I love the effect of two melodies together. That nursery rhyme feeling shows itself in a lot of the songs I've written, like 'Ashes To Ashes' and … 'Thursday's Child'."

The lyric establishes the introspective mood of the *'hours…'* album. "I guess Thursday's Child is somebody that maybe felt that he'd achieved anything that he was ever going to achieve in his life," said Bowie, "and that the way forward looked as bleak as much of his past had done … until it was changed by meeting this particular person that he falls in love with. So it's like a glimmer of salvation in his own life." Although Bowie advised against autobiographical interpretations of the *'hours…'* material, it's difficult to dissociate this analysis from his own redemptive happiness after years of social alienation ("Something about me stood apart … Maybe I'm born right out of my time") and the ambivalent relationship with "tomorrow" that had infused so much of his early writing. In place of the spiritual anguish of *The Man Who Sold The World* or *Diamond Dogs*, the narrator of 'Thursday's Child' is approaching an inner peace, redeemed by love and content to relinquish "my past" without regret and reach for "tomorrow" without trepidation.

Another line in the lyric, "Lucky old sun is in my sky", recalls Ray Charles's 'That Lucky Old Sun' (a US hit in 1964, when The Manish Boys covered several Charles numbers) and also paraphrases "Busy old fool, unruly sun", the opening line of John Donne's *The Sun Rising* – another celebration of love's invincibility in the face of time and circumstance which includes the remarkably comparable line: "Love, all alike, no season knows, nor clime / Nor hours, days, months, which are the rags of time."

The 'Thursday's Child' video was directed by Bowie newcomer Walter Stern, whose previous credits

included The Prodigy's 'Firestarter' and Madonna's 'Drowned World'. Shot in August 1999 at Broadway Stages Studio in New York, it was described by David as "a strange and slow-moving piece that wanders between a present and a past in a bewildering fashion." One of the most low-key and sombre videos Bowie has made, it eschews the fast cutting and distorted images of his previous 1990s work to capture him in reflective mood – literally. Gazing at himself in a bathroom mirror, he travels back in time as his reflection changes into that of a young man, while the image of his partner, removing her contact lenses, undergoes a similar transformation. Reflection and reality interact as Bowie and his *alter ego* muse on what is, what was and what might have been.

Excerpts from three different mixes were previewed on BowieNet in August 1999, with the chosen favourite destined to appear on single formats. The first disc of the two-CD set featured the standard single edit, while the other substituted the so-called 'Rock Mix'. Released on 20 September, 'Thursday's Child' entered the UK chart at its number 16 peak, later receiving a Grammy nomination for "Best Male Rock Vocal Performance". The song featured throughout the *'hours…'* tour, during which numerous performances appeared on American, French, German, Spanish, Italian and Swedish television shows. The *Top Of The Pops* appearance on 24 September was pre-recorded in New York the previous month. The second CD single included a PC-playable version of the video, although some CD2 mispressings erroneously played the CD1 tracks, making them instant collectors' items fetching handsome sums. A live version recorded in Paris on 14 October 1999 was later released as a B-side, and a further so-called "easy listening" version (marginally slower, but otherwise very similar to the *'hours…'* cut) appears in *Omikron: The Nomad Soul*. 'Thursday's Child' made a one-off reappearance on the first of the summer 2000 dates.

TIME

• Album: *Aladdin* • Live: *Motion, Rarest* • Bonus: *David, Aladdin (2003)* • Live Video: *Ziggy, Glass*

Like *Aladdin Sane*'s title track, 'Time' is a showcase for new arrival Mike Garson, whose 1920s New Orleans stride piano dominates the track. "It was an almost swing or Dixieland style," Garson told the Gillmans, "and [David] liked my concept on that because it had to do with time, and I was playing in another time-zone, and he was talking about time." Mick Ronson lifts and explores Garson's riff on guitar, at one point quoting from Beethoven's ninth symphony, from which The Spiders' pre-show music originated. Bowie, meanwhile, howls his way through a lyric of existential ennui and galloping mortality, reviving the dread of time already witnessed in lyrics like 'An Occasional Dream' and 'Changes'. His palpable disillusion ("I had so many dreams, I made so many breakthroughs … but all I have to give is guilt for dreaming") catches Bowie responding to his first flush of success with unmitigated bleakness, while the anguished and simultaneously suggestive burst of heavy breathing during the break in the second verse introduces a positively Brechtian sense of theatricality.

As in so many *Aladdin Sane* lyrics, there are veiled references to figures significant to David at the time. Billy Murcia, the New York Dolls' original drummer and sometime liaison of Angela Bowie, drowned in his bath on 6 November 1972, probably as a result of an overdose of Mandrax and alcohol. David had socialized with the band after their New York gig in October, hence his image of the Grim Reaper, "in Quaaludes and red wine, demanding Billy Dolls and other friends of mine". The song was written in New Orleans on 14 November, within days of Murcia's death.

In January 1973 David spoke, as he often did at this stage, about his lyrics acquiring a life of their own: "I've written a new song on the new album which is just called 'Time', and I thought it was about time, and I wrote very heavily about time, and the way I felt about time – at times! – and I played it back after we recorded it and, my God, it was a gay song! And I'd no intention of writing anything at all gay. When I listened to it back I just could not believe it."

'Time' is inevitably notorious for its barefaced use of the word "wanking" which, coming from a dandified middle-class pop singer still being marketed very much at a young teen audience, gave *Aladdin Sane* terrific parent-shocking value. The BBC banned the song from its playlist and David later altered the word to "swanking" for NBC's *The 1980 Floor Show* (although the dancers behind him left little doubt as to what the line should have been). Fans of great comedy will recall Stephen Fry's apoplectic headmaster attempting to unravel schoolboy Hugh Laurie's prize-winning poem: "Time fell wanking to the floor? Is this just put in to shock, or is there something personal you wish

to discuss with me? … A quotation? What from? It isn't Milton, and I'm pretty sure it can't be Wordsworth…" Interestingly, Stateside ignorance of this peculiarly British profanity meant that the offending word remained intact in the edited 3'38" US single, released in April 1973 in place of the UK's 'Drive In Saturday'. Ken Scott, who nominated 'Time' as his favourite track on *Aladdin Sane*, would later remark upon the curious fact that American radio stations were prone to censor the word "Quaaludes" but would happily allow the "wanking" to proceed unchecked.

'Time' was added to Bowie's live repertoire in 1973, and reappeared for the Diamond Dogs and Glass Spider tours. On the Earthling tour Mike Garson would occasionally play the song's opening piano chords at the tail-end of 'Battle For Britain (The Letter)', as can be heard on *liveandwell.com*. The *1980 Floor Show* version, recorded on 19 October 1973, later appeared on *RarestOneBowie*, while the single mix was included on 2003's *Aladdin Sane* reissue.

TIME WILL CRAWL
• Album: *Never* • A-Side: 6/87 [33] • Video: *Collection, Best Of Bowie*

Never Let Me Down's second track is in many estimations the album's finest moment. Bowie forsakes his mid-1980s croon in favour of the Cockney theatrics of yore, and an admirably restrained guitar break – another rarity on this album – allows room instead for a hauntingly effective trumpet solo. The lyric, too, is among the album's best, a pleasing return to a non-linear approach that paints a desolate landscape of poisoned rivers, nuclear devastation and genetic mutation reminiscent of *Diamond Dogs*. Bowie explained that the lyric was about "science and humanity, basically, the idea of the bright kid who turns into a demonic scientist and creates this catastrophe." Only fleetingly are there suggestions that he might be grasping at straws, with a rather cheesy topical reference to "a Top Gun pilot" and an unwelcome hint of preachiness ("We'll give every life for the crackpot notion"), but without doubt 'Time Will Crawl' is among his strongest mid-1980s work.

As the album's second single it failed to deliver a hit, stalling at a paltry 33. Things might have been different had the BBC opted to show the *Top Of The Pops* performance, Bowie's first in ten years, which was pre-recorded in June during the UK leg of the Glass Spider tour. At the time *Top Of The Pops* adhered to the precept of never featuring songs on their way down the chart, and when 'Time Will Crawl' dropped from the top 40 in the week of its intended transmission, the clip was pulled. A minute-long glimpse of this otherwise unscreened performance – showcasing David with a dummy guitar and sporting a transparent PVC jacket stuffed with pages from newspapers (apparently a political comment about pornographic pin-ups) – was included in BBC2's retrospective *Eighties*, transmitted on New Year's Eve 1989. The full-length clip has since found its way onto bootleg videos.

Meanwhile the official 'Time Will Crawl' video was directed by Tim Pope, a newcomer to the Bowie stable whose reputation rested primarily on a superb run of promos for The Cure. Masquerading as a fly-on-the-wall rehearsal film, the video was a taster for the Glass Spider tour's extravagant stage choreography, featuring Bowie and his backing troupe working through the elaborate stage routines which would accompany 'Fashion', 'Loving The Alien' and 'Sons Of The Silent Age'. Although tour guitarist Peter Frampton doesn't play on the studio track, he appears in the video to mime to Sid McGinnis's solo, which he recreated for the Glass Spider tour.

TIN MACHINE (*Bowie/T.Sales/H.Sales/Gabrels*)
• Album: *TM* • A-Side: 9/89 [48]

The signature tune of Bowie's much-reviled rock outfit is actually one of their better offerings, a *Scary Monsters* retread laying a series of violent images over a furious guitar riff. The fragmented protest lyric offers an early taste of the album's didactic tone, as Bowie rails against "humping Tories, spittle on their chins, carving up my children's future"; the only promise of escape from "this psycho time-bomb planet" is to "make some new computer thing that puts me on the moon". There's a reminiscent hint of the room-retreats of 'Sound And Vision' and 'All The Madmen', a song Bowie had recently been performing live: "Burning in my room … I'm not exactly well" is remarkably close to "talking to my wall, I'm not quite right at all". Sadly the track is marred by Bowie's decision to affect a rather silly American rock'n'roll accent, perhaps to match the momentary invocation of 'Blue Suede Shoes'.

The album cut was released as a double A-side with 'Maggie's Farm'. Julien Temple's Tin Machine promo film includes a stage-managed "live" performance in which fans storm the stage, Bowie spitting blood in the ensuing riot. The song was performed live throughout the first Tin Machine tour, and occasionally on the second.

TINY GIRLS (*Pop/Bowie*)

Produced and co-written by David for Iggy Pop's *The Idiot*, 'Tiny Girls' is worthy of attention for one of Bowie's finest saxophone performances.

TINY TIM : see **ERNIE JOHNSON**

TIRED OF MY LIFE

Probably taped at Haddon Hall around May 1970, this frail 3'05" acoustic demo features Bowie and his acoustic guitar supported by some raucous backing vocals – possibly Mick Ronson – and is the fascinating prototype for 'It's No Game', a song that would not be recorded until ten years later. The opening lines ("I don't know why, but I'm tired of my life / Pain is over me, overloading / I don't know why, but you're trying to be kind") indicate the depressive introspection of the same period's 'Conversation Piece', but we soon reach the familiar "Throw a rock against the road and it breaks into pieces … Put a bullet in my brain, and I make all the papers."

Several sources have claimed that 'Tired Of My Life' was composed in 1963, but it should be noted that the only corroboration of this is a comment once made by Tony Visconti that David wrote 'It's No Game' at the age of sixteen.

TO KNOW HIM IS TO LOVE HIM (*Spector*)

Shortly before the *Diamond Dogs* sessions in late 1973, Bowie recorded a guest saxophone solo for folk-rock combo Steeleye Span, who were recording at Morgan Studios in Willesden while he was completing sax overdubs on Lulu's single 'The Man Who Sold The World'. Steeleye Span, whose bassist Rick Kemp had played in one of Mick Ronson's early bands and had been briefly mooted as bass player for the *Hunky Dory* sessions, were now recording their sixth album, appropriately entitled *Now We Are Six*. Bowie's dissonant alto sax break appears on the closing number, a cover of The Teddy Bears' 1958 hit, ending with a ragged dying honk remarkably similar to the one he would later employ on the *"Heroes"* track 'Neuköln'. David's guest appearance initiated a Steeleye Span tradition of enlisting unlikely stars to close their albums: the follow-up, *Commoner's Crown*, ended with the appearance of Peter Sellers on ukulele.

TONIGHT *(Bowie/Pop)*
• Album: *Tonight* • A-Side: 11/84 [53] • Live Video: *Tina Live – Private Dancer Tour (Tina Turner)*

Premiered on the 1977 Iggy Pop tour, 'Tonight' was subsequently recorded for *Lust For Life*, with co-writer/producer Bowie on piano and backing vocals. Iggy's version begins with a cod angelic chorus of backing vocals provided by David and the Sales brothers, over which the opening lyric establishes that the song is addressed to a lover dying of a heroin overdose: "I saw my baby, she was turning blue, I knew that soon her young life was through / And so I got down on my knees, down by her bed, And these are the words to her I said…"

Needless to say, Bowie's decision to excise this prologue from his 1984 re-recording utterly changes the intention of the piece. "That was such an idiosyncratic thing of Jimmy's that it seemed not part of my vocabulary," he said at the time. "There was that consideration, and I was also doing it with Tina [Turner] – she's the other voice on it – and I didn't want to inflict it on her either. It's not necessarily something that she would particularly agree to sing or be part of. I guess we changed the whole sentiment around. It still has that same barren feeling though, but it's out of that specific area that I'm not at home in. I can't say that it's Iggy's world, but it's far more of Iggy's observation than mine."

Bowie's reading of 'Tonight', set to a lilting reggae arrangement and featuring special guest Tina Turner low in the mix, has come in for a lot of stick, although at the time *Rolling Stone*'s Kurt Loder hailed it as "one of the most vibrantly beautiful tracks he's ever recorded," noting that it "displays Bowie's voice at its sweetest and most human." Like much of Bowie's mid-1980s work it's perfectly accomplished and difficult actively to dislike, but it's sorely lacking in bite. With

no video to support it the single stiffed dramatically, climbing no higher than a shocking number 53 to make it the first chart indication that all was not well post-*Let's Dance*.

Other than backing Iggy Pop on keyboards in 1977 Bowie has only once performed 'Tonight' live, as a duet with Tina Turner at her Birmingham concert on 23 March 1985 (see Chapter 3); this performance later appeared on Tina's 1988 album *Live In Europe*, and in the same year was released as a 12" single in various European countries, even topping the chart in the Netherlands. It was subsequently included on the 1994 CD/video box set *Tina Live – Private Dancer Tour*. On a couple of occasions on 1990's Sound + Vision tour, Bowie inserted a short snippet of the number into 'The Jean Genie'.

TOO BAD

The performing rights organization BMI lists this otherwise unknown Bowie composition, published by the Embassy Music Corporation and almost certainly dating from the mid-1960s.

TOO DIZZY *(Bowie/Kizilcay)*
• Album: *Never*

Never Let Me Down's penultimate track was deleted from the 1995 reissue, and at Bowie's behest it has remained absent from subsequent pressings. The precise reason is unclear but there are a couple of obvious possibilities: in the first place 'Too Dizzy' is quite simply one of the feeblest tracks even on this album, a shabby Robert Palmeresque pop-rocker laying a tiresome guitar break and a yakkety-yak saxophone over a chord sequence almost identical to 'Zeroes'. It's tempting, however, to conjecture that the song's eradication might be down to justified embarrassment over its lyrical content. In a jealous harangue addressed to an imagined girlfriend, Bowie badly oversteps his usual boundary of playful sexism: "you're just pushing for a fight … I'm a-shakin' in anger … I'm not letting you out of my sight … who's this guy I'm gonna blow away, what kind of love is he giving you?" From the one-time author of 'Repetition', this is cause for concern.

"It's a throwaway," said David in 1987, already sounding as if he wanted to disown the number. "I always thought it was better for Huey Lewis! I was unsettled with that song, but it's on the album anyway. It's one of the first songs that Erdal Kizilcay and I wrote together, a sort of try-out to see how we sparred together as writers. I thought a real fifties subject matter was either love or jealousy, so I thought I'd stick with jealousy because it's a lot more interesting!"

In 1987 'Too Dizzy' was briefly mooted for single release, appearing as an American promo. Its removal from *Never Let Me Down* has rendered it a latter-day collector's item, but few will feel impelled to hunt it down.

TOO FAT POLKA

This legendary out-take, also known by the outrageous alternative title 'You Can Have Her, I Don't Want Her, She's Too Fat For Me', was recorded during the Sigma *Young Americans* sessions in August 1974. An apocryphal story has it that the master tape was ceremonially burned at the end of the sessions, but this is a myth; it is understood to remain in Bowie's possession.

TOY : see YOUR TURN TO DRIVE

TRUTH *(Goldie)*

Bowie recorded lead vocals for this track on *Saturnzreturn*, the second album by drum'n'bass architect Goldie, during London rehearsals for the Earthling tour in May 1997. When the two were introduced at the time of the Outside tour, Bowie was already familiar with Goldie's early recordings and was impressed by his 1995 debut *Timeless*. "I liked his stuff," David said later. "I thought that was a nice first album." The following year Goldie's studio collaborator A Guy Called Gerald remixed 'Telling Lies', and in June 1997 Goldie was present at London's Hanover Grand to witness the beginning of the Earthling tour. "I still think that Bowie can go a bit further with this music," he told *Q* after the first warm-up gig, "but it's up to him to experiment. He should take it somewhere it hasn't been before, outside the realm of linear drum'n'bass, so that no-one can judge it."

Saturnzreturn, which also featured contributions from Noel Gallagher of Oasis, was released in two dif-

ferent formats: 'Truth' appears only on the full-length two-disc version. The album treads dark, intimate and unsettling territory not unlike some of Bowie's own early work, and its grandiosity and perceived self-indulgence were later credited with hastening the death of drum'n'bass. 'Truth' is characteristic of the album, a protracted environment of sonic effects that make even the weirdest noises on Bowie's Berlin albums sound fairly conventional. David's echo-laden and barely comprehensible vocal resounds across a backing of phased and reversed synthesizers, layered whispers and echoing bass piano notes, creating a texture of sadness, foreboding and barely concealed panic that is replicated in varous forms throughout the album. In 1998 Bowie co-starred with Goldie in the film *Everybody Loves Sunshine* and contributed to the Channel 4 documentary *When Saturn Returnz*.

TRY SOME, BUY SOME *(Harrison)*
• Album: *Reality* • Live Video: *Reality*

"I love this song so much," Bowie told the Riverside Studios audience on 8 September 2003. "I hope I do it justice." For *Reality*'s second cover version he had turned to a major British songwriter whose work, perhaps surprisingly, he had never recorded before. George Harrison originally wrote 'Try Some, Buy Some' for the ex-Ronettes vocalist Ronnie Spector, whose version was released as a single in April 1971, inexplicably failing to chart on either side of the Atlantic. "At that time," Bowie recalled, "it was the only single by a solo artist that actually had all four Beatles on it. The Beatles had kind of disbanded, but they all loved Ronnie, and it was George Harrison producing it, so they all crept in at different times to put parts on it." Bowie had already paid tribute to the single many years earlier when he included it in the choice of records he played on BBC Radio 1's *Star Special* back in 1979. On that occasion he described Ronnie Spector's recording as "absolutely incredible", remarking that it "made me fall in love with the singer ... my heart went straight out to her." He also recalled that the track was co-produced by the singer's then husband Phil Spector: "I may be wrong but I think it's the last single he ever made, because he was so depressed that it didn't do anything, that nobody bought it." Some years later, on 1990's Sound + Vision tour, David would ocasionally insert a snippet of the song into performances of 'The Jean Genie'.

Bowie was keen to emphasize that it was Ronnie Spector who had originally drawn him to 'Try Some, Buy Some' and that, despite *Reality* being the first album he had recorded since George Harrison's death in November 2001, the connection was purely coincidental: "It didn't really occur to me until I sat down to do the credits for the album that in fact it was a George Harrison song," he admitted, "and I thought, well, that's really lovely, cos it was kind of like doing a tribute to George, but unwittingly." Harrison had included his own version of 'Try Some, Buy Some' on his 1973 album *Living In The Material World*, but Bowie's cover takes most of its cues from the Ronnie Spector original. "We were pretty true to the original arrangement," David observed, "but the overall atmosphere is somewhat different. It's a dense piece."

This is certainly true: the song's lilting 3/4 time and retro production style recall some of the stylistic experimentation of The Beatles' later work, and the multiple layers of synthesizers, drums and strumming mandolins create a richly textured soundscape against which Bowie delivers one of the album's most brilliant vocal performances, gradually building from frail beginnings to a full-blown, heroic finale. The retrospective, older-and-wiser lyric seems signally appropriate both to *Reality* and, in a broader sense, to Bowie himself: lines like "Through my life I've seen grey sky / Met big fry / Seen them die to get high" might have been tailor-made for him, while the sense of an erstwhile iceman's emotional redemption ("Not a thing did I feel / Not a thing did I know / Till I called on your love") covers much the same ground as many of the lyrics from David's later career. "When I first heard that song it had a very different narrative to it," he admitted in 2003. "Now my connection to the song is about leaving a way of life behind me and finding something new. It's overstated about most rock artists leaving drugs, it's such a bore to read about it. But when I first heard the song in '74 I was yet to go through my heavy drug period. And now it's about the consolation of having kicked all that and turning your life around."

'Try Some, Buy Some' was one of the rarer numbers performed on A Reality Tour.

TRYIN' TO GET TO HEAVEN *(Dylan)*

Recorded in 1998 and originally intended as a bonus track for the proposed Earthling tour live album,

Bowie's rather pedestrian 4'58" cover of this song from Bob Dylan's 1997 album *Time Out Of Mind* was unofficially leaked to Spanish radio station DOS 84 in October 1999, and released in downloadable form on the station's website. Otherwise, excepting its appearance on a very rare Virgin promo CDR, the recording remains unavailable.

TUMBLE AND TWIRL *(Bowie/Pop)*
• Album: *Tonight* • B-Side: 11/84 [53]

Credit where credit's due: 'Tumble And Twirl' is one of the most undervalued of Bowie's 1980s recordings, and although its middle-of-the-road arrangement fails to repeat the success of *Lodger*'s 'African Night Flight' or 'Red Sails', its absurdist sense of a musical culture-clash attempts something very similar. In this case the inspiration was Bowie's holiday with Iggy Pop in Bali and Java at the end of 1983. "The very rich oil magnates of Java have these incredible colonial-style houses with sewage floating down the hills into the jungle," Bowie explained the following year. "That stayed with me, and watching films out in the garden projected on sheets. It felt so bizarre to sit there in the jungle watching movies at the end of the garden through monsoon weather with rain pouring down. Images of Brooke Shields ... it was quite absurd." Like several *Tonight* tracks, the composition emerged from Bowie's free-association partnership with Iggy Pop. "I think it worked out around fifty-fifty lyrics on most of the songs, but Jimmy's work stands out most obviously on 'Tumble And Twirl'," said David. "I think that's obviously his line of humour. The lines about the T-shirts and the part about the sewage floating down the hill..."

This isn't a comedy song, though; with its repeated refrain of "I like the free world", it's also an outsider's reaction to Indonesian society. Bowie: "I guess those circumstances make one quite fond of the 'free world' because a country like Java or Singapore is most definitely not free. There's an extraordinary split between one class and another, far more exaggerated than any class system in the West. If I had the choice between Singapore or Java, I'd pick England! That's what I meant by that line, but when put in a musical structure these things take on a life of their own – as we know from past experience."

Like most of *Tonight* 'Tumble And Twirl' has dated badly; its spinning Latino arrangement, false endings and trumpet pips sound uncomfortably like the sort of thing you'd expect to hear coming from Kid Creole And The Coconuts or Wham! at around the same time. But the choppy rhythm guitar, the tumbling clatter of percussion, the tongue-in-cheek lounge-music backing vocals and the marvellous acoustic break make for an immensely likeable excursion into world music. And who could dislike a song that has the audacity to rhyme "dusky mulatto" with "nylons and tattoos"?

TURN BLUE *(Pop/Lacey/Bowie/Peace)*

An early version of 'Turn Blue' was attempted in Los Angeles in May 1975 by Bowie, Iggy Pop and Warren Peace (see 'Moving On'). Two years later the song was furnished with a new lyric and performed during Iggy's 1977 tour (a version appears on *Suck On This!*), before being re-recorded for *Lust For Life* with Bowie on piano and backing vocals. That the original composition dates from the *Young Americans* period is obvious from the outset: 'Turn Blue' is a sprawling soul ballad in the style of 'It's Gonna Be Me'.

TVC15
• Album: *Station* • A-Side: 4/76 [33] • Live: *Stage*

'TVC15' is *Station To Station*'s odd man out, with a lyric of surreal comedy rather than existential angst borne on a wave of honky-tonk piano and chirpy backing vocals. It's apparently indebted to a story David was told by Iggy Pop, some time during 1975's hallucinatory madness, about his girlfriend being swallowed by a television set. A more sinister inspiration may have been the images of mesmeric TV screens prevalent in *The Man Who Fell To Earth*, but there's nothing ominous about this jaunty, cartoonish confection, which is a jarring burst of exuberance among *Station To Station*'s more anguished moments. The "transmission / transition" bridge not only recalls the silver-screen metaphors of many earlier compositions, but offers a playful alternative to the sinister transubstantiation of the title track's "magical movement".

Carlos Alomar later recalled that the rough-and-ready nature of the track was a deliberate strategy, revealing that Bowie "really wanted it fucked up like when we did 'Boys Keep Swinging', kind of loose and stupid. But then when it got to the end, he really

wanted it to drive home."

'TVC15' is something of a forgotten single: released in edited form to coincide with the European leg of the 1976 tour, it stalled at number 33. It featured throughout the Station To Station, Stage, Serious Moonlight and Sound + Vision tours, on the first and last of which David played sax for the number. 'TVC15' resurfaced in the December 1979 *Saturday Night Live* set and again at 1985's Live Aid, where it rose to the occasion with some marvellously sleazy sax from Clare Hurst and a crazed piano line from Thomas Dolby. Among several cover versions is a rendition in the 'Bowie Medley' from the Mike Flowers Pops' 1996 CD single 'Light My Fire'.

TV EYE *(The Stooges)*

From The Stooges' *Fun House*, 'TV Eye' was performed during the 1977 Iggy Pop tour, from which a version featuring Bowie can be heard on *TV Eye* and *Suck On This!*.

20TH CENTURY BOY *(Bolan)*

On 16 February 1999 Bowie teamed up with Placebo for a live performance of the 1973 T Rex hit at the Brit Awards ceremony at London's Docklands Arena. Placebo had previously covered the song for the *Velvet Goldmine* soundtrack, but press coverage of the duet put the emphasis on Bowie's friendship with Marc Bolan. "When he lived in LA in the mid-seventies, we spent a lot of time jamming '20th Century Boy'," David told reporters. A month later on 29 March, the duet was reprised for a Placebo gig at New York's Irving Plaza. Tony Visconti, who had produced Bolan's original, mixed the Brits version for possible release as a B-side to 'Without You I'm Nothing', but the idea was dropped.

UNCLE ARTHUR
• Album: *Bowie*

The opening track of *David Bowie* was recorded at the initial album session on 14 November 1966. It's an eccentric tragicomedy about a socially inadequate thirtysomething who "still reads comics" and "follows Batman", repents getting married and returns to his mother's bosom. Interestingly, the precise circumstances of our hero's domestic tribulations ("Round and round goes Arthur's head, hasn't eaten well for days / Little Sally may be lovely, but cooking leaves her in a maze") would be revisited with a little less of the storybook charm on 1979's 'Repetition'. In 1967 Bowie's American publisher offered 'Uncle Arthur' without success to Peter, Paul and Mary.

UNCLE FLOYD : see SLIP AWAY

UNDER PRESSURE
(Bowie/Mercury/Taylor/Deacon/May)
• A-Side: 11/81 [1] • A-Side: 11/88 • Compilation: SinglesUK, SinglesUS, Best Of Bowie • Bonus: Dance • B-Side: 2/96 [12] • A-Side: 12/99 [14] • Video: Box Of Flix (Queen), Greatest Video Hits 2 (Queen) • Live Video: The Freddie Mercury Tribute Concert

1981 was a quiet year for David Bowie – the first, indeed, since 1970 in which no new album was released in Britain. But while both RCA and Decca went into reissue overdrive, David successfully maintained the momentum of recent hit singles with his sole new release of the year, a one-off collaboration which was to take him once again to the top of the charts.

In July 1981 he was at Mountain Studios in Montreux, recording 'Cat People (Putting Out Fire)' with Giorgio Moroder, a single that would not be released until the following year. In the adjacent studio Queen were recording their album Hot Space. Although there were broad parallels between David Bowie and Freddie Mercury – both projected flamboyantly theatrical, sexually ambiguous personae and were justly fêted for their brilliant live acts – the two had seldom crossed paths during the 1970s. In retrospect a collaboration was both appropriate and overdue, but it came about quite spontaneously; so rapid was the process that only one song was written and recorded, initially under the title 'People On Streets'. Queen's producer David Richards, who had co-engineered "Heroes" and would go on to work with Bowie on many subsequent albums, recalled the impromptu recording as "a complete jam-session and madness in the studio."

The speed with which 'Under Pressure' was created lends the recording its vital edginess; it's not unlike Lennon and McCartney's 'A Day In The Life' in that you can tell a mile off who wrote which bits. Freddie Mercury's scat-singing intro is pure Queen, the "insanity laughs" break is unadulterated Bowie, the "give love one more chance" chorus is Queen in full stadium-anthem mode, and the final "This is our last dance" refrain steals a melodic phrase straight from Bowie's early single 'You've Got A Habit Of Leaving' ("Sometimes I cry, sometimes I'm so sad"). Throughout, the pendulum repeatedly swings between Bowie's preening art-rock and Queen's pumped-up glam. This is the track's strength: it sounds like both a duet and a duel. "To have his ego mixed with ours was a very volatile mixture," said Brian May later, recalling that Bowie was "very aloof" during the session; "It made for a very hot time in the studio." An interesting qualification of that memory is provided by Bowie's particular friend in the group, Roger Taylor, who said in 1999 that "We'd never actually collaborated with anybody before, so certain egos were slightly bruised along the way."

'Under Pressure' was mixed by Queen in New York, and opinions differed as to the final result. Roger Taylor loved the session and, despite opining that "we never actually finished the record to my satisfaction," considered 'Under Pressure' "one of the very best things Queen have ever done ... an incredibly original and unusual song." David himself later admitted that "it stands up better as a demo. It was done so quickly that some of it makes me cringe a bit."

Neither party was initially convinced that 'Under Pressure' should even be released, but the recording was immediately embraced by Queen's label EMI, who were convinced it was a sure-fire hit. It wouldn't have taken a genius to deduce that a single featuring both Bowie and Queen, each boasting a separate constituency of loyal followers, would guarantee massive combined sales. As no other viable collaborative tracks had been recorded during the session (save Bowie's abandoned backing vocals for 'Cool Cat'), Queen's 'Soul Brother' was selected as the B-side, and as a result Queen were given first billing on the single as a whole.

Neither Queen nor Bowie felt inclined to promote the single, and instead Bowie's favoured director David Mallet was given free rein to create a video in which neither party would appear. Mallet concocted a tumbling bricolage of images culled from newsreel footage and silent movies: Greta Garbo, John Gilbert and Nosferatu intercut with images of mass unemployment, tower-blocks collapsing, poverty-stricken slums and the Wall Street Crash. Mallet's use of silent movie footage prefigured the superb *Metropolis*-based 'Radio Ga Ga' promo he made with Queen three years later, by which time he had become, on Bowie's recommendation, their director of choice.

The BBC promptly banned the 'Under Pressure' video because it included scenes of IRA bombings in Belfast, but in Britain at least there was little need for a video to ensure the single's success. Released in November, 'Under Pressure' entered the chart at number 8 and knocked the Police's 'Every Little Thing She Does Is Magic' off the top spot the following week, remaining at number 1 for a fortnight. In America the single reached a more modest 29, nonetheless Bowie's best US placing since 'Golden Years' six years earlier. Queen's immense popularity in South America led to chart dominance in several countries including Argentina, where 'Under Pressure' remained at number 1 throughout the Falklands War in the spring of 1982. The Argentine leader General Galtieri, whose grasp of the time-scale involved was evidently less vivid than his imagination, publicly denounced 'Under Pressure' as a piece of British propaganda cooked up for the occasion.

The recording of 'Under Pressure' gave Bowie the opportunity to discuss his career with Freddie Mercury, whose artistic and financial freedoms with EMI entranced him. An engineer at the Montreux session tells Christopher Sandford that "David was all over him for details ... David had reached the end of his rope with his label." Although Bowie's next few singles would fall under RCA's jurisdiction, the writing was on the wall. He was more than happy for 'Under Pressure' to be released by Queen's label (and later on *Hot Space*, released in May 1982), and in 1983 he would sign to EMI himself.

Queen performed 'Under Pressure' live throughout the remainder of their career, but Bowie would not return to the song until ten years later, when he performed it as a duet with Annie Lennox at the Freddie Mercury Tribute concert on 20 April 1992. 'Under Pressure' was revived for the Outside, Earthling, summer 2000 and A Reality tours, with bassist Gail Ann Dorsey brilliantly taking over the Mercury/Lennox part. "Queen is my favourite band of all time," she revealed in 1998, "and I remember being so overwhelmed at David's suggestion that I cried. To sing a part originally sung by Freddie Mercury so far has

been the greatest honour of my life." A live version recorded on 13 December 1995 (and mixed, appropriately enough, at Mountain Studios), was included on the 'Hallo Spaceboy' CD single.

Lest we forget, the distinctive bass and piano line of 'Under Pressure' were viciously sampled by Vanilla Ice for his chart-busting masterpiece 'Ice Ice Baby', which spent four weeks at number 1 in 1990. Eight years later, Roger Taylor raised the spectre of the song once again with his solo single 'Pressure On', which featured a B-side called 'People On Streets'. Also in 1998, the original cut featured in the movie soundtracks *Stepmom* and *Grosse Pointe Blank*. 'Under Pressure' later featured in the Queen-based stage musical *We Will Rock You*, which opened at London's Dominion Theatre in May 2002.

Since its original release 'Under Pressure' has reappeared in a baffling variety of remixes, although most are practically identical and will be of interest only to the most rabid collector. The original 4'09" single/*Hot Space* version was reissued on a 3" CD single in 1988, whereas the version that appears on Bowie's UK *Singles Collection*, *Best Of Bowie* and *Queen Greatest Hits 2* is a marginally shorter 3'58" edit. Meanwhile *Classic Queen*, the 1995 reissue of *Let's Dance*, and the US compilation *The Singles 1969-1993* all feature a 4'01" remix. December 1999 saw the release of the superfluous 'Rah Mix' single from the "Queen +" album *Greatest Hits III*, taking 'Under Pressure' back into the top 20. The video, by Queen favourites the Torpedo Twins, was of greater interest than the remix, blending footage of Freddie Mercury at Wembley in 1986 with shots of Bowie's performance at the tribute concert to create the illusion that they are performing together. The second CD single's enhanced material included the video and behind-the-scenes footage of its creation.

UNDER THE GOD
• Album: *TM* • A-Side: 6/89 [51] • Live: *Oy* • Live Video: *Oy*

Tin Machine's first single is one of the more conventional tracks from their debut album. Driven by pelting drums and furious garage guitars flagrantly cannibalizing the sub-Stones riff of Bowie's *Pin Ups* cover 'I Wish You Would', it's an efficient but unsophisticated return to the basics of Americanized rock. The lyric is Tin Machine in a nutshell: an unambiguous all-out offensive on the international rise of neo-Fascist politics during the late 1980s. Just as 'Crack City' over-throws the drug subtext of Bowie's 1970s work, so 'Under The God' can be read as as a final exorcism of the Thin White Duke's flirtation with the far right ("Fascist flare is fashion cool"). In 1989 Bowie told *Melody Maker* that the intention was the same as that of 'Crack City': "I wanted something that had the same simplistic, naïve, radical, laying it down about the emergence of a new Nazi so that people could not mistake what the song was about."

Although propelled by Julien Temple's ferocious "performance" video, featuring Tin Machine sur-rounded by a caged mob of rioters, 'Under The God' failed to crack the UK top 50. In America, like every Tin Machine single, it failed to chart at all. The poor showing can partly be attributed to the fact that, despite being the debut single and identical to the album edit, it was foolishly released *after* the album and with no exclusive tracks – save for a 12-minute interview on the extended formats, originally broad-cast on New York's DIR radio show *The World Of Rock*. As well as the CD and 12" singles, a 10" version appeared in some territories. 'Under The God' was performed live on both Tin Machine tours.

UNDERGROUND

• A-Side: 6/86 [21] • Soundtrack: *Labyrinth* •
Compilation: *Best Of Bowie (New Zealand)* • Video:
Collection, Best Of Bowie

Following the 1950s synthesis of 'Absolute Beginners', Bowie's theme song for *Labyrinth* was an unexpected foray into gospel music. "The film essentially deals with a girl's emotions and what she's going through, discovering about herself and her parents and her relationship to her family," he explained at the time, "so I wanted something very emotional, and for me the most emotional music I can think of is gospel."

For 'Underground' Bowie was joined by a 14-strong troupe of backing vocalists who not only reunited him with his *Young Americans* collaborator Luther Vandross, but also included Chaka Khan, Chic's Fonzi Thornton (later to reappear on *Black Tie White Noise*) and the Radio Choir of the New Hope Baptist Church. Lead guitar was taken by veteran bluesman Albert Collins. "I really wanted a guitar player who wasn't used to a studio approach," said David, "and Albert works mainly live gigs, but he's got a history of nearly fifty years of blues playing."

Collins's contribution was described by David as "a very savage, rough, aggressive sound which goes against some of the maybe superficial slickness of the synthesizers."

With Collins providing a gutsy top layer to a bar-rage of programmed keyboards and Hammond organs, 'Underground' is a blast of exuberant fun, making it the second in a trio of really excellent 1986 film themes which stole the march on Bowie's album-based work of the period. Despite being written for a Muppet movie, the lyric can quite feasibly be inter-preted as one of Bowie's withdrawal-and-alienation classics in the tradition of 'All The Madmen' or 'Sound And Vision'. There's an emotive depth to the "lost and lonely" scenario ("no-one can blame you for walking away..."), and Bowie's theatrical yell of "Daddy, daddy, get me out of here!" resonates back across his early songwriting.

The soundtrack album features two versions: the full closing theme and the re-scored opening title on which Bowie also sings. The remixed single failed to repeat the success of 'Absolute Beginners', heralding a long run of disappointing UK chart performances – Bowie wouldn't go top ten again until 'Jump They Say' in 1993. It's interesting to note, however, that three years later an almost actionable facsimile of the gun-shot percussion, synthesized basslines and gospel vocals of 'Underground' would provide Madonna with her number 1 hit 'Like A Prayer'. The single mix made its CD debut on the New Zealand edition of 2002's *Best Of Bowie*.

The video was an interesting creation directed by Bowie newcomer Steve Barron, the man behind some of the most technically brilliant clips of the period including Michael Jackson's 'Billie Jean' and A-ha's 'Take On Me'. Barron's videos for 'Underground' and 'As The World Falls Down' so impressed Jim Henson, who cooperated on the sequences involving the Muppet characters, that he was recruited to direct Henson's major television project *The Storyteller*. Opening as a routine performance video, 'Under-ground' takes off at the first chorus as Bowie melts through the floor amid a fusillade of flash-frame images of his past selves: Ziggy Stardust, the Thin White Duke and Baal all put in appearances, as do shots from *The Man Who Fell To Earth*, *Just A Gigolo*, *Into The Night*, the sleeve artwork of *Diamond Dogs* and many others. As he is transformed into a cartoon fig-ure, the lines in Bowie's animated forehead become the convolutions of Jareth's labyrinth, wherein we find him dancing with the Muppet characters while the film's "helping hands" mime to the gospel backing vocals. At the climax Bowie rips away his real face to become a cartoon for ever. Although he would later dismiss 'Underground' as "just not my kind of video," it offers a satisfying continuity with the mask-wearing that runs through his work from its earliest days.

UNTITLED NO.1

• Album: *Buddha*

This brilliantly unusual number marries a shuffling dance beat with an Eastern melody, synthesized mandolins and obscure vocals. The result is suggestive of a disco-friendly 'Subterraneans' and is clearly indebted to 'No One Receiving' from Brian Eno's 1977 album *Before And After Science* (or, in the Bowie chronology, before *Lodger* and after *"Heroes"*). Bowie sings "It's clear that some things never change," and sure enough his phased vocals and closing "Ooohs" sound – no doubt deliberately – like Brett Anderson impersonating Marc Bolan. Like much of its parent album, this is a really fine Bowie song awaiting discovery.

UNWASHED AND SOMEWHAT SLIGHTLY DAZED

• Album: *Oddity* • Live: *Beeb*

This long and ferocious track is one of several *Space Oddity* numbers smacking of a Dylanesque world of peaceniks, hippies and protest songs. It features some of Bowie's most striking early lyrics and a blistering harmonica solo from Benny Marshall, lead singer with Hull-based outfit The Rats. Tony Visconti invited Marshall to make his contribution when he was brought along to Trident one day by drummer John Cambridge, himself a former Rat. Over the next year Bowie's destiny would become inextricably entwined with other members of the band.

In style and content 'Unwashed And Somewhat Slightly Dazed' anticipates the studies in alienation and madness to be found on Bowie's next two albums, seething with the most violent imagery yet encountered in his songwriting. It's a splenetic diatribe in which "my tissue is rotting and the rats chew my bones" while "my head's full of murders". The targets of his bile seem to be the symbols of capitalism and privilege scattered through the song – bankers,

credit cards, expensive Braque paintings and the porcelain toilet bowl in the many-floored "father's house". As with most of Bowie's songs of the period, the lyric has prompted specific readings. Some have interpreted it as an account of a bad trip, contrasting the sublimity of the potential heroin reading of 'Space Oddity' with a hallucinatory "brainstorm" and a graphic vomiting scene.

At the time, however, Bowie offered some clues of his own. His father Haywood Jones had passed away during the *Space Oddity* sessions, and in November 1969 David told George Tremlett that "'Unwashed And Somewhat Slightly Dazed' describes how I felt in the weeks after my father died." Much of the lyric, though, seems more concerned with a boy racked by insecurity about how he is perceived by his upper-class girlfriend, which inevitably steers thoughts once again in the direction of Hermione Farthingale, the muse of two other *Space Oddity* compositions. Several witnesses have told biographers that class difference was a source of some friction in the relationship, and in October 1969 Bowie told *Disc & Music Echo* that 'Unwashed And Somewhat Slightly Dazed' was "a rather weird little song I wrote because one day when I was very scruffy I got a lot of funny stares from people in the street. The lyrics are what you hear – about a boy whose girlfriend thinks he is socially inferior. I thought it was rather funny really." Although this explanation doesn't rule out the subject of his father's death, it's certainly at variance with what he told Tremlett only three weeks later, offering a salutary early instance of the hazards inherent in taking Bowie's analyses of his own songs at face value and to the exclusion of other readings.

Four minutes into the track comes an impersonation of Marc Bolan's famous vibrato bleat, a trick repeated on the next album's not dissimilar 'Black Country Rock'. Rumours that the original American album featured an extended version of 'Unwashed And Somewhat Slightly Dazed' are unfounded, arising from the fact that the track was segued with 'Don't Sit Down' on the sleeve notes. A new recording was included in the BBC session taped on 20 October 1969, while a third, splendidly energetic and Ronson-enhanced, appeared in the concert set taped on 5 February 1970. This last version now appears on *Bowie At The Beeb*.

UP THE HILL BACKWARDS
• Album: *Scary* • A-Side: 3/81 [32] • Live Video: *Glass*

The superb 'Up The Hill Backwards' is one of the more uncompromising *Scary Monsters* tracks, and when RCA chose to release it as an unlikely fourth single its combination of group singing, screeching guitar and tricksy Bo Diddley rhythms unsurprisingly failed to ignite the chart.

The song was originally called 'Cameras In Brooklyn' and boasted an entirely different set of lyrics. It's always risky to over-interpret Bowie's writing, but 'Up The Hill Backwards' appears to address the simultaneous emotions thrown up by private developments and intrusive press scrutiny in the aftermath of his messy and public divorce, which became absolute a week before the *Scary Monsters* sessions began. Hence, perhaps, the musing on "the vacuum created by the arrival of freedom, and the possibilities it seems to offer", the repeated refrain of "it's got nothing to do with you", the bleak observation that "we're legally crippled, it's the death of love", and the notion that the participants in the song are "more idols than realities". This would certainly make sense of the ironic misquotation of Thomas Harris's 1967 self-help book *I'm OK – You're OK*, a fashionable American bestseller which applied the "transactional analysis" theory to marriage relationships.

A fascinating 3'21" demo has appeared on bootlegs, featuring a funky bass playout, a softer, close-to-the-mike lead vocal and slightly different lyrics ("skylights are falling" instead of "witnesses falling"); it also lacks the discordant Robert Fripp guitar swoops which dominate the finished version. Although the full song has never been included in a live set, extracts were lip-synched by Bowie's dance troupe during the prolonged build-up to his big entrance at the beginning of the Glass Spider show.

V-2 SCHNEIDER
• Album: *"Heroes"* • B-Side: 9/77 [24] • B-Side: 8/97

The opening track on side two of *"Heroes"* is whipped into life by some superb drumming from Dennis Davis and one of Bowie's most accomplished saxophone performances. During recording he accidentally began playing his sax off the beat, but duly submitted to a prior instruction on one of Brian Eno's "Oblique Strategies" cards to "Honour thy errors for

their hidden intentions". The vocoder-style phasing of the vocal line was achieved on what Tony Visconti described as "a cheap little synthesizer in the studio" which provided the vowel sounds only ("ee-oo-i-er"), while David's voice was recorded through an electronic filter to isolate the consonants ("v-t-schn-d"). According to Visconti, "it kind of worked, although one reviewer at the time sussed that this was the way we really did it!"

The title refers to Kraftwerk founder member Florian Schneider, whose impact on Bowie's work is jokingly compared with that of a V-2 rocket. "We just put the two words together," said Visconti later, insisting that the title was meaningless.

'V-2 Schneider' received its first live performance twenty years later during the Earthling tour, becoming the object of much stylistic experimentation as the dates progressed. A limited edition 12" vinyl release credited to "Tao Jones Index" (the name under which the Earthling band advertised secret gigs) featured an excellent live version recorded in Amsterdam on 10 June 1997. In the same year Philip Glass adapted 'V-2 Schneider' as the final movement of his *"Heroes" Symphony*.

VARIOUS TIMES OF DAY :
see **ERNIE JOHNSON**

VELVET COUCH *(Bowie/Cale)* : see **PIANOLA**

VELVET GOLDMINE
• B-Side: 9/75 [1] • Bonus: *Ziggy, Ziggy (2002)*

This superb and undervalued *Ziggy Stardust* out-take was recorded at Trident on 11 November 1971. It's an interesting hybrid; the tight, electric Spiders sound and the quickfire lyric inhabit the same lip-smacking territory as 'Sweet Head', but there's half an eye still on the piano-led clapalongs and exuberant backing vocals of *Hunky Dory*. The title bears further witness to Bowie's preoccupation with a certain Lou Reed-fronted group. Originally titled 'He's a Goldmine', it was slated for side two of *Ziggy Stardust* as late as 15 December 1971. The following month Bowie mentioned its removal in a radio interview, describing it as "a lovely tune, but probably a little provocative."

'Velvet Goldmine' remained unreleased until

1975's reissue of the 'Space Oddity' single, when it was mixed by RCA without consultation. "The whole thing came out without my having the chance to listen to the mix," Bowie remarked later. "Somebody else had mixed it – an extraordinary move." Subsequently the track turned up on *Bowie Rare* (complete with a hilariously inaccurate set of lyrics presumably scribbled down by someone at RCA after a couple of listens), before appearing on both the 1990 and 2002 *Ziggy Stardust* reissues. 'Velvet Goldmine' also gave its name to Todd Haynes's 1998 film (see Chapter 9).

VICIOUS *(Reed)*

Co-produced by Bowie for Lou Reed's *Transformer*. Like two other songs on the album, 'Vicious' was originally drafted in 1968 for an aborted Broadway musical to be co-produced by Andy Warhol and Yves Saint Laurent. "Andy said, 'Why don't you write a song called 'Vicious'?" recalled Reed. "I said, 'Well, Andy, what kind of vicious?' 'Oh, you know, like I hit you with a flower.' And I wrote it down, literally. Because I kept a notebook in those days."

VIDEO CRIME *(Bowie/T.Sales/H.Sales)*
• Album: *TM*

This track is referred to as 'Video Crimes' on the sleeve of *Tin Machine*, but remains in the singular on the disc and lyric sheet. It's a none-too-subtle broadside against the desensitizing effect of video nasties, including the immortal line "Late-night cannibal, cripples decay / Just can't tear my eyes away." The rest of the lyric is equally rough-hewn, but does at least contain a passable pun ("I've got dollars, I've got sense"). Bowie's numbed Berlin-era vocal goes some way toward rescuing the unpromising material, and the relentless robotic march and pseudo-'Fame' rhythm guitar are not without potential, but as usual the whole thing is swamped by an unremitting onslaught of drums and guitars.

An excerpt of 'Video Crime' was included in Julien Temple's 1989 Tin Machine film, set to the unsightly spectacle of women boxers slugging it out in a ring. It's the only track on the first Tin Machine album never to have been performed live.

VOLARE (NEL BLU DIPINTO DI BLU)
(Modugno/Migliacci)
• Soundtrack: *Absolute Beginners*

The coffee-bar culture of 1958 London commemorated in *Absolute Beginners* was played out against a soundtrack not just of rock'n'roll but also of Italian be-bop, one of the year's popular fads. The star attraction was a song called 'Volare' ("to fly") which became a hit phenomenon, charting in no fewer than four different versions during the autumn. The original, by Domenico Modugno, had been Italy's entry in that year's Eurovision Song Contest, but the most successful of the chart versions was by Dean Martin, who took it to number 2.

'Volare' was among the memories of 1958 Bowie recalled during the *Absolute Beginners* shoot, and the re-recording was apparently his suggestion: his character hums along to the song as it plays on the car radio. It's an affectionate recreation, and is therefore a piece of "easy listening" that will have many fans fleeing for the hills in terror and confusion. Once more Bowie proves himself something other than a conventional rocker: he's also a superb *pasticheur*.

The track marks Bowie's first credited collaboration with multi-instrumentalist Erdal Kizilcay, who had worked on pre-production for *Let's Dance* and was soon to become a full-time sessioner and tour musician. During Tin Machine's It's My Life tour several years later, David occasionally sang a few lines from 'Volare' during the extended rendition of 'Heaven's In Here'. Trivia buffs will be pleased to know that 'Volare' is one of the 'Reasons To Be Cheerful (Pt 3)' rattled off by the much-missed Ian Dury in his brilliant 1979 hit.

THE VOYEUR OF UTTER DESTRUCTION (AS BEAUTY) *(Bowie/Eno/Gabrels)*
• Album: *1.Outside* • Live: *liveandwell.com*

As if its unashamedly preposterous title weren't enough, this track finds Bowie singing in the guise of "the Artist/Minotaur", the ghostly figure lurking behind *1.Outside*'s murder-for-art's-sake. But the context matters little, because 'The Voyeur' is an accomplished piece of speeding ambient funk straight from the *Lodger* era ('Look Back In Anger' and 'Red Sails' spring immediately to mind) overlaid by Mike Garson's dissonant piano. Carlos Alomar's insistent rhythm figure and Bowie's "Turn and turn again" underscoring stress the album's cyclical time-frame. The Minotaur appears to get a spiritual/sexual kick from his victims' plight, unleashing some of the most ghoulish images on the album: "The screw is a tightening atrocity / I shake, for the reeking flesh is as romantic as hell."

Plans to release a Tim Simenon remix single in 1995 were dropped, but the song became one of the most successful live recreations for the Outside and Earthling tours, also featuring at Bowie's fiftieth birthday concert. He described it as "fairly hard-nosed and not the most commercial of pieces," and delighted in being able to perform it for various television shows including Channel 4's *The White Room* in December 1995. A version recorded in Rio de Janeiro on 2 November 1997 later appeared on *liveandwell.com*.

WAGON WHEEL *(Reed)*

Co-produced by Bowie for Lou Reed's *Transformer*, this track is grounded in the classic Velvet Underground riff Bowie had already plundered for 'Queen Bitch' and 'Suffragette City'. It has long been rumoured that 'Wagon Wheel' was co-written by David, but there is no proof of this.

WAITING FOR THE MAN *(Reed)*
• Live: *SM72, BBC, Beeb* • B-Side: 4/94

When Bowie first heard Kenneth Pitt's acetate of the then unreleased *The Velvet Underground And Nico* in December 1966, the song that clearly besotted him the most was Lou Reed's classic snapshot of a seedy Harlem heroin score, which would go on to become one of his perennial cover versions. "I literally went into a band rehearsal the next day, put the album down and said, 'We're gonna learn this song,'" David later recalled. "We learned 'Waiting For The Man' right then and there, and we were playing it on stage within a week." In a 2003 article for *Vanity Fair* he added, "In December of that year, my band Buzz broke up, but not without my demanding we play 'Waiting For The Man' as one of the encore songs at our last gig. Amusingly, not only was I to cover a Velvets song before anyone else in the world, I actually did it before the album came out. Now that's the essence of Mod."

Bowie's first studio stab at 'Waiting For The Man' was recorded the same month during the *David Bowie*

sessions: taken at a rather sedate pace and featuring sax and harmonica breaks alongside David's slavish impersonation of Lou Reed, this endearing 4'04" take has surfaced on bootlegs.

Although Bowie has never cut an "official" studio version, four further recordings were made during BBC sessions on 5 February and 25 March 1970, and 11 and 18 January 1972. The earliest of these was edited from *The Sunday Show* before broadcast, and is now believed to be lost forever. The second, recorded by Hype with a rougher hard-rock edge than The Spiders' later versions, was released on the *BBC Sessions 1969-1972* sampler, while the last, a tighter rendition and perhaps the best of the bunch, now appears on *Bowie At The Beeb*.

'Waiting For The Man' made regular live appearances during the 1972 Ziggy Stardust tour, most memorably as a duet with Lou Reed at the Royal Festival Hall on 8 July. The *Santa Monica '72* version appeared as a B-side in 1994, and again on the soundtrack of Cameron Crowe's 2000 film *Almost Famous*. The song reappeared on the Station To Station and Sound + Vision tours, and made a one-off appearance in Vancouver during Tin Machine's It's My Life outing. David was reunited with Reed for a splendid live duet at his fiftieth birthday concert.

WALK ON THE WILD SIDE *(Reed)*

Lou Reed's classic has its roots in a proposed US theatre adaptation of Nelson Algren's 1956 novel *A Walk On The Wild Side*, a searing portrayal of heroin addiction and prostitution. Reed had been asked to compose the music, and although the project was cancelled in 1971 it sowed the germ of Reed's sharpshooting portrait of the characters who passed through Andy Warhol's Factory. "I always thought it would be kinda fun to introduce people to characters they maybe hadn't met before, or hadn't wanted to meet, y'know," he said. "The kind of people you sometimes see at parties but don't dare approach. That's one of the motivations for me writing all those songs in the first place." Thus 'Walk On The Wild Side' acquaints us with a colourful parade of Warhol's "superstars" – Holly Woodlawn, Candy Darling, Joe Dallesandro, the Sugar Plum Fairy and Jackie Curtis.

Co-produced by Bowie, the *Transformer* track is equally renowned for Herbie Flowers's laid-back bassline and for one of pop's all-time great saxophone solos. This was provided by Bowie's former tutor Ronnie Ross, who had never heard of Lou Reed and had no idea that the red-haired rock star who had hired him was the same David Jones who had come for lessons at his Orpington home twelve years earlier. The penny dropped only when David emerged from the control room after Ross had recorded his solo. "I said, 'Hello, how have you been?'" Bowie recalled in 2003. "He said, 'Uh, all right, you're that Ziggy Stardust, aren't ya?' I said, 'You know me better as David Jones.' He said, 'I don't know you, son.' I said, 'See if you remember this: "Hello, I'm David Jones and my dad's helped me buy a saxophone"' – and Ronnie goes, 'My God!' That was so great that I was able to give him a gig. He had absolutely no idea that I had been that little kid who had been over to his house." Ross told the Gillmans that "He had make-up on and it didn't register at first. I was amazed."

Bowie later described 'Walk On The Wild Side' as "a classic, a wonderful song – absolutely brilliant", and it was on his insistence that the track was released as a single. Reed was opposed to the idea, convinced that the references to drugs, transvestism and "giving head" would guarantee airplay bans, and in some quarters he was right. "What kind of repressive culture would ban a song?" enquired Reed later. "There were versions in the United States that were only 14 seconds long, it'd just go 'Bleep-bleep-bleep, do-do-do-do-do-do-do, bleep-bleep-bleep'." Nevertheless the 1973 single reached number 10 in Britain and number 16 in America; in both countries it remains Reed's only major hit. "I probably never would have had a hit with 'Wild Side' if David didn't produce it," he said in 1997. "I haven't had a hit since then, so I assume it's because David produced it…"

WALKING THROUGH THAT DOOR :
see **MADMAN**

WAR (Strong/Whitfield) : see **FAME**

WARSZAWA (Bowie/Eno)
• Album: Low • Live: Stage

The first of the ambient instrumental tracks that make up Low's second side was an attempt to capture the mood of the Polish landscape Bowie had experienced when travelling through the country by train in 1976. "'Warszawa' is about Warsaw and the very bleak atmosphere I got from the city," he explained. Brian Eno's funereal synthesizers against Bowie's wailing, quasi-Gregorian nonsense-vocals conjure up a heady, almost Russian Orthodox atmosphere.

The genesis of 'Warszawa' is usually attributed to Brian Eno, who often worked alone at the Château d'Hérouville during the Low sessions. "When he was finished making his 'sonic bed' David and I came back to do our bits," Tony Visconti explained. One day while Bowie and Visconti were attending a meeting in Paris regarding David's split from his manager Michael Lippman, Eno remained at the studio to look after Visconti's four-year-old son Delaney. Visconti later learned that Delaney had been "playing the notes A, B, C, repeatedly on the piano. Eno sat next to him and finished the phrase which became the opening notes of 'Warszawa'."

The completed track was achieved via a musical equivalent of the lyrical cut-up technique Bowie had been using for years. He told Brian Eno that he wanted to compose an "emotive, almost religious" instrumental piece; Eno suggested that they begin by recording a track of finger clicks. "He laid down I think it was 430 clicks on a clean tape," Bowie explained, after which he and Eno divided the result into arbitrary portions, changing chords at the dividing lines to create a random and unpredictable backing.

As was the case throughout Low, the vocals were recorded after all but Bowie and Visconti had departed; Brian Eno would later express surprise at discovering that Bowie had elected to add voices to 'Warszawa'. According to Tony Visconti, the vocal performance was inspired by "an old recording of a boys' choir from one of the Balkan countries" which Bowie had discovered. "To make him sound like a boy I slowed the tape down about three semitones and he sang his part slowly. Once it was back up to speed he sounded about eleven years old!"

'Warszawa' was performed live throughout the Stage tour. It made a one-off reappearance courtesy of Mike Garson on Dutch TV's Karel in February 1996, before being revived once again for the 2002 Heathen concerts. The Low version featured briefly in 1984's Jazzin' For Blue Jean, while Philip Glass adapted the composition as the final movement of his 1993 Low Symphony. Nina Hagen recorded a cover of 'Warszawa' on her 1987 album Love, and avant-garde saxophonist Simon Haram included a version on his 1999 album

Alone…. Joy Division, fronted by big-time Bowie fan Ian Curtis, were at one stage called Warsaw in honour of Bowie's track; they also included a song called 'Warsaw' on their 1978 debut EP *An Ideal For Living*.

WATCH THAT MAN
• Album: *Aladdin* • Live: *David, Motion* • Live Video: *Ziggy*

Written in New York during the 1972 tour, 'Watch That Man' is as different an album-opener from the Home Counties apocalypse of 'Five Years' as it's possible to imagine. It's a sleazy garage rocker owing a debt to The Rolling Stones' 'Brown Sugar', but the most startling change since *Ziggy Stardust* is the ascendancy of Mick Ronson's storming guitar over Bowie's vocal, which apes the style of *Exile On Main Street* by lying so low in the mix as to be barely audible. Bowie was consciously chasing a rawer, Stones-influenced sound to shake off the tightly-produced Bolanisms of the *Ziggy* album; Ken Scott has confirmed that RCA initially asked him to remix the track with a more up-front vocal, before changing their minds and going with the original. Although outclassed by other songs on the album, 'Watch That Man' can be read as one of Bowie's most calculated changes of direction.

In 1973 Bowie said that the lyric was an attempt "to pinpoint and exaggerate the incident" of an after-show bash he had attended the previous autumn, when his initiation into the drug-addled rock'n'roll Babylon of his first American tour had overwhelmed him with the notion that civilization was collapsing. Such a despondent view of American society makes it an ideal opening gambit for *Aladdin Sane*. The Velvet Underground-style figure of the "Man" who is "only taking care of the room" may indeed be the archetypal supplier, coke-spoon in hand, while the panic-attack at the song's climax ("I was shaking like a leaf, for I couldn't understand the conversation / Yeah, I ran into the street") might describe the classic bad trip of the drugs novice. Some have opined that the song is a paean to Mick Jagger, while another theory has it that 'Watch That Man' commemorates David Johansen's performance at a New York Dolls gig at the Mercer Arts Center in October 1972.

'Watch That Man' featured in 1973's Ziggy Stardust dates and on the Diamond Dogs tour. January 1974 saw the release of Lulu's Bowie-produced cover version, recorded back-to-back with 'The Man Who Sold

The World' (of which it was the B-side) and again featuring David on backing vocals and Mick Ronson on guitar. This recording later appeared on *David Bowie Songbook*.

WATERLOO SUNSET *(Davies)*
• Download: 11/03 • Bonus: *Reality (Tour Edition)* • Japanese B-Side: 3/04

At the Tibet House Benefit concert on 28 February 2003, Bowie joined the legendary Ray Davies for a duet of The Kinks' much-covered 1967 hit. Following this collaboration Bowie found time during the *Reality* sessions to record his own studio version of 'Waterloo Sunset', which was released as the B-side of the 'Never Get Old' cyber-single, and as a bonus track on the 'Tour Edition' of *Reality*. It may not be the most radical recording of Bowie's career, but it's a faithful, affectionate cover of an eternally wonderful song.

WATERMELON MAN *(Hancock)*

The Herbie Hancock blues classic was played live by The Manish Boys.

WE ALL GO THROUGH *(Bowie/Gabrels)*
• B-Side: 9/99 [16]

Described by Bowie as a "faux-psychedelic chanting drone", this B-side (a bonus track on the Japanese release of *'hours…'*) resurrects the minor-key melodies and tricksy chord changes of Tin Machine numbers 'Amlapura' and 'Betty Wrong', setting the ghosts of both in a 'Thursday's Child' instrumental backing. Guitarist Reeves Gabrels later claimed that the composition began life as an instrumental track intended for his 1999 album *Ulysses (della notte)*. The lyric revisits Bowie's sci-fi cut-ups with its "skeletal city" and "lunarscape", but returns to the parent album's embrace of the present, insisting that "we'll all be right in the now". A so-called "easy listening" version, which seems to be identical to the B-side recording, appears in *Omikron: The Nomad Soul*.

WE ARE HUNGRY MEN
• Album: *Bowie*

Originally entitled 'We Are Not Your Friends', this number has been subjected to particular scrutiny owing to its embryonic dabbling in soon-to-be familiar themes of Messiah-worship and Orwellian totalitarianism. The theme is the rise of a dictatorship prepared to take drastic steps to combat overpopulation, but despite some lively lyrics juxtaposing serio-comic extremes of ideology and gratification ("Who will buy a drink for me, your Messiah?"), this is in truth a rather conservative-minded piece of juvenilia: the interjections of a comic-book Nazi and a Kenneth Williams soundalike are more knockabout than chilling, while the implicit suggestion that abortion is some sort of nameless sci-fi horror betrays the suburban values that were still informing Bowie's songwriting at this stage. The track was recorded on 24 November 1966, and omitted from *David Bowie*'s American release.

WE ARE THE DEAD
• Album: *Dogs* • B-Side: 4/76 [33]

Perhaps because it's the only *Diamond Dogs* track never to have been performed live, 'We Are The Dead' remains one of the most criminally underrated songs in the entire Bowie canon. Belonging to the album's original conception as a musical *Nineteen Eighty-Four*, the lyric eavesdrops on Winston Smith's doomed love for Julia. In Orwell's novel the lovers repeat "We are the dead" to one another as the Thought Police approach to arrest Winston, but like all Bowie's best work the song transcends its original source to provoke other, less tangible resonances. When David whispers "I hear them on the stairs" we are reminded not only of Orwell ("There was a stampede of boots up the stairs"), but of 'The Man Who Sold The World' ("We passed upon the stair").

The lyric occupies the same brutalized territory as 'Sweet Thing', moving from one ravaged tableau to the next and offering the album's most sinisterly evocative phrases: "Heaven is on the pillow, its silence competes with hell … It's the theatre of financiers – count them, fifteen round the table, white and dressed to kill…" The hushed tread of the electric keyboard, the roaming guitar feedback and the melodramatic multi-track vocal establish a nightmarish environment that is

right at the heart of *Diamond Dogs* – which at one point was to be called *We Are The Dead*.

The track was later included on the 'TVC15' single as part of RCA's mid-1970s policy of short-changing fans with ancient B-sides. Cover versions have been recorded by a number of bands, including Psychotics and The Passion Puppets.

WE PRICK YOU *(Bowie/Eno)*
• Album: *1.Outside*

Recorded in January 1995, 'We Prick You' offers early evidence of Bowie's dabbling in drum'n'bass styles, although it's still a far cry from the Prodigy-style squall of 'Little Wonder'. Instead the track is loaded with extraordinary buzzes and bleeps from the Eno camp while Bowie throws in an edgy, rhythmically slapstick vocal apparently "to be sung by members of the Court of Justice". This is a track that uses words as rhythmic and sonic information rather than as mere lyrics; Bowie described the result as "dotty". There's an air of sexual desperation in the face of impending apocalypse ("Wanna be screwing when the nightmare comes … wanna come quick then die"), and a hectoring, shouted chorus reminiscent of the trial climax of Pink Floyd's *The Wall*. According to Brian Eno's diary the original refrain was "we fuck you", while the track's working title was 'Robot Punk'. Eno also praises Carlos Alomar's "amazing contribution. He plays like a kind of liquid – always making lovely melodies within his rhythm lines, and rhythms within his melody lines."

The treated loop of Bowie snapping "You show respect, even if you disagree" was originally intended to be a sample of Camille Paglia. "She never returned my calls!" laughed Bowie. "She kept sending messages through her assistant saying, 'Is this really David Bowie, and if it is, is it important?' and I just gave up! So I replaced her line with me." Brian Eno added, "Sounds pretty much like her." The song was performed on the Outside tour.

WE SHALL GO TO TOWN *(Bowie/Gabrels)*
• B-Side: 9/99 [16]

Funereal rhythms, phased vocal effects and programmed synthesizers herald another Berlin-era pastiche from the *'hours…'* sessions. The lyric reiterates the album's banishment of past regret ("Never forget who you've been," advises David, but "Don't bring your things ... only the fool turns around"). Presumably owing to confusion with 'We All Go Through', the track was incorrectly labelled 'We Shall All Go To Town' on the 'Thursday's Child' CD sleeve.

WE'LL CREEP TOGETHER
(Bowie/Eno/Gabrels/Garson/Kizilcay/Campbell)

The Electronic Press Kit issued in advance of *1.Outside* includes footage of Bowie and Brian Eno improvising this suitably nonsensical piece (the title is by no means official), which begins with David addressing an imaginary concert audience in a style recalling the opening of 'Diamond Dogs', only this time in the character of an over-precious ham, adopting a plummy accent to declare "We are surely on our way upon the superhighway of information – as far as I'm concerned you are all number one packet-sniffers!" He then sings a short passage ("We'll creep together, you and I / Under a bloodless chrome sky") over a moody synthesizer backing not unlike some of the 'Segue' accompaniments on the album.

A full-length, five-minute version of 'We'll Creep Together', which reveals the number to be a genuinely beautiful song, was among the tracks leaked onto the Internet by a private collector in 2003 (see 'The *Leon* Tape' for further details).

THE WEDDING
• Album: *Black*

On 24 April 1992, David Bowie and Iman Abdulmajid were married in a private ceremony at Lausanne's city hall. A little over a month later, on 6 June, the wedding was solemnized at St James's Episcopal Church in Florence. Exclusive access to the ceremony was enjoyed by *Hello!* magazine, which ran a lavish 24-page feature capturing the world's most photogenic bride and groom alongside best man Joe (who had celebrated his twenty-first birthday with his father in Mustique the previous week) and guests including David's 78-year-old mother Peggy, Iman's family, Yoko Ono, Brian Eno, Bono and Eric Idle (who later remarked, "There's a gag waiting to happen – Eno, Ono and Bono..."). Childhood friend and sometime backing vocalist Geoff McCormack read

Psalm 121 during the service.

As the families were of different religious backgrounds, and as neither David nor Iman, though believers, practised any orthodox faith, it was decided that the music for the ceremony should be nonsectarian. "We both loathed 'Here Comes The Bride', which is one of the least likeable bits of music that I have ever heard in my life," explained Bowie. "So for the entrance of the bride we chose a tranquil piece of music called 'Evening Gathering', by a Bulgarian group. And I wanted it to be a personalized service, so Iman allowed me to take the lead and write music for the rest of the service – which I did."

The result, intended to combine David's own cultural and spiritual sensibilities with those of his bride's native Somalia, was an instrumental composition later reworked in funkier form as the opening track of *Black Tie White Noise*. 'The Wedding' fuses dance beats, distant backing vocals and Eastern-influenced saxophone cadences to create a sure-footed template for the album. "I had to write music that represented for me the growth and character of our relationship," David told *Rolling Stone*. "It really was a watershed. It opened up a wealth of thoughts and feelings about commitment and promises and finding the strength and fortitude to keep those promises. It all came tumbling out of me while I was writing this music for church. And I thought, 'I can't stop here. There's more that I have to get out.' For me it was a tentative step toward writing from a personal basis. It triggered the album."

WEDDING BELL BLUES *(Nyro)*

Laura Nyro's 1966 number, a hit for Fifth Dimension in 1970, was included in David's medley on CBS's *The Cher Show* in November 1975.

THE WEDDING SONG
• Album: *Black*

After the fashion of *Scary Monsters*, Bowie closes *Black Tie White Noise* with a reworking of the opening track. It's dedicated to his "angel for life" Iman, and in his own words is "every bit as saccharine as you might want it to be." The ambient backbeats of the instrumental version are topped by the touchingly simple pledge that "I'm gonna be so good, just like a good boy should" – another of the album's subliminal throwbacks to the Berlin period, echoing a line from 'Beauty And The Beast'.

WEEPING WALL

• Album: *Low*

Although some sources claim that an early version of 'Weeping Wall' was recorded at Cherokee Studios in 1975 for the aborted *The Man Who Fell To Earth* soundtrack, Bowie was adamant in 1977 that the composition featured on *Low* is "about the Berlin Wall, the misery of it." On 'Weeping Wall' Bowie plays every instrument himself, combining guitar, piano, xylophones and vibraphones in a piece indebted to the repetitious "accumulative" work of Philip Glass. The piece was realized in a similar manner to 'Warszawa', Bowie marking a tape with numbers from 1 to 160 and introducing the instrumental sequences at arbitrary points. 'Weeping Wall' made its concert debut during the complete performance of *Low* at the Roseland Ballroom warm-up show on 11 June 2002, appearing thereafter as Bowie's entrance music at the Meltdown concert a fortnight later before disappearing from the Heathen tour repertoire.

WHAT IN THE WORLD

• Album: *Low* • Live: *Stage* • Live Video: *Moonlight*

This is one of *Low*'s catchier efforts at uniting art-rock with straightforward pop, setting a wall of synthesizer bleeps against a barrage of guitar sound, distorted percussion effects and some droning backing vocals from Iggy Pop – his only *Low* credit. Marking out similar territory to 'Sound And Vision', the lyric reeks of insecurity and withdrawal ("Deep in your room, you never leave your room") and ends with another Bowie staple, the suggestion that his latest persona is finally authentic ("What you gonna be to the real me?"). The reiterated cry of "for your love" echoes the title of a 1965 hit by Bowie's sometime idols The Yardbirds.

A reggae-style reworking featured throughout the Stage and Serious Moonlight tours, and the number was later revived for some of the Outside and Heathen concerts.

WHAT KIND OF FOOL AM I? *(Newley)*

Anthony Newley's song was played live by The Buzz.

WHAT'D I SAY *(Charles)*

Ray Charles's 1959 US hit was played live by The Manish Boys.

WHAT'S GOING ON *(Gaye/Cleveland/Benson)* : see BLACK TIE WHITE NOISE

WHAT'S REALLY HAPPENING?

(Bowie/Gabrels/Grant)
• Album: *'hours…'*

In October 1998 Bowie announced that the lyrics for one of his forthcoming tracks would be completed by the winning entry in a songwriting competition. The half-finished lyric of 'What's Really Happening?' was duly posted on BowieNet, and it was revealed that the winner would receive not only a co-writing credit and a trip to New York for the recording, but also a $15,000 contract with Bowie's publishing company Bug Music. The press loved the story and devoted numerous column inches to irreverent speculation. It later transpired that among the 80,000 hopeful entrants were various members of The Cure.

On 20 January 1999 the winner was named as Alex Grant of Ohio. "Opening my initial thoughts on 'What's Really Happening?' for input on the web was a unique songwriting experience," Bowie declared in a press release. "Now, I am looking forward to the next step where I share the final formation of the cyber song with my co-writer, Alex Grant, and the web at large with a 360-degree interactive adventure." With backing tracks already laid down in Bermuda, the vocal and overdub recording took place at Looking Glass on 24 May 1999. The three-hour session, which was webcast live on BowieNet, culminated in Alex Grant joining Bowie to record backing vocals. David declared that "The most gratifying part of the evening for me was being able to encourage Alex and his pal Larry to sing on the song that he had written." He later revealed that Grant, "a born writer", was using his earnings to put himself through college on a literature course.

'What's Really Happening?' is the first of two comparatively hard-edged numbers after the softer opening tracks of 'hours...', piling layers of rock guitar over a steely vocal melody borrowed from The Supremes' 'You Keep Me Hangin' On'. The title reasserts the album's mistrust of reality and memory, while Grant's quasi-cyberpunk lyrics chime in remarkably well with the album's chronometric theme (but would David ever have written a line quite so 1970s Pink Floyd as "Hearts become outdated clocks / Ticking in your mind"?). There are further echoes of past compositions: the wailing backing vocals are straight from 'Scary Monsters', while the repeated chorus line "what tore us apart?" is recycled from the Tin Machine number 'One Shot'.

Busch for the planned German transmission of Love You Till Tuesday, but in the event 'Mit Mir In Deinem Traum' ("With Me In Your Dream", rather contrarily) was never released; the 3'51" track has since appeared on bootlegs. On 25 July 1969 David performed the number at the Malta Song Festival, and five days later it won the Best Produced Record award at the Italian Song Festival.

Two further unreleased versions have appeared on bootlegs. The first simply features a different vocal sung over the backing of Deram's 'Version 2', while the second, a shorter 3'35" version, is a wavery demo accompanied on organ, thought to have been made for the 1970 television show The Looking Glass Murders.

WHEN I LIVE MY DREAM
• Album: Bowie • Compilation: Deram • Video: Tuesday

'When I Live My Dream' became a familiar item in Bowie's early repertoire from the moment the album version was recorded on 25 February 1967. The subsequent array of different versions indicates that the song was highly regarded by both David and Kenneth Pitt, and certainly it's one of the most assured pieces of songwriting on David Bowie. There's a dark undercurrent of pain in what initially sounds like an innocuous love lyric, and the notion of Bowie dramatizing his emotions as a fiction on the silver screen ("Tell them that I've got a dream and tell them you're the starring role"), prefigures the cinematic fantasies of many later lyrics.

A second version, rearranged by Ivor Raymonde and recorded on 3 June 1967 just two days after the album's release, was proposed as a single in October following Deram's rejection of 'Let Me Sleep Beside You'; it too was turned down. This second version was subsequently used in the Love You Till Tuesday film, which remained unreleased until 1984. Both versions appear on The Deram Anthology 1966-1968.

In 1967 the composition was unsuccessfully offered to Peter, Paul and Mary, while Bowie included a new recording in his first BBC radio session on 18 December 1967. Around the same time he was regularly performing the song in Lindsay Kemp's Pierrot In Turquoise, and it was included in David's abandoned cabaret act the following year. On 29 January 1969 David recorded a German vocal translated by Lisa

WHEN I'M FIVE
• Compilation: Tuesday • Video: Tuesday

This 1968 composition is the kind of early Bowie song that divides critics, depending on how prepared they are to swallow its sugar-coated sentimentality. It takes the form of a little boy's monologue as he ponders the mysteries of the world, complete with a customary hint of mundane tragedy familiar from David's lyrics of the period: "I wonder why my Daddy cries, and how I wish that I were nearly five." The reference to "my grandfather Jones" is interesting if hardly revelatory.

A rough-and-ready demo dating from early 1968, in which David sings an octave lower than on the later version, has appeared on bootlegs. Not long afterwards 'When I'm Five' was aired in a BBC radio session recorded on 13 May 1968, which remains the only full studio recording Bowie ever made of the song. Later that year he included it in his short-lived cabaret showcase, and in 1969 the BBC version appeared in the Love You Till Tuesday film, for which David showcased his movement skills by adopting an infant physicality as he wandered among the candles on top of a giant birthday cake. A subsequent 2'22" demo made with John Hutchinson around April 1969 suggests that 'When I'm Five' was still under consideration for the Space Oddity album.

In January 1969, while David was filming Love You Till Tuesday, Kenneth Pitt's protégés The Beatstalkers released a cover of 'When I'm Five' as the B-side of their 'Little Boy' single. David had been present at the recording the previous April, but contrary to some reports he did not contribute to the track.

WHEN I'M SIXTY-FOUR *(Lennon/McCartney)*

The classic Beatles number, then only a year old, was included as a comedic sequel to 'When I'm Five' in Bowie's 1968 cabaret show.

WHEN THE BOYS COME MARCHING HOME
• European B-Side: 6/02 • B-Side: 9/02 [20] • Bonus: *Heathen (SACD)*

Released on some formats of the 'Slow Burn' and 'Everyone Says 'Hi'' singles, this out-take from the *Heathen* sessions is a slow and melodic number awash with strings, piano and plangent bass, creating a moody soundscape not unlike that of 'Slip Away'. The lyric revisits the album's themes of isolation, abandonment and disappointment, perhaps most closely echoing '5.15 The Angels Have Gone' as Bowie sings a melancholy lyric about stormy skies, foreign shores and disintegrating relationships, seemingly set against the background of soldiers bidding farewell to their loved ones as they set off to fight in a far-away war: "Making for some innocence and peace of mind, while the moon pulls up its net of souls / The sun presses down on my brave new world, but in truth I don't feel brave at all." There is a weary sense of history repeating itself while the defeated outsider looks on in despair: in an interview for the *Daily Mirror* in June 2002, Bowie pointed out that the events of recent months had demonstrated that "There's nothing to learn from history. As we've repeatedly shown, we're not willing to learn." At one point in the song David paints a melancholy self-portrait ("While I and the cobbled nag I ride stumble down another weary mile") which is strongly reminiscent of his identification with the nursery rhyme 'This Is The Way The Old Men Ride', which he mentioned at length in an interview at the time of *Heathen*'s release (see Chapter 2). This is a beautiful song, and without a doubt one of the saddest and prettiest recorded during the *Heathen* sessions.

WHEN THE CIRCUS LEFT TOWN :
see **THE DAY THE CIRCUS LEFT TOWN**

WHEN THE WIND BLOWS *(Bowie/Kizilcay)*
• A-Side: 11/86 [44] • Bonus: *Never*

The title song for Jimmy Murakami's animated feature completes Bowie's 1986 hat-trick of brilliant movie themes, this one built around a suitably ominous loop-the-loop guitar riff courtesy of co-writer Erdal Kizilcay. It's a mystery why this splendidly melodramatic number, which echoes the powerhouse style of Bowie's contemporaneous Iggy Pop collaboration *Blah-Blah-Blah*, didn't achieve greater chart success. The video, directed by Steve Barron with Murakami, superimposed Bowie's animated face and silhouette over a montage of clips from the film. It remains in obscurity, thus far omitted from video compilations, and the song itself has fared little better: to date its only reissues are on the short-lived 1995 re-release of *Never Let Me Down*, and the Chilean and German/ Swiss/Austrian editions of *Best Of Bowie*. The version used in the film itself, incidentally, is a shorter 3'05" edit.

WHERE HAVE ALL THE GOOD TIMES GONE!
(Davies)
• Album: *Pin*

Unusually among the *Pin Ups* set, 'Where Have All The Good Times Gone!' (the exclamation mark was added by Bowie on the sleeve notes) was not a chart hit in its original version. Originally a 1965 B-side for The Kinks, the song's instantly identifiable Ray Davies riff is ideal for Mick Ronson's scrunchy style, while Bowie is well suited to a domestic-disenchantment lyric of the kind so beloved of his own mid-1960s songwriting. During renditions of 'Aladdin Sane' on the 1996 Summer Festivals tour (notably at the Loreley Festival on 22 June), Gail Ann Dorsey would occasionally sing the title, while Bowie responded with a snatch of The Kinks' 'All Day And All Of The Night'.

WHERE'S THE LOO : see **ERNIE JOHNSON**

WHISTLING

The performing rights organization BMI lists this mysterious title as a Bowie composition.

WHITE LIGHT/WHITE HEAT *(Reed)*
• Live: *Motion, Beeb* • A-Side: 10/83 [46] • Live Video: *Ziggy, Moonlight, Glass*

The Velvet Underground classic, originally from their 1968 album of the same name, achieved an even greater impact on Bowie's career than 'Waiting For The Man'. It's become one of his perennial live standards, rivalling the likes of '"Heroes"' and 'Rebel Rebel' for sheer staying power in his concert repertoire. It's also the song referred to in the scrawled sleeve-notes of *Hunky Dory*, where David dedicates 'Queen Bitch' to Lou Reed with the words "Some V.U. White Light returned with thanks".

Eminently suited to The Spiders' raucous live sound, 'White Light/White Heat' was played regularly throughout the Ziggy Stardust tour, including a notable performance with Lou Reed at the Royal Festival Hall on 8 July 1972. Two studio versions were cut for BBC radio sessions on 16 and 23 May 1972; the first of these, a tight and exuberant rendition benefiting from Nicky Graham's madcap boogie-woogie piano, can now be heard on *Bowie At The Beeb*. A third version, begun during the following year's *Pin Ups* sessions but abandoned at the backing-track stage, was later resuscitated by Mick Ronson, who added his own vocal for his 1975 album *Play Don't Worry*.

In 1983 the live cut of 'White Light/White Heat' from the final Ziggy concert was released as a single to promote *Ziggy Stardust: The Motion Picture*, doubtless in an attempt to cash in on the fact that the song had just been revived for the same year's Serious Moonlight tour. Thereafter it reappeared on the Glass Spider, Sound + Vision, 1996 Summer Festivals, Earthling, Heathen and A Reality tours. Further versions featured in Bowie's Bridge School benefit set on 20 October 1996, his *ChangesNowBowie* BBC session, and at the fiftieth birthday concert, for which he was joined on guitar by Lou Reed.

WHO CAN I BE NOW?
• Bonus: *Americans*

Dropped to make way for the John Lennon collaborations, this is one of the most dramatic products of the Sigma *Young Americans* sessions, building from fragile beginnings to a majestic gospel-choir climax. The lyric is vintage Bowie, a meditation on self-identity and role-playing, and possibly a love song too: "If it's all a vast creation, putting on a face that's new / If someone has to see a role for him and me, someone might as well be you." The concluding refrain of "Now can I be real?" reflects Bowie's assertions in contemporary interviews about the unmasked authenticity of his *Young Americans* persona. 'Who Can I Be Now?' was never performed live, and although the studio recording was bootlegged during the 1980s, it was denied an official release until the album's 1991 reissue.

WHO WILL BUY? *(Bart)* : see **FAME**

THE WIDTH OF A CIRCLE
• Album: *Man* • Live: *David, Motion, SM72, Beeb* • Live Video: *Ziggy*

'The Width of a Circle' was captured in its earliest form at Bowie's BBC concert session recorded on 5 February 1970. This recording, now available on *Bowie At The Beeb*, is a shorter four-minute affair, lacking the instrumental passages and raunchy second section familiar from the album version. Another BBC session from 25 March reveals the next stage in the song's development: although not yet the epic it would become, already Mick Ronson's guitar had staked its claim on the number.

During the *Man Who Sold the World* sessions at Trident in April, the song was augmented by the addition of what Tony Visconti called "the boogie beat part". He and Mick Ronson dramatically reworked the composition to include lashings of feedback and squealing rock'n'roll breaks, bringing Bowie's music closer to Deep Purple or Black Sabbath than at any time before or since. Even so David's familiar acoustic guitar, together with an ever-shifting melodic landscape and a cryptic narrative meandering through Eastern spiritualism, hardcore sex and a paraphrase of 'The Teddy Bears' Picnic' ("You'll never go down to the Gods again"), ensure that this is a true Bowie original.

In 1971 Bowie told an American interviewer that the song was about his "experiences as a shaven-headed monk," and certainly there are sufficient echoes of his 1967 Buddhist dabblings to support this remark. Opening with the same rejection of doctrinaires and gurus he had suggested in 'Cygnet Committee' ("I would sit and blame the master first and last"), Bowie embarks on a series of allegorical encounters which confirm that Friedrich Nietzsche was at the top of his reading list in early 1970. First he meets "a monster who was sleeping by a tree" who, on closer inspection, "was me" – a direct echo of *Jenseits von Gut und Böse*: "He who fights with monsters might take care lest he become a monster. And if you gaze for long into an abyss, the abyss gazes also into you."

Bowie's next point of reference is Kahlil Gibran, the Lebanese-born mystic whose 1926 treatise *The Prophet* had been much prized by the hippy movement. The book consists of the Prophet answering a series of questions posed by his disciples, but when Bowie and his *doppelgänger* ask "a simple blackbird" to solve their identity crisis, their faith in his wisdom appears to be mocked: "he laughed insane and quipped Kahlil Gibran." His trust in moral leadership further cautioned by the realization that "God's a young man too", Bowie next finds himself "laid by a young bordello … for which my reputation swept back home in drag". This leads into a final, darkly violent homoerotic tryst with God: "His nebulous body swayed above, his tongue swollen with devil's love".

This unsettling and elusive composition has inspired endless speculation about Bowie's intentions. Certainly it establishes *The Man Who Sold The World*'s running motif of travelling to the edge of a personal and emotional abyss, and as the tempo increases Bowie recklessly disregards the repeated cries of "turn around, go back!" Predictably, the Gillmans advance a detailed hypothesis relating to the schizophrenic visions of Terry Burns and what they term David's "dance with the spectre of mental illness", and while any such readings should be approached with caution, it's worth observing that in 1993 Bowie recalled one of Terry's seizures in terms precisely mirroring 'The Width Of A Circle': "he collapsed on the ground and he said the ground was opening up and there was fire and stuff pouring out of the pavement, and I could almost see it for him, because he was explaining it so articulately." Compare and contrast with "he struck the ground, a cavern appeared, and I smelled the burning pit of fear".

Although never released as a single, the song played a pivotal role in the Ziggy Stardust and Diamond Dogs tours. During the former, the mid-song instrumental break was expanded into a hard-rock workout during which David departed for a costume change while The Spiders moved into an almost shamanic cacophony of strobe lights, feedback and drums. Mick Ronson's extended guitar solo was adapted from one he had previously used in live perform-

ances of 'I Feel Free'. For the stout-hearted the full rendition is in the *Ziggy Stardust and The Spiders From Mars* film, where the number runs to a staggering fourteen minutes. For the original 1983 *Motion Picture* album, the same performance was mixed down to a more modest nine and a half minutes, but a brand new mix of the full-length version was reinstated for the album's 2003 reissue. Another live version by The Spiders From Mars, fronted by Joe Elliott, appears on the 1997 album of *The Mick Ronson Memorial Concert*. The slow-building intro of 'The Width of a Circle' made a brief return during a few concerts on the Earthling Tour, when it was used as an intro to 'The Jean Genie'.

WILD EYED BOY FROM FREECLOUD

• B-Side: 7/69 [5] • US B-Side: 7/69 • Album: *Oddity*
• Live: *Motion, Beeb* • Compilation: *S+V, S+V (2003)*
• Live Video: *Ziggy*

The predominantly acoustic original version of 'Wild Eyed Boy From Freecloud', recorded in little more than twenty minutes at Trident on 20 June 1969, gives little indication of the song's full potential. Released as the B-side of 'Space Oddity', it remained a rarity until its appearance on *Sound + Vision* in 1989 (the 2003 reissue includes Bowie's spoken introduction to the number; still rare is the American 7" mix, which omitted the first verse altogether). But it was the operatic grandeur of the subsequent album version, combining flutes, cello, harp and a soaring brass arrangement with Bowie's bravura performance of perhaps his finest lyric yet, which created an undisputed early masterpiece.

Not unlike 'Space Oddity' the song is a mystical narrative embracing thoughts of isolation, persecution and the supernatural, all perennial Bowie themes finding a new prominence in his 1969 work. "This feeling of isolation I've had ever since I was a kid was really starting to manifest itself through songs like that," he recalled in 1993. The lyrical *milieu* of mountains, eagles and reincarnation reiterates Bowie's preoccupation with Buddhist iconography, while the obvious Messianic/prophetic overtones are a template for what was to come later. In November 1969 David told George Tremlett that he considered the song "one of the best" on the album, while in *Disc & Music Echo* a month earlier he explained the storyline: "The Wild Eyed Boy lives on a mountain and has developed a beautiful way of life. He loves the mountain and the mountain loves him. I suppose in a way he's rather a prophet figure. The villagers disapprove of the things he has to say and they decide to hang him. He gives up to his fate, but the mountain tries to help him by killing the village. So in fact everything the boy says is taken the wrong way – both by those who fear him and those who love him, and try to assist."

Tony Visconti has described the ambitious orchestral arrangement, which took him five days to write, as his "greatest pride" of the *Space Oddity* sessions. "I set up the studio of fifty musicians with David sitting right in the middle playing his 12-string. I was standing in front of him conducting the orchestra. We were both very nervous. What we didn't foresee was that Trident had only just received their new 16-track machine, the first one in England, and there was no test tape included! So the house engineer frantically tried to calibrate it whilst we were rehearsing the song over and over again." Unfortunately the results were flawed: "The playback was diabolical – there was more hiss than music on the tape. The fifty musicians were very expensive, and there was no way we could afford to go into overtime. Eventually, with five minutes to spare, we got a take on tape that had about equal amounts of music and hiss. It was hell to mix. The original vinyls and the re-released RCA CDs all had that terrible hiss on the track. But when Rykodisc remastered the Bowie albums, a new technology had been invented which removed hiss from old recordings, and 'Wild Eyed Boy From Freecloud' finally sounded as brilliant as it did on the day we recorded it…"

It was during the mixing of *Space Oddity* that Visconti (and possibly Bowie himself) were introduced by drummer John Cambridge to his guitarist friend Mick Ronson. For many years it was believed that Ronson's first appearance on an official Bowie release was on the 1970 single version of 'Memory Of A Free Festival', but Tony Visconti has since revealed that Ronson's debut in fact came during the mixing of 'Wild Eyed Boy From Freecloud', when he played "a little guitar line in the middle part and joined in the handclaps in the same section."

An early and surprisingly rocked-up live version, firmly stamped with Ronson trademarks, was included in the BBC session recorded on 5 February 1970; an excellent second BBC version, which followed on 25 March, is now available on *Bowie At The Beeb*. During a few UK dates of the 1973 Ziggy Stardust tour, including the famous final concert, a truncated version of the song was included in a medley with 'All the Young Dudes' and 'Oh! You Pretty Things'.

WILD IS THE WIND *(Tiomkin/Washington)*
• Album: *Station* • A-Side: 11/81 [24] • Live: *Beeb* •
Video: *Collection, Best Of Bowie*

'Wild Is The Wind' was originally recorded by Johnny Mathis as the Oscar-nominated theme for the 1956 Western of the same name. Written by Tin Pan Alley lyricist Ned Washington and *High Noon* composer Dimitri Tiomkin, 'Wild Is The Wind' was later recorded by Nina Simone, an artist greatly admired by Bowie. The two met in Los Angeles during 1975, and although rumours of a studio collaboration remain only rumours, the encounter inspired David to record the number for *Station To Station*. "Her performance of this song really affected me," he recalled in 1993. "I thought it was just tremendous, so I recorded it as an *hommage* to Nina." Bowie's rendition, with its lovely acoustic guitars and fabulously melodramatic vocal performance, is one of his greatest cover versions and provides perhaps the most torridly romantic finale to any of his albums.

'Wild Is The Wind' was edited in 1981 as a single release to promote *ChangesTwoBowie*, accompanied by David Mallet's handsomely shot monochrome video depicting Bowie and his musicians sitting in a circle against a black backdrop, faithful to the 1976 tour's expressionist aesthetic. "I think what we were trying to do when we were filming this was to keep in mind the style of the fifties jazz programmes that were on American television at that time," Bowie explained. 'Wild Is The Wind' was subsequently played on a few early dates of the Serious Moonlight tour, and revived magnificently as the opening number for the summer 2000 concerts. A performance was taped on 23 June 2000 for Channel 4's *TFI Friday*, while an excellent recording from the BBC Radio Theatre concert on 27 June opens the *Bowie At The Beeb* bonus disc.

WILD THING *(Taylor)* :
see **HEAVEN'S IN HERE**

WILDERNESS :
see **ARE YOU COMING ARE YOU COMING**

WIN

• Album: *Americans*

This stately ballad, awash with Philly saxophone breaks and soulful backing vocals, is often mentioned in dispatches even by those who don't much care for *Young Americans*. Despite its laid-back atmosphere it appears to be a veiled attack: in 1975 Bowie described it as "a 'get up off your backside' sort of song really – a mild, precautionary sort of morality song. It was written about an impression left on me by people who don't work very hard, or do anything much, or think very hard – like, don't blame me because I'm in the habit of working hard."

Although work on the track began at Sigma Sound in August 1974, recording was not completed until December at New York's Record Plant. As a result 'Win' wasn't performed until the end of the Philly Dogs tour, the earliest known live version dating from the final show in Atlanta on 1 December. That the song was nevertheless on David's mind during the earlier stages of the tour is suggested by the fact that he would often cry "All you gotta do is win!" during the climax of 'Rock'n'Roll Suicide'.

The song has since been performed live by other artists – notably Beck – but it has yet to return to David's live repertoire, although his latter-day bassist Gail Ann Dorsey has revealed that 'Win' is one of her all-time favourite Bowie tracks. "My favourite Bowie album is *Young Americans* and it was at this time that I really got into David the heaviest," she said in 1998. "We never perform this song. Maybe the next tour, I hope." 'Win' was among the numbers rehearsed for A Reality Tour, even appearing at the occasional soundcheck, but at the time of writing it remains unperformed.

WINNERS AND LOSERS *(Pop/Jones)*

Co-produced by Bowie for Iggy Pop's *Blah-Blah-Blah*, this was the B-side for the album's initial flop single 'Cry For Love'.

WISH I COULD SHIMMY LIKE MY SISTER KATE
(Piron) : see **FOOTSTOMPIN'**

WISHFUL BEGINNINGS *(Bowie/Eno)*

• Album: *1.Outside*

This is the second *1.Outside* track "to be sung by the Artist/Minotaur," and even by comparison with 'The Voyeur' it's a sinister affair, as Bowie breathes his vocal over a heartbeat of bass drum, tambourine and distorted voices. The lyric eavesdrops on the killer's ruminations as he slowly lays out his victim: "Breathing in, breathing out, breathing on only doubt, the pain must feel like snow … Sorry, little girl … There you go, there you go…" This lacks the reassuring absurdism that tempers much of the album, and is one of the more disturbing works in Bowie's later career. 'Wishful Beginnings' didn't make the transition to the Outside tour, and further ignominy beckoned when it was cut from the reissued *1.Outside Version 2* in favour of the Pet Shop Boys remix of 'Hallo Spaceboy'.

WITH A LITTLE HELP FROM MY FRIENDS
(Lennon/McCartney)

Bowie began singing the Beatles' 1967 classic during the encores of his final Sydney concert on 25 November 1978.

WITHIN YOU

• Soundtrack: *Labyrinth*

Not to be confused with 'Without You', this song accompanies Bowie's final showdown with Jennifer Connelly in *Labyrinth*; he sings it on a gigantic optical-illusion set based on M C Escher's *Relativity*, moving impossibly through a series of gravity-defying planes to declare his passion. Reviving the Berlin albums' penchant for pounding synthesizer effects, it's an undervalued number which finds Bowie in splendidly declamatory form, and with its self-lacerating lyric ("You starve and near exhaust me / Everything I've done I've done for you, I move the stars for no-one / Your eyes can be so cruel, just as I can be so cruel…"), it wouldn't be out of place on side two of *"Heroes"*.

WITHOUT YOU

• Album: *Dance*

Distinguished only by the guest appearance of Chic's

Bernard Edwards on bass guitar, 'Without You' is probably the low point of *Let's Dance*, a throwaway love song deploying Bowie's least inspiring croon and a lyric that half-heartedly clutches at the intriguing friction of the album's better songs. Backed by 'Criminal World', it was released as a single in America, Holland, Japan and Spain in November 1983, but for some merciful reason Britain was spared.

WITHOUT YOU I'M NOTHING *(Placebo)*
• A-Side: 8/99

On 29 March 1999 Bowie recorded a vocal overdub for a remix of Placebo's album track 'Without You I'm Nothing', released as a limited-edition CD single on 16 August. Of the four versions, the 'Flexirol Mix' isolated David's vocal contribution. The CD's excessive running time disqualified it from the UK singles chart, although it topped the Budget Albums listing. The sleeve photographs featured Bowie posing with the band and even included a shot of Tony Visconti, who mixed the single. The CD's interactive material included shots of Bowie and Placebo performing at New York's Irving Plaza on the day of recording, when David joined the band for encores of 'Without You I'm Nothing' and '20th Century Boy'.

WOOD JACKSON
• European B-Side: 6/02 • B-Side: 9/02 [20] • Bonus: *Heathen (SACD)*

Released as a B-side on some formats of the 'Slow Burn' and 'Everyone Says 'Hi'' singles, 'Wood Jackson' is a hypnotic and intriguing out-take from the *Heathen* sessions. The funereal Hammond organ, shuffling drums and split-octave vocal, delivered in David's most pronounced mockney, achieve a sinister atmosphere evocative of the cryptic spookiness of classic tracks like 'All The Madmen' and in particular 'The Bewlay Brothers', whose menacing conclusion is echoed in the "Just wants to play" fade-out. The lyric appears to relate the story of a singer-songwriter ("Jackson made twenty tapes in a day, to give away") whose work is scorned ("The tunes they'd call creative when they're running out of names ... the names that hurt poor Jackson"), bringing about destruction to its listeners ("Jackson stole twenty souls in a day"); but

whether Jackson actually murders his critics, or whether the song is a rather more elliptical examination of the moral responsibility of the artist, is at best obscure.

It's possible that Bowie took his protagonist's name from an obscure writer of 1930s science-fiction who was indeed called Wood Jackson (his work included the splendidly titled *The Bat-Men Of Mars*), while the inspiration for the character of the troubled songwriter may possibly be Daniel Johnston, the cult artist from West Virginia who was plagued by mental illness and famed for his bedroom demo tapes (performed on a toy chord organ – hence, perhaps, the prominent Hammond organ on 'Wood Jackson'), which showcased a strange lyrical world of Biblical apocalypse, comic-book superheroes and unrequited love. "He was in different institutions and hospitals all his life," Bowie said of Johnston, who performed at the Meltdown Festival in June 2002, "and would make funny little cassettes of all his songs, on an out-of-tune piano or guitar: beautiful, poignant, sad little pieces. And he'd take them into the local comic shop and swap the cassettes for comics." However, as one of the more cryptic and impenetrable lyrics from the *Heathen* sessions, 'Wood Jackson' is likely to remain open to interpretation.

WORD ON A WING
• Album: *Station* • US B-Side: 7/76 • Bonus: *Station*

This thoroughly beautiful and unusually religious Bowie composition was described by its creator as a "hymn". In 1980 he told the *NME* that it was born out of the coke-addled spiritual despair he had experienced during the filming of *The Man Who Fell To Earth*. "There were days of such psychological terror when making the Roeg film that I nearly started to approach my reborn, born again thing. It was the first time I'd really seriously thought about Christ and God in any depth, and 'Word On A Wing' was a protection. It did come as a complete revolt against elements that I found in the film. The passion in the song was genuine ... something I needed to produce from within myself to safeguard myself against some of the situations that I felt were happening on the film set."

The result is one of the dramatic highlights of *Station To Station*, moving beyond the title track's conflict of belief systems with a shockingly vehement howl of desperation. Against Roy Bittan's beautifully histrionic piano Bowie repeats insistently that he is "trying hard to fit among your scheme of things"; it was during the *Station To Station* period that he began carrying a silver crucifix which he still wears today, despite having little truck with conventional worship. 'Word On A Wing' articulates his suspicion of the blind faith he had seemed to embrace in 'Golden Years' ("I believe all the way" here becomes "Just because I believe don't mean I don't think as well") but, as he later admitted, "There was a point when I very nearly got suckered into that narrow sort of looking … finding the cross as the salvation of mankind around the Roeg period." In 1995 he added: "What was it somebody said? A wonderful analogy: 'Religion is for people who believe in hell; spirituality is for people who've been there.' That for me makes a lot of sense, you know."

An edited mix appeared on the B-side of the 'Stay' single released in America and some other territories. A superb live version recorded at Nassau Coliseum on 23 March 1976 was included on 1991's *Station To Station* reissue. After regular appearances on the 1976 tour 'Word On A Wing' remained under wraps for over twenty years. It was spectacularly revived in 1999, when David reaffirmed that it was a product of "the darkest days of my life … I'm sure that it was a call for help."

WORKING CLASS HERO *(Lennon)*
• Album: *TM*

Their cover of John Lennon's bilious classic (originally from 1970's *Plastic Ono Band*) sums up all that's good and bad about Tin Machine. On an entirely basic level it's a successfully rootsy piece of R&B, but the gimlet-eyed venom of Lennon's lyric is ill served by the adversarial, rackety style of delivery. Those familiar with the original will find little of value in this thumping version, save for the implicit acknowledgement that Tin Machine's socially conscious manifesto is grounded in the legacy of Bowie's one-time collaborator. "That's always been a really favourite song of mine," explained David. "I like that first John Lennon album a hell of a lot. I think all the songs are really beautifully written … very straight from the shoulder. There's an honesty in the lyrics there. And that particular song, I thought, would sound great as a rock song. It seemed very worth doing." Lennon's son Sean, then 13, was present in the studio during

much of the recording of *Tin Machine* and apparently approved of 'Working Class Hero'. "I think he likes it a lot," said Bowie. "He's followed this album almost from the start, from the second week. He's a big Reeves fan."

An excerpt of 'Working Class Hero' was included in Julien Temple's 1989 Tin Machine video, featuring the band dressed in dinner jackets before a plush red curtain. The song was played live on the first Tin Machine tour.

YASSASSIN
• Album: *Lodger* • Dutch/Turkish A-Side: 1979

As *Lodger*'s sleeve-notes obligingly explain, "Yassassin" is Turkish for "Long Life", although in 1979 Bowie claimed he didn't know this when he wrote the song: "I just saw the word written on a wall." This sounds suspiciously like one of the self-deprecating porkies he occasionally enjoys throwing to the press, because the title is integral to the lyric. Like the previous album's 'Neuköln', 'Yassassin' is inspired by the racial tensions to which Bowie's Turkish neighbours in Berlin were subjected, but this time it's lyrically direct: "We came from the farmlands to live in this city … You want to fight but I don't want to leave … Don't say nothing's wrong 'cause I've got a love and she's afeared."

Musically 'Yassassin' is atypical *Lodger* experiment: "An interesting thing about this track was putting two ethnic sounds together," explained Bowie. "We used the Turkish things and put them against a Jamaican backbeat." The latter was a new addition to Bowie's style-book in 1978: the same year's live reworking of 'What In The World' was his first significant attempt at reggae, a style he would later subvert for 'Fashion' before exploiting it more commercially on *Tonight*. Violinist Simon House tackled the Turkish melody, and Bowie later recalled that "He understood the notation immediately, even though he had no experience with Turkish music before." Like most of *Lodger*, 'Yassassin' has remained in relative obscurity, although an edited version was released as a single in Holland and Turkey.

YELLOW SUBMARINE *(Lennon/McCartney)*

The Beatles song was included in Bowie's short-lived

1968 cabaret show.

YOU AND I AND GEORGE (*Traditional*)

The traditional romantic standby, as covered by everyone from Stan Kenton to The Muppets, was performed by Bowie on a couple of the American Sound + Vision dates, and later at the second of his 1996 Bridge School concerts. It was also among the numbers interpolated into 'Heaven's In Here' during the second Tin Machine tour.

YOU BELONG IN ROCK N'ROLL (*Bowie/Gabrels*)
• A-Side: 8/91 [33] • Album: *TM2* • B-Side: 10/91 [48]
• Live: *Oy* • Live Video: *Oy*

Although scarcely an epoch-making classic, Tin Machine's 1991 relaunch single is a spirited attempt at a commercial art-rock sound far removed from the unappealing racket previously associated with the band. The remixed single version is superior to the album cut, featuring some fine phased drum effects to enhance the lolloping rhythm which, in tandem with the honking saxophone breaks, is mildly reminiscent of T Rex's 'Get It On'. Bowie's edgy, close-to-the-mike vocal is one part Bolan to three parts Presley, and the splendidly trashy lyric is pure post-ironic glam: "I love the bad luck that you bring … I love the cheap street in your walk." Its ancestry in Bowie's own work is obvious, the latest in a long line of music-as-consummation metaphors like 'Beat Of Your Drum', 'Rock'n Roll With Me' and 'Sweet Head'.

The single was supported by Julien Temple's video, in which the band larked about in a cluttered studio environment, taping one another with camcorders. It was this video that premiered Bowie's standard *Tin Machine II* image as a clean-shaven crooner with short-cropped hair, unprecedented suntan and ubiquitous lime-green Thierry Mugler suit. The same outfit turned up for a thrillingly unlikely mimed appearance on BBC1's *Wogan* on 14 August 1991, during which Reeves Gabrels played his guitar with a vibrator and a brief post-performance interview dissolved into thinly veiled hostility after one too many of the host's inanities. "I suppose that's not a real guitar," Wogan bumbled at one point, to which Bowie replied, "No, it's my lunch, Terry." (In his 2000 autobiography *Is It Me?*, Wogan records his displeasure at Bowie's uncom-

municative behaviour, even going so far as to boast that the singer didn't know how close he came to being slapped.) There were further performances on *Paramount City* (3 August) and *Top Of The Pops* (29 August), but despite this exposure 'You Belong In Rock N'Roll' went no further than an unimpressive number 33 – nonetheless Tin Machine's highest placing in the singles chart. One of the two CD singles was a limited edition which came in an unwieldy metal and cardboard tin; apparently these were purchased from the US Navy in California and had originally been used to store computer components. The tinned CD and the 12" also boasted a pull-out "streamer" of band portraits.

'You Belong In Rock N'Roll' was performed on the It's My Life tour, from which a live version appears on *Oy Vey, Baby*.

YOU CAN HAVE HER, I DON'T WANT HER, SHE'S TOO FAT FOR ME :
see **TOO FAT POLKA**

YOU CAN'T SIT DOWN (*Clark/Muldrow/Mann*)

Paul Revere & The Raiders' number was covered live by The Manish Boys.

YOU CAN'T TALK (*Bowie/Gabrels/H.Sales/T.Sales*)
• Album: *TM2* • Live Video: *Oy*

First 'I Can't Read', now 'You Can't Talk'. Sadly this is no match for its predecessor, a tuneless window-rattler reminiscent of the equally inessential 'Sacrifice Yourself'. However, the experimental spirit – rhythmic trick-shots and bursts of funk guitar alternating with disorientating vocal effects – prefigures some of the inspired lunacy of *1.Outside*. There are hints, too, of Bowie's earlier Eno collaborations: there's a 'Beauty and the Beast' reference, and the pseudo-rap vocal recalls 'Blackout' and 'African Night Flight'. 'You Can't Talk' was performed during the It's My Life tour.

(YOU CAUGHT ME) SMILIN' (*Stewart*) :
see **HEAVEN'S IN HERE**

YOU DIDN'T HEAR IT FROM ME : see **DODO**

YOU DO SOMETHING TO ME *(Porter)* :
see **HEAVEN'S IN HERE**

**YOU GOT TO HAVE A JOB
(IF YOU DON'T WORK – YOU DON'T EAT)**
(Brown/Reed)

During the early Ziggy concerts in 1972 The Spiders occasionally performed a cover version of this little-known James Brown funk number, in a medley with Brown's more familiar 1971 hit 'Hot Pants'. Written by Brown and his occasional songwriting partner Waymon Reed, 'You Got To Have A Job' was original-ly recorded in 1969 as a duet between Brown and his backing vocalist Marva Whitney, whose solo record-ings were promoted and produced by the soul legend in the late 1960s. In this form it appeared as a Marva Whitney single and on Whitney's 1969 album *It's My Thing*, later resurfacing on various compilations. A fur-ther single version was released by Brown's right-hand man Bobby Byrd in 1970.

The one extant recording of Bowie's live version, bootlegged at Kingston Polytechnic on 6 May 1972, makes for fascinating listening: The Spiders' discom-fort is palpable as Bowie, saxophone to the fore, attempts with limited success to drag them in an all-out shimmying funk direction which, after dropping the song shortly afterwards, he wouldn't attempt again for another two years.

YOU'LL NEVER WALK ALONE
(Rodgers/Hammerstein)

The *Carousel* standard, a number 1 for Gerry And The Pacemakers in 1963, was David's regular finale during the 1966 Bowie Showboat gigs at the Marquee.

YOU'VE BEEN AROUND *(Bowie/Gabrels)*
• Album: *Black* • B-Side: 6/93 [36] • Bonus: *Black (2003)* • Video: *Black*

"We wrote it together, initially to record with Tin Machine, but it never worked out satisfactorily so it got shelved," recalled Bowie in 1993 of 'You've Been

Around', co-written with Reeves Gabrels and essayed only once by Tin Machine on the opening date of their 1989 tour. After gathering dust for three years, the song was revamped for *Black Tie White Noise*. "I resurrected that particular piece and rewrote it," said David. "And what I like about it is the fact that for the first half of the song there's no harmonic reference. It's just drums, and the voice comes in out of nowhere, and you're not sure if it's a melody line or a drone. There's a really ominous feel to it that I like a lot."

Although at the time of *Black Tie White Noise* Bowie was still talking of plans to revive Tin Machine, a further tongue-in-cheek comment would seem to hint at his dissatisfaction with band democracy: "I had the chance, as it was my album, not Tin Machine's, to mix Reeves way into the background, so I knew that that would doubtlessly really irritate him, which indeed it did!" Accordingly 'You've Been Around' submerges Gabrels's guitar beneath layers of choppy bass, jazz trumpet and heavily treated vocals to create a thrilling hybrid superior to anything released under the Tin Machine banner. The sinister soundscape is clearly indebted to The Walker Brothers' *Nite Flights* (whose title track is of course covered on the same album) and Scott Walker's 1984 solo work *Climate Of Hunter*. The lyric also seems to take its cue from the surreal urban dreamscape of 'Nite Flights', prefiguring the fractal images later found on *1.Outside*: "Where the flesh meets the spirit world, where the traffic is thin, I slip from a vacant queue." And the line "you've changed me, ch-ch-ch-ch-ch-ch-changed" is one of the album's many direct references to Bowie's early milestones.

'You've Been Around' was treated to an unremark-able video performance shot by David Mallet for the *Black Tie White Noise* documentary. A Jack Dangers remix appeared on the 'Black Tie White Noise' CD single, and later on the 2002 compilation album *Pro.File Vol. 1: Jack Dangers Remix Collection* and, in extended form, on 2003's *Black Tie White Noise* reis-sue. A 2'55" version, reworked from the original Tin Machine demo and featuring new vocal overdubs from Gary Oldman, appeared on Reeves Gabrels's 1995 solo album *The Sacred Squall Of Now*. Not sur-prisingly this cut overturns Bowie's previous subver-sion, creating a guitar-heavy interpretation which betrays the song's Tin Machine origins.

YOU'VE GOT A HABIT OF LEAVING

• A-Side: 8/65 • Compilation: *Early* • European B-Side: 6/02 • B-Side: 9/02 [20]

David's third single, and his first with The Lower Third, was produced by Shel Talmy at IBC Studios in Portland Place. The band was joined for the session by an anonymous pianist, probably Talmy's favourite Nicky Hopkins. Released on 20 August 1965, the single was credited to the singer alone (no longer "Davie" but "Davy" for this one release) – to the chagrin of the band, who would receive a full credit for their next and last single.

'You've Got A Habit Of Leaving', with its angsty teenage lyric and mid-song thrash-up, is clearly inspired by The Who – in particular their 1965 debut hit 'I Can't Explain', also produced by Talmy and later covered by Bowie on *Pin Ups*. "We had a thing about The Who," David recalled many years later. "In fact, we used to play second support to them down in Bournemouth. That was the first time I met Townshend and got talking to him about songwriting and stuff. I was hugely influenced by him. We had songs called 'Baby Loves That Way', 'You've Got A Habit Of Leaving' – some really duff things. Townshend came into our soundcheck and listened to a couple of things and said, You're trying to write like me! ... I don't think he was very impressed."

Equally unimpressed was the record-buying public, who failed to take the single into the chart despite (or perhaps because of) a breathless press release from Parlophone which proclaimed that Davy Jones and The Lower Third were into Sammy Davis Jnr, barley wine, rump steak, John Steinbeck and kinky boots. Nonetheless, they were now playing a steady stream of live dates and building up a modest coterie of supporters, and just around the corner for Davy Jones lay a new record deal, a new manager and, most significantly of all, a new name.

'You've Got A Habit Of Leaving' was among the songs re-recorded during the *Toy* sessions in 2000. This excellent new version appeared on some formats of 2002's 'Slow Burn' single and later as a B-side of 'Everyone Says 'Hi''.

YOU'VE GOT IT MADE

The performing rights organization BMI lists this otherwise unknown Bowie composition, published by the Embassy Music Corporation and almost certainly dating from the mid-1960s.

YOUNG AMERICANS

• Album: *Americans* • A-Side: 2/75 [18] • Compilation: *74/79, Best Of Bowie* • Live Video: *Moonlight, Glass, Best Of Bowie*

Recorded at Sigma Sound on the first night of the *Young Americans* sessions – 11 August 1974 – the exuberant title track mixes gospel and soul backings with a quickfire lyric sketching an Englishman's impressionistic portrait of twentieth-century America. There are references to the Watergate scandal (given that Richard Nixon's resignation had occurred just three days earlier on 8 August, Bowie's disingenuous "Do you remember your President Nixon?" is hugely topical), the McCarthy witch-hunts ("Now you have been the un-American") and a famous episode in the struggle for black equality ("Sit on your hands on a bus of survivors, blushing at all the afro-sheeners"). Lurking alongside are the tacky totems of Westernization ("Ford Mustang", "Barbie doll", "Cadi" and "Chrysler") and an undercurrent of violence and despair ("would you carry a razor in case, just in case of depression?" and, more graphically, "ain't there a woman I can sock on the jaw?"). For a song often construed as a bouncy slice of pop, the lyric cuts at least as deep as 'I'm Afraid Of Americans' twenty years later.

The opening verse also carries a cynical revision of the celebrated "Wham bam, thank you ma'am" of 'Suffragette City': this time the passionless sexual encounter "took him minutes, took her nowhere". In 1975 Bowie explained that the song was "about a newly-wed couple who don't know if they really like each other. Well, they do, but they don't know if they do or don't. It's a bit of a predicament." In the context of his career path at the time, it's difficult to see this "newly-wed couple" as anything other than Bowie on the one hand and America herself on the other.

David eagerly added the syncopated "Young American" backing vocals at the suggestion of Luther Vandross. Quite coincidentally, the song also preempts Bowie's imminent collaboration with John Lennon via the quotation, musical as well as verbal, of the line "I heard the news today, oh boy" from The Beatles' 'A Day In The Life' (in fact, this is Bowie's second curiously prescient lyric in this respect: back in 1971 he had sung "the workers have struck for *fame* /

'Cause Lennon's on sale again").

'Young Americans' received its stage premiere in Los Angeles on 2 September 1974 at the opening of the Philly Dogs tour, when David introduced it under its working title 'The Young American'. The British single release in February 1975 was identical to the five-minute album cut, whereas the American single was edited to a radio-friendly 3'11". The latter's number 28 chart peak raised Bowie's profile significantly in America; although the albums since *Aladdin Sane* had charted respectably in the States, his previous best single performance was a lowly 64 for 'Rebel Rebel'. The "rare" but inessential US single edit later appeared on *Bowie Rare*, *The Best Of David Bowie 1974/1979*, and some editions of *Best Of Bowie*.

'Young Americans' continued to feature throughout the Philly Dogs tour. The 2 November performance on Dick Cavett's *Wide World Of Entertainment* was used to promote the single, appearing on *Top Of The Pops* on 21 February 1975 and later surfacing on the *Best Of Bowie* DVD. The song returned for the Serious Moonlight, Glass Spider and Sound + Vision tours, invariably prompting Bowie to pick up his acoustic guitar. From 1983 onwards he would tend to update the lyrics, changing "Nixon" to "Reagan", "Lincoln" or even "Anyone". On the early leg of the Sound + Vision tour, the number would often expand into a blues jam into which David would interpolate snippets from a wide variety of old numbers, including jazz and blues standards like 'Drown In My Own Tears', 'Just Walking In The Rain', 'Jailhouse Blues', 'First Time I Met The Blues', 'Fingertips', James Brown's 'Please Please Please', Bessie Smith's 'I Need A Little Sugar In My Bowl', Alvin Lee's 'Going Back To Birmingham', and, rather more unusually, Iggy Pop's 'Sister Midnight'. Since 1990 the song has remained absent from Bowie's repertoire, despite the best efforts of bassist Gail Ann Dorsey: "I would just die and go to heaven if we would do 'Young Americans' one time," she revealed in 2003. "That has been my one request for the last eight years."

Luther Vandross continued to perform 'Young Americans' on stage, while The Cure recorded an unusual cover for the 1995 release *104.9 An XFM Compilation Album*. During U2's Elevation tour, Bono occasionally added lines from the song to 'Bullet The Blue Sky'. In October 2003 Liberal Democrat leader Charles Kennedy included 'Young Americans' among his choices on Radio 4's *Desert Island Discs*, and in the same year the song provided the soundtrack to the powerful closing montage sequence of Lars Von Trier's film *Dogville*.

YOUNGBLOOD *(Lieber/Stoller)*

The Coasters' 1957 US hit was included in David's medley with Cher on *The Cher Show* in November 1975.

YOUR FUNNY SMILE

This mysterious out-take from the *David Bowie* sessions is often listed in Bowie documentation as 'Funny Smile', but the performing rights organization BMI confirms 'Your Funny Smile' as its correct title. See 'Bunny Thing' for further details.

YOUR PRETTY FACE IS GOING TO HELL
(Pop/Williamson)

Mixed by Bowie for Iggy And The Stooges' 1973 album *Raw Power*, this track was recorded under the working title 'Hard To Beat'.

YOUR TURN TO DRIVE
• Download: 9/03

The most obscure of the *Reality* bonus tracks was originally slated to appear on the album's extra disc but was ultimately released only as a download, initially as an exclusive for those who purchased *Reality* from HMV online, and later via Apple's iTunes Music Store.

The decision to omit 'Your Turn To Drive' from the official *Reality* release is understandable when it becomes apparent that the track was in fact recorded during 2000's *Toy* sessions (indeed, the song's BMI registration reveals that its original title was indeed 'Toy'). The track's soundscape has little in common with the tight, spacious production of *Reality*, instead displaying many of the attributes found in the post-*'hours...'*, pre-*Heathen* sound of the *Toy* recordings. A multitude of breathy, ambient vocals sit atop lush layers of rippling piano, wah-wah guitars, a prominent Stylophone and, tellingly, a trumpet solo (Cuong Vu played trumpet during the *Toy* sessions, but the instrument doesn't appear anywhere on *Reality* or

Heathen). Meanwhile the vocal melody is strongly reminiscent of the opening lines of the *'hours...'* B-side 'We All Go Through'. It's an interesting track, but it's certainly out of place among Reality's other offerings and, if the truth be told, it's not of the same standard.

YOUTHQUAKE

One of the US radio jingles recorded by The Lower Third in May 1965 (see Chapter 3).

ZEROES

• Album: *Never*

Following the title track's John Lennon styling, *Never Let Me Down* concludes its superior first side with another nod to The Beatles, this time setting a George Harrison-style sitar over a backing borrowed in part from their 1964 classic 'Eight Days A Week' ("the chord changes at the end are real derivative," said David at the time, "I wanted to get as close as I dare but not make it overly silly"). Bowie is often at his best when his roots are showing, and 'Zeroes' is one of the better tracks on this album largely by virtue of being a blatant concoction of undisguised sources. "I remember enjoying 'Zeroes'," guitarist Carlos Alomar said many years later, "as it was intentionally meant to reproduce those good old Beatle days."

Traffic's 1967 hit 'Paper Sun' is another obvious point of reference, as is Prince's 1983 single 'Little Red Corvette', openly referred to in the lyric. At the Glass Spider tour's London press launch, Bowie responded to a leading question by agreeing that Prince was "sort of the eighties version" of himself, "in terms of the more exhibitionist forms of theatricality and musicianship." He hastily went on to insist that "I've moved on to a different area now, and I don't think anybody else could handle the job better." It's both touching and a little tragic to hear Bowie admitting in 'Zeroes' that "my little red Corvette has driven by" – thankfully he would later conquer such defeatism and resume his place at the experimental vanguard.

'Zeroes' bares the nerve-ends of various stages in Bowie's career. The title inevitably recalls '"Heroes"', while the faked-up live audience at the intro harks back to 'Diamond Dogs'. As in 'Ashes To Ashes' Bowie is clearly in career-retrospective mood, noting glumly that "a toothless past is asking you how it feels" and

hinting at every artist's feelings on unveiling a new work: "Don't you know we're back on trial again today?" There's even an elegant witticism against himself in the line "Something good is happening, I don't know what it is", which is a paraphrase of Bob Dylan's 1965 track 'Ballad Of A Thin Man', whose refrain goes: "Something is happening here, but you don't know what it is, do you, Mr Jones?"

The song eventually erupts into an affirmation of love via a sort of lightweight metaphysical pun ("You are my moon, you are my sun, heaven knows what you are") and the repetitive closing mantra of "Doesn't matter what you try to do / Doesn't matter who we really are" sounds enticingly like Bowie thumbing his nose at whatever critical reaction awaits him. Examine the album credits and you'll see that among the backing vocalists on 'Zeroes' are "Coco" and "Joe". There's no concrete proof of who these two might be, but if they're the obvious candidates, 'Zeroes' begins to make sense as a self-help exercise, a fortress of positivity and a defence against critical intrusion. "I think it had to do with the realization that all the things that are supposed to come from superstardom let you down, and the real thing you've got to live with is yourself," said David in 1987. "That's why the 'little red Corvette' is driven by, all really naïve ... Also I wanted to put in every sixties cliché I could think of! 'Stopping and preaching and letting love in', all those things. I hope there's a humorous undertone to it. But the subtext is definitely that the trappings of rock are not what they're made out to be."

'Zeroes' was performed on the European leg of the Glass Spider tour.

ZIGGY STARDUST

• Album: *Ziggy* • B-Side: 11/72 [2] • Live: *Stage, Motion, SM72, BBC, Beeb* • B-Side: 11/78 [54] • Bonus: *Ziggy, Ziggy (2002)* • A-Side: 4/94 • Live Video: *Ziggy, Best Of Bowie*

The title track of the *Ziggy Stardust* album is also its central piece of narrative, Bowie's richly allusive lyric riding over one of his finest guitar-rock melodies as he charts the rise and fall of the sci-fi superstar himself. Tantalizing clues as to Ziggy's identity blur the Marc Bolan resonances conjured up earlier on the album: there are obvious suggestions of Jimi Hendrix in the guitar hero who "played it left hand" while "jiving us that we were voodoo" and was "killed" by "the kids", but the cryptic observation that "he was the Nazz" suggests a host of other possibilities. The Nazz was a name shared by erstwhile backing bands of both Todd Rundgren and Alice Cooper (who had also fronted a group called The Spiders in the mid-1960s), while some have suggested that the word implies both "Nazarene" (hence Christ) and "Nazi" (dovetailing nicely with the album's totalitarian undertones and Bowie's later evaluation of Hitler as "one of the first rock stars").

The "leper Messiah" might refer to the stage delusions of Vince Taylor or Peter Green (see Chapter 2), while "well-hung and snow-white tan" suggests the coked-up sexuality of Iggy Pop's stage persona. There are hints of Lou Reed: "came on so loaded man" reminds us of The Velvet Underground's latest album, while "Ziggy sucked up into his mind" reprises the Reed-style 'Queen Bitch' line "your laughter is sucked in their brains". As for "making love with his ego", the list of applicants is still growing, although Jim Morrison and Mick Jagger seem the most likely of the original candidates. But all the potential references – and there are plenty of others – defer to the nebulous character of Ziggy himself: the point is not *who* he is, but the fact that he is a construct of rock's archetypes.

'Ziggy Stardust' was completed at Trident on 11 November 1971. Bowie's earlier acoustic demo was included on both the 1990 and 2002 *Ziggy Stardust* reissues. In 1972 three further versions were recorded for BBC radio sessions, on 11 and 18 January and 16 May. The latter two both appear on *Bowie At The Beeb*, while the third is also on the *BBC Sessions 1969-1972* sampler. Despite its pivotal position in Bowie's career and its ubiquitous appearance on singles compilations, 'Ziggy Stardust' has never actually been a hit: the only time it's ever been an A-side was as a live version released to promote *Santa Monica '72* in 1994. This version was accompanied by a video compiled from live footage shot at Dunstable Civic Hall on 21 June 1972, offering fascinating glimpses of an early Ziggy show in action. Another live version, this time from 1978, appeared on *Stage* and the accompanying 'Breaking Glass' single. For such an iconic number 'Ziggy Stardust' has appeared in surprisingly few live sets: aside from the Ziggy Stardust and Stage tours, its only revivals have been for 1990's Sound + Vision outing, the summer 2000 dates and the Heathen and A Reality tours – although David did occasionally add the line "Ziggy played guitar!" to the end of 'Star' on

the Serious Moonlight tour.

'Ziggy Stardust' has, however, been a hit single in a cover version: Bauhaus had their biggest success with a rendition that reached number 15 in October 1982. This recording later appeared on *David Bowie Songbook*, while a further Bauhaus version appears on the 1989 release *Swing The Heartache: The BBC Sessions*. Among the host of other artists who have performed the song are Hootie And The Blowfish, Nina Hagen and Def Leppard, whose singer Joe Elliott also fronted the live Spiders From Mars rendition which appears on the 1997 album of *The Mick Ronson Memorial Concert*. In April 2003 David Baddiel and Frank Skinner "sang" a version on ITV's *Baddiel & Skinner Unplanned*. Touring with The Indigo Girls in 1998, Bowie's bassist Gail Ann Dorsey performed 'Ziggy Stardust' every night, and even Madonna has been known to perform the number at concert soundchecks.

ZION

This rambling 6'01" demo, dating from 1973, has variously appeared on bootlegs under the titles 'Zion', 'Aladdin Vein', 'Love Aladdin Vein' and 'A Lad In Vein'. Adaptations of the central piano phrase and guitar workout would later appear on *Diamond Dogs* as the bridging passage between 'Sweet Thing (reprise)' and 'Rebel Rebel', while snatches of the melody are not unlike parts of *Aladdin Sane*'s title track. Mick Ronson's instantly identifiable swathes of guitar are topped by Mike Garson's piano and a prominent flute line (perhaps from *Aladdin Sane*'s Brian Wilshaw), while Bowie "la las" his way through a vaguely Eastern melody, evidently bereft of lyrics at the time of recording.

Amid the uncertainty over the track's correct title there exists the possibility that 'Zion' might be the name of an altogether different song – either one that has never come to light, or one we know by another name. The common assumption that the track was recorded at Trident during the *Aladdin Sane* sessions has never been authenticated, and one piece of evidence strongly suggests a later date. Martin Hayman, who interviewed Bowie at the Château d'Hérouville towards the end of the *Pin Ups* sessions in the summer of 1973, was played a sneak preview of a new demo for David's next album by the eager singer himself. Explaining that "There are no vocals on it yet, just my la-la-la-ing. It's going to be a musical in one act called *Tragic Moments*, probably running straight through two sides," David played back what Hayman described as "perhaps seven minutes of ... highly arranged, subtly shifting music with just a touch of vaudeville: Mike Garson's piano flashes through like quicksilver. Perhaps the closest approximation to what has gone before would be the title track of *Aladdin Sane.*" This sounds exactly like the track we now know as 'Zion', which perhaps ought to be regarded more as a *Diamond Dogs* demo than an *Aladdin Sane* out-take.

2   tHE ALBUMS

(i) OFFICIAL ALBUMS

The first part of this chapter covers the official canon of David Bowie's studio and live albums. Catalogue number, release date and, where applicable, highest chart placing appears for every major UK release and reissue. Overseas and specialist reissues (such as Rykodisc's AU20 series of gold CDs, EMI's 1990s vinyl re-pressings, and Simply Vinyl's high-quality 2001 vinyl reissues) are ignored.

DAVID BOWIE
Deram DML 1007, June 1967
Deram DOA 1, August 1984
Deram 800 087 2, April 1989 *(CD)*

'Uncle Arthur' (2'07″) / 'Sell Me A Coat' (2'58″) / 'Rubber Band' (2'17″) / 'Love You Till Tuesday' (3'09″) / 'There Is A Happy Land' (3'11″) / 'We Are Hungry Men' (2'58″) / 'When I Live My Dream' (3'22″) / 'Little Bombardier' (3'24″) / 'Silly Boy Blue' (3'48″) / 'Come And Buy My Toys' (2'07″) / 'Join The Gang' (2'17″) / 'She's Got Medals' (2'23″) / 'Maid Of Bond Street' (1'43″) / 'Please Mr Gravedigger' (2'35″)

• *Musicians:* David Bowie *(vocals, guitar)*, Dek Fearnley *(bass)*, Derek Boyes *(organ)*, John Eager *(drums)* • *Recorded:* Decca Studios, Hampstead, London • *Producer:* Mike Vernon

The chart failure of Bowie's third Pye single 'I Dig Everything' in August 1966 compounded his disenchantment with a label that had done little to promote or encourage his work. In September, David took his grievances to his new part-time manager Kenneth Pitt, who arranged for him to be released from his Pye contract. Almost immediately, David began recording.

On 18 October David was joined at R G Jones Studios in Surrey by Dek Fearnley, Derek Boyes and John Eager, three members of his current band The Buzz. Together with two unknown session musicians, they embarked on a four-and-a-half-hour session that produced three new recordings: a revamped version of the previously rejected Pye track 'The London Boys', and two new compositions, 'Rubber Band' and 'Please Mr Gravedigger'. On 24 October Pitt played acetates of the three tracks to Hugh Mendl, A&R Manager of Decca's new subsidiary label, Deram, which had just signed the up-and-coming Cat Stevens. In turn, Mendl played the tracks to Decca staff producer Mike Vernon, whose first production work had been for The Yardbirds in 1963. A deal was struck at once: in addition to purchasing the three recordings, Decca contracted Bowie to make an album to be produced by Mike Vernon, paying £150 plus a royalty agreement for the three tracks, and a further advance of £100 against royalties on the album. Kenneth Pitt considered it "a good deal". It was also a most unusual arrangement for the time – for an artist to win an album contract before proving his commercial value with a hit single or two was rare indeed.

After a delay caused by Derek Boyes's suspected appendicitis, sessions began on 14 November with the recording of 'Uncle Arthur' and 'She's Got Medals' in Decca's Studio No. 2 in West Hampstead. This would remain the venue throughout the sessions, which were slotted in around The Buzz's rapidly depleting gig schedule. November 24 saw the recording of 'There Is A Happy Land', 'We Are Hungry Men', 'Join The Gang' and the B-side 'Did You Ever Have A

Dream'. The Buzz played their last gig on 2 December, and on the same day Deram released their first David Bowie single, the October recording of 'Rubber Band'.

Recording continued for the next fortnight. 'Little Bombardier', 'Sell Me A Coat', 'Silly Boy Blue' and 'Maid Of Bond Street' were cut on 8 December, with 'Come And Buy My Toys' and the album version of 'Please Mr Gravedigger' following on December 12 and 13 respectively.

Mike Vernon found the sessions "a lot of fun" and David "the easiest person to work with," adding that "Some of the melodies were extremely good, and the actual material, the lyrics, had a quality that was quite unique." He was assisted by studio engineer Gus Dudgeon, who also admired the work, telling David Buckley that "the music was very filmic, all very visual and all quite honest and unaffected and therefore unique."

Dek Fearnley, who assisted David with the arrangements, recalled a collaborative working method broadly similar to the process Bowie would still be using more than thirty years later. "He had a song in its basic form," Fearnley told the Gillmans, "and we would just work it out. He would say, 'I'd like to have a violin,' and I'd say, 'Yes, let's keep a soulful feel, let's have a trombone,' and he'd say that'd be a great idea. He was so bloody inspiring ... he spurred me on to things I could never otherwise have done." With only the most rudimentary training between them – neither could read music – the pair furnished themselves with the Observer's Book Of Music in an attempt to read up on the terms used by Vernon's session musicians, many of whom were from the London Philharmonic Orchestra. "It was awful," Fearnley recalled of the embarrassing gaffes they committed, "and David left all that to me."

Kenneth Pitt, who had been absent from the sessions due to a major promotional tour of America and Australia with his client Crispian St Peters, returned to London on 16 December. Months of financial mismanagement finally prompted Bowie to approach Pitt over his concerns about Ralph Horton who, after a series of mutual discussions, willingly relinquished all managerial responsibility on 19 January. Initially overseeing David's affairs on an unofficial basis, Pitt would take over as his full-time manager in April.

Meanwhile, recording at Decca resumed on 26 January with both sides of the forthcoming single, 'The Laughing Gnome' and 'The Gospel According To Tony Day'. A month later on 25 February the album versions of 'Rubber Band', 'Love You Till Tuesday' and 'When I Live My Dream' completed the sessions.

David Bowie was released on 1 June 1967 in a sleeve photographed by Dek Fearnley's brother Gerald. The photo-session took place in Gerald's basement studio beneath a church in Bryanston Street near Marble Arch, where David and Dek had also conducted rehearsals during the album sessions. "That military jacket, I was very proud of that ... it was actually tailored," Bowie recalled many years later of the outfit he had chosen to complement his Robert James pageboy haircut. The sleeve also included some elegantly written hype from the pen of Kenneth Pitt, describing Bowie's vision as "straight and sharp as a laser beam. It cuts through hypocrisy, prejudice and cant. It sees the bitterness of humanity, but rarely bitterly. It sees the humour in our failings, the pathos of our virtues." Thanks to the Deram label's progressive leanings, David Bowie was one of the first albums to be released in both mono and stereo. The American release, which omitted 'We Are Hungry Men' and 'Maid Of Bond Street', appeared in August 1967.

Reviews, although thin on the ground, were extremely positive. The NME's Allen Evans hailed the record as "all very refreshing" and Bowie as "a very promising talent. And there's a fresh sound to the light musical arrangements by David and Dek Fearnley." Disc & Music Echo called the album "a remarkable, creative debut album by a 19-year-old Londoner" and declared, "Here is a new talent that deserves attention, for though David Bowie has no great voice, he can project words with a cheeky 'side' that is endearing yet not precocious ... full of abstract fascination. Try David Bowie. He's something new." Kenneth Pitt, who sent copies of David Bowie to numerous showbusiness contacts in an attempt to drum up interest in his client, received letters of congratulation from figures as diverse as Bryan Forbes and Franco Zeffirelli.

Nonetheless David Bowie was not a success, and its commercial fate was sealed by Deram's lack of interest in promoting it. Decca's head of promotion Tony Hall, a long-time friend of Pitt's who had been instrumental in securing Bowie's contract, had left for another company in May. Even before the album's release it became apparent that David had lost his champion within the company, but the miserably low profile accorded to his Deram releases reached its nadir a year later when Pitt and Bowie attended a

Decca promotion at Selfridge's. Seeing no evidence of Bowie on display, they innocently asked a saleswoman about his album; having rifled through her files, she informed them that David Bowie was not with Decca but with Pye.

By this time, David had recorded various other tracks for Deram, most of which are now collected on the *The Deram Anthology 1966-1968*. With the exception of the second version of 'Love You Till Tuesday' (recorded on 3 June 1967 with the second version of 'When I Live My Dream', and released as a single in July), the remainder of David's Deram material had been systematically rejected by the label, and rumours of a planned second album are no more than supposition. In May 1968, shortly after the Selfridge's incident, Deram turned down David's latest putative single 'In The Heat Of The Morning' and Hugh Mendl told Pitt, "I cannot blame you if you wish to leave us." They did, and from a promising mid-1967 peak David's career went into freefall until the arrival of 'Space Oddity' eighteen months later. It was not time wasted, however; although lacking apparent direction, this was the period during which David forged his associations with Lindsay Kemp and Tony Visconti, both essential participants in what was to come.

In the long run the failure of *David Bowie*, while disheartening to its creator at the time, was in all probability a blessing. One of the most astonishing twists in the story of Bowie's early career was a monstrous blunder made by Ralph Horton at the time of the album sessions in December 1966, without which David's life might have mapped out very differently. Before departing on his trip to America, Kenneth Pitt had negotiated an advance of £1000 as part of a publishing deal with Essex Music but, certain that he could do better, had declined to close the deal and told the company he would reconsider the offer on his return. In America he pulled off a major coup, negotiating with another company (believed to be Koppelman & Rubin) a three-year deal with an advance of $30,000 for exclusive worldwide publishing rights to David's songs. When he returned to London in December to break the good news, Pitt found that in his absence Ralph Horton had signed a contract with Essex Music for an advance of £500 – half of what Pitt had already agreed and a fraction of the amount that would have come with the now invalidated American deal. It was a crushing blow, and after confiding in David's father Pitt elected not to tell David about it until several years later. What might have happened in 1967 with a $30,000 publishing deal to fall back on is matter for conjecture, but with sufficient finance for a major publicity push it's perfectly conceivable that *David Bowie* might have become a substantial hit, and the ensuing years of struggle that eventually bore the fruit of Bowie's 1970s career might have been entirely bypassed. "I'd probably be in *Les Misérables* now," said Bowie in 1996. "Oh, I'm sure I would have been a right little trouper on the West End stage. I'd have written ten Laughing Gnomes, not just one!"

Bowie's Deram recordings, of which *David Bowie* is the most substantial legacy, have instead acquired their own almost mythological status. Mercilessly mocked as music-hall piffle derived from a passing Anthony Newley fad, the album is routinely passed off as, in David Buckley's words, a "cringe-inducing piece of juvenilia" only to be braved by "those with a high enough embarrassment threshold." The Deram period has long since been played down, if not disowned, by David himself. "Aarrghh, that Tony Newley stuff, how cringey," he said in 1990. "No, I haven't much to say about that in its favour. Lyrically I guess it was striving to be something, the short story teller. Musically it's quite bizarre. I don't know where I was at. It seemed to have its roots all over the place, in rock and vaudeville and music hall and I don't know what. I didn't know if I was Max Miller or Elvis Presley."

In their efforts to exonerate Bowie from what has long been considered an aberration, many fans have tried to put the "blame" on Kenneth Pitt, often portrayed as the man who sought to turn David into an all-singing, all-dancing, all-round entertainer. This theory holds no water whatsoever: the album was made before Pitt played any more than an administrative role in David's affairs, and he was absent from the country when the majority of it was written and recorded. For his part, David himself told Mike Vernon during the album sessions that he was a fan of Anthony Newley and, as Gus Dudgeon told David Buckley, "it bothered Mike Vernon and me because we'd say, 'Bowie's really good and his songs are fucking great, but he sounds like Anthony Newley'."

In his memoir, Pitt insists that he "was never happy with David sounding like Newley on some of his records and the decision to do so, conscious or not, was David's alone." Certainly it was Pitt who undertook to broaden David's education with trips to the West End theatre to see variety acts, and it was Pitt's library that exposed David to works like Oscar Wilde's *The Picture Of Dorian Gray* and Antoine de Saint-Exupéry's *The Little Prince*, elements of which emerge in the overall tone of the Deram material. But the idea that Pitt represented some sort of throwback to the Edwardian nursery-room has been unfairly and inaccurately fostered. He managed Bob Dylan on his UK tours, and was responsible for introducing Bowie to some of his key influences. When Pitt returned from abroad in December 1966 it was fresh from meeting Andy Warhol and Lou Reed in New York, and among his luggage was an acetate of *The Velvet Underground And Nico*. As yet unreleased, it was a record that would immediately have a profound effect on Bowie's artistic development. Writing in the *New Yorker* in 2003, David would describe the album's impact on him as "shattering. Everything I both felt and didn't know about rock music was opened to me on one unreleased disc … with the opening, throbbing, sarcastic bass and guitar of 'I'm Waiting For the Man', the lynchpin, the keystone of my ambition was driven home. This music was so savagely indifferent to my feelings. It didn't care if I liked it or not … It was completely preoccupied with a world unseen by my suburban eyes … I played it again and again and again." Studio out-takes from the Deram sessions reveal a side to Bowie's musical palette only hinted at on the *David Bowie* album: they include his first version of 'Waiting For The Man' and the demented 'Venus In Furs' makeover 'Little Toy Soldier'.

Another record Pitt brought back from New York was the eponymous third LP by The Fugs, a Greenwich Village beatnik outfit whose work included setting the poetry of William Blake to hardcore avant-garde backings. The Fugs had a similar impact on Bowie's imagination (he later described them as "one of the most lyrically explosive underground bands ever"), and their 'Dirty Old Man' was co-opted into his live repertoire in 1967 alongside 'Waiting For The Man'. Other sources have confirmed that Bowie was one of Britain's few Frank Zappa fans at the time, even attempting live cover versions of Zappa's early numbers in his Riot Squad concerts. The widely accepted perception of Bowie's Deram period as some sort of Cockney knees-up begins, thankfully, to recede.

In any case, the standard summation of *David Bowie*'s musical achievement as sub-Newley vaudeville whimsy is entirely inadequate. For one thing, the much-vaunted resemblance to Anthony Newley only really surfaces on a handful of tracks like 'Love You Till Tuesday', 'Little Bombardier' and 'She's Got Medals' – and, in keeping with the methodology that would characterize Bowie's later career, the vocal affectation is merely one ingredient in the album's synthesis of ideas. "I got into Anthony Newley like crazy," David recalled in 2002. "Before he came to the States and did the whole Las Vegas thing, he really did bizarre things over here – a television series he did called *The Strange World Of Gurney Slade*, which was so odd and off the wall. And I thought, I like what this guy's doing, where he's going, he's really interesting. And so I started singing songs like him. But I was reading a lot of stuff by the Angry Young Men generation, Keith Waterhouse and John Osborne and stuff like that, and so I was writing these really weird Tony Newley-type songs, but the lyrics were about lesbians in the army, and cannibals, and paedophiles, and things like that. I thought, yeah, this is my bag, this is what my career's gonna be like. And the first album really is the most extraordinary piece of work in that way. I mean – utterly forgettable, but there's no faulting its ambitions."

Furthermore, Gus Dudgeon's oft-quoted description of the *David Bowie* album as "about the weirdest thing any record company have ever put out" has inadvertently fostered the notion that there was nothing else like it in the 1967 charts. This is, of course, untrue. It takes no great leap of the imagination to realize that the album's blend of folk and short-story narrative took many of its cues from the more commercial end of the burgeoning British psychedelia scene of 1966-7. The album's motif of wartime nostalgia, its Blakeian evocations of childhood innocence, and above all its rogues' gallery of lonely misfits and social inadequates, are all very much of a piece with contemporary work by the likes of Syd Barrett's Pink Floyd, The Bonzo Dog Doo-Dah Band, and, by no means least, The Beatles themselves.

Revolver had appeared in August 1966, bringing its tales of lonely people and yellow submarines to a mass audience. *Sgt Pepper's Lonely Hearts Club Band* was recorded at the same time as *David Bowie* and released on the same day, 1 June 1967. *Sgt Pepper* went on to sell rather more copies and is generally acknowledged to be the better album of the two, but it's always been something of a nonsense that the same people who rubbish *David Bowie* for being "whimsical" and "music-hall" are happy to consider

'Being For The Benefit Of Mr Kite!' a stunning piece of experimental pop. Despite *Sgt Pepper*'s obvious superiority, the two albums have a great deal in common. Direct comparisons are hardly the point (although the oompah fairground waltz of 'Mr Kite' is matched precisely on 'Little Bombardier'), but 'Uncle Arthur', 'She's Got Medals' and 'Sell Me A Coat' have more than a whiff of 'Eleanor Rigby', 'Lovely Rita' or 'She's Leaving Home' about them. It has even been suggested that 'Rubber Band', released as a single in December 1966, might have given The Beatles the idea for *Sgt Pepper*'s title. "I have no grounds for believing that," wrote Kenneth Pitt, but he adds that it was a view "widely held" in 1967.

Meanwhile, although the Bonzo Dog Doo-Dah Band had only notched up a couple of flop singles by the time of the *David Bowie* sessions, they were a ubiquitous presence on the pub-gig circuit then being played by The Buzz, and although they have never been acknowledged as a direct influence there can surely be no reasonable doubt. Their debut single 'My Brother Makes The Noises For The Talkies', released in April 1966, allowed the Bonzos to indulge a penchant for crazed *Goon Show* sound effects of the kind that saturated Bowie recordings like 'We Are Hungry Men', 'Please Mr Gravedigger' and 'Little Toy Soldier'. Their second was a cover of the Hollywood Argyles' novelty hit 'Alley Oop', later cited by David as among his favourite singles and directly quoted in 'Life On Mars?'. In January 1968 Bowie had several meetings with Ray Williams of Liberty Records to discuss the possibility of the Bonzos covering one of his songs. Although the band dropped the "Doo-Dah" from their name at around this time, it seems more than a little suspicious that "the doo-dah horn" should turn up in Bowie's 'Ching-a-Ling' later the same year, by which time Gus Dudgeon had become their producer. It must be one of the more amusing coincidences in pop history that both Bowie and the Bonzos should ultimately find their 1960s work overshadowed and sorely misrepresented by a runaway number 5 hit about a spaceman.

As with the juvenilia of any major artist, there is a temptation to over-interpret *David Bowie* in the pursuit of tenuous parallels with the mature canon. Certainly 'We Are Hungry Men' foreshadows Bowie's interest in Orwellian and Messianic themes; certainly 'She's Got Medals' anticipates his stock in trade of gender confusion; certainly 'Come And Buy My Toys' is a pointer to the acoustic folk territory of his next

album; certainly there are plenty of lyrics about playacting and the silver screen; and certainly a preoccupation with the lonely, forsaken individual on the outside of society would remain a motif on every subsequent Bowie album. However, the attempts of some biographers to expose specific lyrics as a catalogue of dark secrets from David's family vault should be taken with a large pinch of salt.

Whatever we find in its fourteen tracks, it seems a pity that *David Bowie* is only ever considered in terms of what we can extrapolate from it, what light it may or may not shed on the important stuff ("picking through the peppercorns of my manure pile," as Bowie put it in 1999, "Looking for something that might indicate I had a future"). Thankfully, it does seem that pop musicologists are at last beginning to regard *David Bowie* not just as a quirky set of embryonic twitterings, but as an album that's actually worth considering in its own right. Nearly twenty years after the sessions, Dek Fearnley told the Gillmans that the album was "the most satisfying thing I have done in my life," and while Bowie is unlikely to join him in that sentiment, there is absolutely nothing here for him to be embarrassed about. *David Bowie* justifiably resides in the shadow of his later work, but those with open ears and open minds know it as a sweet, clever album that has borne nearly four decades of derision with consummate dignity.

SPACE ODDITY

Philips SBL 7912, November 1969
RCA Victor LSP 4813, November 1972 [17]
RCA PL 84813, October 1984
EMI EMC 3571, April 1990 [64]
EMI 7243 5218980, September 1999

'Space Oddity' (5'14") / 'Unwashed and Somewhat Slightly Dazed' (6'10") / 'Don't Sit Down' (0'39") / 'Letter to Hermione' (2'30") / 'Cygnet Committee' (9'30") / 'Janine' (3'19") / 'An Occasional Dream' (2'56") / 'Wild Eyed Boy From Freecloud' (4'47") / 'God Knows I'm Good' (3'16") / 'Memory Of A Free Festival' (7'07")

Bonus tracks on 1990 reissue: 'Conversation Piece' (3'05") / 'Memory Of A Free Festival Part 1' (3'59") / 'Memory Of A Free Festival Part 2' (3'31")

• *Musicians:* David Bowie *(vocals, 12-string guitar,*

Stylophone, kalimba, Rosedale electric chord organ),
Keith Christmas (guitar), Mick Wayne (guitar), Tim
Renwick (guitar, flutes, recorders), Tony Visconti (bass,
flutes, recorders), Herbie Flowers (bass), John "Honk"
Lodge (bass), John Cambridge (drums), Terry Cox
(drums), Rick Wakeman (mellotron, electric harpsi-
chord), Paul Buckmaster (cello), Benny Marshall and
Friends (harmonica) • Recorded: Trident Studios,
London • Producer: Tony Visconti ('Space Oddity':
Gus Dudgeon)

The filming of Love You Till Tuesday marked the effective end of Kenneth Pitt's reign as Bowie's mentor.
Although David briefly moved back to Pitt's
Manchester Street flat in the wake of his split from
Hermione Farthingale in February 1969, new
acquaintances were already propelling his life and
career in a fresh direction. Snapshots of this annus
mirabilis were captured on his second album, which
he would begin recording in June.

Wildly differing accounts have emerged of the
events which conspired to secure Bowie his new contract with Mercury Records, not least because of the
personal stakes of the individuals involved, but the
framework seems to be as follows: by the end of 1968
a nineteen-year-old American emigrée called Mary
Angela Barnett was dating Lou Reizner, the London
head of Mercury Records. Through Reizner she met
the company's glamorous Assistant European
Director of A & R, Calvin Mark Lee. Lee had first met
David Bowie some time in 1967, and remains a shadowy figure in some accounts for the very reason that
David had purposely kept him away from Kenneth
Pitt, knowing that the two were unlikely to be kindred
spirits.

It appears that Calvin Mark Lee was, however
briefly and opportunistically, involved with David on
a level that went beyond friendship; he tells the
Gillmans that he "overlapped for a time with
Hermione". He retains a place in Bowie history as the
man who wore red and silver "love jewel" discs on his
forehead – an image subsequently adopted by the
late-period Ziggy Stardust – and, rather more sub-
stantially, as the man responsible for introducing
David to Angela Barnett, after a Feathers gig at the
Roundhouse on 4 January 1969. This was the ménage-
à-trois to which David referred many years later when
he flippantly told an interviewer that he had met his
future wife when "we were both going out with the
same man." His relationship with Angela didn't begin

until some time later, under the less formal circumstances of a King Crimson gig at the Speakeasy on 19
April. Abetted by Angela, Lee spent the spring of 1969
talking up David's potential to Lou Reizner and forg-
ing useful contacts at Mercury.

Unaware of these goings-on, Kenneth Pitt perse-
vered in trying to win Bowie a contract by more conventional means. In March he unsuccessfully played a
demo of 'Space Oddity' to Atlantic Records, while the
following month, at Bowie's urging, he arranged to
meet Mercury Records' New York director Simon
Hayes, who was on a trip to London. On 14 April Pitt
gave Hayes a private screening of Love You Till Tuesday
(attended, much to Pitt's chagrin, by Calvin Mark Lee,
whom he still didn't realize was on the Mercury staff).
Hayes expressed some interest and suggested George
Martin as a potential producer.

A fascinating glimpse of the genesis of the Space
Oddity album is afforded by a ten-song acoustic demo
tape recorded by David and his Feathers partner John
"Hutch" Hutchinson, probably in mid-April 1969. In
addition to the 'Space Oddity' demo later included on
Sound + Vision, the tape features early versions of
'Janine', 'An Occasional Dream', 'Conversation Piece',
'Letter To Hermione' (here called 'I'm Not Quite'),
and 'Cygnet Committee' (with very different lyrics
and called 'Lover To The Dawn'). There are also ren-
ditions of the Feathers staples 'When I'm Five',
'Ching-a-Ling', 'Love Song' and 'Life Is A Circus'.

Exactly when and where this demo tape was
recorded remains difficult to pinpoint. It was almost
certainly after Kenneth Pitt's meeting with Simon
Hayes on 14 April, and the presence of Hutch means
that it can't have been a great deal later, for he bowed
out and returned to Yorkshire the same month. It has
been suggested that the demos were recorded on professional equipment at Mercury Records' headquarters in Knightsbridge, but this seems highly unlikely
considering Bowie's apologies on the tape for the
"very bad tape recorder and microphone" and for the
noises coming from the piano teacher upstairs; the
usual consensus is that the venue was his new flat in
Foxgrove Road, Beckenham, where he moved on 14
April. From here he would go on to establish the
Beckenham "Arts Laboratory" which held the first of
its regular Sunday gatherings at the Three Tuns pub
on 4 May.

In mid-May Pitt successfully negotiated a one-year
contract with Simon Hayes whereby Bowie was to
receive royalties and production costs for a new

album, while Mercury retained two one-year renewal options. The record would be distributed on the Mercury label in America, and its affiliate Philips in the UK.

The George Martin plan came to nothing after Pitt's approaches were rebuffed and word eventually came back that the fabled fifth Beatle didn't like 'Space Oddity'. Pitt wrote "GEORGE MARTIN IS FALLIBLE" in his diary and turned instead to Tony Visconti, who had produced Bowie's later Deram sessions. 'Space Oddity' had already been tabled as a lead-off single for the forthcoming album, but Visconti famously considered the song a gimmick and deputed it to Bowie's former engineer Gus Dudgeon. Since his work on *David Bowie*, Dudgeon had produced two of the Bonzo Dog Band's albums and, with Visconti, had recently completed production on The Strawbs' eponymous debut. "I listened to the demo and thought it was incredible," Dudgeon recalled. "I couldn't believe that Tony didn't want to do it … he said, 'That's great, you do that and the B-side, and I'll do the album.' I was only too pleased."

Recording began on 20 June 1969 at Trident Studios in Soho, where Dudgeon oversaw 'Space Oddity' and the original B-side version of 'Wild Eyed Boy From Freecloud'. David had recorded 'Ching-a-Ling' at the same venue the previous October, but the *Space Oddity* sessions cemented the beginning of a long-term relationship with Trident that would last until the completion of *Aladdin Sane*. It was a day that also saw the debut of several figures who would populate Bowie's music in future years. Save for a few in-house BBC recordings it was apparently the first ever studio session for bassist Herbie Flowers, who later played on *Diamond Dogs* and Lou Reed's *Transformer*, and whose subsequent credits would include backing work for Marc Bolan and Paul McCartney, writing Clive Dunn's novelty hit 'Grandad', and being a core member of the classical-rock outfit Sky.

Rick Wakeman, who played Mellotron, was still an unknown – The Strawbs and Yes lay in the future, and 'Space Oddity' was only his second time in a recording studio. "I asked Visconti if he knew a Mellotron player," explained Dudgeon, "and he said he knew a bloke who played in a Top Rank ballroom … We did one take and he made a mistake. Apologized. We did another one – and that was it. Pretty good really – the second session in his life and take two is the master." Drummer Terry Cox was borrowed from folk group Pentangle, while Junior's Eyes guitarist Mick Wayne

("he did that great solo and the rocket take-off effect") came at Visconti's recommendation. Bowie himself played acoustic guitar and Stylophone, and the session also made use of a total of eight violins, 2 violas, 2 celli, 2 double basses and 2 flutes to orchestral arrangements by Paul Buckmaster, a classically trained musician who had scored arrangements for Marsha Hunt and William Kimber. "It's possible Bowie was the first person to call Buckmaster," said Dudgeon, "I can't recall, but the first sessions he did were with me and he was great, the perfect choice."

While Mercury and Philips set about promoting the rush-released single on both sides of the Atlantic in time for the Apollo 11 moonshot, the album sessions proper commenced at Trident on 16 July. Tony Visconti recruited further members of Junior's Eyes, the cult underground band whose June 1969 album *Battersea Power Station* he had recently produced. They were guitarist Tim Renwick (later to join the post-Roger Waters Pink Floyd), bassist John "Honk" Lodge and drummer John Cambridge, formerly of Hull band The Rats. Their vocalist Benny Marshall would drop by at a late stage in the sessions and contribute a harmonica solo, while Bowie also drafted in Beckenham Arts Lab regular Keith Christmas on additional guitar. Another new arrival was studio engineer Ken Scott, who had cut his teeth at Abbey Road with George Martin and The Beatles, working on *Magical Mystery Tour* and *The Beatles* as well as Jeff Beck's seminal *Truth*.

"I must confess that my work was naïve, bordering on sloppy, on this album," said Visconti many years later. "I really didn't know too much about the quality control of sound and how to turbo-charge the sound of instruments for rock … I am, however, proud of several tracks where I felt more comfortable in my capacity of bass player and recorder player, as in 'Letter To Hermione' and 'An Occasional Dream'." One of Visconti's personal triumphs was the lavish fifty-piece orchestral rearrangement of 'Wild Eyed Boy From Freecloud'.

The sessions continued on and off until mid-October, punctuated by David's Sunday gigs at the Beckenham Arts Lab and by various interruptions, some more serious than others. The first was David's Mediterranean trip with Kenneth Pitt to perform at the Maltese and Italian Song Festivals at the end of July. They arrived home on 3 August to the news that David's father Haywood Jones was seriously ill. He died two days later, never to know his son's great success, and David's grief was channelled in part into a new song, 'Unwashed And Somewhat Slightly Dazed'. On 16 August came the open-air event at Beckenham Recreation Ground which David commemorated in 'Memory Of A Free Festival'. By the autumn, however, his disillusion with the slack attitude of his hippy peers would bring forth the boiling anger of 'Cygnet Committee'.

The album's original UK sleeve depicted David against a blue polka-dot background taken from a design by Victor Vasarely, a pop artist whose work was enthusiastically collected by Calvin Mark Lee. The back cover was a piece of flower-power artwork by David's old friend George Underwood emerging from aspects of the album's lyrics, and conspicuously similar in style to the cover he had painted (at Bowie's recommendation) for the previous year's Tyrannosaurus Rex album *My People Were Fair And Had Sky In Their Hair ... But Now They're Content To Wear Stars On Their Brows*. Underwood's painting notably included an unmistakable portrait of Hermione Farthingale, together with an astronaut, a smouldering joint, and a weeping woman (presumably the shoplifter in 'God Knows I'm Good') being comforted by a Pierrot remarkably similar in appearance to the 'Ashes To Ashes' character David would adopt a decade later. Bowie's original sketch for this illustration apparently also included portraits of Kenneth Pitt and Calvin Mark Lee; although neither appeared in the finished picture, the legend "CML33" commemorated 33-year-old Lee's input as layout designer. Pitt, whose relations with Lee were by now mutually hostile, later recalled, "I had had nothing to do with the album's sleeve and when I saw the final product my heart sank."

The album was released in Britain on 14 November 1969. "This has been a good writing period for me and I'm very pleased with the outcome," David told *Disc & Music Echo*. "I just hope everyone else is too." Certainly his interviewer Penny Valentine seemed so, describing the album as "rather doomy and un-nerving, but Bowie's point comes across like a latter-day Dylan. It is an album a lot of people are going to expect a lot from. I don't think they'll be disappointed." *Music Now!* hailed the album as "Deep, thoughtful, probing, exposing, gouging at your innards ... This is more than a record. It is an experience. An expression of life as others see it. The lyrics are full of the grandeur of yesterday, the immediacy of today and the futility of tomorrow. This is well worth

your attention." Others were less impressed. Under the headline "Over ambitious Bowie is a disappointment", *Music Business Weekly* declared that "Bowie seems to be a little unsure of the direction he is going in and has written a collection of numbers ranging from folk through R&B to Indian chant. He is far better at folk – both writing and singing – and should have concentrated on developing this talent. In other words, over ambitious."

This may well be the earliest recorded instance of a syndrome that has dogged Bowie's critical reception throughout his career – the inability of reviewers to discard their entrenched familiarity with his previous musical identity (this critic admits elsewhere in the review that he liked the hit 'Space Oddity' and was hoping for more of the same). Nevertheless this is, by Bowie's standards, an unusually unfocused album. Poised midway between the vaudevillean psychedelia of his debut and the first stirrings of glam on *The Man Who Sold the World*, it presents a folk-rock sensibility, preoccupied chiefly with the fortunes of David's 1969 dalliance with the hippy movement and the misfortunes of his relationship with Hermione Farthingale. The autobiographical element of the lyrics is demonstrably greater than in his earlier work, and while subsequent albums may have addressed deeper, darker areas of David's psyche, few of his songs have ever offered the same air of frank confessional as those on *Space Oddity*. Musically there is every sign that Bowie was still casting about in search of his own voice. Following the Bee Gees pastiche of 'Space Oddity' itself, there are distinct traces of Simon And Garfunkel and even José Feliciano on tracks like 'Letter To Hermione' and 'An Occasional Dream', occasional nods to the ever-present Marc Bolan, and a Beatles-flavoured 'All You Need Is Love'/'Hey Jude' singalong to end 'Memory Of A Free Festival'. In the meandering melodies and classical instrumentation there are hints of the progressive rock movement then enjoying its first flowering, although mercifully the album is devoid of the pomposity and bombast so often associated with the genre. But without doubt the overriding influence is Bob Dylan, echoes of whose early work ring throughout the album's environment of acoustic guitars, harmonica solos and folksy protest lyrics. *Disc & Music Echo*'s Penny Valentine reported that David himself had claimed "he sings like Dylan would have done if he'd been born in England," revealing much about Bowie's perception of himself in pop's stylistic marketplace at the time of the album's release. For his part Kenneth Pitt disliked David's latest affectation, observing later that "Having finally rid himself of the Newley influence, it would be a serious blow if he now faced the charge of being the new Dylan…" When Pitt attempted to broach the subject after hearing the album, David apparently burst into tears and left the room: another wedge had been driven between artist and manager.

Pitt may have had a point, but *Space Oddity* is still a remarkable step forward from anything Bowie had recorded before. Augmented by the excellent playing of Junior's Eyes and the immensely clever orchestrations of Paul Buckmaster and Tony Visconti, Bowie at last sounded like a major artist making a major album. In Radio 2's *Golden Years* documentary in 2000, Bowie described *Space Oddity* as "kind of iffy, in that musically it never really had a direction … I don't think that I, as the artist, had a focus about where it should go." But regardless of his still embryonic musical identity, several tracks – notably 'Unwashed And Somewhat Slightly Dazed', 'Wild Eyed Boy From Freecloud' and the arguable highlight 'Cygnet Committee' – offer the most compelling evidence yet of his burgeoning talent as a lyricist. These are great songs, without doubt the best he had so far written.

Opinions differ as to whether *Space Oddity* deserves recognition as the first essential Bowie album or whether that accolade should be held over for its successor, but certainly the monolithic reputation of its title track does the album more harm than good. 'Space Oddity' is a classic song to be sure, but it's the least representative track on offer here. In this respect Tony Visconti was absolutely right; a novelty hit, however good, was no way to boost the credibility of an album of serious-minded songwriting, particularly at a time when the ascendancy of progressive rock was widening the gulf between the single and album markets.

This was not the only reason for the album's failure to chart; behind the scenes there was a disheartening repeat of David's experiences with Decca. In mid-November 1969, precisely the time of the single's chart peak and the album's release, the management of Philips Records underwent a major staff shake-up, losing Bowie some of his key supporters within the company and, so Pitt believed, adversely affecting the album's promotion. Alongside the mismanagement of November's showcase concert at the Purcell Room (see Chapter 3), this was a serious blow at a time when David's profile should have been significantly

raised. Nonetheless 1969 ended with a few crumbs of comfort: Bowie found himself voted the year's Best Newcomer in a readers' poll for *Music Now!*, and the ever-supportive Penny Valentine of *Disc & Music Echo* named 'Space Oddity' her record of the year. All the same, by March 1970 the album had sold a meagre 5025 copies in Britain.

The story was even bleaker in America, where Mercury's Ron Oberman was a lone voice attempting to champion a hit single that never came. The album had its US release in February 1970, but sales were minimal and reviews few and far between. *Zygote* commended 'Space Oddity' and 'Memory Of A Free Festival' (indeed, it was the latter's widely favourable reception in America that resulted in the recording of a single version), but complained that the rest of the album suffered from "a lack of flow" and was "very awkward to the ear", finding fault with Bowie's "reliance on big productions" and "his repetitious use of Bo Diddley syncopation" (an unusual criticism, as only 'Unwashed And Somewhat Slightly Dazed' and at a stretch 'God Knows I'm Good' could really be accused of such a thing). The review concluded that "Bowie is erratic. When he succeeds, he's excellent; when he fails, he's laborious." A year later Nancy Erlich of the *New York Times* would discover the album and praise it as "a good collection of rock material full in its variety, melodically interesting, flawlessly and interestingly arranged and produced," appreciating the lyrics for their "almost endless layers of meaning". But this was too little too late. Bowie had yet to make any impact in America.

While the original UK release was called *David Bowie*, the American version (which featured slightly different sleeve artwork) was re-titled *Man Of Words/Man Of Music*. In 1972, as part of RCA's repackaging of Bowie in the wake of *Ziggy Stardust*, the album was re-released as *Space Oddity*, the title by which it has since become known (in Spain RCA called it *Odisea Espacial* – "Space Odyssey"). This version featured new front and rear sleeve photography shot at Haddon Hall in 1972 by Mick Rock, and boasted some breathtakingly pretentious sleeve notes, erroneously claiming that the title track was recorded in 1968 before going on to explain that the album "was NOW then, and it is still now NOW: personal and universal, perhaps galactic, microcosmic and macrocosmic." The third track, the studio horseplay of 'Don't Sit Down', was removed from the 1972 version and remained absent until Rykodisc's 1990 reissue, whose packaging included a reproduction of the original US artwork. To confuse matters still further, EMI's 1999 reissue restored the original UK artwork to the front cover, but retained the title *Space Oddity*.

THE MAN WHO SOLD THE WORLD
Mercury 6338 041, April 1971
RCA Victor LSP 4816, November 1972 [26]
RCA International NL 84654, November 1984
EMI EMC 3573, April 1990 [66]
EMI 7243 5219010, September 1999

'The Width Of A Circle' (8'05") / 'All The Madmen' (5'38") / 'Black Country Rock' (3'32") / 'After All' (3'51") / 'Running Gun Blues' (3'11") / 'Saviour Machine' (4'25") / 'She Shook Me Cold' (4'13") / 'The Man Who Sold The World' (3'55") / 'The Supermen' (3'38")

Bonus tracks on 1990 reissue: 'Lightning Frightening' (3'38") / 'Holy Holy' (2'20") / 'Moonage Daydream' (3'52") / 'Hang On To Yourself' (2'51")

• *Musicians:* David Bowie *(vocals, guitar)*, Mick Ronson *(guitar)*, Tony Visconti *(bass)*, Mick Woodmansey *(drums)*, Ralph Mace *(synthesizer)* • *Recorded:* Trident & Advision Studios, London • *Producer:* Tony Visconti

When *The Man Who Sold the World* began recording at Trident Studios in April 1970, David Bowie was in the middle of a period of unprecedented professional and personal upheaval. The attention brought to him by the previous year's hit 'Space Oddity' had died down and the follow-up, 'The Prettiest Star', had flopped. The three members of his new outfit Hype were now living at Haddon Hall, where another regular visitor was his half-brother Terry Burns. Although now a voluntary resident at Cane Hill Hospital in south London, Terry would stay at Haddon Hall for up to four weeks at a time during the early part of 1970. Meanwhile David's professional relationship with his manager Kenneth Pitt was rapidly deteriorating, and with the ascendancy of Angela Barnett and Mick Ronson (see "Hype" in Chapter 3), change hung heavy in the air.

In an interview for *Disc & Music Echo* in February 1970, Bowie had intimated that a new long-player was on the way. "The next album will be more solid," he promised. "As the first side will be completely augmented it means specially writing a whole set of new material. The second side will be just me with guitar." The album that eventually appeared bore no resemblance to such a pattern, but it's interesting to note that the live BBC session recorded on 5 February did: Bowie played the first four numbers on acoustic guitar and was then joined by the electric band for the remainder of the performance.

During February and March Tony Visconti and Mick Ronson constructed a makeshift studio beneath the stairwell at Haddon Hall, and it was here that Bowie would demo much of his early 1970s material. "We wrote the original stuff for *The Man* in that little room under the stairs," he confirmed many years later. In mid-April, just prior to the commencement of the album sessions, Hype convened at Advision Studios in Gosfield Street to record the single version of 'Memory Of A Free Festival'. It was to be drummer John Cambridge's final Bowie credit.

Work on the record that would become *The Man Who Sold The World* began at Trident at 1.00am on 18 April 1970, continuing on and off until 1 May. Thereafter the sessions moved to Advision from 12-22 May.

Tony Visconti, who played bass on the album as well as producing it, says that *The Man Who Sold the World* was intended to be "our *Sgt Pepper* – anything goes, no matter how far-fetched." However, Visconti would soon discover that the majority of the sessions would be spent trying to coax the newly-wed David out of his apparent apathy for the project. "This man would just not get out of bed and write a song," said Visconti later. "…we just laid down the chords, the arrangement, the guitar solos, the synthesizers, and David would be out in the lobby of Advision holding hands with Angie and going coochie-coochie-coo … we had about three days left and I said, 'David, you're going to have to throw some lyrics on these songs, and vocals … I was totally infuriated with him that I had to work so close to the deadline and of course we had hardly any time left to mix that album. David wasn't around for most of the mixes, either. He came up with a lot of clever bits, like the little talking section in the middle of 'All the Madmen', but really the album was me and Mick Ronson. David just wasn't there."

Strong words and, perhaps, not entirely fair: 'The Width of a Circle' and 'The Supermen', to name two, were certainly in existence before the sessions began, as was the basic melody of 'Black Country Rock'. Visconti and Ronson may have dominated the arrangements and mixes, but Bowie's role in the actual songwriting is not in question: "I really did object to the impression given in some articles that I did not write the songs on *The Man Who Sold The World*," he said in 1998. "You only have to check out the chord changes. *No-one* writes chord changes like that."

John Cambridge's involvement in the album was short-lived: he was sacked early in the sessions after having difficulties with the percussion part in 'The Supermen', and receives no credit on the finished record. "John was ousted at Ronno's request," says Visconti. "Little by little, Ronno replaced the group with other mates from Hull." Cambridge was replaced by Mick "Woody" Woodmansey, another member of Ronson's former band The Rats. "Mick was a very fundamental drummer," Bowie recalled many years later. "He was quite open to direction and in a way sort of carried out what I wanted done much more than most of the other drummers I've worked with. His strengths definitely were in the area of British rock and British rhythm & blues."

The group swelled to five with the arrival of keyboardist Ralph Mace, a Philips executive who had become the label's Bowie man at the time of January's 'Prettiest Star' session. "Ralph was a virtuoso and a dear, supportive friend," says Visconti. "He worked in the classical department and was about 45 at the time. He looked very straight, with short hair and business suits, but what a lovely soul and concern he had for our music!" Mace, whose keyboard contributions would prove crucial to some of the album's more unsettling moments, described the sessions as "a creative build-up, a synthesis", and disagreed with Visconti's account of Bowie's approach to the sessions. "David would bounce ideas off people," he told the Gillmans. "I thought that David knew what he wanted and what he didn't. There was often a grey area in between when he was searching, but when he was right he knew."

Although it has its quieter moments, the hard-rock arrangements and unrestrained guitar heroics on *The Man Who Sold The World* make it unquestionably Bowie's "heaviest" album until *Tin Machine*, and stylistically something of an aberration between the predominantly acoustic sensibilities of the two albums on either side of it. This turn of events can be laid largely at the door of Mick Ronson. "Mick's idols were Cream," said Visconti. "He coached Woody to play like Ginger Baker and me to play like Jack Bruce. David was loving the sound of his new band."

Speaking in 1976, Bowie described the making of *The Man Who Sold the World* as "a nightmare", also calling it "the most drug-oriented album I've made", and adding that it was recorded "when I was the most fucked up" and "holding onto some kind of flag for hashish". Curiously, neither Visconti nor anyone else interviewed about this period recalls David taking drugs at the time, and bearing in mind that Bowie's comments were made at the depth of his coke-addled Thin White Duke phase – a period when he was far more evidently "fucked up" than in 1970 – they should be taken with a pinch of salt. More lucidly, David once explained that "With *The Man Who Sold the World* I wanted to work in some kind of strange micro-world where the human element had been taken out, where we were dealing with a technological society. That world [was] an experimental playground where you could do dangerous things without anybody taking too many risks, other than ideas risks." On another occasion he described the album's content as "very telling for me – it was all family problems and analogies, put into science-fiction form."

Even those with little stomach for prurient theorizing tend to agree that this album covers what, by Bowie's standards, is highly intimate territory. Although the lyrics are less straightforwardly autobiographical than those on the *Space Oddity* album, there is an unsettling darkness about the material which appears to proceed from the darkening of David's personal world over the previous year. The death of his father, his disillusion with the Beckenham Arts Lab hippies, the souring of some close friendships, and above all the continuing deterioration of his half-brother's mental health, are manifested on *The Man Who Sold The World* in a series of sinister excursions into a netherworld of paranoia, manic depression, quasi-religious ecstasy, violent homoeroticism and schizoid hallucination. In 1999 he explained that "I'd been seeing quite a bit of my half-brother during that period, and I think a lot of it, obviously, had been working on me … I think his shadow is on quite a lot of the material in a way … knowing about the fragility of mental stability in my family generally, on my mother's side particularly, I think I was going through an awful lot of concern about exactly what my mental condition was, and where it may lead."

Notwithstanding the "science-fiction" remark, part of what makes these songs so disturbing is that they are largely devoid of the glitzy sci-fi sheen which renders *Ziggy Stardust* or even *Diamond Dogs* almost cosy by comparison. Few Bowie songs are scarier than 'All The Madmen', 'After All' or the title track itself. Nor can 'Saviour Machine' or 'The Supermen' be dismissed as mere comic-strip, tunnelling as they do into a darkly Nietzschean cavern of the subconscious. Bowie had been reading the German philosopher in early 1970, and the introduction of Nietzsche into his customary environment of subverted fairytale and self-lacerating introspection results in some uncomfortably intimate confrontations with what David later described as the "devils and angels" within himself. He would certainly have been aware not only of Nietzsche's proposals about the affirmation of the Superman and the doctrine of power, but also that the philosopher himself had died virtually insane.

The "devils and angels" remark exposes another *leitmotif*, surely connected with the album's title. Many of the songs include variants on a central image of the narrator climbing to a high vantage-point and undergoing an unexpected, disturbing or, in the case of 'Black Country Rock', "crazy" experience. The same thing happens, in one form or another, in 'All The Madmen' ("It's pointless to be high"), 'The Width Of A Circle' ("He struck the ground, a cavern appeared"), 'She Shook Me Cold' ("We met upon a hill"), 'The Supermen' ("mountain magic"), and the title track itself ("We passed upon the stair"). The common link is surely the key Gospel passage in which Christ is tempted by the Devil into becoming, in effect, the man who sold the world: "The Devil taketh him up into an exceeding high mountain, and showeth him all the kingdoms of the world, and the glory of them; and saith unto him, All these things will I give thee, if thou wilt fall down and worship me. Then said Jesus unto him, Get thee hence, Satan." (Matthew 4: 8-10). There can be little doubt that in 1970 Bowie's own inner demons were battling it out on just such an apocalyptic plane.

During the break between the Trident and Advision sessions came a pivotal moment in Bowie's career. Unhappy with the direction in which Kenneth Pitt was attempting to steer his work but anxious not to destroy a close friendship, Bowie had already sought the advice of Olav Wyper, the General Manager at Philips Records. Unwilling to intervene between an artist and his manager, Wyper had referred David to a legal firm in Cavendish Square. On 7 May Bowie arrived for a meeting at Pitt's flat

accompanied by a young litigation clerk called Tony Defries who, according to Pitt's account, proceeded to do all the talking while David sat silently on the chaise longue. Pitt agreed to dissolve forthwith any professional obligations between himself and David. The pair parted amicably if sadly, and not long afterwards Tony Defries resigned his job to become Bowie's full-time manager. David's final commitment to Pitt was his appearance at the Ivor Novello Awards on 10 May. Two days later he was at Advision, working once again on his album.

It was an episode of the utmost significance. In retrospect the difference in business practice between the prudent, old-school Pitt and the hard-boiled huckster Defries could not have been more acute. They remain two of the most influential figures in Bowie's story, and despite the fact that each tended to polarize the opinions of contemporary eyewitnesses, from the point of view of David's career there was good and bad in both. It's extremely doubtful whether Pitt's cautious approach would ever have broken America or launched Bowie as a global superstar, let alone do so with such spectacular results as those later achieved by the machinations and methods of Defries. Furthermore, Defries brought with him the kind of resources that had previously been unavailable to David. Over the years Pitt had staked a considerable personal investment in his client, but the amounts involved were negligible by comparison with the funds made available by Defries's colleague Laurence Myers, who had recently formed a management company called Gem Productions (which also took The New Seekers and Gary Glitter onto its books in 1970). Gem would under-write most of the expenses incurred over the next couple of years, until Bowie's success led to the formation in 1972 of MainMan, Defries's business empire.

Countless facts, figures and contradictory quotes about Tony Defries have filled the middle chapters of many a Bowie biography, but they are not the subject of the present book. It is sufficient to say that the contractual small-print of MainMan's financial dealings and the profligate insanity of the 1972-1975 period, which under Defries's stage-management were part and parcel of what made Bowie a star, also ensured that individuals other than David banked the lion's share of his earnings until the beginning of the 1980s – by which time Defries himself had long since been ousted under far more acrimonious circumstances than those attending Pitt's departure. But all this lay far in the future; for the time being Defries, like Angela, provided essential support, strategies and resources. As Tony Visconti has since suggested, "Angie and Defries are often maligned by critics and cronies of David, but without their constant support and input, there would never have been a Ziggy, or an Aladdin, or a future Bowie for that matter."

In the last days of his professional association with Bowie, Kenneth Pitt had drawn up ambitious plans to approach a major artist to design the new album sleeve, his shortlist including Andy Warhol, David Hockney and Patrick Procktor. These plans came to nothing, but it seems likely that Pitt's intentions influenced Bowie's first choice of sleeve design. It is commonly believed that the original sleeve was the famous photo of Bowie in a dress, but this appears not to be the case. David initially asked Mike Weller, a familiar face at the Beckenham Arts Lab whose work echoed the pop-art style of the likes of Warhol and Roy Lichtenstein, to design a cover reflecting the album's ominous atmosphere. Weller proposed a painting of Cane Hill Hospital, where a friend of his was a patient – apparently he was unaware that it was also where Terry Burns lived – and Bowie received the idea enthusiastically. Weller's cartoon design, which he entitled "Metrobolist" (after Fritz Lang's *Metropolis*), featured a gloomy rendition of Cane Hill's main entrance block with a shattered clock-tower. In the foreground stood a cowboy figure copied from a photograph of John Wayne, carrying a rifle in reference to 'Running Gun Blues'. At Bowie's suggestion, Weller added his "exploding head" trademark, a device he had previously used on his posters for the Arts Lab, so that fragments of the cowboy's ten-gallon hat were seen breaking away from his head. The speech-bubble, later blanked out by Mercury, apparently contained a pun on "arms" encapsulating references to guns, drug-taking and record-players.

Weller tells the Gillmans that David was "very pleased" with the finished design, but it appears that not long afterwards Bowie changed his mind and persuaded Philips's art department to commission Keith Macmillan to photograph him instead in the "domestic environment" of the Haddon Hall living-room. For this celebrated photo-session, Bowie reclined on a chaise longue in a cream and blue satin dress – a man's dress, he later explained – purchased from the Mr Fish boutique. With one hand dropping the last of a scattered pack of playing cards and the other toying

effeminately with his wavy locks (by now his 'Space Oddity' perm was growing out in favour of a luxuriant post-hippy style), he resembled nothing so much as Lauren Bacall in her prime. He later explained that the photo, overlaid with a canvas texture, was intended to mimic the style of the Pre-Raphaelite painter Dante Gabriel Rossetti. At the time it was a deeply provocative image, and the most brazen enactment of gender-confusion Bowie had yet undertaken.

In America, Mercury had already given the go-ahead for the printing of the "cartoon" sleeve and, much to Bowie's displeasure, the "dress" cover was only used in the UK. It should be added that some sources, including Angela Bowie, dispute this account and insist that the cartoon artwork was only commissioned *after* a shocked Mercury refused to release the "dress" cover in America. However, bearing in mind that the American album preceded the UK release by a matter of five months, and that Angela Bowie claims elsewhere in her book that the idea for Ziggy Stardust's hair colour in 1972 came from David's collaboration with Lulu two years later, her grasp of chronology is to be approached with extreme caution. It's certain, however, that Bowie's initial enthusiasm for the cartoon cover had evaporated. The Gillmans produce a witness from Bowie's early American fan base who was told by David in 1972 that the cartoon sleeve was "horrible … I don't know what that cover was all about." With splendid contradiction, Bowie said in 1999 that "I actually thought the cartoon cover was really cool … for me it had lots of personal resonance about it."

When RCA reissued *The Man Who Sold The World* in 1972 both countries replaced the sleeve with a black and white shot by Brian Ward, showing David performing a high kick in his early Ziggy gear. Like the same year's reissue of *Space Oddity*, the RCA version came with a set of breathlessly polysyllabic sleeve notes informing the listener that Bowie's music was "Neither metaphor nor analogue … Phantasmagoria is its reality; the preternatural its unsettling truth." The "kick" photo remained the album's official sleeve until the 1990 reissue reinstated the "dress" picture and obligingly included the various alternative covers in its packaging, including the artwork for the original German release, which was again entirely different: a curious Pythonesque cartoon of a winged Bowie on the front, and an androgynous beret-wearing portrait on the back. Most recently, the booklet of EMI's 1999 reissue included further shots from the "dress" photo-session.

The American version of *The Man Who Sold The World* was released in November 1970, while in Britain it didn't appear until April 1971, almost a year after the sessions themselves. Although nowhere a huge success on its initial release, it sold better in America than in Britain, benefiting from an energetic publicity push by Mercury whose American head of A&R, Robin McBride, gushed over the album as an "extraordinary creation in rock music". Its critical success even led to a promotional tour in February 1971 – Bowie's first trip to America, where the reviews eclipsed anything written about *The Man Who Sold The World* in Britain. In the *Los Angeles Free Press*, Chris Van Ness declared that "What happens to a flower-child, when all of the world around him is going slightly crazy and power struggles are taking over everything, including his music, is that he harnesses his genius, conforms to the insanity, outpowers the loudest group around, and does it all just a little better than anybody else ... There is a fine edge of madness that runs throughout the album ... The concepts of the title song, 'The Supermen' or 'Saviour Machine' are not your normal song themes, but then David Bowie is not your normal writer." *Rolling Stone* found the album "uniformly excellent" and "an experience that is as intriguing as it is chilling, but only to a listener sufficiently together to withstand its schizophrenia ... Tony Visconti's use of echo, phasing and other techniques on Bowie's voice to achieve a weird and supernatural tone ... serves to reinforce the jaggedness of Bowie's words and music, the latter played in an intimidatingly heavy fashion by an occasionally brilliant quartet guided by Visconti's own maniacally sliding bass".

Accounting for the album's American success in a 1971 interview for *Disc & Music Echo*, Bowie explained, "For one thing it got massive airplay, and I suppose in a way it's more palatable than things I've done in the past because of its heavy backing. It's not that I have a very strong feeling for heavy music – I don't. In fact I think it's fairly primitive as a music form. I look for sensation rather than quality, and heavy music seems to be full of musicians who have quality rather than musicians who for some reasons can chill your spine." This sounds suspiciously as though Bowie was already distancing himself from the album's intermittent Led Zeppelin pretensions; certainly when he re-entered the studio a few months later to record *Hunky Dory*, the results were noticeably

more acoustic and, in places, even more spine-chilling.

Reports of *The Man Who Sold The World*'s American success should not be exaggerated, however. By the end of June 1971 a mere 1395 copies had been sold in the US, and the story of "massive" American sales in the run-up to the UK release smacks more of hype than of accuracy. Michael Watts was exaggerating wildly in both directions when he commented in *Melody Maker* in January 1972 that *The Man Who Sold the World* had cleared 50,000 copies in the States and about five in Britain, "and Bowie bought them." But sales of the first UK release were indeed disastrous, and as a result the British "dress" sleeve is now a real collector's item, fetching around £200, while the ultra-rare German sleeve can command considerably more.

Despite its poor sales, *The Man Who Sold The World* garnered decent reviews in Britain. *Melody Maker* called it "a surprisingly excellent album" with "some tremendous flashes of brilliance" among the "inventive and unusual" writing. The *NME* found "a bit of horror in 'All The Madmen', some quiet folk on 'After All', and much drive in 'The Width Of A Circle'", but considered the overall tone "rather hysterical".

By the time the album was released in Britain, Bowie had shaken off a year of comparative lethargy and was demoing new material at a breakneck pace. Tony Visconti, however, disliked Tony Defries and had had enough of David's "poor attitude and complete disregard for his music". He had quit at the end of the *Man Who Sold The World* sessions and transferred his energies into producing the early successes of David's friendly rival Marc Bolan. Visconti didn't see Bowie again for three years, but would later return to collaborate on some of his finest albums.

On the eve of Bolan's success, Visconti oversaw a fascinating interlude which would prove crucial to Bowie's future. Keeping alive the name Hype from Bowie's pre-*Man Who Sold The World* live outfit, Visconti enlisted The Rats' vocalist Benny Marshall, who joined the trio of Ronson, Visconti and Woodmansey to record new material for the Vertigo label in November 1970. Re-named Ronno, the band released a solitary single called 'Fourth Hour Of My Sleep'. Although material for a proposed Ronno album was beginning to accumulate, Visconti's duties in the Bolan camp soon forced him to bow out. His replacement on bass was Trevor Bolder, yet another Hull acquaintance of Ronson's. "We were in rival bands," Bolder later explained. "I was playing Muddy Waters-type R&B in the Chicago Star Blues Band, while The Rats were closer to The Yardbirds or even Cream." Thus it was that by the spring of 1971 there existed a four-piece band that was effectively Benny Marshall and The Spiders From Mars. Marshall, however, was not destined to front the group for long; in May 1971, a year after the dissolution of the *Man Who Sold The World* sessions, Ronson received a telephone call from Bowie that would provide the springboard for everything that was to follow.

Meanwhile *The Man Who Sold The World* went on to belie its initially indifferent reception to become one of the most highly regarded of all Bowie's albums. Artists as diverse as Kurt Cobain and Boy George have cited *The Man Who Sold The World* as a major influence. "It wasn't until years later that it was recognized for its forward-thinking sound and songwriting concepts," says Tony Visconti, who has described it as "almost a textbook in how to make an alternative album" and often cites it alongside *Scary Monsters* as his joint favourite Bowie collaboration. Viewing *The Man Who Sold The World* dispassionately one might argue that the fine balance had yet to be perfected, and that the hard-rock leanings just occasionally topple over into self-indulgence – but in the face of the album's panoramic sweep, and the sheer quality of its finest moments, this is a minor consideration. When all is said and done, *The Man Who Sold The World* is one of the best and most important albums in the history of rock music.

HUNKY DORY

RCA Victor SF 8244, December 1971 [3]
RCA International INTS 5064, January 1981 [32]
RCA BOPIC 2, April 1984
RCA International NL 83844, November 1984
EMI EMC 3572, April 1990 [39]
EMI 7243 5218990, September 1999 [39]

'Changes' (3'33") / 'Oh! You Pretty Things' (3'12") / 'Eight Line Poem' (2'53") / 'Life on Mars?' (3'48") / 'Kooks' (2'49") / 'Quicksand' (5'03") / 'Fill Your Heart' (3'07") / 'Andy Warhol' (3'58") / 'Song For Bob Dylan' (4'12") / 'Queen Bitch' (3'13") / 'The Bewlay Brothers' (5'21")

Bonus tracks on 1990 reissue: 'Bombers' (2'38") / 'The Supermen (Alternate Version)' (2'41") / 'Quicksand

(Demo Version)' (4'43") / 'The Bewlay Brothers (AlternateMix)' (5'19")

• *Musicians:* David Bowie *(vocals, guitar, saxophone, piano)*, Mick Ronson *(guitar)*, Trevor Bolder *(bass, trumpets)*, Mick Woodmansey *(drums)*, Rick Wakeman *(piano)* • *Recorded:* Trident Studios, London • *Producers:* Ken Scott, David Bowie

Following the completion of *The Man Who Sold The World* in May 1970, Bowie's activities both on stage and in the studio slowed to a virtual standstill for nearly a year. There were a number of practical reasons for this, not least the series of contractual challenges confronting David's new manager Tony Defries. In mid-1970 Bowie was without a publishing contract. His deal with Essex Music had expired the previous June, and Kenneth Pitt had rejected a renewal offer as unacceptably low. In October 1970 Defries negotiated a publishing deal with Chrysalis, then a young company whose major signings were Jethro Tull and Ten Years After. Impressed by David's new recording 'Holy Holy' (produced by Herbie Flowers at Trident in June 1970) and seduced by Defries's grandiose assurances, Chrysalis agreed to a fifty-fifty royalty split and a shockingly generous upfront payment of £5000. The interpretation of an additional royalty clause would later be disputed by Chrysalis, leading to lawsuits with both Defries and Essex Music in 1973. Like Defries's ongoing financial dispute with Kenneth Pitt, these were just some of the aggravations that would dog the endlessly litigious MainMan years.

Meanwhile, Bowie had been channelling his energies into a period of intensive songwriting. Bob Grace, the Chrysalis partner who had courted him on the strength of 'Holy Holy', hired Radio Luxembourg's London studios for the recording of Bowie's new demos. It was here that David – sometimes alone, sometimes with friends – essayed much of the material that would eventually find its way onto *Hunky Dory*. Angela Bowie attests that by the end of 1970 David's songwriting had undergone a development which would infuse the flavour of the new album: he was now composing not on acoustic guitar, but on the piano. One of the demos recorded around December was 'Oh! You Pretty Things', enthusiastically seized by Bob Grace and farmed out to Peter Noone, who made it a hit the following spring.

After his promotional tour of America in February 1971, David returned to Haddon Hall and Radio

Luxembourg, where he churned out new demos with insatiable speed. Among those providing instrumental backings during these sessions was a group of schoolboys from Dulwich College who called themselves Runk. It was with these musicians (guitarist Mark Carr Pritchard, bassist Polak de Somogyl and drummer Ralph St Laurent Broadbent) that David recorded early versions of 'Moonage Daydream' and 'Hang On To Yourself'. Bob Grace proposed releasing the tracks as a single to recoup some of the costs of the demo sessions, and in order to bypass David's Mercury contract it was decided to do so under an assumed name. Thus it was that Runk were re-named Arnold Corns – apparently after David's favourite Pink Floyd song 'Arnold Layne' – and the single was released on B&C Records in May.

Although the Arnold Corns project made no commercial impact it gave Bowie the chance to indulge in a spot of Warholian star-manufacture. Freddi Burretti (real name Frederick Burrett) was a flamboyant, openly gay 19-year-old fashion designer whom David had met at the Sombrero, then London's trendiest gay nightclub. Burretti, who was now providing David and Angela with some of their extravagant apparel, was re-styled "Rudi Valentino" and presented as the group's lead singer, even though he hadn't even been present at the sessions. "I believe that the Rolling Stones are finished and that Arnold Corns will be the next Stones," Bowie declared preposterously. In an interview for *Curious* magazine "Rudi" camped it up in a manner that made Bowie's subsequent gay revelations seem positively tame. "On Saturday I was very stoned and I dressed up like a little boy and looked quite cute," he declared, going on to add that "I always wear just my own hair and just a little make-up." His pet hates were apparently "spots, snobs, closet queens and big mouths," and he intimated that a full-length album entitled *Looking For Rudi* was on the way. In fact the Arnold Corns project went no further than two more tracks recorded in June, 'Looking For A Friend' and 'Man In The Middle', on which Burretti did sing alongside contributions from the *Hunky Dory* band; but these were shelved and only released in the wake of Bowie's fame.

At around the same time, Bowie was working in the studio with another of Burretti's circle, a male prostitute called Mickey King who took lead vocal on the infamous out-take 'Rupert The Riley', recorded in April 1971. Shortly afterwards David began writing songs for his old friend Dana Gillespie, who had been

introduced to Tony Defries and was hoping to launch a singing career.

Some Bowie chroniclers have found it inexplicable that these excursions into anonymity should have coincided with the preparation of an album as strong and definitive as *Hunky Dory*. Others have suggested that Bowie's assumption of the role of starmaker was nothing more than a narcissistic attempt to emulate the methods of his idol *du jour* Andy Warhol without appreciating that he'd need to be a celebrity himself before such a scheme was likely to work. But there was another, more significant reason for David to hide behind flimsy pseudonyms while he honed his new material: Tony Defries was adamant that Mercury would never release another David Bowie record.

David's contract with Mercury was due to expire in June 1971, but the company had every intention of taking up its renewal option and was even planning to offer David improved terms. In May, however, Tony Defries informed the company's representative Robin McBride – who had flown to London from Chicago specifically to offer a new three-year deal – that "under no circumstances would David record another note for Mercury." McBride tells the Gillmans that Defries went on to explain that if Mercury pursued their renewal option and insisted on a new album, "we will deliver the biggest piece of crap you have ever had. That's not a direct quote. But that's pretty much what he said." In theory, Mercury could have called this bluff; in practice, they agreed to terminate David's contract. Through Gem Productions Defries paid off David's outstanding debts to Mercury, who in turn surrendered their copyright on the previous two albums.

While Defries pursued another, better record deal, David prepared to take his new material into the studio. Several of the musicians who had dropped in and out of the Haddon Hall circle over the preceding months were considered for the forthcoming sessions. Arnold Corns guitarist Mark Carr Pritchard was one; *Space Oddity* drummer Terry Cox was another, as was David's former Turquoise colleague Tony Hill. However, by May 1971 David had arrived at the conclusion that there was one colleague he could not do without. He telephoned Mick Ronson.

Since the end of the *Man Who Sold The World* sessions and the short-lived attempt to continue under the name Ronno, Mick Ronson had returned to Hull and, he later revealed, sunk into a deep depression. Now Bowie asked him to return to London, bringing with him Woody Woodmansey and a bassist to replace Tony Visconti. Some sources suggest that Ronson's first choice was his former King Bees colleague Rick Kemp, with whom he had played on Michael Chapman's *Fully Qualified Survivor*, but if this was ever a serious proposition it didn't last long: according to some reports Defries vetoed Kemp on the grounds of his receding hairline. Kemp instead joined the emerging folk-rock outfit Steeleye Span, and in his place came Ronno bassist Trevor Bolder.

The three musicians moved into Haddon Hall to rehearse David's new material. Led by Ronson, they also assisted David on the recording of tracks by Dana Gillespie at Trident, including 'Mother, Don't Be Frightened' and the original 'Andy Warhol'. Meanwhile Bowie elected to exploit his forthcoming 3 June BBC session as a showcase for his growing circle of performers and a clutch of new songs, one of them freshly composed to commemorate the birth of his son on 30 May (see Chapter 4). A few days after David's appearance at Glastonbury Fayre on 23 June, the band decamped to Trident to begin recording the new album.

The title *Hunky Dory*, which had been revealed at the BBC gig (almost uniquely: Bowie usually leaves the naming of his albums until the last minute), was suggested by Bob Grace of Chrysalis, who tells the Gillmans of an ex-RAF pub landlord he knew in Esher, "one of those classic Battle of Britain types" whose vocabulary was peppered with upper-crust jargon "…like 'prang' and 'whizzo'; another was 'everything's hunky-dory'. I told David and he loved it."

In the absence of Tony Visconti David recruited Ken Scott, the studio engineer on his Mercury albums, to produce and mix the sessions. Scott had recently completed work on George Harrison's *All Things Must Pass*, whose acoustic textures were not far removed from the eventual sound of *Hunky Dory*. The first hint of a co-production credit for David himself would be manifested in the sleeve-note "assisted by the actor". Meanwhile Visconti's arranging role was taken over by Bowie and Ronson who, together with Bob Grace, shortlisted the tracks one night at Ken Scott's house. Among the rejected demos were 'How Lucky You Are' and 'Right On Mother' (although the latter was recorded the same year by Peter Noone), while others, like 'Bombers' and 'It Ain't Easy', would be recorded at Trident but dropped from the final album.

Bowie is understood to have taken an active interest in the sound of his new recordings which could not have presented a greater contrast with his attitude during the previous album's sessions. A late addition to the studio band was pianist Rick Wakeman, who had won acclaim since his work on 'Space Oddity' as the player who had transformed The Strawbs into a major chart proposition. "He invited me round to his flat in Beckenham, which I used to call Beckenham Palace," recounted Wakeman later. "He told me to make as many notes as I wanted. The songs were unbelievable – 'Changes', 'Life On Mars?', one after the other. He said he wanted to come at the album from a different angle, that he wanted them to be based around the piano. So he told me to play them as I would a piano piece, and that he'd then adapt everything else around that. And that's what happened. We went into the studio and I had total freedom to do whatever I liked throughout the album. Everyone literally played around what I was playing. I still rate it as the finest collection of songs on one album."

The Trident sessions began with a serious hiccup, when it transpired that certain band members had failed to learn the songs. As Wakeman recalled on Radio 2's *Golden Years* documentary, David was forced to call a halt: "He said, you've had good rehearsal facilities, you're being paid, this is a wonderful opportunity – and you haven't learned them. He said, you can pack your stuff up, go and practise them, and we'll come back in the studio when you've learned them … if you want to go back and be a small band up in Hull or whatever, that's fine." When the sessions reconvened a week or two later, Wakeman recalled, "the band were hot! They were so good, and the tracks just flowed through."

The actual piano played by Wakeman on *Hunky Dory* (and later by Mick Ronson on *Ziggy Stardust*) was a celebrity in itself: it was the same instrument used for The Beatles' 'Hey Jude' and many of the early albums by Elton John and Harry Nilsson. Under Wakeman's tutelage, Bowie and Ronson deferred to the piano-led nature of the compositions in a predominantly acoustic set of arrangements from which the only major deviations were the Lou Reed guitar pastiche of 'Queen Bitch' and the plangent electric solo on 'Song For Bob Dylan'. But Mick Ronson's talents were by no means being suppressed; in place of the heavyweight guitar workouts he had brought to *The Man Who Sold The World*, he was now showing the mettle of his classical training with sumptuous string orchestrations on tracks like 'Fill Your Heart', 'Life On

Mars?' and 'Quicksand'. Ken Scott was besotted by Ronson's ability, not only as a guitarist ("he was better than any of The Beatles") but as an instinctively talented arranger: "he didn't really know what he was supposed to do, so he was much freer."

Recording continued through July. In August Defries arranged the pressing of 500 promo discs ("with my stuff on one side and some of David's songs on the other," recalled Dana Gillespie later) to use as bait for record companies. This now ultra-rare promo (BOWPROMO 1A-1/1B-1) included 'Oh! You Pretty Things', 'It Ain't Easy', 'Queen Bitch', 'Quicksand' and – of particular interest to collectors – early mixes of 'Bombers' and 'Kooks', a different vocal take of 'Eight Line Poem', and a shorter early mix of Dana Gillespie's 'Andy Warhol'. In August, while Ken Scott mixed the album, Tony Defries flew to New York with some of the new recordings. Within days he had secured a deal with RCA, whose head of A&R, Dennis Katz, was "knocked out" by the material: "It was theatrical, musical, the songs were excellent, there was real poetry, it seemed to have everything," he told the Gillmans. Defries accepted Katz's offer of $37,500 per album, a major improvement on Bowie's fortunes but small beer by the standards of RCA, who were accustomed to paying their artists well into six figures per album. In subsequent years Defries would manœuvre the terms of the deal to his greater favour, and it has been speculated that he initially favoured RCA as Bowie's label because of its reputation for the kind of internecine strife that allowed quick-witted operators to manipulate its executives. David needed little persuasion that Elvis Presley's label was his natural home, and Defries, who made no secret of his admiration for the methods of Presley's notorious manager Colonel Tom Parker, was no less entranced by the idea.

It was during the latter stages of the *Hunky Dory* sessions that another crucial element of Bowie's future career fell into place. A *succès de scandale* on London's theatre scene in the summer of 1971 was an imported American production called *Pork* which played at the Roundhouse (the scene of Hype's coming-out party a year earlier) for 26 nights from 2 August. Adapted from Andy Warhol's collection of taped conversations with the New York *demi-monde*, *Pork* was presented by the LaMaMa Experimental Theatre Company who, under the direction of Tony Ingrassia and his assistant Leee Black Childers, constituted a Warholian freakshow of the first order. There

was Wayne (later Jayne) County, a transvestite who played a character called Vulva, obsessed with different kinds of excrement; the huge-breasted Geri Miller, who gave herself a douche on stage; the similarly endowed Cherry Vanilla, who played the title role (based on Warhol's superstar Brigid Polk); and Tony "Zee" Zanetta, who held court as Warhol himself, a voyeur who dressed his friends up just for show. To a British theatre released only three years earlier from the Lord Chamberlain's censorship restrictions, *Pork's* parade of masturbation, homosexuality, drugs and abortion offered a thrilling onslaught of bad taste. Predictably, the production was granted acres of free publicity by the affronted splutterings of the press. The *News Of The World* obligingly announced that it made *Hair* and *Oh! Calcutta* look like the proverbial "vicar's tea party", while the *Times* judged it "repellently narcissistic … a witless, invertebrate, mind-numbing farrago". The *Daily Telegraph* declared that "It's nude, it's crude and it's a heap of rubbish." Wayne County later recalled that "…there was someone else who said '*Pork* is nothing but a pigsty. *Pork* is nothing but nymphomaniacs, whores and prostitutes running around naked on stage.' The next night we were packed to the rafters!"

A few days before *Pork* opened at the Roundhouse, Leee Black Childers led a delegation of the company to see Bowie perform at the Country Club in Haverstock Hill. According to County, "We were all dressed up: glitter, ripped stockings, make-up … Leee had done his hair with magic marker, and David was just fascinated with us. We were freaks, and that was where he started thinking, 'Oh, I'll be a freak as well.'" There is undoubtedly an element of truth in this, but over the years County and his colleagues have overplayed their influence; his assertion in 1996 that "Without any of that, David would have just continued having long floppy hair and singing folk songs" is pushing it a bit. It's instructive to note that the *Pork* veterans have tended over the years to champion Angela Bowie's role in the story, and vice versa. Angela's appetite for kooky outrage drew her like a magnet to the *Pork* company and it was she, not David, who fraternized with them. Bowie, as ever, assimilated much of what he saw, but County's claim that "If it hadn't been for *Pork*, there would never have been a MainMan, or for that matter a Ziggy Stardust" is frankly ridiculous. "Many of my influences were primarily British – Lindsay Kemp and his coterie," Bowie said in 2002. "Much as I enjoyed the Warhol crowd, my map was already drawn."

All the same, David saw *Pork* night after night, and wasted no time in introducing the cast to Tony Defries on his return from America. Ronson considered the New Yorkers "a bunch of loonies", but Bowie was entranced by their outrageousness, their sleazy sexuality, their New York street cool, their connections with Warhol, and above all their dedication to superficiality and role-playing. When Defries took David to New York in September to sign his RCA contract, it was Tony Zanetta who engineered Bowie's first audience with Warhol himself. And when, the following year, Defries set up his management company MainMan, it was the cast of *Pork* who were enlisted to run the office. Their contribution to the madness that followed cannot be underestimated.

For *Hunky Dory*'s sleeve image, David turned to photographer Brian Ward. "I did a lot of trying out of images with Brian around this time," he later recalled. Among the concepts mooted for *Hunky Dory* was the image of an Egyptian pharaoh, an idea David had first trailed in his *Rolling Stone* interview earlier that year ("He plans to appear on stage decked out rather like Cleopatra," reported John Mendelsohn). It was a topical enough idea; in late 1971 the media were whipping themselves into a frenzy with their coverage of the British Museum's forthcoming Tutankhamun exhibition, and for a few weeks Britain went Egypt-mad. Although the Bowie photos, in which he posed both as a sphinx and in the lotus position, have survived (one of them appears, entirely misleadingly, in the packaging of the 1990 reissue of *Space Oddity*) the image, thankfully, did not. "We didn't run with it, as they say," Bowie commented later. "Probably a good idea."

Instead he opted for a simpler image reflecting the album's preoccupation with the silver screen. By the late summer of 1971 David had foregone his predilection for frocks in favour of flowing shirts, fluffy blouses, loose flares and floppy hats, his latest accessory an affected cigarette holder. "I was into Oxford bags, and there are a pair, indeed, on the back of the album," said David later, explaining that he was attempting "what I presumed was kind of an Evelyn Waugh Oxbridge look." The front cover image was a close-up of Bowie living out his Bacall/Garbo fantasies, gazing wistfully into space as he pushes the flowing locks back from his forehead. The photograph was re-coloured by David's old friend George Underwood, suggesting a hand-tinted lobby-card from the days of the silent cinema and, simultaneously, Warhol's famous *Marilyn Diptych* screen-prints. At a time when many album sleeves were locating the artist as a diminutive figure in an artfully contrived landscape of post-psychedelic paraphernalia, Bowie tellingly chose to emphasize the notion of his own iconic, ironic star status.

Hunky Dory was released by RCA on 17 December 1971, by which time David was halfway through recording his next album. Presented with the sleeve image as a *fait accompli* and informed that Bowie was already planning a further change of both image and musical style, RCA's marketing department was at a loss over how to promote the album. There were disagreements over the amount of money already being spent on an artist regarded by many as an unproven one-hit wonder, and the resulting campaign was something of a damp squib. Even so, *Hunky Dory* rapidly found admirers. The *NME* called it Bowie "at his brilliant best", while *Melody Maker* considered it "not only the best album Bowie has ever done, it's also the most inventive piece of song-writing to have appeared on record for a considerable time." The same review went on to dub David "Mick Jagger's heir".

American critics were similarly impressed: the *New York Times* hailed *Hunky Dory* as evidence that Bowie was "the most intellectually brilliant man yet to choose the long-playing album as his medium of expression", while *Rock* magazine considered him "the most singularly gifted artist making music today. He has the genius to be to the 70's what Lennon, McCartney, Jagger and Dylan were to the 60's." Despite such glowing notices the sales figures were poor, and it was not until after the impact of its successor that *Hunky Dory* was widely heard; belatedly entering the UK chart in September 1972, the album went two places higher than even *Ziggy Stardust*. "*Hunky Dory* gave me a fabulous groundswell," Bowie recalled in 1999. "I guess it provided me, for the first time in my life, with an actual audience – I mean, people actually coming up to me and saying, 'Good album, good songs.' That hadn't happened to me before."

Much of *Hunky Dory*'s background, from its early titling to the fact that most of the songs were written and demoed prior to the sessions, stands in contrast not only with Bowie's previous album, but with the instinct for spontaneous studio improvisation that has dominated his career. And it shows; *Hunky Dory* is by no means an aberration, but more than any other

Bowie album it is first and foremost the coherent, polished work of a songwriter. A glance at the dense black type of its lyric-sheet reveals what is for Bowie an unusually verbose collection of songs, while the richness and sophistication of the music – notably the extraordinary fluidity of Bowie's chord changes – is something entirely new. Crucially, he had also perfected a voice of his own at last, a unique high baritone slipping imperceptibly in and out of the deranged falsetto, music-hall Cockney and affected Americanisms of earlier recordings but underscoring them all with a strong sense of its own identity: embedded even in the album's most blatant impersonations of Dylan and Reed can be heard a timbre that is quintessentially Bowie. Mick Ronson's scintillating orchestral arrangements and the helter-skeltering virtuosity of Rick Wakeman's piano (without doubt the album's defining feature) provide the finishing touches to a work staggeringly superior to anything Bowie had produced before. Tony Visconti, a great admirer of the album, later said that "there was no indication that he had this one in him when we parted after *The Man Who Sold The World*." For some *Hunky Dory* remains Bowie's finest album, and its influence on the history of pop music continues to be felt in the work of countless artists as diverse as Suede, Blur, Kate Bush and Eurythmics. "*Hunky Dory* – I love the sound of it," confirmed Dave Stewart in 1999. "I still kind of use it as a sort of reference-point". Boy George has gone further, citing *Hunky Dory* as the record that changed his life: "The album as a whole is so unusual, so far removed from anything you heard on the radio," he said in 2002. "It's so complete, it all fits together." *Hunky Dory*'s status as one of rock's milestone albums is borne out by the fact that reissues have charted in every decade since the 1970s (most recently in 2002, when a post-*Heathen* summer sale of Bowie albums by high street chains carried the 1999 reissue to number 39 in the UK chart).

Hunky Dory stands at the first great crossroads in Bowie's career. It was his last album until *Low* to be presented purely as a sonic artefact rather than a vehicle for the dramatic visual element with which he was soon to make his name as a performer. It was also perhaps the last album ever on which he was not, to a greater or lesser degree, playing out a role – although this, given the album's silver-screen fixation and David's description of himself as "the actor" on the sleeve, might be contested. "This album is full of my changes and those of some of my friends," he

announced in a press release in 1971, and certainly *Hunky Dory* stands alongside its predecessor as arguably the most intimate and revelatory of Bowie's recordings.

"The album got a lot out of my system, a lot of the schizophrenia," David later admitted. Precise readings are to be attempted at the listener's discretion, but there can be no doubt that this is an album which bristles with cryptic significance and resonates with provocative imagery. In January 1972 Bowie told *Melody Maker*'s Michael Watts that his songs "can be compared to talking to a psychoanalyst. My act is my couch." Built into *Hunky Dory*'s dense lyrical landscape is a host of suggestive *leitmotifs* and recurring obsessions. The pursuit of musical pastiche, already a strong element in Bowie's work but previously restricted to momentary effects, is here consolidated in a systematic series of cross-references: he incorporates masses of quotations and allusions to rock lyrics both famous and obscure, but even more obviously, the second side of the album opens with a cover version – albeit one impeccably crafted to the style of the surrounding songs – heralding a succession of *hommages* to Bowie's American heroes Andy Warhol, Bob Dylan and Lou Reed. "The whole *Hunky Dory* album reflected my new-found enthusiasm for this new continent that had been opened up to me," said David in 1999, explaining that "It all came together because I'd been to the States ... that was the first time that a real outside situation affected me so 100 per cent that it changed my way of writing and changed the way that I looked at things."

Lyrically *Hunky Dory* is also the most openly "gay" album Bowie had yet recorded. In August 1970 The Kinks had reached number 2 with their subversive transsexual hit 'Lola', heralding a revival of pop's dalliance with a fringe of society that had fascinated Bowie since the days of the Manish Boys. The spring of 1971, when he wrote most of *Hunky Dory*, was a period which saw him embracing London's gay subculture, with regular trips to the Sombrero and much socializing with Freddi Burretti's exotic coterie. According to Angela, "The Sombrero people began supplying the fuel very quickly; the material on *Hunky Dory* ... came directly from their lives and attitudes". David and Angie pursued a cross-dressing policy, he in a succession of gowns from Mr Fish, she in pinstripe suits and a haircut taken, in David's words, "one hundred per cent" from Burretti's friend Daniella Parmar. On 24 April, spurred on by the then current release of *The Man Who Sold The World* in its transvestite sleeve, the *Daily Mirror* photographed David in his dress on the Haddon Hall lawn. Pre-dating his famous "I'm gay" interview by nine months, he happily told the *Mirror* that he was "queer and all sorts of things," declaring that "I cannot breathe in the atmosphere of convention … I find freedom only in the realms of my own eccentricity." By January 1972, just as *Hunky Dory* was garnering its good reviews, the scene was set for the final push.

Play-acting or not, David's new-found gay sensibility feeds directly into *Hunky Dory*. The album contains his most obviously gay lyric yet in the form of 'Queen Bitch', while the contemporaneous Arnold Corns out-take 'Looking For A Friend' pushes back the barriers even more ostentatiously. Some have detected similar coding elsewhere on the album, notably in 'The Bewlay Brothers' and 'Oh! You Pretty Things', but the gay pose is merely part of the wider conceit of theatrical role-playing which Bowie was rapidly propelling to its logical conclusion. His fascination with artifice and insincerity – his own and others' – is manifested in the opening and closing tracks of *Hunky Dory*, both of which see David pondering others' perception of him as a "faker".

There are other, perhaps less superficial motifs running like seams through *Hunky Dory*'s lyrics. A new kind of fantasy existence is much in evidence, perhaps spurred by David's trip to America in 1971: 'Life On Mars?' and 'Andy Warhol' both refer directly to the "silver screen" which, alongside the observation that "I'm living in a silent film", ushers in a parade of cinematic icons from Greta Garbo to Mickey Mouse. There is a continuation of previous albums' ambivalent approaches to self-appointed leaders, icons, and "prophets", some more disturbing than others: Dylan, Lennon, Himmler, Churchill, Crowley. The occultist poet, sometime member of the Hermetic Order of the Golden Dawn and scourge of the Edwardian moral majority would exert a more tangible grip on Bowie's work four years later, but in the meantime the notion of "Crowley's uniform" of cultivated notoriety is just another allusive ingredient in *Hunky Dory*'s eclectic melting pot. "I used him because he was such an obvious symbol," said Bowie later, "it's an in-built icon." Such figures inform the album's troubled awareness of man's slender grasp on relationships and morality which are all that raise him above barbarism. Alongside the "cavemen" of 'Life On Mars?' and the "stone age man" of

'Quicksand', there are repeated references to "Homo Sapiens" and "children", "mothers", "fathers", "brothers" and "friends". The ultimate plea of 'Song For Bob Dylan' is "Give us back our family". Bowie has confirmed that the most impenetrable lyric of all, 'The Bewlay Brothers', addresses his relationship with his half-brother. The Nietzschean notions of *The Man Who Sold The World* are also back with a vengeance, and a further species of *Übermenschen* is introduced on 'Oh! You Pretty Things' with its references to Bulwer-Lytton's *The Coming Race*. Above and beyond the mortal figures there are reappearances by the "superman" and "devil" who had figured so heavily on *The Man Who Sold The World*, part and parcel of Bowie's rapidly refining but always obscure blend of religious imagery, Nietzschean philosophy and sci-fi apocalypse. *Hunky Dory*'s cathedral floors, cracks in the sky and "bullshit faith" provide a thematic bridge between the previous album and the next.

But if *Hunky Dory* has a principal theme then perhaps it is the Wildean dread of "impermanence", the knowledge that youth and urgency will be consumed by the inevitability of change and decay as Bowie stumbles into "a million dead-end streets" and begins to fear that he "ain't got the power anymore," becoming a "king of oblivion" while a new generation of "strangers" and "Pretty Things" inherits the earth. Bowie later described *Hunky Dory* as a "very worried" album, and a persistent thread appears to be his anxiety that the creative well is running dry, that in the absence of inspiration he is killing with intellect a talent he has always regarded as instinctive: "sinking in the quicksand of my thought" when he should be following the advice of the album's only cover version: "forget your mind and you'll be free". The process of writing, and its loss, permeate the album. In 'The Bewlay Brothers', "the solid book we wrote cannot be found today"; in 'Oh! You Pretty Things' "some books are found" in "a world to come"; in 'Song For Bob Dylan' the "old scrapbook" is renewed by the arrival of "the same old painted lady from the brow of the superbrain" – presumably Pallas Athena, the goddess of the creative arts who emerged from the brow of Zeus; and an early demo of the out-take 'Bombers' even concludes on a plaintive line about how "you used to look in my holy book". And over it all hangs the threat that "pretty soon now, you're gonna get older."

Of course *Hunky Dory* covers more ground than Bowie's creative angst – we must not dismiss the optimistic edge introduced by 'Kooks', whose subject matter puts a more positive construction on 'Oh! You Pretty Things' and 'Changes' – but it's difficult to hear David's cry of "Oh God, I could do better than that!" on 'Queen Bitch' without concluding that part of the game-plan is a severe spring-cleaning in preparation for the birth of a superstar. Having exorcised some of the most frighteningly withdrawn and introspective material he had ever written, Bowie could free his mind to concentrate on the conquest of pop. Perhaps ironically, in the process he produced in *Hunky Dory* an album that occupies a privileged place at the very heart of his recorded legacy.

THE RISE AND FALL OF ZIGGY STARDUST AND THE SPIDERS FROM MARS

RCA Victor SF 8287, June 1972 [5]
RCA International INTS 5063, January 1981 [33]
RCA BOPIC 3, April 1984
RCA International NL 83843, October 1984
EMI EMC 3577, June 1990 [25]
EMI CD EMC 3577, June 1990 [25]
EMI 7243 5219000, September 1999
EMI 539 8262, July 2002
    (30th Anniversary 2CD Edition) [36]
EMI 7243 5219002, September 2003 *(SACD)*

'Five Years' (4'42") / 'Soul Love' (3'33") / 'Moonage Daydream' (4'37") / 'Starman' (4'16") / 'It Ain't Easy' (2'57") / 'Lady Stardust' (3'21") / 'Star' (2'47") / 'Hang On To Yourself' (2'38") / 'Ziggy Stardust' (3'13") / 'Suffragette City' (3'25") / 'Rock 'n' Roll Suicide' (2'57")

Bonus tracks on 1990 reissue: 'John, I'm Only Dancing' (2'43") / 'Velvet Goldmine' (3'09") / 'Sweet Head' (4'14") / 'Ziggy Stardust (demo)' (3'38") / 'Lady Stardust (demo)' (3'35")

Bonus tracks on 2002 reissue: 'Moonage Daydream (Arnold Corns version)' (3'53") / 'Hang On To Yourself (Arnold Corns version)' (2'54") / 'Lady Stardust (Demo)' (3'33") / 'Ziggy Stardust (Demo)' (3'38") / 'John, I'm Only Dancing' (2'49") / 'Velvet Goldmine' (3'13") / 'Holy Holy' (2'25") / 'Amsterdam' (3'24") / 'The Supermen' (2'43") / 'Round And Round' (2'43") / 'Sweet Head (Take 4)' (4'52") / 'Moonage Daydream (New Mix)' (4'47")

• *Musicians:* David Bowie *(vocals, guitar, saxophone)*, Mick Ronson *(guitar, piano, vocals)*, Trevor Bolder *(bass)*, Mick Woodmansey *(drums)*, Dana Gillespie *(backing vocals on 'It Ain't Easy')* • *Recorded:* Trident Studios, London • *Producers:* Ken Scott, David Bowie

The Rise And Fall Of Ziggy Stardust And The Spiders From Mars was Bowie's first hit album and his ticket to superstardom. The central conceit – a visionary poet who, with a little extraterrestrial assistance, becomes a rock star in a world teetering on the brink of apocalypse – was an exotic consummation of David's life-long absorption of disparate elements of the zeitgeist. Andy Warhol, Little Richard, Marc Bolan, Lou Reed, Iggy Pop, T S Eliot, Christopher Isherwood, *Pork*, *A Clockwork Orange*, *Metropolis*, *2001*, *Quatermass* – all went into the melting pot. A cross between "Nijinsky and Woolworth's" was how David described the juxtaposition of high art and delicious banality embodied in Ziggy Stardust, a character who pushed to new extremes Bowie's fascination with the nature of celebrity. The work achieved its fullest expression on stage, where outlandish costumes, make-up, mime, pantomime, *commedia dell'arte* and kabuki theatre crystallized in a thrilling exploration of the artificial relationship between performer and audience. "It's no surprise that Ziggy Stardust was a success," David later explained. "I packaged a totally credible plastic rock-'n'roll singer – much better than the Monkees could ever fabricate. I mean, my plastic rock'n'roller was much more plastic than anybody's. And that was what was needed at the time."

For a while in late 1972 and early 1973 Bowie and Ziggy were practically indistinguishable from one another. Part of the album's enduring mystique is that the self-mythologizing pretensions of the songs themselves ("I could make a transformation as a rock-'n'roll star / So inviting, so enticing to play the part") operate as a parallel enactment of the process that simultaneously launched Bowie himself as a major artist. "You listen to the album, and he wrote about desiring stardom," photographer Mick Rock observed thirty years later. "He had stars in his eyes and on his mind, for sure. He was projecting, heavily, before it actually happened – that's the fascinating part. How prescient he was. Because it did all come to pass. In retrospect, he knew. He had an acute sense of the moment, and rode it brilliantly." It was during the early stages of the *Ziggy Stardust* campaign that, with the encouragement of Tony Defries, David began to live out the MainMan nostrum that in order to become a star, one must learn to behave like one. Publicists were hired to ensure that doors were always held open for him. He had a bodyguard and travelled everywhere by limousine. Photography was controlled and plans laid to restrict press access to David himself – and all at a time when, to the majority of the record-buying public, David Bowie was nobody. "Tony Defries had this idea that if we just told the world that I was super-huge, and then treated me as though I were, then something might happen," David later explained. As we know, Defries was right.

This appropriation of a specific set of behavioural conventions in order to manipulate the real world would become a template for Bowie's career. Before *Ziggy Stardust* his work as a songwriter and performer, however experimental, had maintained a monolithic aspect, a conventional view of the artist as Olympian observer at the centre of a creative web of assimilated influences and abilities. After *Ziggy Stardust* Bowie, like Warhol, would achieve the status of a postmodern artefact, a blank canvas, styling his creative output in response to the shifting sands of fashion and experience. "I'm really just a photostat machine," he told journalists in 1973, "I pour out what has already been fed in. I merely reflect what is going on around me." Thus the music on *Ziggy Stardust*, which rarely comes first in any dissection of the mythology built up around the album, is a vigorous restatement of the three-minute pop perfected by Bowie's childhood heroes of the 1950s, filtered through the electric soundscape of the early 1970s. It is an eloquent plea for the pop song, in all its gimcrack cheapness, as a valid artform, and an energetic dismissal of the increasingly pompous quest for neoclassical "sophistication" in rock.

Bowie's red hair, make-up and space-age costumes were more than just an eye-catching gimmick – although of course they were that too, and did their job well. Ziggy's multi-referential appearance circumscribed its own superficiality, injecting a sense of exotic decadence and pantomimic ritual into a popular culture dominated by the T-shirt-and-jeans norm of "progressive" rock. Glam was about cherishing uncertainty, anxiety and change, and it did so via a heady combination of nostalgia and futurism.

It's a common mistake, as it is with any creative school, to assume that glam was some kind of "movement", but if there was one consistent aim it was the diversification of culture and the dismantling of trib-

al allegiances. Bowie asserts that he, and other glam pioneers like Roxy Music, attempted "to broaden rock's vocabulary. We were trying to include certain visual aspects in our music, grown out of the fine arts and real theatrical and cinematic leanings – in brief, everything which was on the exterior of rock. As far as I was concerned, I introduced elements of Dada, and an enormous amount of elements borrowed from Japanese culture. I think we took ourselves for avant-garde explorers, the representatives of an embryonic form of postmodernism. The other type of glam rock was directly borrowed from the rock tradition, the weird clothes and all that. To be quite honest, I think we were very elitist. I can't speak for Roxy Music, but as far as I'm concerned, I was a real snob … I believe there were these two kinds of glam, one high and the other situated lower. I think we were more in the first category!"

Roxy Music's Brian Eno concurs: "I think all those things were a sort of reaction to what had happened before, which was an idea of musicianship where you turned your back on the audience and got into your guitar solo," he tells Barney Hoskyns in his book *Glam!*, "I think all of those bands – us and Bowie and the others – were turning round towards the audience and saying, 'We are doing a show.'"

The 1970s have long since been repackaged as a decade of gloriously amusing tastelessness, but the popular portrayal of glam as nothing more than a groovy fancy-dress party is superficial and inadequate. Glam allowed the charts to be re-colonized by a teenage consumer-culture for the first time in a decade. It forced changes in direction for artists as mainstream as Rod Stewart, Elton John and The Rolling Stones. It brought its own sexual revolution and sowed the seeds for punk and new wave. Through the emergence of bands like Queen and Kiss it helped to fashion the future of hard rock, and filtered through the space-age extravagance of "black glam" performers like George Clinton and Bootsy Collins it beat a direct path to the hermaphrodite disco chic of 1980s giants like Prince and Madonna. But amid all the brow-furrowing analysis of Ziggy and his contemporaries, what is often overlooked is their sense of triviality, irony and fun. "Whatever came out of early seventies music that had any longevity to it generally had a sense of humour underlying it," said Bowie twenty years later. "The Sweet were everything we loathed; they dressed themselves up as early seventies, but there was no sense of humour there … there was a real sense of irony about what we were doing … I remember saying at the time that rock must prostitute itself, and I'll stand by that. If you're going to work in a whorehouse, you'd better be the best whore in it."

Naturally, there were those in the media who opposed the new music on the very grounds that it was a plastic fabrication. On hearing 'Get It On' John Peel famously withdrew his long-standing loyalty to Marc Bolan, and "Whispering" Bob Harris denounced Roxy Music on *The Old Grey Whistle Test*. But as 1972 grew old, even the critics began realizing that glam's inauthentic gesture was its very point.

Of the many individual influences on the character of Ziggy Stardust perhaps the most obvious is Iggy Pop, the pre-punk rocker from Michigan who was introduced to David during his September 1971 trip to New York. Iggy was virtually unknown in Britain although, ever ahead of the pack, David had already described him as his favourite singer in a *Melody Maker* interview the previous December. Upon his return to England, Bowie told producer Ken Scott that his new record was going to be "much more like Iggy Pop" ("I had never even heard of Iggy Pop," Scott confesses to the Gillmans). Iggy's uninhibited and often violent stage act – "unleashing the animalistic parts of rock", as Bowie put it – was a crucial ingredient in the *alter ego* David was now crafting for himself. MainMan's Leee Black Childers later suggested that "Bowie's infatuation with Iggy had to do with Bowie wanting to tap into the rock'n'roll reality that Iggy lived, and that Bowie could never live because he was a wimpy little south London art student and Iggy was a Detroit trash bag. David Bowie knew he could never achieve the reality that Iggy was born into. So he thought he'd buy it." Iggy represented what David later called "the wild side of existentialist America, and of course, being a real nutcase about America and American music, that was everything that I thought we should have in England." The same was equally true of Lou Reed, already a major influence on Bowie's songwriting: "He gave us the environment in which to put our more theatrical vision," explained Bowie. "He supplied us with the street and the landscape, and we peopled it."

But the Lou/Iggy axis was qualified by another vital influence: Marc Bolan. By the time of the *Ziggy Stardust* sessions, Bowie's old friend had achieved his breakthrough, reinventing his songwriting with a new vocabulary of trashy urban sci-fi which usurped the Tolkienesque folk-fantasies of old. At the same time

he had revamped his band as an electric outfit, and despite the outrage of some of his former fans the commercial effect was immediate and decisive. In the spring and summer of 1971 T.Rex notched up a total of ten weeks at number 1 with 'Hot Love' and 'Get It On'. Bolan's fey, diffident public persona, not to mention the breathy, soft-spoken and close-to-the-mike style of his studio vocals, were assimilated into the *Ziggy Stardust* gestalt. So, too, were the 1950s throwback elements of Bolan's rock'n'roll act and, of course, his make-up. Bolan could hardly have known what he was starting when he decided at the last minute to daub glitter on his cheeks for an appearance on *Top Of The Pops* in March 1971.

In the ongoing and ultimately pointless debate about which of the two glam architects deserves the greater recognition, it can't be ignored that Bolan made the decisive move from acoustic folk-rock to glitter-clad electric pop a full year before Bowie – but, lest we forget, he did so with the help of a post-*Man Who Sold The World* Tony Visconti. Bolan had been present at Hype's legendary "birth of glam" performance back in February 1970, and Visconti, who believes that "the Roundhouse gig planted the seed in Marc's head," has suggested that Bolan and Bowie "simultaneously kind of invented" the glitter movement. Perhaps the most perceptive judgement comes from photographer Mick Rock: "If David Bowie was the Jesus Christ of glam, then Marc Bolan was John the Baptist!"

"I don't think he would be pleased to be associated purely with glam rock," Bowie said of Bolan in 1998. "He didn't see himself as a glam artist but more as something else. The concept of a bridge or of a missing link works well for him – it's exactly how he felt."

The word "Stardust", which in the wake of Bowie's success would be appropriated by one Shane Fenton (and, later, by an unappealing David Essex movie), derived originally from the 1929 Hoagy Carmichael standard, and had been popularized recently by Joni Mitchell's iconic 'Woodstock'. However, Bowie poached the word specifically from a much-ridiculed 1960s act called the Legendary Stardust Cowboy. Born Norman Carl Odam and remembered for his novelty single 'Paralyzed', the Legendary Stardust Cowboy's renown was largely based on being booked for an "ironically"awful appearance on *Rowan & Martin's Laugh-In*. "They all laughed at him and he walked off and cried," said David. In 1990 he told *Q* that the singer "was on Mercury Records along with me in the 'Space Oddity' days, and he sang things like 'I Took A Trip (In A Gemini Spacecraft)' … He was a kind of Wild Man Fisher character; he was on guitar and he had a one-legged trumpet player, and in his biography he said, 'Mah only regret is that mah father never lived to see me become a success'. I just liked the Stardust bit because it was so silly." In 2002 Bowie renewed his acquaintance with Odam, booking him to appear at the Meltdown Festival and unexpectedly covering 'Gemini Spaceship' on *Heathen*.

The fact that the Legendary Stardust Cowboy sang songs about spacemen and rocket-ships goes some way towards explaining why Bowie was attracted to his stage-name. Meanwhile, David explained that "The Ziggy bit came from a tailor's that I passed on the train one day. It had that Iggy connotation, but it was a tailor's shop, and I thought, Well, this whole thing is gonna be about clothes, so it was my own little joke calling him Ziggy. So Ziggy Stardust was a real compilation of things."

But if one figure is to be isolated as the model for Ziggy, it is the wayward second-division rock'n'roller Vince Taylor. Not an expatriate American as Bowie has sometimes stated, but a Middlesex-born boy whose family had moved to the States in the 1940s, Taylor released a couple of flop singles for Parlophone (including his only composition of any renown, 'Brand New Cadillac'), before finding his niche on the Continent in 1961 as the so-called "French Elvis". Signed to the French label Barclay, Taylor's eccentric and temperamental disposition was fuelled by an increasing intake of wine, amphetamines and LSD. "As soon as I get on stage, I go out of myself, I lose control," he once declared, "often I lose consciousness." His incipient mania and excessive lifestyle made an immediate impact on the young Bowie, who met him in London around 1966. "I went to quite a few parties with him," David recalled thirty years later, "…and he was out of his gourd, totally flipped. I mean, the guy was not playing with a full deck at all. He used to carry maps of Europe around with him, and I remember very distinctly him opening a map out on Charing Cross Road, outside the tube station, putting it on the pavement and kneeling down with a magnifying glass. I got down there with him, and he was pointing out all the sites where UFOs were going to be landing over the next few months. He had a firm conviction that there was a very strong connection between himself, aliens and Jesus Christ."

Back in France in 1967, Taylor's grasp of reality progressively fell away amid a series of troubled stage incidents uncannily mirroring the decline of Syd Barrett at around the same time. Tales of his bizarre antics – not necessarily reliable ones – filtered back to England, until one night, according to Bowie, "he came out on stage in white robes and said that the whole thing about rock had been a lie, that in fact he was Jesus Christ – and it was the end of Vince, his career and everything else. It was his story which really became one of the essential elements of Ziggy and his world-view." After some years of recuperation Taylor did in fact rebuild a modest career, even releasing an album called *Vince Is Alive, Well And Rocking In Paris* in June 1972, the very month that *Ziggy Stardust* appeared. But fame was never to be his, and he died in 1991. The previous year, Bowie told Q magazine that Taylor had "…always stayed in my mind as an example of what can happen in rock'n'roll. I'm not sure if I held him up as an idol or as something not to become. Bit of both, probably. There was something very tempting about him going completely off the edge. Especially at my age then, it seemed very appealing: Oh, I'd *love* to end up like that, totally nuts. Ha ha!"

The citing of obscure and underground influences has, consciously or not, always been a key ingredient in Bowie's strategy, but by 1972, rock history had provided no shortage of other, more obvious models for Ziggy's rise and fall: in addition to Syd Barrett, recent casualties included Jim Morrison, Peter Green (another white-robed stage Messiah who succumbed to deteriorating mental health), Janis Joplin, Brian Jones and Jimi Hendrix. The wider conceit of an album peddling a fictional band-within-a-band was nothing new in the post-*Sgt Pepper* landscape, while the idea of a "leper Messiah" visiting a spiritually hungry society has its roots in The Who's *Tommy*; indeed, David's sometime idol Pete Townshend is another contender for the guitar hero so memorably portrayed in *Ziggy*'s title track.

The first *Ziggy Stardust* track to be recorded was the Ron Davies cover 'It Ain't Easy', which was cut at Trident Studios on 9 July 1971 and originally slated for inclusion on *Hunky Dory*. This was only one instance of the considerable overlap between the two albums, which were effectively recorded back-to-back, punctuated only by Bowie's trip to America in September to sign his RCA contract. Out-takes from this prolific period which would end up as B-sides or latter-day bonus tracks include 'Velvet Goldmine', 'Round And Round', 'Sweet Head', 'Amsterdam', the revamped arrangement of 'The Supermen' and the superior second version of 'Holy Holy'. Other, less familiar rejects include 'Shadow Man', 'Only One Paper Left', 'It's Gonna Rain Again', and an abandoned re-recording of the Arnold Corns number 'Looking For A Friend'. The attendant *Ziggy*-era single 'John, I'm Only Dancing' would be recorded some months later, in June 1972.

The *Ziggy Stardust* sessions proper began at Trident on 8 November 1971, the main body of the album being recorded over the next fortnight. 'Hang On To Yourself' was committed to tape on that first day, as was an initial attempt at 'Star', which was completed on 11 November along with 'Ziggy Stardust', 'Velvet Goldmine' and 'Sweet Head'. 'Moonage Daydream', 'Soul Love', 'Lady Stardust' and the new version of 'The Supermen' were all completed the following day, and 'Five Years' followed on 15 November. "We recorded quickly, just as we always did," recalled Ken Scott later. "We generally worked Monday through Saturday, 2.00pm until we finished, generally midnight-ish." Woody Woodmansey confirms that the pace of recording was unprecedented: "We'd already done a couple of albums very quickly with David, but this one really was wham, bam, thank you ma'am!" he said in 2003. "We went in one day, did most of the basic backing tracks, then listened to them and went, 'Nah, that's not quite captured it.' So we tried again the next day, and that was it, we'd got it. Then, listening back to it, we all went: 'Hell, there's nothing else around like this.' It was the first time it'd hit all of us that this really was something new." January 1972 saw work begin on 'Rock'n'Roll Suicide' and 'Suffragette City', which were completed on 4 February along with 'Starman', the final track to be written. Composed specifically with the singles market in mind, 'Starman' ousted 'Round And Round' from the album at the last moment – the titles are swapped on the box of a master tape dated 9 February.

An earlier master dated 15 December 1971, before the recording of those vital last three tracks and evidently prior to a re-think regarding 'It Ain't Easy', reveals a fascinating glimpse of the album's original track-listing. Side one was to be 'Five Years', 'Soul Love', 'Moonage Daydream', 'Round and Round' and 'Amsterdam', while side two ran 'Hang On To Yourself', 'Ziggy Stardust', 'Velvet Goldmine', 'Holy Holy', 'Star' and 'Lady Stardust'. The album itself was apparently to be called *Round And Round*.

By all accounts, Bowie's sense of purpose during the Trident sessions was decisive and absolute. "He knew what he wanted musically," recalled Ken Scott, "and he didn't want to know any of the technicalities." With some tracks being recorded almost entirely live, Bowie often dictated the exact content of the band's contributions. "There was just no room for anything else," he recalled later. "I had to – at least in *my mind* I had to – hum a lot of Ronson's solos to him. It got to the point where every single note and every part of the song had to be exactly as I heard it in my head … that's not true of, say, *The Man Who Sold The World*, which was very much Ronson. But say the more melodic solos that Ronson did, an awful lot of that was just me telling him what notes I wanted. But that was cool. He's very laid back and he'd just go along with it." Ken Scott is keen to stress the significance of Ronson's contribution: "Mick Ronson was important," he tells Mark Paytress. "Like me, he had the job of trying to anticipate what David wanted, and then translating that into musical terms. In that respect he was very good. They were both on the same wavelength. He knew exactly what David wanted at that time."

By comparison with the lengthy pre-session composition periods for *Space Oddity* and *Hunky Dory*, there is every indication that the construction of *Ziggy Stardust* was a piecemeal affair: indeed, the early track-listing of the December master suggests that the entire concept of Ziggy's rise and fall was a last-minute notion grafted on after the arrival of 'Starman' and 'Rock'n'Roll Suicide'. In his first major interview about the album, for American radio in January 1972, David was eager to dispel the notion which still persists today that *Ziggy Stardust* attempts a coherent narrative: "It wasn't really started as a concept album. It got kind of broken up because I found other songs that I wanted to put in the album that wouldn't fit in with the story of Ziggy … what you have on that album when it finally comes out is a story which doesn't really take place. It's just a few little scenes from the life of a band called Ziggy Stardust and The Spiders From Mars, who could feasibly be the last band on earth, because we're living the last five years of earth … It depends which state you listen to it in. Once I've written an album, my interpretations of the numbers on it are totally different afterwards than when I wrote them. And I find that I learn a lot from my own albums about me." It was only with his subsequent emergence in the guise of the iconic Ziggy character in the spring of 1972 that the album itself would pull together as a cohesive whole.

Eighteen months later, in a 1973 interview for *Rolling Stone*, David held forth at length to William Burroughs about his latest reading of the Ziggy story, based on his short-lived plans to stage the album as a West End musical and TV spectacular. While his own accounts may have varied over the years, in this particular version he makes it clear that, contrary to popular belief, Ziggy Stardust himself is not an extra-terrestrial. He is a human who inadvertently makes contact with forces from another dimension via his radio (as related in the lyric of 'Starman') and, mistaking their messages for spiritual revelation, adopts a Messianic role on Earth while the passionless alien "infinites" use him as their channel for an invasion that will destroy the world. Very little of this story is apparent on the original album, but this in itself is instructive: throughout his career Bowie has led by example, reinterpreting his own work to suit the mood of the moment. In the same interview, he claims to be "rather kind of old school, thinking that when an artist does his work it's no longer his … I just see what people make of it."

Just as the album's unifying concept did not spring fully-formed from the brow of its creator, so the iconic appearance of Ziggy Stardust himself underwent a protracted gestation: in early publicity photographs Bowie bears little resemblance to the strutting peacock of popular legend. The first step came in early January 1972 with the cutting of his luxuriant *Hunky Dory*-style tresses: "Remember, we recorded *Ziggy* immediately after *Hunky Dory*, so David still had the long flowing locks and all that," said Ken Scott in 2003. "His move into the Ziggy persona came after we'd recorded the album." At around the same time Bowie began wearing a tight-fitting, open-chested jumpsuit designed by Freddi Burretti and made from what David described as "a quite lovely piece of faux-deco material" which he had found in a Cypriot street market a year earlier. Together with a custom-made pair of red lace-up wrestling boots, this became his standard early Ziggy uniform, later imitated by everyone from The Sweet to Suzi Quatro. It was in this outfit that Bowie made his most significant early Ziggy appearances: in the pages of *Melody Maker* in January 1972, on *The Old Grey Whistle Test* the following month, and most notably on the cover of the *Ziggy*

Stardust album itself. The photo shoot was conducted by *Hunky Dory* veteran Brian Ward outside the K West furrier's offices at 23 Heddon Street, a little cul-de-sac just off London's Regent Street near to Ward's own studio. "We did the photographs outside on a rainy night," Bowie recalled later, "and then upstairs in the studio we did the *Clockwork Orange* lookalikes that became the inner sleeve."

Although the K West sign has long since gone, the location remains a place of pilgrimage for Bowie fans. The famous image is a notable oddity among Bowie's album covers which otherwise, almost without exception, feature a studio close-up of David in his latest guise. For *Ziggy Stardust*, Bowie/Ziggy is instead a diminutive figure dwarfed by the shabby urban landscape, picked out in the light of a street-lamp, framed by cardboard boxes and parked cars. As on the cover of *Hunky Dory*, David's flesh-tones, hair and gaudy jumpsuit have been artificially re-tinted, enhancing the adventitious impression that the guitar-clutching visitor to this unglamorous twilit backstreet has just touched down from another dimension altogether.

Even the K West sign, so glaringly prominent above David's head on the album sleeve, has aroused speculation: certainly it provides Bowie with a ready-made visual pun on "quest" – his own and Ziggy's. The rear sleeve stresses the sci-fi overtones with what is surely a tongue-in-cheek reference to *Doctor Who*: with one hand on his hip and a cigarette in the other, David gazes at the camera from inside the incongruous setting of a public telephone box, the mode of interplanetary travel favoured by the BBC's Time Lord since his first appearance in the early 1960s. And, perhaps indebted to Slade's 1970 album *Play It Loud*, the rear sleeve also carries the celebrated injunction "To be played at maximum volume".

Not long after the photo shoot, Bowie's hair underwent a second and definitive change in appearance, apparently inspired by a magazine article David had seen about the Japanese designer Kansai Yamamoto, whose stylized work was taking the fashion world by storm and who would take over from Freddi Burretti a year later as Bowie's principal costume designer. "The Ziggy hairstyle was taken lock, stock and barrel from a Kansai display in *Harpers*," Bowie later recalled. "He was using a kabuki lion's wig on his models which was brilliant red. And I thought it was the most dynamic colour, so we tried to get mine as near as possible … I got it to stand up with lots of blow-drying and this dreadful, early lacquer." What the 'Ziggy Stardust' lyric had already prophetically described as a "screwed-down hairdo, like some cat from Japan" was created at Haddon Hall in late February by Angela's hairdresser Suzi Fussey. By the time the year's most celebrated coiffure appeared on *Top Of The Pops* in July the Ziggy Stardust tour was well into its stride, and for David Bowie there was no turning back.

But before the red hair and the stage show came the advance publicity, which generated one of the decisive interviews of Bowie's career. In the wake of *Hunky Dory*'s critical garlands, music journalists were already touting David Bowie as the great hope of 1972, and the *Melody Maker* interview published on 22 January was proof that he knew it. "I'm going to be huge, and it's quite frightening in a way," he told Michael Watts, who confirmed that "Everyone just knows that David is going to be a lollapalooza of a superstar throughout the entire world this year." But, famously, it was another aspect of Watts's interview that grabbed all the limelight. Headlined "Oh You Pretty Thing", it described David's new "yummy" appearance and dutifully reported his latest bombshell: "'I'm gay,' he says, 'and always have been, even when I was David Jones.'"

Latter-day accounts of Bowie's career have sometimes approached this crucial moment with an ingenuousness that surpasses all understanding. Contrary to widespread assumption, very few people at the time were genuinely taken in by Bowie's brilliantly timed shock tactic – least of all Watts himself, whose response in the article itself was to note that "there's a sly jollity about how he says it, a secret smile at the corners of his mouth … if he's not an outrage, he is, at the least, an amusement." Watts appreciated and clearly enjoyed the fact that Bowie's declaration was simply the most headline-grabbing yet of his attempts to project a sense of his own otherness. Taboo subjects have always appealed to David's appetite for sensation, and his desire to operate outside traditional systems naturally attracted him to homosexuality's sub-culture. "I liked the idea of these clubs and these people and everything about it being something that nobody knew about," he explained later. "So it attracted me like crazy. It was like another world that I really wanted to buy into."

This in itself didn't make him gay; indeed, anecdotal evidence amassed by manifold sources confirms that the Ziggy period was one of energetic heterosexuality at every opportunity. In later years David's

remarks on the subject were nothing if not inconsistent. "It's true I am bisexual," he said in 1976, only to respond to an interviewer's question a few years later with the retort, "Bisexual? Oh Lord, no. Positively not. That was just a lie. They gave me that image so I stuck to it pretty well for a few years." During the New Zealand tour in 1978 he told a chat-show host, "Yes, I am bisexual, that was a genuine statement." Launching himself on a mass market in 1983, Bowie was at pains to recant his former declaration to anyone who'd listen – particularly in America. He told *Time* magazine that it had been a "major miscalculation" and in *Rolling Stone* he called it "the biggest mistake I ever made." When pressed on the question by *Smash Hits* in 1987, Bowie amusingly underscored the whole saga by occasioning them to print: "Ha ha! You shouldn't believe everything you read."

There can be little doubt that David dabbled ("I was physical about it, but frankly it wasn't enjoyable," he said in 1993, "It wasn't something I was comfortable with at all, but it had to be done,") but ultimately the question of his own sexual orientation is splendidly irrelevant. In the *Melody Maker* interview he was doing something far more fundamental: he was embracing the spirit of Camp according to its truest definition, which is not about sex but about the elevation of the aesthetic above the purely practical. Just so, David's relentless habit of editing his personality, appearance, vocabulary and frames of reference to present a succession of "new" Bowies, each fashioned for effect and exclusivity, follows the manifesto of Camp established by Oscar Wilde and Susan Sontag. Camp invested Bowie/Ziggy with a useful air of ironic detachment, placing the received image of the star on a pedestal aloof from the mundane reality of studio sessions, tour buses, and the wife and baby at home. David himself would later insist that the revelation was not premeditated: "I was starting to build Ziggy, he was starting to come together and I was naturally falling into that role," he told Watts in 1978, "… you sort of pick up on bits of your own life when you're putting a role together. Bang! It was suddenly there on the table. It was as simple as that."

According to Angela Bowie, even Tony Defries was "profoundly shocked" by the revelation, but as the music papers fell over one another to follow up the story he "realized the full commercial potential of David's sex-role games". For his part, producer Ken Scott has opined that Defries was actually behind the declaration in the first place, devising it as a publicity coup.

Inevitably, reactions to the "I'm gay" interview were inconsistent and far-reaching. There were those who condemned Bowie's stance in reactionary terms – later the same year Cliff Richard denounced him as being instrumental in the disintegration of society's moral fibre. In America, a country famously ill at ease with the concept of irony, most Bowie coverage now began and ended with the question of his sexuality, while the few American performers of the 1970s who sought to emulate Bowie, like the entertaining but forgettable Jobraith, did so within a stiflingly gay context. As late as 1976 many American critics still regarded David primarily as a gay icon, which is unsurprising given that Cherry Vanilla, MainMan's publicity officer, had swamped the press with enthusiastic and lurid details of David's sexual adventures in advance of his first US tour in 1972. As the occasionally hostile reception to the tour demonstrated, America was not yet ready for homosexuality as a marketing strategy. "Alice Cooper had to stop wearing ladies' sling-back shoes and false eyelashes and dresses and get more into horror," remarked Jayne County later. "People could understand horror and blood and dead babies, but they couldn't understand male/female sexuality, androgyny or, as little American boys would say, fag music." Bowie later intimated that he had disapproved of Cherry Vanilla's tactics from the start: "All the time that was going on, I was in another country, so it was very hard for me to keep any sort of control … when I got to America and found out how I'd been set up, I thought, 'My God, I can't fight this enormous snowball, I'll have to work with it and gradually push it down into something more manageable.'" In some quarters it would take until 1983's 'China Girl' video for the sceptics to concede that David Bowie might not be quite the raving queen he had once cracked himself up to be.

In both Britain and America David was eagerly adopted as a figurehead by gay-lib activists; in the summer of 1972 Gay News welcomed him as "probably the best rock musician in Britain" and "a potent spokesman" for something called "gay rock". But Bowie's long-standing refusal to politicize himself or "be a cause" for anyone – a protestation he had long ago made to Kenneth Pitt – inevitably resulted in some of the flag-wavers experiencing a misplaced sense of betrayal when he turned out not to be everything they had projected onto him. But this is not to deny the impact of Bowie's projection of a gay sensibility before a mainstream pop audience, which was positively seismic. In 1972 the decriminalization of homosexuality was only five years old, and notwithstanding the provocative bisexual innuendoes of Mick Jagger and Ray Davies, there were no openly gay role-models in the country. Bowie was the first star to challenge the reactionary perception of homosexuality as the preserve of limp-wristed shop assistants in mediocre sitcoms. Instead he rubbed the nation's nose in the idea that homosexuals could be young, attractive, talented and successful. He was the first "gay" man marketed to both girls and boys. He undermined walls of bigotry simply by providing a pretext for debate. As Dead Or Alive's Pete Burns pointed out in 1984, "that was a real breakthrough. You used to hear dockers saying, 'Ah, I'd give Bowie one.' That was great, but it'll never happen again." In the coming months Bowie's stage relationship with Mick Ronson would subvert the standard macho interplay between rock singer and lead guitarist, and within a year of Bowie's pivotal 'Starman' appearance on Top Of The Pops, most British groups pitched at the teenage market boasted at least one gratuitously effeminate member – Sweet's bassist Steve Priest and Mud's guitarist Rob Davis being only the most prominent. And Bowie was already setting the agenda for the pop music of the future: the teenage audience of the Ziggy Stardust tour included not only Pete Burns but Boy George, Holly Johnson and Marc Almond.

By the time The Rise And Fall Of Ziggy Stardust And The Spiders From Mars was finally released on 6 June, Bowie had been touring Britain for four months and was already the talking-point of the year. "Of course there's nothing that Bowie would like more than to be a glittery super-star," noted the NME, "and it could still come to pass. By now everybody ought to know he's tremendous and this latest chunk of fantasy can only enhance his reputation further." In Melody Maker Michael Watts found the album "a little less instantly appealing than Hunky Dory" but admitted that "the paradox is that it will be much more commercially successful … because Bowie's bid for stardom is accelerating at lightning speed." The warmest reviews came from America, where Cashbox enthused that "The songs are uniformly brilliant and the production by Bowie and Ken Scott is virtually flawless. It's an electric age nightmare. It's a cold hard beauty. It's another example of the shining genius of David Bowie. An album to take with you into the 1980's." Phonograph Record praised "a self-contained rock and roll album about rock and roll" which showcases "one of the most distinctive personalities in rock … Should he become a star of the *Ziggy Stardust* magnitude, he will deserve it, and hopefully his daydreams won't be forced to turn to suicide when it's all over." Hmm. The *Philadelphia Inquirer* declared that "David Bowie is one of the most creative, compelling writers around today." *Rolling Stone* hailed *Ziggy Stardust* as "David Bowie's most thematically ambitious, musically coherent album to date, the record on which he unites the major strengths of his previous work", concluding that Bowie "has pulled off his complex task with consummate style, with some great rock & roll … with all the wit and passion required to give it sufficient dimension and with a deep sense of humanity that regularly emerges from behind the Star façade. The important thing is that despite the formidable nature of the undertaking, he hasn't sacrificed a bit of entertainment value for the sake of message."

This last comment is perhaps the bottom line on *Ziggy Stardust*: after all is said and done, it remains at the end a tremendously entertaining piece of pop music. The themes and motifs are all there for the taking, and of course they are endlessly fascinating: the nature of stardom, the ongoing extraterrestrial *shtick*, the end of the world, the false Messiah and the mistrust of organized religion (there are even more priests and churches in *Ziggy Stardust*'s lyrics than in its predecessor's), the lure of America, rock music and celebrity as metaphors for sexual consummation, decline, defeat, catharsis: all Bowie's pet subjects wrapped in eleven perfect pop songs.

Those who come to the album for the first time, aware of its awesome reputation, are often surprised by what a well-mannered, quietly crafted set of songs they find. Most Bowie enthusiasts will cite other, lesser-known albums in preference, and even David himself has advised caution: "I find the *Ziggy Stardust* record very thin," he said in 1990. "It sounded really powerful then; maybe systems have got better, it sounds kind of weedy." Certainly *Ziggy Stardust*'s chart-friendly string arrangements, polite piano and reined-in guitar solos stand in surprising contrast with the proto-punk assault of The Spiders' live act, but this is part of its winning formula. Midway between the sophisticated acoustic balladry of *Hunky Dory* and the all-out glam slam of *Aladdin Sane*, its contentious visions of alienation and decline are conveyed in a commercial, almost easy-listening idiom. It is a brilliant stroke, appealing across the widest possible spectrum.

It certainly worked. Although *Ziggy Stardust* only made number 75 in America, the critics were won over and the word was out. In Britain the album climbed rapidly to its number 5 peak, remaining in the UK chart for over two years. By January 1973, when RCA presented Bowie with a gold disc for *Ziggy Stardust*, MainMan was feeding reports to the press that the album had sold a million copies, but this was a flagrant exaggeration: at the end of 1972 it had sold 95, 968 units in Britain, and around the same number in America. It remains a big seller to this day; reissues have entered the top 40 on three separate occasions, most recently in July 2002 when the thirtieth anniversary edition, which collected together B-sides, out-takes and related tracks on a bonus disc, entered the UK chart at number 36. In 2003 there followed an SACD version, remixed by Ken Scott in 5.1 surround sound at Abbey Road Studios.

Bowie has certainly made greater records, but none will ever achieve the cultural impact of this one. *The Rise And Fall Of Ziggy Stardust And The Spiders From Mars* made him a household name and left a milestone on the highway of popular music, rewriting the terms of the performer's contract with his audience and ushering in a new approach to artifice and theatre that permanently altered the cultural aesthetic of the twentieth century.

ALADDIN SANE

RCA Victor RS 1001, April 1973 [1]
RCA International INTS 5067, January 1981 [49]
RCA International NL 83890, March 1984
RCA BOPIC 1, April 1984
EMI EMC 3579, July 1990 [43]
EMI 7243 5219020, September 1999
EMI 7243 5830122, May 2003
(30th Anniversary 2CD Edition) [53]

'Watch that Man' (4'25") / 'Aladdin Sane (1913-1938-197?)' (5'06") / 'Drive In Saturday' (4'29") / 'Panic in Detroit' (4'25") / 'Cracked Actor' (2'56") / 'Time' (5'09") / 'The Prettiest Star' (3'26") / 'Let's Spend the Night Together' (3'03") / 'The Jean Genie' (4'02") / 'Lady Grinning Soul' (3'46")

Bonus tracks on 2003 reissue: 'John, I'm Only Dancing (sax version)' (2'41") / 'The Jean Genie (original single mix)' (4'02") / 'Time (single edit)' (3'38") /

'All The Young Dudes' (4'10") / 'Changes' (live in Boston 1/10/1972)' (3'19") / 'The Supermen (live in Boston 1/10/1972)' (2'42") / 'Life On Mars? (live in Boston 1/10/1972)' (3'25") / 'John, I'm Only Dancing (live in Boston 1/10/1972) (2'40") / 'The Jean Genie (live in Santa Monica 20/10/1972)' (4'09") / 'Drive In Saturday (live in Cleveland 25/11/1972)' (4'53")

• *Musicians:* David Bowie *(vocals, guitar, harmonica, saxophone)*, Mick Ronson *(guitar, piano, vocals)*, Trevor Bolder *(bass)*, Mick Woodmansey *(drums)*, Ken Fordham *(saxophone)*, Brian "Bux" Wilshaw *(saxophone, flute)*, Mike Garson *(piano)*, Juanita "Honey" Franklin, Linda Lewis, Mac Cormack *(backing vocals)* • *Recorded:* Trident Studios, London; RCA Studios, London, New York and Nashville • *Producers:* David Bowie, Ken Scott

"My next role will be a person called Aladdin Sane," Bowie told Russell Harty on 17 January 1973, just days before completing the sessions which had begun on tour in America the previous autumn. 'The Jean Genie' had been first off the mark, cut at RCA's New York and Nashville studios in October. Following the end of the tour sessions resumed in New York, where 'Drive In Saturday' and Bowie's studio version of 'All The Young Dudes' were cut on 9 December, but the bulk of the album was recorded back in London between late December and January. Bowie once again co-produced with Ken Scott, assisted by studio engineer Mike Moran (later to enjoy his fifteen minutes of fame duetting with Lynsey De Paul on Britain's 1977 Eurovision entry 'Rock Bottom'). The Trident sessions, which were slotted in around ongoing UK concert commitments, concluded with 'Panic In Detroit' on 24 January 1973. The following day David boarded the *QEII* for America, where the finishing touches were added to the album in New York.

That *Aladdin Sane* is conspicuously "American" by comparison with Bowie's earlier work should come as no surprise. 'The Jean Genie' was only the first in a series of compositions prompted by David's impressions of the country he crossed by train and chartered Greyhound in the autumn of 1972, and the notion of an outsider's travelogue of America was emphasized by the ascribing of a location to each track on the album's label: New York ('Watch That Man'), Seattle-Phoenix ('Drive In Saturday'), Detroit ('Panic In Detroit'), Los Angeles ('Cracked Actor'), New Orleans

('Time'), Detroit and New York again ('The Jean Genie') and RHMS *Ellinis*, the vessel that had carried David home in December 1972 ('Aladdin Sane'). There were also two British locations: London ('Lady Grinning Soul') and, more specifically, Gloucester Road ('The Prettiest Star').

The character of Aladdin Sane was, as Bowie explained, "Ziggy goes to America", and the album supplants its predecessor's aspirational fantasy of America with the harsh reality that David had begun to experience. "Here was this alternative world that I'd been talking about," he recalled many years later, "and it had all the violence, and all the strangeness and bizarreness, and it was really happening. It was real life and it wasn't just in my songs. Suddenly my songs didn't seem so out of place. All the situations that we were going through were duly noted down, and all the remarks I had heard, real Americanisms that caught my ear. Just the look of certain places like Detroit really caught my imagination because it was such a rough city and it almost looked like the kind of place that I was writing about ... I thought, I wonder if Kubrick has seen this town? It makes his kind of world in *Clockwork Orange* look kind of pansy!"

Aladdin Sane's lyrics are riddled with images of urban decay, degenerate lives, drug addiction, violence and death – although, in among the smack-crazed gangsters and raddled roués, there is a touching nostalgia for 1950s rock'n'roll and the golden age of Hollywood. As evidenced by both the title track and 'The Jean Genie', there's also a firm restatement of the pantomimic elements in Bowie's frame of reference; *Aladdin*, the epitome of British pantomime, offers an appropriate model for an album recorded in London over the Christmas period, and the ever more extravagant costumes and make-up adopted by Bowie during 1973 pointed in the same direction.

In many ways *Aladdin Sane* refines the themes of earlier albums: notions of religion shattered by science, extraterrestrial encounters posing as Messianic visitations, the impact on society of different kinds of "star", and the degradation of human life in a spiritual void. "*Aladdin Sane* was an extension of Ziggy on the one hand. On the other, it was a more subjective thing," explained David. "*Aladdin Sane* was my idea of rock and roll America. Here I was on this great tour circuit, not enjoying it very much. So inevitably my writing reflected that, this kind of schizophrenia that I was going through. Wanting to be up on stage performing my songs, but on the other hand not really wanting to be on those buses with all those strange people. Being basically a quiet person, it was hard to come to terms. So *Aladdin Sane* was split down the middle."

The heightened Americanism of Bowie's writing, together with the fast pace of the album's development, gives *Aladdin Sane* a harder, rawer edge than its predecessor. "We wanted to take it that much rougher," Ken Scott later explained. "*Ziggy* was rock and roll but polished rock and roll. David wanted certain tracks to go like The Rolling Stones and unpolished rock and roll." Certainly Bowie's more abandoned vocal delivery and Mick Ronson's dominant guitar both seem influenced by David's increasing interest in that other band of Americanized Brits. Their imprimatur is everywhere on *Aladdin Sane*: besides the rip-roaring cover of 'Let's Spend The Night Together', there is a direct reference to Mick Jagger in 'Drive In Saturday', while 'Watch That Man' is a blatant take-off of 'Brown Sugar', a song inspired by the soul singer Claudia Lennear, to whom Bowie now added his own tribute in the form of 'Lady Grinning Soul'. From *Aladdin Sane* onwards, the two-way pollination and downright poaching of ideas between Bowie and Jagger would continue on and off for well over a decade.

Stones comparisons aside, without doubt the defining feature of *Aladdin Sane* is the arrival of pianist Mike Garson, who had joined The Spiders for the first US tour. Garson's breathtaking jazz/blues inflections forcibly steer *Aladdin Sane* away from pure rock'n'roll, creating a vigorous hybrid somewhere between the Stones and Kurt Weill which dramatically expands Bowie's experimental horizons. "Even though The Spiders were the well-known commodity, I was the one who was getting the attention," Garson later told the Gillmans of the atmosphere in the studio. "He was fascinated – he wanted everything I could do." Bowie later confirmed that he was consciously seeking to subvert the already successful sound of The Spiders. "You wouldn't think of bringing a fringe avant-garde pianist into the context of a straight-ahead rock and roll band, but it worked out well," he said many years later. "It brought some really interesting textural qualities to the album that wouldn't have had quite the same feel on it if Mike hadn't been there."

Alongside Garson came other new faces, some of whom would join The Spiders on stage for the remainder of the 1973 tour: Ken Fordham and Brian "Bux" Wilshaw on saxophones, plus a trio of backing vocalists: Juanita Franklin (a veteran of Lou Reed's *Transformer*), Linda Lewis (soon to have her first solo hit with 'Rock-A-Doodle Doo' and now forever associated with the soul classic 'It's In His Kiss'), and David's long-time friend Geoffrey MacCormack (here credited as "Mac Cormack"), receiving the first of many credits on Bowie's 1970s albums.

The sessions produced a number of unused tracks, including Bowie's studio version of 'All The Young Dudes' and the superior second version of 'John, I'm Only Dancing', which was originally pencilled in as the album's final track. The unfinished demo 'Zion' is often believed to hail from the *Aladdin Sane* sessions, but the evidence points to a later date (see Chapter 1).

The album's punning title was at one stage to have been the less equivocal *A Lad Insane*. An earlier and more cryptic working title was *Love Aladdin Vein*, as Bowie explained to *Disc & Music Echo*: "The album is about the States … Originally, I felt *Love Aladdin Vein* was right, then I thought, 'Maybe I shouldn't write them off so easily' – so I changed it. Also 'Vein' – there was the drugs thing, but it's not that universal." During the sessions he declared that "Ziggy was meant to be clearly cut and well defined with areas for interplay, whereas Aladdin is pretty ephemeral. He's also a situation as opposed to being just an individual."

Shot in January 1973, the *Aladdin Sane* sleeve photo introduced perhaps the most celebrated image of Bowie's long career: the topless shot of the flame-haired singer, his downcast face sliced in two by a vivid red-and-blue lightning streak while an airbrushed tear slides down his collarbone. Photographer Brian Duffy, introduced to David by Tony Defries, believed that Bowie's inspiration for the "flash" design came from a ring once worn by Elvis Presley, but the image has wider implications: Pierre Laroche's elaborate make-up is a deliberate expression of the fractured, "split down the middle" personality Bowie himself described. Delighted with the result, Defries insisted that RCA reproduce the sleeve in an unprecedented seven-colour system which necessitated the use of a printing company in Zürich.

In the year that had elapsed since the recording of *Ziggy Stardust* Bowie had been a busy man, touring almost non-stop while lending his writing, producing and mixing skills to Mott The Hoople (*All The Young Dudes*), Lou Reed (*Transformer*) and Iggy Pop (*Raw Power*). Moreover he had become a star, and to say that expectations were high would be an understatement. Released on 13 April 1973 while Bowie was busy on his first Japanese tour, *Aladdin Sane* entered the UK chart at number 1 – commonplace now but almost unheard of then – with advance orders in excess of 100,000 guaranteeing an instant gold disc and the envied status of Britain's best-selling album since the days of The Beatles. It was Bowie's first chart-topping album, remaining at number 1 for five weeks. Although most of the notices were ecstatic, *Aladdin Sane*'s commercial smash inevitably heralded the first signs of the build-'em-up-and-knock-'em-down tactics so beloved of the British music press. "Take away Bowie's image, and there's nothing left," complained Dave Laing in *Let It Rock*, going on to assert that "His stuff reminds me increasingly of the Beatles just before they split – the aimless doodlings of *Abbey Road*, when they had nothing to say and everything to say it with … still, if he falters, there's always Gary Glitter." Disgruntled loyalists who had supported Bowie in the early days were distressed to see their hero becoming an idol for screaming teenagers, and the letters columns of *Melody Maker* and *NME* began to feature complaints of the "selling out" variety: a sure sign of success.

In America, where David now had three albums in the lower rungs of the chart, *Aladdin Sane* was given a warm reception and climbed to number 17. *Billboard* considered it a combination of "raw energy with explosive rock", noting that "the sonic impact is all-important, and there's plenty of vocal exertion and instrumental exuberance". In *Rolling Stone*, Ben Gerson subjected the album to a close and intelligent analysis (albeit relying too heavily on the assumption of David's homosexuality – where is the evidence that 'Cracked Actor' and 'Let's Spend The Night Together' are explicitly gay?), concluding that through his "provocative melodies, audacious lyrics, masterful arrangements and production", Bowie was now "of major importance."

Aladdin Sane is an album of contradictions, and compared with its immediate predecessors there are times when its restless creativity can't disguise the sense of a rush job. Writing some years later, Charles Shaar Murray noted that "It was all too obvious that the heat was on … The songs were written too fast, recorded too fast and mixed too fast." At its best, however, the album transcends the tightly-produced, freeze-dried glam of *Ziggy Stardust* to explore a richer, more textured style of production, with 'Drive In Saturday', 'Lady Grinning Soul' and the title track

itself the obvious jewels.

"It was almost like a treading-water album," Bowie remarked 20 years later, "but funnily enough, in retrospect, for me it's the more successful album, because it's more informed about rock'n'roll than *Ziggy* was." Indeed, *Aladdin Sane* remains one of the most urgent, compelling and essential of Bowie's albums, its historical value running deeper than its commercial success. The very fact that it's less disciplined than *Ziggy Stardust* discloses the album's tantalizingly unhinged personality, as the rococo elaborations of Mike Garson's piano run counter to the tight efficiency of The Spiders' rock act. In its often deranged musicality *Aladdin Sane* not only exposes the nature of its title character, but hints at the pressures already incumbent on its creator. In retrospect it's clear that Bowie was moving far beyond the derivative Bolanisms of his previous album, producing in *Aladdin Sane* an energetic moment of transition between the glam sound he had helped to pioneer – here staunchly represented by effortless classics like 'The Jean Genie' – and, as evidenced by 'Drive In Saturday' and 'Panic In Detroit', the first stirrings of a fascination with the more voluptuous textures of American soul.

PIN UPS

RCA Victor RS 1003, October 1973 [1]
RCA International INTS 5236, February 1983 [57]
RCA BOPIC 4, April 1984
EMI EMC 3580, July 1990 [52]
EMI 7243 5219030, September 1999

'Rosalyn' (2'27") / 'Here Comes the Night' (3'09") / 'I Wish You Would' (2'40") / 'See Emily Play' (4'03") / 'Everything's Alright' (2'26") / 'I Can't Explain' (2'07") / 'Friday On My Mind' (3'18") / 'Sorrow' (2'48") / 'Don't Bring Me Down' (2'01") / 'Shapes Of Things' (2'47") / 'Anyway, Anyhow, Anywhere' (3'04") / 'Where Have All the Good Times Gone!' (2'35")

Bonus tracks on 1990 reissue: 'Growin' Up' (3'26") / 'Amsterdam' (3'19")

• *Musicians:* David Bowie (*vocals, guitar, saxophone*), Mick Ronson (*guitar, piano, vocals*), Trevor Bolder (*bass*), Aynsley Dunbar (*drums*), Mike Garson (*piano*), Ken Fordham (*saxophone*), G A MacCormack (backing vocals) • Recorded: Château d'Hérouville Studios, Pontoise • Producers: Ken Scott, David Bowie

On 5 July 1973, the day after Ziggy Stardust's wake at the Café Royal, David and Angela attended the royal premiere of the latest James Bond movie, Live and Let Die. Three days later David took the boat train for Paris en route to the Château d'Hérouville Studios in Pontoise, where he was to begin work on his new album.

Formerly Chopin's house and much favoured as a recording venue since Elton John's Honky Château had popularized it two years earlier, the studio was recommended to David by Marc Bolan, who had just used it to record Tanx. The Bowie sessions actually took place in the George Sand Studio, located in the converted stables.

Although Bowie had apparently intended to keep The Spiders From Mars together for the new LP, his failure to warn Trevor Bolder and Woody Woodmansey in advance of Ziggy's "retirement" speech had quickly led to a rift. Mike Garson received a telephone call from the MainMan office on the morning of Woodmansey's wedding (over which he was presiding as an official of the Church of Scientology), asking him to inform the bridegroom that his services would not be required on the new album. "Woody was devastated," Garson told the Gillmans. "This was his life and he thought he was going to the top with David."

Both Garson and Mick Ronson were assured their place on the new album alongside Aladdin Sane veterans Ken Fordham and Geoffrey MacCormack, but Trevor Bolder initially seemed to be facing the same fate as Woodmansey. Invitations were issued to ex-Cream bassist Jack Bruce and to drummer Aynsley Dunbar, whose previous employers included the Bonzo Dog Band, Frank Zappa and Jimi Hendrix. Dunbar accepted but Bruce did not, and Trevor Bolder was wooed back after all. "Trevor also sensed that he was going to lose his gig and so he went along," Garson told Jerry Hopkins; "Mick [Ronson] felt the same insecurity. So there was tension between them and David." This doesn't quite square with Bowie's later recollection that Ronson himself had suggested Aynsley Dunbar, having entertained mixed feelings about continuing with The Spiders' rhythm section: in Moonage Daydream, Bowie reveals that he and Ronson had discussed their respective solo

prospects during the latter stages of the Ziggy tour, and that Ronson had "asked me not to mention our plans to either of the others yet, as he hadn't made up his mind whether or not he would have them in his [solo] band."

Whatever the case, any such tension seems only to have sharpened the results, for Pin Ups exudes a technical confidence and accomplishment that often exceeds Aladdin Sane. Bowie described the Château d'Hérouville as "a good place for nostalgia", and hence an ideal venue for his latest project. Conceived as a stop-gap while David recharged his creative batteries (and possibly, according to Tony Zanetta, as a stalling manoeuvre while MainMan resolved a royalty dispute with David's publisher Chrysalis), Pin Ups was Bowie's tribute to the bands who had inspired him in his teenage years. "These are all bands which I used to go and hear play down the Marquee between 1964 and 1967," he explained. "I've got all these records back at home." Significantly, however, home is where he left them; the songs on Pin Ups are subjected to radical Bowie/Ronson makeovers, liberally sprinkled with the avant-glam additions of Mike Garson's jazz piano and Ken Fordham's saxophone. "We just took down the basic chord structures and worked from there," David explained. "Some of them don't even need any working on – like 'Rosalyn' for example. But most of the arranging I have done by myself and Mick, and Aynsley too."

One of David's more surprising plans was to include a re-recorded version of his 1966 B-side 'The London Boys' interspersed, a verse at a time, between the main tracks. "That dates from the first Deram album," he told Rock magazine, not entirely accurately. "It's about a young boy who comes up to London, gets pilled out of his head, all those things." The idea was dropped, perhaps because 'The London Boys' provided too cynical a setting for the exuberance of the cover versions themselves.

The sessions, which continued until early August, also included abandoned versions of the Beach Boys' 'God Only Knows' and the Velvet Underground's 'White Light/White Heat'. Rumours persist of an abandoned "Pin Ups II" album supposedly begun at the Château sessions, and leaning more heavily on American music: it may have included these aborted numbers along with rumoured versions of The Stooges' 'No Fun', Lovin' Spoonful's 'Summer in the City' and Roxy Music's 'Ladytron'. The abandoned 'White Light/White Heat' backing track was later used by Mick Ronson on his 1975 solo album *Play Don't Worry*, while 'God Only Knows' was revived in October 1973 for the Astronettes album and re-recorded many years later for *Tonight*.

Also laid down during the *Pin Ups* sessions were backing and vocal tracks for the Lulu covers 'Watch That Man' and 'The Man Who Sold The World'. Lulu spent several days at the Château, although the tracks would not be completed until later in the year. Other studio visitors included Nico, Ava Cherry and future *Young Americans* vocalist Jean Millington. While in France, David and Angela posed in a series of fashion shots for the *Daily Mirror* based on that year's Paris collections; David gave Angela the greater prominence in the feature, as she was now attempting to launch a career as a model and actress. By the end of 1973 it was being reported that she was to play the title role in *Wonder Woman* and appear in *Hawaii Five-0* and *FBI*. She never did.

The cover photo of *Pin Ups* pursued the album's swinging London theme with an appearance by Twiggy, already enshrined in 'Drive In Saturday' as "Twig the Wonder Kid". Taken at the Château by her then partner Justin de Villeneuve, the shot was originally intended for the cover of *Vogue*. "I was really quite nervous," Twiggy recalls in her autobiography *In Black And White*, "as I was a huge fan and as starstruck as anyone else would be … He immediately put me at ease. He was everything I could have hoped for and more, witty and funny and incredibly bright; into films, directors, literature, art." A clash in skin tones created problems for the photographer, and *Aladdin Sane*'s make-up designer Pierre Laroche came to the rescue. "I had just come back from California and was as brown as a nut," explains Twiggy, "while Bowie looked like he'd never seen the sun. So they had this idea to whiten my face down – leaving my neck and shoulders brown and bare – and colour Bowie up. Anyway, the result was fabulous." Meanwhile, *Vogue*'s circulation manager was having second thoughts: "'We can't have a man on the cover of *Vogue*,' he announced. I couldn't believe it … Bowie was as knocked out by the picture as we were. As Justin owned the copyright Bowie said 'while they're pissing about arguing' he'd like to use it for the cover of the album he was recording. In the end *Vogue* never used it. Pathetic really." Promoted to the *Pin Ups* sleeve, the photo was assured a far larger market: "Strange to think that it's possibly the most widely distributed photograph ever taken of me," concludes Twiggy,

"and yet it was done right at the end of my modelling career."

The rear sleeve consisted of two of Mick Rock's concert shots from the Ziggy tour and a new photo of Bowie in a double-breasted suit, cradling his saxophone in the crook of his arm. "I chose the performance photos for the back cover as they were favourite Rock shots of mine," Bowie writes in *Moonage Daydream*. "I also did the back cover layout with the colour combination of red writing on blue as it again hinted at Sixties psychedelia." Meanwhile, it seems that the Twiggy photo pushed out another intended sleeve: photographer Alan Motz tells Christopher Sandford that he "wanted to shoot Bowie metamorphosing into an animal" for the cover of *Pin Ups*. If this is true, Motz's idea would soon be recycled.

Sandford's biography also claims that *Pin Ups* was nearly the subject of an injunction by Island Records, who wanted to prevent RCA from rush-releasing it ahead of Bryan Ferry's covers album *These Foolish Things*; apparently Ferry had referred to Bowie's album as "a rip-off" of his own idea. In the end no action was taken, and both albums were hits. Indeed *Pin Ups* remains one of Bowie's biggest sellers, matching *Aladdin Sane*'s record of five weeks at UK number 1. It secured his status as the best-selling album artist of 1973, clocking up a new record of 182 individual weeks on the chart in one year. With *Hunky Dory*, *Ziggy Stardust* and the reissued Mercury albums all doing good business, at the end of the year RCA presented Bowie with a plaque to commemorate his achievement in having five albums simultaneously in the chart over a period of 19 weeks. At the end of 1973 Bowie's total UK sales stood at 1,056,400 albums and 1,024,068 singles.

The sleeve and marketing of *Pin Ups* initiated a brief phase in which David was referred to simply as "Bowie". "*Pin Ups* means favourites, and these are Bowie's favourite songs. It's the kind of music your parents will never let you play loud enough!" ran the American advertising campaign. Despite its huge UK success, critical response was lukewarm: *Sounds* declared that David "used R&B as a prop, not a springboard". In America *Billboard* was more accommodating, commenting that "There's humor in this music if you want to take it as a look back in musical time."

That's exactly the spirit in which *Pin Ups* should be approached: it remains perhaps glam rock's most cogent expression of its own inherent nostalgia, an affectionate reminder of the process that had led to the charts of 1973. It's unsurprising that both Bowie and Bryan Ferry hit upon the same idea for, as the cocktail-party glamour of Roxy Music and the ersatz Teddy Boy pose of chart acts like Mud and Showaddywaddy demonstrated, by the end of 1973 pop was embarking on its first great embrace of its own history. Set in this climate, *Pin Ups* is entirely in keeping with Bowie's penchant for what he once called "future nostalgia". Being a collection of cover versions, it will never have the compelling allure of his other 1970s work, but it remains a superb, energetic and greatly underrated throwaway, showcasing a band of musicians operating at the height of their powers.

DIAMOND DOGS

RCA Victor APLI 0576, April 1974 [1]
RCA International INTS 5068, May 1983 [60]
RCA International NL 83889, March 1984
RCA BOPIC 5, April 1984
EMI EMC 3584, August 1990 [67]
EMI 7243 5219040, September 1999
EMI 07243 577857 2 3, June 2004
  (30th Anniversary 2CD Edition)

'Future Legend' (1'05") / 'Diamond Dogs' (5'56") / 'Sweet Thing' (3'39") / 'Candidate' (2'40") / 'Sweet Thing (reprise)' (2'31") / 'Rebel Rebel' (4'30") / 'Rock'n Roll With Me' (4'00") / 'We Are the Dead' (4'58") / '1984' (3'27") / 'Big Brother' (3'21") / 'Chant of the Ever Circling Skeletal Family' (2'00")

Bonus tracks on 1990 reissue: 'Dodo' (2'55") / 'Candidate' (5'05")

Bonus tracks on 2004 reissue: '1984/Dodo' (5'27") / 'Rebel Rebel (US Single Version)' (2'58") / 'Dodo' (2'53") / 'Growin' Up' (2'23") / 'Candidate' (5'05") / 'Diamond Dogs (K-Tel Best Of Edit)' (4'37") / 'Candidate (Intimacy Mix)' (2'57") / 'Rebel Rebel (2003 Version)' (3'10")

• *Musicians:* David Bowie *(vocals, guitar, saxes, moog, mellotron)*, Mike Garson *(keyboards)*, Alan Parker *(guitar on '1984')*, Herbie Flowers *(bass)*, Tony Newman *(drums)*, Aynsley Dunbar *(drums)*, Tony Visconti *(strings)* • *Recorded:* Olympic & Island Studios, London; Studio L Ludolf Machineweg 8-12,

Hilversum • *Producer:* David Bowie

At the Château d'Hérouville in the summer of 1973 Bowie had told a journalist that his next album would be "a musical in one act called *Tragic Moments*", but when he told others in the autumn that it would be called *Revenge, or The Best Haircut I Ever Had*, and that it would feature protest songs about "how bad the food in Harrods is these days", it was clear that he was just enjoying himself. "There were a lot of changes going on around that time," Mick Ronson later recalled. "David had all these little projects ... [he] wasn't quite sure what he wanted to do." While Ronson began work on his solo debut *Slaughter On 10th Avenue*, Bowie entered a period of transition. No longer able to brave the fans who regularly beat a path to the doors of Haddon Hall, he and Angela took the decision to leave Beckenham. They moved briefly into Diana Rigg's flat in Maida Vale, and thence to a five-storey Georgian terraced house in Chelsea's fashionable Oakley Street. "You can't really be rock-and-roll royalty without a rock-and-roll palace," explained Angela in her autobiography, and from their opulent new residence the Bowies entertained Rod Stewart and Ronnie Wood of The Faces, together with the Jaggers, Bianca and Mick.

In October Bowie recorded a studio version of the '1984/Dodo' medley premiered in *The 1980 Floor Show*, marking not only his last work with producer Ken Scott (who departed to work on Supertramp's *Crime Of The Century*) but also his final recording at Trident, the studio that had borne the majority of his work for the last five years. Trident's reputation as a state-of-the-art venue waned during the late 1970s, and the studio eventually closed its doors, ironically enough, in 1984. During October and November David was often at Olympic Studios in Barnes, producing tracks for a planned album by The Astronettes, the three-piece group devised as a showcase for his new girlfriend, the eighteen-year-old American Ava Cherry. The project was shelved, although a twelve-track compilation called *People From Bad Homes* eventually appeared in 1995. Among the songs were early versions of numbers that would later surface on *Young Americans*, *Scary Monsters* and *Tonight*.

Further extra-curricular activities in the autumn of 1973 included the completion of Lulu's single 'The Man Who Sold The World' and a guest appearance on Steeleye Span's *Now We Are Six*. At around the same time Bowie declined a request to produce Queen's second album; their only collaboration would come eight years later. There were also plans to collaborate on *Oktobriana: The Movie*, a film adaptation of the Iron Curtain comic-book superheroine which would have starred another of David's new girlfriends, Amanda Lear.

Meanwhile, other forces were shaping David's career plans. On 17 November, at the instigation of *Rolling Stone* journalist Craig Copetas, David entertained the legendary beat poet William Burroughs at Oakley Street. The resulting double interview ("Beat Godfather Meets Glitter Mainman", published in *Rolling Stone* the following February) reveals a fascinating snapshot of David's intentions and aspirations as 1973 drew to a close. Fascinated by Burroughs's working methods and impressed by his 1964 novel *Nova Express*, David now revealed that he was experimenting in the "cut-up" technique favoured by writers like Burroughs and Brion Gysin, marvelling at the "wonder-house of strange shapes and colours, tastes, feelings" it created. His immediate plans centred on the West End stage. First he spoke of a full-scale rock musical telling the Ziggy Stardust story: "Forty scenes are in it and it would be nice if the characters and actors learned the scenes and we all shuffled them around in a hat the afternoon of the performance and just performed it as the scenes come out." Next he revealed, almost as an aside, that "I'm doing Orwell's *Nineteen Eighty-Four* on television."

The exact origins of Bowie's interest in staging Orwell's novel remain a moot point. He had clearly been working on the idea well over a month earlier, as evidenced by the Orwellian '1984/Dodo' medley. MainMan president and Bowie biographer Tony Zanetta later claimed that the impetus came from Tony Ingrassia, the director of *Pork*: "In September [1973] Defries had dispatched Tony Ingrassia to England to co-write and direct a musical production of George Orwell's *Nineteen Eighty-Four*, one of David's favourite books. David loathed doing anything on assignment … They worked together for a few days, then David refused to get out of bed … Nonetheless, David's discussions with Ingrassia had stimulated his imagination." In November Bowie claimed to have written twenty new songs for *Nineteen Eighty-Four*, which would be "almost a kitchen-sink kind of thing. I shall look very different in it, and there's a lot of good music in the show. Some of it is as much as three years old. I kept a lot of songs back because I knew I wanted them for some kind of show."

Neither project came to fruition: the *Ziggy Stardust* show was rejected as a retrograde step, although two of its new songs, 'Rebel Rebel' and 'Rock'n Roll With Me', were salvaged for use on the next album. At the end of 1973 George Orwell's widow, Sonia, withheld permission for the *Nineteen Eighty-Four* project. Undeterred, David relocated his new enthusiasms in a creation of his own: the urban wilderness of Hunger City, where his Orwellian compositions would form the basis of the dystopian post-apocalypse nightmare of *Diamond Dogs*. "It still implied the idea of the breakdown of a city," said Bowie in 1999, "a disaffected youth that no longer had home-unit situations, but lived as gangs on roofs and really had the city to themselves." For a time the album's working title was *We Are The Dead* – a key quotation from *Nineteen Eighty-Four* – but the work that finally emerged had moved beyond the margins of Orwell's novel. Both the fragmented lyrics and the portrait of urban America's sordid meltdown were clearly indebted to Burroughs, while the music was a four-way tussle between the receding sounds of glam, the rising influence of black soul, the synthesized nightmares of *The Man Who Sold The World*, and the ubiquitous rock-'n'roll swagger of Jagger. A significant innovation was the introduction of a brand new Bowie voice – 'Sweet Thing' and 'Big Brother' unveil the sonorous *basso profundo* that would become a key element in David's vocal armoury, and a fundamental influence on the goth bands of the 1980s.

Diamond Dogs was also a product of material necessity. By the end of 1973 Tony Defries's MainMan organization had become a colossus of extravagance: its American division now retained over twenty employees and had moved into palatial premises in New York's Park Avenue. Everything, from the Dom Perignon and the Bloomingdale's expense accounts to the custom-made gold-tipped MainMan matchsticks, was being paid for by Bowie's earnings. David, apparently heedless of what was being done with his money, was living on a monthly cash allowance and signing everything else to MainMan's credit accounts – which Defries deducted from his earnings. Meanwhile MainMan's London office was besieged by creditors. In December 1973 the Château d'Hérouville began gathering affidavits in preparation for action over non-payment for the *Pin Ups* sessions. It was small wonder that Defries was anxious for the goose to deliver another golden egg at the earliest opportunity.

At the height of its excess MainMan unwittingly sowed one of the seeds of its own downfall. In late 1973 the company's London office took on a young receptionist of French-American extraction, blessed with an impressive fluency in languages and a hard-nosed approach to business. She would shortly become David's personal assistant and all-purpose fixer, from which position she would play an instrumental role in extricating him from MainMan's clutches when the showdown finally came. Corinne Schwab, or Coco as she is known, remains Bowie's personal assistant to this day.

Diamond Dogs presented Bowie with a daunting prospect: having disbanded The Spiders, for the first time in four years he would have no recourse to Mick Ronson's arrangements and instrumental prowess. It remains to this day the only album on which lead guitar is credited to Bowie himself. "I knew that the guitar playing had to be more than okay," he recalled in 1997. "That couple of months I spent putting that album together before I went into the studio was probably the only time in my life where I really buckled down to learn the stuff I needed to have on the album. I'd actually practise two hours a day." Bowie also produced the album alone, and in an initial burst of enthusiasm – or possibly megalomania – he declared he would play every instrument himself. In the event, despite taking the lion's share of the guitar work and all of the saxophone and synthesizer parts, he relented: Aynsley Dunbar and Mike Garson returned from the *Pin Ups* sessions, and Herbie Flowers, last heard on *Space Oddity*, was re-recruited on bass. Two newcomers were drummer Tony Newman, formerly of the Jeff Beck Group, and Blue Mink's Alan Parker (previously hired by Flowers to play on Clive Dunn's alarming 1971 album *Permission To Sing*), who played guest guitar on '1984' and augmented Bowie's riff on 'Rebel Rebel'.

Recording, which began in December at Olympic Studios, was overseen by Olympic's resident engineer Keith Harwood, whose previous credits included Led Zeppelin's *Houses Of The Holy* and numerous sessions with The Rolling Stones. *Diamond Dogs* was to be Harwood's first Bowie credit, although the two had worked together 18 months earlier on Mott The Hoople's *All The Young Dudes*. "I was kind of in awe of him," David recalled in 1993, "because he'd worked on three Stones albums, so he was really a professional rock'n'roller. He was one of the first people

who was like down-and-out rock'n'roll. He had the greasy hair and the boots and the leather jacket. I'd been used to engineers and producers like Ken Scott, who goes home to his wife at night – tie and shirt and all that."

Recording proceeded at a frenetic pace. Even by comparison with the *Ziggy Stardust* sessions David was now governing his colleagues' contributions like a full-blown control freak. "I just came in and played the parts and he explained some things," Mike Garson told the Gillmans. "It was more like being a session musician." David spent six or seven hours at a time in the studio, and even Ava Cherry had to tread carefully: "He could be very dark. If he was working and you went into the room and started talking, he'd scream, 'Get out! Get out!'"

That *Diamond Dogs* is characterized by what David described as "a quality of obsession … desperate, almost panicked", can be put down to another significant development in his lifestyle at the time of the sessions. Although he later professed to having experimented with most psychoactive drugs while still in his teens, it was not until, in Angela Bowie's words, "the third quarter of 1973" that David embarked on a serious relationship with cocaine. At the time cocaine was something of a status symbol, an emblem of chic favoured by musicians for its ability to stimulate creativity. It was popularly reputed to be harmless and non-addictive, but anyone under such illusions need only look at footage of David Bowie between 1974 and 1976, and observe the alarming decline in his articulacy, disposition and appearance. At the time of the *Diamond Dogs* sessions the early symptoms were already beginning to manifest themselves.

By January 1974, Olympic Studios had followed the example of the Château d'Hérouville and threatened to eject David unless MainMan started paying its fees. While Defries stonewalled, the sessions continued at Ludolf Studios in Holland, where The Rolling Stones were in the process of recording their album *It's Only Rock'n'Roll*. It was here that David recorded 'Diamond Dogs' and the debut single 'Rebel Rebel', which was released in February two months ahead of the album. While in Holland, David recorded a mimed performance of 'Rebel Rebel' for the television show *Top Pop*.

In addition to sundry Rolling Stones, also present at various stages during the *Diamond Dogs* sessions were Pete Townshend and Rod Stewart, although there is no evidence to support any of the several rumours of uncredited celebrity contributions on the album. It is known, however, that Ron Wood (still with The Faces) provided guitar on Bowie's Springsteen cover 'Growin' Up' which, despite being latterly associated with *Pin Ups*, was in fact recorded during the *Diamond Dogs* sessions.

Experiencing difficulty at the mixing stage – a process with which he has never been confident – Bowie elected to complete the reconciliation with his former producer Tony Visconti, whom he called in to arrange the strings on '1984' and oversee the majority of the mix (the exceptions were 'Rebel Rebel', 'Rock'n Roll With Me' and 'We Are The Dead', which David had already mixed with Keith Harwood). The mixing of *Diamond Dogs* was Visconti's first project at his own custom-built studio in Hammersmith, which had only just been completed and was still entirely unfurnished. "I told David we hadn't even got any chairs in, but he said it didn't matter and the next day this big Habitat van arrived and they started unloading chairs, tables, the lot, all so he could complete the album at my place."

"This album again has a theme," David said in 1974. "It's a backward look at the sixties and seventies and a very political album. My protest. These days you have to be more subtle about protesting than before. You can't preach at people any more. You have to adopt a position of almost indifference. You have to be supercool nowadays. This album is more me than anything I've done previously." Later in the year he explained that the cut-up technique, which he had used for "igniting anything that might be in my imagination", had resulted in his "finding out amazing things about me and what I'd done and where I was going ... I suppose it's a very Western Tarot." One result was Bowie's new character: the louche, post-apocalypse lounge lizard Halloween Jack, "a real cool cat" who, according to the title track, "lives on top of Manhattan Chase" in the ravaged urban landscape that provided the album's environment.

Mike Garson found the album "macabre", remarking later that it had "a different vibe, it felt heavier, it was on the dark side," something he put down to David's overwork and drug use. "He didn't look good to me. I remember saying as a friend, 'You'd better watch out.' He was very thin, his face was drawn." *Diamond Dogs* is laden with the customary images of alienation, paranoia and play-acting that inhabit Bowie's work, but there is indeed a darker, nastier twist, suggesting that the fantasy world which was once so alluring has now become a prison. Where once he merely "felt like an actor" and was "hooked to the silver screen", by the time of *Diamond Dogs* Bowie is "locked in tomorrow's double-feature", playing "an all-night movie role" where "my set is amazing, it even smells like a street." As fantasy usurps reality and the apocalyptic omens of 'Five Years' are fulfilled, there are violent images of brutalized sex, bodily mutilation, and "poisonous" journalists circling like vultures ("the streets are full of pressmen" in one song, "spreading rumours and lies and stories they made up" in another, while "tens of thousands found me in demand" in a third). The recurring image of scavengers "like packs of dogs" underlines a persistent, nihilistic negation of "tomorrow", a word that haunts the lyrics like a badge of despair. The only figure who offers comfort in the spiritual wasteland is the Orwellian 'Big Brother' who arrives at the album's climax, reiterating Bowie's ongoing anxieties about leadership, surrender and faith.

Above all else the album is saturated with references to drug-taking. Bowie's earlier compositions had never shied away from the subject, but *Diamond Dogs* finds him lyrically fixated on cocaine, as though he might normalize the taboo by mentioning it at every opportunity. "Is it nice in your snowstorm, freezing your brain?" he enquires in 'Sweet Thing', before bleakly concluding, "It's all I ever wanted, a street with a deal". The rest of the album grimly follows suit: "You'll be shooting up on anything, tomorrow's never there"; "Should we powder our noses?"; "Lord, I'd take an overdose"; and, most graphically of all, "We'll buy some drugs and watch a band, and jump in a river holding hands." Even the innocuous 'Rebel Rebel' is equipped with "cue lines and a handful of ludes". It's worth noting that the lyrics David wrote for Mick Ronson's album at around the same time are stuffed with similar references.

In 1978 David described *Diamond Dogs* as a "very English, apocalyptic kind of view of our city life ... it just coincided with the first economic disasters in New York. [There were] obvious inspirations from the Orwellian holocaust trip. It was pretty despondent." In 1991 he recalled that "The main thing was to make rock and roll absurd. It was to take anything that was serious and mock it ... It seemed to be part of my manifesto at the time."

The original release came in a gatefold sleeve which opened to reveal a photo-montage of fog-shrouded skyscrapers alongside the lyrics of 'Future

Legend'. The photography was by MainMan vice-president Leee Black Childers who, despite being employed as David's official photographer, was usually passed over in favour of bigger names. "I don't think David ever thought of me as a photographer," he said years later. "It wasn't even his idea to use me on *Diamond Dogs*. It was Tony Defries trying to save money." More notorious by far was the album's front sleeve. The Belgian artist Guy Peellaert, whose *Rock Dreams* had been published a year previously and the originals exhibited at Biba's in London, had been engaged by Mick Jagger to design a sleeve for the as yet unfinished *It's Only Rock'n'Roll*. Unwisely given David's magpie tendencies, Jagger told Bowie about the commission. "I immediately rushed out and got Guy Peellaert to do my cover too. He never forgave me for that!" admitted David later. Jagger is supposed to have subsequently remarked that you should never wear a new pair of shoes in front of David.

Peellaert's *Diamond Dogs* painting of Bowie as a half-canine circus freak became a *cause célèbre* when RCA elected to airbrush out an offending portion of its anatomy. A few untreated copies slipped through the net and are now highly prized by collectors: in March 2004 a copy of the pre-airbrushed sleeve was sold on eBay for a staggering US $8988. From 1990 onwards the original artwork was restored for the album's various reissues, which also included Peellaert's rejected design for the inner sleeve, featuring Bowie and a baying hound against a New York backdrop. Both images were developed from studio pictures shot by photographer Terry O'Neill, who had hired a dog in order to photograph its hindquarters in a similar pose to Bowie's, the better to assist Peellaert with his painting. At the end of the session O'Neill suggested that David pose for some shots with the dog, and he later recalled the moment when the hound unexpectedly struck its dramatic pose: "Bowie had the dog on a lead. It was lying down, so I tried to get the dog up. Then suddenly it leapt up. It was an awesome sight because the dog was bloody massive, a Great Dane or something. But David just sat there, cool as a cucumber. He didn't react to the dog at all. I guess he was posing immaculately. Most rock stars would jump a mile if that happened. He probably didn't even notice the dog. Which helped the picture, of course." The *Diamond Dogs* artwork, incidentally, would prove to be the very last appearance of the Ziggy Stardust hairstyle. In keeping with the convention established by *Pin Ups*, David was credited throughout the original album simply as "Bowie".

Diamond Dogs was released in April 1974, boosted in America by a $400,000 advertising campaign that included deluxe press packs, giant billboards in Times Square and Sunset Boulevard, double-page magazine ads, subway posters proclaiming "The Year Of The Diamond Dogs", and even a specially filmed television commercial, one of the first of its kind for a pop album. Although *Diamond Dogs* failed to break the States decisively, its eventual chart peak at number 5 in the late summer established Bowie as an artist of some stature in America, where it was certified gold (marking the sale of a million copies) by August. In the UK it shot to number 1, repeating the success of its predecessors.

In a grandiose stunt Tony Defries refused to issue review copies of the album, instead inviting critics to a preview where they were packed into a hot MainMan office and allowed to listen to the record once through. Tape recorders were banned and no lyric sheets provided. Perhaps not surprisingly, some of the critics were unimpressed. "Most of the songs are obscure tangles of perversion, degradation, fear and self-pity," wrote Eric Emerson in *Rolling Stone*. "It's difficult to know what to make of them. Are they masturbatory fantasies, guilt-ridden projections, terrified premonitions, or is it all merely Alice Cooper exploitation? Unfortunately, the music exerts so little appeal that it's hard to care what it's about. And *Diamond Dogs* seems more like Bowie's last gasp than the world's." Emerson, who went on to describe David's guitar-playing as "cheesy" and the record as "Bowie's worst album in six years", was in the minority, however. *Billboard* noted that "A subtler, more aesthetic Bowie comes to the forefront here" on an album "which should reinforce his musical presence in the 70's". *Rock* magazine found it "a strong and effective album, and certainly the most impressive work Bowie's completed since *Ziggy Stardust*", suggesting that "where *Aladdin Sane* seemed like a series of Instamatic snapshots taken from weird angles, *Diamond Dogs* has the provoking quality of a thought-out painting that draws on all the deeper colors." In Britain the critics were equally pleased; *Melody Maker* considered the album "really good" and drew comparisons with Phil Spector's "wall of sound" production, noting that Bowie albums were now received "with as much awe as a release by the Beatles in the sixties." *Sounds* pronounced the album David's "most impressive work since *Ziggy Stardust*," while *Disc* likened it to "the greatly underrated *The Man Who Sold The World*. It's eerie, bleak, but compelling listening and undeniably brilliant. It contains some of the best music Bowie's ever written … very much Bowie's LP and without doubt the finest he's made so far."

With its manic alternations between power-charged garage rock and sophisticated, synthesizer-heavy apocalyptic ballads, *Diamond Dogs* is now widely accepted as one of Bowie's major works: the spectacular zenith of the paranoid horror themes of his early 1970s albums, a convincing vindication of his abilities as a guitarist, and a vigorous valediction to glam rock. In its finest moments it circumvents the restrictions both of pop music and of the pejorative "concept album" label often applied to it. "A song has to take on character, shape, body and influence people to an extent that they use it for their own devices," David had told William Burroughs in the *Rolling Stone* interview. "The rock stars have assimilated all kinds of philosophies, styles, histories, writings, and they throw out what they have gleaned from that." In tracks like 'We Are The Dead', 'Big Brother' and the supreme 'Sweet Thing/Candidate' sequence, *Diamond Dogs* achieves just this, throwing out some of the most sublime and remarkable sounds in the annals of rock music.

DAVID LIVE

RCA Victor APL 2 0771, October 1974 [2]
RCA PL 80771, 1984
EMI DBLD 1, August 1990

'1984' (3'20") / 'Rebel Rebel' (2'40") / 'Moonage Daydream' (5'10") / 'Sweet Thing' (8'48") / 'Changes' (3'34") / 'Suffragette City' (3'45") / 'Aladdin Sane' (4'57") / 'All The Young Dudes' (4'18") / 'Cracked Actor' (3'29") / 'Rock'n Roll With Me' (4'18") / 'Watch That Man' (4'55") / 'Knock on Wood' (3'08") / 'Diamond Dogs' (6'32") / 'Big Brother' (4'08") / 'The Width of a Circle' (8'12") / 'The Jean Genie' (5'13") / 'Rock'n'Roll Suicide' (4'30")

Bonus tracks on 1990 reissue: 'Band Intro' (0'09") / 'Here Today, Gone Tomorrow' (3'32") / 'Time' (5'19")

• *Musicians:* see *The Diamond Dogs Tour* (Chapter 3)
• *Recorded:* Tower Theatre, Philadelphia; Record Plant Studios, New York • *Producer:* Tony Visconti

Recorded during several nights' residency at the Tower Theatre, Philadelphia, *David Live* is at once a fascinating and frustrating record of the extraordinary Diamond Dogs tour. A major element of the show's impact was visual, and a live album couldn't hope to capture the reality of a spectacular theatrical experience. Even the grainy and unappealing Dagmar sleeve photographs fail to convey the splendour of the set, and serve only to demonstrate how unwell David was looking by this stage in his descent into cocaine addiction.

The recording, which came near the end of the tour's opening leg and a month before the *Young Americans* sessions began, took place under far from ideal circumstances (see Chapter 3). A degree of confusion surrounds the dates of the recordings, which are given incorrectly on some reissues: the correct dates are 8 – 12 July 1974. The live recording was handled by *Diamond Dogs* engineer Keith Harwood, marking the end of his brief association with Bowie. Harwood died a few years later in a car accident while driving home from Olympic Studios in Barnes, apparently hitting the very same tree that claimed Marc Bolan's life.

Even to the most accommodating critic *David Live* is something of a curate's egg. As anyone who's heard an alternative bootleg of the Diamond Dogs tour will confirm, the standard of performance – particularly David's voice – seldom gives an accurate reflection of the show's usual high quality. Furthermore the mix is hard and unforgiving, which Tony Visconti puts down both to shabby recording (for which he wasn't responsible, being involved only at the mixing stage) and hasty post-production decreed by RCA, who wanted to release the album in time for the second leg of the tour. The backing vocals were re-recorded at Record Plant because, according to Visconti, "the singers danced a lot and were out of breath".

Mixing took place at New York's Electric Lady Studios in July, prior to the commencement of the *Young Americans* sessions in Philadelphia. "If you listen to that recording, you'll hear that it's very brittle and lacks depth," said Visconti. "For the twelve musicians or so that he had on stage, it sounds very puny … It was one of the quickest and shoddiest albums I've ever done, and I'm not proud of it at all."

Although it didn't stop the album going top ten on both sides of the Atlantic (securing Bowie's position as top UK album seller for the second year running), press reaction was muted and occasionally hostile. Lester Bangs wrote in *Creem* that "without all the gauche props and stage business the recent live album is a dismal flatulence". In *Melody Maker* Chris Charlesworth found David "hoarse, throaty and often off-key", while Charles Shaar Murray considered the album an example of "outright artifice and self-parody". Bowie himself dismissed *David Live* in a 1977 interview for *Melody Maker*: "God, that album! I've never played it. The tension it must contain must be like a vampire's teeth coming down on you. And that photo on the cover! My God, it looks like I've just stepped out of the grave. That's actually how I felt. That record should have been called *David Bowie Is Alive And Well And Living Only In Theory*" (an ironic reference to the Broadway show, and perennial Bowie influence, *Jacques Brel Is Alive And Well And Living In Paris*).

Despite the grim reaction and the unhappy background associated with the album, *David Live* remains a worthwhile document of the crossover period between *Diamond Dogs* and *Young Americans*. The sound is often tinny and unsatisfying, and some of the re-recorded backing vocals jarringly loud, but in the main it's a fresh, honest record of a great show. The cabaret-style reworkings of 'All The Young Dudes' and 'The Jean Genie' are fascinating, 'The Width Of A Circle' is magnificent, and best of all is the quite brilliant 'Rock'n'Roll Suicide', reinvented as a melodramatic Vegas torch song. A faulty microphone pick-up means that 'Space Oddity' is missing from the set, but the 1990 reissue added the bonus recordings 'Time' and 'Here Today, Gone Tomorrow'. Not included on this re-release was the excellent live version of 'Panic In Detroit' also recorded during the *David Live* concerts but restricted to the B-side of the 'Knock On Wood' single, and subsequently *Bowie Rare*. At the time of writing, Tony Visconti is understood to be working on a brand new remix of *David Live* for a forthcoming reissue.

Early pressings of *David Live* accidentally swapped the second and fourth sides of the double LP. In July 1979 a truncated single album culled from *David Live* was released by RCA in Holland under the title *Rock Concert – Live At The Tower, Philadelphia 1974*. It is understood that this unusual move was the result of *Stage* enjoying particular success on the Dutch market.

YOUNG AMERICANS

RCA Victor RS 1006, March 1975 [2]
RCA PL 80998, October 1984
EMI EMD 1021, April 1991 [54]
EMI 7243 5219050, September 1999

'Young Americans' (5'10") / 'Win' (4'44") / 'Fascination' (5'43") / 'Right' (4'13") / 'Somebody Up There Likes Me' (6'30") / 'Across the Universe' (4'30") / 'Can You Hear Me' (5'04") / 'Fame' (4'12")

Bonus tracks on 1991 reissue: 'Who Can I Be Now?' (4'36") / 'It's Gonna Be Me' (6'27") / 'John, I'm Only Dancing (Again)' (6'57")

• *Musicians:* David Bowie *(vocals, guitar, piano)*, Carlos Alomar *(guitar)*, Mike Garson *(piano)*, David Sanborn *(saxophone)*, Willie Weeks *(bass)*, Andy Newmark *(drums)*, Larry Washington *(conga)*, Pablo Rosario *(percussion)*, Ava Cherry, Robin Clark, Luther Vandross, Anthony Hinton, Diane Sumler *(backing vocals)*, plus (on 'Across The Universe' and 'Fame'): John Lennon *(vocals, guitar)*, Earl Slick *(guitar)*, Emir Ksasan *(bass)*, Dennis Davis *(drums)*, Ralph McDonald *(percussion)*, Jean Fineberg, Jean Millington *(backing vocals)* • *Recorded:* Sigma Sound, Philadelphia; Electric Lady, New York • *Producer:* Tony Visconti *('Across the Universe' and 'Fame':* David Bowie, Harry Maslin)

"I thought I'd better make a hit album to cement myself over here, so I went and did it. It wasn't too hard, really," Bowie told *Melody Maker* in 1976, a year after *Young Americans* had made him a household name in the States.

During his residency at Philadelphia's Tower Theater in July 1974, David made his first visit to the city's Sigma Sound Studios to work with Michael Kamen on some new Ava Cherry recordings. Sigma was the home of Kenny Gamble and Leon Huff's Philadelphia International label, whose roster of artists (The Three Degrees, The O'Jays, The Stylistics, The Spinners) formed the centre of America's black music revolution. Songs like '1984' and 'Rock'n Roll With Me' had already hinted at David's enthusiasm for the soul and funk of the "Philly" sound, and his encounter with guitarist Carlos Alomar the previous April had confirmed his latest musical aspirations. Ten years earlier, during his time with The Manish Boys, David's most treasured album had been James

Brown's *Live At The Apollo*, and when he met Alomar his "great dream in life ... to go to the Apollo" was fulfilled: "I couldn't believe it," he recalled many years later. "Not only did Carlos know the Apollo, he was in the house band there." Sure enough, in April 1974 Bowie had told *Rock* magazine that he had "been going down to the Apollo in Harlem. Most New Yorkers seem scared to go there if they're white, but the music's incredible. I saw The Temptations and The Spinners on the same bill there, and next week it's Marvin Gaye, incredible!" In the spring of 1974 Bowie was singing the praises of Barry White, The Isley Brothers, the Ohio Players (whose 'Here Today, Gone Tomorrow' he would soon introduce into his repertoire) and even The Jackson Five, whom he saw perform at Madison Square Garden.

At the start of the six-week break in the Diamond Dogs tour schedule, Bowie returned to New York to mix *David Live*, giving Corinne Schwab a shopping list of black albums he wanted to hear in preparation for his return to Sigma Sound. In the weeks leading up to the sessions the US chart was topped by The Hues Corporation's 'Rock The Boat' and George McCrae's 'Rock Your Baby', by far the biggest hits yet to emerge from the embryonic disco movement.

David had initially hoped to employ Sigma's resident rhythm group, known as the MFSB ("Mothers, Fathers, Sisters, Brothers"), but with the exception of percussionist Larry Washington they were busy on other projects, so another recruitment drive began in New York. Mike Garson, David Sanborn and Pablo Rosario remained from the tour band, but Earl Slick was now replaced by Puerto Rican-born Carlos Alomar, who had played guitar at the April 1974 Lulu session. In addition to his work at the Apollo with The Main Ingredient, Alomar's credits included touring with James Brown, Ben E King, Chuck Berry and Wilson Pickett. Alomar recommended replacements for Tony Newman and Herbie Flowers: Main Ingredient drummer Andy Newmark, formerly of Sly & The Family Stone, and the legendary black bassist Willie Weeks, a veteran of The Isley Brothers. When David contacted Tony Visconti in London and told him he had Willie Weeks on board, the producer caught the next plane over: "I'm a bass player myself, and he was my idol," Visconti later explained.

Work at Sigma began on 11 August 1974. "The session was booked for four and I arrived at the hotel at five and just ran to the studio, really jetlagged," recalled Visconti, who had just completed work on Thin Lizzy's *Nightlife*. "David arrived at midnight. He was very thin in those days and living sort of reversed hours. He was going to bed at about eleven in the morning and all that. However, on that very first night of recording, there was such an electrifying atmosphere in the air that we recorded, that evening, 'Young Americans'." At David's invitation, Carlos Alomar's wife Robin Clark was enlisted as a backing vocalist for the session, as was the still unknown Luther Vandross, who had dropped by to visit his old schoolmate Carlos.

The sessions proceeded at a hectic pace, taking only two weeks to complete. "David did mostly live vocals, and although all the songs were written, they were being heavily rearranged as time went on," said Visconti. "Nothing was organized, it turned out to be one enormous jam session." Driven by an ever-increasing intake of uppers and cocaine, Bowie became a workaholic even by his own standards, staying awake day and night to record while the band slept in the studio. An anonymous musician later recalled David "waiting several hours for coke to be delivered from New York and he wouldn't perform until it came."

The Sigma sessions were prodigiously productive: among the out-takes which would not see the light of day for many years were 'It's Hard To Be A Saint In The City', 'After Today', 'Who Can I Be Now?', 'It's Gonna Be Me', 'John, I'm Only Dancing (Again)' and the mythical out-take 'Too Fat Polka'. "A small group of fans stood vigil outside the studio listening as hard as they could," Visconti remembered. "On the last day David took pity on them and invited them in for an hour of listening." Many years later Bowie was still affectionately dedicating Philadelphia concert performances of 'Young Americans' to "the Sigma Kids".

Towards the end of the fortnight, the sessions were increasingly marred by disputes with Tony Defries, who disliked David's new material and opposed his intention to scrap the expensive Diamond Dogs set for the forthcoming autumn tour. In an interview for the *Los Angeles Times* in September, when he was supposed to be promoting *David Live*, Bowie openly defied his manager by enthusing instead about the new recordings which would not be released for another six months. "My record company doesn't like me to do this," he said, "But I'm so excited about this one ... and it can tell you more about where I am now than anything I could say." He explained that in the past he had used "science fiction patterns because I was trying to put forward concepts, ideas and theories, but this album hasn't anything to do with that. It's just emotional drive ... There's not a concept in sight." He stressed the album's personal authenticity: "This one is the nearest to actually meeting me since that *Space Oddity* album, which was quite personal," he explained, adding that "the songs on *Diamond Dogs* I got the biggest kick out of, 'Rock'n Roll With Me' and '1984', gave me the knowledge that there was another album at least inside of me that I was going to be happy with." Of his *faux*-black vocal style, he revealed that "It's only now that I've got the necessary confidence to sing like that. That's the kind of music I've always wanted to sing. I mean, those are my favourite artists ... the Jackie Wilsons, that type."

The album's myriad working titles included *Dancin'*, *Somebody Up There Likes Me*, *One Damn Song* (a quotation from the title track), *Shilling The Rubes* (an American slang term that roughly translates as "conning the suckers" – a throwback to the Hype philosophy of 1970) and *The Gouster* (according to Tony Visconti, this was contemporary street slang for "a cool hip guy who walks down the street snapping his fingers", but it's worth noting that *Cassell's Dictionary Of Slang* defines "gowster" as a "habitual user of marijuana, morphine or heroin"). As late as December 1974 David informed *Disc* that the album would in fact be called *Fascination*, a remark which reveals that he had recently completed a new track. Indeed, although it's commonly believed that all but the John Lennon collaborations were finished at Sigma in August, this is in fact far from accurate. At the end of the Philly Dogs tour in December, Bowie would enter New York's Record Plant Studios with Tony Visconti, Carlos Alomar and David Sanborn to complete 'Win' and 'Fascination', the latter adapted from 'Funky Music', a composition Luther Vandross had performed in the tour's support set. An early track-listing of *The Gouster*, compiled by Tony Visconti shortly after the Philadelphia sessions, confirms that neither track had yet been completed: at this stage the album was to open with 'John, I'm Only Dancing (Again)', followed by 'Somebody Up There Likes Me', 'It's Gonna Be Me', 'Who Can I Be Now?', 'Can You Hear Me', 'Young Americans' and 'Right'. The *Fascination* track-listing announced by *Disc* in December sees the newly completed 'Win' and 'Fascination' ousting 'Who Can I Be Now?' and 'Somebody Up There Likes Me'. At this stage 'John, I'm Only Dancing (Again)' was still in the running as the opening track, but cir-

cumstances were about to dictate an altogether more radical rethink. Again, previous accounts have often confused their dates regarding the most famous collaboration on *Young Americans*. Many place it in late 1974 when in fact, as corroborated by Keith Badman's admirable day-by-day chronology *The Beatles After The Break-Up*, the recordings took place in January 1975.

With the title track already mixed in London by Tony Visconti, Bowie and his producer became regular fixtures at Record Plant during December and January, mixing *Young Americans* with the assistance of in-house engineer Harry Maslin. Bowie was renting two suites in New York's Pierre Hotel, where he spent his free time building model sets and shooting test footage for his mooted *Diamond Dogs* film. At the same time John Lennon was working at Record Plant, putting the finishing touches to his covers album *Rock'n'Roll*; he was in the middle of his famous year-long "lost weekend", and had first met Bowie in Los Angeles the previous September. According to Ava Cherry David was "in awe" of Lennon, but as the two began to socialize in New York the prospect of a collaboration reared its head. In early January an impromptu jam led to a one-day session at the nearby Electric Lady Studios, spawning David's cover of 'Across The Universe' and a new number, the iconic 'Fame'. For the session David roped in Carlos Alomar, Emir Ksasan and other members of the Philly Dogs band, giving Earl Slick and Dennis Davis their Bowie studio debuts. Newcomers were drummer Ralph McDonald and backing vocalists Jean Fineberg and Jean Millington, who later married Earl Slick.

Tony Visconti had returned to England with what he believed was the finished album on the very morning of the Electric Lady session. "The three of us, John, David and myself, stayed up until about ten in the morning, and had a great time together, and I wish I'd been in the studio with them," said Visconti. "About two weeks after I'd mixed the album, David phoned to tell me about 'Fame'. He was very apologetic and nice about it, and said he hoped I wouldn't mind if we took a few tracks off and included these." In Visconti's absence David had co-produced and mixed the new tracks with Harry Maslin (whose overall contribution to the album has been given greater credit in recent years: in addition to his acknowledged work on the two Lennon tracks, EMI's 1999 reissue gives Maslin a co-production credit alongside Visconti on every track bar 'Young Americans', and credits the production of 'Can You Hear Me' to Bowie and Maslin alone). To make way for the two new tracks, 'Who Can I Be Now?' and 'It's Gonna Be Me' were dropped from the album. "Beautiful songs," Visconti said later, "and it made me sick when he decided not to use them. I think it was the personal content of the songs which he was a bit reluctant to release, although it was so obscure I don't think even I knew what he was on about in them!" As for missing out on producing the Lennon tracks: "if I said I didn't weep I'd be lying. It hurt. I got on so well with Lennon, it would've been the most wonderful experience of my recording career. Oh well." A lasting result of the encounter was an introduction to Lennon's then girlfriend, May Pang, whom Visconti would later marry. "Never wear a new girlfriend in front of Tony!" joked Bowie many years later.

John Lennon's other contribution to David's career came in the form of some hard advice about how to disentangle himself from his manager: Lennon himself was still fighting a rearguard action against Allen Klein in the wake of the Beatles split. "It was John that sorted me out all the way down the line," David said later. "I realized I was very naïve. I still thought you had to have somebody else who dealt with these things called contracts." Shortly after his discussions with Lennon, Bowie began legal proceedings to separate himself from Tony Defries and MainMan. Corinne Schwab contacted a Beverly Hills lawyer called Michael Lippman, who commenced action against MainMan on David's behalf at the end of January.

RCA understandably sided with the artist (some executives have since told biographers that they relished the opportunity to repay some of the indignities heaped on them over the years by Defries), and the unreleased *Young Americans* became a significant bargaining chip. The label was already confident that the new recordings, boosted by a big-name guest collaboration, would give David his American breakthrough. Bowie had sensibly locked the Sigma Sound masters in a bank vault, and RCA's Geoff Hannington visited Electric Lady Studios "at dead of night with dollar bills" to collect the two Lennon tracks before MainMan got its hands on them. Defries tried, unsuccessfully, to block the album's release. The lawsuit progressed through 1975, becoming one of the most talked-about legal disputes in showbusiness history, and its aftermath was lengthy and unpleasant. A deal would eventually be struck which, in most estimations, left

Defries the victor. It was not until well into the 1980s that David would begin making the sort of money commonly associated with a rock star of his stature. Among the terms of the settlement was the agreement that any new material written or recorded up to 30 September 1982 (the termination of David's original contract with Defries) would be subject to a 16 per cent royalty payment to MainMan. From October 1982 onwards David would assume full rights to his new songs, but Defries retained a percentage of the pre-1982 work in perpetuity: he would receive 16 per cent of all future earnings on work between the severance agreement and September 1982, and an astonishing 50 per cent of all future earnings on everything from the Decca recordings up to and including *David Live*.

Any final analysis of the MainMan controversy must be qualified by an acknowledgement that David had only himself to blame for failing to inspect the small print of the documents he had signed from 1970 onwards. And, of course, the glorious madness of the MainMan circus was instrumental in launching him before a global audience. David told *Melody Maker* in 1978 that "My anger was spent a good couple of years ago, and all the feelings of being used, done-out-of and whatever have more or less melted into the mist ... I certainly would not have achieved that degree of notoriety without all that nonsense going on ... Without some of those initial ridiculous fusses, some of the best things might never have come to light. It did come to light through the efforts of him and the crazies who were running around at the time, so I guess I'm thankful for that period in a way." At the same time, he was quick to emphasize that "I'll never condone what went on."

"We all got ripped off by Defries," photographer Mick Rock told *Uncut* in 2003, "in terms of money and the abuse of intellectual property. Partly because we didn't know what the hell intellectual property was in those days. There was villainy afoot, and it's legitimate for David to criticize him, though as he was facilitating access for me, I had no problem with him. And it was because Defries signed David to his production company, rather than directly to RCA, that David was able to do that amazing Wall Street deal many years later [1997's so-called "Bowie Bonds" flotation], and move his records from one label to another. Long-term, he benefited."

A happier outcome of the short-term ordeal was that Bowie renewed his friendship with Defries's predecessor Kenneth Pitt, who spent many hours giving David sound advice by telephone during late 1974 and early 1975. Pitt's long-standing financial dispute with Defries was settled in the same year, and 20 years later Pitt was still attending Bowie's concerts.

The final touches had been put to *Young Americans* at Record Plant on 12 January 1975. Bowie telephoned the artist Norman Rockwell to invite him to paint the album sleeve but, as David later explained, "His wife explained in this quavering, elderly voice, 'I'm sorry, but Norman needs at least six months for his portraits.' So I had to pass." Another rejected sleeve design was a full-length photograph of David in a flying suit, complete with white silk scarf, standing in front of a Stars and Stripes flag and raising a glass. The eventual choice was a back-lit and heavily airbrushed photo of David by Eric Stephen Jacobs.

The album was released on 7 March to a generally warm reception, particularly from American critics who had never been entirely happy with David's glam period. "It works well. The key here is that Bowie's sophisticated soul … does not sound the least bit put on. The vocals do not sound nearly as strained as they have on some of his more raucous rockers, nor do they sound as camp," noted *Billboard* approvingly, adding that the record "should not only endear Bowie even more to his current fans but should open up an entirely new avenue of fans for him." *Record World* described it as Bowie's "most compelling album to date", while *Cashbox* crowned David "the brightest star in the pop music constellation with this latest RCA release". *Rolling Stone* was more cautious, recommending 'Fame' and lauding the album as "a very successful experiment … certainly much better than many of his other experiments", but describing the vocals as "distorted" and 'Across The Universe' as "just hideous". In Britain, some of Bowie's former champions were similarly unconvinced. Michael Watts, whose *Melody Maker* interview had helped launch David to stardom in 1972, noted disparagingly that the album was "designed to cast our hero in the mould of soul superstar", but that "I get a persistent picture of nigger patronisation as Bowie flips through his soul take-offs at Sigma Sound like some cocktail-party liberal … he patently lacks any deep emotional commitment to his material."

David himself has since been less than complimentary about *Young Americans*, although his famous description of the album as "plastic soul" has been quoted out of context for decades. What he actually told the *NME*, only a few months after the album's release, was that he was attempting to comment on the media's appropriation of musical forms: "My statement is 'rock and roll is walking all over everybody'," he explained, "Like, I tried to do a little stretch of how it feels musically in this country, which is sort of the relentless plastic soul basically. That's what the last album was." On another occasion he described *Young Americans* as "the squashed remains of ethnic music as it survives in the age of muzak rock, written and sung by a white limey." Elsewhere he exclaimed, "It's the phoniest R&B I've ever heard. If I ever would have got my hands on that record when I was growing up I would have cracked it over my knee." In 1976 he told *Melody Maker* that "I don't listen to it very much. I don't like it very much. It was a phase."

More recently, David has moderated his opinion. "I shouldn't have been quite so hard on myself, because looking back it was pretty good white, blue-eyed soul," he told *Q* magazine in 1990. "At the time I still had an element of being the artist who just throws things out unemotionally. But it was quite definitely one of the best bands I ever had … And I was like most English who come over to America for the first time, totally blown away by the fact that the blacks in America had their own culture, and it was positive and they were proud of it … and to be right there in the middle of it was just intoxicating, to go into the same studios as all these great artists." In 1978 he explained, "I wanted to get into that Warholism of Polaroiding things … *Young Americans* was my photograph of American music at the time."

To this day *Young Americans* splits Bowie fans down the middle. Some deplore its inauthentic soul-boy pretensions and view it as an aberration by an artist whose talents lie elsewhere. Others revel in its deft embrace of funk and soul, marvelling at how a man under such terrible personal and professional pressures could produce a record of such limpid beauty and consummate musicianship. Certainly Visconti's production, the band's playing and in particular Bowie's soaring vocals have seldom been bettered. It's not without justification that some of the lyrics have been regarded as superficial and woolly by comparison with the rest of Bowie's 1970s work, but on closer inspection the familiar anguish penetrates the album's soft-focus trappings: the violent underbelly of the title track, the minatory tone of 'Somebody Up There Likes Me', and in particular the blistering spite of 'Fame' are sorely undervalued. "*Young Americans* is a fantastic soul record, but soul with something else going on," says admirer Bob Geldof. "There's an edginess to it."

Whatever else it was, *Young Americans* was the album that finally broke the US market, going top ten, spawning a number 1 single in 'Fame', and transforming Bowie from a mildly unsavoury cult artist to a chat-show friendly showbiz personality. More importantly, by jumping on the Stax/George McCrae bandwagon, Bowie had undertaken the first significant excursion into black soul by a mainstream white artist and, despite the ridicule he invited by doing so, had broken down barriers on the path to the forthcoming disco explosion. In the wake of Bowie's Sigma sessions Elton John recorded 'Philadelphia Freedom', which (backed by a duet with John Lennon!) charted alongside 'Young Americans' in March 1975. Other British releases that followed Bowie's example during 1975 included Roxy Music's 'Love Is The Drug' and Rod Stewart's *Atlantic Crossing*.

In the longer term Bowie's white translation of soul and funk, and the accompanying pose of finger-snapping cool in a tailored suit, would provide a keynote for 1980s bands as diverse as ABC, Talking Heads, Spandau Ballet and Japan. Michael Jackson would buy it all back again – as a black artist singing white man's black music – with devastating commercial success. And if 'Space Oddity' had originally borrowed from the sound of the early Bee Gees, Bowie was now more than repaying the debt, paving the way for a commercial atmosphere that would foster the Gibb brothers' biggest successes. In this light at least, the importance of *Young Americans* is beyond question. Of course, by the time the disco craze arrived, David Bowie had moved somewhere else altogether.

STATION TO STATION
RCA Victor APLI 1327, January 1976 [5]
RCA PL 81327, 1984
EMI EMD 1020, April 1991 [57]
EMI 7243 5219060, September 1999

'Station To Station' (10'08") / 'Golden Years' (4'03") / 'Word On A Wing' (6'00") / 'TVC15' (5'29") / 'Stay' (6'08") / 'Wild Is The Wind' (5'58")

Bonus tracks on 1991 reissue: 'Word On A Wing (Live)' (6'10") / 'Stay (Live)' (7'24")

• *Musicians:* David Bowie *(vocals, guitar, saxophone),*

Carlos Alomar *(guitar)*, Roy Bittan *(piano)*, Dennis Davis *(drums)*, George Murray *(bass)*, Warren Peace *(vocals)*, Earl Slick *(guitar)* • *Recorded:* Cherokee & LA Record Plant Studios, Hollywood • *Producers:* David Bowie, Harry Maslin

When *The Man Who Fell To Earth* completed shooting in August 1975 Bowie returned to Los Angeles, where Coco Schwab had found him a house in Stone Canyon Drive. Ava Cherry had departed for Trinidad following a quarrel before the film shoot. Angela Bowie remained on the sidelines, occasionally helping to pick up the pieces during the depths of David's drug dependency, but the end of the marriage was now only a matter of time.

May 1975 had seen an abortive collaboration in Los Angeles with Iggy Pop (see 'Moving On' in Chapter 1), and there are unreliable rumours of uncredited contributions to recordings by Marc Bolan and Keith Moon during the same period. In April, however, Bowie had famously announced his departure from rock music. "I've rocked my roll," he said. "It's a boring dead end. There will be no more rock-'n'roll records or tours from me. The last thing I want to be is some useless fucking rock singer." Later in the year he declared that rock music had been emasculated by absorption into the mass media, leaving it "dead. It's a toothless old woman. It's really embarrassing." Those who remembered as far back as 1973 knew that such statements were always subject to retraction, and in this case the retirement lasted six months.

In October 1975 David contacted Harry Maslin, who had co-produced the John Lennon tracks on *Young Americans*, and asked him to come to Los Angeles to work on a new album. Carlos Alomar, Earl Slick, Dennis Davis and Warren Peace were re-convened, and the band was completed with two new recruits: Weldon Irvine's bass player George Murray – bringing together for the first time the Murray/Davis/Alomar rhythm section who would play on every Bowie album up to *Scary Monsters* – and Bruce Springsteen's E-Street Band pianist Roy Bittan, who had worked with Slick in the group Tracks. "I needed a pianist because Mike Garson was off being a Scientologist somewhere," said David. "Roy impressed me a lot." Garson's version of events is rather different: he tells the Gillmans that after exchanging Christmas presents with David in 1974 and being told "I want you to be my pianist for the next twenty years", he simply never heard from Bowie again, considering himself a victim of David's purge of the MainMan era. He wouldn't re-enter Bowie's career until the *Black Tie White Noise* sessions in 1992.

According to Tony Zanetta's *Stardust*, Deep Purple bassist and co-vocalist Glenn Hughes was also present during the early stages of *Station To Station* and was invited by David to sing on the album, but Deep Purple, who had already lost Ritchie Blackmore, apparently objected. If this story is true, nothing came of it.

After two weeks' rehearsal, the band entered Hollywood's Cherokee Studios in October. Both the split from Tony Defries and the commercial success of *Young Americans* conspired to create an unfamiliar atmosphere of artistic freedom: "I loved those sessions," Harry Maslin tells Jerry Hopkins, "because we were totally open and experimental in our approach. We weren't trying to create a hit single ... I think he felt this was time to feel free. He wanted to do the music the way he heard it and we didn't worry about RCA." Earl Slick would similarly recall that David "had one or two songs written, but they were changed so drastically that you wouldn't know them from the first time anyway, so he basically wrote everything in the studio." Carlos Alomar concurs, telling David Buckley that "It was one of the most glorious albums that I've ever done ... We experimented so much on it."

The album was provisionally entitled *The Return Of The Thin White Duke* and then *Golden Years*, after the first track to be completed. 'Golden Years' was premiered on ABC's *Soul Train* on 4 November, and released as a single later the same month while the sessions continued, interrupted only by David's appearances on *The Cher Show* and *Russell Harty Plus*.

After returning from New Mexico looking healthier than at any time since 1973, Bowie had once again stepped back into the abyss. Lasting nearly three months and fuelled by David's obsessive perfectionism and prodigious cocaine intake, the sessions sometimes continued for over 24 hours non-stop. On one occasion work began at 7.00am and continued until nine the following morning, when a halt was called only because another artist was booked into Cherokee. Within 90 minutes David had recommenced recording at the nearby LA Record Plant, where he worked until midnight. "He liked to work four days or so, very strenuous hours, then take a few days off to rest and get charged up for another sprint," confirmed Maslin.

Today Bowie confesses that he was so addled that he can hardly remember making the album. "I remember working with Earl on the guitar sounds," he recalled in 1997, "And screaming the feedback sound that I wanted at him ... I also remember telling him, 'Take a Chuck Berry riff and play it all the way through the solo, don't deviate from it, just play that one riff over and over and over again, even though the chords are changing underneath, just keep it going.' ... And that's about all I remember of it. I can't even remember the studio. I know it was in LA because I've read it was." Contemporary footage of Bowie bears witness that the *Station To Station* sessions were probably his darkest hour. "I was flying out there – really in a bad way," he told *Q* in 1996. "I listen to *Station To Station* as a piece of work by an entirely different person ... It's an extremely dark album."

The compelling and often sinister atmosphere was a by-product of David's increasingly unhealthy state of mind: his long-term interest in obscure occultism had now reached obsessive levels. "It was unreal, absolutely unreal," he recalled in 1983. "Of course, every day that you stay up longer – and there's things that you have to do to stay up that long – the impending tiredness and fatigue produces that hallucinogenic state quite naturally. Well, *half*-naturally. By the end of the week my whole life would be transformed into this bizarre nihilistic fantasy world of oncoming doom, mythological characters and imminent totalitarianism. Quite the worst. I was living in LA with Egyptian décor. It was one of those rent-a-house places but it appealed to me because I had this more-than-passing interest in Egyptology, mysticism, the Kabbalah, all this stuff that is inherently misleading in life, a hotchpotch whose crux I've forgotten."

The distressing depths to which David plummeted in 1975 are recalled in a host of notorious anecdotes, many of which derive from the same source: a 17-year-old reporter called Cameron Crowe who had successfully penetrated Bowie's inner circle and gathered spool upon spool of interview footage. Crowe's subsequent articles in *Playboy* and *Rolling Stone* were so sensational that they rapidly became the stuff of legend, but while there is no doubt that Bowie got up to some frighteningly unhinged behaviour during the period, we would do well to remember that he has always enjoyed playing with interviewers, and that his performance may have been embellished for Mr Crowe's benefit. Tales abound of black candles, bottled urine, bodies falling past windows, witches stealing David's semen, demons attacking him in photographs, the exorcism of his swimming pool, the CIA infiltrating his movie-making plans, and The Rolling Stones sending him hidden messages in their record sleeves. Angela Bowie has corroborated some of these stories, but the point, surely, is that David Bowie was not a well man. Existing on a diet of red and green peppers, with the curtains constantly drawn because, as he later recalled, he "didn't want the LA sun spoiling the vibe of eternal now", Bowie was wasting away both mentally and physically. "At some points I almost reached 80lbs," he recalled in 1997. "It was really, really painful. And also my disposition left a lot to be desired. I was just paranoid, manic depressive, it was all the usual emotional paraphernalia that comes with abuse of amphetamines and coke and all that."

Into the spiritual void came the areas of interest that infused *Station To Station*. "A lot of them were, I guess, considered taboos," he explained in 1996, "they were things that most people would leave alone and not bother with, because the results of investigating them might be quite dodgy ... like the whole Fascist thing." What David later referred to as his "wayward spiritual search" had begun in New York in early 1975 when he met Kenneth Anger, the author of *Hollywood Babylon* whose film *Inauguration Of The Pleasure Dome* was an exploration of the neo-pagan warlock Aleister Crowley, a figure who famously attracted the attention of Led Zeppelin's Jimmy Page at around the same time (a groundless suspicion that Page meant him harm was reportedly another of Bowie's myriad neuroses during the period). David embarked on a long trawl through Crowley's magic treatises and texts by Madame Blavatsky and the Armenian mystic Gurdjieff, together with MacGregor Mathers's *The Kabbalah Unveiled* and a host of fashionable conspiracy paperbacks on subjects like the Tarot, numerology, the Golden Dawn's connections with Nazi iconography, Himmler's alleged search for the Holy Grail in pre-war England, and prehistoric visits from spacemen. The contents of this unwholesome melting pot, together with a substantial dose of his alienated *Man Who Fell To Earth* character Thomas Newton, congealed in the creation of David's latest *alter ego*: an emotionless Aryan superman called The Thin White Duke.

Station To Station marks a precise halfway point on the journey between *Young Americans* and *Low*. There are enough finger-snapping grooves to keep the American market buoyant, but elsewhere the album prefigures the glacial mechanization of David's imminent "European canon". The chilly Teutonic beat of the title track is partially inspired by Bowie's growing enthusiasm for the ground-breaking sounds of German techno bands like Neu!, Can and Kraftwerk. The austere tone is fixed by the unspaced sleeve lettering and Steve Shapiro's monochrome cover photo from *The Man Who Fell To Earth*. Latter-day reissues have reinstated the full-colour version originally planned for the album, but for the official release Bowie decided at the eleventh hour to use a cropped black-and-white copy of the same photograph, cut adrift within a huge white border, reflecting the stark monochrome aesthetic of the Thin White Duke character and the 1976 tour. The photo shows Bowie as Newton entering a soundproof chamber whose walls eliminate extraneous and ambient sound, leaving only heartbeat and electrical brain activity audible – a resonant link with the sensory-deprivation themes of *The Man Who Fell To Earth*.

At the time David spoke of the album as "a plea to come back to Europe for me ... one of those self-chat things one has with oneself from time to time." In 1999 he described his state of mind during the sessions as "psychically damaged. I mean, the words themselves, *Station To Station*, have a significance inasmuch as they do refer to the Stations of the Cross, but then I took that further and it was actually about the Kabbalistic Tree of Life, so for me the whole album was symbolic and representative of the trip through the Tree of Life." The album, he explained, was conceived as a kind of aural spell: "It had a certain magnetism that one associates with spells. There's a certain charismatic quality about the music ... that really eats into you. I still don't know what I think about that album. I find it, at times, probably really quite beautiful, and at other times extraordinarily disturbing."

Station To Station certainly sounds like the cry of an unsettled soul, torn between cocaine, occultism and Christianity, most starkly in the oppositions of the title track and the devotional content of 'Word On A Wing'. There is also a hunger for beauty and tenderness, nowhere clearer than in the desperate yearning of 'Wild Is The Wind'. The twin search for love and belief underpins much of the album: David's reiteration in 'Word On A Wing' that he is "ready to shape the scheme of things" sounds like a breath of cautious optimism on both the spiritual level (in 1976 he began the slow journey back to recovery) and the material (the *Station To Station* sessions coincided with the last gasp of his Faustian pact with MainMan). In a wasteland of shattered faith and broken relationships Bowie finds himself "searching and searching, and oh what will I be believing, and who will connect me with love?" But it's easy to exaggerate the album's darker elements. Alongside the desperation of 'Stay' and 'Word On A Wing' are the bouncy nonsense of 'TVC15' and the romantic optimism of 'Golden Years', which realigns the title track's uncertainties with an affirmation that "I believe, oh Lord, I believe all the way".

Although describing *Station To Station* in 1976 as "devoid of spirit, very steely", Bowie later confessed to reservations about its commercial sheen: "I compromised in the mixing. I wanted to do a dead mix ... All the way through, no echo ... I gave in and added that extra commercial touch. I wish I hadn't." But the decision to go for a mainstream polish made sense. The US market knew little of David Bowie before *Young Americans*, and his much-vaunted changes in musical style meant nothing to them. To *Billboard*'s reviewer, *Station To Station* was therefore "a disco dance album" from an artist "who seems to have found his musical niche following the success of 'Fame' and now 'Golden Years'"; the observation that "the lyrics don't seem to mean a great deal, and the 10-minute title cut drags" merely underlines the extent to which America remained unprepared to consider Bowie's intellectual challenges and stylistic restlessness. *Station To Station* was a commercial success in America – indeed, more so than in Britain, where it peaked at number 5 against America's number 3 – but in the fickle US marketplace it was to be the end of Bowie's flirtation with the mainstream until the 1980s.

In Britain, the *NME* found the album "a strange and confusing musical whirlpool where nothing is what it seems", and while admitting that "the significance of the lyrics remains elusive", concluded that it was "one of the most significant albums released in the last five years." For "five" we can now read "thirty-five": *Station To Station* is now regarded by many as one of Bowie's most important works, a multi-textured experience illuminated, but not diminished, by an awareness of the anguish that attended its creation.

In December 1975, hard on the heels of the *Station To Station* sessions, Bowie began work on his proposed incidental soundtrack for *The Man Who Fell To Earth*. Harry Maslin again produced at Cherokee, and David flew in his old *Space Oddity* colleague Paul Buckmaster to collaborate on the project. With Bowie's guitar and Buckmaster's cello accompanied by synthesizers and some of the earliest drum machines, the compositions were strongly influenced by Kraftwerk's latest album *Radio-Activity*, released the previous month. However, the soundtrack was destined not to see the light of day. "When I'd finished five or six pieces, I was told that if I would care to submit my music along with other people's..." Bowie recalled later. "I just said, 'Shit, you're not getting any of it.' I was furious, I'd put so much work into it. Actually though, it was probably as well. My music would have cast a completely different reflection on it all. It turned out for the better and it did prompt me in another area – to consider my own instrumental capabilities, which I hadn't really done very seriously before. The area was one that was suddenly exciting me ... And that's when I got the first inklings of trying to work with Eno."

This account doesn't quite tell the whole story. "David was so burned out by the end of *Station To Station*," Harry Maslin tells Jerry Hopkins, "he had a hard time doing movie cues. The movie was complete and we had all the videotapes and that's what we were working with ... He was in bad shape. He had no concentration on the music." David was now quarrelling with Michael Lippman, the lawyer who had become Tony Defries's short-lived replacement as manager. Paul Buckmaster recalls the sessions being blighted by cocaine abuse, and matters came to a head when David, overcome by emotional and physical stress, all but collapsed in the studio. "There were pieces of me laying all over the floor," he later said. It was a turning-point of sorts: over the next few days he sacked Michael Lippman, abandoned the film soundtrack (which was handled instead by John Phillips of The Mamas and The Papas), and laid immediate plans to leave Los Angeles for good.

LOW

RCA Victor PL 12030, January 1977 [2]
RCA International INTS 5065, June 1983 [85]
RCA International NL 83856, March 1984
EMI EMD 1027, August 1991 [64]
EMI 7243 5219070, September 1999

'Speed Of Life' (2'45") / 'Breaking Glass' (1'42") / 'What In The World' (2'20") / 'Sound And Vision' (3'00") / 'Always Crashing In The Same Car' (3'26")

/ 'Be My Wife' (2'55") / 'A New Career In A New Town' (2'50") / 'Warszawa' (6'17") / 'Art Decade' (3'43") / 'Weeping Wall' (3'25") / 'Subterraneans' (5'37")

Bonus tracks on 1991 reissue: 'Some Are' (3'24") / 'All Saints' (3'35") / 'Sound And Vision (Remixed version, 1991)' (4'43")

• *Musicians:* David Bowie *(vocals, ARP, tape horn, bass-synthetic strings, saxophones, cellos, tape, guitar, pump bass, harmonica, piano, percussion, Chamberlain, vibraphones, xylophones, ambient sounds)*, Brian Eno *(Splinter mini-moog, Report ARP, Rimmer EMI, guitar treatments, Chamberlain, vocals on 'Sound and Vision')*, Carlos Alomar *(guitar)*, Dennis Davis *(percussion)*, Ricky Gardiner *(guitar)*, Eduard Meyer *(cellos on 'Art Decade')*, George Murray *(bass)*, Iggy Pop *(vocals on 'What in the World')*, Mary Visconti *(vocals on 'Sound and Vision')*, Roy Young *(piano, Farfisa organ)*, Peter and Paul *(pianos and ARP on 'Subterraneans')* • *Recorded:* Château d'Hérouville Studios, Pontoise; Hansa Studios, Berlin • *Producers:* David Bowie, Tony Visconti

The genesis of *Low*, one of Bowie's most iconic and influential albums, lay in compositions originally intended for the soundtrack of *The Man Who Fell To Earth*. "We all had pressures, deadlines," recalled Nicolas Roeg in 1993. "Eventually we brought in John Phillips to do the score. Then six months later David sent me a copy of *Low* with a note that said, 'This is what I wanted to do for the soundtrack'. It would have been a wonderful score."

But *Low* was more than a rejected movie soundtrack: it was a form of creative therapy and one of Bowie's definitive changes in direction. Ravaged by cocaine and already fascinated by the avant-garde electronic music of German groups like Kraftwerk, Neu! and Tangerine Dream, David elected in the summer of 1976 to relocate to the Continent where, with the mutual support of the similarly afflicted Iggy Pop, creative rebirth would run parallel with physical recovery. "I was in a serious decline, emotionally and socially," he said in 1996. "I think I was very much on course to be just another rock casualty – in fact, I'm quite certain I wouldn't have survived the seventies if I'd carried on doing what I was doing. But I was lucky enough to know somewhere within me that I really was killing myself, and I had to do something drastic to pull myself out of that."

Although referred to ubiquitously as the first of Bowie's "Berlin" albums, the majority of *Low* was in fact recorded at the Château d'Hérouville near Paris, where *Pin Ups* had been made three years earlier and where Iggy Pop's *The Idiot* had just been completed. Although there was a certain amount of overlapping, the *Low* sessions proper began at the Château on 1 September 1976. Carlos Alomar, George Murray and Dennis Davis were recalled from *Station To Station*, and were joined by keyboardist Roy Young, formerly of The Rebel Rousers. Bowie had initially hoped to secure the services of Neu! guitarist Klaus Dinger, but when the offer was declined ("in the most polite and diplomatic fashion," David later recalled), the job went instead to former Beggar's Opera guitarist Ricky Gardiner, who had originally been recommended by Tony Visconti to play on *The Idiot* (he didn't, but would subsequently work on *Lust For Life*). "He was totally left-field and completely savvy with special effects," Visconti later said of Gardiner. "I was in awe of him."

The most significant new arrival was Brian Eno, the erstwhile Roxy Music member whose remarkable solo albums had impressed David immensely. Roxy Music had supported several Bowie gigs in the summer of 1972, and the pair had met up again the following year when recording simultaneous solo projects (*Diamond Dogs* and *Here Come The Warm Jets*) at Olympic Studios. Acquaintance deepened into friendship after Bowie's Wembley shows in May 1976, as Eno recalled: "I went backstage and then we drove back to where he was living in Maida Vale. He said that he'd been listening to *Discreet Music* [Eno's November 1975 album], which was very interesting because at that time that was a very out-there record which was universally despised by the English pop press. He said he'd been playing it non-stop on his American tour, and naturally flattery always endears you to someone." Likewise Eno considered *Station To Station* "one of the great records of all time … I thought it was very strong, a real successful joining of that American urban funk scene with the kinds of things we had been doing in the early seventies."

Eno, with his neoclassical allegiances to minimalist composers like John Cage and Philip Glass, and his antipathy to every established convention of rock music, provided a stimulating contrast to Bowie. He has often stated that his ultimate aim is the subsumption of the individual, the effacement of the artist's personality from the music. By contrast Bowie's work had hitherto thrived on the traditional dynamics of performed music and the fabrication of a succession of *Übermenschen* to perform it. As Eno wrote many years later during the *1.Outside* sessions, "I become the sculptor to David's tendency to paint. I keep trying to cut things back, strip them to something tense and taut, while he keeps throwing new colours on the canvas. It's a good duet."

Shortly before the Château d'Hérouville sessions Bowie contacted Eno and invited him to join him on what he explained would be a purely experimental album, originally to be called *New Music, Night And Day*. "What I think he was trying to do was to duck the momentum of a successful career," Eno later explained. His influence on the work that became *Low* would be difficult to exaggerate, but contrary to widespread belief he was not the album's producer. "It amazes me how so-called responsible journalists don't even bother to read the credits on the album," said Tony Visconti many years later. "Brian is a great musician, and was very integral to the making of those three albums [*Low*, *"Heroes"* and *Lodger*]. But he was not the producer." Bowie has been equally keen to stress this fact: "Over the years not enough credit has gone to Tony Visconti on those particular albums," he said in 2000. "The actual sound and texture, the feel of everything from the drums to the way that my voice is recorded, is Tony Visconti."

Visconti, with whom David had last worked on *Young Americans*, had been called in to mix *The Idiot* and took the producer's chair for the *Low* sessions. He later explained that Bowie "wanted to make an album of music which was uncompromising and reflected the way he felt. He said he didn't care whether or not he had another hit record, and that [the recording would be] so out of the ordinary that it might never get released." Among the innovations Visconti brought to the studio was a new gadget called the Eventide Harmonizer which, as he explained to David, "fucks with the fabric of time!" The Harmonizer was the first machine capable of altering pitch while maintaining tempo, its influence most obvious in the speeded-up vocals on Bowie's later recording 'Scream Like A Baby'. It was this gadget that would engineer the drop in pitch on the tight, buzzing snare-drum sound that became one of *Low*'s revolutionary characteristics.

By the time Brian Eno joined the *Low* sessions the rest of the band had already begun laying down backing tracks. "Brian was there to programme different keyboard instruments for David, Roy and himself," explained Ricky Gardiner. Despite Bowie's unprecedented embrace of electronic processes, he was reluctant to use synthesizers merely to imitate other instruments: "I don't want to reproduce violin sounds – I'd much rather use the synthesizer as a texture," he revealed. "If I need a sound that I haven't heard in my head, then I require the assistance of a synthesizer to give me a texture that doesn't exist. If I want a guitar sound, I use a real guitar, but then I might mistreat it by putting it through the synthesizer afterwards and deforming the sound."

This approach was key to Bowie's methodology: as ever, he was less interested in mimicking the new European music than in hybridizing it with other forms. In this respect, as he himself has pointed out, the oft-cited connection with groups such as Kraftwerk was no more than a starting point: "What I was passionate about in relation to Kraftwerk was their singular determination to stand apart from stereotypical American chord sequences and their wholehearted embrace of a European sensibility displayed through their music," David explained in 2001. "This was their very important influence on me." However, "Kraftwerk's approach to music had in itself little place in my scheme. Theirs was a controlled, robotic, extremely measured series of compositions, almost a parody of minimalism. One had the feeling that Florian and Ralf were completely in charge of their environment, and that their compositions were well prepared and honed before entering the studio. My work tended to expressionist mood pieces, the protagonist (myself) abandoning himself to the zeitgeist (a popular word at the time), with little or no control over his life. The music was spontaneous for the most part and created in the studio. In substance too, we were poles apart. Kraftwerk's percussion sound was produced electronically, rigid in tempo, unmoving. Ours was the mangled treatment of a powerfully emotive drummer, Dennis Davis. The tempo not only 'moved' but also was expressed in more than 'human' fashion. Kraftwerk supported that unyielding machine-like beat with all synthetic sound generating sources. We used an R&B band. Since *Station To Station* the hybridization of R&B and electronics had been a goal of mine."

The experimental techniques brought to the studio by Brian Eno included the use of the "Oblique Strategies" cards which he had developed in 1975 with Peter Schmidt. The cards would be turned over by musicians at random during recording to reveal instructions such as "Emphasize the flaws", "Fill every beat with something" or even "Use an unacceptable colour". The results were a staggering departure for Bowie; with Eno's encouragement, he was now subjecting the music itself to the kind of randomization he had already visited on the lyrics of previous albums. "I would put down a piano part, say," David explained in 1993, "and then take the faders down so you could only hear the drums and [Eno] only knew what key it was in. Then he would come in and put an alternative piece in, not hearing my part … we would leapfrog with each other, each not hearing each other's parts, and then at the end of the day put each other's parts up and see what happened."

Carlos Alomar was initially suspicious of Bowie's new off-the-wall approach: "I fought it for a second," he told Radio 2's *Golden Years*, "but, respecting his curiosity and his innovativeness, I said, 'Well, let me try this, maybe something will come of it.' And I'll tell you one thing – it was the best of all that I've ever done with David Bowie. I love the trilogy more than anything else."

Lyrically, too, Bowie was moving beyond the cut-ups of previous albums into an entirely impressionistic, non-linear concept. Eno, he explained, "got me off narration, which I was so intolerably bored with … Brian really opened my ideas to the idea of processing, to the abstract of communication." In sharp contrast with the verbosity of *Diamond Dogs* or *Young Americans*, *Low* is a lyrically sparse album; six tracks are instrumentals embellished at most by pseudo-Gregorian chants, while the remainder have only brief, fragmentary, repetitive lyrics charting the introspective isolation of Bowie's healing process.

During the sessions David had to go to Paris to attend a court hearing as part of his proceedings against Michael Lippman. While he was away, Eno continued working on the understanding that if David liked the result he could use it on *Low*. This, Eno explained to the *NME*, "meant I could work without any guilty conscience about wasting somebody else's time, because if he hadn't wanted them I would have paid him for the studio time and used them on my own album. As it happened, I did a couple of things that I thought were very nice and he liked them a lot." One result was the basic framework of 'Warszawa'.

By all accounts the Château d'Hérouville sessions were traumatic, interrupted by an episode of food poisoning and a succession of unhappy scenes arising from Bowie's conflicts with Lippman and with Angela, who arrived at the studio to introduce David to her new boyfriend. Visconti later called the session "a horrible experience" compounded by a "really antagonistic" relationship with the studio staff, one of whom turned out to be an undercover journalist who had infiltrated the building to spy on proceedings for the French music press. Even so, there were lighter moments: Carlos Alomar recalls ending each evening watching videos of the BBC's new hit *Fawlty Towers*, and Visconti confirms that "despite the outside pressures, when Bowie, Eno and I were in the studio working at our peak, it was magic."

Most of the band were present for the first five days only, after which Eno, Alomar and Gardiner remained to play overdubs. By the time Bowie wrote and recorded the lyrics everybody but Visconti and the studio engineers had departed. David had initially suggested that the first fortnight's recordings should be treated as demos but, Visconti later recalled, "after the two weeks had gone I said, 'We have much more than demos here, why do we have to re-record all this lovely stuff?' So we listened back, and the lesson learnt from that is that we keep the machines running while we're creating and we do all the demos on 24-track, just in case." After years of differing approaches, it was the *Low* sessions that saw Bowie plumping for the three-phase studio methodology he still favours to this day: backing tracks first, followed later by guest overdubs and instrumental solos, followed finally (sometimes weeks or even, in the case of *Lodger* and *Scary Monsters*, months later) by the composition of lyrics and the taping of vocals. It was a process he had used as far back as *The Man Who Sold The World*, but from hereon it became the established norm.

At the end of September, with most of the album already recorded, Bowie and Visconti left the Château in favour of the Hansa Studios in West Berlin (but not, contrary to popular belief, the Hansa By The Wall premises where *Low* would later be mixed and *"Heroes"* recorded). It was to prove a decisive step: despite Angela's attempts to coax David back to his tax-exile residence in Switzerland, Berlin would become his new adoptive home. After a short spell in the Hotel Gehrhus he moved into a seven-room flat at 155 Hauptstrasse, an area of tattered nineteenth-century finery in the city's unfashionable Schöneberg district, which remained his base for the next two years. "It was the antithesis of Los Angeles," he later said. "The people in Berlin don't give a damn about your problems. They've got their own … I thought if I could survive in Berlin without being mollycoddled, then I had a chance of surviving." After years of living in the relentless glare of celebrity David revelled in the anonymity Berlin offered. For the first time since early 1972 he had stopped dyeing his hair; he gave away his designer clothes and wore jeans and checked shirts. Disguised by a wispy moustache and a short back and sides administered by Tony Visconti, he rediscovered the joys of exploring a city on foot and by bicycle.

But Berlin was more than just a conveniently anonymous recharging station. It was the city of Fritz Lang, Christopher Isherwood and Bertolt Brecht, the adoptive home of George Grosz, Marc Chagall and the Brücke group, the melting pot of European modernism that had informed Bowie's work from the very beginning. "We just dug the whole idea that this was Berlin," said Iggy Pop later. "This is a war-zone, this is no man's land." In a sense Berlin was the very pattern of the post-apocalyptic urban landscape David had already envisaged in *Ziggy Stardust* and *Diamond Dogs*. As an arrested crossroads between East and West, and between past and future, 1970s Berlin was the ideal spiritual home for Bowie. He referred to the city as "the artistic and cultural gateway into Europe in the twenties", saying that "virtually anything important that happened in the arts happened there."

David had now been painting on and off for over a year – Tony Visconti recalls him sketching portraits of John Lennon in early 1975, and by the time of *The Man Who Fell To Earth* and *Station To Station* it had become his favourite pastime. Now, inspired by the city's cultural heritage and his encounters with its exotic *demi-monde*, he began painting in earnest. Berlin was home to all manner of minorities – artists, immigrants, punks, drag queens – who appealed to Bowie's affinity with outsiders. After his Berlin concert in April 1976 he had befriended Romy Haag, the most celebrated of the city's drag artists, who now became a semi-permanent fixture. His off-duty adventures in Berlin's art galleries, drag clubs and late-night drinking haunts provided the backdrop of the withdrawn, post-traumatic soundscapes of *Low* and *"Heroes"*.

"The first side of *Low* was all about me, 'Always Crashing In The Same Car' and all that self-pitying crap," explained David a year later, summing up the prevailing mood as "isn't it great to be on your own, let's just pull down the blinds and fuck 'em all." But he went on to explain that "side two was more an observation in musical terms: my reaction to seeing the East bloc, how West Berlin survives in the midst of it, which was something I couldn't express in words. Rather it required textures…"

Contrary to popular belief, however, Berlin's mythical "decadence" was not the quality which primarily attracted David to the city. "Berlin was my clinic," he said some years later. "It brought me back in touch with people. It got me back on the streets; not the street where everything is cold and there's drugs, but the streets where there were young, intelligent people trying to get along, and who were interested in more than how much money they were going to make a week on salary. Berliners are interested in how art means something on the streets, not just the galleries." In 1977 he declared that he had become "incapable of composing in Los Angeles, New York, London or Paris. There's something missing. Berlin has the strange ability to make you write only the important things. Anything else you don't mention, you remain silent, and write nothing … and in the end you produce *Low*."

At Hansa Bowie recorded the final tracks, 'Weeping Wall' and 'Art Decade', and added vocals to some of the Château recordings. The tail end of the sessions coincided with what was effectively the last gasp of David's marriage with Angela, who visited him in November 1976 to discuss their relationship. The stresses of recent times culminated in a dramatic incident on 10 November when David collapsed with a suspected heart attack and was rushed by Angela to the city's British military hospital. His condition was diagnosed rather less sensationally as an irregular heartbeat brought on by excessive drinking, and by the time the story broke Angela was back in London, appearing in a fund-raising revue called *Krisis Kabaret* with her boyfriend Roy Martin. The end came not long afterwards on another visit to Berlin, when David refused Angela's demand that he fire Coco Schwab. "I went into Corinne's room," writes Angela in her biography, "gathered up her clothes and some of the gifts I'd given her in better times, threw them out of the window into the street, and called a cab and caught a flight to London." Angela and David met only once more to exchange legal documents, and their divorce became final in February 1980.

Low lives up to its name, offering in its few sparse lyrics a numbing parade of private neuroses, from the agoraphobic ("wait until the crowd goes", "pale blinds drawn on day") to the isolated ("sometimes you get so lonely", "you never leave your room") to the violent ("breaking glass in your room again", "always crashing in the same car") to the out-and-out nihilistic ("nothing to read, nothing to say"). Bowie's apprehension that the album might never be released was not without foundation. Horrified RCA executives expecting another *Young Americans* or *Station To Station* pulled the album from the Christmas 1976 schedule and, as David later recalled, one of them offered to buy him a house in Philadelphia "so he can write some more of that black music". Tony Defries, whose royalty settlement ensured that he retained a keen interest in David's commercial stock, did his best to stop *Low* being released at all.

The album eventually appeared in January 1977, a week after David's thirtieth birthday, adorned with a heavily treated cover photograph from *The Man Who Fell To Earth* showing Bowie in profile. He later confirmed that the visual pun – "low profile" – was deliberate: not only was *Low* his least commercial album yet, but he did practically nothing to promote its release, preferring instead to tour as Iggy Pop's keyboard player. Only later did he speak of the album's "terribly important" position in his career, explaining in 1983 that *Low* offered "a world of relief, a world that I would like to be in. It glowed with a pure spirituality that hadn't been present in my music for some time. Mine had in fact almost become darkly obsessed ... That album, more than any of the others that we did, was responsible for my cleaning up musically, and my driving for more positive turns of phrase, if you will, in my music. Except for a slight relapse in *Scary Monsters*." Similarly, in 2001 he remarked that "I get a sense of real optimism through the veils of despair from *Low*. I can hear myself really struggling to get well."

Low garnered mixed reviews from a truly baffled press. In *Melody Maker* Michael Watts hailed it as "a remarkable record and certainly the most interesting Bowie has made. It's so thoroughly contemporary, less in its pessimism, perhaps, though that's deeply relevant to these times, than in its musical concept: the logic of bringing together mainstream pop ... and experimental music perfectly indicates what could be the popular art of the advanced society we are moving into." *Creem*'s Simon Frith unexpectedly called the

album "a fun record, such a refreshing *jeu d'esprit* ... *Low* made me laugh a lot," while *Billboard* praised the "well defined, laid-out instrumental journeys into some brooding, mysterious lands."

Most critics, however, were united in their distaste. Another writer in *Creem* considered the record "inaccessible", while the *Boston Phoenix* dismissed it as "experiments in drone, repetition and time annulment". Long-time Bowiephile Charles Shaar Murray, reviewing the album very much in the shadow of punk, told *NME* readers that *Low* was "so negative it doesn't even contain emptiness", branding it "a totally passive psychosis, a scenario and soundtrack for total withdrawal ... Futility and death-wish glorified, an elaborate embalming job for a suicide's grave ... an act of purest hatred and destructiveness ... it stinks of artfully counterfeited spiritual defeat and emptiness ... comes to us at a bad time and doesn't help at all." Few albums have ever elicited such a savage response, and none has ever deserved it as little. The album confounded its detractors (whom Eno described as "bloody thick"), reaching number 2 in the UK chart and, perhaps even more impressively, number 11 in America. Despite the hostile reaction it received from many critics at the time, it is now widely regarded as one the most brilliant and influential albums ever recorded.

Low was also a spectacularly clever record for Bowie to release at a time when rock journalism was obsessed with one group and one group only: The Sex Pistols. Punk offered nothing essentially new for Bowie, as anyone who has heard the live thrash-outs of The Spiders From Mars will testify. "When Ziggy Stardust fell from favour and lost all his money," David said at the time, "He had a son before he died, Johnny Rotten." Certainly Bowie had patented Johnny Rotten's punk archetype on the sleeve photo of the re-released *Space Oddity* album four years earlier – flimsy jumper, dazed stare, dishevelled red hair, bad teeth and all. In his book *Glam!*, Barney Hoskyns presents a persuasive analysis of punk as "glam ripping itself apart", and more than one commentator has remarked on the obvious connection between glam's colourful aliases (Ziggy Stardust, Gary Glitter, Ariel Bender) and punk's (Sid Vicious, Rat Scabies, Polly Styrene). Wisely for a 30-year-old riding the wave of a new generation, Bowie left punk well alone: by sidestepping it he avoided becoming either a fogey or a father-figure. In any case, David's hermetic isolation throughout much of 1976 and 1977 meant that punk was all but finished by the time he encountered it: "Whether it was my befuddled brain or because of the lack of impact of the English variety of punk in the US, the whole movement was virtually over by the time it lodged itself in my awareness," he admitted many years later. "Completely passed me by. The few punk bands that I saw in Berlin struck me as being sort of post-1969 Iggy, and it seemed like he'd already done that."

The contribution of new-wave guitarist Ricky Gardiner, once described by Visconti as *Low*'s "unsung hero", has often been underestimated, but it is the album's swathes of electronic sound, trailblazing percussion effects and deadpan, emotionally burned-out vocals that demand the attention. They were not merely the touchstone for up-and-coming acts like Gary Numan, but a major influence on talents from such diverse ends of the spectrum as Joy Division, Soft Cell, Depeche Mode and Trevor Horn. As Bowie later said, "the position we adopted on *Low* coloured what was to happen in English music for some time … [especially] in terms of ambience and drum sounds. That 'mash' drum sound, that depressive gorilla effect, set down the studio drum fever fad for the next few years." Speaking of the so-called "triptych" of *Low*, *"Heroes"* and *Lodger* in 2001, he added: "For whatever reason, for whatever confluence of circumstances, Tony, Brian and I created a powerful, anguished, sometimes euphoric language of sounds. In some ways, sadly, they really captured, unlike anything else in that time, a sense of yearning for a future that we all knew would never come to pass. It is some of the best work that the three of us have ever done. Nothing else sounded like those albums. Nothing else came close. If I never made another album it really wouldn't matter now, my complete being is within those three. They are my DNA."

Although Brian Eno receives only one co-writing credit on *Low* and plays on just six of the eleven tracks, he has been given increasing credit over the years by revisionists, including Bowie himself. When Philip Glass reworked sections of the music as the *"Low" Symphony* in 1992, the credit was to "the music of David Bowie and Brian Eno". Glass himself has hailed the original album as "a work of genius", and he is not alone in his opinion. Few participants in modern music can fail to be touched, enthralled and irrevocably influenced by *Low*. Most Bowie fans, this one included, consider it one of the pinnacles of his career.

"HEROES"

RCA Victor PL 12522, October 1977 [3]
RCA International INTS 5066, June 1983 [75]
RCA International NL 83857, November 1984
EMI EMD 1025, August 1991
EMI 7243 5219080, September 1999

'Beauty And The Beast' (3'32") / 'Joe The Lion' (3'05") / '"Heroes"' (6'07") / 'Sons Of The Silent Age' (3'15") / 'Blackout' (3'50") / 'V-2 Schneider' (3'10") / 'Sense Of Doubt' (3'57") / 'Moss Garden' (5'03") / 'Neuköln' (4'34") / 'The Secret Life Of Arabia' (3'46")

Bonus tracks on 1991 reissue: 'Abdulmajid' (3'40") / 'Joe The Lion' (Remixed version, 1991) (3'08")

• *Musicians:* David Bowie *(vocals, keyboards, guitars, saxophone, koto)*, Carlos Alomar *(guitar)*, Dennis Davis *(percussion)*, George Murray *(bass)*, Brian Eno *(synthesizers, keyboards, guitar treatments)*, Robert Fripp *(guitar)*, Antonia Maass, Tony Visconti *(backing vocals)* • *Recorded:* Hansa by the Wall, Berlin • *Producers:* David Bowie, Tony Visconti

Following the completion of Iggy Pop's *Lust For Life* in May 1977, Bowie summoned Tony Visconti and Brian Eno to Berlin to begin work on his new album. Hansa By The Wall Studio 2, a spacious converted dance hall that had once been used for social functions by the Gestapo, offered a less claustrophobic environment than that of the *Low* sessions. "It was more expansive," said Visconti later. "He used a bigger studio. Just five hundred yards from East Berlin, from the Wall, and every afternoon I'd sit down at that desk and see three Russian Red Guards looking at us with binoculars, with their Sten guns over their shoulders, and the barbed wire, and I knew that there were mines buried in that wall, and that atmosphere was so provocative and so stimulating and so frightening that the band played with so much energy – I think they wanted to go home, actually." Carlos Alomar confirms that both the proximity of the Wall and the studio's history affected the creative process: "These things are hanging in the air," he tells David Buckley, "and when things get darker physically, you kind of think of darker themes too. Berlin was a rather dark, industrial place to work."

Joining *Low* veterans Alomar, Davis, Murray and Eno were backing vocalist Antonia Maass and ex-King

Crimson guitarist Robert Fripp, who had been an occasional acquaintance of Bowie's since 1969. Above all else it is Fripp's unique guitar sound which sets *"Heroes"* apart from its predecessor. "Fripp did everything in about six hours, straight off the plane from New York," Eno later told the *NME*. "He arrived at the studio at 11pm, and we said, 'Do you fancy doing anything?' ... So I plugged him into the synthesizer for treatments and we just played virtually everything we'd done at him and he'd just start up without even knowing the chord sequence. By the next day he'd finished, packed up and gone home. It was all first takes, incredible." Many years later Bowie recalled, "The only premise that I gave him was to play with total abandonment, and in a way that he would never consider playing on his own albums. I said 'Play like Albert King,' and he would look puzzled for a few moments, and then he'd go in and try his damnedest to get somewhere near it, but it would come out his way. So things like 'Joe The Lion' were him really having a bash at the blues. He was great like that – he really got into the swing of it."

The initial recording process was rapid, with the majority of the instrumental backings laid down during the first two days. "We did second takes, but they weren't nearly as good," said Eno. "We'd sort of say, 'Let's do this, then,' and we'd do it, then someone would say 'Stop' and that would be it, the length of the piece. It seemed completely arbitrary to me. David would say, 'OK, it's that, that twice as long as that and then that. Then do this a couple of times, then come back to that.' And in that tiny space of time, Carlos Alomar would have worked out this lovely melody line. All of those little melody parts are his, and he thinks them out at lightning speed. He's quite remarkable." Equally spontaneous was Bowie's vocal work, as Visconti later attested: "He'd never have a clue what he'd sing about until he actually walked in front of the microphone." Bowie confirmed that the songs were written with "absolutely no idea of the consequences, and no preconceptions of any kind." Eno later remembered an unusual aspect of the studio methodology: "My recollection is, for some reason, we slipped into the Peter Cook and Dudley Moore characters – Bowie was Pete and I was Dud ... It was hilarious, I don't think I've ever laughed so much making a record. Which is funny, when you think how the album sounds, but I often think you make music to be the place that you aren't in." Bowie later confirmed Eno's recollection: "We certainly had our share of schoolboy giggling fits ... Brian and I did have Pete and Dud done pretty pat. Long dialogues about John Cage performing on a 'prepared layer' at the Bricklayers Arms on the Old Kent Road and suchlike. Quite silly."

Visconti later described *"Heroes"* as "a very positive version of *Low*. It was such a positive period of his life. He was, in fact, a hero. We all felt like heroes. It was a heroic album." The sense of heroism was qualified, however, by David's insistence on the ironic quotation marks around the album's title, which he admitted was chosen at random. "I thought I'd pick on the only narrative song to use as the title," he told the *NME* in 1977. "It was arbitrary, really, because there's no concept to the album ... It could have been called *The Sons Of Silent Ages*. It was just a collection of stuff that I and Eno and Fripp had put together. Some of the stuff that was left off was very amusing, but this was the best of the batch, the stuff that knocked us out."

One particularly affirmative development was that the *"Heroes"* sessions more or less coincided with the decisive severance of Bowie's dependence on cocaine, although he later admitted that it would be several more years before he was entirely clean. "I would have days where things were moving in the room," he recalled in 1983, "and this was when I was totally straight. It took the first two years in Berlin to really cleanse my system. Especially psychically and emotionally." (Quite when Bowie finally renounced cocaine remains a moot point, but it was later than is often assumed. Certainly more than one musician has confirmed that there were lapses at after-show parties during 1983's Serious Moonlight tour, while David himself recently confessed that "I slipped around *Let's Dance*," and elsewhere made a cryptic but surprising remark to the effect that 1987's *Never Let Me Down* was "a drug album"; but to all intents and purposes the hardcore dependency was over by the end of 1977.)

In contrast with the breakneck pace of *Low* and *Lust For Life*, following the initial burst of recording the sessions progressed at a more leisurely pace, with vocals, overdubs and mixing continuing on and off until August. The final mixes took place at Mountain Studios in Montreux, on the shores of Lake Geneva – Bowie's first visit to a studio that would become one of his regular haunts. Among the engineers at Mountain was Dave Richards, a new name in the Bowie roll-call who would make his mark on many future productions. His assistant, Eugene Chaplin, was a neighbour of David's in Switzerland and the son of a rather well-known silent comedian.

During the sessions David made several trips to Paris (to give interviews, shoot the video for 'Be My Wife' and attend the French premiere of *The Man Who Fell To Earth*) and took a holiday in Spain with Bianca Jagger. In early September he returned to Britain to record his appearances on *Marc* and *Bing Crosby's Merrie Olde Christmas*, and to participate in a barrage of interviews. Having done almost nothing to sell *Low*, he went to the other extreme for *"Heroes"*, performing the title track on *Top Of The Pops* and various Continental counterparts. In Germany and France the album was released with customized versions of the title track re-recorded in the appropriate languages. There were even whispers – sadly unfounded – that David was preparing to perform the song on ATV's *The Muppet Show*. "I didn't promote *Low* at all and some people thought my heart wasn't in it," he explained. "This time, I wanted to put everything into pushing the new album. I believe in the last two albums, you see, more than anything I've done before. I mean, I look back on a lot of my earlier work and, although there's much that I appreciate about it, there's not a great deal that I actually like … There's a lot more heart and emotion in *Low* and, especially, the new album." To *Melody Maker* he added: "*"Heroes"* is, I think, compassionate. Compassionate for people and the silly desperate situation they've got themselves into. That we've all got ourselves into, generally by ignorance and rash decisions."

Propelled by a marketing slogan that read "There's Old Wave, there's New Wave and there's David Bowie", *"Heroes"* climbed to number 3 in the UK chart and generated a flush of admiring notices. The *NME* welcomed the album as "among the most mature and trenchant Bowie has achieved" and his "most moving performance in years". *Melody Maker*, which made *"Heroes"* its album of the year, hailed it and its predecessor as "among the most adventurous and notably challenging records yet thrust upon the rock audience. Inevitably controversial, these albums have combined the theories and techniques of modern electronic music with lyrics that have found Bowie dispensing with traditional forms of narrative in pursuit of a new musical vocabulary adequate to the pervasive mood of despair and pessimism that he has divined in contemporary society." In America, where *Low* had already taken a pasting, *"Heroes"* stalled at number 35 and the single sank without

trace. *Billboard* cautiously reviewed the album as "a musical excursion into a realm only Bowie himself can define", adding that "Bowie's lyrics are filled with dark forebodings buried in synthesizer electronics."

The persuasive but single-minded hypothesis advanced by the Gillmans in their influential biography, combined with Visconti's quotes and of course the undeniably uplifting title track itself, have led to a common perception of *"Heroes"* as a triumphant burst of optimism. Even the most rudimentary inspection reveals precious little evidence of this: the music is often colder and bleaker than anything on *Low*. Certainly the lyrics show a change of tack, being wittier and more plentiful than on the previous album, and the decision to play out with the pop-friendly 'Secret Life Of Arabia' instead of the more obvious dying fall of 'Neuköln' suggests a brightening agenda. But it would be misleading to describe *"Heroes"* as a happy album. "It's louder and harder and played with more energy in a way," Bowie mused in 2001, "but lyrically it seems far more psychotic. By now I was living full time in Berlin, so my own mood was good. Buoyant even. But those lyrics come from a nook in the unconscious. Still a lot of house-cleaning going on, I feel." Indeed, the lyrics systematically return to a running theme of drunkenness – something to which Bowie later admitted he had succumbed in Berlin during the long recovery from cocaine addiction – and although at times the music is serene and emotionally positive, at others it is almost demented in its darkness. Sukita's sleeve photograph, based like that of *The Idiot* on Erich Heckel's paintings *Roquairol* and *Young Man*, shows a wild-eyed Bowie locked in a rigid pose of serio-comic agitation, raising a flat palm as though he has just mimetically lifted the final mask of artifice from his face. In 1983 David suggested that the album was about "looking at the street life in Berlin … there's a serious quality to the people, a resistance to silliness."

Another theme foregrounded by *"Heroes"* – one which Bowie would take to greater extremes on *Lodger* – is its sense of cultural cosmopolitanism. The "Japanese influence" in the lyric of 'Blackout' and the koto in 'Moss Garden' indicate that his thoughts were once again with the country that had inspired him during the Ziggy period. The Middle Eastern undertones of 'Neuköln' and 'The Secret Life Of Arabia' seal the sense of *"Heroes"* as an aural Berlin. The conflicts inherent in the city's ramshackle diversity – the enriching quality of multi-racial life set against its social inequities and the displacement of the individual – make for an album with a bittersweet flavour.

Although at the time of its release *"Heroes"* was greeted as a work that made sense of *Low* and artistically superseded it, the pendulum of history has tended to swing back in favour of *Low*'s more dangerously experimental achievements. *"Heroes"* repeats the pattern of keeping the more conventional songs on the first side and the ambient instrumentals on the second, and ultimately it stands as a consolidation and a refinement of its trailblazing predecessor rather than a definitive new work in its own right. All the same, *"Heroes"* is a very fine album indeed, and remains one of Bowie's most influential works. The great Patti Smith eulogized the album in a long poem for the *Hit Parader* in 1978, and it was in deference to *"Heroes"* that U2 chose to record 1991's *Achtung Baby* with Brian Eno at Hansa By The Wall. And shortly before his death, John Lennon admitted that he had approached *Double Fantasy* with the ambition to "do something as good as *"Heroes"*." Few albums in the annals of rock can stake as impressive a claim as that.

STAGE

RCA Victor PL 02913, September 1978 [5]
EMI EMD 1030, February 1992

'Hang On To Yourself' (3'26") / 'Ziggy Stardust' (3'32") / 'Five Years' (3'58") / 'Soul Love' (2'55") / 'Star' (2'31") / 'Station to Station' (8'55") / 'Fame' (4'06") / 'TVC15' (4'37") / 'Warszawa' (6'50") / 'Speed of Life' (2'44") / 'Art Decade' (3'10") / 'Sense of Doubt' (3'13") / 'Breaking Glass' (3'28") / '"Heroes"' (6'19") / 'What in the World' (4'24") / 'Blackout' (4'01") / 'Beauty and the Beast' (5'08")

Bonus track on 1992 reissue: 'Alabama Song' (4'00")

• *Musicians:* see *The Stage tour* (Chapter 3) •
Recorded: Spectrum Arena, Philadelphia; Civic Center, Providence; New Boston Garden Arena, Boston • *Producers:* David Bowie, Tony Visconti

After the unsatisfactory *David Live*, Bowie appointed Tony Visconti in overall charge of recording and mixing his 1978 live album. The recordings were made at four US concerts: two in Philadelphia (28-29 April), and one each in Providence (5 May) and Boston (6 May). "What makes the sound of the album so con-

sistent," explained Visconti, "was the fact that RCA loaned us their excellent mobile studio, which we parked outside each venue … Each show was miked exactly the same way and no one was permitted to change the settings on the console from show to show." Visconti considered many of the numbers too fast after the first night's recording in Philadelphia, and the band re-rehearsed on the afternoon of 29 April to re-establish the original studio tempi. So consistent were the band's performances thereafter, explained Visconti, "that we were able to use the intro and outro of 'Station To Station' from Boston and the bulk from Rhode Island. The edits are practically imperceptible."

While the tour continued, Visconti mixed the album in May at Good Earth Studios in London. Unlike *David Live*, on which studio overdubs had been deemed necessary, *Stage* is in Visconti's words "a truly live album – nothing was 'fixed' in the studio later on". Nothing, that is, except an almost excessive favouring of the band sound over that of the crowd. "I just used the audience tracks in the intros and endings to prove that they were there," explained Visconti, "but cut them completely during the bulk of the recording. The sound was so pristine that we were accused of substituting studio recordings for these. I can assure you that they were totally live and very difficult to play, deserving clean sound unfettered by jeers."

Another decision taken at the mixing stage was a radical reshuffle of the original playing order, to arrange the vintage crowd-pleasers on the first disc and the new material from *Low* and *"Heroes"* on the second. "It was an idea of mine," says Visconti, "and David approved." Sadly, this does rather demolish the dynamic of the original concerts, but this is not to suggest that *Stage* lacks impact. There's nothing here to rival the tormented melodrama of *David Live* or the historical significance of *Ziggy Stardust: The Motion Picture*, but the sheer quality of performance and production make for an icily perfect memento of the 1978 tour. Among the highlights are superb renditions of 'Fame', 'Breaking Glass' and '"Heroes"', but sadly missing are 'Be My Wife', 'The Jean Genie', 'Stay', 'Suffragette City' and 'Rock'n'Roll Suicide', all of which were performed at one or more of the recorded dates. A splendid 'Alabama Song' was, however, added to Rykodisc's 1992 reissue.

With sleeve photography by Gilles Riberolles, *Stage* was released on 25 September 1978, during the four-month break in the tour while Bowie was recording *Lodger* in Montreux. In Britain a limited run was pressed in yellow vinyl (coloured discs being all the rage in 1978), while in Holland it appeared in both yellow and blue. The original cassette release inadvertently switched the second and fourth sides.

Despite a respectable UK performance *Stage* was a relative flop in America, peaking at number 44. As Bowie's relationship with RCA cooled during 1978, a disagreement arose about whether *Stage* constituted one or two albums towards fulfilling his contract. Backed up by the precedent of *David Live* RCA won the dispute, but by the end of the year Bowie had resolved to complete his obligations as soon as possible and move to a new label.

LODGER

RCA BOW LP 1, May 1979 [4]
RCA International NL 84234, March 1984
EMI EMD 1026, August 1991
EMI 7243 5219090, September 1999

'Fantastic Voyage' (2'55") / 'African Night Flight' (2'54") / 'Move On' (3'16") / 'Yassassin' (4'10") / 'Red Sails' (3'43") / 'D.J.' (3'59") / 'Look Back In Anger' (3'08") / 'Boys Keep Swinging' (3'17") / 'Repetition' (2'59") / 'Red Money' (4'17")

Bonus tracks on 1991 reissue: 'I Pray, Olé' (3'59"); 'Look Back In Anger' (6'59")

• *Musicians:* David Bowie *(vocals, piano, synthesizer, Chamberlain, guitars)*, Carlos Alomar *(guitar, drums)*, Dennis Davis *(percussion)*, George Murray *(bass)*, Sean Mayes *(piano)*, Adrian Belew *(mandolin, guitar)*, Simon House *(mandolin, violin)*, Tony Visconti *(mandolin, backing voices, guitar)*, Brian Eno *(ambient drone, prepared piano and cricket menace, synthesizers and guitar treatments, horse trumpets, Eroica horn, piano)*, Stan *(saxophone)*, Roger Powell *(synthesizer)* • *Recorded:* Mountain Studios, Montreux; Record Plant Studios, New York • *Producers:* David Bowie, Tony Visconti

In September 1978, midway through the four-month break in the Stage tour, Bowie took his band to Montreux to begin work on a studio album with Brian Eno and Tony Visconti. Although *Lodger* is now widely referred to as the third album in Bowie's "Berlin trilogy", it was in fact recorded in Switzerland and New York, which had become Bowie's twin homes by the time it was released.

Working titles for the album included *Despite Straight Lines* and *Planned Accidents*, both clues to Bowie's latest methodology. He would later remark that a mistake repeated three times becomes an arrangement, and for *Lodger* he went out of his way to create conditions under which such mistakes might bear fruit. With basic tracks already laid down by the rhythm section the remaining members of the tour band were shipped in. "When I arrived," Adrian Belew recalled, "they had about twenty tracks already done: bass, drums, rhythm guitar, but no vocals. They said, 'Adrian, we're not going to let you hear these songs. We want you to go into the studio and play accidentally – whatever occurs to you' … I would just suddenly hear 'One, two, three, four' in the headphones and a track would start … I didn't even know what keys the songs were in or anything. The one particular song where I remember I lucked out on was 'Red Sails', 'cos I started the guitar feeding back and it was right in key. Anyway, they would let me do this maybe two or three times and by then I might know something about the song, so it was over."

Some tracks were spliced into loops and re-used as backing information. "Often when [David] chose a section for looping," wrote Sean Mayes, "He would pick the part with the most mistakes, which when repeated became an integral part of the song." Famously, Bowie instructed the band to swap instruments for 'Boys Keep Swinging'. "David was very keen on spontaneity," explained Mayes. "He liked everything to be recorded in one or two takes, mistakes and all." Several tracks, notably 'African Night Flight', 'Yassassin' and 'Red Sails', were constructed around a melodic clash of disparate cultures. Nobody spoke of "world music" at the time, but *Lodger*'s intercontinental eclecticism steals the march on the 1980s work of Peter Gabriel and Paul Simon. David described the album as a "sketchpad" of his experiences among other cultures.

Tony Visconti recalls that Brian Eno was given far more leeway during the *Lodger* sessions than previously: "The first two, *Low* and *"Heroes"*, were a delicate balance, but on this one, Brian was very much in control." The recording session for 'Look Back In Anger' (another working title for the album) was a case in point. According to Visconti, Brian Eno "made a chart of his eight favourite chords and stuck them on the studio wall and he had a teacher's pointer and he pointed. He told the band, 'Just get into a funky groove, boys.' He was telling these three black guys who came from the roughest part of New York, 'Just play something funky.'" Sean Mayes later confirmed that "There was some grumbling about this 'back to school' session!", and Carlos Alomar tells David Buckley that he considered the experiment "bullshit … I totally, totally resisted it. David and Brian were two intellectual guys and they had a very different camaraderie, a heavier conversation, a 'Europeanness'. It was too heavy for me." Bowie later admitted that "Brian and I did play a number of 'art pranks' on the band. They really didn't go down too well though. Especially with Carlos who tends to be quite 'grand'."

All the same, Eno's presence is less keenly felt on *Lodger* than on the previous two albums, and indeed he neither co-wrote nor played on four of the ten tracks. Adrian Belew believes that Bowie's working relationship with Eno was "winding down" by the time of the *Lodger* sessions, and similar reservations are shared by Tony Visconti, who has always regarded *"Heroes"* as the peak of the period. "I don't think [David's] heart was in *Lodger*," he once remarked, adding on another occasion that "We had fun, but nevertheless an ominous feeling pervaded the album for me."

Despite the experimental spirit of the sessions, Bowie's songwriting was in fact becoming more conventional. Gone were the sprawling instrumental tracks and half-finished vignettes; according to Visconti, "We dropped the ambient-side-two concept and just recorded songs!" In an interesting development, most of the lyrics remained unwritten at the time of the three-week Montreux sessions. Sean Mayes recalls that David was already singing snatches of 'Yassassin' and 'Red Sails', but others merely had working titles like 'This Tangled Web' and 'Portrait Of The Artist'. Rather than improvise on the mike as he had for the previous two albums, Bowie elected to write the lyrics later, and *Lodger* remained unfinished until March 1979, when the vocal tracks, instrumental overdubs and mixing were completed at New York's Record Plant in the space of a week.

Alongside *Lodger*'s cultural diversity is evidence that Bowie's lyrics are becoming politicized on individual issues: 'Fantastic Voyage' tackles the nuclear arms race and 'Repetition' addresses domestic violence. For Brian Eno such linear concepts represented a step in the wrong direction; he was less than happy

with the sessions and has often denigrated *Lodger* in subsequent interviews. "It started off extremely promising and quite revolutionary and it didn't seem to quite end that way," he once said, admitting that he and Bowie "argued quite a lot about what was going to happen" on individual tracks.

"I never took what would be called world beat to its fruition," said Bowie. "Brian Eno did. I think some of what we wrote together, like 'African Night Flight', probably gave him the impetus to get on with things like *My Life In The Bush Of Ghosts*, which followed on from *Lodger*. He found the idea of combining different ethnic music against a Westernized beat fairly stimulating."

Despite the apparent tensions, *Lodger* boasts what Bowie called "a kind of optimism". Promoting the album in May 1979, he said, "I think it would have been terribly depressing if this one had been down. I'm so pleased it has been so up. You never know until you come out of the studio exactly what you've done." RCA's rather crass internal publicity quoted executive Mel Ilberman as saying, "It would be fair to call it Bowie's *Sergeant Pepper*, a concept album that portrays the Lodger as a homeless wanderer, shunned and victimized by life's pressures and technology."

By contrast with the almost universal praise for *"Heroes"*, reviews were mixed. The *New York Times* considered it David's "most eloquent" record in years, but *Rolling Stone* dismissed it as "just another LP, and one of his weakest at that: scattered, a footnote to *"Heroes"*, an act of marking time." *Billboard* was noncommittal, noting merely that "the tone of the album is less foreboding than his more recent musical excursions". *Melody Maker*'s Jon Savage dismissed it as "a nice enough pop record, beautifully played, produced and crafted, and slightly faceless", and wondering in conclusion, "will the eighties really be this boring?" Savage also found time to discuss *Lodger*'s unusual gatefold sleeve design, a wrap-around photograph by Brian Duffy showing Bowie spreadeagled in a contorted, Egon Schiele-like pose, inside a tiled bathroom (or is it a mortuary?) with what looks like a comb (or is it a cut-throat razor?) clutched in his bandaged right hand, his nose and mouth squashed up against an imagined window or mirror. The lettering, scrawled on a postcard marked with the album's title in four languages, sets the travelogue motif and suggests stitched-up lacerations: "a part of that childlike autistic edge of unease that Bowie likes to keep", noted Savage, adding that the cover pose was reflected in the sleeve's inner photographs, omitted from subsequent reissues: "a carefully kept baby, a mortuary corpse, a shrouded Christ, a carefully killed Che Guevara."

Notwithstanding Eno's reservations, *Lodger* is far from being a conventional rock album. On the contrary, its daring collision of musical influences and downright strange noises is if anything even less compromising than either *Low* or *"Heroes"*. It lacks their icy clarity and has been accused of being over-cluttered and overproduced, while the oddly obscure and muffled mix contributes to the initial inaccessibility. "My only regret is that we went to New York to finish this album," said Visconti later, "and it suffered at the mixing stage because New York studios simply were not as versatile or well-equipped as their European counterparts in those days." Bowie concurs: "I think Tony and I would both agree that we didn't take enough care mixing," he mused many years later. "This had a lot to do with my being distracted by personal events in my life, and I think Tony lost heart a little because it never came together as easily as both *Low* and *"Heroes"* had."

But *Lodger* repays close attention. The opening side's insistent quest theme ('Move On', 'African Night Flight', 'Red Sails', 'Fantastic Voyage') revives a perennial motif retreating through Bowie's Berlin albums ("I've lived all over the world, I've left every place") and his Los Angeles exile ("got to keep searching and searching"), right back to his very earliest compositions ("I've gotta pack my bags, leave this home, start walking"). The journey is metaphorical as well as geographical: the frenzied chant of "we're going to sail to the hinterland!" at the climax of 'Red Sails' is a bold announcement of Bowie's studious avoidance of the creative mainstream. On its second side *Lodger* moves from philosophical travelogue to a skewed critique of Western society, setting the totems of the American dream ("you can buy a home of your own, learn to drive and everything") against capitalism's oppressive underbelly in the claustrophobic nightmares of 'D.J.' and 'Repetition'.

Lodger is also a challenging step forward from an artist who could so easily have settled for a second helping of *"Heroes"*. Unlike Eno, Bowie was a face as well as a sound, and he had already sensed the need to discard his airbrushed, bomber-jacketed, back-lit *"Heroes"* persona. He was right. In the very week that 'Boys Keep Swinging' peaked at number 7 in June 1979, Tubeway Army's brilliant but hugely derivative

'Are Friends Electric?' entered the chart, heralding an avalanche of ersatz Berlin-Bowie androids posing behind their synthesizers in eyeliner and *Blake's 7* jumpsuits. By the time it happened, David had already moved on. The drainpipe schoolboy suit he sported for the *Lodger* sleeve and the 'Boys Keep Swinging' video suggested that he was now aligning himself with new wave acts like Elvis Costello, The Jam and Blondie (whose male members had sported the same uniform on the sleeve of the band's 1978 classic *Parallel Lines*). But above and beyond the trappings, Bowie had now colonized a different musical landscape entirely. Like all his best moves, *Lodger* kept him one step ahead of the pack: undervalued and obscure practically from the moment of its release, its critical re-evaluation is long overdue.

SCARY MONSTERS (AND SUPER CREEPS)

RCA BOW LP 2, September 1980 [1]
RCA PL 83647, 1984
EMI EMD 1029, June 1992
EMI 7243 5218950, September 1999
EMI 7243 5433182, September 2003 *(SACD)*

'It's No Game (No. 1)' (4'15") / 'Up The Hill Backwards' (3'13") / 'Scary Monsters (And Super Creeps)' (5'10") / 'Ashes To Ashes' (4'23") / 'Fashion' (4'46") / 'Teenage Wildlife' (6'51") / 'Scream Like A Baby' (3'35") / 'Kingdom Come' (3'42") / 'Because You're Young' (4'51") / 'It's No Game (No. 2)' (4'22")

Bonus tracks on 1992 reissue: 'Space Oddity' (4'57") / 'Panic In Detroit' (3'00") / 'Crystal Japan' (3'08") / 'Alabama Song' (3'51")

• *Musicians:* David Bowie *(vocals, keyboards)*, Dennis Davis *(percussion)*, George Murray *(bass)*, Carlos Alomar *(guitar)*, Robert Fripp *(guitar on 'It's No Game', 'Up the Hill Backwards' 'Scary Monsters', 'Fashion', 'Teenage Wildlife', 'Kingdom Come')*, Chuck Hammer *(guitar on 'Ashes to Ashes', 'Teenage Wildlife')*, Roy Bittan *(piano on 'Up the Hill Backwards', 'Ashes to Ashes', 'Teenage Wildlife')*, Andy Clark *(synthesizer on 'Ashes to Ashes', 'Fashion', 'Scream Like a Baby', 'Because You're Young')*, Pete Townshend *(guitar on 'Because You're Young')*, Tony Visconti *(backing vocals, acoustic guitar on 'Up the Hill Backwards', 'Scary Monsters')*, Lynn Maitland, Chris

Porter *(backing vocals)*, Michi Hirota *(voice on 'It's No Game (No. 1)')* • *Recorded:* Power Station Studios, New York; Good Earth Studios, London • *Producers:* David Bowie, Tony Visconti

On 8 February 1980, while he was on an Alpine skiing holiday with his son Joe, David's divorce from Angela became absolute. A week later, Joe returned to school in Britain and David arrived at New York's Power Station Studios to begin work on his new album. Tony Visconti was once again in the producer's chair, and recalls that Bowie intended from the outset that this would be his first conscious attempt since *Young Americans* to cut a record with commercial potential. "There was a certain degree of optimism making that album," said Bowie in 1999, "because I'd worked through some of my problems, I felt very positive about the future, and I think I just got down to writing a really comprehensive and well-crafted album."

A few early versions of the tracks had already been taped at Keith Richards's Ocho Rios studio in Jamaica, previously used for the Station To Station tour rehearsals. As before, the backing tracks were laid down by Bowie and his Alomar/Davis/Murray rhythm section, for whom this was the fifth and final consecutive studio album: only Carlos Alomar would work with David hereafter. It is rumoured that Bowie began the project with Tom Verlaine on lead guitar, while *Lodger* guitarist Adrian Belew claims that he was paid an advance for the album months earlier, and was surprised to learn that the sessions had gone ahead without him. In the event, most of the lead guitar parts were played by *"Heroes"* veteran Robert Fripp, with additional overdubs by newcomer Chuck Hammer and, on one track, by special guest Pete Townshend. Keyboardist Andy Clark was joined by *Station To Station* pianist Roy Bittan, who was recording Bruce Springsteen's *The River* in an adjacent studio. Tony Visconti recalled an occasion in the lounge at Power Station when "Dennis Davis actually turned to Bruce Springsteen … and asked, 'What band are you in?'"

Recording at Power Station continued for two and a half weeks, during which only the closing track, 'It's No Game (No. 2)' was completed in its entirety. The remaining tracks were left as instrumentals and, as Visconti later recounted, "Instead of immediately writing finished melodies and lyrics, David begged to take a long break to think it all out, so we adjourned

until two months later in London." When the pair reconvened in April at Good Earth Studios, "David had written great lyrics and carefully thought-out melodies, something he hadn't done on the triptych albums." Thus 'Jamaica' became 'Fashion', 'Cameras In Brooklyn' was re-titled 'Up The Hill Backwards', 'It Happens Every Day' was now 'Teenage Wildlife', and 'People Are Turning To Gold' had transformed into 'Ashes To Ashes'. The album's title track was apparently indebted to an advertising campaign for Kellogg's Corn Flakes, who were offering novelty gifts of "Scary Monsters and Super Heroes".

At Good Earth the remaining vocal tracks were completed, including the Japanese narration by actress Michi Hirota. Some of the instrumental tracks recorded in New York, including a cover of Cream's 'I Feel Free', were abandoned before any vocals were recorded. Also at the Good Earth sessions, David was reunited with Chimi Youngdong Rimpoche, the Buddhist monk he had befriended in the late 1960s. Now working at the British Museum, David's former guru was invited to the studio by Visconti, who was aware of plans to stage a rock concert in Lhasa where it was hoped that Bowie might headline. Nothing came of the proposal.

Bowie later described *Scary Monsters* as "some kind of purge. It was me eradicating the feelings within myself that I was uncomfortable with. You have to accommodate your pasts within your persona. You have to understand why you went through them. You cannot just ignore them or put them out of your mind, or pretend they didn't happen, or just say, 'Oh, I was so different then.' It's very important to get into them and understand them. It helps you reflect on what you are now." *Scary Monsters*, then, is an act of controlled exorcism, a therapeutic head-to-head with the inner demons who had appeared so prominently on earlier albums like *The Man Who Sold The World*. This time, though, the intention is not self-laceration but self-help.

Scary Monsters is also Bowie's wordiest album since *Young Americans*, a development reflected in the songwriting process. David was no longer improvising on the mike but preparing fully crafted songs which combined to evince a rather grim end-of-term report on his rite of passage through the 1970s; he reworks the old Astronettes number 'I Am A Laser' for 'Scream Like A Baby', revisits Major Tom as an emblem of his own career in 'Ashes To Ashes', takes what appears to be an almost embarrassingly upfront look at the aftermath of his divorce in 'Up The Hill Backwards', offers parental advice to Joe in 'Because You're Young', and harshly addresses those who would seek to put him on a pedestal in both 'Fashion' and the undervalued 'Teenage Wildlife'. These last two songs also hint at the totalitarian undertones of earlier roles, while 'It's No Game' berates "Fascists" and 'Scream Like A Baby' projects an Orwellian future in which "faggots" and other minorities are oppressed. Appropriately, the whole is framed by two variants of 'It's No Game', developed from a composition about world-weariness and the vagaries of talent and celebrity apparently written when David was only sixteen.

Even the cover version, Tom Verlaine's 'Kingdom Come', fits perfectly into what Bowie described as the album's "scattered scheme of things": in his hands Verlaine's pseudo-spiritual lyric becomes a dogged affirmation that the artist is both destined and doomed to pursue his creative muse ("I'll be breaking these rocks until the Kingdom comes / And cuttin' this hay until the Kingdom comes ... It's my price to pay"). In 1980 David confessed to the *NME*'s Angus MacKinnon that he was plagued by a sense of "inadequacy" as an artist, that "I have this great long chain with a ball of middle-classness at the end of it which keeps holding me back ... my vision gets blinkered and becomes narrowed all the time", and that his talent "comes and goes, it hides, it gets lost and it reappears, rather like a stream that you come across when you're walking through a wood. You see it sometimes and it sparkles and then it disappears ... that is the most frustrating feeling of all."

In another interview to promote the record, Bowie rather curtly described it as "painless", an interesting choice of adjective for an album that appears to be one of the most sustained personal statements of his career. Its attempt to set a mood of downbeat retrospection within a progressive musical framework appears to be confirmed by his suggestion to MacKinnon that "I don't think I would try to revitalize the same area of energy and sensibilities that, say, Ziggy had. I wouldn't attempt that again, because I haven't got that same positivism within my make-up any more. I mean, the very juvenile sort of assertiveness and arrogance of that period ... I can't write young." In the same interview he explained that "I can do no more than write about how I feel about things ... what dubious kind of thoughts I have about where I am and what I've done."

Sean Mayes, the pianist on *Lodger* and the Stage tour, later recalled a social visit from Bowie just after the album's final mixes had been completed: "I sat on the floor in a Knightsbridge flat and heard *Scary Monsters*. David was depressed – as he always is after completing a project. He was sure it was terrible and would be a failure. But then he laughed and said this was how he always felt!"

Scary Monsters (And Super Creeps) was released on 12 September 1980 in one of Bowie's finest album sleeves: a grainy photograph of David in his 'Ashes To Ashes' Pierrot outfit overlaid with a garish painting of the same by Edward Bell. The retrospective mood was reinforced by the back cover's torn-up glimpses of the sleeve designs for *Aladdin Sane*, *Low*, *"Heroes"* and *Lodger*. Although the cover apparently upset photographer Brian Duffy, who felt that his picture was marginalized by the cartoon artwork, it attracted widespread acclaim. The ink-blot lettering, an adaptation of the Gerald Scarfe style popularized a few months earlier by Pink Floyd's *The Wall*, would be replicated on countless sleeve designs over the next few years. Such was the success of the image that David released a similar painting by Bell for a 1982 Bowie calendar: this painting, in which he runs his hand through his hair in a style reminiscent of the *Hunky Dory* sleeve, was included in the packaging of subsequent reissues. The *Scary Monsters* distressed-clown look, advanced most potently by David Mallet's 'Ashes To Ashes' video, remains one of Bowie's most enduring images.

The album received universal praise (in *Record Mirror*, Simon Ludgate awarded it seven stars out of a maximum five), and saw Bowie garlanded with awards: the *Daily Mirror*/BBC Radio Rock And Pop Awards voted him the best male singer of 1980, as did the *Record Mirror* readers' poll, which also voted 'Ashes To Ashes' and 'Fashion' the best videos of the year. Even in America *Scary Monsters* restored Bowie's flagging commercial stock sufficiently to take it to number 12 in the chart ("Though the LP begins with a song in Japanese, this should be the most accessible and commercially successful Bowie LP in years," *Billboard* predicted correctly). Even so, the singles flopped completely in the States. 'Ashes To Ashes', a UK number 1, failed to chart at all, while 'Fashion' (UK number 5) made a feeble 70.

In Britain the album's performance was spectacular, spawning four hit singles, becoming Bowie's first UK number 1 since *Diamond Dogs*, and staying in the chart longer than any album since *Aladdin Sane*. Its success can be attributed partly to good timing:

'Fashion' became the national anthem of the burgeoning New Romantic movement, composed largely of former Ziggy kids who had come of age and were strutting their brightly-coloured stuff in London joints like Billy's and The Blitz. With its massively influential video, 'Ashes To Ashes' provided the record-buying public with its first mainstream taste of a Bowie-inspired phenomenon of which he himself was now partaking. "You have to remember that Bowie was the reason we were all there anyway," said former Blitz kid Boy George in 1999. "The Blitz was a homage to what Bowie had created, so it was fair enough if he came in and said, ooh, I'll have some of that!"

In this light, *Scary Monsters* was the ultimate in self-reflexivity even by Bowie's standards. He had, in effect, pastiched what was already a pastiche of all his former selves – each of which had been, in its own time, a collage of other influences. Never before had he worn such a multi-layered mask, and it's one of the album's master strokes that in the midst of capitalizing on his figurehead status, Bowie simultaneously renews his old distaste for "movements" and disowns his parade of imitators – the "same old thing in brand-new drag", as he pointedly articulates in 'Teenage Wildlife'.

Another factor in the success of *Scary Monsters* was, quite simply, the groundwork put in by Bowie's previous three studio albums. As he remarked a decade later, "By the time of *Scary Monsters* the kind of music that I was doing was becoming very acceptable … it was definitely the sound of the early eighties." He also remarked that the album was "the epitome of the new wave sound at the time; from bubbling synthesizers to erratic and unconventional guitar playing, it had all those elements that are, by definition, the young way of playing music."

Above all else, its success can be put down to the sheer quality of the songwriting and recordings. "We kind of felt that we'd finally achieved our *Sgt Pepper*," said Visconti, "a goal we had in mind since *The Man Who Sold The World*." But the album's spectacular success was qualified by its aftermath. *Scary Monsters* was David's last major collaboration with Tony Visconti for twenty years, and – the facts are not entirely unconnected – his last truly great album for a very long time. Greater commercial success lay ahead, but *Scary Monsters* signalled the end of Bowie's golden run of cutting-edge albums. That it arrived at the start of a new decade, and was David's most retrospective

recording for some time, has tended with hindsight to seal the impression that *Scary Monsters* really does, in the words of its final track, "draw the blinds on yesterday".

Today *Scary Monsters* sounds as fresh and dynamic as ever, the triumphant culmination of Bowie's steely art-rock phase and a crucial doorway into early 1980s British pop; it comes as little surprise that it was one of the first Bowie albums selected by EMI for release on SACD in 2003. Its reputation has a tendency to rest on three classic singles, which overshadow its enormously rewarding second side and the elegant framing device of 'It's No Game', but even so this is an album which towers over Bowie's career and is considered by many to be his masterpiece. *Scary Monsters* remains the benchmark by which every subsequent Bowie recording is judged.

LET'S DANCE

EMI America AML 3029, April 1983 [1]
EMI America AMLP 3029, October 1983 (*picture disc*)
Virgin CD VUS 96, November 1995
EMI 493 0942, 1998
EMI 7243 5218960, September 1999
EMI 7243 5433192, September 2003 (*SACD*)

'Modern Love' (4'46") / 'China Girl' (5'32") / 'Let's Dance' (7'38") / 'Without You' (3'08") / 'Ricochet' (5'14") / 'Criminal World' (4'25") / 'Cat People (Putting Out Fire)' (5'09") / 'Shake It' (3'49")

Bonus track on 1995 reissue: 'Under Pressure' (4'01")

• *Musicians:* David Bowie (*vocals*), Carmine Rojas (*bass*), Omar Hakim (*drums*), Tony Thompson (*drums*), Nile Rodgers (*guitar*), Stevie Ray Vaughan (*guitar*), Rob Sabino (*keyboards*), Mac Gollehon (*trumpet*), Robert Arron (*tenor sax, flute*), Stan Harrison (*tenor sax, flute*), Steve Elson (*baritone sax, flute*), Sammy Figueroa (*percussion*), Bernard Edwards (*bass on 'Without You'*), Frank Simms, George Simms, David Spinner (*backing vocals*) • *Recorded:* Power Station Studios, New York • *Producers:* David Bowie, Nile Rodgers

Before the filming of *Merry Christmas Mr Lawrence* in mid-1982, Bowie spent a sabbatical in the South Pacific in the company of a collection of home-made compilation tapes. "I wanted something to listen to and I found that my natural inclination was to choose mainly rhythm and blues from the fifties and sixties," he said later. "I wanted to find stuff that I could play over and over again, because in the South Pacific it can get very boring. I really was doing my Desert Island Discs in a way, and I found it was interesting to see what in fact I did choose – everything from James Brown to the Alan Freed Rock & Roll Orchestra, Elmore James, Albert King, Red Prysock, Johnny Otis, Buddy Guy, Stan Kenton … there was just about nothing representing the last fifteen or twenty years. I asked myself, why have I chosen this music? … it was very non-uptight music and it comes from a sense of pleasure and happiness. There is enthusiasm and optimism on those recordings."

David's renewed acquaintance with the artists who had inspired his earliest recordings would profoundly influence the new album – his first in over two years. Having returned to New York after the film shoot, he discovered that RCA's policy of milking his back catalogue had now extended as far as releasing his five-year-old duet with Bing Crosby, alongside a heavily promoted and beautifully packaged picture-disc set of vintage singles under the title *Fashions*. Apparently concluding that this was part of an attempt to butter him up ahead of the impending expiry of his RCA contract, he was heard to comment that it would have been nice if he could have had similar advertising budgets for *Low* and *"Heroes"*. Despite David's increasingly unhappy relationship with RCA during the preceding few years, the label was eager to sign him again. He, however, had other ideas, and entered into negotiations with several record companies: in late 1982 an unofficial bidding war began between RCA, Geffen, Columbia and EMI.

Bowie's dissatisfaction with RCA was not the only reason for the long delay since *Scary Monsters*: he had also been awaiting the expiry of his severance agreement with Tony Defries. As of 30 September 1982 David would assume full rights to his new songs; royalties from anything he wrote before that date would be due to his former manager. Having bided his time, Bowie now prepared to begin work on his new album which, he told one reporter with tongue firmly in cheek, had the provisional title *Vampires And Human Flesh*.

Originally Tony Visconti was to have produced the sessions. "I was hurt," he said later, "because I was booked to do *Let's Dance* and he blew me out two weeks before … for three months he kept saying,

'Keep December free, we're going to go in and record then.' Getting close to that month, I phoned up Coco, and she said, 'Well, you might as well know – he's been in the studio for the past two weeks with someone else. It's working out well and we won't be needing you, he's very sorry.'"

The "someone else" was Nile Rodgers, whose phenomenally successful group Chic had put him at the cutting edge of New York's club scene in the late 1970s with massive international hits like 'Le Freak' and 'Good Times'. His writing and production work for other artists had spawned dance classics like Sister Sledge's 'We Are Family' and Diana Ross's 'Upside Down'. Rodgers, who was putting the finishing touches to his solo debut *Adventures In The Land Of The Good Groove*, chanced to meet Bowie at a bar in New York's Carlisle Hotel. The two apparently sat next to each other for twenty minutes before Rodgers introduced himself. "I was expecting Ziggy Stardust," he later admitted, and had failed to recognize the "average-looking guy" sitting quietly at the bar. David later recalled that "We started talking about old blues and rhythm & blues stuff and found we'd both had the same artists as strong influences. I guess that triggered me off thinking it might be fun working with him."

"David could have had any producer – white or black – he wanted," Rodgers told *Musician* in 1983. "He could have gone with Quincy Jones and a more sure-fire chance at a hit. But he called me up, and for that I feel honoured." Keen to secure a healthy advance from a new label and on the point of recovering his royalty entitlement from MainMan, Bowie was acutely conscious of the need to deliver a commercial hit. Rodgers would later confirm on Radio 2's *Golden Years* that this was what Bowie asked of him when he arrived in Montreux to cut pre-production demos: "When I got to Switzerland, he told me that he wanted me to do what I did best – 'Nile, I really want you to make hits.' And I was sort of taken aback, because I'd always assumed that David Bowie did art first, and then if it happened to become a hit, so be it!"

In Montreux Bowie played Rodgers his new songs on a twelve-string guitar. "If I was going to make hits, I could only use the formula I knew," Rodgers explains in *Strange Fascination*, "Which was, you call a song 'China Girl', it better sound Asian. You call a song 'Let's Dance', you damn well better make sure people dance to it." Assisting on the three-day demo session was a young Turkish expatriate called Erdal

Kizilcay, whose multi-instrumental reputation had reached Bowie's ears in 1982. Kizilcay would later become a full-time member of the Bowie retinue, but on this occasion his contribution extended no further than pre-production.

Rodgers described the demos as "merely a template, little maps to say okay, great, well, we have a song now, big deal! Now let's go back to America and make a hit!" Bowie had booked four weeks at New York's Power Station, previously the venue for *Scary Monsters*, and in December he and Rodgers began recording what Bowie declared would be a warm, optimistic and funky album. "I felt I was becoming a little static with the kind of synthesizer-techno stuff I'd been doing," he told the press at the time. "I wanted to break away from that. Every few years I have to redefine what I'm writing. I had to do it when I moved to Berlin and I had to do it again just recently."

In keeping with the spirit of renewal, *Let's Dance* saw the recruitment of all-new personnel: for the first time since *Space Oddity* there was no continuity with the previous album's musicians. "I wanted to have a little relief from the guys that I usually work with," he explained. "I wanted to try people that I'd never worked with before, so that I couldn't predict how they were going to play." David had already booked Stevie Ray Vaughan, an unknown 28-year-old blues guitarist from Austin, Texas, whom he had heard playing at the 1982 Montreux Jazz Festival. "Stevie is just dynamite," said David at the time. "He thinks Jimmy Page is a modernist! Stevie's back there with Albert King. He's the whiz kid."

The remaining musicians were chosen by Rodgers who, having taken over the producer's chair, also stepped into Carlos Alomar's accustomed place on rhythm guitar (Alomar was originally asked to play on the album, but Bowie's new hirers-and-firers refused his customary request for a rise, instead offering worse terms than before; he declined). Chic's drummer Tony Thompson and bassist Bernard Edwards were drafted in, as were regular Chic sessioners Rob Sabino and Sammy Figueroa. Brothers George and Frank Simms had provided backing vocals for Rodgers on several projects. The rest of the band were top New York session men, including Omar Hakim from Weather Report ("a fascinating drummer with impeccable timing", David later remarked) and Puerto Rican Carmine Rojas, who had played bass for Stevie Wonder and Nona Hendryx. The trumpeter and three-man saxophone section

came from the jazz outfit Asbury Jukes, and between them boasted experience with the likes of Diana Ross, Dave Edmunds, Klaus Nomi and Boz Scaggs.

For the first time, David himself didn't play a single instrument. "This is a singer's album," he declared. Nile Rodgers described the production as "modern big band rock", and David agreed, telling *Musician* magazine that "I really wanted that same positive optimistic rock'n'roll big band sound that was very impressionistic for me back when. It's got a hard cut, very high on treble – it *sears* through."

The sessions were completed in twenty days during December 1982, under a civilized 10.30am-6.00pm schedule. "This is the fastest I've ever worked in my life," Rodgers said afterwards. "Bowie said he likes to work this way and I plan to do the same for the rest of my career. It's just the most energetic way to make records. The musicians were really pumped up because of the fast pace, and as a result we got some great performances." He later recalled that "Almost everything was one take. Stevie Ray Vaughan played everything in a matter of a couple of days. David sang all of his vocals on the entire album in a matter of two days." At the time Bowie declared that he had seldom enjoyed recording so much, although the band's attempts to turn him into a fan of American football were apparently a failure. He was particularly effusive in his praise of Stevie Ray Vaughan, whose lead guitar overdubs were laid down towards the end of the sessions. "In the third week of December Stevie strolled into the Power Station and proceeded to rip up everything one thought about dance records," David later wrote. "In a ridiculously short time he had become midwife to a sound that I had had ringing in my ears all year. A dance form that had its melody rooted in a European sensibility but owed its impact to the blues." *Let's Dance* was to be Vaughan's big break, and with his group Double Trouble he signed to the Epic label in the wake of the album's success.

"Unlike some of the groups I've worked with in the past, where Bernard and I had to take charge in the studio, David has a deep understanding of music," said Nile Rodgers in 1983. "He knows a lot more than he gets credit for." After the demo stage, however, the creative responsibility was left largely to the producer. "I wrote the arrangements based on the demos," Rodgers explained. "When they were played against the tracks, David and I would make some alterations, but nothing very radical. We heard the music the same way and didn't have a major disagreement over any musical point, as happened when we produced Diana Ross."

After a Christmas holiday in Acapulco (during which he filmed his cameo in *Yellowbeard*), David returned to New York to finish post-production and close a deal with his chosen label, who had originally taken his fancy during the Queen collaboration in 1981. Bowie signed a five-year contract with EMI America on 27 January 1983, for an undisclosed sum variously reported as between $10 and $20 million. He delivered the masters of *Let's Dance* and promptly set off for Australia to film the videos for the first two singles. They, like the fashionable album packaging (Greg Gorman's sleeve photo depicts Bowie shadow-boxing against a city skyline, while Derek Boshier's accompanying artwork apes the cartoon graffiti of street artist Keith Haring), would provide the heavy ammunition for a well-oiled, all-out commercial assault.

It worked. Preceded by the smash-hit title single that topped the charts on both sides of the Atlantic, *Let's Dance* was released on 14 April 1983 to unprecedented commercial success. In Britain it entered at number 1, and although it spent only three weeks there – a feat surpassed by *Aladdin Sane*, *Pin Ups* and *Diamond Dogs* – it remained in the chart for over a year. Crucially, it was also a US number 1: having largely ignored Bowie since the mid-1970s, the American market exploded. *Billboard* hailed the album as "Bowie's most accessible music in years … bracing, state-of-the-art urban dance rock", while *Commonweal* called it "some of the most exciting R&B-based dance music in years". Delighted with its latest investment, EMI declared *Let's Dance* its fastest-selling album since *Sgt Pepper*. Six million copies were sold as the album spawned two more hit singles and trailed the massive Serious Moonlight tour which ran from May to December. EMI issued a picture disc version to tempt collectors, while the jilted RCA got in on the act by re-releasing Bowie's back catalogue at a budget price, meaning that by July he had no fewer than ten albums in the UK top 100. This feat, unique for a living artist, contributed to Bowie's record for the highest number of individual album-weeks on the chart in 1983 – a staggering 198. In the all-time stakes this is second only to the 217 weeks clocked up three years later by Dire Straits.

"It was an album he had to make," said Tony Visconti a year later. "He told me when I last saw him, 'I'm sorry I didn't use you, but I wanted one of those economical New York type of albums. It was very important, a new record label.'" Visconti admitted that he "liked 'Ricochet' and 'Modern Love' very, very much", but was less impressed with the remainder of the album. The first signs of dissent among the British music press came from Michael Watts, who had conducted the famous "I'm gay" interview back in 1972. "His new album seems to be a step sideways," Watts wrote. "He's not doing anything particularly new and I suspect for the first time ever his fans are up there with him and he's not ahead of the game."

Success came at a price. *Let's Dance* rocketed Bowie into the premier league of wealth and global superstardom, but it had an immediate and detrimental effect on him as an artist. It is a classy, beautiful, precision-tooled pop record, but its solid professionalism is its defining feature, and artistically it remains perhaps Bowie's least challenging album of all. More even than his later 1980s offerings, *Let's Dance* is an album on which anything remotely resembling a rough edge has been sanded down and polished up until the glare is dazzling. At least during his much derided Glass Spider and Tin Machine periods Bowie was willing to stick his neck out and risk ridicule; on *Let's Dance* he plays it safe in every department, projecting a sun-tanned, hair-bleached revision of himself for the MTV generation. There are worrying signs, too, that his creative well is running dry; of the eight tracks, three are covers or reworkings, heralding the descent into cover version hell that was to follow on the next album. Nothing on *Let's Dance* is truly awful, but seldom had a previous Bowie album included anything quite as nugatory as 'Without You' or 'Shake It'.

Within three years Bowie had begun distancing himself from the album, glad of its success but admitting that it had hemmed him in as an artist. "*Let's Dance*, I think really, was more Nile's album than mine," he told one interviewer. "It was Nile's vision of what my music should sound like, and I provided the songs." Nile Rodgers is not about to disagree: "[Bowie] spent the entire record sitting on the sofa while I made his record," he said in 1998. "Then he walked in the studio and he sang. It was the perfect marriage."

But on closer inspection *Let's Dance* is not without its surprises. There is little doubt that the healthy, drug-free family figure Bowie presented in 1983 concealed a more complex set of truths, and there are signs that he is smuggling some surprisingly controversial material in beneath the shiny dance-floor veneer. Even the ostentatious heterosexuality, rammed home by the famously explicit 'China Girl' video, is counterpointed by the ambiguities of Metro's 'Criminal World'. The themes seem to be the fear of surrendering selfhood and the death of spirituality – hardly the sort of ideas you'd expect to find on a party album. Iggy Pop's threat of destructive love in 'China Girl' ("I'll ruin everything you are") is developed through the anxious title track ("Because my love for you would break my heart in two if you should fall into my arms…"), and the notion of cultural invasion is highlighted by the videos of both songs. 'Modern Love' posits a world of "no confession" and "no religion", while 'Ricochet' suggests that we "turn the holy pictures so they face the wall" against the "sound of the Devil breaking parole".

Bowie's only solution is the one he had previously adopted in 'Because You're Young' – to "dance my life away", or in this case to "put on your red shoes and dance the blues". In 'Modern Love' the concept that "terrifies me" also "makes me party" so that, far from being an exuberant slice of optimism, the album's title seems like a cry of desperation. The sense of fiddling while Rome burns is made explicit on the final track, 'Shake It': "I could take you to heaven, I could spin you to hell / But I'll take you to New York, it's the place that I know well." Out of context, the themes are every bit as dark as those on *Scary Monsters*; married with the upbeat, funky shimmer of Nile Rodgers's production, they are entirely submerged. Whether this is the album's downfall or its subversive triumph is a matter of opinion. Few would disagree that the title track is one of Bowie's great songs, setting a bellowing delivery of an angst-ridden lyric against a monumental dance backing; but otherwise only 'Ricochet' escapes being buried beneath the high-gloss finish.

But then, 1983 was like that. It was the year of Spandau Ballet's *True*, Paul Young's *No Parlez*, Culture Club's *Colour By Numbers*, and Michael Jackson's all-conquering *Thriller* which, incidentally, beat *Let's Dance* to win the Album of the Year Grammy. The chill theatrics, gender-meltdowns and fashion experiments of Bowie's 1970s career had been repackaged with huge success by acts as diverse as Eurythmics, The Human League, Yazoo, Heaven 17, Kajagoogoo, Howard Jones, Thompson Twins and Duran Duran. It was a year of shiny, trivial pop in pastel suits and peroxide hair. Bowie was a common ancestor to many of 1983's big hitters and, as godfather to the rising "Goth" phenomenon, he was also revered on the fringes of the mainstream, as Bauhaus had demonstrated by taking 'Ziggy Stardust' into the top 20 the previous October. The club kids who had championed *Scary Monsters* three years earlier were now topping the charts with their own bands, and perhaps we shouldn't begrudge Bowie gatecrashing the party with such a suitable record. From its foot-tapping backbeats to its scribble-chic sleeve design *Let's Dance* is, ultimately, 1983 in a bottle.

ZIGGY STARDUST: THE MOTION PICTURE

RCA PL-84862, October 1983 [17]
EMI 0777 7 80411 22, September 1992
EMI 72435 41979 25, March 2003
(30th Anniversary Special Edition)
EMI ZIGGYRIP 3773, March 2003
(limited edition red vinyl 30th Anniversary Special Edition)

1983/1992 version: 'Hang On To Yourself' (2'56") / 'Ziggy Stardust' (3'09") / 'Watch That Man' (4'10") / 'Wild Eyed Boy From Freecloud/All the Young Dudes/Oh! You Pretty Things' (6'35") / 'Moonage Daydream' (6'17") / 'Space Oddity' (4'51") / 'My Death' (5'42") / 'Cracked Actor' (2'51") / 'Time' (5'12") / 'The Width of a Circle' (9'36") / 'Changes' (3'34") / 'Let's Spend the Night Together' (3'09") / 'Suffragette City' (3'02") / 'White Light/White Heat' (4'06") / 'Rock'n'Roll Suicide' (4'20")

2003 version: 'Intro' (1'06") / 'Hang On To Yourself' (2'55") / 'Ziggy Stardust' (3'19") / 'Watch That Man' (4'14") / 'Wild Eyed Boy From Freecloud' (3'15") / 'All the Young Dudes' (1'38") / 'Oh! You Pretty Things' (1'46") / 'Moonage Daydream' (6'25") / 'Changes' (3'36") 'Space Oddity' (5'05") / 'My Death' (7'21") / 'Intro' (1'02") / 'Cracked Actor' (3'03") / 'Time' (5'31") / 'The Width of a Circle' (15'45") / 'Let's Spend the Night Together' (3'02") / 'Suffragette City' (4'32") / 'White Light/White Heat' (4'01") / 'Farewell Speech' (0'39") / 'Rock'n'Roll Suicide' (5'17")

• *Musicians:* see *The 1973 Ziggy Stardust tour* (Chapter 3) • *Recorded:* Hammersmith Odeon, London; The Hit Factory, New York • *Producers:* David Bowie,

Mike Moran, Tony Visconti .

The live recording of the last Ziggy Stardust concert was released over ten years later by an ex-label eager to cash in on Bowie's success with *Let's Dance*. Although by no means sparklingly produced, the 1983 version of *Ziggy Stardust: The Motion Picture* is a fascinating document of the most celebrated gig in Bowie's career, and an eye-opener for those accustomed only to the tight, well-mannered studio style of The Spiders From Mars. In order to arrange the tracks on vinyl 'Changes' was moved from its correct place in the running order, while 'The Width Of A Circle' was edited down from its 14-minute-plus entirety. 'White Light/White Heat' was released as a single to promote the album; if RCA had wanted a hit, the three-cornered medley would have been a far better idea.

The concert was recorded by Ken Scott and an early mix completed in 1973 with the help of *Aladdin Sane* engineer Mike Moran. In late 1981 Bowie remixed the album at The Hit Factory with Tony Visconti, resulting in what some considered an unpalatable over-emphasis on backing vocalists, saxophones and organ. Visconti, who described the process as "more of a salvage job than an artistic endeavour", explained that "the sound quality was poor and I was called in to beef it up, which also required David and me to re-sing many of the backing vocals. They were simply not recorded well on tape – partly because Trevor Bolder and Mick Ronson didn't sing into the microphones!"

As in the accompanying film, the two encore numbers featuring guest artist Jeff Beck were omitted from the album for reasons which remain unclear: some reports claim that the problem was a dispute over royalties, others simply that Beck was embarrassed by his appearance in the film. "What I was later told from various people is that Jeff kind of felt out of place in the show," said Tony Visconti many years later. "He came on stage with his flared trousers and just an ordinary jacket, and he felt a bit lacklustre, and he felt like he didn't fit in the film." Beck had also expressed dissatisfaction with his guitar solo, and even recorded a brand new overdub for Visconti and Bowie in December 1981 before his contribution was vetoed. "We could view the film and play to the film – it was a nice set-up," Visconti later recalled of the overdub session. "It was CTS Studios, I think, in north London, and they could lock up film and tape. Jeff played his solo and it sounded great ... He was really, really happy with it. We all went home, I went back to bed, and the next day David phoned me and he said Beck still didn't want to be in the film!"

In 2002 Tony Visconti oversaw a brand new stereo mix of the album, released in March 2003 under the elongated title *Ziggy Stardust And The Spiders From Mars: The Motion Picture Soundtrack*. This two-CD (and two-LP) version, which accompanied the 5.1 surround sound re-release of D A Pennebaker's concert film, was universally hailed as a vast improvement on the 1983 original. Not only is Visconti's new mix spectacularly sharper and brighter, but considerably more of the concert is included. There are no new numbers as such (the Jeff Beck encores are, alas, still absent), but the 2003 edition proudly includes such delights as the *Ode To Joy* intro, the full-length 'The Width Of A Circle', and Bowie's unexpurgated farewell speech. 'Changes' has been restored to its proper place in the running order and there is a wealth of between-song banter, most notably the preamble to 'My Death', which David introduces as "a quiet song – shhhh!", stopping after a couple of bars to silence the audience before beginning the number afresh. The deluxe packaging of the 2003 reissue included a replica ticket, an essay by D A Pennebaker, and a fold-out poster backed by press cuttings about the famous concert. Thus a mildly disappointing live album was transformed into a handsome and inestimably valuable record of a great occasion.

TONIGHT

EMI America DB 1, September 1984 [1]
Virgin CD VUS 97, November 1995
EMI 493 1022, 1998
EMI 7243 5218970, September 1999

'Loving The Alien' (7'10") / 'Don't Look Down' (4'09") / 'God Only Knows' (3'05") / 'Tonight' (3'43") / 'Neighborhood Threat' (3'11") / 'Blue Jean' (3'10") / 'Tumble And Twirl' (4'58") / 'I Keep Forgettin''(2'34") / 'Dancing With The Big Boys' (3'34")

Bonus tracks on 1995 reissue: 'This Is Not America' (3'51") / 'As The World Falls Down' (4'50") / 'Absolute Beginners' (8'00")

• *Musicians:* David Bowie (*vocals*), Carlos Alomar

(guitar), Derek Bramble *(bass, guitar, synthesizer)*, Carmine Rojas *(bass)*, Sammy Figueroa *(percussion)*, Omar Hakim *(drums)*, Guy St Onge *(marimba)*, Robin Clark, George Simms, Curtis King *(backing vocals)*, Tina Turner *(vocals on 'Tonight')*, Iggy Pop *(vocals on 'Dancing With The Big Boys')*, Mark Pender *(trumpet, flugelhorn)*, Stanley Harrison *(alto sax, tenor sax)*, Steve Elson *(baritone sax)*, Lenny Pickett *(tenor sax, clarinet)* • *Recorded:* Le Studio, Morin Heights, Canada • *Producers:* David Bowie, Derek Bramble, Hugh Padgham

Following the Serious Moonlight tour, Bowie took a holiday in Java and Bali with Iggy Pop and his girl-friend Suchi. Since their last brief collaboration in 1979 Iggy's fortunes had taken another dip, and until David's success with 'China Girl' he had been forced to tour almost incessantly. It would be misleading to write off *Tonight* purely as an exercise in generating songwriting royalties for Iggy Pop, but Bowie's wish to help out his friend certainly had a bearing on the end result.

Nile Rodgers was not invited back to follow up *Let's Dance*, a fact he attributes to Bowie's need to prove that his music could stand up without assistance from a celebrated hit-maker. His replacement nonetheless reaffirmed David's interest in black music: Derek Bramble, a comparatively unproven British producer then working with ex-Linx singer David Grant, was formerly the bass guitarist with Heatwave who had scored hits with 'Boogie Nights' and 'Always And Forever' in the late 1970s. *Let's Dance* engineer Bob Clearmountain was unavailable but suggested British producer Hugh Padgham, who had worked with XTC, Peter Gabriel and most successfully The Police; his production credits included their huge 1981 hit *Ghost In The Machine*. Padgham later admitted to feeling "a bit iffy about doing it just as engineer", but he swallowed his pride for the chance to work with Bowie. It was he who suggested the venue – previously used by The Police – and in May 1984 Bowie and Iggy Pop began recording *Tonight* in the unfamiliar surroundings of Le Studio in Morin Heights, near Montreal.

Derek Bramble was joined on guitars by Carlos Alomar and a band of *Let's Dance*/Serious Moonlight personnel, together with new additions Mark Pender, Curtis King and Guy St Onge, whose contributions on marimba (an instrument popularized during 1983 by the Thompson Twins, culminating in their anthemic Christmas hit 'Hold Me Now') provide *Tonight* with its most distinctive instrumental identity. String arrangements were by Arif Mardin, whose work with Aretha Franklin had attracted Bowie's attention; he would later co-produce the *Labyrinth* songs. Keeping continuity with the Serious Moonlight tour brochure, the sax section was again dubbed "The Borneo Horns". The saxophones exert a particularly omnipresent influence on *Tonight*, marking the apotheosis of Bowie's 1980s "horn section" preoccupation. The Borneo Horns would continue to flourish as an outfit: as well as reappearing on *Never Let Me Down*, they would play on Duran Duran's *Notorious* and release their own 1987 album, *Lenny Pickett And The Borneo Horns*, before returning to the Bowie stable many years later on 2002's *Heathen*.

Tonight features only two new Bowie compositions ('Loving The Alien' and 'Blue Jean'), alongside two fresh Bowie/Pop numbers ('Tumble And Twirl' and 'Dancing With The Big Boys'); the remaining five tracks are cover versions of songs by Iggy Pop and others. The dearth of new material seems sadly symptomatic of the creative blight that seized David in the wake of 1983. "I suppose the most obvious thing about the new album is that there's not the usual amount of writing on it from me," he told the *NME*. "I didn't really feel as if I had enough new things of my own because of the tour. I can't write on tour," – (says the author of *Aladdin Sane* and *Young Americans*) – "and there wasn't really enough preparation afterwards to write anything that I felt was really worth putting down. I didn't want to put out things that 'would do', so there are two or three that I felt were good things to do, and the other stuff. What I suppose I really wanted to do was to work with Iggy again … We're ultimately leading up, I hope, to me doing his next album." This prediction would be fulfilled with Iggy's *Blah-Blah-Blah* two years later. Despite Bowie's reservations there was, according to Hugh Padgham, "a bunch of songs" with "real possibilities" from the *Tonight* sessions which failed to reach the final cut.

One of the cover versions, The Beach Boys' 'God Only Knows', had been shortlisted for *Pin Ups* a decade earlier. "I think that this album gave me a chance, like *Pin Ups* did a few years ago, to do some covers that I always wanted to do," explained Bowie. The new collaborations with Iggy Pop were a little more experimental. "We worked very much the way we did on *Lust For Life* and *The Idiot*," Bowie revealed. "I often gave him a few anchor images that I wanted him to play off and he would take them away and start free-associating and I would then put that together in a way I could sing." Iggy contributed backing vocals on 'Dancing With The Big Boys', while David was joined on the title track by Tina Turner, whose massively successful comeback album *Private Dancer* was released in June, featuring a cover of '1984' that was the first of several Turner/Bowie crossovers during the period.

David maintained the *Let's Dance* policy of playing no instruments himself. "I very much left everybody else to it," he confessed at the time. "I just came in with the songs and the ideas and how they should be played and then watched them put it all together. It was great! … Hugh Padgham and Derek put the sound together between them. It was nice not to be involved in that way." For long-term fans this sort of talk was guaranteed to set alarm bells ringing. Another warning sign was the unusual length of the sessions. "*Let's Dance* was done in three weeks," Bowie later recalled. "*Tonight* took five weeks or something, which for me is a really long time. I like to work fast in the studio." At the time David claimed that *Tonight* was a genuine attempt to create a new kind of sound. "I've got to a point that I really wanted to get to where it's an organic sound, and it's mainly saxophones. I think there's only two lead guitar solos on it. No synthesizers to speak of, though there are probably a couple of *twing* sounds or something. It's really got the *band* sound that I wanted, the horn sound."

It appears, however, that the sessions were less than harmonious; in *Strange Fascination* Hugh Padgham reveals that Derek Bramble was in the habit of asking for unnecessary retakes: "I was trying to keep quiet and I could see David going 'Why?' Then I eventually said, 'Look, Derek, there's nothing wrong with that vocal, it's not out of tune. What are you doing?' I don't think Derek was used to anyone being able to do a vocal in one take … Eventually it did get to a bit of siding up, with David and me on one side and Bramble, the producer, on the other." Carlos Alomar is less equivocal: "Derek Bramble was a really nice guy, but he didn't know jack-shit about producing." Whether Bramble was actually fired remains uncertain, but in Radio 2's *Golden Years* Padgham confirmed that there was "a bit of a falling-out", and he took over as producer for the tail end of the sessions. Padgham disliked many of the recordings (he "hated" 'Blue Jean' and 'Tonight', preferring the "more left-field" compositions that had been abandoned), and

now regrets that he "didn't have the balls" to suggest that Bowie finish off the other songs. "But it is difficult," he tells David Buckley. "Who am I to say to Mr David Bowie that his songs suck?"

The combined successes of *Let's Dance*, the Serious Moonlight tour and *Merry Christmas Mr Lawrence* meant that Bowie's commercial stock had never been higher; *Tonight* entered the UK album chart at number 1 in September 1984. Mick Haggerty's rather attractive sleeve portrays a blue-skinned David set against a riot of photomontage, oil-paint daubs and stained glass lilies and roses, indebted to the work of Gilbert and George. At the time, most critics were happy with the album. In the *NME* Charles Shaar Murray commended the "dizzying variety of mood and technique," while *Billboard* noted that "the once and future Mr Jones takes yet another turn, saving more edgy, passionate dance-rock for the second side while throwing the spotlight on surprisingly restrained ballads and midtempo rockers, replete with dreamy rhythms and even lush strings courtesy of Arif Mardin." *Rolling Stone* was less accommodating, announcing that "This album is a throwaway, and David Bowie knows it." The album hit number 11 in America.

Posterity has not been kind to *Tonight*, now widely regarded as the first in a string of follies set to continue with *Never Let Me Down*. Certainly the album lacks anything approaching the quality of Bowie's 1970s work, and it's with some justification that it has been written off as a slapdash act of appeasement aimed at his new mainstream audience. He later admitted as much: "I really liked the money I was making from the touring, and it seemed obvious that the way that you make money is give people what they wanted, and the downside of that is that it just dried me up as an artist completely, because I wasn't used to doing that. What I'm used to doing is being very stubborn, obscure, confrontational in my own indulgent way."

Even in the act of promoting *Tonight* in 1984, Bowie seemed almost apologetic: "Recently I've used an *accepted vocabulary*, as Eno would say … I feel on the whole fairly happy about my state of mind and my physical being and I guess I wanted to put my musical being in a similar staid and healthy area, but I'm not sure that that was a very wise thing to do." By the time of *Never Let Me Down*, David was already dismissing *Tonight*. "It didn't have any concept behind it, it was just a collection of songs," he said in 1987. "It sounded sort of jumbled, it didn't hold together well at all … though if you take a song out of context and play it, it sounds pretty good. But if you play it as an album it doesn't work, and that was unfortunate."

In later years Bowie would effectively disown his entire 1984-1987 period. "I wasn't really interested and I let everyone tell me what to do," he said in 1993. "I let people arrange my songs. I let photographers choose stylists who brought along what they thought were great, trendy clothes. And I really couldn't be bothered … A wave of total indifference came over me." In 1989 he described *Tonight* and *Never Let Me Down* as "great material that got simmered down to product level. I really should have not done it quite so *studio-ly*. I think some of it was a waste of really good songs. You should hear the demos from those two albums. It's night and day by comparison with the finished tracks. There's stuff that I could really kick myself about. When I listen to those demos it's, 'How did it turn out like that?' You should hear 'Loving The Alien' on demo. It's *wonderful* on demo, I promise you! But on the album, it's not as wonderful."

Nonetheless, despite its obvious flaws *Tonight* is often a more interesting and rewarding album than its predecessor. Clearly there is nothing here as brilliant as the title track of *Let's Dance*, but while the rest of that album is little more than beautifully produced fluff, *Tonight* at least offers evidence of an experimental spirit. Bowie's unexpected reggae reworkings of 'Don't Look Down' and 'Tonight' are surprisingly successful, and while some of the remaining cover versions are mediocre in the extreme, the new songwriting is arguably superior to anything on *Let's Dance*. One is left with a frustrating sense of what might have been: 'Loving The Alien' in particular is a superb piece of writing all but demolished by insipid performance and meddlesome overproduction. What emerges is certainly less of a commercial bullseye than *Let's Dance*, but at least it's a little less obvious into the bargain.

Significantly, *Tonight* was the first Bowie album that was manifestly behind its time: it may have reached number 1 but, unlike *Let's Dance*, it made little connection with what was cutting-edge in 1984. The sensation of the year was yet another Bowie-indebted act: fronted by long-time fan Holly Johnson, Frankie Goes To Hollywood combined scandalous cartoon-strip homoeroticism with razor-sharp Trevor Horn production to redefine pop almost overnight. Frankie were the new cheerleaders in a tidal wave of openly gay outrages whose assault on Thatcher's Britain left family-friendly heterosexuals like the new-look David Bowie stranded on the shore: Bronski Beat, Boy George and the newly solo Marc Almond were among the darlings of 1984's pop aristocracy. Meanwhile Bowie's more cerebral heartlands had been claimed by the suburban angst-rock of The Cure and The Smiths, while the inexorable rise of Prince presented a colourful and credible successor to Ziggy Stardust. It was against just such acts that Bowie's music might have been evaluated in any previous year. Instead, on the basis of *Tonight*, he seemed content to compete with the likeable, unchallenging pop of Duran Duran, Wham! and Nik Kershaw. The results speak for themselves.

NEVER LET ME DOWN

EMI America AMLS 3117, April 1987 *(LP)* [6]
EMI America CDP 7 46677 2, April 1987 *(CD)* [6]
Virgin CD VUS 98, November 1995
EMI 7243 5218940, September 1999

'Day-In Day-Out' (5'35") *(Vinyl: 4'38")* / 'Time Will Crawl' (4'18") / 'Beat of Your Drum' (5'04") *(Vinyl: 4'32")* / 'Never Let Me Down' (4'05") / 'Zeroes' (5'45") / 'Glass Spider' (5'31") *(Vinyl: 4'56")* / 'Shining Star (Makin' My Love)' (5'04") *(Vinyl: 4'05")* / 'New York's In Love' (4'32") *(Vinyl: 3'55")* / ''87 And Cry (4'19")' *(Vinyl: 3'53")* / 'Too Dizzy' (4'00") / 'Bang Bang' (4'29") *(Vinyl: 4'02")*

Bonus tracks on 1995 reissue: 'Julie' (3'40") / 'Girls' (5'35") / 'When The Wind Blows' (3'32")

• *Musicians:* David Bowie *(vocals, guitar, keyboards, mellotron, moog, harmonica, tambourine)*, Carlos Alomar *(guitar, guitar synthesizer, tambourine, backing vocals)*, Erdal Kizilcay *(keyboards, drums, bass, trumpet, backing vocals, guitar on 'Time Will Crawl', violins on 'Bang Bang')*, Peter Frampton *(guitar)*, Carmine Rojas *(bass)*, Philippe Saisse *(piano, keyboards)*, Crusher Bennett *(percussion)*, Laurie Frink *(trumpet)*, Earl Gardner *(trumpet, flugelhorn)*, Stan Harrison *(alto sax)*, Steve Elson *(baritone sax)*, Lenny Pickett *(tenor sax)*, Robin Clark, Loni Groves, Diva Gray, Gordon Grodie *(backing vocals)*, Sid McGinnis *(guitar on 'Bang Bang', 'Time Will Crawl' and 'Day-In Day-Out')*, Coco, Sandro Sursock, Charuvan Suchi, Joe, Clement, John, Aglae *(backing vocals on 'Zeroes')*,

Mickey Rourke (*rap on 'Shining Star (Makin' My Love)'*) • *Recorded:* Mountain Studios, Montreux; Power Station Studios, New York • *Producers:* David Bowie, David Richards

Following Bowie's success at Live Aid, EMI were impatient to release another album. *Dance*, a compilation of 12" mixes from *Let's Dance* and *Tonight*, reached the sleeve-design stage in late 1985 but was scrapped. At the end of 1986, after more than two years spent channelling his energies into film soundtracks, acting, producing for Iggy Pop and putting off his label's repeated requests to generate more "product", Bowie finally returned to Mountain Studios in Montreux. The result of the month-long session was the album now commonly regarded as his creative nadir.

Received wisdom has it that *Never Let Me Down* is the last gasp in a downward spiral of mediocrity half-heartedly aimed at Bowie's new "Phil Collins" audience, a blind-alley trajectory that would be brought to a juddering halt by the drastic shake-up of Tin Machine. What is now forgotten is that in 1987 Bowie was already admitting that he had become "lost", and spoke optimistically of *Never Let Me Down* in precisely the terms he would later apply to Tin Machine: he described the album as "linear and rock-oriented," going on to explain that "When you get lost you go back to point one … and it just goes back to the guitar again, and so it became a guitar-oriented album." He called *Never Let Me Down* "a progression from *Scary Monsters* rather than my last two records," a claim he would later repeat almost verbatim for *Tin Machine*. Another taste of things to come is the demonstrative air of post-Live Aid social conscience: *Never Let Me Down* is riddled with images of urban poverty, prostitution, drug addiction and nuclear meltdown. "The subject matter on the album seems to be split between personal romance, personal feelings of love, and some kind of statement or indictment of an uncaring society, particularly a response to what's happening in the major cities in terms of the homeless," said Bowie.

The band assembled for the album was the usual combination of old and new. Carlos Alomar, Carmine Rojas and "The Borneo Horns" were back from *Tonight*. They were joined by Erdal Kizilcay, who had worked on and off with David on various projects since 1982. "He can switch from violin to trumpet to French horn, vibes, percussion, whatever," enthused David. "His knowledge of rock music begins and ends with the Beatles! His background is really jazz." Lead guitar was mainly entrusted to Peter Frampton, a former classmate of David's at Bromley Technical High School whose own taste of fame had come and gone with two hit albums in the mid-1970s. Newcomer Sid McGinnis, a sometime member of David Letterman's studio band, took Frampton's place on lead guitar for three tracks, while Bowie himself played lead on 'New York's In Love' and "87 And Cry'.

Bowie's co-producer was David Richards, an engineer since the days of *"Heroes"* who had co-produced Iggy Pop's *Blah-Blah-Blah*. "By the time we started in the studio [Bowie] had written over twelve songs with all the arrangements completed," recalled Richards. As ever, Bowie encouraged a collaborative effort: "I made demos of everything before we went in, and I played them to everybody and I said, 'I want it to sound exactly like this, but better!'"

During the first two weeks Bowie, Richards and Kizilcay cut the basic tracks at Mountain Studios. Next Carlos Alomar and Peter Frampton flew in to record their guitar parts, and thereafter the sessions moved to New York's Power Station. According to Richards this enabled Bowie to "add on the sounds you can only get in New York – The Borneo Horns, the girl backing vocalists, and a great percussionist called Crusher Bennett. Crusher set all his 'bangers' and 'scrapers' on a table, which I miked at each end. So whenever he moved around, the sounds would pan with him, creating some strange spatial effects."

While some of Bowie's vocals were recorded in New York, the majority were taken from guide vocals he had already cut in Switzerland. "David always sang a guide vocal very early on in the recording process," explained Richards, "Most of these vocals were so good and had such great spontaneity that they ended up on the record." A notable exception was the title track, a last-minute addition written, recorded and mixed at Power Station in 24 hours. The mix was handled by *Let's Dance* engineer Bob Clearmountain, who was responsible for what Bowie called the album's "great, forceful sound … It's fascinating watching him work; he's like a painter."

David promoted *Never Let Me Down* as an eclectic hybrid of long-standing influences and personal nostalgia, explaining that there was "a lot of reflection on the album. The whole reflective thing about it was totally unconscious. I realized how much it drew from the sixties and early seventies when I'd finished. It gives it an overall atmosphere that I hadn't intended, but it's quite nice. It doesn't seem to be a bitter look back; it seems to be quite energetic and up."

"We had the most fun doing this album that we ever had, because it was really coming back to just us and not all the outside influences," said Carlos Alomar in 1987. "The first thing you notice is David's voice. He sounds marvellous! He sounds refreshed, he's singing very high as he did before, as opposed to that very low baritone. This lends itself to … a different, high energy music." Alomar would later revise his opinion, telling David Buckley that Bowie was "at a loss during the whole album", that the music was over-rehearsed and the demos an imposition (he resented being asked to reproduce Erdal Kizilcay's demo parts: "why do you want me to play something played by a guy trying to imitate *me* and who sounds horrible playing me?"). Alomar also believes that EMI had effectively forced Bowie into the studio against his wishes: "Bowie felt let down. He discussed EMI constantly and talked about how horrible they were." If Bowie did indeed feel "let down", the album's title was supremely ironic.

"It's a pompous little title, isn't it?" David laughed in a pre-release interview for *Music & Sound Output*. "Seen out of context it's quite abrasive, but in the context of the songs on the album I think it's rather tongue-in-cheek to use it as the title. Also there's a vaudevillean thing about the cover. The two combined are rather comical."

In March 1987 Bowie and his band performed a series of eight press shows to announce the forthcoming Glass Spider tour. "I realized it was just a tremendous album to be touring," gushed Bowie, later adding that "A lot of it was written consciously with performance in mind: what kind of songs do I want to do night after night that I can enjoy playing? That brought the energy up on everything. It stopped it getting too reflective…"

Never Let Me Down was released on 27 April 1987 in a variety of different formats, all of which included the "vaudevillean" cover shot of the newly long-haired David leaping in a circus ring surrounded by elements from the songs: a drum, a skyscraper, a candyfloss cloud, one of the voyeuristic angels from the 'Day-In Day-Out' video, and a lot more besides. It was the first Bowie album to enjoy simultaneous release on vinyl and CD, and in an unusual move the two formats featured different edits – all but four of the tracks are anything up to a minute longer on CD. A blue vinyl version appeared in Australia, while in Japan the album included a Japanese vocal version of the out-take 'Girls'.

What might come as a surprise after all these years of counter-publicity is that some of the reviews were positively glowing. *Billboard* hailed the album as "A welcome return to form for the ever-ambitious Bowie," with a "superb title cut" and work from Frampton that "bodes well for Bowie's creative spirit". But such opinions were in the minority. The lead-off single 'Day-In Day-Out' had already performed its unspectacular slide out of the top 40 and the British critics were waiting with knives sharpened. The devastatingly irreverent and then highly influential teenybop magazine *Smash Hits* had recently coined a new nickname for Bowie which it deployed in a scathing review. "If Dame David Bowie is such a bleeding chameleon," pondered Tom Hibbert, "Why, pray, can't he change into something more exciting than the skin of an ageing rock plodder?" Despite a barrage of publicity, sales were no more than middling. Most artists would celebrate a number 6 chart placing, but it was Bowie's worst performance with a new album since *The Man Who Sold The World*.

Of all the mementoes of the wilderness years between *Scary Monsters* and *Black Tie White Noise*, none has been so systematically panned as *Never Let Me Down*. Nobody has a good word for it. Bowie has often allowed himself to be browbeaten by popular reaction, and in recent years he has colluded with critical opinion and assimilated the trashing of *Never Let Me Down* into his own view of his work, describing it as "a bitter disappointment". In 1993 he remarked that "There were some good songs on it, but I let go and it became very soft musically, which wasn't the way I would have done it if I had been more involved," adding later that "I was letting the guys arrange it, and I'd come in and do a vocal, and then I'd bugger off and pick up some bird." It's the only album not even mentioned in the official career biography posted on BowieNet in 1998. The notion that *Never Let Me Down* is an irredeemable disaster, serving only to illustrate how the mighty are fallen, has pretty much entered the realm of established fact.

The chances that this album will one day be reclaimed as a misunderstood classic are certainly remote, but in consigning it to the sacrificial altar as the scapegoat of all Bowie's 1980s misfortunes, both he and his critics have done it a serious disservice. *Never Let Me Down* in fact shows encouraging signs of recovery after the half-hearted apathy of Bowie's previous two albums. For a start he is writing more songs; they may not be masterpieces, but to its credit *Never Let Me Down* features ten new Bowie compositions, which is more than *Let's Dance* and *Tonight* put together. Furthermore, 'Julie' and 'Girls' make this the first Bowie session in many long years prolific enough to produce extra B-side material. In the second place, for better or worse, one can already hear Bowie feeling his way towards Tin Machine, marginalizing *Tonight*'s overbearing saxophone harmonics in favour of a surprisingly hard guitar sound. And thirdly, for the first time since *Scary Monsters* David contributes more than just his voice to the recordings, taking an active role with contributions on keyboards, harmonica and guitar – *lead* guitar on two tracks.

The results are far from brilliant. *Never Let Me Down* is hideously overproduced and suffers from fiddly, overwrought arrangements and a nasty, tinny drum acoustic. The uncluttered spontaneity of the title track, recorded in a few hours as an afterthought, positively shines beside some of its overcooked bedfellows. All three lead guitarists veer dangerously close to the sort of hoary, clichéd rock agenda so nimbly avoided by Bowie's previous roster of classic soloists. Even the shoddy cut-and-paste logo and the dismal sleeve artwork, conceived by Mick Haggerty and photographed by Greg Gorman, seem to have been designed by committee. If you sit down with the lyric sheet and half an hour to spare, you can spot all the "clever" references included in the cluttered photo, but what's the point? It's a picture of David Bowie jumping through hoops, and that tells us all we need to know.

But Alomar was right about Bowie's voice, which is in top flight, and the vocal pastiches (Neil Young on 'Time Will Crawl', Smokey Robinson on 'Shining Star', John Lennon on the title track) yield interesting if not always successful results. The alternation of clammy rock'n'roll love songs with over-sincere social comment is no more appealing here than on *Tin Machine*, but when Bowie chooses to inject the lyrics with his more accustomed collisions of non-linear imagery, as in 'Zeroes', 'Glass Spider' and 'Time Will Crawl', he reminds us that he is a major songwriting talent. Sadly, these tracks suffer the same fate as 'Loving The Alien' – grandiose and ambitious material cut adrift by maddeningly mediocre production – but at least they offer a genuine taste of the melodramatic panache we'd always expected of David Bowie until 1983. His self-reflexive habit is back in force,

with a series of verbal and musical echoes of past albums, in particular *Diamond Dogs*. Titles like 'Glass Spider' and 'Zeroes' speak for themselves. Whether this is a continuation of the self-sampling triumph of *Scary Monsters* or simply a hollow trading on former glories is a matter for debate. Whatever the case, Bowie struggles to keep up the momentum: after a reasonably promising first side and the near-greatness of 'Glass Spider', expectations fade away.

Not Bowie's finest hour, then, but by no means his worst. There's nothing here as outstanding as the title track of *Let's Dance*, but neither is there anything quite as thumb-twiddling as 'Without You' or as unwelcome as a clapped-out Beach Boys cover. Even on the dreariest tracks there's an energy of performance and a sense of commitment to the music and that simply isn't there on *Tonight*. Even Carlos Alomar has relented of late: "After not hearing it for a while, I went back and listened to it," he posted on his website in 2003. "Remarkably I did enjoy it. One of the things that popped up was the fact that I had started diving into the synthesizer guitar at the time, and I do remember all the experimentation that went on. It's funny about Bowie albums – after a few years they all fall into place as you see the progressions of his musical endeavours." Alomar is quite right of course. This is scarcely a great or even a satisfactory album, but coming to it again one finds to one's surprise that *Never Let Me Down* sounds more like a David Bowie record than either of its predecessors, and for many it remains a happier listening experience than what came next.

TIN MACHINE

EMI USA MTLS 1044, May 1989 *(LP)* [3]
EMI USA CDP 7919902, May 1989 *(CD)* [3]
Virgin CD VUS 99, November 1995
EMI 493 1012, 1998
EMI 7243 5219100, September 1999

'Heaven's in Here' (6'01") / 'Tin Machine' (3'34") / 'Prisoner of Love' (4'50") / 'Crack City' (4'36") / 'I Can't Read' (4'54") / 'Under the God' (4'06") / 'Amazing' (3'04") / 'Working Class Hero' (4'38") / 'Bus Stop' (1'41") / 'Pretty Thing' (4'39") / 'Video Crime' (3'52") / 'Run' (3'20") *(CD only)* / 'Sacrifice Yourself' (2'08") *(CD only)* / 'Baby Can Dance' (4'57") *Bonus track on 1995 reissue:* 'Country Bus Stop' (1'52")

• *Musicians:* David Bowie *(guitar, vocals)*, Reeves Gabrels *(guitar)*, Hunt Sales *(drums, vocals)*, Tony Sales *(bass, vocals)*, Kevin Armstrong *(rhythm guitar, Hammond B3)* • *Recorded:* Mountain Studios, Montreux; Compass Point Studios, Nassau • *Producers:* Tin Machine, Tim Palmer

Desperate situations require desperate measures, and by the end of 1987 Bowie was all too aware that he was in danger of becoming a laughing stock. The residual goodwill of even the most loyal fans was wearing a little thin, and there was a growing sense that the shining light of 1970s rock was a spent force. Bowie later admitted that the feeling was not confined to onlookers: "More than anything else, I thought I should make as much money as I could, and then quit," he said in 1996. "I didn't think there was any alternative. I thought I was obviously just an empty vessel and would end up like everyone else, doing these stupid fucking shows, singing 'Rebel Rebel' until I fall over and bleed." He considered retiring from music altogether to concentrate on his painting. Instead, just as he had done a decade earlier, he chose a radical course of action to drag himself bodily out of the mainstream, and in the process took one of the most controversial and massively derided leaps of his career.

Bowie's first attempt at a new sound involved a brief collaboration with Bon Jovi producer Bruce Fairbairn (see 'Like A Rolling Stone' in Chapter 1), but the session was not adjudged a success. Another, far more influential figure was about to appear in the story.

At the end of the Glass Spider tour in November 1987, Bowie's American press officer Sarah Gabrels gave him a demo tape recorded by her 31-year-old husband Reeves, whom David had befriended backstage on the American leg of the tour without ever knowing that he was a musician. "He was very clever – he'd picked out all the best bits of guitar playing he'd done," said Bowie later. "I loved the tape, so I got hold of him immediately." In May 1988 Gabrels, who was then giving guitar lessons to students in Kensington, was flown out to Switzerland where he stayed with Bowie for nearly a month. "He was at a crossroads," Gabrels tells David Buckley. "Either he became Rod Stewart and played Las Vegas, or he followed his heart." Gabrels, who by his own admission had nothing to lose, "was naïve enough to point out the obvious", telling Bowie that "I've never had the

drug of commercial success. The only barrier between you doing what you want and you doing what you think you should do, is *you*."

A graduate of Berklee College of Music, Gabrels was an art-school experimentalist whose favoured guitar style, a hardcore squall somewhere between the sounds of Robert Fripp and Earl Slick, rapidly found favour with Bowie. The first fruits of the new relationship came in July 1988 at the "Intruders At The Palace" concert (see Chapter 3), after which the pair returned to Montreux to begin work on what was envisaged as a David Bowie solo project. The first idea was a concept album based on Steven Berkoff's *West*, but this was scrapped after yielding only one demo, 'The King Of Stamford Hill'. Widening their horizons, the pair began working on embryonic versions of 'Heaven's In Here', 'Bus Stop', 'Baby Can Dance' and even 'Baby Universal'. To produce the forthcoming sessions Bowie appointed newcomer Tim Palmer, whose previous clients included British goth-guitar outfits like The Mission, Gene Loves Jezebel (who would later support some of Bowie's UK dates in 1990) and The Cult, whose guitarist Billy Duffy had recommended him to David.

At this stage it is conceivable that the project might have evolved into experimental art-rock in the vein of *Scary Monsters* (one of Gabrels's favourites) or *Lodger* (the last Bowie album that Palmer had "really enjoyed"). However, Bowie was about to deliver another of his customary curve balls, one which would arguably redirect a valuable experiment in a more regressive direction. A rhythm section was needed, and both he and Gabrels were eager to avoid using polished session-men. Bowie had floated possible names, including Frank Zappa's drummer Terry Bozzio and Brian Eno's bassist Percy Jones (both direct links to Bowie's Berlin period; the former was playing with Zappa when David enlisted Adrian Belew in 1978, while the latter played on Eno's mid-1970s albums including *Another Green World*). Instead Bowie settled upon the ultimate in unreconstructed rock'n'rollers: at a party in Los Angeles he chanced to meet bassist Tony Sales who, with his percussionist brother Hunt, had provided the rhythm section on Iggy Pop's *Lust For Life* back in 1977. Sales later recalled: "I went up to say hey, how you doing. He went, Tony! Hey, listen, I was thinking about this project…"

The Sales brothers joined Bowie and Gabrels at Mountain Studios at which point, according to Tim

Palmer in *Strange Fascination*, "all hell broke loose. The sessions took on a completely different feel; it was much more chaotic." Bowie declared that his wish was to return to the basics of rock'n'roll – something he'd been claiming to do in one way or another as far back as *Let's Dance* – but this time without resort to studio processing of any kind. The keynotes were spontaneity and, as David would later reiterate, an egalitarian band effort. "To be able to write like this with other people," he enthused, "it's been something I haven't been able to do for a long time." Ten years later he explained that the band dynamic forced a reassessment of his role in the studio. "All three of them were very canny, masters of the put-down – the Sales brothers, being the sons of Soupy Sales, were born stand-ups. So I wasn't allowed to lord it, which I recognized as a situation I wanted. To be part of a group of people working towards one aim."

Bowie remembered a "strange period of feeling each other out" during the first week of the sessions. Gabrels recalled: "When I first got there, Hunt has got a knife on his belt and he's wearing a T-shirt that says, 'Fuck You, I'm From Texas,' so I think, oh *shit*. And whenever I played something they'd say no, you play it like this, kid. And after a week of being a nice guy – walking that fine line between ignoring what people were telling me and being gracious about it – I did it how I wanted."

Also on board for the sessions was Bowie's Live Aid/Intruders At The Palace rhythm guitarist Kevin Armstrong. Since 1985 he had toured with Iggy Pop, played in Jonathan Ross's house band, worked with Elvis Costello and Paul McCartney, and played the guitars – uncredited – on Transvision Vamp's imminent album *Velveteen*.

After a few months' break recording recommenced at Compass Point Studios in Nassau, where the sessions were long and prolific. Bowie was adamant that he wanted an authentic live sound, and any tracks that required embellishment were rejected out of hand: "That's why we did something like thirty tracks. We just wrote them and played them as they came, as they hit the deck … there's very little overdubbing on it at all." Some tracks, including 'I Can't Read', were recorded completely live. "It took a certain leap of faith on the part of the engineers to trust us in the way we wanted to record," said Gabrels. "They kind of looked at us funny because we wanted to play all at the same time and David wanted to sing, which is generally not done any more."

The songwriting was also handled on the hoof; Bowie was improvising on the microphone in a way he hadn't done since *"Heroes"*. "It was impressionistically written," he revealed. "The very first things that came into my mind and what suited the feeling of the music." He was egged on in this approach by the band: "They were there all the time saying, don't wimp out, sing it like you wrote it. Stand by it. I have done and frequently do censor myself in lyrics. I say one thing and then I think, Ah, maybe I'll just take the edge off that a bit. I don't know why I do that. I'm English."

The subject matter, too, saw a retrenchment of sorts as Bowie discarded his celebrated detachment and wrote from a position of first-person frankness. "Things like 'I Can't Read' came from my own desperations, not from watching or observing other people," he said. "'Crack City' is because of my own very intense and dangerous liaison with cocaine in the mid-seventies … I'm making my art serve me and not having me serve my art, which is just another way of working. People say, 'Why can't he be like he used to be? It's more fun for us to watch him fucking up.' Fuck 'em. I'm not interested."

The new sound was a combination of Bowie's back-to-basics imperative, Gabrels's guitar experiments and the Sales brothers' crashing roadhouse blues style. Bowie cited the influence of Jimi Hendrix and Cream along with guitar maestro Glenn Branca and jazz heroes John Coltrane and Miles Davis; he told one reporter that "There's a lot of Mingus and Roland Kirk in some of the more free pieces." Gabrels added that "There was almost an architectural reference – deconstructivism and things like that, letting the ends of the music dangle. You know, if the guitar makes noises when you plug it in, why can't that go on tape as well?" This sounds enticingly like a return to the spirit of the Eno collaborations, and Bowie intimated that this was a period to which he had turned for inspiration. "[I] spent a long time with my old albums. *"Heroes"*, *Lodger*, *Scary Monsters*, *Low*, to push myself back into why I was writing." He also repeated an assertion he had made regarding *Never Let Me Down* two years earlier: "This, for me, is like catching up from *Scary Monsters*. It's almost dismissive of the last three albums I've done. Getting back on course, you could say."

Both album and band were christened *Tin Machine* after one of the new songs. Even here, Bowie assumed an air of rock'n'roll indifference: "We really weren't interested in what kind of band name we had, so it was almost arbitrary – ah, let's just pick a song title." Reeves Gabrels recalls that the Sales brothers favoured *Tin Machine* "because it was like The Monkees, having your own theme song!" His own suggestion was *The Emperor's New Clothes*, although he later admitted that this would have been "a little too much like setting yourself up; giving your critics ammunition."

When *Tin Machine* was launched it was made clear to the press that anyone wanting to interview David would get the rest of the band as well. Although he played the part to the hilt, few onlookers were truly convinced that this new, anonymous Bowie was quite as sincere about band democracy as he was keen to suggest. Growing a beard and letting your drummer do all the talking was no way for a superstar to behave, and the laddishness that dominated interviews would soon be written off by critics as a piece of calculated stage management, the latest in a long line of pretentious blunders by a self-reinventor fallen on hard times. "I think the context annoyed and angered, and really gave the critics the excuse they needed to humiliate somebody, which is what they really look for more than anything else," he observed ten years later.

As a defensive tactic while Bowie recharged his creative batteries Tin Machine clearly served its purpose. It forcibly jettisoned the mainstream audience which had threatened his well-being as an artist in recent years. It allowed him to escape the pressures of stadium tours and play his songs in tiny clubs in front of a few hundred people at a time. It returned him to a predicament – creatively if not financially – of having to work for his supper. It was good for him. Whether it was any good for the rest of us is an entirely separate matter.

When *Tin Machine* was released at the end of May 1989, the initial response was one of cautious enthusiasm. *Rolling Stone* described the album as "Sonic Youth meets *Station To Station*," going on to note approvingly that *"Tin Machine* effectively reconciles the bracing noise of a full-tilt electric band with the nuances of Bowie's writing craft." *Q* declared that the album "revives [Bowie's] energy levels and all-round excitement quota by recalling some of the bolder moments of his musical history," resulting in "the loudest, hardest, heaviest effort of his whole career … an experience that's not unlike allowing your head to be used as a punchbag. Stranger still, you'll come to find you kind of like it." The album shot to number 3

in the UK chart – three places higher than *Never Let Me Down*. But its subsequent fall – both from the billboards and in critical estimation – was swift.

At the end of 1989 *Tin Machine* appeared in *Q*'s fifty best albums of the year; to give some sense of perspective, The Cure's masterpiece *Disintegration* did not. Only seven years later *Tin Machine* appeared in the same magazine's "Fifty Albums That Should Never Have Been Made". In 1998 a panel of pop stars, DJs and journalists voted *Tin Machine* 17th in a *Melody Maker* poll of the worst albums of all time. The following year, when Glasgow's hardcore post-punk artist Rico was making waves with his debut album *Sanctuary Medicines*, he revealed to *Q* that the opening track featured the sound of a copy of *Tin Machine* being smashed to smithereens. "I was looking for a shit album," he explained, "so I bunged it on the turntable and gave it a good fucking beating. I thought that was fair enough." Critical abuse seldom comes any less equivocal than that; *Tin Machine* is now widely regarded as one of the greatest follies of Bowie's recorded output.

The initial reviews were right to note that *Tin Machine* boasts a raw energy that Bowie's work had lacked since *Scary Monsters*. That aside, it's not an easy or even a particularly likeable album. An abiding characteristic of Bowie's career is his willingness to absorb and assimilate whatever external influences are at hand, often with superb results. He once famously described himself as a photostat machine. On this occasion, it seems that his susceptibility to outside stimuli turned against him: in Reeves Gabrels he had found a collaborator with the potential of another Eno or Fripp, but any experimental aspirations seemed in constant conflict with the no-nonsense rock instincts of the rhythm section. Many years later Gabrels revealed that, despite the financial advantage it offered him, he had tried to dissuade Bowie from the democratic band concept "because I thought the Sales brothers were nuts! I didn't want to be in a band any more. Bands are a nightmare, and democracy doesn't work as well as benevolent dictatorships in rock'n'roll in my opinion."

Gabrels is surely right. Re-reading contemporary interviews with Tin Machine, it's ghoulishly clear that Bowie was allowing himself to be dragged into the prevailing "Fuck You, I'm From Texas" mentality, and forcibly encouraged to disown whichever bits of his back catalogue proved too highbrow for his colleagues' tastes. The band's refusal to let David rewrite his lyrics results merely in the most half-baked set of songwords he's ever allowed onto an album. With a few notable exceptions, *Tin Machine* is saddled by a one-dimensional element of hectoring demagoguery as Bowie unleashes unsophisticated polemics on drugs ('Crack City'), splatter-movies ('Video Crime') and neo-Nazism ('Under The God'). On tracks like 'Pretty Thing' there's an entirely unwelcome injection of posturing rock'n'roll sexism, and throughout the album there's a ridiculous overdose of embarrassingly misplaced swearing. When the word "wanking" appeared amid the delicately preening glam of *Aladdin Sane*'s 'Time', a delighted taboo-breaking shudder ran down the collective spine of a generation of teenagers. When the line "don't look at me you fuckheads" turns up in 'Crack City', it's as though someone has accidentally let Roy Chubby Brown into a meeting of the Fabian Society. Matters aren't helped by the sleeve photography (by *"Heroes"* veteran Sukita), which reveals the bearded Bowie and his three sidemen posing uncomfortably in double-breasted suits like a gaggle of insipid estate agents.

But despite all reservations, *Tin Machine* is by no means the atrocious write-off its reputation suggests. Gabrels at his best provides guitar work on a par with the past achievements of Robert Fripp and Adrian Belew. "I would have gone for a somewhat more technically proficient and aggressive rock thing," he tells Buckley, "rather than a garage thing, which is what we got with the Sales brothers." More than once Bowie has leapt to the defence of *Tin Machine*'s undisputed highlight, the superb 'I Can't Read', a song that sidesteps all the album's problems to emerge as a genuine classic, offering a sophisticated lyric and a textured sonic discretion quite unusual amid the surrounding crash-bang-wallop delivery. The entirely ignored 'Amazing' is another highlight, while the title track and 'Baby Can Dance' both hint at what the album might have sounded like with a less wilfully fuzzy, horribly drum-heavy mix. 'Bus Stop' offers a welcome spot of light relief, and 'Heaven's In Here' is genuinely exhilarating until it disintegrates into an unconvincing attempt at Hendrix-style demolition.

And although, at the time, *Tin Machine* was greeted by many with incredulity, historically it now makes complete sense. Bowie's accustomed art-rock territory was all but extinct in 1989; the charts were ruled by trivial pop-rappers who had nothing to offer him, the British indie renaissance had yet to take off and the dominant sounds from America were coming

from new heavy metal giants like Guns N'Roses. Most of the rising acts Bowie was citing with enthusiasm (Dinosaur Jnr, Sonic Youth and in particular Pixies, whose breakthrough album *Doolittle* was released at the same time as *Tin Machine*) inhabited the proto-grunge hinterland as yet unknown to the mainstream. It would be pushing credibility to suggest that Tin Machine paved the way for Nirvana, but if nothing else David was once again moving with the tide.

Bowie's retreat to Berlin in 1976 to dismantle his first period of mainstream success resulted in some of the finest albums in rock history. While the same will never be said of *Tin Machine*, it's worth bearing in mind that the project was evidently an invaluable process of creative therapy. "Some people liked it, some didn't like it, but for me, that band was absolutely necessary," David would say in 2003. "It accomplished exactly what it was supposed to do, which was bring me back to my absolute roots and set me back on the right course of what I do best." If the project ultimately unlocked the door to *The Buddha Of Suburbia*, *1.Outside* and *Earthling* then it was surely worth it. But as an album in its own right, *Tin Machine* must remain one of the least satisfactory listening experiences in Bowie's recorded legacy. "Some nights it just blew me away," he said five years later of the band in general. "It was so adventurous and so brave. When it worked, it was unbeatable, some of the most explosive music that I've been involved in or even witnessed. But when it was bad, it was so unbelievably awful you just wanted the earth to open up and take you under."

TIN MACHINE II

London 828 2721, September 1991 *(LP)* [23]
London 828 2722, September 1991 *(CD)* [23]

'Baby Universal' (3'18") / 'One Shot' (5'11") / 'You Belong in Rock N'Roll' (4'07") / 'If There Is Something' (4'45") / 'Amlapura' (3'46") / 'Betty Wrong' (3'48") / 'You Can't Talk' (3'09") / 'Stateside' (5'38") / 'Shopping For Girls' (3'44") / 'A Big Hurt' (3'40") / 'Sorry' (3'29") / 'Goodbye Mr. Ed' (3'24") / 'Hammerhead' (0'57")

• *Musicians:* David Bowie *(vocals, guitar, piano, saxophone)*, Reeves Gabrels *(guitar, backing vocals, vibrators, Drano, organ)*, Hunt Sales *(drums, percussion, vocals)*, Tony Sales *(bass, backing vocals)*, Tim Palmer *(additional piano, percussion)*, Kevin Armstrong *(piano on 'Shopping for Girls', rhythm guitar on 'If There Is Something')* • *Recorded:* Studios 301, Sydney; A&M Studios, Los Angeles • *Producers:* Tin Machine, Tim Palmer *('One Shot':* Hugh Padgham)

Most of Tin Machine's second album was recorded in Sydney in the autumn of 1989, hard on the heels of the band's inaugural tour. The project was reactivated at the end of 1990, following a year's hiatus in which Bowie had diverted his energies to his Sound + Vision tour and *The Linguini Incident*. Before recording resumed, news broke that David had finally parted company with EMI.

In a joint statement in December 1990 both parties announced that the split was amicable, but other sources have spoken of a serious row over Bowie's increasingly uncommercial work and the continued attempts of exasperated EMI executives to secure another *Let's Dance*. It is believed that the label refused point-blank to market another Tin Machine album, whereupon Bowie elected to sever the alliance. The Rykodisc/EMI reissue programme remained unaffected (at the time of the split, the albums from *Young Americans* onwards were yet to be re-released), but Bowie's new material needed a new home.

In March 1991 Tin Machine negotiated a deal with Victory Music, a new label launched by the electronics giant JVC and distributed worldwide by London Records and Polygram. In the same month the band reconvened in Los Angeles to record a further three tracks for *Tin Machine II*. The studio line-up of the first album, including guest instrumentalist Kevin Armstrong and co-producer Tim Palmer, were joined in Los Angeles by *Tonight*'s Hugh Padgham, now renowned for his production work with Phil Collins and Sting. Padgham considered 'One Shot' "a bloody great song" but was unimpressed by the Tin Machine ethos; he tells David Buckley that "The Sales brothers were basically mad", but that "Reeves was a master of his instrument in an Adrian Belew kind of way."

Another blast from the past was sleeve illustrator Edward Bell, creator of the classic *Scary Monsters* artwork. Bell's sleeve design was a charcoal sketch of four *kouroi*, Greek statues dating from the sixth century BC, which were once believed to represent Apollo but are now understood to be idealized figures lacking individual identity – and therefore entirely in keeping with Bowie's fallen-god, one-of-the-boys Tin Machine ethos. *Kouroi* are represented as athletic, naked youths, and with tiresome predictability *Tin Machine II* became the second album sleeve in Bowie's career to undergo castration. British buyers were left to the mercy of the original artwork, but in America the terrifying organs of generation were airbrushed away and civilization was saved.

Tin Machine II was released on 2 September 1991, less than a month after EMI's reissues of the Berlin albums; comparisons were inevitable and none of them were in *Tin Machine II*'s favour. There were those who applauded the album – the *NME* gave it a surprising thumbs-up and *Billboard* approved of the "lashing axe-fueled Hugh Padgham-produced track 'One Shot'" among other "potent rockers" – but they were in the minority. The album only reached number 23 in the UK chart, while in America it scraped to number 126. As Tony Horkins of *International Musician* stoically hypothesized, "maybe, like the rest of Bowie's career, it'll all make a lot more sense in a few years' time." Even in 1991 Bowie was speaking of *Tin Machine II* primarily as a therapeutic work-in-progress manoeuvre. "The band became my obstacle," he explained to Horkins. "They re-present me with ideas and also problems that I wouldn't encounter working on my own, telling people what to do. You start to learn how to tell people how to do things, and that becomes a system. And once you've got a system you're really fucked up … I needed to break it! Fortuitously, this band has done that for me. My system has been broken."

Tin Machine II is a record of extremes. Its best moments are an improvement on much of the band's previous output, but its worst moments are simply unspeakable. From the outset of the Tin Machine project it was clear that much of the band's character would be defined by its irrepressible and outspoken drummer Hunt Sales, who established himself from the earliest interviews as the joker in the pack. By the time of *Tin Machine II* he had been promoted to the status of band mascot, his "It's My Life" tattoo prominently displayed on the back cover artwork (a rear-view of Bell's charcoal *kouroi* with a ripped photo of Hunt's shoulders overlaid, *Scary Monsters*-style, onto one of the four figures). In an alarming development of Tin Machine's pretensions to band democracy, Hunt Sales sings lead vocal on two of the album's tracks, one of them entirely self-penned. There's no denying the man's credentials as a musician, but on the evidence of these tracks his no-frills, no-irony, southern blues agenda is simply the antithesis of everything we associate with David Bowie. "I always felt that he would have been more in tune with a big band set-up," admitted David in 1997. "The whole thing about him is that slouch and mood of the big band drummers." Similar collisions have fuelled some of Bowie's finest work; here, the temptation to over-indulge a colleague threatens to bring *Tin Machine II* to its knees. 'Stateside' and 'Sorry' rank among the most frighteningly bad songs ever to find their way into the Bowie canon.

Far more promising are the signs that David was tiring of *Tin Machine*'s indiscriminate rocked-up style and seeking to inject a degree of sophistication into the proceedings; he described the new album as "sensitively aggressive". *Tin Machine II* offers a more balanced and polished production style than its predecessor, and boasts a greater variety of instrumentation, including some of Bowie's best saxophone work in years. The experimental element is wilfully eccentric – Reeves Gabrels plays his guitar with a vibrator on some tracks – but there's no denying that the results are all the better for it. On the first album the tendency was for every track to degenerate into a guitar-and-drums demolition; here, thankfully, such urges are reined in. Better still, Bowie's lyrics are a massive improvement on the half-baked posturings of *Tin Machine*, returning to his more accustomed territory of allusive, fragmented imagery. The best tracks, notably 'Baby Universal', 'Shopping For Girls' and the genuinely brilliant 'Goodbye Mr. Ed' (with music co-written, to give him his due, by Hunt Sales), deserve a wider audience than they are ever likely to reach.

But ultimately no amount of songwriting can compensate for the lack of governance that consigns *Tin Machine II* to mediocrity. Long before the end one yearns for Bowie to overthrow what remains of the band's autonomy, seize the reins of power and get on with the serious business of making a proper solo album. "Even taking in The Spiders or whoever, I've never been in a band," he told *The Irish Times* in August 1991. "I've never been *in* a band. I've always led a band. It's probably the only band I'll ever be in, because it's fulfilling everything I ever thought you could do with a band and I would see no necessity for being with another one." Thus, even before *Tin Machine II* was released, there were hints aplenty that the end was in sight.

TIN MACHINE LIVE: OY VEY, BABY
London 828 3281, July 1992 *(LP)*
London 828 3282, July 1992 *(CD)*

'If There Is Something' (3'55") / 'Amazing' (4'06") / 'I Can't Read' (6'25") / 'Stateside' (8'11") / 'Under The God' (4'05") / 'Goodbye Mr. Ed' (3'31") / 'Heaven's In Here' (12'05") / 'You Belong in Rock N'Roll' (6'59")

• *Musicians:* see *The It's My Life tour* (Chapter 3) • *Recorded:* Orpheum Theater, Boston; Academy, New York; Riviera, Chicago; NHK Hall, Tokyo; Kouseinenkin Kaikan, Sapporo • *Producers:* Max Bisgrove, Tom Dubé, Reeves Gabrels, Dave Bianco, David Bowie

Released on a wave of indifference in the summer of 1992, Tin Machine's final assault on the market has the ignominious distinction of being the only new Bowie album since 1967 not to have entered even the lowest reaches of the UK chart. A live Tin Machine album was hardly likely to tempt the casual buyer, but even the most devoted fan might have hoped for a more imaginative track-listing. During the It's My Life tour the band had performed covers of 'Debaser', 'I've Been Waiting For You' and 'Go Now' which, had they been included here, might at least have loosened the wallet of the completist. Instead the album was dominated by a sprawling eight-minute rendition of the dreaded 'Stateside' and a *twelve*-minute 'Heaven's In Here', ensuring that even the most patient loyalists thought twice before buying it.

The album's ill fortune was compounded by ugly, indistinct packaging and an unspeakably misconceived title ("Hunt Sales's title, I might add," revealed Bowie in 1997, "the whole Soupy Sales link"). Reeves Gabrels later explained that the title was "a play on the fact that there are no original ideas," but taking a pot-shot at U2's universally acclaimed *Achtung Baby* was entirely unworthy of Bowie, and even if it was meant in jest it backfired disastrously. The reviews, where they appeared at all, were the most vitriolic he had ever had (*Melody Maker* declared that Bowie hereby "ceases to exist as an artist of any worth whatsoever") and the album sank like a stone. Plans to release a second instalment called *Use Your Wallet* (presumably a hilarious reference to *Use Your Illusion*, the two-album set released in 1991 by Guns N'Roses) were forgotten.

Oy Vey, Baby was recorded at five different venues: first to be taped was 'I Can't Read' in Boston on 20 November 1991, with 'Stateside' and 'Heaven's In Here' following in New York later the same month. 'Amazing' and 'You Belong In Rock N'Roll' were recorded in Chicago on 7 December, while the remaining three tracks were taped on the Japanese leg in February 1992: 'If There Is Something' and 'Goodbye Mr. Ed' in Tokyo, and finally 'Under The God' in Sapporo. Bowie is said to have described the mix, overseen by Reeves Gabrels and the tour's engineer Max Bisgrove, as "deconstructionist R&B." Frankly, that makes it sound more interesting than it really is. It's not actually a *bad* album – say what you like about them, Tin Machine could play live – but Gabrels is in a minority of one when he reveals that this is his favourite Tin Machine record.

Still, there's one reason to be grateful for *Oy Vey, Baby*. From the earliest Tin Machine interviews, Bowie had repeatedly asserted that the band intended to produce at least three albums. The third turned out not to be another time-consuming and self-subverting studio effort, but a live set apparently turfed out so that David could resume his solo career without delay. And so he did; within a month of *Oy Vey, Baby*'s appearance Bowie had released 'Real Cool World', his first new solo single since 1987, and the more substantial pleasures of *Black Tie White Noise* were already in the works.

BLACK TIE WHITE NOISE

Arista 74321 13697 2, April 1993 [1]
EMI 7243 5 8481402 (7243 5 8333824 / 7243 5
    8481327 / 7243 4 9063495), August 2003
(limited edition 10th anniversary reissue)

'The Wedding' (5'04") / 'You've Been Around' (4'45") / 'I Feel Free' (4'52") / 'Black Tie White Noise' (4'52") / 'Jump They Say' (4'22") / 'Nite Flights' (4'30") / 'Pallas Athena' (4'40") / 'Miracle Goodnight' (4'14") / 'Don't Let Me Down & Down' (4'55") / 'Looking For Lester' (5'36") / 'I Know It's Gonna Happen Someday' (4'14") / 'The Wedding Song' (4'29") / 'Jump They Say (Alternate Mix)' (3'58") *(CD & cassette only)* / 'Lucy Can't Dance' (5'45") *(CD only)*
Bonus tracks on 2003 reissue: 'Real Cool World' (5'25") / 'Lucy Can't Dance' (5'48") / 'Jump They Say (Rock Mix)' (4'04") / 'Black Tie White Noise (3rd

Floor US Radio Mix)' (3'40") / 'Miracle Goodnight (Make Believe Mix)' (4'28") / 'Don't Let Me Down & Down (Indonesian Vocal Version)' (4'53") / 'You've Been Around (Dangers 12" Remix)' (7'39") / 'Jump They Say (Brothers In Rhythm 12" Remix)' (8'22") / 'Black Tie White Noise (Here Come Da Jazz)' (5'32") / 'Pallas Athena (Don't Stop Praying Remix No 2)' (7'26") / 'Nite Flights (Moodswings Back To Basics Remix)' (9'52") / 'Jump They Say (Dub Oddity)' (6'13")

• *Musicians:* David Bowie *(vocals, guitar, saxophone, dog alto)*, Pugi Bell *(drums)*, Barry Campbell *(bass)*, Sterling Campbell *(drums)*, Nile Rodgers *(guitar)*, Richard Hilton *(keyboards)*, John Regan *(bass)*, Michael Reisman *(harp, tubular bells)*, Dave Richards *(keyboards)*, Philippe Saisse *(keyboards)*, Richard Tee *(keyboards)*, Gerado Velez *(percussion)*, Al B Sure! *(vocals on 'Black Tie White Noise')*, Lester Bowie *(trumpet)*, Reeves Gabrels *(guitar on 'You've Been Around')*, Mick Ronson *(guitar on 'I Feel Free')*, Mike Garson *(piano on 'Looking for Lester')*, Wild T Springer *(guitar on 'I Know It's Gonna Happen Someday')*, Fonzi Thorton, Tawatha Agee, Curtis King Jr., Denis Collins, Brenda White-King, Maryl Epps, Frank Simms, George Simms, David Spinner, Lamya Al-Mughiery, Connie Petruk, David Bowie, Nile Rodgers *(backing vocals)* • *Recorded:* Mountain Studios, Montreux; 38 Fresh Recording Studios & The Hit Factory, New York • *Producers:* David Bowie, Nile Rodgers

Five days after their marriage in April 1992, David and Iman were in Los Angeles when the city erupted in its worst outbreak of civil unrest since the 1960s. A combination of his marriage and his eyewitness experience of urban America's crucible of racial violence would inspire Bowie's next cycle of songs. *Black Tie White Noise* was conceived as a fusion of black and white signifiers, a meeting of intellectual and cultural tempos as well as of musical ones. The title track was a response to the Los Angeles riots, while on a calmer note the opening and closing tracks were developments of the music Bowie had composed for the June wedding ceremony in Florence. Other compositions confronted equally personal subjects, notably touching on the death of David's half-brother Terry in 'Jump They Say'. "I think this album comes from a very different emotional place," he told *Rolling Stone*. "That's the passing of time, which has brought maturity and a willingness to relinquish full control over my emotions, let them go a bit, start relating to other people, which is something that's been happening to me slowly – and, my God, it's been uphill – over the last ten or twelve years." In an interview for MTV he was keen to underplay the idea that the album heralded a new optimism. "I hope there's an edge. I don't think it's like a glowing, kind of 'everybody's sailing into the sunset and life will be roses ever after' – I don't think I would ever write an album like that. But it's probably a lot less bleak than some of my previous albums."

The title itself was a minor masterpiece. "I think *Black Tie White Noise* refers to the very obvious," David explained, "The radical boundaries that have been put up in most of the Western world. It also has a lot to do with the black and white sides of one's thinking. I think it goes a little further than simply the racial situation … I think, at this particular moment in time, it's very important to promote the coming together of the disparate elements of any nation, specifically America, where the record was written, but actually I guess even more so now in Europe." Over and above the album's directly political concerns, the title operates as a multiple pun on Bowie's own musical affiliations and studio techniques. "White noise itself is something that I first encountered on the synthesizer many years ago," he explained. "There's black noise and white noise. I thought that much of what is said and done by the whites is white noise. 'Black tie' is because for me, musically, the one thing that really turned me on to wanting to be a musician, wanting to write, was American black music … for a number of years I worked with rhythm and blues bands, and my participation in them formed my own 'black ties' in that area of music."

To co-produce the album Bowie turned again to Nile Rodgers, who had produced *Let's Dance* ten years earlier, and from the early summer of 1992 recording alternated between Mountain Studios in Montreux and Rodgers's home territory at New York's Hit Factory. The first fruit of the collaboration was the movie theme 'Real Cool World', released as a single in August 1992 and prefiguring the sophisticated dance-floor jazz of the forthcoming album.

Rodgers was instrumental in adding a state-of-the-art club sheen to the more dance-oriented tracks, but otherwise *Black Tie White Noise*, in stark contrast with *Let's Dance*, is dominated not by him but by Bowie.

According to Rodgers, David was "a lot more relaxed this time than he was at the *Let's Dance* sessions, a hell of a lot more philosophical and just in a state of mind where his music was really, really making him happy." The process of harnessing all this positive energy made for a greater challenge: "*Let's Dance* was the easiest record I've ever made – three weeks in total. *Black Tie White Noise* was the hardest – one year, more or less." Dramatically colouring these and other contemporary comments, Nile Rodgers later told David Buckley that he did not enjoy making *Black Tie White Noise* at all, complaining that Bowie dismissed any attempt to repeat the formula of *Let's Dance*: "I felt my hands were tied to a large extent … I was playing great commercial licks to Bowie, and he was rejecting them almost across the board … When we finished that record, I knew it wasn't cool. I knew it wasn't nearly as cool as *Let's Dance*. Don't get me wrong. I think there's really clever, interesting stuff on it. But the point is, it ain't as good as *Let's Dance* … he was not budging. It was an exercise in futility."

These sentiments clearly reveal a different set of priorities from Bowie's own. "This time around it was more my vision," David averred in 1993, "And Nile provided the buoyancy and the enthusiasm for the project … If the artist has some quite definite ideas, Nile will roll with those and just help get them activated." This time the outcome was not slick R&B, but a fusion of Middle Eastern melodies, European disco, New York club sounds and freestyle jazz. There are strong echoes of both *Station To Station* and *Low*, harnessed throughout to a relentless dance beat.

If Nile Rodgers provides the groove, trumpeter Lester Bowie gives the album its essential musical identity. "Throughout the eighties there was this nagging idea that somewhere in time I wanted to work with Lester on trumpet, and this really was the opportunity," explained David. "He came in to do one track, 'Don't Let Me Down & Down', and he was such a blast, he was so great to work with, that we just kept him on!" Lending his fierce, brassy freestyle blowing to a total of six tracks, Lester Bowie (who sadly died in 1999) also provides the perfect foil to his namesake's saxophone work. *Black Tie White Noise* finds David's sax more strongly to the fore than on any other album, a result of his renewed commitment to the instrument during the preceding Tin Machine tour. "I think David would be the first to admit that he's not a saxophonist in the traditional sense," Rodgers told *Rolling Stone*. "I mean, you wouldn't call him up to do gigs. He uses his playing as an artistic tool. He's a painter. He hears an idea, and he goes with it. But he absolutely knows where he's going..." The horn arrangements were handled by 70-year-old Afro-Cuban jazz veteran Chico O'Farrill, who had recorded with greats such as Dizzy Gillespie, Stan Kenton and Benny Goodman. *Black Tie White Noise* marked something of a career renaissance for O'Farrill, who recorded with renewed vigour and even received a Latin Grammy nomination a year before his death in 2001.

The title track's guest vocal by Al B Sure!, who had previously enjoyed a few minor hits in collaboration with Barry White and Quincy Jones, sets the seal on the album's streetwise black posture. However, it was the presence of two other guests that drew the greatest attention. Providing instrumental solos on 'Looking For Lester' and 'I Feel Free' respectively were pianist Mike Garson – last heard on *Young Americans* – and guitarist Mick Ronson, making his first appearance on a Bowie album since *Pin Ups*. The presence of the two ex-Spiders and the return of Nile Rodgers led some critics to conclude that Bowie was disowning his recent career and attempting to set the clock back by recording the album that *Let's Dance* always should have been. There's certainly no shortage of surreptitious referencing to Bowie's pre-*Let's Dance* career. The notion of opening and closing the album with variants of the same composition is a direct throwback to *Scary Monsters*. One of David's new drummers, former Duran Duran sessioner Sterling Campbell, had been a teenage pupil of Bowie's veteran percussionist Dennis Davis, who dropped in to visit during the New York sessions. And in different ways, two of the album's cover versions, 'I Feel Free' and 'I Know It's Gonna Happen Someday', hark back to the Ziggy era.

But *Black Tie White Noise* is by no means a clean break with everything post-1983; it has half an eye on Bowie's more recent past, showcasing several talents previously heard on his less admired 1980s recordings: several of the backing vocalists hail from the *Let's Dance* and *Labyrinth* sessions, and there are reappearances by *Never Let Me Down*'s Philippe Saisse and David Richards. Indeed, the retro-imagery of Nick Knight's inlay photography, depicting Bowie in shirtsleeves and Bogey hat, clutching a 1940s microphone, comes straight from the video of 'Never Let Me Down'. Reeves Gabrels guests on 'You've Been Around', itself a rejected Tin Machine composition. As ever, *Black Tie White Noise* is a synthesis of old and new; what's different is that for the first time in a decade, the alchemy is just about right.

Black Tie White Noise heralded yet another new record label: during the sessions Bowie signed a contract with BMG, affiliated with Arista and the small American label Savage, enthusing about the artistic freedom he had been guaranteed. "David Nemran of Savage Records ... encouraged me to do exactly what I wanted to do, without any kind of indication that it would be manipulated, or that my ideas would be changed, or that other things would be required of me," said David. "That made me feel comfortable and that was the deciding factor." In turn, the Savage chairman declared that Bowie was "absolutely the artist to break the label wide open ... He's everything that I would use to describe us."

The album arrived in a blaze of publicity and, in the UK at least, an immensely favourable climate afforded by the explosion of "Britpop". Bands like Blur, The Auteurs and in particular the brilliant Suede were openly acknowledging their debt to Bowie, not only in interviews (Brett Anderson's soundbite about being "a bisexual man who's never had a homosexual experience" was a self-conscious repackage of Bowie's famous 1972 outing, and was equally successful in courting publicity), but also in their blatantly referential post-glam singles and live acts. In the run-up to the releases of *Black Tie White Noise* and, a week earlier, Suede's eponymous debut, the *NME* pulled off the coup of introducing David to Brett for a double interview in which the two singers discussed influences and exchanged compliments (Bowie: "Your playing and your songwriting's so good that I know you're going to be working in music for quite some time". Anderson: "Lots of things that we rip you off for like, well, specifically like the octave lower vocals and things like that, I just love what it does to the song, how it makes it darker"). The mutual appreciation benefited, in different ways, the credibility of both. Suede's music continued to pay homage to Bowie: their second album, released eighteen months later, was named *Dog Man Star* after three of his classic early LPs, while 1999's *Head Music* plundered the art-rock territory of *Scary Monsters* and included tracks called 'Elephant Man' and 'She's In Fashion'.

In March 1993 the preview single 'Jump They Say' was released in an array of formats featuring numerous remixes by fashionable producers like Brothers In Rhythm and Leftfield, setting a precedent that would prevail for most of Bowie's singles during the 1990s.

'Jump They Say' became Bowie's biggest hit in seven years, and the good omens continued with his best reviews in a decade. "*Black Tie White Noise* is an album which picks up where *Scary Monsters* left off in 1980, and if any collection of songs could reinstate his godhead status, this is it," declared *Q*, adding that the album was full of "imagination and charm", with a title track "as heartfelt and socially relevant as anything Bowie has recorded." *Billboard* considered the album "trail-blazing and brilliant", boasting "inspired covers" and "echoes of *Let's Dance*, *Scary Monsters* and *Ziggy Stardust*." *Vox* was more cautious with the praise, admitting that the "radio-friendly pillage of Bowie's musical history" was "both well-timed and familiar enough to re-establish his commercial appeal" and that Bowie's sax playing "doesn't quite top the bizarre foghorn sounds he produced on "*Heroes*", but its bent, ethnic-sounding notes create the album's most atmospheric moments."

The album was released on 5 April 1993 in a variety of formats. The Japanese CD boasted 'Pallas Athena (Don't Stop Praying Mix)' as a third bonus track, while buyers of the Singaporean CD were treated to an otherwise unavailable Indonesian version of 'Don't Let Me Down & Down'. Sales were spectacular in Britain, where *Black Tie White Noise* entered the album chart at number 1, deposing *Suede* in the process. The news from America was not so good: in June 1993 Savage Records went into liquidation, severely curtailing the album's distribution in America and several other territories. It peaked at number 39 in the US chart before becoming temporarily unavailable. Savage filed for bankruptcy and even attempted to sue Bowie and BMG to recover funds, although the case was dismissed.

Nor was this the only blow to the album's commercial potential. 'Jump They Say' was an exceptional song and deservedly a top ten hit, but few who heard the album could believe that the immensely catchy 'Miracle Goodnight' – a potential international smash if ever there was one – had been passed over as the debut single. Furthermore Bowie declined to take the new material on tour ("It takes up so much time … I really want to involve myself in my own life again"), instead releasing the *Black Tie White Noise* video shot in May 1993. The only other promotional outings for the album were a pair of appearances on American television in the same month. Bearing in mind that his next studio ventures would see a marked swing away from the commercial, it's instructive to note that

later in the year Bowie turned down a request to perform on MTV's *Unplugged*. They required the greatest hits; he firmly declined.

In August 2003 EMI released a beautifully packaged three-disc tenth anniversary edition of *Black Tie White Noise*, comprising the original album, a bonus CD of remixes and rare tracks (including such delights as 'Real Cool World', the Indonesian 'Don't Let Me Down & Down' and several promo-only remixes, but not the 'Alternate Mix' of 'Jump They Say' that had featured on the original CD), and an accompanying DVD of 1993's *Black Tie White Noise* video.

Whereas many Bowie albums have been undervalued in their day and only later rehabilitated, it seems with hindsight that *Black Tie White Noise* was, if anything, over-praised at the time of its release. It's a supremely confident, professional and commercial piece of work, and its best moments are exceptional; without a doubt it was, at the time, Bowie's finest record since *Scary Monsters*. But although it was a massive and exhilarating step in the right direction, there were far better things to come. Even before the album was released Bowie had begun working on a forthcoming soundtrack project, and despite making the occasional claim that his next plan was to revive Tin Machine, he was in fact heading for new territory once again. The full-scale artistic renaissance was just around the corner.

THE BUDDHA OF SUBURBIA
Arista 74321 170042, November 1993 [87]

'Buddha Of Suburbia' (4'28") / 'Sex And The Church' (6'25") / 'South Horizon' (5'26") / 'The Mysteries' (7'12") / 'Bleed Like A Craze, Dad' (5'22") / 'Strangers When We Meet' (4'58") / 'Dead Against It' (5'48") / 'Untitled No.1' (5'01") / 'Ian Fish, U.K. Heir' (6'27") / 'Buddha Of Suburbia' (4'19")

• *Musicians:* David Bowie *(vocals, keyboard, synths, guitar, alto and baritone sax, keyboard percussion)*, Erdal Kizilcay *(keyboards, trumpet, bass, guitar, live drums, percussion)*, Mike Garson *(piano on 'South Horizon' and 'Bleed Like a Craze, Dad')*, 3D Echo *(drum, bass and guitar on 'Bleed Like a Craze, Dad')*, Lenny Kravitz *(guitar on 'Buddha of Suburbia', second version)* • *Recorded:* Mountain Studios, Montreux; O'Henry Sound, Burbank • *Producers:* David Bowie, David Richards

In February 1993 Bowie was interviewed by the novelist Hanif Kureishi for an American magazine. Kureishi took advantage of the meeting to seek permission to use some of Bowie's early songs in the incidental score of BBC2's forthcoming dramatization of his Whitbread Prize-winning novel *The Buddha Of Suburbia*. "And then I said, Oh, maybe you'd fancy doing a bit for it," recalled Kureishi, "and he said, I thought you were never going to ask!"

The choice of composer could scarcely have been more appropriate. Kureishi's irreverent, semi-autobiographical rite of passage follows the adventures of Karim, a Bromley teenager who navigates a path through the bogus mystics, racial collisions and sexual ambivalences of the 1970s, carving out a career as an actor while his friend Charlie becomes a fabricated rock star somewhere between Bowie, Sid Vicious and Billy Idol. *The Buddha of Suburbia*'s cultural satire, historical pastiche and philosophical analysis of the journey from suburbia to stardom offered the perfect stimulus for Bowie's music.

For the title song David created a blissful pastiche of his own early sound but the remainder of his incidental score was carefully understated, at pains to avoid what he called "the usual pitfalls of over-arranging against small ensemble theatre." With Kureishi in attendance in Montreux, Bowie completed the forty-plus soundtrack pieces by the early summer of 1993. The score was later nominated for a BAFTA, but long before that Bowie took the compositions into Mountain Studios where, sharing instrumental duties with his long-time collaborator Erdal Kizilcay, he began work on a new solo album using the score as his point of origin.

Recorded in a mere six days and mixed over the following fortnight, *The Buddha Of Suburbia* is a radical extrapolation of the original soundtrack, employing methodologies seldom seen on a Bowie album since the Berlin period. "I took each theme or motif from the play and initially stretched or lengthened it to a five or six minute duration," Bowie explained. "Then, having noted which musical key I was in and having counted the number of bars, I would often pull down the faders leaving just the percussive element with no harmonic informations to refer to. Working in layers I would then build up reinforcements in the key of the composition, totally blind so to speak. When all faders were pushed up again a number of clashes would make themselves evident. The more dangerous or attractive ones would then be isolated and repeated…"

Mike Garson, recently reunited with Bowie on *Black Tie White Noise*, was enlisted for two piano overdubs which he improvised in a three-hour session in a Los Angeles studio. Three tracks remained entirely instrumental, while the non-linear lyrics accompanying most of the others furthered the impression that Bowie had re-adopted the working methods of Brian Eno, who had no involvement with the album but whose influence is acknowledged in the occasionally overwrought sleeve notes. Here Bowie outlines his belief that the narrative form is "almost redundant", explaining his preference for using "the rhythmic element as an armature of sorts, placing, rather like decorations on a Christmas tree, blobs of arcane information … Having said that, I am completely guilty of loading in great dollops of pastiche and quasi-narrative into this present work at every opportunity." His declaration that artists like himself "have been parading a numbed, self-degrading affair over the last decade" and should now "rebalance the often loutish nadir into which we have blundered" sounds remarkably like an apology for the 1980s in general and Tin Machine in particular.

As Bowie's sleeve notes also explain, "This collection of music bears little resemblance to the small instrumentation of the BBC play". In other words, *The Buddha Of Suburbia* is not a soundtrack album at all but a fully-fledged opus. With the exception of the theme song the music doesn't feature in the serial at all, nor was it ever intended to. Bowie's lyrics, re-orchestrations and textural additions render the album a tight and coherent work in its own right. Unfortunately, few critics or consumers realized as much at the time, but this was hardly their fault: *The Buddha Of Suburbia* was marketed as a TV soundtrack rather than as a Bowie album. David's name was almost unnoticeable on the original sleeve and his face was absent altogether. Aside from a photocall with Hanif Kureishi and the seldom-seen video of the title track, he did little to promote the album. EMI's *The Singles Collection* was released only a week later and went top ten, further eclipsing the new work. Despite some excellent reviews (*Q* gave it four stars, noting approvingly that "Bowie's music walks a knife-edge once again"), *Buddha* stalled at number 87 in the UK chart.

Ten years later, Bowie cited *The Buddha Of Suburbia* as his personal favourite of all his studio projects. "I really felt happy making that album" he recalled.

"Overall, it was just myself and Erdal Kizilcay working on that. Erdal was a fellow musician, Turkish, living in Switzerland. He had studied at an Istanbul conservatory, and for his degree had to become proficient on every instrument in the orchestra. This led to a lot of testing on my part. I would produce an oboe from my jacket pocket: 'Hey, Erdal, don't you think oboe would be nice there?' He would trot off to the mic and put down a beautiful solo, then say, 'That's quite good but how about if I doubled it with the North Albanian Frog-Trembler?' And he would. The album itself only got one review, a good one as it happens, and is virtually non-existent as far as my catalogue goes – it was designated as a soundtrack and got zilch in the way of marketing money. A real shame."

The Buddha Of Suburbia, then, remains one of the choicest treasures awaiting discovery among Bowie's less familiar work. It represents the vital missing link between *Black Tie White Noise* and *1.Outside*, showcasing Bowie at his most bravely experimental, mingling acoustic guitars, synthesizer pop and long, ambient instrumentals in a style immediately reminiscent of *Low* and *"Heroes"*. It is also the first album since *The Man Who Sold The World* on which Bowie composes every track unassisted, and the amazingly rapid recording time – another aspect unheard of since the 1970s – delivers a work of vitality and excitement.

In October 1995 *The Buddha Of Suburbia* received its first official release outside the UK, boasting vastly improved sleeve artwork. The original image, a scene from the BBC serial's stage production of *The Jungle Book* clumsily overlaid on a map of Beckenham, was replaced by a monochrome shot of Bowie sitting on a bed.

SANTA MONICA '72
Trident Music International/Golden Years GY002, April 1994 [74]
Intermusic APH 102804, 1995

'Intro' (0'15") / 'Hang On To Yourself' (2'47") / 'Ziggy Stardust' (3'24") / 'Changes' (3'32") / 'The Supermen' (2'57") / 'Life On Mars?' (3'28") / 'Five Years' (5'21") / 'Space Oddity' (5'22") / 'Andy Warhol' (3'58") / 'My Death' (5'56") / 'The Width Of A Circle' (10'39") / 'Queen Bitch' (3'01") / 'Moonage Daydream' (4'38") / 'John, I'm Only Dancing' (3'36") / 'Waiting For The Man' (6'01") / 'The Jean Genie' (4'02") / 'Suffragette City' (4'25") / 'Rock'n'Roll Suicide' (3'17")

• *Musicians:* see *The Ziggy Stardust tour (US)* (Chapter 3) • *Recorded:* Civic Auditorum, Santa Monica

Recorded on 20 October 1972 during Bowie's first US tour, this Ziggy Stardust gig was originally broadcast on American FM radio. It was a favourite among bootleg collectors for many years, before receiving an official release from the MainMan stable in 1994. Many consider *Santa Monica '72* to have the edge on *Ziggy Stardust: The Motion Picture*; certainly, despite its inferior sound quality, it's a very valuable record of an earlier phase in the Ziggy Stardust era. The playing is tighter and more R&B-styled than the later gig, with the lush excesses of both Mick Ronson's guitar and Mike Garson's piano not yet fully indulged. There's an early rendition of 'The Jean Genie' (whose video was shot only eight days later), and there are plenty of songs later dropped from the repertoire.

Also of note is the delightful packaging of the original release, which includes a replica ticket for the Santa Monica concert and a plethora of material from the MainMan archives: rare photos, backstage passes, equipment invoices, RCA telegrams and even payslips for the band, which reveal the disparity between the wages (none of them large) doled out to Bowie, Ronson, Bolder and Woodmansey. By contrast, a 1995 European reissue arrived in desperately ugly packaging under the clumsy title *Ziggy Stardust And The Spiders From Mars "Live"*.

1.OUTSIDE
RCA 74321 310662, September 1995 [8]
    (*CD: card sleeve*)
RCA 74321 307022, September 1995 [8]
    (*CD: jewel case*)
RCA 74321 307021, September 1995
    (*LP: 'Excerpts From 1.Outside'*)
BMG 74321 369002, March 1996
    (*CD: '1.Outside Version 2'*)
Columbia 511934 2, September 2003

'Leon Takes Us Outside' (1'24") *(Vinyl: 0'24")* / 'Outside' (4'04") / 'Hearts Filthy Lesson' (4'56") / 'A Small Plot of Land' (6'33") / 'Segue – Baby Grace (A Horrid Cassette)' (1'40") / 'Hallo Spaceboy' (5'13") / 'The Motel' (6'49") *(Vinyl: 5'03")* / 'I Have Not Been to Oxford Town' (3'48") / 'No Control' (4'32") / 'Segue – Algeria Touchshriek' (2'02") / 'The Voyeur of Utter Destruction (As Beauty)' (4'20") / 'Segue – Ramona A. Stone/I Am With Name' (4'01") / 'Wishful Beginnings' (5'08") / 'We Prick You' (4'34") / 'Segue – Nathan Adler' (1'00") / 'I'm Deranged' (4'29") / 'Thru' These Architects Eyes' (4'20") / 'Segue – Nathan Adler' (0'28") / 'Strangers When We Meet' (5'06")

• *Musicians:* David Bowie *(vocals, saxophone, guitar, keyboards)*, Brian Eno *(synthesizers, treatments & strategies)*, Reeves Gabrels *(guitar)*, Erdal Kizilcay *(bass, keyboards)*, Mike Garson *(piano)*, Sterling Campbell *(drums)*, Carlos Alomar *(rhythm guitar)*, Joey Barron *(drums)*, Yossi Fine *(bass)*, Tom Frish *(guitar on 'Strangers When We Meet')*, Kevin Armstrong *(guitar on 'Thru' These Architects Eyes')*, Bryony, Lola, Josey & Ruby Edwards *(backing vocals on 'Hearts Filthy Lesson' and 'I Am With Name')* • *Recorded:* Mountain Studios, Montreux; The Hit Factory, New York • *Producers:* David Bowie, Brian Eno, David Richards

On the evidence of Bowie's 1993 albums, a studio reunion with Brian Eno was now only a matter of time. In fact the two had already discussed the possibility at Bowie's wedding reception the previous year, while David was still in the early stages of recording *Black Tie White Noise*. In March 1994, after Eno had heard and "got really excited about" *The Buddha Of Suburbia*, the pair convened at Mountain Studios. Although fifteen years had passed since the *Lodger* sessions, Bowie recalled that it was "almost as though no time had been wedged in, like we were carrying on from the third album together." There was still a crucial disparity between their approaches, however: "I'm actually very nineteenth-century – a born Romantic, unlike Brian, who's terminally end-of-twentieth century ... Brian is someone who will take things from low art and elevate them to high art, whereas I do precisely the opposite: I'll take things from high art and demean them down to the street level." From this creative collision was to emerge the most fully imagined, beautifully crafted Bowie album in many a long year, and arguably his 1990s masterpiece.

Bowie assembled a core band of names from various stages of his career. Reeves Gabrels returned on lead guitar, marking his arrival as a permanent member of the Bowie ensemble. Erdal Kizilcay returned on

bass, and having guested on David's last two albums Mike Garson resumed a central role on piano. The principal drummer, Soul Asylum's Sterling Campbell, had previously played on *Black Tie White Noise* and was described by David as "spontaneous and extremely inventive. Sterling plays a song differently every time; there are definite shades of his teacher, Dennis Davis."

Emboldened by Eno's unorthodox approach to studio work, Bowie kept "paints, charcoal, scissors, paper and canvas" on hand throughout the sessions, "to give us something to fly on when not playing." Eno had devised a complex series of role-playing games which are explained in his 1995 diary, *A Year With Swollen Appendices* – essential reading for the Bowie enthusiast. Having observed his family the previous Christmas, Eno explained that "It occurred to me that the great thing about games is that they in some sense free you from being yourself: you are 'allowed' forms of behaviour that otherwise would be gratuitous, embarrassing or completely irrational. Accordingly, I came up with these role-playing games for musicians." Detailed character studies were issued to each player so that "individuals were in different cultural universes", while Eno's lengthy *Notes on the vernacular music of the Acrux region* was a kind of sci-fi fantasy designed "to imagine a new musical culture, and to invent roles for musicians within it." This bizarre tract, reproduced in full in Eno's book, casts the *1.Outside* band as eccentric characters with anagram names like "Elvas Ge'beer", "G. Noisemark", "Azile Clark-Idy" and "P. Maclert Singbell", who "carries around an enormous library of recordings of fatal gunshot sounds for use as percussion elements."

Mike Garson later told David Buckley that "It was one of the most creative environments I have ever been in. We would just start playing. There was no key given, no tonal centre, no form, no nothing." On Radio 2's *Golden Years* he recalled another experiment: "In our earphones we would listen to some Motown music, some Marvin Gaye or different artists ... and we'd be playing over the top of that, but that would never land on the tape." Eno later revealed that Bowie "almost sat out the first few days of that record. He set up an easel in the studio and was just painting. We were creating musical situations and occasionally he would join in if it became interesting."

When rehearsals began in earnest, the "Oblique Strategies" employed for the Berlin albums were again in evidence. Individual musicians were handed cards with instructions like "You are the last survivor of a catastrophic event and you will endeavour to play in such a way as to prevent feelings of loneliness developing within yourself," or "You are a disgruntled ex-member of a South African rock band. Play the notes you were not allowed to play." As Eno later explained, "There are certain immediate dangers to improvisation, and one of them is that everybody coalesces immediately. Everyone starts playing the blues, basically, because it's the one place where everyone can agree and knows the rules. So in part they were strategies to stop the thing becoming over-coherent. The interesting place is not chaos, and it's not total coherence. It's somewhere on the cusp of those two."

Thematically Bowie was eager to address his interest in contemporary art, which by 1994 had led him to join the editorial board of *Modern Painters* magazine. He was becoming particularly fascinated by the more macabre end of the performance art spectrum, notably Rudolf Schwartzkögler, leading light of the "Viennese Castrationists" who had cut off his own penis, and Ron Athey, an HIV-positive New Yorker whose 'Four Scenes In A Harsh Life' involved impaling himself with knitting needles and carving patterns into a fellow performer's back before hanging blotting-paper prints of the blood over his audience's heads. Bowie was also drawn to the neo-brutalism of young British artists like Damien Hirst, who had recently made waves with his famous series of dead animal exhibits.

From such lurid origins grew the germ of a concept about death as art. "Apart from this unhealthy, almost obsessive interest in ritualistic artists," Bowie told *Vox*, "The album also has some sort of a feeling of this new paganism that seems to be springing up with the advent of scarifications, piercings, tribalisms, tattoos and whatever. It's like a replacement for a spiritual starvation that's going on. It's like a tribe with dim memories of what their rituals used to be. They're sort of being dragged back again in this new, mutated, deviant way, with so-called gratuitous sex and violence in popular culture and people cutting bits off themselves. For me, it seems like a natural kind of thing." David himself had recently submitted to the tattooist's needle (a dolphin on his calf as a love token for Iman), and the Outside tour would see him dripping with earrings for the first time in twenty years. The "new paganism" he had identified was closely connected with the pre-millennial tension that every philosopher and chat-show host had begun

discussing in the mid-1990s; the idea that an imagined milestone in time creates dangerous ripples through society was a beguiling subject for Bowie, whose lyrics have always been preoccupied by time as a pitiless constant in human existence. *1.Outside* would reopen such territory, expressing anxiety about "now, not tomorrow" as the "twentieth century dies".

Bowie was also keen to explore a growing preoccupation with one of the monsters of classical antiquity: "I had a thing about the Minotaur for the last couple of years," he explained in 1995. "I'd been drawing and painting it a lot and didn't really know why until about four or five weeks ago in the *New York Times* there was an article on the new cave paintings in the south of France – the most sophisticated cave paintings that have ever been found … The most remarkable thing of all is one composite of a human being with a bull's head – 26,000 years before the Greeks came up with it." The Minotaur is a motif not only in *1.Outside*, but also in several of Bowie's painterly pursuits of the period: he contributed to 1994's *Minotaur Myths And Legends* show, and the character dominated his 1995 solo exhibition.

Another kind of art was informing Bowie's muse: in early 1994 he and Eno visited the Guggin psychiatric hospital near Vienna, where the painters' wing was, he explained, "an Austrian experiment to see what happens when you allow people with mental disabilities to give free rein to their artistic impetuses … It's quite obvious that these outsider artists don't have the parameters that are placed on most artists … Their motivation for painting and sculpting comes from a different place than that of the average artist who's sane on society's terms." As 'Jump They Say' had intimated a year earlier, and as the new album's title would reiterate, Bowie was ready to position himself as an "outsider artist" once again.

Another influential ingredient was Bowie's fascination with computers and in particular the Internet, which he had embraced with the same missionary zeal that had accompanied his conversion to the cutting-edge technologies of earlier eras. A new AppleMac program designed by a friend enabled David to shuffle and randomize his lyrics in a high-tech variant of the cut-up technique he had used as long ago as *Diamond Dogs*. "I used bits of poems and articles out of magazines and newspapers, and I retyped them out and put them into the computer," he explained. "And it spews it all back out again, and I make of it what I will." It's a misapprehension, incidentally, that the aim of Bowie's randomizing and cutting-up sprees is to produce gibberish; in fact he uses the results merely as starting points for the actual writing process. Relating his methods to the structural practices of James Joyce and William Burroughs, he told *Time Out*: "I come from almost a traditional school now, of deconstructing phrases and constructing them again in what is considered a random way. But in that randomness there's something we perceive as a reality – that in fact our lives aren't tidy, that we don't have tidy beginnings and endings."

Further to this was Bowie's interest in the breakdown of society's hierarchy of significant information. Mentioning to *Ikon*'s Chris Roberts the equal weight given by current press reports to the O J Simpson trial and the Middle East crisis, he suggested, "When you get that lack of stress upon what's important and what isn't, the moral high ground seems to disappear as well. You're left with this incredibly complex network of fragments that is our existence … There's no point in pretending, well, if we wait long enough everything will return to what it used to be and it'll all be saner again and we'll understand everything and it'll be obvious what's wrong and what's right. It's *not* gonna be like that. So the album deals with all that to an extent. That kind of … surfing on chaos."

A year earlier, while promoting *Black Tie White Noise*, he had admitted that he was becoming tempted by "the idea of one more time developing a character. I do love the theatrical side of the thing – not only do I enjoy it, I also think I'm quite good at it." Now Bowie was immersing himself in the most complex fictional world he had yet created, fashioning not one but seven protagonists in what he labelled the "non-linear Gothic Drama Hyper-cycle" of *1.Outside*. "One of the days that we worked," he later recalled, "– it was 12 March 1994, I'll never forget – we had a blindingly orgiastic session where it just didn't stop. Almost the entire genesis for this album is contained in those three and a half hours, but it's nearly all dialogue and narrative description and wandering off into characters. I play out a character for maybe five minutes at a time: I mean, I developed an entire interior life for him whilst I was on mike…"

Thus emerged the fictional setting of Oxford Town, New Jersey, and its outlandish, *Twin Peaks*-style inhabitants: Detective Professor Nathan Adler (born 1947, we are told), a gumshoe from the bureau of Art-Crime Inc, a police department based in the studio that had once belonged to the painter and suicide Rothko; Baby Grace Blue, a 14-year-old girl whose dismembered body is discovered draped across the doorway of the Oxford Town Museum of Modern Parts; Ramona A Stone, a "no-future priestess of the Caucasian Suicide Temple" who deals in body-parts jewellery and "interest-drugs"; Algeria Touchshriek, a 78-year-old loner who deals in "art-drugs and DNA prints"; Leon Blank, a mixed-race "Outsider" with convictions for "plagiarism without license"; Paddy, one of Nathan Adler's informants; and The Artist/Minotaur, a shadowy figure lurking behind "the art-ritual murder" at the centre of the impenetrable narrative. "With *1.Outside*, placing the eerie environment of a *Diamond Dogs* city now in the nineties gives it an entirely different spin," explained Bowie. "It was important for this town, this locale, to have a populace, a number of characters. I tried to diversify these really eccentric types as much as possible … The narrative and the stories are not the content – the content is the spaces in between the linear bits. The queasy, strange textures."

The backing tracks for *1.Outside* were completed at Mountain Studios in ten days, but embellishments continued on and off until November 1994. Among the vast amount of recorded material were 'Get Real' and 'Nothing To Be Desired', released as single B-sides in some territories.

The first public intimation of the new project came in December 1994 when *Q* magazine published an Internet conversation between Bowie and Eno, in which they discussed the latest mixes and David confided that "I really feel we are in an extremely exciting and uninvestigated area. Same goose bumps as 1976…" The same edition featured an extraordinary three-page article by Bowie, entitled *The Diary Of Nathan Addler, or The Art-Ritual Murder Of Baby Grace Belew: An occasionally on-going short story*. This, give or take a couple of differently spelt names (note "Belew", the name of one of David's ex-guitarists), was the same darkly comic piece of fiction that would later appear in *1.Outside*'s inlay booklet. As fragmented and non-linear a narrative as might be expected from Bowie in full flow, the story opens on 31 December 1999 with the gruesome dismemberment and cybernetic rebuilding of Baby Grace's corpse by "a dark spirited pluralist". There is gallows humour aplenty and a strong recollection of 1987's 'Glass Spider': "The limbs and their components were then hung up on the splayed web, slug-like prey of some unimaginable creature … It was definitely murder – but was it art?" The Sam Spade-style narrator Nathan Adler reminisces about Damien Hirst, Ron Athey and Chris Burden (the "nail-me-to-my-car" performance artist formerly commemorated in 'Joe The Lion'). There are dissertations on a fabled Korean artist whose audience watched him undergo voluntary amputations ("By the dawning of the'80s, rumour had it that he was down to a torso and one arm … I suppose you can never tell what an artist will do once he's peaked"), and even a passing thought about "Bowie the singer" in his Berlin days. The linking thread is an obsession with pain, death and blood: "We're mystified by blood. It's our enemy now. We don't understand it. Can't live with it. Can't, well … y'know?"

Although the Montreux sessions were completed by November 1994 and the results mixed at London's Westside Studios, the release of the album was delayed by more of the contractual wrangling that had hamstrung Bowie's releases in recent times. He later explained that he was unable to interest any record label in releasing the original version, envisaged as a double or even triple CD which, at this stage, went under the working title of *Leon*. Reeves Gabrels would later indicate that in its original form, the album would have been over three hours in length: "We hoped that it would have come out intact and uncompromised by financial/commercial pressures," Gabrels recounted on his website in 2003. "It would have been a very serious musical statement, and maybe pissed more people off than Tin Machine." Faced with record company hostility towards the uncompromising nature of the *Leon* album, Bowie elected to remove much of the original material and record some more conventional additions. Sessions took place at New York's Hit Factory in January and February 1995, when several of the more linear numbers were recorded, including the title track itself; thus *Leon* gave way to *1.Outside*. Other new cuts included 'Thru' These Architects Eyes', 'We Prick You', 'I Have Not Been To Oxford Town', 'No Control' and 'Strangers When We Meet', while 'Hallo Spaceboy' and 'I'm Deranged' were refashioned from the previous year's raw material. For the New York sessions the band was joined by veteran rhythm guitarist Carlos Alomar, now entering the twentieth year of his relationship with Bowie. Another old face was Kevin Armstrong, last heard on *Tin Machine II*, while drummer Joey Barron was a newcomer for the New York

sessions – "Metronomes shake in fear, he's so steady," said David.

Brian Eno's diary reveals that he spent early January at his Brondesbury Villas studio in Kilburn, working alone on "vocal support structures for David's voice samples", which included "a sad Touchshriek piece" and "Ramona Was So Cold" (the second 'Nathan Adler' segue). On 11 January he joined Bowie in New York, where they spent the next three days working on 'Dummy' (the prototype version of 'I'm Afraid Of Americans' destined for the soundtrack of *Showgirls*), before moving on to the other New York recordings.

In June 1995 Bowie signed a new deal with Virgin America, who also purchased the rights to his back catalogue from *Let's Dance* to *Tin Machine*; these albums would be reissued with bonus tracks during 1995. In Britain he entered into a new agreement with BMG, who had released his last two albums in the UK but were now affiliated to RCA, the label with whom he had parted company back in 1982.

1.Outside – The Nathan Adler Diaries: a hyper cycle was finally released on 25 September 1995. In Britain the CD arrived in a cardboard digipak (replaced in later pressings by a standard plastic jewel case) adorned with the *Diary Of Nathan Adler* text and a series of astonishing computer-enhanced images in which, alongside gruesome shots of offal, severed fingers and dismembered hands, Bowie's face morphed into the features of each of the album's characters: the mixed-race Leon Blank, the septuagenarian Algeria Touchshriek, even the Minotaur and 14-year-old Baby Grace. The cover image was *Head Of DB*, an acrylic painting on canvas made by David in 1995.

The album was promoted almost exclusively on CD, the only vinyl version being a single LP called *Excerpts From 1.Outside* from which 'No Control', 'Wishful Beginnings', 'Thru' These Architects Eyes', 'Strangers When We Meet' and a couple of the segues were missing altogether, while 'Leon Takes Us Outside' and 'The Motel' were shortened edits by Kevin Metcalfe. The Japanese CD included the outtake 'Get Real'. Six months later came the European CD *1.Outside Version 2*, which has 'Hallo Spaceboy (Pet Shop Boys Remix)' instead of 'Wishful Beginnings'. Double-CD reissues in Australia and Japan included various remixes and B-sides, while Columbia's 2003 UK reissue restored the original track-listing, and Sony's 2004 US version (LEGACY 092100) included 'Get Real'.

Following a muted reaction to the lead-off single 'The Hearts Filthy Lesson', the press gave the album almost unqualified approval. "Bowie's scalpel is certainly closer to the pulse than for years," said the *NME*, while *Melody Maker* thrilled to "the brilliant speeding electronic funk of 'The Voyeur Of Utter Destruction (As Beauty)'" and announced that Bowie "is poised to be a healthy influence once more on a fifth generation of glamorous chameleons." In the *Daily Telegraph* Charles Shaar Murray welcomed "an excellent David Bowie album, a genuine creative rebirth. Threatening and murky … His gift for the charismatically disturbing seems to have reasserted itself." The *Guardian* hailed *1.Outside* as "a very fine thing, containing Bowie's best music of the past 15 years," a sentiment echoed by *Time Out*, for whom the "edifice of sounds, cultures, rhythms, samples and textures, with randomised lyrics that don't so much tell a story as create word-moods, rewards the open-minded listener with Bowie's best album for 15 years." *Q* commended it as "a bold and fascinating trip … undoubtedly Bowie's most dense and uncompromising work since *Scary Monsters* … it's clear that he is once again imaginatively sparking with life." There were, of course, dissenting voices, including *Ikon*'s Taylor Parkes who complained that "Bowie's desperate desire to be considered 'highbrow' has snuffed out any potential of accidental alchemy" and peremptorily dismissed the album as a "sorry sack of shit … facile, confused and immature … quite simply, rubbish." Across the Atlantic *Billboard* described it as "a dark concept album that is alternately tedious and inspired, but always musically challenging." In Britain the album peaked at number 8; in America, where Bowie's profile had been significantly raised by recent citations from bands like Nirvana and Nine Inch Nails, it reached number 21 – his best US album performance since *Tonight* and no mean achievement for such a wilfully uncommercial work.

After the round of broadly favourable reviews a backlash was inevitable, and by the time the Outside tour arrived in Britain in November, members of the music press were falling over one another to rubbish an album hitherto praised by their colleagues. The *NME*'s Simon Williams found the English language a sadly inadequate medium in which to launch his assault: "El Bowza's latest lurch away from reality is entitled *Outside* [sic], which is kind of about 'outsiders' and involves all these strange neo-futuristic characters running around El Bowza's head and it's

sort of a concept album blah blah bollocks blah blah ARSE!!!!!!!" A perceptive analysis. Certainly *1.Outside* presents a soft target for anyone who seriously believes Bowie hadn't noticed that impersonating a 78-year-old man called Algeria Touchshriek was going to be rather silly, but it seems more likely that he was in on the joke.

What counts is that the music is Bowie's finest in years, combining viscerally exciting Nine Inch Nails-flavoured rock ('Hallo Spaceboy', 'The Hearts Filthy Lesson') with Scott Walker-esque freefall jazz madness ('A Small Plot Of Land'), frightening, multi-textural soundscapes that could only be the work of the Bowie/Eno partnership ('Wishful Beginnings', 'The Motel'), and prototype drum'n'bass stylings ('I'm Deranged', 'We Prick You') which point the way forward. With each song ascribed to a particular character the album shifts through subtly different moods: the lyrics are by turns poetic, violent and comical, creating impressionistic tone-pictures rather than a coherent narrative. Indeed, *1.Outside*'s linking concept has been over-stated. The five spoken "segues", in which Bowie's heavily treated voice delivers monologues by the various characters, are both brilliant and ridiculous, but the album functions perfectly well with or without them. "You can take it as you want," David insisted. "It's not necessary to follow the narrative. I've sort of left that way behind."

A particular triumph of *1.Outside* is the way it enmeshed itself in the cultural fabric of its time. Veteran artists like Paul Weller and Adam Ant were surfing the Britpop wave in 1995 with successful comeback albums, but *1.Outside* placed Bowie elsewhere, aligning him with the industrial art-rock of Nine Inch Nails and the fringes of the trip-hop/techno schools of Tricky, Goldie and The Chemical Brothers. But the album's affinity with the cultural landscape of 1995 went far beyond the confines of pop music. It arrived in a world still squirming at the fate of John Wayne Bobbitt and the glamorous cruelty of *Pulp Fiction*. It inhabited the trashy cyberpunk *milieu* of movies like *Judge Dredd*, *Tank Girl* and *Twelve Monkeys*, and tapped into the popular diet of extraterrestrial conspiracy theories exemplified by the so-called Roswell Incident and American TV's latest sensation *The X-Files*. It was one of the first great albums of the Internet age and danced to the same pre-millennial angst as Pulp's Christmas 1995 hit 'Disco 2000'. It provided an ideal soundtrack to Damien Hirst's bisected cows and became the literal soundtrack to

David Fincher's black-hearted film thriller *Seven*, an orgy of razor blades, drip-tubes and mutilation that hit British cinemas in December 1995 and played 'The Hearts Filthy Lesson' over its closing credits. The following year 'A Small Plot Of Land' became the theme music of BBC2's *A History Of British Art*. For the first time since *Scary Monsters*, Bowie had released an album that accessed the zeitgeist at all levels.

Noticeably, *1.Outside* was also the first album since *Scary Monsters* on which Bowie decisively threw off the shackles of his middle-aged "just say no" persona and revelled once again in the artful unwholesomeness that was the stock-in-trade of his 1970s work. This is a triumphantly queasy, deliciously unpleasant album, and by the time of its release Bowie had dropped the black-and-white attitude that had brought forth the likes of 'Crack City', and was once again prepared to explore areas of moral complexity. "I'm not suggesting for one small minute that you rush out and get your junkie kit together," he told one interviewer in 1996, "Not at all. It's just interesting that people who make those explorations, if they go through the cusp of those experiences, they do tend to come out the other side in a way better people for it, you know? That's a dangerous thing to say, but it's true in my case. I'm glad I did everything I did, I really am." He would never have said anything like that in the 1980s.

At an epic 75 minutes *1.Outside* is far and away Bowie's longest studio album; he has since remarked that he "never should have made it as long as it is", a view echoed by Eno in his diary. It will appeal to fans of *Low*, *Lodger* and *Diamond Dogs*, the three albums it most closely resembles, more readily than to lovers of *Let's Dance*: "Accessibility is not its keynote!" David laughed at the time. But critics who complained that the album was pretentious were rather missing the point, because the first person to describe it as such was Bowie himself. "Brian and I decided in the late seventies that we had developed a new school of pretension," he said in 1996. "*We* gave it the title. Other people may bandy it around, but we *knew* … We saw nothing wrong with that. We rather saw pretension, or the idea of pretending – the playfulness that has any kind of evocative feeling in art – actually something to go for." A year later he told journalists in Buenos Aires that "When I made the *Low* album with Brian Eno, I got a telegram from the managing director of the record company, giving the advice that I really shouldn't waste my money and that I should go

back to Philadelphia and make *Young Americans II*. So when I heard similar comments about *1.Outside*, I knew that I'd done a good album."

The Diary Of Nathan Adler ends on a cliffhanger and the promise "To be continued…" At the time Bowie intimated that he saw *1.Outside* as the first episode in a five-album sequence that would carry him up to the millennium. There was even talk of the project culminating in an opera devised with Eno and director Robert Wilson for the 1999 Salzburg Festival (some years later, in October 2000, David admitted that "I know there was talk of it being presented at Salzburg, Austria, but I didn't get on with the artistic director there at all. It was rather gratifying to hear that he was removed from the festival this year!"). Bowie later revealed that a staggering 27 hours of extra material existed from the Montreux sessions: "Some of it I'd like to put out as a companion piece to *1.Outside*, a sort of archival, limited-edition album," he said, and in 2000 he confirmed that he was continuing post-production on the material, to be called *2.Contamination*. Meanwhile, in March 2003 a series of previously unheard extracts from the final mix of the original *Leon* album were leaked onto the bootleg circuit (see 'The *Leon* Tape' in Chapter 1), offering a fascinating glimpse of what might have been. Intriguing stuff indeed; but we'd be unwise to expect any official release of the Montreux material to maintain continuity or resolve the plot of *1.Outside*. In Q's Internet chat in 1994, Bowie had said: "Our expectations of an ending or conclusion … learned from repeated story-film-narrative culture, gives us a completely unjustified set of expectations for life," to which Brian Eno replied that "the big breakthrough is accepting that fade-outs happen at both ends of whatever you are doing. I always liked records that faded up as well as down, so you felt that what you were hearing was part of a bigger and unknowable thing that existed somewhere out in the ether, but to which you couldn't have access."

As we know, the immediate follow-up never materialized. Bowie slipped sideways, just as he's always done, and *1.Outside* remains as brilliant and intriguingly inconclusive as it was surely always supposed to be.

EARTHLING

RCA 74321 449442, February 1997 *(CD)* [6]
RCA 74321 449441, February 1997 *(LP)* [6]

Columbia 511935 2, September 2003

'Little Wonder' (6'02") / 'Looking For Satellites' (5'21") / 'Battle For Britain (The Letter)' (4'49") / 'Seven Years In Tibet' (6'22") / 'Dead Man Walking' (6'50") / 'Telling Lies' (4'50") / 'The Last Thing You Should Do' (4'58") / 'I'm Afraid of Americans' (5'00") / 'Law (Earthlings on Fire)' (4'48")

• *Musicians:* David Bowie *(guitar, vocals, alto sax, samples, keyboards)*, Reeves Gabrels *(programming, synthesizers, real and sampled guitar, vocals)*, Zachary Alford *(drum loops, acoustic drums, electronic percussion)*, Gail Ann Dorsey *(bass, vocals)*, Mike Garson *(keyboards, piano)*, Mark Plati *(programming loops, samples, keyboards)* • *Recorded:* Looking Glass Studios, New York; Mountain Studios, Montreux • *Producer:* David Bowie

Earthling was a celebration of Bowie's exceptional relationship with the band he had gathered together for the Outside tour. "They're probably the most enjoyable set of musicians I've worked with," he told Alan Yentob in 1996. "It's the greatest fun and satisfaction I've had with a band since The Spiders." In April of that year he recorded 'Telling Lies' alone in Montreux as a template for the sound he wanted, and the song was premiered during the Summer Festivals tour. In late August Bowie took the band to Looking Glass, the Manhattan studio owned by Philip Glass where, incidentally, the *Low* and *"Heroes"* symphonies were also recorded.

An important new arrival was engineer Mark Plati, a New Yorker who had cut his teeth at Arthur Baker's Shakedown Studios before working with Prince on *Graffiti Bridge* and, at Looking Glass, with artists such as Deee-Lite. In addition to engineering and co-writing several tracks, he and Reeves Gabrels took second billing as co-producers – behind Bowie himself, for whom *Earthling* was the first self-produced album since *Diamond Dogs*. "I knew exactly what I wanted," David explained. "We didn't have any time to pull in a co-producer ... so I just sort of went for it." Speed and spontaneity were the keynotes of the sessions: "There was no aforethought. It was very immediate, very spontaneous, and it virtually put itself together. Writing and recording, two and a half weeks, and then a couple of weeks of mixing ... it was really very fast."

Earthling was a development of the techno stylings that had emerged on *1.Outside* tracks like 'I'm

Deranged' and 'We Prick You', which Bowie described as "almost a quite moderate version of jungle", alongside the Outside tour's experimental realignments of numbers like 'Andy Warhol' and 'The Man Who Sold The World'. The new songs pushed further into a territory that had first captured his attention in 1993 when a friend sent him a tape of "the original Caribbean London guys like General Levy ... I found it so exciting, as exciting as any new rhythm that's going to become the vocabulary of that time." As ever, Bowie was intent on adapting and subverting his source material: "We came into the studio specifically with the idea of trying to juxtapose all the dance styles that we'd been working with live," he explained. "Jungle, aggressive rock and industrial." Also back in force were the computer-randomized cut-ups of *1.Outside*. David had now co-designed the Verbasizer, a refinement of his previous program which formulated random but actual sentences out of the words fed into it.

The experimental spirit of the *1.Outside* sessions fed directly into the new work, as David later explained: "Back when we did *1.Outside* [Gabrels and I] had the idea of transferring little bits of guitar to sampling keyboards and constructing riffs from those pieces. It's real guitar, but constructed in a synthetic way. But Brian Eno got in the way – in the nicest possible way – so we didn't get to that until this album." Zachary Alford's percussion samples were similarly home-made, as Bowie told *Modern Drummer*: "He would take, like, half a day and work out loops of his own on the snare, and create patterns at 120 bpm that we would then speed up to the requisite 160 ... And then over the top of that he would improvise on a real kit. So what you had was a great combination of an almost robotic, automaton approach to fundamental rhythm, with really free interpretative playing over the top of it." In the same interview he explained that "What I really wanted to do was not so very dissimilar to what I did in the seventies, and something I've repeatedly done, which is to take the technological and combine it with the organic. It was very important to me that we didn't lose the feel of real musicianship working in conjunction with anything that was sampled or looped or worked out on the computer."

In addition to 'Telling Lies' and an overhaul of the *1.Outside* out-take 'I'm Afraid Of Americans', seven new compositions emerged as album tracks. Also recorded during the *Earthling* sessions were a revamped (and as yet unreleased) version of 'Baby Universal', which had been revived on stage earlier in the year, and a new acoustic rendition of 'I Can't Read', originally intended for the album but ousted by 'The Last Thing You Should Do'. It later appeared as a single and featured in the soundtrack of *The Ice Storm*.

In early September 'Little Wonder' and 'Seven Years In Tibet' were added to the band's repertoire for the "East Coast Ballroom" tour, while 'Telling Lies' was previewed on the Internet in the same month. Work on the album continued through October, interrupted only by Bowie's appearances at the Bridge School benefit concerts, where the spectacle of Neil Young's headlining set inspired the lyrics of 'Dead Man Walking'. 'Telling Lies' was officially released as a single in November. The album was given a live preview in early January when all but two of the songs were included in Bowie's fiftieth birthday concert. The 'Little Wonder' single followed on 27 January and, riding the wave of fiftieth birthday publicity, *Earthling* itself was released on 3 February.

As usual the overseas markets offered various alternative formats. The Japanese issue included a poster and lyric sheet, and offered 'Telling Lies (Adam F Mix)' as an extra track. In Hong Kong the Mandarin version of 'Seven Years In Tibet' was included on a bonus CD, while the French release came with a limited-edition promo disc featuring live versions of 'The Hearts Filthy Lesson' and 'Hallo Spaceboy' from the 1996 Phoenix Festival. Sony's 2004 US reissue (LEGACY 092098) would later include 'Telling Lies (Adam F Mix)', 'Little Wonder (Danny Saber Dance Mix)', 'I'm Afraid Of Americans (V1)' and 'Dead Man Walking (Moby Mix 2)'.

Earthling garnered Bowie's best reviews for many years, surpassing even the widely favourable reaction to *1.Outside*. "There is something about Bowie's perennial dilettante enthusiasm that's rather engaging this time around," wrote John Mulvey in the *NME*, "as he grafts careering backbeats onto his familiar portentous tracts ... it's not the future, but it's pretty fine." *Q* found the album "shot through with a gnarly atmospheric chill not encountered since *Scary Monsters*," while *Mojo* commended Bowie for "offering refined mainstream applications of cutting-edge experimentation," noting that "the use to which he puts those pulsating jungle rhythms here is considerably more interesting than 90 per cent of purist drum'n'bass ... Far from slowing down and mellowing out with age, Bowie seems more energised by the passing years, moving faster and faster to accommodate the ever-growing sum of influences and cultural contradictions operating on his muse. He'll undoubtedly come in for some stick for using young folks' musical forms, but wouldn't it be wonderful if all 50-year-old rockers retained such an interest in the future?"

There were indeed many who accused Bowie of merely jumping on the latest musical bandwagon, as if this were something he'd never done before. Unhelpfully, both the mainstream press and the music papers elected on the strength of 'Little Wonder' to brand *Earthling* a "drum'n'bass" or "jungle" album, a description that crystallized into a common consensus despite being demonstrably inaccurate. Certainly the sonic assaults of 'Little Wonder' and 'Battle For Britain' are heavily influenced by acts like Tricky, Goldie and in particular The Prodigy, but the album is firmly grounded in a conventional songwriting sensibility that can be heard just as clearly beneath the fashionable drum-loop trappings of 'Little Wonder' as anywhere else. Nobody would describe 'Looking For Satellites' or 'Seven Years In Tibet' as jungle: they're just classic Bowie. "I'd hate the impression to be that it's overridingly jungle," said David at the time, adding elsewhere that "This record owes a debt to drum'n'bass in the use of rhythm, but I don't have much interest in the top information; what we are doing is a million light years away from what, say, Goldie would be doing or any number of other drum'n'bass purist artists."

After the often brutal cynicism of *1.Outside*, the lyrical content marks a cautious return to the spiritual realms of *Station To Station*: 'Looking For Satellites' and 'Dead Man Walking' in particular address man's universal predicament with a touching poignancy. "I guess the common ground with all the songs is this abiding need in me to vacillate between atheism or a kind of Gnosticism," Bowie told *Q*. "I keep going backwards and forwards between the two things, because they mean a lot in my life. I mean, the church doesn't enter into my writing, or my thoughts; I have no empathy with any organized religions. What I need to find is a balance, spiritually, with the way I live and my demise. And that period of time – from today until my demise – is the only thing that fascinates me." Of the music itself, he concluded that "it feels really good-hearted and uplifting ... I get all happy when I hear it." As for the album's title: "it was supposed to describe the Earth; man and his pure habitat on Earth. And I suppose the irony isn't lost on me that it's sort of me in maybe my most worldly kind of human guise to date."

Even though it was recorded in New York with a band consisting entirely of Americans, *Earthling* is also arguably Bowie's most "British" album since the 1970s. After years spent name-dropping American or European influences, David appeared to have turned his attention instead to young British artists, and the album's undercurrent of transatlantic friction is by no means restricted to 'I'm Afraid Of Americans'. Since 1993 there had been a growing sense that Bowie was a homecoming hero of British rock, and with the release of *Earthling* timed to coincide with his fiftieth birthday, his critical rehabilitation by the British music papers was all but complete. Asked in late 1996 whether he still felt British, Bowie replied, "More so than ever before." During the Summer Festivals tour he had taken to wearing a Union Jack frock-coat he co-designed with Alexander McQueen, inspired by Gavin Turk's exhibit *Indoor Flag*. It was hardly an original gesture; the Union Jack was already a standard accessory of the music papers' "Britpop" hype, and more than one band had draped itself in the flag for *Melody Maker* or the *NME*. Post-*Earthling* the trend would become a craze, with everyone from the Spice Girls to Eurythmics turning up at the Brit Awards in tailor-made Union Jack outfits.

Earlier in the decade Morrissey had courted controversy with his ambivalent flag-waving, but Bowie was not about to repeat the mistakes of 1976. In its own quiet way *Earthling*'s sleeve artwork puts a twist on his revived sense of national identity. Back to the camera in his Union Jack coat, he gazes out over the garishly tinted rolling fields of a pastoral England, a Blakeian "green and pleasant land" nostalgically evoking cricket, cream teas and the last night of the Proms. His Colossus-of-Rhodes stance suggests both the proud eighteenth-century landowner in a Gainsborough portrait and, simultaneously, the isolated visitor in an alien landscape evoked many years earlier by the *Ziggy Stardust* sleeve. "Frank Ockenfels took the photograph," explained Bowie, "And then Dave De Angelis, who's a really good computer designer in England, squeezed in a bit of England in front of me, as I was in New York when I shot that." Amid the inner sleeve's distorted band portraits are images that hark back to Bowie's Los Angeles exile in the mid-1970s. The blurred George Pal-style flying

saucer is, David explained, "a satellite made out of silver foil from a Marlboro packet … part of an art movie I made in 1974," while the swirling pattern also used on the sleeve of the 'Little Wonder' single is a Kirlian photograph of David's fingertip and crucifix, also dating from the Los Angeles period. Kirlian Energy, he explained, is "a force that you find around the whole body, and may help to explain the idea of auras and healers, the energy that they have. There was a woman doctor called Dr Thelma Moss who had a research department at UCLA which was backed by the Pentagon to fund the exploration of Kirlian Energy, because they'd heard the Russians were investigating it. So she developed a machine, and made me one." This particular experiment had involved the taking of two Kirlian photographs. The first, shot just before David set to work on a particularly large helping of cocaine, shows the fingertip and crucifix in simple outline. The second, taken thirty minutes later, is the sizzling image that appears on the *Earthling* sleeve.

Earthling is a faster, rockier, more exuberant album than its predecessor, and its immediacy and ostensible lack of pretension proved more critic-friendly and more commercial. It out-performed *1.Outside* with a number 6 peak in the UK chart, earning a Grammy nomination for Best Alternative Music Performance (which it lost to Radiohead's *OK Computer*). "There's nothing complex about the album at all," said Bowie at the time. "This one is pretty primitive in a way." The studied artistry of *1.Outside* remains arguably a more substantial feast, but there's no denying that the furious broadside offered by *Earthling* makes for a very fine album indeed. Both are essential purchases for those willing to partake of Bowie's creative rebirth.

'HOURS…'
Virgin CDVX 2900, October 1999
   (lenticular sleeve) [5]
Virgin CDV 2900, October 1999 [5]
Columbia 511936 2, September 2003

'Thursday's Child' (5'24") / 'Something In The Air' (5'46") / 'Survive' (4'11") / 'If I'm Dreaming My Life' (7'04") / 'Seven' (4'04") / 'What's Really Happening?' (4'10") / 'The Pretty Things Are Going To Hell' (4'40") / 'New Angels Of Promise' (4'35") / 'Brilliant Adventure' (1'54") / 'The Dreamers' (5'14")

• *Musicians*: David Bowie (*vocals, keyboards, acoustic*

guitar, Roland 707 drum programming), Reeves Gabrels *(guitars, drum loops, synth and drum programming)*, Mark Plati *(bass, guitar, synth and drum programming, mellotron on 'Survive')*, Mike Levesque *(drums)*, Sterling Campbell *(drums on 'Seven', 'New Angels Of Promise', 'The Dreamers')*, Chris Haskett *(rhythm guitar on 'If I'm Dreaming My Life')*, Everett Bradley *(percussion on 'Seven')*, Marcus Salisbury *(bass on 'New Angels Of Promise')*, Holly Palmer *(backing vocals on 'Thursday's Child')* • *Recorded:* Seaview Studios, Bermuda; Looking Glass & Chung King Studios, New York • *Producers:* David Bowie, Reeves Gabrels

Despite Bowie's decisive rejection of the commercial mainstream in the mid-1990s, by the time the Earthling tour came to an end his personal fortune had reached a new peak. During 1997 the papers were full of stories about his asset flotation, referred to by the tabloids as "Bowie Bonds". The scheme involved David staking the royalties on his back catalogue as security against a loan of $55 million, to be repaid over an agreed period after which the royalty rights would revert to him. Prudential Securities purchased all the "Bowie Bonds" on the opening day of sale; it was the first such deal struck by a rock musician, establishing a precedent followed by artists such as Elton John.

Also in 1997, Bowie resold his back catalogue to EMI for a reported advance of $28.5 million, paving the way for yet another reissue programme which would begin with EMI's *Best Of…* CDs before moving on to the albums proper in the autumn of 1999. Bowie spent some of his new-found funds buying out a share of the publishing rights retained by his former manager Tony Defries. Other investments meant that by the end of the 1990s he was routinely appearing in the upper reaches of speculative lists of the entertainment industry's wealthiest figures.

In 1998 David retreated from the limelight to devote his attention to a number of new ventures: his fine-art publishing company 21, film roles in *Everybody Loves Sunshine*, *Il Mio West* and *Mr Rice's Secret*, and the establishment of his ISP BowieNet. The year was not without its musical endeavours: he mixed the Earthling tour album eventually released two years later as *liveandwell.com*, recorded 'A Foggy Day In London Town' for the *Red Hot + Rhapsody* charity CD, and the most exciting news was that he had patched up his differences with producer Tony Visconti; in August the two entered the studio for the

first time in 17 years (see 'Safe' in Chapter 1).

Much of late 1998 was spent working on new compositions with Reeves Gabrels in Bermuda, which for a short time in the late 1990s was Bowie's residence and base of operations (in 1995 he had sold the Mustique house he had owned for a decade, while in May 1998 the press reported that his Lausanne residence was on the market for 4.5 million Swiss francs). The duo began amassing a stockpile of coherent songs – rather than studio experiments – in a manner Bowie had seldom done since the mid-1980s. Demos were recorded on guitar or, in the case of 'Thursday's Child' and 'The Dreamers', on keyboards. "There was very little experimentation in the studio," David explained. "A lot of it was just straightforward songwriting. I enjoy that; I still like working that way." Reeves Gabrels was about to become the first Bowie collaborator to share the songwriting credits throughout an entire album. "I think we just agreed to do that," David explained, "and he certainly didn't blanch at it!"

At the beginning of 1999 the two spent some time in London and at the George V Hotel in Paris, writing and demoing material for the Eidos Interactive computer game *Omikron: The Nomad Soul* (see Chapter 8). The Paris-based company's invitation to provide soundtrack material for the game would provide the springboard for the album sessions proper, and eight of the songs on *'hours…'* would also be included in *Omikron*. Gabrels later explained that the requirements of the *Omikron* project influenced the style of the new songs: "Firstly, we sat down and wrote songs with just guitar and keyboard before going into a studio. Secondly, the characters we appear as in the game, performing the songs, are street/protest singers and so needed a more singer-songwriter approach. And lastly it was the opposite approach from the usual cheesy industrial metal music one would normally get."

February and March saw Bowie's live collaborations with Placebo in London and New York, where he also recorded his contribution to the Placebo single 'Without You I'm Nothing'. At around the same time he was asked to produce both Marilyn Manson and Red Hot Chili Peppers, but by now he was too busy to consider either offer.

In the spring Bowie and Gabrels entered Seaview Studios in Bermuda to begin recording. In May, a month before the album was officially announced, David told reporters that he and Gabrels had "been writing enormous amounts of material for several months" – as many as 100 songs, many of them in an acoustic vein. "We're recording most of the stuff ourselves," he said, "and Reeves and I are playing most of the instruments and programming drums, etc. But I think you'll be surprised at the actual intimacy of it all." Gabrels would later reveal that three songs – 'Survive', 'We All Go Through' and 'The Pretty Things Are Going To Hell' – were originally intended for his 1999 solo album *Ulysses (della notte)*. He also explained that "Because the album was taking a decidedly more introspective turn, it meant that I needed to approach the guitar-playing in a different way in order to wrap around the vocals and support the mood of the song in the solos. As co-writer and co-producer I had to be extra careful that the guitar player in me was responding to the lyric content of the songs."

For the album sessions Bowie recalled *Earthling*'s Mark Plati and *1.Outside*'s Sterling Campbell, but otherwise *'hours...'* featured a clutch of newcomers. Mike Levesque of Dave Navarro's band provided most of the percussion while Chris Haskett, formerly of The Rollins Band, played guest guitar on 'If I'm Dreaming My Life'.

Much attention had already been given to 'What's Really Happening?', a Bowie/Gabrels composition whose lyric was completed by Alex Grant, winner of BowieNet's "cyber-song" contest. With a backing track already laid down in Bermuda, the vocal and instrumental overdubs were added at New York's Looking Glass Studios on 24 May 1999. A remixed version of another track, 'The Pretty Things Are Going To Hell', was destined for inclusion in the film *Stigmata*, whose incidental score was being masterminded by Mike Garson and Billy Corgan of The Smashing Pumpkins.

After the left-field extremities of *1.Outside* and *Earthling*, the new work marked a conscious return to more traditional elements of songwriting. The acoustic textures and conventional melodic sensibilities led to pre-release rumours that *'hours...'* might be considered a successor to *Hunky Dory*. David avoided such comparisons, but agreed that retrospection was a keynote. "I wanted to capture a kind of universal angst felt by many people of my age," he explained. "You could say that I am attempting to write some songs for my generation." The album finds Bowie embarking on an exploration of memory, dreams and relationships with a frankness unparalleled since the 1970s; a recurring motif is the melancholy conflict between how things are and how things might have been. "The 'what if?' approach to life has always been such a part of my personal mythology," David told *Uncut*, "and it's always been easy for me to fantasize a parallel existence with whatever's going on. I suspect that dreams are an integral part of existence, with far more use for us than we've made of them, really. I'm quite Jungian about that. The dream state is a strong, potent force in our lives ... That other life, that *doppelgänger* life, is actually a dark thing for me. I don't find a sense of freedom in dreams; they're not an escape mechanism. In there, I'm usually, 'Oh, I gotta get outta this place!' The darker place. So that's why I much, much prefer to stay awake." He revealed that the album's original title had been *The Dreamers*, an idea quashed when Reeves Gabrels asked, "As in Freddie And...?".

Accordingly 'Something In The Air' and 'Survive' both dissect old relationships that have turned sour, while 'If I'm Dreaming My Life' and 'Seven' are both riven with doubt about the persistence and reliability of memory. 'What's Really Happening?', 'The Dreamers' and 'The Pretty Things Are Going To Hell' consider the impotence of age beneath the weight of personal history. What's surprising, though, is the album's sense of optimism. Whereas the relentless tread of "time" and the pitiless advance of "tomorrow" were totems of anxiety in Bowie's early work, *'hours...'* achieves at least a partial sense of reconciliation with the inevitable. 'Thursday's Child' banishes "regret" with its stoic plea to "throw me tomorrow / seeing my past to let it go".

Integral to this newly philosophical streak is the fact that *'hours...'* is shot through with the most overt religious imagery of any Bowie album to date. The oblique spiritualism of *Earthling* is still in evidence, but the sheer amount of Christian iconography is unparalleled except perhaps by 'Word On A Wing' – a song David chose to resurrect for live performance in 1999. The album contains paraphrases from the Bible and even the poetry of John Donne. There are countless references to life and death, heaven and hell, "gods", "hymns" and "angels". Most obvious of all is the title itself: Bowie explained that *'hours...'* was "about reflecting back on the time that one's lived, and how long one has left to live. Also, it's about shared experience, so there's the obvious double punning of 'ours'." The Book of Hours is the medieval prayer book which separates the day into the *Horae*, canonical hours to which are allocated devotions, readings and hymns. That this particular collection of devotions is both "hours" and "ours" reflects Bowie's conviction that "A belief system is merely a personal support system really. It's up to me to construct one that isn't carved in stone, that may change overnight. My songs do that."

Another delve into Christian symbolism is the sleeve photograph. It depicts not one but two Bowies, articulating the album's dialogue between past and present selves but also creating a deliberate echo of *La Pietà*, the image of the Virgin cradling the dead Christ which is a staple of medieval and Renaissance art (and is one of the Stations of the Cross, the formal Passion tableaux which provided the basis of 'Station To Station'). A long-haired and vaguely angelic-looking Bowie cradles his former self (goatee beard, spiky *Earthling* hair and all), suggesting not only a new musical incarnation but, perhaps, a requiem for another closing phase of life and career. "I was inspired by *La Pietà*," David confirmed, "but since I didn't want to wear a dress any more, we made it a man. It can be visualized as life and death, past and present." Meanwhile the back cover recalls medieval images of the Fall of Man: a trio of Bowies echo Adam, Eve and the central figure of God, while a Serpent writhes centre stage. Thus the bookends of 'hours…' suggest Fall and Redemption, constants in every belief system and certainly in Bowie's.

The sleeve was photographed by Tim Bret Day at Big Sky Studios in Ladbroke Grove, where another elaborate set-up, this time depicting Bowie burning on a crucifix, was also completed. "We shot Bowie and then made a dummy of him and set the whole thing alight," explained Bret Day later. "Lee Stewart did the rest in post-production. It's the whole thing of burning the old – that was then, but this is what I'm doing now. Deep down, he doesn't particularly want to talk about the past or hear his old records. He's not interested in anything prior to what he's doing today. I think that's the best thing about him." One of the crucifixion shots appeared inside the 'hours…' booklet. Meanwhile, graphic designer Rex Ray created the new Bowie logo, in which letters and numerals swapped roles over a multi-coloured bar-code design.

The retrospective tone of the new material, and its frequent references to families and relationships, raised the inevitable question of whether 'hours…' might be considered autobiographical. David was quick to dismiss such suggestions: "It's a more personal piece," he told *Uncut*, "but I hesitate to say it's autobiographical. In a way, it self-evidently isn't. I also hate to say it's a 'character', so I have to be careful there. It is fiction. And the progenitor of this piece is obviously a man who is fairly disillusioned. He's not a happy man. Whereas I am an *incredibly* happy man! … I was trying to capture elements of how, often, one feels at this age … There's not much concept behind it. It's really a bunch of songs, but I guess the one through-line is that they deal with a man looking back over his life." To the *New York Daily News* he added that "I've had twelve of the most buoyant years of my life. It's been fabulous. But I can't stand happy albums. I don't own any happy albums and wouldn't want to write one."

In another interview, this time for *Q*, Bowie added that "Obviously I am totally aware of how people read things into stuff like this. I'm quite sure some silly cow will come along and say, 'Oh, that's about Terry, his brother, and he was very disappointed about this girl back in 1969, whenever he got over her…' That sort of thing comes with the territory, and because I have been an elliptical writer, I think people have – quite rightly – gotten used to interpreting the lyrics in their own way."

From August 1999 onwards, a so-called "building hours" promotion saw excerpts from the album previewed on BowieNet, while the sleeve image was revealed a square at a time over successive days. On 21 September the entire album was made available to download from BowieNet and participating record store websites, making Bowie the first major-label artist to sell a complete album over the Internet.

'hours…' was released into the shops on yet another new label, Virgin, on 4 October 1999. The initial release came in a limited-edition "lenticular" case, whose grooves allowed the *Pietà* image to move through three dimensions depending on the angle at which it was viewed. The Japanese issue included 'We All Go Through' (elsewhere a single B-side), while a limited-edition French release included a second CD containing the same extra track and a video charting the making of 'hours…'. However, a 12" vinyl picture disc version which appeared in 2000 is, despite its Virgin logo and catalogue number, no more than a semi-legal collector's item. Sony's 2004 US reissue (LEGACY 092099) included five bonus tracks: 'We All Go Through', 'Something In The Air (*American Psycho* Mix)', 'Survive (Marius De Vries Mix)', 'Seven (Beck Mix 2)', and 'The Pretty Things Are Going To Hell (*Stigmata* Film Version)'.

Bowie's legendary status was once again on the up: he was appearing in the top tens of numerous "millennium" polls, and had been voted the *Sun*'s 'Music Star Of The Century' and *Entertainment Weekly*'s 'Classic Solo Artist Of All Time'. However, critical reaction to the new album was decidedly mixed, the music press for once proving more enthusiastic than the dailies. *Mojo*'s Mark Paytress announced that the album was "no masterpiece" but nonetheless "crowns a trilogy that represents significantly more than a mere coda to a once-unimpeachable career." *Record Collector*'s Steve Pafford noted that "An artist sometimes needs to produce a more public-pleasing album in order to pursue less popular and more experimental endeavours, and *'hours…'* firmly falls into this category … a well-structured album, full of little reminiscences, and disarmingly honest in its approach." The *Independent On Sunday* made the "solid album of slow-burning rock ballads" its CD of the week, while *Q* gave four stars to what it considered "a richly textured and emotionally vivid set", adding that "This time around, Bowie sounds influenced by nobody except himself, and he couldn't have picked a better role model."

The *Guardian*, on the other hand, found the album "sludgy and laborious", while the *Independent* considered it "as bad as anything he's done, including the Tin Machine albums". *Select* complained that "Bowie seems to have transformed himself into a more highbrow Sting" with "a lack of urgency that suggests that the 'confessional' is just another style Bowie's trying out for size", while *Time Out* dismissed the album as "Bowie's most pointless and desultory record since *Tin Machine II*." The *NME* considered 'Thursday's Child' "splendid, sweeping stuff," but complained that "the rest of the album is a pale imitation of the same moody magnificence" let down by "mediocre songwriting." In the *Sunday Times* Mark Edwards praised the writing but made no bones about his distaste for Reeves Gabrels, declaring that throughout the 1990s "Bowie has been capable of writing songs with all the melodic brilliance and lyrical quirkiness of his glorious 1970s peak. Unfortunately, he then lets Gabrels smother them in unnecessary layers of guitar. Possibly Gabrels thinks he is avant-garde. He isn't. He just makes pointless noise."

It wasn't all bad news; the *Scotsman* admitted that the songs "will grow in stature with further listens, even if they are far more delicate blooms" than Bowie's classics, and Mark Paytress confessed to "a

sneaking suspicion that *'hours…'* will be remembered with at least as much affection" as many of the EMI reissues that had appeared a fortnight earlier.

Tony Visconti considered *'hours…'* a throwback to Bowie's early recordings: "I think it's a very nineties sound," he told reporters, "but his songwriting has returned to that more melodic sound with accessible lyrics". Visconti believed that the new material revealed not "that weirded-out Bowie whose [lyrics] were harder to understand, but one that has beautiful lyrics about relationships and life experiences and, like in the sixties, a vast sonic panorama."

As usual, Visconti's remarks are perceptive: yes, the proliferation of twelve-string acoustic intros and the ravishing melodies may superficially suggest a throwback to the *Hunky Dory* days, but *'hours…'* nevertheless offers a very modern sound: programmed synthesizers, vocodered vocals and Reeves Gabrels's whizzing guitar effects are never far from the top of the mix. In Britain the album was a success, its number 5 chart peak putting it higher than any album since *Black Tie White Noise*. In America it made less impact, peaking at number 47 by comparison with *Earthling*'s 39. Commercially, yet again reservations abound over the choice of lead-off single: the complex and multi-layered 'Thursday's Child' was perhaps too challenging a proposition for the charts, whereas the instant acoustic impact of either 'Seven' or 'Survive', two beautiful songs subsequently released as singles, just might have launched the album with a smash hit.

Despite its comparative commercial success, *'hours…'* ultimately failed to win the widespread critical approval accorded to its immediate predecessors, and after the sensory assaults of *1.Outside* and *Earthling*, its gentler tone certainly came as a surprise and perhaps a disappointment to some. In both writing and production the album is unusually cluttered and indistinct, lacking the focus and attack of the best Bowie albums and betraying unwelcome signs of padding. But few would deny that its best moments – like the magnificent 1970s throwback 'Survive' and the stunning techno-ballad 'Something In The Air' – offer a convincing reminder that this is still the work of one of rock's finest songwriters. *'hours…'* makes a less aggressive artistic statement than any Bowie album since the mid-1980s, but on its own terms it's a success: a collection of lush, melancholic and often intensely beautiful music, and a necessary stepping-stone towards a new maturity of songwriting which would soon yield more spectacular results.

LIVEANDWELL.COM

Virgin/Risky Folio, September 2000

Disc One: 'I'm Afraid Of Americans' (5'19") / 'The Hearts Filthy Lesson' (5'33") / 'I'm Deranged' (7'11") / 'Hallo Spaceboy' (5'11") / 'Telling Lies' (5'18") / 'The Motel' (5'44") / 'The Voyeur Of Utter Destruction (As Beauty)' (5'48") / 'Battle For Britain (The Letter)' (4'35") / 'Seven Years In Tibet' (6'19") / 'Little Wonder' (6'15")
Disc Two: 'Fun (Dillinja Mix)' (5'52") / 'Little Wonder (Danny Saber Dance Mix)' (5'30") / 'Dead Man Walking (Moby Mix 1)' (7'31") / 'Telling Lies (Paradox Mix)' (5'10")

• *Musicians:* see *The Earthling Tour* (Chapter 3) • *Recorded:* Radio City Music Hall, New York; Paradiso, Amsterdam; Phoenix Festival, Stratford-upon-Avon; Metropolitan, Rio de Janeiro • *Producers:* David Bowie, Reeves Gabrels, Mark Plati

On the heels of 1997's Earthling tour, Bowie's guitarist Reeves Gabrels was hopeful that the band might record "a follow-up *Earthling*-type album, much in the same way that *Aladdin Sane* followed *Ziggy*, an extrapolation of the previous album. The music had evolved, the band was playing great and the window of opportunity time-wise was there." Bowie, however, wished instead to compile a live album from the many recordings made during the Earthling tour, and it was on this project that he embarked in the early weeks of 1998. In addition to mixing the live recordings with Gabrels and Mark Plati, he reconvened the band to cut two new studio tracks: the elusive drum'n'bass composition 'Fun', and a cover of Bob Dylan's 'Tryin' To Get To Heaven'.

The album was originally intended to receive a full commercial release but, as Gabrels later explained, "Unfortunately Virgin refused to put it out after it was submitted in late winter 1998. Aside from the obvious, the bad news was that in the amount of time spent by David, Mark Plati and myself compiling and editing, we could have written and recorded the follow-up *Earthling* album that I'd hoped we'd do." Instead, Bowie and Gabrels moved on to begin work on 'hours…'.

Various tracks from the cancelled release were sub-

sequently offered to BowieNet members in downloadable form, before a revised version of the album finally materialized as a limited-edition double CD on 13 September 2000, when free copies were distributed exclusively to BowieNet subscribers. With no discernible catalogue number, and its artwork and liner notes executed by BowieNet members, *liveandwell.com* is something of an oddity; but despite the unusual circumstances of its release it is undoubtedly an "official" album.

Culled from four dates on the 1997 tour, Disc One's track details are as follows: 'I'm Afraid Of Americans' and the last three tracks hail from the *GQ* Awards in New York on 15 October; 'The Hearts Filthy Lesson' is from the Phoenix Festival on 19 July; 'Hallo Spaceboy' and 'The Voyeur' are from Rio on 2 November; and the remaining three tracks are from Amsterdam on 10 June (the gig from which the live 'Pallas Athena' and 'V-2 Schneider' had already been released).

liveandwell.com is a beautifully mixed and hugely impressive memento of the Earthling tour, and is well worth hunting down. It's only a pity that there wasn't room for some of the tour's rarer delights, such as 'O Superman' and 'V-2 Schneider'. The bonus disc includes some of David's favourite mixes of the Earthling singles, plus the otherwise unavailable 'Dillinja Mix' of 'Fun'. Of the studio version of Bob Dylan's 'Tryin' To Get To Heaven' there is no sign; to date the recording has only received a one-off airing on Spanish radio.

TOY

(Unreleased)

• *Musicians:* David Bowie *(vocals, keyboards, Stylophone, mandolin)*, Earl Slick *(guitar)*, Gail Ann Dorsey *(bass)*, Mark Plati *(bass, guitar)*, Sterling Campbell *(drums)*, Lisa Germano *(acoustic and electric violin, recorder, mandolin, accordion)*, Gerry Leonard *(guitar)*, Cuong Vu *(trumpet)*, Holly Palmer *(backing vocals)*, Emm Gryner *(backing vocals)* • *Recorded:* Sear Sound Studios, New York; Looking Glass Studios, New York • *Producers:* David Bowie, Mark Plati

Before his triumphant Glastonbury homecoming in June 2000, Bowie had already confirmed his intention to record a new album with the tour band. "I've pulled together a selection of songs from a somewhat unusual reservoir and booked time in a studio," he revealed that same month, fuelling speculation that his next project would find him re-recording the 1960s songs he had begun performing the previous year. "Not so much a *Pin Ups II* as an *Up Date I*," he explained.

Sure enough, in July 2000 work began on a new album which soon acquired the working title of *Toy*. Producer Mark Plati later recalled that "we pretty much just bundled the live band into Sear Sound in New York, set everyone up, and let rip. A number of the songs had been rehearsed, so we were somewhat prepared this time. The idea was to keep it loose, fast, and not clean things up too much or dwell on perfection. As a result, we had 13 basic tracks cut in around nine days. In this period we managed a few overdubs on each tune, including Tony Visconti conducting a 14-piece section for the string arrangements he did on two of the songs."

Among the vintage numbers re-recorded for *Toy* were 'The London Boys', 'I Dig Everything', 'Can't Help Thinking About Me', 'You've Got A Habit Of Leaving', 'Baby Loves That Way', 'Conversation Piece', 'Let Me Sleep Beside You', 'Silly Boy Blue', 'In The Heat Of The Morning' and 'Karma Man'. This last was later dropped from the projected track-listing in favour of a song listed as 'Secret 1', apparently Gail Ann Dorsey's favourite of the recordings; it seems likely that this was the superb new recording of the legendary Ziggy-era demo 'Shadow Man'. In addition to the archive revivals, the *Toy* sessions included two new songs, 'Afraid' and 'Uncle Floyd' – both written, according to David, in the style he "may have written them in, in the sixties". Both songs would later be resurrected for *Heathen*, with 'Uncle Floyd' now retitled 'Slip Away'. Intriguingly, Bowie also told fans that "some of the songs from the sixties were never recorded, let alone released, so will be as new to you as any of the new ones that I've written." These were possibly the elusive 'Miss American High', 'Hole In The Ground' and 'Toy'; the first is registered as a title by Bowie's publishing company Nipple Music and appears to have been recorded during the sessions; the second remains no more than a rumoured title; while 'Toy' would be re-titled 'Your Turn To Drive' and receive a limited online release three years later.

After the initial sessions at Sear Sound, recording took a two-month break for the happiest of reasons: just after 5.00am on 15 August 2000, David and

Iman's daughter Alexandria Zahra Jones was born in New York. David assisted with the delivery, cutting the baby's umbilical cord. "This has to be the happiest of times in my life," Iman told readers of *Hello!* magazine, for whom the couple granted an inevitable but very beautiful photo-session the following month. "I have my whole family around me. Alexandria has been the force around whom everyone has gathered. And my soul feels complete." David concurred, saying that "Overnight, our lives have been enriched beyond belief." Finding themselves inundated by gifts for the baby, David and Iman issued a request that fans and well-wishers should instead make donations to Save The Children.

Meanwhile, during the two-month break in the *Toy* sessions, Mark Plati attended a New York gig by the Eels, whose live ranks had recently been swelled by multi-instrumentalist Lisa Germano. "After listening to a few songs, and being familiar with some of Lisa's solo records and her work with other artists," Plati later explained, "I knew I needed to get her on the Bowie album." At Plati's suggestion Lisa Germano, whose other credits included work with Sheryl Crow and John Mellencamp, sent some samples of her work to Bowie. He contacted her immediately, and in late September the pair convened at Plati's home studio to record a series of instrumental overdubs. "Lisa really took to the material," Plati later recalled, "putting down all sorts of parts on an arsenal of eccentric instruments, including an electric violin tuned one octave lower than usual, a 1920s Gibson mandolin, and an old, tiny tortoiseshell blue-green Hohner accordion, with a strap so old and tired we had to beg it to stay together (assisted by duct tape) for the duration of a song.

"David was completely into these sessions – we worked at my place for two days this time – as he'd not done any work on the album since August, nor listened to it much. He seemed just plain ready to work, and he was thrilled with how great and fresh the songs were. It was a lot of fun, and very exciting – David kept pulling ideas out of the air for Lisa to play, and it was great to see how well they got on and how musically in sync they were from the first few minutes." For Plati, the addition of Germano's overdubs was the icing on the cake: "Her playing – especially violin – was simply magical and made some of the songs truly complete. It was as if she was a part of the band from the conception of the record, and not grafted on afterwards."

Also contributing overdubs was the Irish-born ambient art-rock guitarist Gerry Leonard, whose previous session work included recordings with Laurie Anderson, Cyndi Lauper and Sophie B Hawkins, and who records his own material under the name Spooky Ghost. It was also during the October sessions that Bowie, Plati and Sterling Campbell recorded 'Pictures Of Lily' for the tribute album *Substitute: The Songs Of The Who*.

On 20 October David took a break from recording to make a surprise appearance at the VH1 Fashion Awards at Madison Square Garden, presenting Stella McCartney with the "Fashion Designer Of The Year" award. It was at this ceremony that Ben Stiller filmed spoof interviews and scenes of himself accepting an award for his forthcoming movie *Zoolander*.

Mixing began at Looking Glass Studios on 30 October 2000, with David now predicting a release date of March 2001: "And there will definitely be some supporting gigs," he said at the end of October. "No tour, mind. But definitely some supporting gigs, at least in New York." He revealed that he was designing the "very odd" sleeve artwork, and of the album itself he declared that "It really has surpassed my expectations already. The songs are so alive and full of colour, they jump out of the speakers. It's really hard to believe that they were written so long ago." He described the music as "dreamy, a little weird at times, it rocks, it's sad, it's got passion, it... it... it's really good."

On 18 July 2000, just as the *Toy* sessions were getting under way, EMI had reaffirmed its enthusiasm for Bowie's back catalogue by reissuing 20 studio albums (*Space Oddity* to *Tin Machine*, and *1.Outside* to *'hours...'*) for commercial download on the Internet. However, by early 2001 it was becoming clear that all was not well between Bowie and his record label. In February (the same month that David performed 'Silly Boy Blue' at the Tibet House Benefit Concert – the nearest he would come to the mooted gigs), the release of *Toy* was rumoured to have been postponed until May, and thereafter it seemed to disappear from the schedules altogether. In June Bowie revealed that "EMI/Virgin seem to have a lot of scheduling conflicts this year, which has put an awful lot on the back burner. *Toy* is finished and ready to go, and I will make an announcement as soon as I get a very real date." By July he was referring darkly to "unbelievably complicated scheduling negotiations" with his label, and in October, he announced that "Virgin/EMI have had scheduling problems and are now going for an album of 'new' material over the *Toy* album. Fine by me. I'm extremely happy with the new stuff. I love *Toy* as well and won't let that material fade away. If you've been following the newspapers you will have seen that EMI/Virgin are having major problems themselves. This has not helped. But all things pass."

Tony Visconti would later say that Bowie was "hurt terribly" by the label's refusal to release *Toy*. By the beginning of 2002 David's departure from Virgin/EMI had been confirmed, and in March came the announcement that he had negotiated with Columbia Records to launch the new album *Heathen* via his own ISO label. *Toy* remains unreleased as an album, but several of the tracks have appeared as B-sides and bonus tracks: 'Conversation Piece' appeared on the *Heathen* bonus disc, while 'Shadow Man', 'You've Got A Habit Of Leaving' and 'Baby Loves That Way' were released as B-sides on various single formats in 2002. 'Uncle Floyd' and 'Afraid' were reworked for *Heathen*. Excerpts from 'The London Boys' were made available as a limited download for BowieNet members, while in 2003 'Your Turn To Drive' was offered as an exclusive HMV download for online purchasers of *Reality*. "*Toy* has actually started now to become a reservoir of B-sides and bonus tracks, so it's much depleted," Bowie said in 2003. "From the original 14 or so that I did, I think seven are now out there. I think there's still enough in the past to be able to pop some more back and top it up, so to speak, but you know what? New writing just takes precedence. It always does."

HEATHEN

ISO/Columbia 508222 9, June 2002 [5]
  (CD: limited edition card case with bonus disc)
ISO/Columbia 508222 2, June 2002 [5]
  (CD: jewel case)
ISO/Columbia 508222 1, June 2002 [5] *(vinyl)*
ISO/Columbia 508222 6, December 2002 *(SACD)*

'Sunday' (4'45") / 'Cactus' (2'55") / 'Slip Away' (6'04") *(SACD: 6'14")* / 'Slow Burn' (4'40") *(SACD: 5'04")* / 'Afraid' (3'28") / 'I've Been Waiting For You' (3'00") *(SACD: 3'16")* / 'I Would Be Your Slave' (5'14") / 'I Took A Trip On A Gemini Spaceship' (4'05") / '5.15 The Angels Have Gone' (5'00") *(SACD: 5'25")* / 'Everyone Says 'Hi'' (3'59") / 'A Better Future' (4'11") / 'Heathen (The Rays)' (4'17")

Bonus Disc: 'Sunday (Moby Remix)' (5'09") / 'A Better Future (Remix by Air)' (4'56") / 'Conversation Piece' (3'52") / 'Panic In Detroit' (3'00")

Bonus tracks on SACD version: 'When The Boys Come Marching Home' (4'46") / 'Wood Jackson' (4'48") / 'Conversation Piece' (3'52") / 'Safe' (5'53")

• *Musicians:* David Bowie *(vocals, keyboards, guitars, saxophone, Stylophone, drums)*, Tony Visconti *(bass, guitars, recorders, string arrangements, backing vocals)*, Matt Chamberlain *(drums, loop programming, percussion)*, David Torn *(guitars, guitar loops, Omnichord)*, The Scorchio Quartet: Greg Kitzis *(first violin)*, Meg Okura *(second violin)*, Martha Mooke *(viola)*, Mary Wooten *(cello)*, Carlos Alomar *(guitar)*, Sterling Campbell *(drums and percussion)*, Lisa Germano *(violin)*, Gerry Leonard *(guitar)*, Tony Levin *(bass)*, Mark Plati *(guitar, bass)*, Jordan Ruddess *(keyboards)*, The Borneo Horns: Lenny Pickett *(baritone saxophone)*, Stan Harrison *(alto saxophone)*, Steve Elson *(tenor saxophone)*, Kristeen Young *(backing vocals, piano)*, Pete Townshend *(guitar on 'Slow Burn')*, Dave Grohl *(guitar on 'I've Been Waiting For You')*, Gary Miller *(additional guitar on 'Everyone Says 'Hi'')*, Dave Clayton *(keyboards on 'Everyone Says 'Hi'')*, John Read *(bass on 'Everyone Says 'Hi'')*, Solá Ákingbólá *(percussion on 'Everyone Says 'Hi'')*, Philip Sheppard *(electric cello on 'Everyone Says 'Hi'')* • *Recorded:* Allaire Studios, New York; Looking Glass Studios, New York; Sub Urban Studios, London • *Producers:* Tony Visconti, David Bowie *(except 'Afraid': David Bowie, Mark Plati; 'Everyone Says 'Hi': Brian Rawling, Gary Miller)*

While Virgin vacillated over the release of *Toy*, the early months of 2001 saw Bowie begin work on a new studio project which would reunite him with producer Tony Visconti for their first full-length album since *Scary Monsters*. After years of silence, apparently occasioned by Visconti's frankness with interviewers in the early 1980s, the two had become reconciled in 1998 and had already worked on various one-off studio projects including Placebo's 'Without You I'm Nothing', The Rustic Overtones' *Viva Nueva*, and the 1998 Bowie recordings 'Safe' and 'Mother'. Visconti, who had also contributed string arrangements during the *Toy* sessions, was delighted to be working with Bowie again. "It was only in very recent years, around the time he made contact again, that I realized how much I missed him," he said. "We had both grown

and changed, so the time was right to open the channels again. However, I've discovered how sensitive he is about his privacy and I've learned to respect that."

Bowie was equally pleased by the long-awaited reunion. "Although we've been friends off and on forever, over the last few years we haven't actually done any work together," he said in October 2000, "so the beginning of next year's album will be critical for both of us, as I'm sure that we've both learnt a lot over the ensuing years. Maybe we've gotten into some bad recording habits as well. What Tony and I always found to be one of our major strengths is the ability to free each other up from getting into a rut. So no doubt there will be some huge challenges, but also some pretty joyous occasions."

Although writing and demoing began as early as January 2001, David's domestic life demanded that the new sessions proceed at a more leisurely pace than usual: his daughter Alexandria was now the undisputed centre of attention, and he assured journalists that he was not about to repeat the errors of the 1970s. "I don't want to start doing what I unfortunately did with my son, inasmuch as I spent an awful lot of time on tour when he was a young child," David later told the *Observer*. "I really missed those years, and I know he did too. Fortunately we were together by the time he was six and I brought him up from that point on. It was a one-parent family. I don't want to repeat the same mistakes with Lexi." Speaking of becoming a father for the second time, he remarked elsewhere that "I really, really love it. To be honest, I really have to pull myself together weekly to focus on my music, that sometimes it almost feels like a distraction. The music, I mean. But I think I'm beginning to find a sense of balance between daddy-fying and workifying. Mind you, the next album might have lyrics like 'the wheels on the bus go round and round..'"

Despite David's evident joy, it was sadly a period of mixed fortunes for the Bowie family. On 2 April 2001 the news emerged that David's 88-year-old mother Peggy Jones had died peacefully at the St Albans nursing home where she had lived for some years. Only a month later came the news that David's friend and colleague Freddi Burretti had died in Paris at the age of 49. The emotional upheavals of 2001 would be reflected in Bowie's new songs, many of which meditated on such weighty topics as bereavement, faith, mortality and the uncertainty of the future.

"In coming into this album," David later explained, "I thought, 'What's the best way of approaching big questions without being too grand?'" His solution was to approach the project with the aim of creating a collection "of serious songs to be sung". He also wanted to ensure that the reunion with Tony Visconti would not "smack of trying to recapture anything we'd done before", and as a result "it was very important to me to make sure that we had some very good musical structures" before the sessions began. "I went in with the idea of creating a personal, cultural restoration," David later explained to *Interview* magazine. "I wanted to capture everything – all the ideas, all the techniques that I've used over the years – while working within this prism called the zeitgeist. In the process, I wanted to create a timeless piece that didn't owe to the past, present or future, but just floated in its own autonomous kind of place."

Tony Visconti recognized a marked development in Bowie's approach to songwriting since the days of *Scary Monsters*: "His knowledge of harmonic and chordal structure had vastly improved," Visconti would say later. "This had already been good when I last worked with him, but now there was more depth to his melodic and harmonic writing. I had developed too, so we'd kind of moved in a parallel way along the same route. We were definitely on the same wavelength. A part of him wants commercial success, but there's a bigger part of him that has great artistic integrity, and it was therefore important to him for *Heathen* to make a great artistic statement."

For the first time since *The Buddha of Suburbia*, all of the new material was written by David alone. "It's increasingly evident to me that my needs to make music change periodically," he said in 2002. "There's the narrative, crafted song type; then the experimental ideas and situational type; and thirdly a theatrical-motivated, scenario type. I guess *Heathen* owes a lot to the first type, with a little of the second as seasoning."

Preparatory work was carried out at New York's Looking Glass Studios, where David assembled "a lot of music that I really liked, almost 40 pieces, maybe even more. They were just sort of motifs; they weren't finished, established pieces of work." The intention of these initial sessions, he explained, was "to re-establish myself as a writer and a putter-together of sounds", and to establish a framework for the subsequent sessions. "Tony and I wanted to give each song its own identity and character without getting lost in a hailstorm of musical ideas."

A decisive moment in the album's development came in the Spring of 2001 when, as Bowie later recalled, guitarist David Torn recommended a new studio venue. "He said 'David, you must go and see this new place.' He said the atmosphere is unlike any other studio that he'd ever been to." The venue in question was Allaire Studios, a new facility created by photographer and musician Randall Wallace at Glen Tonche in the Catskill mountains, some two hours' drive north of New York City. "It was almost an epiphany that I had," Bowie told *Interview* of his first visit to Allaire. "Walking through the door, everything that my album should be about was galvanized for me into one focal point. Even though I couldn't express it in words right that second, I knew what the lyrics were already. They were all suddenly accumulated in my mind. It was an on-the-road-to-Damascus type of experience, you know? It was almost like my feet were lifted off the ground."

Glen Tonche is a luxury estate built in the 1920s by the wealthy industrialist Raymond Pitcairn. "He'd obviously knocked around a lot with nautical types," said Bowie, "because the whole place has a kind of yacht feel that you get from Eisenhower-era yachts – those very American but aristocratic pieces of work. The whole thing is wood, with great, vast main rooms, and the grounds are full of deer, pigs and bears. The dining room that we ended up using as our studio has 40-foot tall ceilings, with 25-foot windows that look out over a reservoir and the mountains." The picturesque but barren surroundings offered an unusual source of creative inspiration for Bowie, who generally prefers to work in urban settings like New York and Berlin, but he was keen to point out that "this is not cute, on top of this mountain: it's stark, and it has a Spartan quality about it. In this instance, the retreat atmosphere honed my thoughts … I don't know what happened up there, but something clicked for me as a writer."

Tony Visconti later revealed that Bowie was "writing furiously" within days of arriving at Allaire. "This studio was just amazing and it also had a vibe about it," he recalled. "We were really high, about 2000 feet above sea level, overlooking this big reservoir. And we'd see hawks in the sky, saw an eagle one day. We'd see deer and wild turkeys and all that. David would get up every morning at six and go in and write that day's work. He'd finish up some of his ideas. And then Matt [Chamberlain] and I would hit the studio about 10:30 or 11 in the morning and start recording the first song."

During his free time David would listen to music as diverse as Moby, Air, Richard Strauss, Gustav Mahler and the Comedian Harmonists, a six-part harmony group from the 1930s. Crucial lyrics like 'Sunday' and 'Heathen (The Rays)' were inspired directly by Bowie's new surroundings, and were among the first to be composed. "The heavier-weighted things, the keystones to the album, were written in the earlier part," David explained later. "I wanted to get those done. And I got lighter after I felt that I'd made my breakthrough."

Recording continued in Allaire's Neve Room during August and September. "We're putting in a modest 10-hour day," revealed Tony Visconti at the time, "but we cut 19 tracks in two weeks." The initial recordings were laid down by Bowie and Visconti with input from two newcomers, percussionist Matt Chamberlain and guitarist David Torn. Chamberlain's extensive credits included Macy Gray's *On How Life Is* and Elton John's *Songs From The West Coast*, and he had also worked with the likes of Garbage, Peter Gabriel, Tori Amos and The Corrs. Most recently he had played on Natalie Merchant's 2001 album *Motherland*, which had also been recorded at Allaire. "I knew his work by reputation, and he had been working with Natalie when we had gone to look at the place, so I was able to meet and talk with him a little," Bowie later explained. Multi-instrumentalist and guitar "texturalist" David Torn, who recorded his contributions to *Heathen* in September 2001, had twice won the Experimental category in *Guitar Player*'s poll awards. His previous credits included work with Laurie Anderson, David Sylvian, kd lang and Ryuichi Sakamoto, as well as his own Splattered Cell recordings and contributions to numerous film soundtracks including *Three Kings*, *Velvet Goldmine* and *The Big Lebowski*.

"I was keen to work with musicians neither of us had worked with before," Bowie explained to *Time Out*, "so I told my band, whom I've worked with for seven years now, 'You're all sacked, fuck off', ha ha. No, that's not true. I said: 'Listen, guys, for artistic reasons we won't be working together on the next album, but we'll pick up when I've finished and go back out as a band!'" It wasn't the first time that Bowie had chosen to wipe the slate clean and record with a fresh group of musicians, and Visconti would later express his admiration at David's ability to "stage" an album by assembling an unpredictable and exciting combination of performers, "knowing what characters to put together to make something wonderful and odd." Bowie's own instrumental contribution was greater than on any album in recent memory, encompassing guitars, saxophone, Stylophone, keyboards (including Theremins and the EMS AKS briefcase synth previously featured on *Low*) and even drums. In October 2001 he declared excitedly that he had "played probably more on this album than any other that I've done since *Diamond Dogs* or maybe *Low*." This was a development actively encouraged by Visconti. "With most producers, I get the feeling I'm being judged when I play something," David explained. "If I have an option of playing something myself or turning it over to a qualified, card-carrying musician, I'll usually opt for the latter. Then I'll kick myself, because it never quite sounds the way I would have done it."

Visconti would later reveal that "On some tracks, like 'Sunday' and 'I Would Be Your Slave', we decided to resurrect the '"Heroes"' vocal sound." Just as he had done in Berlin 25 years earlier, Visconti set up three microphones at increasing distances from the singer, their gates adjusted to open only when David sang above a certain volume. "You need a big studio, and Allaire's room is huge and not treated – other than a few carpets and tapestries judiciously placed on the floors and walls."

In addition to the core band, a succession of guest musicians travelled to Allaire to provide overdubs. Among them was the Irish-born textural guitarist Gerry Leonard, who had previously contributed to the *Toy* sessions and would soon go on the become a key member of Bowie's live band, as would backing vocalist Catherine Russell, a jazz, gospel and R&B singer whose previous credits included a number of stage musicals and session work with Madonna, Cyndi Lauper, Chaka Khan, Steely Dan and Paul Simon. St Louis-born singer-songwriter Kristeen Young had been contacted by Tony Visconti after he heard her 2000 album *Enemy*; having already arranged to record solo tracks with Visconti, she was delighted to be asked to work on the Bowie album, and in the wake of the *Heathen* sessions David would contribute a guest vocal on her Visconti-produced album *Breasticles*.

Keyboardist Jordan Ruddess, whose *Heathen* contributions were recorded in late August, had previously played on 'Mother' and 'Safe', and had more recently worked with Tony Visconti on Prefab Sprout's 2001 album *The Gunman And Other Stories*. "David Bowie doesn't like a lot of options," Ruddess revealed at the time of the *Heathen* sessions. "He has a good idea of how he wants the end result to sound, so practically what's on his demo is close to what he wants."

It appears that Jordan Ruddess may have replaced Bowie's original choice, jazz singer and pianist Annette Peacock. At the launch in October 2000 of her long-awaited comeback album *An Acrobat's Heart*, Peacock had told reporters that Bowie had asked her to record with him the following January and even suggested that she accompany him on tour. Bowie is known to be a long-time admirer of Peacock: back in 1973 she had turned down his invitation to play synthesizers on *Aladdin Sane*, but he had nevertheless been instrumental in getting her signed to MainMan, where her songs were covered by both The Astronettes and Mick Ronson. Another reunion that went no further than the planning stages was with guitarist Robert Fripp, who had met David in New York during the final stages of King Crimson's 2000 tour. In December 2000 Fripp's wife, Toyah Willcox, wrote in her online diary that "Robert is in talks to possibly do some work with David Bowie" – but, for the time being at least, this was not to be.

Heathen did, however, see Bowie reunited with no fewer than three of his former guitarists. Nirvana veteran and Foo Fighter Dave Grohl, who had backed Bowie at his fiftieth birthday concert, provided a suitably aggressive solo on 'I've Been Waiting For You'. "He just called and asked if I'd play guitar on a song." Grohl later recalled. "And I said, yes, sure; he sent me the copy of the songs, I played guitar and sent it back." Meanwhile Carlos Alomar, who had also worked with Visconti on the Prefab Sprout album, was reunited with Bowie for the first time since the Outside tour and recorded his overdubs in mid-October. The attention of most reviewers, however, was concentrated on Pete Townshend's contribution to 'Slow Burn'. Following Bowie's cover version of The Who's 'Pictures Of Lily', recorded during the previous year's *Toy* sessions, the pair met in New York in October 2001 during preparations for the Concert For New York City. Armed with Bowie's backing tapes, Townshend recorded his 'Slow Burn' overdubs later the same month, telling fans that Bowie's album was "surprising, moving, poetic, in a musical and visionary sense."

Mixing took place in October at Looking Glass Studios, where Tony Visconti reworked elements of the Mark Plati-produced 'Afraid', originally recorded

for *Toy* in 2000, to bring it in line with the new tracks. Another song from the *Toy* sessions, 'Uncle Floyd', had been entirely re-recorded at Allaire under its new title 'Slip Away'. It was also at Looking Glass that vocals and guitars for 'Everyone Says 'Hi'' were recorded by Bowie, Visconti and Carlos Alomar, before the track was completed at London's Sub Urban Studios by guest producers Brian Rawling and Gary Miller. Outtakes from the *Heathen* sessions included the B-sides 'Wood Jackson' and 'When The Boys Come Marching Home'. Bowie later intimated that the sessions had been very prolific, remarking that "the hard part was knowing which songs not to include."

Overdubbing continued on and off into the New Year, with Visconti adding work by the Scorchio Quartet, who had accompanied Bowie at the Tibet House Benefit Concert the previous February, and saxophone trio The Borneo Horns, returning to the Bowie stable for the first time since *Never Let Me Down*, who recorded their contribution to 'Slow Burn' on 29 January 2002.

December 2001 saw two entirely separate but significant developments for David. Firstly, after a couple of false starts over the preceding two years, the lifelong smoker finally quit his 60-a-day habit, this time apparently for good. Secondly, on 15 December came an announcement which onlookers had been expecting for some time, as a press release revealed that David had parted company with Virgin Records. "On Thursday morning Bowie's business representatives, RZO, sent a letter to Virgin Records stating that 'We respectfully decline your attempts to negotiate a new contract in light of the missed option pick-up of a year ago.'" Instead, Bowie had taken the step of forming his own independent label, ISO. "I've had one too many years of bumping heads with corporate structure," he explained. "Many times I've not been in agreement with how things are done and as a writer of some proliferation, frustrated at how slow and lumbering it all is. I've dreamed of embarking on my own set-up for such a long time and now is the perfect opportunity." It transpired that Bowie had registered ISO as a record label over a year earlier, and was now ready to begin operations at once. "I want to keep the whole experience at a human level," he said. "To characterize ISO, I think I would use guitarist Robert Fripp's phrase and describe it as aiming to be 'a small, mobile, intelligent unit'."

In March 2002 came the announcement that Columbia Records had entered into a multi-album deal with ISO for the marketing and distribution of Bowie's work, beginning with *Heathen*. Columbia chairman Don Ienner declared that "David Bowie is simply one of the most distinctive, influential and exciting artists of our time, and *Heathen* is a remarkable addition to his incredible body of work. The album is filled with amazing songs and performances that evoke vintage Bowie without ever looking backward, and I think it's the album that his worldwide audience has been waiting for. Music needs David Bowie right now, and we couldn't be more proud that he has chosen Columbia as his new home." David later told *Billboard* that "Absolutely no attempt was made on their part to guide me into making a chart-oriented record. What I brought them is what they took – and with great enthusiasm."

Meanwhile, other influences were shaping the creative progress of *Heathen*. November 2001 had seen the publication of Iman's autobiographical portfolio *I Am Iman*, a fascinating visual essay on the politics of beauty and ethnicity in Western society. David wrote a touching foreword for the book, which was adorned by the work of photographers such as Annie Liebowitz, Herb Ritts, Helmut Newton and Norman Parkinson. Initial copies came with a limited-edition CD of tracks selected by David and Iman, offering an intriguing insight into the place David's work occupies in the couple's lives: 'The Wedding', 'Wild Is The Wind', 'Loving The Alien', 'As The World Falls Down' and 'Abdulmajid'. The book's stunning cover photograph was taken by the Swiss photographer Markus Klinko, a New York resident who would soon take his place in Bowie lore as *Heathen*'s sleeve photographer. Klinko's striking *Heathen* portraits were shot in early 2002 and computer-enhanced by his partner Indrani. Bowie then enlisted Jonathan Barnbrook, the British designer of *I Am Iman*, to create the album's idiosyncratic upside-down typeface.

As its title suggests, *Heathen* continues to pursue the troubled spirituality of 1990s albums like *1.Outside, Earthling* and *'hours…'*, and its core themes maintain a sense of strong continuity with Bowie's earlier work. "My entire career, I've only really worked with the same subject matter," he remarked in 2002. "The trousers may change, but the actual words and subjects I've always chosen to write with are things to do with isolation, abandonment, fear and anxiety – all of the high points of one's life." Although *Heathen*'s assertive tone seems considerably less weary and resigned than that of its immediate predecessor

'hours…', the sense of the darkness that comes with an ageing perspective is even stronger. "There are times in our quiet lives when we're very happy," Bowie told *Interview*, "but there comes a point where you're not growing any more, and your body's strength is diminishing. Especially in one's mid-fifties, you're very aware that that's the moment you have to leave the idea of being young. You've got to let it go." But of the album, he explained that "I didn't want it to become pathetic either, like, you know, 'Here's an old man's recollections' or something. Still, I had no embarrassment about expressing the thoughts and experiences of an old man. There's a British nursery rhyme I carry with me. The first line is 'This is the way the young men ride – clip-clop, clip-clop, clip-clop, clip-clop,' and it ends with 'This is the way the old men ride – hobbledy, hobbledy, hobbledy, down into the ditch'. I had it in my mind that I'm in the 'This is the way the old men ride' part. I wanted to give some sense of what happens when you arrive at this age – do you still have doubts, do you still have questions and fears, and does everything burn with as much luminosity as it did when you were young? As a kickoff to get me going, I used the songs of Richard Strauss, which have influenced me for such a long time. There is a certain sense of universality in those songs that Strauss wrote at the end of his life, when he was 84 [the *Four Last Songs*]: they're the most terribly romantic, sad, poignant pieces that I think have ever been written. I kind of used them as a template for songs on the new album like 'Sunday', 'Heathen (The Rays)', 'I Would Be Your Slave' and '5.15 The Angels Have Gone'." David would later describe Gundula Janowitz's 1973 recording of the *Four Last Songs* as "…transcendental. It aches with love for a life that is quietly fading. I know of no other piece of music, nor any performance, which moves me quite like this."

However, Bowie was at pains to stress that his interest in the pathos of age had nothing to do with self-pity. "I don't find it a problem being old and I don't mind not thinking like I used to think when I was young," he told Tim Cooper in the *Observer*. "I don't have that thing about 'I'm old but I feel like an 18-year-old inside!' I don't. I feel like exactly what I am, which is 55 going on 56, and it seems to be a pretty cool age to be. I've experienced a lot and have a sense of who I am that maybe I didn't have a few years ago." In another interview he suggested that he now had "fewer and fewer questions about life", which in turn allowed him to concentrate on "the questions that are unresolvable. I'm approaching those questions in the new songs. At first I thought, 'Well, if I write about this, I won't have anything left to write about.' But then I realized that what life is about is quite a subject to take on. And at the moment, I feel like I've only scratched the surface."

It is this continuing philosophical quest which invests *Heathen* with its overpowering atmosphere of darkness and spiritual despair. "Probably my greatest strength as a writer is an ability to capture transitory, nagging fear," David suggested. "I don't do political worldview very well, but I'm good at capturing ephemeral pockets of doubt and underlying anxiety." The air of world-weary reminiscence which had dominated *'hours…'* is supplanted on *Heathen* by a more immediate sense of existential dread in songs like 'Sunday', 'Afraid', and in particular the mortal angst of the title track. "Obviously the idea of fear is very strong within the album," Bowie told Radio 4's *Front Row*. "I think one of the major fears actually, that underlines it all for me personally, is the fear that there is no spiritual life … I confront it every day of my life. It's something I've always thought about. I'm a very spiritual person, inasmuch as I've had this awful bloody journey searching for a spiritual life."

As so often in his work, Bowie subverts the traditional dialogue of the love song to create a series of philosophical meditations which tackle more profound and abstract concepts. 'I Would Be Your Slave' is far from being the submissive love lyric it first appears to be, while 'A Better Future' finds Bowie making demands not of a lover, but of God. "They're stubborn, they're naïve declarations," he explained, "that if you're not going to do anything about our world, you know, you're not going to have any support for your plans in the future, God!" Even the ostensibly cheery 'Everyone Says 'Hi'' is a meditation on bereavement, while the title track addresses the moment when the narrator feels his life ebbing away. "Anxiety and spiritual searching have been consistent themes with me, and that figures into my worldview," he said. "But I tend to make my songs sound like relationship songs."

"David was very jovial," Visconti later told the *Guardian*. "But he would go somewhere in the mornings when he was writing these songs. You could see he was really struggling with questions. After a few weeks I said: 'It seems like you're addressing God himself.' The concept of *Heathen* is a godless century. He was addressing the bleakness of our soul … and maybe his own soul."

Another recurrent motif on the album, starkly expressed in tracks like 'Slow Burn', was what Bowie described as "fear forward about my daughter, more than anything else. Since my daughter's been born I am changing as a writer. There has been a shift in the weight of my responsibilities, relinquishing my own concerns about myself and Iman as a couple, and instead thinking about Lexi and what her world is going to be like." This anxiety on the behalf of his daughter's generation is nowhere more clearly expressed than in Bowie's demand for 'A Better Future'. "I had rosy expectations for the twenty-first century, I really did," David told the *Observer*. "The whole idea was lifting my spirits quite a lot during 1998 and 1999. But it has become something other than what I expected it to be. And it's obviously a pretty typical parental concern to wonder what type of a world you have brought your child into."

Given the timing of its release, and the fact that Bowie lives and works in New York, it was inevitable that many commentators would also suggest that *Heathen*'s doom-laden subject matter was in part a response to the events of 11 September 2001. Although he acknowledged that a retrospective resonance was unavoidable, David denied that it was intentional. "It was all written before," he told *Entertainment Weekly*, "every single song … I don't want it to reflect that situation particularly at all, because in fact that crock of songs came out of a general feeling of anxiety I've had in America for a number of years. It wasn't that localized – bang! – thing that happened in September." As Visconti later explained, the album was in the middle of recording on the day of the terrorist attacks. "For that whole day we lost contact with our loved ones. Iman was very close to it. He got hold of her for 10 minutes and the phones went down. My son lived very close. His business partner lived across the street and managed to get out five minutes before the building collapsed. All of us have stories like that. Did it influence the album? Undoubtedly, but a lot of those lyrics are very prophetic. I swear to you only a few lines were amended after September 11." In another interview Bowie remarked that "Probably a half-dozen of my albums you could have put out just after September 11 and people would have thought they were commenting on that tragedy. I think a general state of angst was there before anything happened in September, in all honesty. There's always disaster and near-disaster in life."

Indeed, Bowie's love of New York seemed to grow rather than to diminish in the aftermath of 11 September. Shortly after his daughter's birth, David had intimated that he and Iman were planning to relocate to London. "There is no way I'm bringing up my child in America," he had told GQ magazine in 2000. "No way. We'll be back over to London, without a doubt." A year later, he appeared to have changed his mind. "New York has always been a terrific place," he said in November 2001, "and we both really adore living here. Somehow, if it's possible, it seems to be an even tighter community than it was before. I don't think either of us would want to trade places with anywhere else at the moment." This was a point of view to which he would repeatedly return during promotional interviews in 2002. Echoing the sentiments he had expressed at the time of *The Elephant Man* over 20 years earlier, he compared London's paparazzi-infested streets with the relaxed atmosphere of New York: "There are certain cities – London, LA, Paris – where I don't have a good time. I have a great time here: we can go where we want, eat where we want, walk out with our child, go to the park, ride the subway, do the things that any other family does … In London it's more excitable and becomes more event-oriented, but here the recognition is almost at a community level. It's like, 'Hi Dave, how ya doing!' It's a very friendly thing over here."

The anxiety expressed throughout *Heathen* is not, then, the same anxiety that had brought forth the paranoid eschatology of *Diamond Dogs* or the desperate clutching at spiritual straws of *Station To Station*. It was the anxiety of a happy, fulfilled mind struggling to come to terms with intimations of mortality. "It's a head-spinning dichotomy," David confessed to Ingrid Sischy in her excellent piece for *Interview*, "of the lust for life against the finality of everything. It's those two things raging against each other, you know? And that produces these moments that feel like real truth … It's like, how do you come to terms with that situation? Is there any comfort factor to be found in here at all? What is the point of all this? And that's kind of what *Heathen* is. I love this work. I love this life. I'm so greedy not to want to give it up. I just don't want to give it up. It's hard to give it up. This album is about that." In another statement, he defined the protagonist of *Heathen* as "One who does not see his world. He has no mental light. He destroys almost unwittingly. He cannot feel any of God's presence in his life.

He is the 21st-century man."

The album's concerns are reflected in its richly allusive sleeve packaging, which ranks among the most beautiful and intriguing of any Bowie album. The trio of leather-bound books whose spines are prominently displayed offer a forthright announcement of the album's themes. *The General Theory of Relativity* was Albert Einstein's 1915 thesis on the nature of gravity and acceleration which paved the way for modern man's understanding of the nature of the universe. Similarly ground-breaking was Sigmund Freud's *The Interpretation Of Dreams* (written 1897, published 1900), which galvanized the whole notion of interpretation by suggesting that dreams were a form of wish-fulfilment whose "manifest content" disguised a "latent content". It would be difficult to imagine a more fundamental description of the process of reading Bowie's lyrics, and it should be noted that countless Bowie songs directly address the Freudian approach to dreams, from early compositions like 'Did You Ever Have A Dream' and 'When I Live My Dream' to 'hours…' tracks like 'The Dreamers' and 'If I'm Dreaming My Life'. Most resonant of all is the inclusion of *Die Fröhliche Wissenschaft* (*The Gay Science*), the revolutionary 1882 work in which Bowie's long-time muse Friedrich Nietzsche set forth his famous proclamation that "God is dead" and proposed the doctrine of "eternal recurrence" – the idea that man may be fated to relive every moment in his life throughout eternity. Both proposals were motivated by Nietzsche's rejection of the idea of a divine, omniscient and judgmental authority, and his desire to redirect man's attention from the fantasy of an afterlife to the inherent freedom of the world in which he exists. The relevance of such proposals to the songwriting on *Heathen* speaks for itself. It's also worth noting that the title of *Die Fröhliche Wissenschaft* was inspired by the troubadour songs of medieval Provence, some of which were included in the appendix of Nietzsche's 1887 edition, thus making it a doubly appropriate choice for Bowie's *Heathen* library.

More immediately striking than the literary references are the stark images of medieval and Renaissance paintings defaced by splatters of paint and knife-slashes. Given that the paintings are of specific and obviously relevant Christian subjects, the images offer a graphic and literal enactment of the iconoclasm proposed by Nietzsche's "murder of God". Bowie's fear for his child's future, and indeed the tragedy of September 11, are inevitably reflected in the detail from Guido Reni's *Massacre of the Innocents* (1611), while Duccio di Buoninsegna's *Madonna and Child with Six Angels* (1300-05) suggests a similar theme (in the inverted detail used it's presumably no coincidence that, to coin a phrase, the angels have gone). The ripped canvases are an inverted detail from Carlo Dolci's *Magdalene* (1660-70) and an engraving copied from an undated *Christ and St John with Angels* by Peter Paul Rubens (1577-1640), one of Bowie's favourite painters. The booklet in the standard jewel-case CD version boasted an additional ripped canvas, this time of Raffaello Sanzio's *St Sebastian* (1501-02). "I think one of the subtexts for the word "heathen" is one that is barbaric or Philistine," David commented; hence "the idea of the iconoclastic pieces in it, like the ripping of paintings and destruction of religious things." In keeping with the defaced images, the album's idiosyncratic crossed-out typeface evokes the writings of Jacques Derrida, another of Bowie's favoured philosophers whose experiments with crossed-out text propose the cancellation of the written word and the end of discourse. Markus Klinko's photographs reinforce the sense of spiritual and discursive negation: Bowie sits at a Spartan schoolroom desk, his pen hovering over a blank page, his face wiped clean from the picture. Close-up shots show him slicing through the pages and ripping them from the book, while his crucifix is scratched out of another photo. The cover portrait's blank, silvery eyes offer a multiplicity of interpretations, suggesting a state both human and celestial, of both blindness and transcendence. In both style and subject matter, the photographs are also clearly indebted to the surrealists who had influenced Bowie's work since the days of *Station To Station*: "The actual imagery is nicked from Man Ray and Buñuel," he explained. "Those are the old Dali eyes in *Un Chien Andalou* and all that."

Heathen was released in Europe on 10 June 2002, and in America the following day. The initial limited-edition CD came in a deluxe cardboard digipak with a bonus disc featuring two remixes, the *Toy* re-recording of 'Conversation Piece', and the 1979 version of 'Panic In Detroit'. This edition also boasted an enhanced PC feature offering online access to the album's lyrics, some of the rejected cover designs and, for those lucky enough to have compatible software, two otherwise unavailable audio tracks (an extract from the *Toy* version of 'The London Boys' and the

1998 track 'Safe'). A standard jewel-case CD, minus the bonus disc and enhanced features, was released simultaneously. As usual the Japanese release carried an extra track, in this case the single B-side 'Wood Jackson'. Six months later, in December 2002, *Heathen* became the first Bowie album to be issued in the new-fangled SACD format, Tony Visconti having remixed the album to 5.1 sound. The SACD version included slightly longer versions of four tracks, and also 5.1 remixes of 'When The Boys Come Marching Home', 'Wood Jackson', 'Conversation Piece', and an extended 'Safe' that was over a minute longer than the B-side version.

The album was hyped by the usual exhaustive round of TV appearances and interviews, a series of pre-release "listening parties" organized by BowieNet, and an advertising campaign which promoted *Heathen* as Bowie's 25th studio album (which, accommodating the Tin Machine releases and *The Buddha of Suburbia*, it was). In America there was even a specially-shot TV commercial featuring Bowie with a young girl: this, too, was later made available via the enhanced CD. "I use a parent-child situation," David explained. "The child wanders around as Dad sings in the booth. At the very end, the viewer is taken to the window and sees Earth in all its glory. There's a sense of abandonment on both the album and commercial." The campaign was a success, and *Heathen* matched its predecessor's performance with a number 5 peak in the UK chart. It fared well throughout Europe, reaching number 3 in France and Germany, number 2 in Norway and number 1 in Denmark and Malta. In America it hit number 14, Bowie's best showing in the US chart since *Tonight* in 1984.

The reviews were noticeably better than for *'hours...'*, and indeed better than for any album of recent times. "*Heathen* achieves a balance noticeably lacking in Bowie's output of the past 20 years," said the *Guardian*, which found the album "strident, confident, lush with melodies ... packed with fantastic songs, liberally sprinkled with intriguing touches, *Heathen* is the sound of a man who has finally worked out how to grow old with a fitting degree of style." *Music Week* called the album "a stunning return to form", while *Vanity Fair* rejoiced in "a real David Bowie album – his first collaboration in 20 years with producer Tony Visconti, and by far his best in ages." *Rolling Stone* praised the "splendid, often moving effect" of "his least affected album in a decade ... A loose theme runs through these songs, covers included: the search for guiding light in godless night. But the real story is *Heathen*'s perfect casting: Bowie playing Bowie, with class."

Naturally, there were a few dissenting voices, but even those who qualified their praise were largely won over. "*Heathen* is a return to form," conceded the *Sunday Times*, "but not quite a return to *that* form." The *Mail On Sunday* praised Bowie's success in "writing powerful tunes and resonant phrases, singing with verve and drama and throwing interesting musicians together", but noted that "Bowie made his reputation by breaking new ground but now he is borrowing from his brilliant past." Only *Uncut*'s Ian MacDonald seemed wholly dissatisfied, complaining that "none of the 12 tracks on *Heathen* displays anything memorable in the way of melody or chorus, their phrasing short-breathed and tired, their sequences energyless. There's no commanding feeling of arrival or departure. The album drifts in and drifts out, as do many of its tracks, without any evident conviction … It's a melancholy task to have to speak about a Bowie album in such terms of disappointment and dissatisfaction." So melancholy was MacDonald's task that he was alone in undertaking it: such opinions were heavily outnumbered. The *Times* hailed *Heathen* as "the artist's most cohesive album in a decade" and praised its "total attention to songs that come impressively arranged and brilliantly sung." The *Daily Express* described *Heathen* as "easily his best album for the best part of 20 years", while the *Independent On Sunday* declared that "If Bowie's 90s dabblings with techno-pop left you cold, this is the comeback for you." The *Independent*'s David Gill noted that the return of Tony Visconti had resulted in "a much more assured sound than on recent albums, one reminiscent of, but not beholden to, those earlier successes", and also found the time to praise *Heathen*'s challenging subject matter: "Bowie is a pop icon from a time when stars weren't afraid to brandish their intellectual interests, rather than their ignorance. Don't bother searching for similar concerns on the new Oasis album." (In an unfortunate piece of timing, Oasis's similarly named *Heathen Chemistry* was released only three weeks after *Heathen*, to be greeted by more brickbats than bouquets.)

The *Evening Standard*'s guest reviewer Boy George hailed "a real return to form", while the *Daily Mail* announced that "David Bowie harks back to the well-crafted songs of his golden era" and "sings impressively throughout." The *NME*'s Sarah Dempster con-

sidered *Heathen* "a largely unaffected anniversary waltz through the velvet-lined vaults of his past. And it's great. All of it." *Time Out* welcomed Bowie's "most enjoyable album since *Scary Monsters* – a collection of strong, melodic songs executed with playful primitivism and sung with a force and passion that would be remarkable in a man half his age." *Q*'s David Quantick praised *Heathen* for offering "the beefiest sound of a Bowie record since 1980's *Scary Monsters*, which is the album it most resembles", and went on to rejoice in the fact that "David Bowie, always much more than just a Greatest Hits, still makes music that no-one else has heard before, and still does it well. And *Heathen*? A return to form. Definitely."

A combination of good omens (the return of Tony Visconti was the album's most talked-about feature) and good timing (its release coincided with widespread press coverage of the Meltdown Festival and the 30th anniversary of *Ziggy Stardust*) made *Heathen* the most hotly anticipated Bowie album in recent years. It swiftly garnered a nomination for the Mercury Music Award, and the acclaim continued with numerous appearances in 2002's "albums of the year" lists and a Grammy nomination for 'Slow Burn' in the "Male Rock Vocal Performance" category. Its initial run of 20 consecutive weeks in the UK album chart was the longest sustained chart presence by any Bowie album since *Let's Dance*. "It's been very positively received," David noted happily, at the same time wryly noting the ubiquity of one particular critical cliché: "It seems to be traditional now that every album since *Black Tie White Noise* is the best album I've put out since *Scary Monsters*. Inevitably, that's what I get. But this one just seems to have caught people's imaginations."

Thankfully the enthusiastic reception accorded to *Heathen* was more than justified. Bowie's songwriting seems both more substantial and more committed than on '*hours…*', and his vocal performance is a revelation. In place of the ironic distancing of *1.Outside* or the studied cool of *Black Tie White Noise* (approaches which were nonetheless perfect for those albums), *Heathen* finds Bowie singing with genuine passion and depth, immediately recalling his bravura performances on albums like "*Heroes*" and *Scary Monsters*. Apparently without effort, he hits high notes whose like have rarely been heard on a Bowie album since the 1970s, while elsewhere his rich baritone suggests that he has once again turned for inspiration to the more experimental work of his idol Scott Walker, in particular the textured atmospherics of 1995's *Tilt*. "Of course they recall Scott," Bowie declared. "I'm a huge fan." Tony Visconti's production reaps immediate rewards, investing *Heathen* with the richest, strongest sound of any Bowie album in years, striking a perfect balance between uncluttered space and the baroque additions for which the producer's work is justly noted. The sumptuous string arrangements in 'Afraid' and 'I Would Be Your Slave' are quintessential Visconti, as are the layered backing vocals and tightly controlled synthesizers and horns which permeate the album. The ominous electronics of the opening and closing tracks update the sinister ambiences of *Low* without ever sounding retrogressive, and perhaps best of all, the majestic soundscape of the outstanding ballad 'Slip Away' offers a virtual masterclass in how to capture a classic Bowie sound without chasing after past glories.

Heathen may not be Bowie's most obviously melodic album, but then neither are *Low* or *"Heroes"*, and those few critics who dismissed it as lacking in tunes were making the same mistake as their counterparts 25 years earlier. After three or four hearings, *Heathen*'s melodic subtlety and harmonic brilliance emerge to scintillating effect. Combined with superb performances, not to mention some of the finest and most probing lyrics Bowie has ever written, the result is a positive triumph. The only remotely uncertain note is that when the new material is this good, the inclusion of three cover versions seems a trifle excessive. All three are excellent recordings, but the suitably spiky 'Cactus' and the delightfully tongue-in-cheek 'Gemini Spaceship' would have been ample, so perhaps Neil Young's 'I've Been Waiting For You' might have been relegated to a B-side and replaced by one of Bowie's originals. But in the face of the album's other achievements this is a minor cavil. Since the dissolution of Tin Machine in 1992, Bowie's decade of experimentation had resulted in some fine albums. But it is *Heathen* that finds him finally emerging from the shadow of his 1990s collaborators with an impressive collection of songs which evoke the classic Bowie of old, but are at the same time convincingly modern in style, intent and execution. It's fitting, then, that *Heathen* appears to have reinvigorated Bowie as an artist. "I know how good this album is," he said in 2002. "It's an incredibly successful album for me creatively. I wouldn't change a note of it. I really adore it. And it's given me an unbelievably buoyant kind of confidence about what I am as a writer. And I almost

feel that I will be writing some of my very best work over the next few years."

REALITY

ISO/Columbia COL 512555 9, September 2003 [3]
    (CD: limited edition card case with bonus disc)
ISO/Columbia COL 512555 2, September 2003 [3]
    (CD: jewel case)
ISO/Columbia COL 512555 3, November 2003
    (CD: Tour Edition with bonus DVD)
ISO/Columbia CS 90752 6, December 2003 *(SACD)*
ISO/Columbia CN 90743, February 2004
    (DualDisc CD/DVD-Audio Edition)

'New Killer Star' (4'40") / 'Pablo Picasso' (4'05") / 'Never Get Old' (4'25") / 'The Loneliest Guy' (4'11") / 'Looking For Water' (3'28") / 'She'll Drive The Big Car' (4'35") / 'Days' (3'19") / 'Fall Dog Bombs The Moon' (4'04") / 'Try Some, Buy Some' (4'24") / 'Reality' (4'23") / 'Bring Me The Disco King' (7'50")

Bonus Disc: 'Fly' (4'10") / 'Queen Of All The Tarts (Overture)' (2'53") / 'Rebel Rebel' (3'09")

Bonus track on Tour Edition: 'Waterloo Sunset' (3'28")

• *Musicians:* David Bowie *(vocals, guitar, keyboards, Stylophone, baritone sax, percussion, synths, backing vocals)*, Sterling Campbell *(drums)*, Gerry Leonard *(guitar)*, Mark Plati *(bass, guitar)*, Mike Garson *(piano)*, Gail Ann Dorsey *(backing vocals)*, Catherine Russell *(backing vocals)*, Matt Chamberlain *(drums on 'Bring Me The Disco King' and 'Fly')*, Tony Visconti *(bass, guitar, keyboards, backing vocals)*, David Torn *(guitar)*, Carlos Alomar *(guitar on 'Fly')*, Mario J McNulty *(additional percussion, drums on 'Fall Dog Bombs The Moon', additional engineering)* • *Recorded:* Looking Glass Studios, New York; Allaire Studios, New York; The Hitching Post Studio, Bell Canyon • *Producers:* David Bowie, Tony Visconti

As the Heathen tour drew to a close in October 2002, Bowie was already eager to return to the studio. He would later recall that he began writing new songs "immediately after leaving the road after doing the Five Boroughs tour … I was back at home with the baby and wife and doing daily things, and I started writing immediately. Because I have a loose and comfortable contract with my new record company, it was great to be able to go in and start recording as it was percolating."

In stark contrast to the frustrations of Bowie's relationships with various record labels in the 1990s and early 2000s, Columbia's enthusiasm for his natural recording pace was evidently suiting David very well: for the first time in recent memory, he was back to making an album a year. "They said they would agree to this when I first took my ISO label to them," he explained in 2003. "I said, 'Look, I will require that I can put out stuff when I want to, and I don't want to have one of those sell-through dates inflicted on me,' which is what you usually get: 'Oh, we've got another 18 months until you can do that.' They've been great so far, and when I hit them with a new album they're ready for it."

Following the success of *Heathen*, there was no question that Bowie's renewed partnership with Tony Visconti would continue. "We made *Heathen* our kind of debut reunion album," David explained. "The circumstances, the environment, everything about it was just perfect for us to find out if we still had a chemistry that was really effective. And it worked out. It was perfect, not a step out of place, as though we had just come from the previous album into this one. It was quite stunningly comfortable to work with each other again." In November 2002 Bowie and Visconti reunited to lay initial plans for their next studio project. The recent concerts had invigorated David's appetite for touring, and the challenge on this occasion was to create an album that would be, as he later put it, "built to play live". The result was *Reality*, a more muscular, rock-based album than its predecessor, fashioned with an eye to the major world tour that would begin in the autumn of 2003 and continue well into the following summer.

One of the fundamental creative resolutions that would shape the development of *Reality* was Bowie's decision not to return to the remote mountain surroundings of Allaire Studios that had played host to *Heathen*; instead, the new album would be recorded at Looking Glass Studios in New York City, previously the venue for most of the *Earthling* and *'hours...'* sessions. David had by no means lost interest in the rural setting of Allaire; on the contrary, in January 2003 he even purchased the neighbouring 64-acre Little Tonche Mountain in Shokan, with a view to building a country retreat. "I love mountains," he told the *New York Post*. "I'm a Capricorn. I was born to be gallivanting on a peak somewhere." For a confirmed city-dweller who had always seemed the most reluctant of mountain residents during his years in Switzerland, this was a remarkable turn of events. "I was never a Woodstocky kind of person, at all, ever," he admitted, "but when I got up there, I flipped at how beautiful it is. There's a barrenness and sturdiness in the rugged terrain that draws me."

Notwithstanding this newfound affinity for the wilderness, the new album was to see a wholehearted return to the more familiar streetwise milieu of Bowie's lyrical and musical world; as ever, his songwriting and music would be directly affected by his surroundings. "I'm terribly influenced by geography and where I am," he remarked. "My albums are pretty good snapshots of where I was and what I was going through when I was there. You can feel the Catskill Mountains in *Heathen*. You can feel the spirituality." By way of contrast, *Reality* would prove to be as urban a record as any he has made.

Following a couple of days' preliminary work in November 2002, the *Reality* sessions proper began at Looking Glass in early January 2003. Bowie initially brought in four or five demos that he had prepared on his home equipment, but these were very basic: "I don't want my home to be taken over by the recording process," he told *Sound On Sound*. "I'm very wary of that. I really saved everything for working over at Looking Glass."

Although Looking Glass Studio A offers the most spacious of the facilities at Philip Glass's venue, Bowie opted to record *Reality* in the more cramped surroundings of Studio B, which is rented by Tony Visconti on a semi-permanent basis. "We wanted the record to have a real tight New York sound," said Visconti. "David loves the sound of Studio B. We did a little bit of work in there at the end of *Heathen*, and it was because we liked it so much that I started to rent it. Then, when he wanted to work at Looking Glass again for these latest sessions, I assumed we were going to book Studio A, but he said, 'No, I want to do as much as I can in your room.' The monitoring in there is terrific, and anything that I bring out of that room sounds really good."

The studio band assembled for the *Reality* sessions reflected the success of the 2002 live dates, replacing many of the less familiar *Heathen* personnel with a tighter line-up composed largely of Bowie's touring musicians: Earl Slick and Gerry Leonard on guitar, Sterling Campbell on drums, Mike Garson on piano, and Mark Plati on guitar and bass. Bowie's live bassist

Gail Ann Dorsey and multi-instrumentalist Catherine Russell contributed only backing vocals to the *Reality* sessions. Further guitar overdubs would be provided by *Heathen* veterans David Torn and Carlos Alomar, while 'Bring Me The Disco King' and the bonus track 'Fly' utilized drum parts recorded by Matt Chamberlain during the *Heathen* sessions two years earlier.

Before the band arrived, the new compositions were demoed at Looking Glass by Bowie and Visconti, with the help of assistant engineer Mario J McNulty. "We talk an awfully large amount when we make a record," Visconti said later. "We can talk for hours without recording anything, then suddenly, we strike when the iron is hot and record at a relentless pace for several hours." In keeping with the spontaneity that Bowie and Visconti have always enjoyed in the studio, much of the demo material survived on the final album. "Inevitably, we'd hardly redo anything," Visconti recalled. "I always record things carefully in the first place, because I know we're not going to redo them, and so a lot of the demo parts ended up on the final version." As a result, several of the bass parts on *Reality* were played by Visconti himself rather than by Mark Plati, who had originally been lined up to record them: "Before the band came in, I'd played bass on all of the demos," explained Visconti, "and some of my bass parts eventually made it all the way to the album in preference to Mark Plati's. This was the case on 'New Killer Star' – Mark had a go at it, but there was some kind of personality in my bass playing that David preferred, and the same applied to 'The Loneliest Guy', 'Days' and 'Fall Dog Bombs The Moon'. It's Mark's bass on all of the other tracks, including the part I wrote for 'Looking For Water'." Similarly, Mario McNulty's percussion on 'Fall Dog Bombs The Moon' would be retained on the final album.

Bowie continued in the tradition of *Heathen* by playing many of the instruments himself, including guitar, saxophone, Stylophone and keyboards. Mike Garson would be entrusted with the prominent piano parts on tracks like 'The Loneliest Guy' and 'Bring Me The Disco King', but the lion's share of the more textural synthesizer work was played by Bowie himself. "He loves his Korg Trinity," said Visconti. "He knows it intimately, and he can just dial up sounds at will. When he was writing his songs he made notes of certain sounds that he wanted to use, and he ended up playing most of the sonic landscape parts; the big

string parts, choirs and so on." However, Bowie's favourite new toy was not a keyboard but a striking white 1956 Supro Dual Tone guitar, which he had purchased on eBay and entrusted to the Staten Island instrument restorer Flip Scipio, the result being an instrument which, in Visconti's words, "was never meant to sound so good." This guitar was of the same make used by Link Wray on his 1958 single 'Rumble', a groundbreaking early classic of avant-garde rock which became something of a band favourite during the *Reality* sessions and the subsequent tour.

"There's a sense of freedom working with Tony that I rarely find with other producers," David enthused. "A non-judgemental situation where I can just fart about and play quite badly on all manner of instruments, and Tony doesn't laugh! I can't tell you how important it is to feel that free in the studio, and that somebody isn't judging your musical abilities. Often, when I've done something with Tony, it just sounds right. It might not be played perfectly – there's no virtuosity on the keyboards or anything – but there's a certain way that I'll put a B flat into a chord that nobody else would, probably because they've been trained properly, and it just sounds interesting. Well, Tony can spot that, whereas a lot of other producers will say, 'Whoo, that B flat's a bit suspect.' I'll be thinking, 'Ah, shit! No, that sounds good, Mr Producer!'"

For his part, Visconti praised Bowie's intuitive ability to get the best out of his producer, noting that Bowie "hasn't forgotten a thing. He'll suddenly just turn around and, referring to a very tight digital delay, he'll say, 'You know that sound you got on my voice on *Young Americans*? I want that for the chorus.' He's got a good mental picture of how something should sound."

As usual, the bass, percussion and rhythm guitar parts were cut live to create the initial rhythm tracks before the addition of vocals and overdubs. "The melodies were sketchy, the lyrics were sketchy, and so there was no point in recording lead guitars and other things at that stage," explained Visconti. "Sterling, Mark and David would often play along to a click track that we had on the demos, consisting of a basic drum loop from a drum box, together with a scratch keyboard or scratch guitar and David's vocal." As on *Heathen*, Visconti's preference for old-fashioned analogue recording had a bearing on the sessions: "We initially recorded to 16-track analogue tape because I just love the sound," he explained. "I'd talked David into working that way on *Heathen* – I told him it was really worth doing, because we'd capture the analogue compression and warmth on digital. When we'd transfer it, the sound would still be there, and that proved to be right on *Heathen*, so we started this new album in exactly the same way."

An initial eight-day session yielded eight basic tracks, after which rhythm guitars and vocals were added. "Very odd chord sequences on this new stuff," David revealed to BowieNet as recording progressed. "Definitely, on a couple of songs, patterns that I've not used before." At this stage the spirit was still firmly one of experimentation. "We would record vocals and have no idea as to whether we'd keep them," explained Visconti. "By the end of the album I'd have at least three different vocal sessions for each song." Although the majority of David's vocals were selected from single takes, they were occasionally composited on the final album: "Any vocals that we did in February were matched up with any vocals we did in May," said Visconti. "We could easily cut from one vocal track to another. Each time, David would usually do two passes and call it quits, because he goes for feel and passion. He sings great, he's always singing in tune, he always sings full voice, so there's never any need for eight or nine David Bowie vocal takes. I know it and he knows it."

Visconti was full of praise for Bowie's vocal technique. "He's gifted and he's also intuitive," the producer told *Sound On Sound*. "Sometimes I would coach him if I needed to remind him about something he'd done earlier, or I might make a suggestion – some line might require more angst or whatever – and he's receptive to anything like that. He's a consummate professional, and I'm really blessed to be working with such a great singer. Also, he recently gave up smoking, so he's recaptured some of his high range. He'd lost at least five semitones, and he's now gained most of them back." Indeed, by the time of the *Reality* sessions Bowie had succeeded in staying off the cigarettes for over a year. "It's hard," he remarked in 2003, "and it's still going to be hard in 10 years"; elsewhere he declared that smoking had been "without doubt the toughest thing to quit in the world", more so than drink and drugs. David now satisfied his addictive urges with nothing more life-threatening than herbal tea-tree sticks, which duly appeared in several photo-shoots during the *Reality* period and on which, he freely confessed, he was now hooked.

While lead guitar was entrusted to Earl Slick, the more ambient guitar overdubs were provided by *Heathen* veterans David Torn, whose contributions include the trilling riff underpinning 'New Killer Star', and Gerry Leonard, whose madcap Spanish guitar lends an idiosyncratic touch to 'Pablo Picasso'. Once the guitar overdubs had been added, Bowie and Visconti became concerned that the percussion tracks lacked the ambience and impact of those on the previous album, a fact which they concluded was down to the acoustic quality of the spacious Allaire Studios where *Heathen* was recorded. They decided to take the remarkable if logical step of carrying the Looking Glass drum recordings to Allaire Studios and playing them back through the monitors, thus capturing the unique ambience of the *Heathen* venue. The resulting tracks were mixed with the untreated Looking Glass recordings to varying degrees. "The result is that there might be a slight difference, but overall it sounds as if the drum kit was at Allaire," concluded Visconti. "This is especially so on 'Pablo Picasso', while about 40 per cent of the drums on 'Looking For Water' was captured in the Allaire room. It's got a nice one-second decay in there, which is ideal for drums."

In April David revealed in his BowieNet journal that he had written 16 songs for the album, eight of which he was "mad for". The songwriting process was as eclectic as ever: some pieces were created by fashioning a melody over a series of looped chords, while others began life as more conventional pieces of songwriting. "I guess something that was virtually looped on this album was 'Looking For Water', and so a secondary consideration was the melodic content on top," David revealed, "whereas 'She'll Drive The Big Car' was specifically a written piece. It's self-evident when you know that and then hear the songs."

As has always been the case, Bowie's new songs were written from the diverse points of view of a cast of characters, each existing at a remove from the songwriter himself. "I think this album is more anecdotal, and there's past glimpses of people that I felt I might have known, or that I did know," he explained, "amalgams of people from New York really." Thus 'She'll Drive The Big Car' eavesdrops on the emotions of a disappointed heroine just as 'Life On Mars?' had done many years earlier, while 'Fall Dog Bombs The Moon' is, in Bowie's words, "an ugly song sung by an ugly man". The narrator of 'The Loneliest Guy' is an isolated soul whose ancestry can be traced back through compositions as diverse as 'Algeria Touchshriek', 'Sound And Vision' and 'Conversation

Piece'. "I guess it's just this Greco-Roman notion of turning something nebulous into a personification that you can recognize, like a deity," Bowie mused. "You know, back then, they would transform a set of emotions into a god. I just convert ideas into people. It's just easier to handle them that way."

The sessions continued on and off until late May 2003, with mixing continuing at Looking Glass. As with *Heathen*, Visconti created an additional 5.1 mix of the album for release on SACD and related formats. As mixing got under way, David announced to the world in June that the new album was to be called *Reality*, and told *Blender* magazine that "This album is a bit thrusty. I'm not sure if being thrusty is a great thing at age 56, but I suppose it's better than being dead – or limp."

"There's a part of David Bowie that definitely does not want to repeat himself, so we were committed to avoiding the *Heathen* formula," said Visconti. "We realized that we'd created this kind of genre for *Heathen*, and we wanted to go in another direction. I'd referred to that album as his 'magnum opus' – I told him, 'That was more like a symphony, and you can't write too many of those.' I mean, the great composers didn't write a new symphony every couple of months. *Heathen* consisted of very broad strokes and a grand sonic landscape – there were layers and layers of overdubs – whereas for *Reality* he wanted to change to something that he and his live band could play on stage with great immediacy, without the need for synthesizer patches and backing tracks. He wanted to make this more of a band album."

Bowie concurred: "As I knew that we were going to continue touring this year, I was looking for something that had a slightly more urgent kind of sound than *Heathen*, but I think the mainstay of the album is that I was writing it and recording here in downtown New York. It's very much inspired by where I live and how I live and the day-to-day life down here. There is a sense of urgency to this town. The engine of it is therefore a lot more street-beat than, say, *Heathen*, which by virtue of the fact that it was written in the mountains, had a much deeper, more majestic, tranquil kind of quality to it."

That *Reality* is steeped in the atmospheres, moods and environs of New York is apparent from even the most cursory glance at the lyrics: many of the songs find Bowie's characters struggling with the pressures and challenges of urban America – there are "city spires", "streets", "buildings", "sidewalks", "chrome",

"glass" and "metal" wherever you look, and the string of specific local references is unparalleled by any other collection of Bowie songs since perhaps *Aladdin Sane*: the lyrics on *Reality* bristle with references to Battery Park, Riverside Drive, the Hudson River, Ludlow and Grand, and New York itself, which is even name-dropped in Jonathan Richman's obligingly appropriate lyrics for 'Pablo Picasso'. "Downtown was always mythological," Bowie told the *Miami Herald* in 2003. "This is where the beatniks were, and the Beat poets, and the early songwriters, and the Dylans, and jazz started here as well. It's a musician writer's dream to go and live in the Village."

A strong sense of place has been a key creative priority throughout Bowie's career. "The albums that I've written out of character with the place where I'm living have often been failures," he mused. "They don't work so well, it's very odd. Still, [*Reality*] is not my 'New York album'. I didn't want it to be saying 'This is what New York's like right now.' There really was no through-line; it is just a collection of songs. Because of the way that Tony and I work together, there's some kind of continuity throughout, but that's more in the style of production. There was very little struggle to find out what would be right for the album. In all, I think we only left off two or three songs."

Given the wider geopolitical background against which the album was written and recorded, the resonance of 9/11 and its wide-ranging after-effects could not help but be felt on *Reality*. "The irrational feelings that you get on a day-to-day basis, living here since 9/11, have left a decided mark on this record," Bowie told *Blender*, but at the same time he was keen to point out that *Reality* was not "about" the terrorist attacks any more than it was about New York. "I didn't want to get crippled by all the events of the last couple of years," he told *Interview* magazine. "I didn't want what was going on in the world to overtake me and carry me to a place where I just couldn't work anymore. I've seen that happen before to people around me. I felt like I was becoming a passive spectator of everything that was happening, so there was an urgency to my need to pin down this particular moment in time."

Over and above specific circumstances of geography and politics, *Reality* approaches many of the ideas already explored by *Heathen*, albeit in a different, perhaps more optimistic spirit. "This album is a counterpoint to the idea of a spiritual search," David explained. "It started off as a random collection of songs – just whatever I was writing at the moment – that express how I feel right now, in this time. But afterwards, reflecting on the work itself, there are recurrent themes: the sense of anxiety about the times that we're living through and a strong sense of place. It was unwitting, though, because I wasn't planning on doing that."

And so, once again, *Reality* finds Bowie dismantling and reassembling the imponderable questions he has addressed throughout his career as a writer. "Writing this record … was almost like remaking something out of the bits and pieces that have been left after this great, awful upheaval," he explained. "I'm doing it metaphysically with my songs, grabbing these artefacts and putting them together in a quite substantial manner so that there's something there that I recognize as a truth. It's just a human trait to want to continually make a bridge between separate things, to want to forge links. It comes from our desperate need to find a truth to get us through to the next day. But these days, everything we create and put together as true is almost immediately debunked. That's what's so slippery. I suppose the positive thing about creating these anchors and watching them be torn apart is that the process helps us understand the chaos that is the actuality of our existence."

A prevalent theme on the album appears to be the debasement of the very concept of "reality" in western culture. Bowie has always been fascinated by the media's provocatively corruptible relationship with real events, a syndrome pushed to new extremes during the early years of the 21st century by the televising of wars and terrorist atrocities between the commercial breaks. More than ever, reality has become a subjective commodity in the hands of the headline-makers and politicians who massage the facts into whatever shapes suit their requirements; and, amid an atmosphere of galloping disenfranchisement which shrugs impotently as an unelected president declares war on the basis of an expedient fiction, the only democratic process for which the populace seems to retain any enthusiasm is to be found in the mind-numbing bread and circuses of 'Reality TV', which purports to convey unmediated truth but is, for any number of reasons, anything but real.

"I feel that reality has become an abstract for so many people over the last twenty years," Bowie told *Sound On Sound*. "Things that they regarded as truths seem to have just melted away, and it's almost as if we're thinking post-philosophically now. There's

nothing to rely on any more. No knowledge, only interpretation of those facts that we seem to be inundated with on a daily basis. Knowledge seems to have been left behind and there's a sense that we are adrift at sea. There's nothing more to hold onto, and of course political circumstances just push that boat further out." This, as he explained to *Interview* magazine, was a concern that informed the ironic title and subject matter of *Reality*: "This is probably a period when, more than any other time, the idea that our absolutes are disintegrating is manifest in real terms. Truths that we always thought we could stand by are crumbling before our eyes. It really is quite traumatic."

David also reiterated the musings about the chaotic breakdown of the hierarchy of information that he had first mentioned at the time of *1.Outside*: "We live in a world where every headline is famous for 15 minutes. You know: 'At War With America', 'Britney Spears Wears A T-Shirt', 'Saddam Is Still On The Loose' – they all get the same space, the same time. It creates a situation where all news seems equally important. I don't know whether that's a good thing or a bad thing. If you have an inquiring mind, you can really pick through it all and find some semblance of the things that you want to find. But I think, for most people, the process is just so fundamentally overwhelming that they'll accept whatever they happen to be looking at that evening."

From these considerations arise the vignettes of stranded individuals, bewildered lives and disappointed dreams that make up much of *Reality*. "I wonder about the great sense of indifference that seems to be creeping into the culture," Bowie mused. "I think at least partially it has to do with the paralyzing factor of having to wade through so much information to arrive at some approximation of what is really happening. But it also has something to do with this feeling amongst people that the power has totally been taken away from them, that whatever they say is not going to affect the course of events. I imagine part of the appeal of 'reality shows' is that people suddenly feel like they have a voice – they can say 'Number three is a good dancer,' 'Number four has a better ass!'"

Despite this bleak outlook, Bowie was at pains to stress that he intended *Reality* to be a more positive album than *Heathen*, even while describing the defiant optimism of 'New Killer Star' as "essentially just something to hang onto." The impulse to discover a renewed sense of optimism was, he told *Interview*, a result of becoming a parent for the second time: "You see, as much as the album is trying to create anchors that I know actually aren't there, there are also these devices that I need to put into my life so that my daughter has the impression from her dad that she has some kind of future. I can't talk about negativity in the same way as I would have done before she was born – every time I say, 'The world is fucked up and not worth living in,' she's going to look at me and say, 'Well, thanks for bringing me into it.' I'm morally obliged to find whatever out there is worth living for." This was a theme to which Bowie returned repeatedly in interviews during 2003. In the *Miami Herald* he confessed: "To be quite honest, I don't feel particularly positive or optimistic about things, but I try to redirect that energy," while in *Word* magazine he insisted that the album was "not 'woe is me', it's not a *Diamond Dogs*. I want the ultimate feeling after hearing it to be a good feeling. That there is something to be said for our future and it will be a good future." In *Performing Songwriter* he pondered: "Maybe I wouldn't have bothered so much, or maybe this album wouldn't have had that half-hearted attempt to find the silver lining, if I didn't have my daughter. Because it's very easy for me to be quite nihilistic … I think that things are pretty much as they always have been for the last 25,000 years. I don't think we're really evolving much above the caveman sensibility. It's still about surviving and killing and looking after one's immediate family. Not much more than that has happened, frankly. Technologically, obviously things have moved along at a speed that we don't understand, nor can control, because our emotional and spiritual sides are so far behind our abilities to manufacture stuff. So I'm not very positive, but I have to change all that."

In all of these statements can be seen evidence of a new identity that had been gradually emerging in David Bowie since his full-time return to New York at the end of the 1990s: as had been demonstrated by his work for the Tibet House Trust, the Robin Hood Foundation, Artists For Literacy, War Child and a dozen other charitable organizations, by his increasing distaste for the Bush administration, and indeed by Iman's prominent role as ambassador for the United Nations High Commission for Refugees, the Bowies had by now become central figures among New York's liberal-intellectual elite. In this respect there was a growing sense that David's work, although seldom polemic in nature, was beginning to take its place alongside that of artists like Lou Reed and Woody Allen, as part of the humanitarian conscience of Manhattan culture.

However, as always, Bowie was at pains to point out that *Reality* makes no pretence to be a coherent or premeditated manifesto of ideas. "The album has no big point," he told *Interview*'s Ingrid Sischy. "It is an impression of quite fast snapshots. I'm still just feeling my way through. The problem I'm having is actually trying to find those flecks of light that I can truly believe in, and not just throw them in for the sake of trying to make my work a bit lighter. You know, in a few years my daughter is going to be asking, 'Is there a God, Dad?' Am I going to be able to resolve that issue for myself before then? I don't think so. Do I tell her about what obstacles I am confronting and how I stumble around in the dark about it? Do I present her with this kind of obstacle course right from the beginning? It's really hard to be able to tell the truth to your child when you're not absolutely sure what the truth is yourself."

When asked by the *Boston Globe* about his religious beliefs, Bowie intimated that the spiritual struggle that had been so manifest on *Heathen* was continuing unabated. "It's cowardly," he admitted of his own wavering conviction. "It's 'I believe in you, I don't believe in you, I believe in you, I don't believe in you.' I think, 'Make up your mind! Get off the fence!' But you know what? That kind of vacillation is just a byword in my spiritual life. It's terrible and I get racked with stress about this, but it always has been that way with me. Ever since I was a teenager, there has been this endless search. And as I get to those days of finality, it becomes less and less clear. The only thing I know is that none of the questions I ever ask will be answered, not in this lifetime. But it still doesn't stop me from asking." If *Reality*'s keynote is a determination to battle onward and upward in defiance of the spiritual anxiety that had dominated *Heathen*, then it might be argued that the album's key line is the couplet from 'New Killer Star': "All my idiot questions / Let's face the music and dance".

"*Reality*, to me, is about the lack of consciousness in people's lives these days; in other words, the denial of what is reality," suggested Tony Visconti. "Or maybe it's about being spiritually empty. But I can assure you he doesn't phone me up and say, 'Let's make an album about spiritual emptiness today.'"

The sense of our (and Bowie's, and the album's) endlessly ambiguous relationship with reality is emphasized by the strikingly odd packaging design, the result of a collaboration between *Heathen* typographer Jonathan Barnbrook and graphic artist Rex Ray, who had previously worked on the cover designs of 'hours...' and 2002's *Best Of Bowie*. Ray's artwork rejects the airbrushed cool and ostentatious intellectualism of the *Heathen* imagery in favour of a garish anime-style cartoon of Bowie, his familiar features distorted by the simplified lines, exaggerated hairstyle and outsized saucer eyes that are the trademarks of Japanese animation. The cartoon Bowie strides forward from an abstract background of scribbled shapes, ink-blots, daubs of paint, blobs, balloons and clip-art stars. "The album's packaging has a *Hello Kitty* feel to it," explained Bowie, referring to the kitsch Japanese cartoon character franchise. "It's an anime- or a manga-type character in an abstract background that plays off the whole inappropriateness and lovability of that whole cartoony world, with the word 'Reality' slapped against it. It is kind of a cheap punch, but it looks right. The typography for the album, too, looks almost hammy. It's just this idea that the word 'reality' has become so devalued. It's like it has been damaged, so we reconcile it, or we put the word 'virtual' in front of it to give it any sense. I don't know – maybe the word 'reality' has outlived its use." Asked about the album cover in another interview, he remarked more bluntly that "The whole thing has a subtext of 'I'm taking the piss, this is not supposed to be reality.'"

In the weeks prior to its release the album was promoted by BowieNet's "*Reality* Jukebox", which showcased online excerpts of each track, and by various publicity stunts like a CD-ROM feature released by the *Sunday Times*. However, in keeping with the vicissitudes of 2002's *Heathen* campaign, in most territories *Reality* was not supported by conventional single releases. 'New Killer Star' appeared as a CD single in Italy and Canada, but in the UK and elsewhere it was confined to a DVD-only single which appeared two weeks after the album's release. 'Never Get Old', originally intended as the second single, went no further than the promo CD stage before being reassigned as a downloadable "cyber-single" in the UK. Bowie gave every indication that he had lost interest in the singles market and was increasingly disdainful of the transient chart-fodder that dominated it. In 2002 he had made disparaging remarks about the British appetite for "Kylie and Robbie and *Pop Idol* and stuff like that. You can't get away from that when you hit the shore, so I know all about the cruise ship entertainment aspect of British pop." In 2003 he told Radio 1's Mark Radcliffe that "I'm not sure that many people these

days want to get something *out* of music – they just want something on in the background, whilst they're walking down the street, you know." In a world in which it had become increasingly difficult for any recording artist beyond the age of 30 to get radio airplay, and in which the singles market had dwindled to the extent that many high-street stores had stopped selling them, it was understandable that Bowie should have opted to turn his back on the world of singles and videos, and was instead keen to promote himself as an album artist for devotees of real music. (Nevertheless, his protest in 2003 that he was "not a singles artist" was somewhat confounded by a Channel 4 documentary in February 2004 which revealed that he was the UK's tenth biggest-selling singles act of all time.)

Reality was released in Europe and most other territories on 15 September 2003, and in America the next day. Following the precedent set by *Heathen*, the album initially appeared in two CD formats: a standard single disc, and a 2CD version in a card sleeve whose bonus disc featured the out-takes 'Fly' and 'Queen Of All The Tarts (Overture)', as well as the new studio recording of 'Rebel Rebel'. The Japanese version boasted an extra track in the form of 'Waterloo Sunset'. In the weeks and months following the initial release there would come a dizzying variety of further versions, beginning with the 'Tour Edition', whose release was staggered to coincide with the arrival of A Reality Tour in each new territory, beginning with the European release in November. This edition added 'Waterloo Sunset' and a DVD of the Riverside Studios cinema performance of *Reality* recorded on 8 September 2003 (December's Canadian 'Tour Version' differed in that the DVD only featured five songs). Next came the SACD release; indeed, 2003 was the year that SACD began to take off, EMI duly reissuing three classic Bowie albums – *Ziggy Stardust*, *Scary Monsters* and *Let's Dance* – with new remixes in September. In February 2004 Columbia released a trial version of *Reality* in the brand new DualDisc format, featuring a normal CD version of the album on one side of the disc and the 5.1 mix in DVD-Audio format on the reverse. Restricted to a trial market in the Boston and Seattle areas of the US, this version was of particular interest to collectors in that the DVD element also included a photo gallery and the otherwise unavailable *Reality* promotional film, featuring filmed clips to accompany 'Never Get Old', 'The Loneliest Guy', 'Bring Me The Disco King' and 'New

Killer Star'.

In Britain *Reality* was an immediate hit, entering the UK chart at number 3 (Starsailor's *Silence Is Easy* was at number 2, while The Darkness topped the chart with *Permission To Land*), marking the highest UK chart position for a new Bowie album since *Black Tie White Noise* a decade earlier. In other territories the news was similarly good: *Reality* went top ten in 20 countries, reaching number 3 in Germany and Austria, number 2 in France, Greece, Portugal, Russia and Norway, and topping the charts in Denmark and the Czech Republic. On *Billboard*'s European Top 100 Albums chart, *Reality* entered at number 1. By contrast, in the US it failed to match *Heathen*'s performance, although its number 29 peak was still a considerable improvement on *'hours…'* and *Earthling*, and 'New Killer Star' rapidly garnered the now seemingly obligatory Grammy nomination for "Male Rock Vocal Performance". A Brit Awards nomination for "Best British Male Artist" followed in 2004.

Critical reaction was overwhelmingly positive. The ever-predictable "best album since *Scary Monsters*" mantra was once again trotted out in reviews everywhere, but on this occasion the critics' short-term memory proved marginally better than usual, many recalling that they had also liked *Heathen* and remarking that *Reality* proved that it was no flash in the pan. "With each listen, *Reality* feels stronger than *Heathen*," said the *Miami Herald*, "That's two good ones in a row." *Dotmusic*'s online review went further, claiming that "If *Heathen* was a little overpraised by relieved critics, then *Reality* is a more deserving case. Now we can all relax a little and get used to Bowie being back in the zone … Not one to miss an opportunity, he doesn't stray far from the template he set up on *Heathen* … But the songs are better." In conclusion: "Bowie's best since *Scary Monsters*, yet again."

Mojo's David Sheppard welcomed "the sound of an artist engaging with his muse rather than desperately wedging his songwriting through this or that stylistic hoop", concluding that *Reality* was "almost certainly Bowie's best album for 20 years." In the *Mail On Sunday*, Tim De Lisle noted approvingly that "this record pulsates with creative vigour", offering "a gleaming showcase for his voice, or rather voices. Bowie has always been several people and most of them are here." Noting the melancholy preoccupations of the lyrics, David Sinclair in the *Times* welcomed "an album which could mark the opening of a rich seam, provided his bleak cast of mind does not

get the better of him". *Q*'s Garry Mulholland noted "the vague references to current violent events contained within the likes of 'Fall Dog Bombs The Moon' and 'New Killer Star'", and concluded that "If Bowie's great '70s era was buoyed by a reckless hedonist adventure followed by an elegantly exhausted ennui, then the best of *Reality* sounds like a man coming to terms with what was lost in those mad years and the saving graces of love and stability." The result, he considered, was "Bowie's best music since *Scary Monsters*."

The *Boston Globe* remarked on the album's sense of spiritual anxiety, noting that "There's a restlessness to much of the music that not only makes for a great album but suggests that Bowie is struggling more than ever for answers." *Rolling Stone*'s Anthony DeCurtis found the album "intriguing", declaring that "With co-producer Tony Visconti, Bowie toughens up his sound, sawing at the edges of Jonathan Richman's 'Pablo Picasso' and, on 'New Killer Star', reclaiming the insinuating guitar propulsion he'd loaned to Lou Reed when he produced *Transformer*." The *NME*'s Tim Wild commended *Reality*'s "sweet collection of songs", singling out 'Bring Me The Disco King' "a true thing of beauty – dark NY jazz, delivered with the confidence of a man who knows he can do exactly what he wants." In the *Guardian*, Caroline Sullivan judged *Reality* "touching, intelligent and – a bonus – listenable", suggesting that "the rocking archness of 'New Killer Star' and the haunted, look-back-in-anger mood of 'Bring Me The Disco King' show why he still merits the consideration not enjoyed by grunts like the Rolling Stones … Bowie's striking vocals are royally raging on a bruising cover of Jonathan Richman's 'Pablo Picasso', then frail and old as 'Disco King' and 'Days' fade out like wisps of smoke."

A rare voice of dissent was Adrian Thrills in the *Daily Mail*, who conceded that "Bowie's loud-and-direct approach is largely a success," but found the cover versions "disappointing" and "lacklustre" and worried that "there are also times when *Reality* veers too closely to Tin Machine, his ill-fated roots-rock band of the early Nineties; the instrumentation, while capably anchored by bassist Gail Ann Dorsey [sic] and drummer Sterling Campbell, is often dense and cluttered. My initial suspicion is that many of these songs might have benefited from a less adorned approach." Even so, he believed that "*Reality* finds Bowie with a renewed sense of purpose" and was "his most passionate offering in years."

More representative of the prevailing critical opinion was an eloquent review by Mim Udovitch in the *New York Times*, who noted approvingly that "*Reality* is more than a bit thrusty", praising "the impeccable production of Tony Visconti", the "buried, exultant background vocals, random discordant touches and vibrant, layered arrangements", and the sense of immediacy that "makes you feel that Mr Bowie and his spectacularly hard-rocking band might be about to materialize in your living room ready for an encore." Udovitch went on to suggest that Bowie's ongoing dialogue with his personal beliefs "conveys the sense of an urgently felt personal communication", asserting that "The burst of bitter energy that results from this struggle is exhilarating rather than depressing. It is also moving," and concluding that "It's a rather singular accomplishment that *Reality* makes the personal contemplation of mortality sound so crashingly, defiantly vital … In short, it has all the alchemy of a great rock record – songs about death that were made to be played loud and live."

Uncut's Chris Roberts rejoiced in Bowie's reclamation of straight-ahead pop-rock as a vessel for his unique songwriting talent: "Over its stomping drums and squalling guitars he drapes lovely, left-handed songs, rich with unexpected angles, daring detours and words which muse over mortality yet emerge seeming upbeat. *Reality* is lyrically mournful; musically euphoric. It's pop, frisky pop, but with plenty of couplets about how everything falls away … the album's littered with quips and sighs about time passing … It's a very, very good sexy-angst album. For real."

As Roberts rightly points out, one of *Reality*'s triumphs is its successful fusion of intelligent songwriting with a reinvigorated sense of rock attack: as Bowie's "thrusty" soundbite had indicated, *Reality* emerges as a more primal piece of work than the delicate, self-consciously artful *Heathen*. It's noticeable that while he had cited such influences as Richard Strauss and Gustav Mahler during the *Heathen* sessions, at the time of *Reality* much of his talk was of The Dandy Warhols, Grandaddy, Radiohead (whom he described as "awesome" and "the best band around") and Blur (whose 2003 album *Think Tank* he judged "a first class piece of work"). In this respect the two albums bear a similar relationship to that between *1.Outside* and *Earthling*, or *Hunky Dory* and *Ziggy Stardust*: as is so often the case in Bowie's career, two consecutive albums share the same thematic and musical bloodline, but once again the second of the pair finds the cerebral and ethereal making certain concessions to the visceral. This certainly doesn't mean that *Reality* is in any way less intelligent or less finely wrought than its predecessor; merely that it catches Bowie in the more instinctive songwriting mode that periodically alternates with his more self-absorbed phases. The result is an album that seems at first sight to offer less complexity and fewer sonic layers than *Heathen*, but at the same time deploys a greater abundance of catchy hooks and buoyant pop-rock atmospherics: *Reality* is Bowie's most immediately melodic album in many a long year, positively bursting with infectious riffs and memorable tunes. The swaggering guitars of 'New Killer Star', the fabulous soul-funk of 'She'll Drive The Big Car', the deliciously catchy hooks of 'Never Get Old', and the final hypnotic brilliance of 'Bring Me The Disco King' effortlessly take their place among the Bowie classics.

But *Reality*'s masterstroke is that despite its warmer, more approachable atmosphere, it sacrifices none of *Heathen*'s artistic sensibility; its lasting value lies not just in its infectious melodies and evocative lyrics, but in the exquisitely judged oddness of its sonic textures, from the deranged guitar wobbles underpinning the riffs to the proliferation of weird and wonderful percussion effects, defiantly strange washes of synthesizer, Stylophone, sax and harmonica, and the joyously brilliant piano virtuosity of Mike Garson. As on *Heathen*, Tony Visconti's guiding hand is much in evidence, giving full rein to Bowie's experimental spirit while simultaneously imposing the discretion, economy and de-cluttering that allow the music to breathe, enabling Bowie to inhabit the songs with a dramatic sense of intimacy and immediacy. The lyrics are by turns dignified, intelligent, funny and moving, the two cover versions converging immaculately with the mood and intent of Bowie's own compositions. *Reality* finds Bowie returning, as he put it, "to the themes that have gnawed at me since I was a teenager – trying to find a spiritual connection, a sense of isolation, and a vague futurism." The result is not just a worthy successor to *Heathen*, but a substantial addition to the canon. *Reality* is a fine, forthright collection of terrific songs, delivered with all the confidence and panache of Bowie's greatest work.

(ii) SOUNDTRACK ALBUMS

The only individual tracks listed are those in which Bowie is directly involved. "Various Artists" compilation soundtracks are only included if they feature otherwise unavailable recordings or mixes.

JUST A GIGOLO
Jambo Records JAM 1, June 1979

'Revolutionary Song' (4'41")

CHRISTIANE F. WIR KINDER VOM BAHNHOF ZOO
RCA BL 43606 (Germany), April 1981
EMI 7243 5 33093 2 9, July 2001

'V-2 Schneider' (3'10") / 'TVC15' (3'32") / '"Helden"' (6'05") / 'Boys Keep Swinging' (3'16") / 'Sense Of Doubt' (3'58") / 'Station To Station' (8'46") / 'Look Back In Anger' (3'05") / 'Stay' (3'21") / 'Warszawa' (6'15")

The soundtrack album from the 1981 German film is compiled from *Station To Station*, *Low*, *"Heroes"*, *Stage* ('Station To Station' only) and *Lodger*. Completists will value the album as the only CD source of the 7" edit of 'Stay' and the full-length '"Helden"'. Despite being heavily imported from Germany and from France (where it was called *Christiane F. 13 Ans, Droguée, Prostituée*), Italy (where it became *Christiana F. Noi Ragazzi Zoo Berlino*), and the United States (rather prosaically, *Christiane F. Children From Zoo Station*), the album was denied an official release in the UK until 2001, when it was finally issued as part of EMI's comprehensive milking of Bowie's back catalogue.

DAVID BOWIE IN BERTOLT BRECHT'S BAAL
RCA BOW 11, February 1982 [29]

'Baal's Hymn' (4'00") / 'Remembering Marie A.' (2'04") / 'Ballad Of The Adventurers' (1'59") / 'The Drowned Girl' (2'24") / 'The Dirty Song' (0'37")

Bowie's studio versions of the *Baal* songs are consid-

erably more elaborate than the sparse banjo-accompanied renditions in the BBC play itself. Recording took place in September 1981 at Berlin's Hansa Studios – Bowie's last major session at the venue to date – and according to producer Tony Visconti the atmosphere was "electrifying. We recorded the songs in the same way as they used to as well, with a German pit band, one player per instrument, all fifteen of them arranged in a semicircle."

Dominic Muldowney, who had composed the music for the BBC production, was hired to score full arrangements. David originally intended to sing live with the band, but according to Visconti "that was a technical impossibility because we didn't hear the arrangements until the last moment. So Muldowney conducted the scores with no vocal, then explained them to us after the event." Visconti adds that Bowie "wanted to record this as a souvenir. David said it wasn't going to be any big deal and probably wouldn't sell, but he felt it should be recorded for posterity." In fact the beautifully packaged EP sold remarkably well, reaching number 29 in the UK singles chart in a startling confirmation of Bowie's post-*Scary Monsters* commercial punch.

Adventurous spirits will find plenty of excitement and value in these recordings, particularly 'The Drowned Girl' with its Brechtian realignment of Gertrude's willow speech, and the heart-rending 'Remembering Marie A.', a bitter paean to the transience of earthly pleasure. The complete *Baal* EP has yet to be released on CD, although 'Baal's Hymn' and 'The Drowned Girl' were included on the 2003 reissue of *Sound + Vision*.

CAT PEOPLE
MCA MCF 3138, April 1982

'Cat People (Putting Out Fire)' (6'41") / 'The Myth' (5'09")

THE FALCON AND THE SNOWMAN
EMI America EJ 2403051, April 1985

'This Is Not America' (3'51")

ABSOLUTE BEGINNERS
Virgin V 2386, April 1986 [19]
Virgin VD 2514, April 1986 [19]

'Absolute Beginners' (8'00") / 'That's Motivation' (4'12") / 'Volare' (3'12")

• *Musicians:* David Bowie *(vocals),* Kevin Armstrong *(guitar),* Matthew Seligman *(bass),* Rick Wakeman *(piano),* Steve Nieve *(keyboards),* Neil Conti *(drums),* Luis Jardim *(percussion),* Janet Armstrong *(backing vocals),* Don Weller *(solo sax),* Gary Barnacle, Paul Weimer, Willie Garnett *(tenor saxes),* Andy MacKintosh, Don Weller, Gordon Murphy *(baritone saxes)* • *Recorded:* Abbey Road Studios, London • *Producers:* David Bowie, Clive Langer, Alan Winstanley *('Volare': David Bowie, Erdal Kizilcay)*

In addition to Bowie's three tracks, recorded in June 1985, *Absolute Beginners* includes an instrumental reprise called 'Absolute Beginners (refrain)', performed by Gil Evans. The single LP version (Virgin V 2386) omits 'Volare'.

LABYRINTH
EMI America AML 3104, July 1986 [38]

'Opening Titles Including Underground' (3'19") / 'Magic Dance' (5'10") / 'Chilly Down' (3'44") / 'As The World Falls Down' (4'50") / 'Within You' (3'29") / 'Underground' (5'57")

• *Musicians:* David Bowie *(vocals, backing vocals),* Robbie Buchanan *(keyboards, synthesizers and programming),* Will Lee *(bass, backing vocals),* Steve Ferrone *(drums, drum effects),* Dan Huff *(guitar on 'Magic Dance'),* Cissy Houston, Chaka Khan, Luther Vandross, Fonzi Thornton, Marcus Miller, Marc Stevens, Daphne Vega, Garcia Alston, Mary Davis Canty, Beverly Ferguson, A Marie Foster, James Glenn, Eunice Peterson, Rennele Stafford, Diva Gray *(backing vocals),* plus *(on 'Underground'):* Richard Tee *(acoustic piano and Hammond B-3 organ),* Bob Gay *(alto sax),* Albert Collins *(lead guitar),* Nicky Moroch *(rhythm guitar),* plus *(on 'As The World Falls Down'):* Nicky Moroch *(lead guitar),* Jeff Mironov *(guitar),* Robin Beck *(backing vocals),* plus *(on 'Chilly Down'):* Kevin Armstrong *(guitar),* Neil Conti *(drums),* Matthew Seligman *(bass),* Nick Plytas *(keyboards),* Charles Augins, Richard Bodkin, Kevin Clash, Danny John-Jules *(lead vocals),* plus *(on 'Opening Titles Including Underground'):* Ray Russell *(lead guitar),* Paul Westwood *(bass guitar),* Harold Fisher *(drums),* David Lawson *(keyboards),* Brian Gascoigne *(keyboards),* Trevor Jones *(keyboards)* • *Recorded:* Atlantic Studios, New York; Abbey Road Studios, London • *Producers:* David Bowie, Arif Mardin *('Opening Titles Including Underground': Arif Mardin, Trevor Jones; 'Chilly Down': David Bowie)*

Released in July 1986 to coincide with the US premiere, *Labyrinth* intersperses the film's six Bowie songs with Trevor Jones's incidental score. "Eye of newt and tongue of mole, David Bowie has become a troll," quipped *Melody Maker*, while the *NME* launched an ironic broadside with the announcement that "Most of us are familiar with David Bowie from his role as Vendice Partners in the sparkling musical comedy *Absolute Beginners*, but how many, I wonder, know that David is also a talented all-round entertainer and singer? While not yet at the stage where he feels confident enough to record and release a fully-fledged long player in its own right, David has been making his own, unmistakable contributions to other people's records since 1982."

"Jim [Henson] gave me a completely free hand," Bowie explained of the *Labyrinth* songs, which he recorded in mid-1985 before filming commenced. One track, 'Chilly Down', features the same core musicians as 'Absolute Beginners'. Typically of Bowie's work of the period, the recordings teeter on the precipice of disastrous over-manning, as a cursory glance at the appropriately labyrinthine credits will testify. Co-produced with *Tonight*'s Arif Mardin, the *Labyrinth* soundtrack is destined to remain on the periphery of Bowie's recorded legacy, which is a pity because its better tracks, like the same year's 'When The Wind Blows', hint at a fresh and energetic synthesizer-led sound of real passion and depth, far worthier of David Bowie than most of the overheated noises he was making on his official albums of the time.

WHEN THE WIND BLOWS
Virgin V 2406, November 1986

'When The Wind Blows' (3'32")

THE CROSSING
Chrysalis CDP 3218262, November 1990

'Betty Wrong' (3'45")

SONGS FROM THE COOL WORLD
Warner Bros 9362 450782, August 1992

'Real Cool World' (3'24")

THE BUDDHA OF SUBURBIA
Arista 74321 170042, November 1993 [87]

Not a true soundtrack album but a fully-fledged studio project, *The Buddha Of Suburbia* is included in section (i) of this chapter.

SHOWGIRLS
Interscope 926612, January 1996

'I'm Afraid Of Americans' (5'09")

LOST HIGHWAY
Interscope INTD 90090, February 1997

'I'm Deranged (Edit)' (2'40") / 'I'm Deranged (Reprise)' (3'49")

BASQUIAT
Island 524 260 2, March 1997

'A Small Plot Of Land' (2'48")

THE ICE STORM
Velvel VEL 79713, October 1997

'I Can't Read' (5'30")

STIGMATA
Virgin CDVUS 161, August 1999

'The Pretty Things Are Going To Hell' (4'45")

AMERICAN PSYCHO
Koch KOC-CD 8164, April 2000

'Something In The Air (American Psycho Remix)' (6'01")

INTIMACY
Virgin 7243 8100582 8 (France), March 2001

'Candidate' (2'57")

The soundtrack of this Anglo-French co-production, released in France as *Intimité*, includes 'The Motel' from *1.Outside*, but its main feature of interest for Bowie collectors is a new edit of 'Candidate', later included on 2004's *Diamond Dogs* reissue.

MOULIN ROUGE
Twentieth Century Fox/Interscope 493 035-2, May 2001

'Nature Boy' (3'25") / 'Nature Boy' (4'09")

In addition to Bowie's two versions of 'Nature Boy' (the second co-credited to Massive Attack), the soundtrack album of Baz Luhrmann's remarkable musical extravaganza features Beck's cover of 'Diamond Dogs' and the 'Elephant Love Medley', incorporating Nicole Kidman and Ewan McGregor's rendition of '"Heroes"'.

TRAINING DAY
Priority Records 7243 8 11278 2 7 (US), September 2001

'American Dream' (5'21")

CHARLIE'S ANGELS: FULL THROTTLE
Columbia/Sony 512306 2, June 2003

'Rebel Rebel' (3'09")

MAYOR OF THE SUNSET STRIP
Shout! Factory DK34096, March 2004

'All The Madmen (Live Intro/Original LP Version)'
(5'36")

The soundtrack album of this Rodney Bingenheimer biopic contains a rarity in the form of a poor-quality snippet of Bowie singing 'All The Madmen' at a private party during his American sojourn in February 1971. The short bootleg-style clip then segues into the original studio version of the track.

(iii) OTHER ARTISTS' ALBUMS

This section covers Bowie's contributions as a performer and producer to other artists' recordings. Catalogue number, release date and highest UK chart placing appear for each release. The only tracks listed are those in which Bowie is directly involved. Some albums, such as those by Lou Reed and Iggy Pop, are of considerable significance in Bowie's career and are discussed accordingly; for others, refer to the entries in Chapter 1.

Also included are albums by the likes of Philip Glass, The Spiders and The Cybernauts, which are of interest despite having no direct Bowie involvement.

ALL THE YOUNG DUDES *(Mott The Hoople)*
CBS 65184, September 1972 [21]

'Sweet Jane' / 'Momma's Little Jewel' / 'All The Young Dudes' / 'Sucker' / 'Jerkin' Crocus' / 'One Of The Boys' / 'Soft Ground' / 'Ready For Love/After Lights' / 'Sea Diver'

The genesis of Bowie's relationship with Mott The Hoople is covered under 'All The Young Dudes' in Chapter 1. Sessions for the album, which was produced by Bowie and Mick Ronson, began on 14 May 1972 at Olympic Studios, resuming at Trident in June and July. 'Dudes' aside, Bowie's influence is less marked than on the contemporaneous *Transformer*, although unsurprisingly the cover of 'Sweet Jane' was his idea. "I thought I was going to have to contribute a lot of material," David told Charles Shaar Murray. "Now they're in a wave of optimism and they've written everything on the LP bar that one Lou Reed song and the 'Dudes' single."

Ian Hunter described Bowie as "one of the few people who can walk in and there is magic in the room. He has a very inquisitive mind, he's fast, and you feel that the guy knows more than you do so you put yourself in his hands." His admiration of Bowie remains undiminished, but their relationship was always tempered by the knowledge that each had something to offer the other: "He sucks, like Dracula," Hunter told the Gillmans. "He sucks what he can get and then he moves on to another victim." In this instance it seems likely that what Bowie craved was the secret of Mott's legendary rapport with a live audience. "I think he was upset because he never had riots," Hunter said. "People were too polite to riot at his concerts." Bowie admitted that when he saw Mott in concert he was impressed by their "integrity and naïve exuberance ... I couldn't believe they could command such an enormous following and not be talked about." Following Bowie's involvement public recognition beckoned, although Hunter's mistrust of Tony Defries put paid to plans for David to produce the band's next single in New York at the end of 1972.

'All The Young Dudes' launched Mott The Hoople before a mainstream audience, and thereafter they proved that their native talent wasn't to be underestimated; their next LP *Mott* reached number 7, by far their biggest hit in the album charts. Having parted company with Bowie and released his own solo debut, Mick Ronson joined the band in 1974, continuing in partnership with Ian Hunter long after the band split in December of the same year.

TRANSFORMER *(Lou Reed)*
RCA Victor LSP 4807, November 1972 [13]

'Vicious' / 'Andy's Chest' / 'Perfect Day' / 'Hangin' Round' / 'Walk On The Wild Side' / 'Make Up' / 'Satellite Of Love' / 'Wagon Wheel' / 'New York Telephone Conversation' / 'I'm So Free' / 'Goodnight Ladies'

Ever since his first meeting with Lou Reed in September 1971, Bowie had been intent on working with his idol. When Reed first heard *Hunky Dory* he declared, "I knew there was somebody else living in the same areas I was." Not surprisingly, he "especially loved" 'Queen Bitch'. As Reed's biographer Victor Bockris explains, "In Bowie, Reed would find a collaborator as important as Warhol – only much more commercial."

Reed had quit the Velvet Underground in September 1970 after finishing work on *Loaded*. In 1971 he signed a deal with RCA's Dennis Katz – the same executive who contracted Bowie to the label – and in January 1972 he was in London to record his solo debut album *Lou Reed*. By general consensus the album was a minor disaster, a collection of warmed-over Velvet Underground rejects on which Reed didn't even play guitar, badly served by Richard Robinson's lacklustre production. *Lou Reed* was coldly received within RCA, but Dennis Katz later explained that the company "had a lot of faith in Bowie, so they were willing to take a shot on another album, assuming he was working with Lou." The result was *Transformer*, one of the classic albums of the 1970s and one of the essential Bowie collaborations.

Reed flew back to London in July 1972, making a guest appearance at David's Royal Festival Hall gig within hours of his arrival. Work began on *Transformer* at Trident later the same month and continued into August, between Bowie's commitments on the Ziggy Stardust tour and Mott The Hoople's *All The Young Dudes*. Like that album, *Transformer* was co-produced by Bowie and Mick Ronson, although several sources,

including Reed himself, have suggested that the governing hand was Ronson's. "*Transformer* is easily my best-produced album," he told the *NME*. "That has a lot to do with Mick Ronson. His influence was stronger than David's, but together as a team they are terrific." For his part, Bowie was keen to dispel the idea (not uncommon at the time) that he was annexing Reed and turning him into an imitation of himself. "All that I can do is make a few definitions on some of the concepts of some of the songs and help arrange things the way Lou wants them," he explained.

The combination of the sensitive, non-confrontational Bowie and the uptight, sarcastic Reed made for a volatile atmosphere in the studio. According to Angela Bowie, Lou "blew up at David and Ronno in the studio one day during the *Transformer* sessions; I made a beeline for the door as soon as he exploded...". Reed later told reporters that working with David had been "a lot of fun, but when he gets drunk he thinks he's Ziggy." At this stage in his career getting drunk was as far as Bowie would go, whereas Ken Scott recalls that Reed was "out of his skull, permanently ... completely wrecked" throughout the *Transformer* sessions.

"I love what he did on *Transformer*," said Reed thirty years later of Bowie's contribution to the album. "That's why it came out that way. What Mick Ronson did, the strings for example, were also pretty good for a little guy from Hull. He was a talented guy ... which was amazing cause you could not understand a word when he was talking."

Musicians were recruited from both the Bowie and Reed camps: the vocal quartet included future *Aladdin Sane* backing singer Juanita "Honey" Franklin. The album also featured 'Space Oddity' bassist Herbie Flowers who, in addition to providing the classic bassline to 'Walk On The Wild Side', played string bass and tuba. David's quondam saxophone tutor Ronnie Ross was enlisted to play on 'Walk On The Wild Side', while Mick Ronson provided guitar, piano and recorders.

"Last time they were all love songs," remarked Reed of the album, "this time they're all hate songs." Emboldened by the down-at-heel glamour and sexual freedoms of Bowie's circle, Reed produced a cycle of sharply observed vignettes of eccentrics, lowlifes and lovers. "Writing songs is like making a play and you give yourself the lead part," he explained at the time, suspiciously echoing David's *modus operandi*. "And you write yourself the best lines that you could. And you're your own director … I'm always checking out people I know I'm going to write songs about. Then I become them. That's why when I'm not doing that, I'm kind of empty. I don't have a personality of my own. I just pick up other people's personalities."

"Lou loved Soho, especially at night," David revealed. "He thought it was quaint compared to New York. He liked it because he could have a good time and still be safe. It was all drunks and tramps and whores and strip clubs and after-hours bars, but no-one was going to mug you or beat you up. It was very twilight." This is the world that drips from every note of *Transformer*, which inhabits a demi-monde of trashy street-life that is an intoxicating melee of Velvet Underground and *Ziggy Stardust*. Indeed, Reed's happy-go-lucky approach to sexuality was quite prepared to drift in a fashionable direction, and *Transformer*, title and all, systematically toys with provocative notions of gender-reversal. Reed briefly reinvented himself as a glammed-up creation in Freddi Burretti suits, black velvet and rhinestones, heavy eye-shadow and black lipstick. Immortalized in Mick Rock's *Transformer* sleeve photo (shot in concert at the King's Cross Happiness Cinema), it was a look that Tim Curry would co-opt for *The Rocky Horror Show* a year later. Before long, however, Reed hardened the glam image into his famous "Phantom of Rock" persona. "I did three or four shows like that, and then it was back to leather," he said some time later. "We were just kidding around – I'm not into make-up."

"People like Lou and I are probably predicting the end of an era," Bowie told journalists. "Any society that allows people like Lou and me to become rampant is pretty well lost. We're both very mixed-up, paranoid people – absolute walking messes."

Transformer was released in November 1972 to mixed reviews. *Fusion* announced that, in Bowie and Ronson, "Lou Reed has found the perfect accompaniment to such flights of fancy that he's been lacking since John Cale went his own way", whereas Nick Kent of the *NME* considered the album "a total parody of Reed's whole style". Many American reviews were stacked against the album because of a personal grievance: Lisa Robinson, the partner of *Lou Reed*'s ousted producer Richard Robinson, was a rock writer who ran a journalists' collective in New York, and she encouraged colleagues to pan the album in print. "What's the matter with Lou Reed?" wrote Ellen Willis in the *New Yorker*. "*Transformer* is terrible – lame, pseu-

dodecadent lyrics, lame, pseudo-something-or-other singing, and a just plain lame band." However, quality will out. *Transformer* reached number 13 in Britain and a respectable enough 29 in America, and is rightly regarded today as one of the great rock albums.

After completing *Transformer* Bowie and Reed drifted apart and, for the next couple of decades, were rarely close. Victor Bockris records a quarrel in New York in 1974, while the pair's very public altercation in a Kensington restaurant in April 1979 is well documented. Happily, all differences had been resolved by the time of Reed's guest appearance at Bowie's fiftieth birthday concert in January 1997. "So many things have changed in both our lives," said David, "and we're both just more open to other people than we were before." David and Iman became close friends with Reed and his partner Laurie Anderson, and Bowie subsequently contributed a guest vocal to Reed's 2003 album *The Raven*.

A 2002 reissue of *Transformer* (RCA 65132) added Lou Reed's previously unreleased acoustic demos of 'Hangin' Round' and 'Perfect Day'.

RAW POWER (*Iggy And The Stooges*)
CBS 32083, May 1973

'Search And Destroy' / 'Gimme Danger' / 'Your Pretty Face Is Going To Hell' / 'Penetration' / 'Raw Power' / 'I Need Somebody' / 'Shake Appeal' / 'Death Trip'

September 1971 saw Bowie's first encounter with James Jewel Osterberg, alias Iggy Pop, the Bacchanalian vocalist with hardcore Michigan-based outfit The Stooges. His stage name was derived from a combination of The Iguanas, the band he had joined in 1964, and a Michigan junkie called Jim Popp. After drumming for a series of acts including Junior Wells, Buddy Guy and The Shangri-Las, he formed The Psychedelic Stooges in 1967 and earned a growing reputation as America's wild man of rock.

Having made two explosive proto-punk albums, The Stooges disbanded in August 1971 amid a slew of "artistic differences" and drug abuse. When Bowie met him, Iggy had already been written off by many as a spent force, infamous merely for his violent stage antics and charges of indecent exposure. In February 1972, at the beginning of the Ziggy Stardust tour, Bowie persuaded Tony Defries to fly Iggy to London, where he became a permanent member of the

MainMan retinue. Together with Lou Reed, Iggy was paraded before American journalists at Bowie's press conference at the Dorchester Hotel on 16 July, by which time David had encouraged The Stooges to re-form (newcomer James Williamson took over from guitarist Ron Asheton, who moved onto bass to replace the sacked Dave Alexander). The previous day the band had played an orgiastic gig at the King's Cross Cinema, which has since been described as the birth of punk rock. "The total effect was more frightening than all the Alice Coopers and *Clockwork Orange*s put together," wrote the *NME*'s Nick Kent, "simply because these guys weren't joking."

Fortified by a management deal with MainMan and a two-album contract with CBS, The Stooges became the third act in succession to be rescued from the doldrums by Bowie's patronage. Tony Defries was keen that Bowie should produce the album but Iggy declined, insisting that it was a project he had to tackle himself. Ensconced in CBS's London studios in August 1972, they began recording a new set of songs which ran the gamut of Iggy's nihilistic proto-punk vision. When Defries heard the maniacal results he was horrified. "Defries freaked!" Iggy later recalled. "It was all far too violent to be associated with David!" The manager decreed that, with the exception of 'Search And Destroy' and the basic riff for 'Tight Pants' (which became 'Shake Appeal'), the band must start again from scratch. "So we went in the studio and did the record, one helluva motherfucking record," Iggy later explained. "I don't think anybody from MainMan ever came down to that studio, we just did it ourselves. Bowie was never in the studio."

The result was *Raw Power*, the hardcore cult classic released in May 1973 under the revised band name "Iggy And The Stooges", featuring cover photography shot by Mick Rock at the King's Cross gig. Bowie's only direct involvement was in mixing the album, a task he undertook with Iggy on 24-25 October 1972 at Hollywood's Western Sound Studios during his first US tour. Iggy's lack of experience at the recording stage had left very few options for mixing. "He brought the 24-track tape in," Bowie recalled. "He had the band on one track, lead guitar on another and him on a third. Out of 24 tracks there were just three tracks that were used. He said, 'See what you can do with this.' I said, 'Jim, there's nothing to mix.' So we just pushed the vocal up and down a lot." Ron Asheton later disowned "Bowie and Iggy's cocaine artsy-fartsy mix", complaining that "We did a rough mix when we recorded the album and it was much, much better," and that Bowie had "just fucked that album up, really fucked it!" On the other hand, Iggy Pop himself was happy with the result, later saying that by comparison with the band's original mix "I think what David and I came up with at those sessions was better … I think he helped the thing. I'm very proud of the eccentric, odd little record that came out." In 1998 Iggy remixed *Raw Power* once again, and the result – an even more frightening hail of noise than the original – was greeted by most reviewers as an improvement. Bowie, however, still prefers the 1972 mix: "It has more wound-up ferocity and chaos," he wrote 30 years later, "and, in my humble opinion, is a hallmark roots sound for what was later to become punk."

Although Bowie's magic touch had worked wonders for Lou Reed and Mott The Hoople, *Raw Power* didn't repeat the success, failing to chart on either side of the Atlantic. It was barely recognized at all until Iggy's post-punk rehabilitation a few years later: reissued in June 1977, *Raw Power* climbed to number 44 in the UK chart. But it was far too late to rescue The Stooges; after a US tour that had redefined the parameters of rock and roll excess, the group had split from MainMan and folded in 1974.

NOW WE ARE SIX *(Steeleye Span)*
Chrysalis CHR 1053, March 1974 [13]

'To Know Him Is To Love Him'

SLAUGHTER ON 10TH AVENUE *(Mick Ronson)*
RCA Victor APLI 0353, March 1974 [9]

'Growing Up And I'm Fine' / 'Music Is Lethal' / 'Hey Ma Get Papa'

Following the dissolution of The Spiders From Mars, Tony Defries was eager to groom Mick Ronson for solo stardom. "Mick always had a lot of girls screaming and reaching for him," recalled MainMan's Leee Black Childers, "and Tony saw this and thought there was money to be made." Ronson confirmed that Defries was more interested in his pin-up potential than in his musicianship: "they told me that I could be the next David Cassidy," he commented ruefully.

Bowie is often said to have had mixed feelings about Ronson's solo career; his then girlfriend Ava

Cherry tells the Gillmans that "Maybe David felt that Mick had betrayed him as far as he was trying to be the star. But he was very upset, very, *very* upset." Sensational though such back-stabbing theories might be, they hardly square with the fact that Bowie collaborated on three tracks for Ronson's album; the real cooling of their relationship came later. Indeed, Bowie was already aware of Ronson's solo aspirations during the latter stages of the Ziggy tour, and it was he who suggested the album's Richard Rodgers-penned title track: "I bought him an album containing it," David later wrote in *Moonage Daydream*, "and he spent some time taking it apart and arranging it for himself while alone in his hotel rooms. He asked me if I'd write a couple of songs for him, as writing wasn't really his forte, to which of course I agreed."

Produced and arranged by Ronson himself, *Slaughter On 10th Avenue* was recorded at the Château d'Hérouville directly after the *Pin Ups* sessions. Ronson enlisted Trevor Bolder, Aynsley Dunbar and Mike Garson to play on the album, but although Bowie was present at some of the sessions in August 1973 he didn't contribute to the recording. He did, however, write 'Growing Up And I'm Fine', and also co-wrote 'Hey Ma Get Papa' with Ronson and provided English lyrics for the Italian number 'Music Is Lethal'.

Slaughter On 10th Avenue was released in March 1974, a month ahead of *Diamond Dogs*, in a blaze of MainMan publicity which included a six-storey billboard in New York's Times Square. Ronson toured extensively to promote the album, which rapidly shot to number 9 in the UK chart. But despite his charisma and talent – the genuine excellence of his lead vocals is seldom acknowledged – Ronson was never comfortable as a frontman. "I'm more of an instrumentalist, more of a musician than I am a singer," he admitted later. "I was sort of fooling myself … and other people too." In February 1974 MainMan had begun filming a documentary about Ronson, capturing him in concert and revisiting old haunts and friends in Hull. The film was never released, stalling with Ronson's solo career. "He was pushed into [going solo] by Tony and the MainMan machine," said Bowie's hairstylist Suzi Fussey, who went on to marry Ronson. "It was a very hard thing to do after coming off something like David, and Mick wasn't ready."

Slaughter On 10th Avenue survives as a fine, upstanding album, handsomely showcasing one of rock's great guitar talents. On the basis of this album

and its admirable follow-up *Play Don't Worry*, the comparative failure of Ronson's solo career was one of marketing and not of talent. According to Childers, "Ronson wasn't Bowie and Tony just didn't know how to sell him."

The 1994 Mick Ronson compilation *Only After Dark* (GY003) included *Slaughter On 10th Avenue* and three live bonus tracks. The DeadQuick label's 1997 reissue of *Slaughter On 10th Avenue* (SMMCD 503) included four bonus live cuts.

WEREN'T BORN A MAN *(Dana Gillespie)*
RCA APL 1 0354, March 1974

'Andy Warhol' / 'Backed A Loser' / 'Mother, Don't Be Frightened'

At the time of the *Pin Ups* sessions David's former girlfriend Dana Gillespie, now a MainMan client, was playing Mary Magdalene in the West End production of *Jesus Christ Superstar*. Busy plugging her role in the forthcoming Ken Russell biopic *Mahler*, Tony Defries decreed that it was time for her to release a solo album. Although mainly produced by Robin Cable and Mick Ronson, *Weren't Born A Man* dusts down three tracks co-produced and arranged by Bowie in 1971, including Gillespie's idiosyncratic rendering of 'Andy Warhol', a song David had originally written for her and on which he provides guitar and backing vocals. Despite MainMan's attempts to market Gillespie as a hardcore lesbian outrage, *Weren't Born A Man* was a total failure which did nothing to ease the disintegration of Bowie's relationship with his management company.

The three Bowie-related tracks later reappeared on the 1994 Golden Years CD *Andy Warhol*.

PLAY DON'T WORRY *(Mick Ronson)*
RCA Victor APLI 0681, February 1975 [29]

'White Light/White Heat'

Mick Ronson's second solo album was recorded at Trident in 1974. This time Bowie's involvement was second-hand only, as Ronson exhumed the abandoned backing track of 'White Light/White Heat' recorded during the *Pin Ups* sessions. *Play Don't Worry* failed to repeat the success of its predecessor, but commands equal respect as a finely crafted album. The 1994 compilation *Only After Dark* (GY003) includes *Play Don't Worry* and three bonus tracks including Ronson's cover of 'Soul Love', recorded in December 1975, while the 1997 reissue on the DeadQuick label (SMMCD 504) adds nine bonus tracks, again including the 'Soul Love' cover.

Touring with Ian Hunter two months after the release of *Play Don't Worry*, Ronson gave an interview to Allan Jones in which he offered some outspoken opinions on his former employer, then holed up in Los Angeles in the depths of his cocaine period. "I just wish Dave would get himself sorted fuckin' out," Ronson said angrily. "He's totally fuckin' confused, that lad. I know he is. What he really needs is some good friends around him … I just wish he could be in this room right now, sat here, so I could kick some sense into him." Few, least of all Bowie himself, would now deny that Ronson's views were entirely justified, but it was as a result of this interview that relations between the two cooled severely for several years.

SPIDERS FROM MARS *(The Spiders)*
Pye NSPL 18479, 1976

Featuring no involvement whatsoever from Bowie or indeed Mick Ronson, and released to a deafening silence in 1976, *Spiders From Mars* saw Mike Garson, Trevor Bolder and Woody Woodmansey joining forces with vocalist Pete McDonald and guitarist Dave Black in an attempt to capitalize on former glories. Proceeds were donated to the Church of Scientology, to which Garson had converted Bolder and Woodmansey during their Bowie days. Despite (or perhaps because of) some remarkable sleeve-notes by *Melody Maker*'s Chris Welch ("Who are these men who bombarded our planet with an intergalactic rhythm? As their cosmic telephone rings, should we answer?"), the album was a flop. It was reissued on CD in June 2000 by Castle Music (ESMCD 894).

Woody Woodmansey went on to release a 1977 solo album called *U-Boat*, and later played on recordings by Art Garfunkel and Dexys Midnight Runners. Trevor Bolder found work with bands including Uriah Heep and Wishbone Ash. The pair were reunited in 1994 at the Mick Ronson Memorial Concert, later teaming up with members of Def Leppard to form The Cybernauts (see below).

THE IDIOT *(Iggy Pop)*
RCA Victor PL 12275, March 1977 [30]

'Sister Midnight' / 'Nightclubbing' / 'Funtime' / 'Baby' / 'China Girl' / 'Dum Dum Boys' / 'Tiny Girls' / 'Mass Production'

Ever since *Raw Power* Iggy Pop had remained a fixture in the MainMan retinue, often financially bailed out by Tony Defries and joining David in his prodigious drug blowouts during the American interlude of 1974-5. Although grateful for Bowie's patronage, Iggy was never happy billed as "a MainMan artist", later telling the *NME* that Tony Defries was "a sort of puppet master" with "this huge Colonel Tom Parker obsession … it was quite impossible for us to work together. He wanted me to be a puppet for stray projects, a film version of *Peter Pan*, things like that, but all he really cared for was making Bowie a star. He only kept me on to keep Bowie happy."

After splitting from Defries and embarking on an American tour commemorated by the live album *Metallic KO*, The Stooges disbanded in early 1974. In May 1975 David and Iggy, both at the height of their chemical insanity, made an abortive attempt to record some new tracks in Los Angeles (see 'Moving On' in Chapter 1). Later the same year, on the verge of a mental breakdown, Iggy voluntarily entered UCLA's Neuropsychiatric Institute with the intention of weaning himself off heroin with a methadone substitute. Bowie was one of his few visitors there, and although it was by no means a squeaky-clean Iggy who accepted David's invitation to join the Station To Station entourage in 1976, it was certainly a healthier one. During tour rehearsals Bowie, Iggy and Carlos Alomar composed 'Sister Midnight', destined for inclusion on Iggy's next album.

In late June, a month after the Station To Station tour ended in Paris, sessions commenced at the Château d'Hérouville Studios. David generally took the musical lead, composing and arranging the instrumental backings while Iggy wrote the lyrics on large sheets of paper on the studio floor, although positions were occasionally reversed: "Contrary to what people think, many ideas for the lyrics came from Bowie and many musical ideas came from me," Iggy later explained. The album was largely a two-man effort, with Bowie providing not only backing vocals but also playing guitar, synthesizers and saxophone. Other contributions came from guitarist Phil Palmer and

Bowie's rhythm section of Dennis Davis and George Murray.

In August the sessions moved briefly to Musicland Studios in Munich, where Bowie met his future collaborator Giorgio Moroder, the man responsible for much of the "Discomotorik" style that was taking Europe by storm and infusing David's new work. From there David and Iggy moved to Berlin's Hansa Studios, where they were joined by Tony Visconti for mixing and post-production. Visconti later recalled that the quality of the recordings was dubious and that the mixing was "a salvage job".

The Idiot marked the beginning of a year of unbridled creativity for both Iggy and David; by the autumn of 1977 they had produced no fewer than four albums. According to Visconti, the pair "just totally inspired each other", enjoying a "creative relationship" that provided mutual support as they embarked on the road to recovery: "They had some kind of pact or agreement to get themselves healthy." When David moved into his flat in Berlin's Hauptstrasse during the subsequent *Low* sessions, Iggy found an apartment in the same building.

"Bowie gave me a chance to apply myself, because he thinks I have some talent," Iggy later said of the sessions for *The Idiot*. "I think he respected me for putting myself in a loony bin." He freely admitted that Bowie "was my last ditch … We didn't have a band, there was just the two of us on that whole album, like a couple of little old ladies with knitting needles or something. David plays better Angry Young Guitar than any Angry Young Guitar Player I've ever heard, including [Stooges player] James Williamson."

Released in March 1977, *The Idiot* reached a modest number 30 in the UK and number 72 in America – Iggy's first chart entries in either country. The album's cover, a black-and-white photograph by Andy Kent (not by Bowie himself, as often reported) showing Iggy striking a tortured, stiff-limbed pose, was inspired by Erich Heckel's painting *Roquairol*, a disturbing image of lunacy housed in Berlin's Brücke museum and much admired by David and Iggy. "Roquairol" was an incurably insane character in *Titan*, a nineteenth-century German novel by Jean Paul, and Heckel's painting used as its model the artist's friend Ernst Ludwig Kirchner, a fellow founder of the Brücke school who also fell victim to mental illness. David would later pose for his own variation on the same picture for the sleeve of *"Heroes"*.

Because of David's unprecedented contribution at all levels, *The Idiot* is an essential acquisition for the Bowie enthusiast. As well as producing the album, he co-wrote and played on every track (offering even more compelling evidence than *Diamond Dogs* of his guitar ability), and provides unmistakable backing vocals throughout. Although imbued with Iggy Pop's unique personality the album sits incongruously among the rest of his work, and in many ways makes more sense as a Bowie project, a stepping stone between *Station To Station* and *Low*. More importantly it's a terrific album, and one that deserves deeper scrutiny than it receives from Bowie fans who know it primarily as the source of the original 'China Girl'.

The Idiot provided an influential template for many artists, most notably Joy Division, whose debut album *Unknown Pleasures* drew heavily on the industrial soundscapes and relentless percussion of tracks like 'Nightclubbing' and 'Mass Production'. When the band's troubled singer Ian Curtis was found hanged at his Manchester home on 18 May 1980, the album on his record player was *The Idiot*.

LUST FOR LIFE (*Iggy Pop*)
RCA PL 12488, September 1977 [28]

'Lust For Life' / 'Sixteen' / 'Some Weird Sin' / 'The Passenger' / 'Tonight' / 'Success' / 'Turn Blue' / 'Neighborhood Threat' / 'Fall In Love With Me'

Following the completion of the Iggy Pop tour in April 1977 (see Chapter 3), Bowie and Iggy convened at Berlin's Hansa By The Wall to begin work on Iggy's next LP. 'Turn Blue', 'Some Weird Sin' and 'Tonight' had been test-driven during the tour, and an album's worth of others soon followed. The *Lust For Life* sessions were completed within two and a half weeks, during which Iggy surpassed even David's reputation as a studio workaholic. Each vocal was cut live in one take.

"During that album, the band and Bowie'd leave the studios to go to sleep, but not me," said Iggy. "I was working to be one jump ahead of them for the next day … See, Bowie's a hell of a fast guy. Quick, quick. Very quick thinker, very quick action, very active person, very sharp. I realized that I had to be quicker than him, otherwise whose album was it gonna be?" There's a tacit implication here that *The Idiot* had not been Iggy's album, and indeed *Lust For Life* immediately proclaims itself a more independent work. The arrangements are freer, rockier and less delicately textured than one might expect from a pure Bowie product. Two of the songs, including the classic 'The Passenger', were written without input from David, although elsewhere the pattern remained that Iggy would write the lyrics to David's music. Bowie plays piano and, as on *The Idiot*, his backing vocals are unmistakable.

The band was retained from Iggy's tour, augmented by Bowie's right-hand man Carlos Alomar. Production was credited to "Bewlay Bros", who on this occasion were David, Iggy and engineer Colin Thurston. The sleeve photo, again by Andy Kent, provided a sharp contrast to the anguished posture on *The Idiot*: the straight portrait of a healthy, grinning Iggy sealed the album's tone of positivity, rebirth and success.

Lust For Life includes the original versions of 'Tonight' and 'Neighborhood Threat' (and of course the title track, which David added to his live set in 1996) and, lest we forget, it boasts three-quarters of the future Tin Machine. That in itself may not be anything to shout about, but *Lust For Life* certainly is – it's an exuberant, driving set of songs and remains Iggy Pop's highest-charting album.

TV EYE *(Iggy Pop)*
RCA PL 12796, May 1978

'TV Eye' / 'Funtime' / 'Sixteen' / 'I Got A Right' / 'Lust For Life' / 'Dirt' / 'Nightclubbing' / 'I Wanna Be Your Dog'

Culled from both stages of Iggy Pop's 1977 tour, *TV Eye* features Bowie on only four tracks ('TV Eye', 'Funtime' and 'Dirt', recorded on 21 March in Cleveland, and 'I Wanna Be Your Dog', recorded on 28 March in Chicago). Bowie co-produced and mixed the entire album at Hansa.

PETER AND THE WOLF
(Eugene Ormandy/Philadelphia Orchestra)
RCA RL 12743, May 1978

In December 1977 Bowie flew to New York to provide the narration for a new recording of Prokofiev's children's classic. He was RCA's third choice for the job behind Peter Ustinov and Alec Guinness, and later described the record as a Christmas present for his son. Released with Benjamin Britten's *The Young Person's Guide To The Orchestra* on side two, the album made number 136 in the US charts. While not to be compared with John Gielgud's definitive recording, Bowie's narration is not unaccomplished, and a fascinating curio from a period in which his other unlikely collaborations embraced figures as diverse as Marc Bolan, Bing Crosby and Marlene Dietrich.

SOLDIER *(Iggy Pop)*
Arista SPART 1117, January 1980 [62]

'Play It Safe'

BLAH-BLAH-BLAH *(Iggy Pop)*
A&M AMA 5145, October 1986 [43]

'Real Wild Child (Wild One)' / 'Baby, It Can't Fall' / 'Shades' / 'Fire Girl' / 'Isolation' / 'Cry For Love' / 'Blah-Blah-Blah' / 'Hideaway' / 'Winners And Losers' / 'Little Miss Emperor'

Between engagements on *Absolute Beginners* and *Labyrinth*, Bowie visited Iggy Pop in New York in November 1985. Impressed by the new songs Iggy had been developing with ex-Pistol Steve Jones, David offered to lend his co-writing and producing services for a new album, apparently declaring: "I can make this as commercial as hell." During a Christmas cruise in the Caribbean and a skiing trip in Switzerland, the two composed a new set of songs ready to take into Mountain Studios in May 1986. "We went to Gstaad with our respective women and had a skiing holiday which went on for three months," recalled David the following year. "I took a four-track up there. We wrote in the evenings and skied in the day, and then went down to Montreux and recorded *Blah-Blah-Blah* there. It worked out so well that I thought I'd record my album [*Never Let Me Down*] the same way."

Although not so heavily stamped with Bowie's influence as *The Idiot*, the third major Bowie/Pop collaboration was strongly informed by David's latest enthusiasms: joining Steve Jones were two of Bowie's recent conscripts, Kevin Armstrong and Erdal Kizilcay. At the time *Blah-Blah-Blah* was generally considered a more convincing demonstration of Bowie's talent than anything to be found on *Never Let Me Down*.

Blah-Blah-Blah charted in America at number 75, Iggy's greatest success in his home country since *The Idiot* a decade earlier. In Britain it was his best showing since *Lust For Life*, and gave him his first ever hit single in 'Real Wild Child'. Once again Bowie had come to his friend's commercial rescue, but many diehard Iggy fans regarded *Blah-Blah-Blah* as a sell-out. In recent years Iggy himself has been less than complimentary about the album, claiming that Bowie's influence was overpowering. There's certainly a sense in which the excellent but over-polished *Blah-Blah-Blah* was his own *Let's Dance*, heralding the dawn of a new, cleaned-up Iggy Pop who was fit to appear on *Top Of The Pops* and record duets with Deborah Harry.

LIVE IN EUROPE *(Tina Turner)*
Capitol ESTD 1, March 1988 [8]

'Tonight' / 'Let's Dance'

This live album includes Bowie's guest appearance at Tina's Birmingham NEC concert on 23 March 1985.

YOUNG LIONS *(Adrian Belew)*
Atlantic 7567 820992, July 1990

'Pretty Pink Rose' / 'Gunman'

In January 1990 Bowie recorded two tracks for his Sound + Vision guitarist Adrian Belew. "I didn't want to be seen as going back to being a sideman for David Bowie," explained the optimistic Mr Belew, "and what we decided was maybe it'd be good if David came and did something on my record to make sense of this touring." It's worth noting that the album also features a Belew composition called 'Looking For A UFO', which may have helped inspire Bowie's 'Looking For Satellites' a few years later.

"LOW" SYMPHONY *(Philip Glass)*
Point Music 438 150-2, 1993
Decca 475 075-2 PM2, August 2003 *(2CD set)*

'Subterraneans' / 'Some Are' / 'Warszawa'

Philip Glass, who had briefly collaborated with Bowie at a John Cale concert in 1979, composed and record-ed his *"Low"* Symphony in the spring of 1992. Glass had never before called one of his works a symphony, and confessed that there was "an implied ideological thrust" in the decision to confer the term on a work derived from a sphere alien to the classical establishment. "Talent and quality have the annoying habit of turning up in the strangest places," he explained. "In the question of Bowie and Eno's original *Low* LP, to me there was no doubt that both talent and quality were evident there – regardless of the fact that the music was written by men who had gone to art school and not a proper music school. My generation was sick to death of academics telling us what was good and what wasn't. So certainly all that was implied in my decision to write the *"Low"* Symphony."

Glass's concerns about the establishment reaction were well founded: several orchestras returned the completed score with comments to the effect that they didn't do rock'n'roll. "So basically, they didn't open the score," Glass observed. "They thought it was bass, drums, and David Bowie singing." The symphony was eventually recorded by the Brooklyn Philharmonic Orchestra at the composer's own Looking Glass Studios in New York, and released in 1993 on his Point Music label.

"I've taken themes from three of the instrumentals on the record and, combining them with material of my own, have used them as the basis of three movements of the symphony," Glass explained. "My approach was to treat the themes very much as if they were my own and allow their transformations to follow my own compositional bent where possible. In practice, however, Bowie and Eno's music certainly influenced how I worked, leading me to sometimes surprising musical conclusions. In the end I think I arrived at something of a real collaboration between my music and theirs."

As Glass's comments made clear, the *"Low"* Symphony acknowledges Brian Eno's contribution on an equal footing with Bowie's, and portraits of all three appear on the album's cover. Bowie was perceptibly flattered that his work had been realigned by an experimental practitioner of classical forms. The *"Low"* Symphony remains not only of interest to the Bowie enthusiast, but of genuine and intrinsic value in itself, playing to the strengths of Bowie's melodic sensibility as well as to Glass's familiar compositional techniques. The interpretation of 'Some Are' in particular is a classic piece of Glassian "accumulative" orchestration in the tradition of *Music In Twelve Parts* or

Koyaanisqatsi.

On 13 June 2002, a performance of the *"Low"* and *"Heroes"* symphonies by the London Sinfonietta at the Royal Festival Hall formed part of Bowie's Meltdown Festival programme. The two symphonies were reissued by Decca as a double CD set in August 2003.

SUCK ON THIS! *(Iggy Pop)*
Revenge TMIMIG 50, August 1993

'Raw Power' / '1969' / 'Turn Blue' / 'Sister Midnight' / 'I Need Somebody' / 'Search And Destroy' / 'TV Eye' / 'Dirt' / 'Funtime' / 'Gimme Danger' / 'No Fun' / 'I Wanna Be Your Dog'

This semi-official bootleg was recorded in Cleveland on 21 March 1977 – the same night as three of the tracks on *TV Eye* – and features Bowie on keyboards throughout. The same recording appears on the Iggy Pop box set *Night Of The Iguana* (Remedy Records REM 991004/3053862/WAG 378).

HEAVEN AND HULL *(Mick Ronson)*
Epic 4747422, May 1994

'Like A Rolling Stone' / 'Colour Me' / 'All The Young Dudes'

Mick Ronson's ferocious talent was destined never to burn as brightly as it had during his four-year association with Bowie, but his ongoing partnership with Ian Hunter and a string of impressive collaborations (lead guitar on Bob Dylan's all-star 1976 tour alongside artists like Joni Mitchell and Leonard Cohen, and later production work for acts as diverse as David Johansen, John Mellencamp and Morrissey) ensured a legacy to be reckoned with. Ronson's final solo album was released posthumously in 1994, featuring Bowie on three tracks alongside contributions from Joe Elliott, Peter Noone, Chrissie Hynde and John Mellencamp. Proceeds went to the T J Martell Foundation, a cancer charity. A promo CD, entitled *The Mick Ronson Story … Heaven And Hull* (Epic 6143) included a short interview with Bowie.

ANDY WARHOL *(Dana Gillespie)*
Golden Years GY001, 1994

'Andy Warhol' / 'Backed A Loser' / 'Mother, Don't Be Frightened'

This compilation, drawn from Dana Gillespie's albums *Weren't Born A Man* and *Ain't Gonna Play No Second Fiddle,* includes all three of the singer's Bowie-related recordings.

ONLY AFTER DARK *(Mick Ronson)*
Golden Years GY003, 1994

'Growing Up And I'm Fine' / 'Music Is Lethal' / 'Hey Ma Get Papa' / 'White Light/White Heat'

This double CD compiles Mick Ronson's solo albums *Slaughter On 10th Avenue* and *Play Don't Worry,* together with selected bonus tracks.

THE SACRED SQUALL OF NOW *(Reeves Gabrels)*
Upstart U20, September 1995 *(US)*

'You've Been Around' / 'The King Of Stamford Hill'

PEOPLE FROM BAD HOMES
(Ava Cherry And The Astronettes)
Golden Years GY005, 1995

'I Am Divine' / 'I Am A Laser' / 'Seven Days' / 'God Only Knows' / 'Having A Good Time' / 'People From Bad Homes' / 'Highway Blues' / 'Only Me' / 'Things To Do' / 'How Could I Be Such A Fool' / 'I'm In The Mood For Love' / 'Spirits In The Night'

From October 1973 until July 1974, Bowie dabbled with a project intended to launch the singing careers of his girlfriend Ava Cherry and schoolmate Geoffrey MacCormack. With the addition of Jason Guess, a friend of Cherry's from New York, the three were dubbed The Astronettes and made their debut as backing vocalists for *The 1980 Floor Show.* In the same month David began producing tracks with the threesome at Olympic Studios, using Aynsley Dunbar, Herbie Flowers and Mike Garson from the *Diamond Dogs* personnel plus *1980 Floor Show* and Arnold

Corns guitarist Mark Carr Pritchard.

The project ran out of steam as David became more involved with *Diamond Dogs,* and recording was postponed until the following year. With Ava Cherry and Geoffrey MacCormack (now billed as "Warren Peace") both permanent members of the Diamond Dogs entourage, recording recommenced at Philadelphia's Sigma Sound in July 1974 with the assistance of Bowie's musical director Michael Kamen. At around the same time it was reported that Ava was to play the role of Dorothy in a Broadway revival of *The Wizard Of Oz* (possibly the all-black adaptation *The Wiz*), but as Bowie's ghostwriter cheerily informed *Mirabelle* readers, "at the last minute she decided against the show and instead is now one of my back-up singer-dancers".

Although both MacCormack and Cherry continued to provide backing vocals at Bowie's concerts, the Astronettes project was abandoned. Over twenty years later MainMan's "Golden Years" range, also responsible for *Santa Monica '72* and *RarestOneBowie,* finally released a collection of the recordings under the title *People From Bad Homes.* The album contains much of interest, notably prototype versions of 'Scream Like A Baby' ('I Am A Laser'), 'Somebody Up There Likes Me' ('I Am Divine', included as a hidden track at the beginning of the CD), and Bowie's first stab at The Beach Boys' 'God Only Knows'. Also scattered throughout the album, and often mixed into the songs themselves, are snippets of studio chat during which David's voice can be heard. In truth, however, the mixing of the unfinished tracks is very basic, and on the evidence of this album Cherry and her male co-stars lack the accomplishment of most of Bowie's singing protégés. This is a fascinating set of recordings, capturing Bowie at a moment of musical transition between the funkier pedal-guitar tracks on *Diamond Dogs* and the softer soul numbers of *Young Americans,* but there's nothing here remotely as urgent or accomplished as his major work of the period.

"HEROES" SYMPHONY *(Philip Glass)*
Point Music PCHP 1824, May 1997
Decca 475 075-2 PM2, August 2003 *(2CD set)*

'"Heroes"' / 'Abdulmajid' / 'Sense Of Doubt' / 'Sons Of The Silent Age' / 'Neuköln' / 'V-2 Schneider'

In 1997 Philip Glass followed up his *"Low"* Symphony with the logical sequel. Again Brian Eno was given equal credit with Bowie, and again all three appeared on the sleeve. Glass, who now described *Low* and *"Heroes"* as "part of the new classics of our time", found himself writing to a different brief. Shortly after commencing work on the project he mentioned it to a friend, the avant-garde New York choreographer Twyla Tharp. "Straight away she wanted *"Heroes"* for her new dance company," Glass explained, "and soon after, we met with David. He immediately shared Twyla's enthusiasm and I found myself writing a symphonic score shortly to become a ballet." As a result of this development, the *"Heroes"* Symphony consists of six comparatively short movements. "I structured it differently," explained Glass. "And probably, without Twyla's needs taken into account, I would have ended the piece quietly. Basically, you write a piece to get everyone up and standing, so that's what I did."

Twyla Tharp's "emotionally charged" ballet opened in New York and embarked on an international tour in 1997. Meanwhile the *"Heroes"* Symphony received its concert premiere at London's Royal Festival Hall on 15 May, while the studio recording by the American Composers Orchestra was released the same month. Conceding that the symphony was "well performed" and "sumptuously recorded", *BBC Music Magazine* was sniffy about the proliferation of "stock Glass clichés ... the tedious arpeggiated triplets, the insistent doodling duplets, the minor mode, the contrary motion scales", and concluded that "only 'Abdulmajid' widens the scope."

Initial pressings of the Japanese release came with a bonus CD single (Point Music SADP-5) featuring a remix of '"Heroes"' by Aphex Twin which matched Bowie's original vocal to Glass's orchestration. In 1997 Bowie revealed that Glass had "asked me if I'll write with him a third symphony, so I think that's exciting. Kind of scary, because he's so in another world." In the ensuing years the two remained in contact through Bowie's use of the composer's Looking Glass Studios during the recording of albums like *'hours...'* and *Reality.* In 2003 Bowie said that "The last time we talked, Philip was quite keen that we actually write something together, or indeed that maybe I would have a go at writing something specifically for him to convert into a symphonic piece, but I haven't gotten round to doing anything like that."

On 13 June 2002, a performance of the *"Low"* and *"Heroes"* symphonies by the London Sinfonietta at the Royal Festival Hall formed part of Bowie's Meltdown

Festival programme. The two symphonies were reissued by Decca as a double CD set in August 2003.

THE MICK RONSON MEMORIAL CONCERT
(Various Artists)
Citadel CIT2CD, August 1997

On 29 April 1994, a year to the day after Mick Ronson's death, friends and colleagues gathered for a tribute concert at the Labbatt's Apollo, Hammersmith – formerly Hammersmith Odeon, venue of the final Ziggy Stardust gig 21 years earlier. Among those taking part were Glen Matlock, Steve Harley, Joe Elliott, Bill Wyman, Rolf Harris, Roger Daltrey, Trevor Bolder, Woody Woodmansey, Tony Visconti, Gus Dudgeon, John Cambridge, Benny Marshall, Dana Gillespie, Roger Taylor, Peter Noone and Ronson's close friend and collaborator Ian Hunter. The compère was Bob Harris, who had introduced many of the early Ziggy Stardust concerts and presented several of Bowie's BBC radio sessions in the 1970s. The event was directed and organized by long-term Bowie fan Kevin Cann, and proceeds went to the building of a stage in Ronson's home town of Hull.

A few feathers were ruffled by the one glaring absence from the concert. "It wasn't big enough, was it?" remarked Ian Hunter later. "Freddie's was big – David knew he'd be seen by a lot of people there." When a journalist from the French magazine *Rock & Folk* asked Bowie in 1998 why he didn't attend, it became clear that the decision hadn't been taken lightly. After a long pause, David replied, "I would rather remain silent on this subject," going on to say that "I'll talk about this absence sooner or later. Truthfully, I wasn't convinced about the real motivations behind this event but, frankly, I'd rather keep quiet for the moment, it's too delicate." He did, however, add that "there were problems with personality conflicts. The only thing I can say is that Ian doesn't have anything to do with it."

Although Bowie had no involvement in the concert, the live album is worthy of mention by virtue of its numerous connections with his work. Tracks include 'It Ain't Easy' by the Rats (including Marshall, Visconti and Cambridge), 'The Width Of A Circle', 'Ziggy Stardust', 'Moonage Daydream', 'White Light/White Heat' and 'Suffragette City' by The Spiders From Mars (including Bolder and Woodmansey, with Joe Elliott on lead vocal), and a final encore of 'All The Young Dudes' led by Ian Hunter and the assembled masses.

SATURNZRETURN *(Goldie)*
FFRR 828990 2, February 1998 [15]

'Truth'

ALL THE YOUNG DUDES – THE ANTHOLOGY
(Mott The Hoople)
Columbia 4914002, September 1998

'All The Young Dudes (David Bowie Vocal)' (4'30")

ALL THE WAY FROM STOCKHOLM TO PHILADELPHIA – LIVE 71/72 *(Mott The Hoople)*
Angel Air SJP CD029, December 1998

'All The Young Dudes' (4'03") / 'Honky Tonk Women' (8'45")

This live compilation includes Bowie's guest appearance at Mott The Hoople's Philadelphia concert on 29 November 1972.

ULYSSES (DELLA NOTTE) *(Reeves Gabrels)*
www.reevesgabrels.com, November 1999
E-Magine EMA-61050-2, October 2000

'Jewel'

Reeves Gabrels's second solo album, recorded concurrently with *'hours…'* in 1999 and featuring Bowie on the track 'Jewel' alongside contributions from Dave Grohl, Frank Black, Robert Smith and *'hours…'* veterans Mark Plati and Mike Levesque, was initially released as an MP3 download from the guitarist's website. After *Yahoo! Internet Life Magazine* named *Ulysses (della notte)* its Internet Album of the Year, Gabrels secured a deal with the fledgling E-Magine label for a conventional CD release in October 2000. "*Ulysses* really needs to be listened to as a whole," Gabrels told *Guitar World* magazine. "On the Internet people tend to download individual songs instead of entire albums, which is why I wanted it to come out in a more traditional format."

CYBERNAUTS LIVE *(The Cybernauts)*
Arachnophobia Records ASO 2001, March 2001

In 1983, when his then band Uriah Heep were sup-porting Def Leppard's Pyromania tour of America, for-mer Spiders bassist Trevor Bolder struck up a friend-ship with Leppard vocalist and long-time Bowie fan Joe Elliott. It was this relationship which led to Elliott's collaboration with Bolder and Woody Woodmansey at 1994's Mick Ronson Memorial Concert (see above). Three years later, Bolder and Woodmansey were invited to arrange a similar per-formance to mark the unveiling of Ronson's memori-al stage in Hull and, as Bolder later explained, "this time we decided to take the band on the road and do a few gigs for fun, and finish off with the memorial concert in Hull." Thus were born The Cybernauts: Bolder, Woodmansey and Elliott were joined by Def Leppard guitarist Phil Collen and keyboardist Dick Decent. Drawing on a repertoire consisting almost exclusively of classic Bowie numbers from the Ziggy days, the band performed five gigs in the summer of 1997, one of which, at Dublin's Olympia Theatre on 7 August, was recorded and later released as a CD. "Joe came up with the idea that we should record the Dublin show," revealed Bolder. "I'm really glad we did it, because it turned out for me to be one of the best live albums I've played on. Playing those great Bowie songs again with Joe, Phil, Woody and Dick was so much fun and something I never thought I would do again."

Cybernauts Live received its only official release in Japan, but later became available by mail order from the band's website www.cybernautsruleok.com. This version comes with a bonus disc entitled *The Further Adventures Of The Cybernauts*, featuring seven studio cuts (of which six are Bowie numbers ranging from the inevitable 'Moonage Daydream' to the more unusual 'Lady Grinning Soul') recorded in August 1997 and January 2001. Although there's no direct contribution from Bowie, this finely performed, well recorded and nicely presented memento will be of obvious interest to collectors.

VIVA NUEVA *(Rustic Overtones)*
Tommy Boy Music TBCD1471, June 2001

'Sector Z' / 'Man Without A Mouth'

Tony Visconti was introduced to the Portland-based Rustic Overtones at a New York gig in February 1999. Impressed by the seven-piece band's "wonderful, sleazy rhythmic feel" and their fusion of "funk, soul, hip-hop and a hint of New Orleans", Visconti offered to produce their album. Recording at New York's Avatar Studios (formerly The Power Station, scene of the *Scary Monsters* sessions) was so fruitful that Visconti "wrote an e-mail to David Bowie that he should come to our studio and check the band out. Much to our surprise he said he would!"

In July 1999 the group convened in Looking Glass Studios, where David recorded vocals for 'Sector Z' and 'Man Without A Mouth'. The latter replaced 'Hit Man', which Bowie considered less suitable for his voice. "We couldn't believe his generosity and our luck," said Visconti. "We blocked his exit long enough for a group photo. What a cool day!" Bowie later described the Rustic Overtones as "a terrific band".

Originally due for release by Arista in early 2000 under the title *This Is Rock And Roll* (a quotation from 'Sector Z'), the album was shelved after a change in record company management, eventually appearing in June 2001 on the Tommy Boy label. During the intervening period two new tracks were produced by David Leonard, and five more by the band them-selves. Nine of the original Visconti-produced record-ings survived the reshuffle, including the two Bowie collaborations. *Viva Nueva* (the title is pidgin Spanish for "new life", reflecting the band's relief that the frus-trating wait for its release was finally over) is an exu-berant, brilliant piece of work, with Bowie's collabo-ration on the truly excellent 'Sector Z' one of many highlights.

THE STRING QUARTET TRIBUTE TO DAVID BOWIE *(Petr Uhlir, Jan Alan, Jiri Masarik, Pavel Malina, Roman Finger)*
Vitamin CD-8668, August 2002

'Ashes To Ashes' / 'Changes' / 'Space Oddity' / 'The Man Who Sold The World' / 'Ziggy Stardust' / 'Golden Years' / 'Let's Dance' / '"Heroes"' / 'Fame' / 'Falling Through Space (original composition)'

As a rule this book disregards "tribute" compilations, but this one is unusual enough to warrant attention. The liner notes promise "a magnificent fusion of utter emotional depth", and while that might be stretching credibility, these classical string rearrangements of familiar Bowie songs are nothing if not arresting, ranging from the serene ('The Man Who Sold The World') to the barking ('Golden Years').

THE RAVEN (Lou Reed)
Warner Bros. 9362 48373-2, January 2003
  (two-disc version)
Warner Bros. 9362-48372-2, January 2003
  (single disc version)

'Hop Frog' (1'46")

Lou Reed's ambitious and unusual 2003 album (recorded under the working title POE-try) commemorates the soundtrack of an elaborate theatrical piece devised with director Robert Wilson and originally presented at Hamburg's Thalia Theatre in 2000. Based on the writings of Edgar Allan Poe, the album features thirteen songs, linked by the spoken dramatization of various short stories adapted for the project by Reed.

"The language is so beautiful," Reed remarked of Poe's work in December 2001, on the eve of the production's revival at the Brooklyn Academy of Music. "I spent so many hours with the dictionary, because some of these words were already arcane when he used them. He was a show-off in that way. My God, what a vocabulary. So I spent time finding out what these things meant, and then making it a little bit – not necessarily contemporary, but what it actually meant. But the word he picked always had a beautiful sound." Reed's compositions radically revise Poe's original stories. "I knew people would say, 'How dare he rewrite Poe?'," Reed observed, "but I thought, here's the opportunity of a lifetime for real fun: to combine the kind of lyricism that he has into a flexible rock format. I really like my version of it. It's accessible, among other things. And I felt I was in league with the master. In that kind of psychology, that interest in the drives and the meaning of obsession and compulsion, in that realm Poe reigns supreme."

Among the guest actors on The Raven are Willem Dafoe, Steve Buscemi, Amanda Plummer and Fisher Stevens. Other collaborators include Laurie Anderson, Ornette Coleman and David Bowie, who recorded his contribution, a vocal duet with Reed on 'Hop Frog', in November 2001. The Raven was released in two different formats: the full-length version was a limited edition two-disc set, while the single disc concentrated more heavily on the songs at the expense of the spoken material. 'Hop Frog' features on both versions.

26 MIXES FOR CASH (Aphex Twin)
Warp Records WarpCD102, March 2003

'"Heroes" (Aphex Twin Remix)' (5'18")

This compilation includes the Aphex Twin remix of '"Heroes"' originally released on a limited edition bonus disc with Philip Glass's "Heroes" Symphony in 1997.

BREASTICLES (Kristeen Young)
N Records ZM 00103, June 2003

'Saviour' (5'24")

Like The Rustic Overtones before her, singer-songwriter Kristeen Young found a champion in Tony Visconti, who recruited her to sing backing vocals on Heathen. Their subsequent studio collaboration resulted in this extraordinary album, for which Bowie provides a guest vocal on 'Saviour'. Also like The Rustic Overtones, Kristeen Young experienced some difficulty in getting her album released. Recorded in mid-2002, Breasticles eventually appeared the following year on the Portuguese label N Records. Fans of Celine Dion will be thoroughly baffled, but lovers of proper music are strongly advised to seek Breasticles out; they will be handsomely rewarded by a fine, intelligent, enthralling piece of work.

DARKNESS AND DISGRACE
(Des De Moor and Russell Churney)
Irregular Records IRR051, October 2003

'Future Legend/Bewitched' / 'Diamond Dogs' / 'It's No Game' / 'The Man Who Sold The World' / 'Look Back In Anger' / 'We Are The Dead' / 'Lady Stardust' / 'The London Boys' / 'Boys Keep Swinging' / 'The Bewlay Brothers' / 'Be My Wife' / 'Always Crashing In The Same Car' / 'Be My Wife (Reprise)' / 'Life On Mars?' / 'Please Mr Gravedigger' / 'Station To Station' / 'All The Madmen' / 'The Buddha Of Suburbia' / '"Heroes"/Kopf Bis Fuß' / 'I Have Not Been To Oxford Town' / 'Time' / 'All The Young Dudes'

This fascinating memento of the critically acclaimed cabaret show *Darkness And Disgrace* (see Chapter 9 for further details) is performed by Des de Moor and Russell Churney with guest vocals from the show's director Barb Jungr. Stripped to the bare minimum of voice, piano and acoustic guitar with occasional bass and percussion, the repertoire veers away from the obvious and towards the intriguing: the down-tempo version of 'I Have Not Been To Oxford Town' is remarkable, while the track billed as 'It's No Game' turns out to be the song's ancestor 'Tired Of My Life'. The results may not be to every rock fan's taste, but there can be no denying that this is one of the most unusual and interesting Bowie cover projects ever undertaken. "To hear these songs in such a personalized context is a real ear-opener," David himself remarked. "I listened as though someone else had written them."

ZIG ZAG *(Earl Slick)*
When!/Sanctuary WENCD216, December 2003

'Isn't It Evening (The Revolutionary)' (4'55")

Recorded in early 2003 alongside the *Reality* sessions, Earl Slick's solo album went under the unusual working title *Newfs* (a term of endearment for Newfoundland dogs, of which Slick is an aficionado). Produced by Mark Plati, the album features work from fellow Bowie veterans Sterling Campbell and Emm Gryner, while David himself co-wrote and sang vocals on 'Isn't It Evening (The Revolutionary)'. Other guest vocalists include Robert Smith, Joe Elliott, Martha Davis and Royston Langdon.

(iv) DAVID BOWIE COMPILATION ALBUMS

A staggering number of Bowie compilations has appeared over the years: what follows is a comprehensive guide to UK releases. Promo albums are generally ignored. Full track-listings are given only for key compilations of otherwise unavailable material, while individual tracks of importance are mentioned in each entry. For those wishing to collect Bowie's juvenilia, the essential purchases are Early On (1964-1966) *and* The Deram Anthology 1966-1968.

The completist will also want to acquire the 1992 CD version of Love You Till Tuesday *and the 1989 CD* The Manish Boys/Davy Jones And The Lower Third. *Of the post-1969 compilations there are significant rarities to be found on* Sound + Vision, RarestOneBowie, Bowie At The Beeb *and the 1993 US import* The Singles 1969 To 1993.

THE WORLD OF DAVID BOWIE
Decca SPA 58, March 1970

Issued in the wake of 'Space Oddity', this compilation of Deram recordings included the first official releases of 'Karma Man', 'Let Me Sleep Beside You' and 'In The Heat Of The Morning'. It was reissued in April 1973 with a Ziggy-era sleeve photo.

IMAGES 1966-1967
Deram DPA 3017/18, May 1975

Another compilation of Deram tracks.

CHANGESONEBOWIE
RCA Victor RS 1055, June 1976 [2]
RCA PL81732, 1984

Bowie's earliest official "greatest hits" compilation saw the first appearance of 'John, I'm Only Dancing' on an album (its first in any format in America); some early pressings erroneously included the *Aladdin Sane* out-take version. The album, which was packaged in austere *Station To Station*-style monochrome with the same unspaced lettering, hit number 10 in America and number 2 in Britain, where it was kept off the top spot by ABBA's *Greatest Hits*.

THE BEST OF BOWIE

K-Tel NE 1111, December 1980 [3]

This very successful post-*Scary Monsters* package included newly edited versions of 'Life On Mars?' (3'36") and 'Diamond Dogs' (4'37"), while 'Fame' and 'Golden Years' were the 7" edits rarely issued on compilations. The track-listing differed on some overseas versions.

ANOTHER FACE

Decca TAB 17, May 1981

Another reissue of Deram material, plus both sides of the 'Liza Jane' single.

DON'T BE FOOLED BY THE NAME

Pye PRT BOW1, September 1981

This 10" EP was the first of numerous repackages of Bowie's three 1966 Pye singles and B-sides.

CHANGESTWOBOWIE

RCA BOW LP 3, November 1981 [24]
RCA PL84202, 1984

RCA's second compilation was assembled without consulting Bowie, and apparently he was far from pleased with the result. He did, however, consent to promote it by filming a video for the six-year-old recording 'Wild Is The Wind', released as a single in November 1981. *ChangesTwoBowie* saw the first appearance of 'John, I'm Only Dancing (Again)' on long-playing format.

THE MANISH BOYS/DAVY JONES AND THE LOWER THIRD

See For Miles CYM 1, October 1982
See For Miles SEA 1, June 1985
See For Miles SEA CD 1, December 1989

Originally released as a 10" EP, then as a 12" single and finally a CD, this four-track compilation of David's two 1965 singles and their B-sides is the only official reissue of the single versions of 'I Pity The Fool' and 'Take My Tip'.

FASHIONS

RCA BOWP 101-110, November 1982

A limited edition of 25,000 packs of ten RCA singles, here reissued as picture discs in a plastic wallet.

BOWIE RARE

RCA PL 45406, December 1982 [34]

A year after *ChangesTwoBowie*, RCA made a cynical grab at the Christmas market with this hotchpotch from the archives. None of the tracks was previously unreleased, although most had appeared only as B-sides and some, like the Italian version of 'Space Oddity' and the American 7" edit of 'Young Americans', had never been released in the UK. Although the album provided a useful round-up for the completist, it was a pretty shabby affair – three of the B-sides had only just been reissued in RCA's *Fashions* set, 'John, I'm Only Dancing (Again)' had appeared on *ChangesTwoBowie*, 'Holy Holy' was the 1972 version rather than the genuinely rare original, and did anyone really need 'Young Americans' with a verse missing? To add insult to injury the lyric sheet was a farrago of inaccuracies. Bowie let it be known that he considered the album "horrendous", "atrocious" and "offensive".

Although most of *Bowie Rare* would be superseded by bonus tracks on subsequent releases, it remains the only UK album to offer 'Ragazzo Solo, Ragazza Sola' and the excellent 1974 live version of 'Panic In Detroit' originally found on the 'Knock On Wood' single.

GOLDEN YEARS

RCA BOWLP 004, August 1983 [33]

After the ill feeling over *Bowie Rare*, David's former label sought his cooperation for this opportunistic package of oldies, all of which featured in 1983's Serious Moonlight set-list. Bowie assented on the condition that no attempt would be made to suggest that the album was a concert recording, and vetoed the use of the words "Serious" and "Moonlight" in the title.

LIFETIMES
RCA, August 1983

Although containing nothing that couldn't be found elsewhere, RCA's individually numbered limited edition promo remains a collector's rarity, containing a representative track from every album between *Space Oddity* and *Scary Monsters* with the exception of *Stage*.

A SECOND FACE
Decca TAB 71, August 1983

Another collection of Deram material.

PRIME CUTS
Decca KMC2 5006, August 1983

Yet another Deram compilation, this time only on cassette and including both sides of the 'Liza Jane' single for good measure.

LOVE YOU TILL TUESDAY
Deram BOWIE 1, April 1984 [53]
Pickwick PWKS 4131P, 1992

Released in 1984 to accompany Kenneth Pitt's unveiling of the *Love You Till Tuesday* film, this compilation features slightly remixed versions of the soundtrack songs, plus a couple of 1960s tracks that don't appear in the film at all. It remains the only official source of the 1968 rarity 'When I'm Five' (3'05"). The 1992 CD reissue has a re-ordered track-listing, includes 'The London Boys' instead of 'The Laughing Gnome', and substitutes the *David Bowie* album versions of 'Love You Till Tuesday', 'Sell Me A Coat' and 'When I Live My Dream'. More importantly, it retains 'When I'm Five' and features the previously unreleased full-length versions of 'Space Oddity' (4'35") and 'Ching-a-Ling' (2'55") – the latter remains unique to this CD. The vinyl version offers the shorter film edits of both tracks, as does *The Deram Anthology 1966-1968*.

FAME AND FASHION
RCA PL84919, April 1984 [40]

Another predictable compilation of RCA material

which, like *Golden Years*, made the top 40. Both albums were among the label's first (and now rarest) Bowie CDs.

DAVID BOWIE: THE COLLECTION
Castle Communications CCSLP 118, November 1985
Castle Communications CCSCD 118, 1992

A double LP of Deram tracks and the three 1966 Pye singles with their B-sides.

RARE TRACKS
Showcase SHLP 137, April 1986

A 12" repackage of the Pye singles and B-sides.

1966
Pye PRT PYE 6001 / PYX 6001, October 1987
Castle Classics CLACD 154, 1989

Yet another reissue of the above. For mad people there was even a 12" picture disc.

SOUND + VISION
Rykodisc RCD 90120/90121/90122/RCDV1018, September 1989
Rykodisc RCD 90330/90331/90332, October 1995
EMI 72439 451121, December 2003

Disc One: 'Space Oddity (Original Demo)' (5'07") / 'Wild Eyed Boy From Freecloud (Rare B-side Version)' (4'48") / 'The Prettiest Star (Single Version)' (3'09") / 'London Bye Ta Ta' (2'33") / 'Black Country Rock' (3'31") / 'The Man Who Sold The World' (3'54") / 'The Bewlay Brothers' (5'20") / 'Changes' (3'30") / 'Round And Round' (2'39") / 'Moonage Daydream' (4'37") / 'John, I'm Only Dancing (Sax Version)' (2'41") / 'Drive In Saturday' (4'27") / 'Panic In Detroit' (4'23") / 'Ziggy Stardust (Live 1973)' (3'14") / 'White Light/White Heat (Live 1973)' (3'57") / 'Rock'n'Roll Suicide (Live 1973)' (4'29") *Disc Two:* 'Anyway, Anyhow, Anywhere' (3'06") / 'Sorrow' (2'53") / 'Don't Bring Me Down' (2'05") / '1984/Dodo' (5'27") / 'Big Brother' (3'18") / 'Rebel Rebel (Rare Single Version)' (2'58") / 'Suffragette City (Live 1974)' (3'48") / 'Watch That Man (Live 1974)'

(5'05") / 'Cracked Actor (Live 1974)' (3'28") / 'Young Americans' (5'10") / 'Fascination' (5'43") / 'After Today' (3'47") / 'It's Hard To Be A Saint In The City' (3'46") / 'TVC15' (5'29") / 'Wild Is The Wind' (5'56")
Disc Three: 'Sound And Vision' (3'02") / 'Be My Wife' (2'55") / 'Speed Of Life' (2'45") / '"Helden" (1989 Remix)' (3'37") / 'Joe The Lion' (3'05") / 'Sons Of The Silent Age' (3'17") / 'Station To Station (Live 1978)' (8'48") / 'Warszawa (Live 1978)' (6'50") / 'Breaking Glass (Live 1978)' (3'34") / 'Red Sails' (3'42") / 'Look Back In Anger' (3'05") / 'Boys Keep Swinging' (3'16") / 'Up The Hill Backwards' (3'13") / 'Kingdom Come' (3'42") / 'Ashes To Ashes' (4'22")

Sound + Vision Plus: 'John, I'm Only Dancing (Live 1972)' (2'40") / 'Changes (Live 1972)' (3'18") / 'The Supermen (Live 1972)' (2'44") / 'Ashes To Ashes (CD Video Version)' (3'34")

Additional tracks on 2003 reissue: 'Wild Eyed Boy From Freecloud (Rare B-side Version)' (4'57") / 'London Bye Ta Ta (Previously Unreleased Stereo Mix)' (2'33") / 'Round And Round (Alternate Vocal Take)' (2'39") / 'Baal's Hymn' (4'00") / 'The Drowned Girl' (2'24") / 'Cat People (Putting Out Fire)' (6'41") / 'China Girl' (5'32") / 'Ricochet' (5'14") / 'Modern Love (Live)' (3'43") / 'Loving The Alien' (7'10") / 'Dancing With The Big Boys' (3'34") / 'Blue Jean' (3'10") / 'Time Will Crawl' (4'18") / 'Baby Can Dance' (4'57") / 'Amazing' (3'04") / 'I Can't Read' (4'54") / 'Shopping For Girls' (3'44") / 'Goodbye Mr. Ed' (3'24") / 'Amlapura' (3'46") / 'You've Been Around' (4'45") / 'Nite Flights (Moodswings Back To Basics Remix Radio Edit)' (4'35") / 'Pallas Athena (Gone Midnight Mix)' (4'21") / 'Jump They Say' (4'22") / 'Buddha Of Suburbia' (4'28") / 'Dead Against It' (5'48") / 'South Horizon' (5'26") / 'Pallas Athena (Live)' (8'18")

In 1986 Bowie's licensing contract with RCA expired, meaning that the pre-*Let's Dance* albums became scarce. In common with many early CD reissues, the mastering and packaging of RCA's *Space Oddity* to *Scary Monsters* CDs had been of indifferent quality, but nevertheless they now command ever-higher sums among collectors.

In 1989 Bowie negotiated a new reissue programme with the small Massachusetts-based company Rykodisc. "What knocked me out about them is the care they take with the product," he explained, "so there really was no question of who I wanted to go with to release all the old stuff." As an added incentive, the Rykodisc reissues were not only to feature remastering and luxury packaging, but bonus tracks comprising rare B-sides and previously unreleased recordings. "I would look for old obscure tracks and demos and so on," said Bowie, "And they had their fingers on stuff I'd forgotten about, so between us we compiled a lot of original things that hadn't seen the light of day – and probably never should have!" The balance shifted from *Low* onwards, as Rykodisc's Jeff Rougvie explained: "Our deal was with Bowie and his former managers, MainMan, who co-owned the bulk of the material. Everything up to *Station To Station* was kept in a shared vault, and we had access to all of that. But Bowie himself has the masters to the Berlin albums, so although he's said that there are 50 cuts left over, we don't have them! He did go in and pull out the bonus tracks for the CDs, but I don't know how much else is really there, or what state it's in."

Between 1990 and 1992, all thirteen studio albums from *Space Oddity* to *Scary Monsters* were reissued, together with the three live albums and the new hits compilation *ChangesBowie*. Initially each release appeared on both CD and vinyl, although the last three (*Scary Monsters*, *Stage* and *Ziggy Stardust: The Motion Picture*) were issued only on CD. Spearheading the campaign was the lavish four-CD (or six-LP) box set *Sound + Vision*. Although officially released only in America, it was widely imported to Britain where the price hovered around the £50 mark. The limited edition of 350 wooden-boxed versions, each containing a certificate signed by David, retailed for a great deal more. *Sound + Vision* remains probably the finest Bowie compilation, offering roughly three tracks from each album session (including three apiece from the live LPs), and boasting some unusually imaginative choices. The main attraction is the array of rarities, including the April 1969 demo of 'Space Oddity', the superior alternative takes of 'John, I'm Only Dancing' and 'Rebel Rebel', the rare original versions of 'The Prettiest Star' and 'Wild-Eyed Boy From Freecloud', and several previously unreleased gems: 'London Bye Ta Ta', '1984/Dodo', 'After Today' and 'It's Hard To Be A Saint In The City'. The CD format included a fourth disc, subtitled *Sound + Vision Plus*, which contained three live tracks recorded in Boston on 1 October 1972, together with a CD video version of 'Ashes To Ashes'.

Both the vinyl and CD formats originally came in an LP-sized plastic box. *Sound + Vision* was reissued in November 1994, this time with a CD-ROM version of 'Ashes To Ashes'. In October 1995 it reappeared as a more modest CD-sized box set, minus the bonus disc.

In December 2003 EMI released a deluxe repackage of *Sound + Vision*, again minus the original bonus disc (whose live 1972 tracks had by now appeared on the *Aladdin Sane* 30th Anniversary Edition). This time *Sound + Vision* was upgraded to four full-length CDs to incorporate the post-*Scary Monsters* material in EMI's reissue catalogue. To confuse matters, the four discs were fuller than before, meaning that although the original track order was maintained intact, Disc Two now began with '1984/Dodo' and Disc Three with 'Station To Station'. The significant new rarities on the 2003 edition included an extended B-side version of 'Wild Eyed Boy From Freecloud' with David's spoken introduction, a previously unreleased stereo mix of 'London Bye Ta Ta', a previously unreleased alternative vocal of 'Round And Round', the first time on CD for two of the *Baal* tracks and the live B-side version of 'Modern Love', and previously unavailable remixes of 'Nite Flights' and 'Pallas Athena'. Every studio album up to 1993 was now represented by an average of three tracks (although only one song from *Never Let Me Down* made the grade), marking the first major appearance of Tin Machine on a Bowie compilation. The termination of 2003's *Sound + Vision* after *The Buddha Of Suburbia* was dictated by the fact that Columbia held the rights to the albums from *1.Outside* onwards, although the set closes with 1997's live 'Pallas Athena'.

CHANGESBOWIE
EMI DBTV 1, March 1990 [1]
EMI BDTV 1, March 1990 [1]

EMI's chart-friendly 1990 companion to the *Sound + Vision* box set was a predictable trip through Bowie's back catalogue distinguished (if that's the word) only by the remix single 'Fame 90'. Not surprisingly *ChangesBowie* did very well, knocking Sinead O'Connor's *I Do Not Want What I Haven't Got* off the number 1 spot and spending 29 weeks in the UK chart.

INTROSPECTIVE
Tabak CINT 5001, 1990

Another reissue of the 1966 Pye singles, with a 1990 interview tacked on as an added incentive.

ROCK REFLECTIONS
Deram 8205492, 1990

A heavily imported Australian CD of Deram tracks.

EARLY ON (1964-1966)
Rhino R2 70526, 1991

'Liza Jane' (2'18") *(CD only)* / 'Louie, Louie Go Home' (2'12") *(CD only)* / 'I Pity The Fool' (2'09") / 'Take My Tip' (2'16") / 'That's Where My Heart Is' (2'29") / 'I Want My Baby Back' (2'39") / 'Bars Of The County Jail' (2'07") / 'You've Got A Habit Of Leaving' (2'32") / 'Baby Loves That Way' (3'03") / 'I'll Follow You' (2'02") / 'Glad I've Got Nobody' (2'32") / 'Can't Help Thinking About Me' (2'47") / 'And I Say To Myself' (2'29") / 'Do Anything You Say' (2'32") / 'Good Morning Girl' (2'14") *(CD only)* / 'I Dig Everything' (2'45") / 'I'm Not Losing Sleep' (2'52")

This diligent compilation is a valuable addition to the archives, amassing on a single CD every official release from Bowie's pre-Deram career – except for 'I Pity The Fool' and 'Take My Tip', which are instead the previously unreleased alternative takes. The only official CD of the single versions can be found on 1989's *The Manish Boys/Davy Jones And The Lower Third*.

Even better are the five exclusive demos unearthed in the 1980s by Bowie's early producer Shel Talmy. 'That's Where My Heart Is', 'I Want My Baby Back', 'Bars Of The County Jail', 'I'll Follow You' and 'Glad I've Got Nobody' all date from 1965, and were unavailable until this release.

THE SINGLES COLLECTION
EMI CDEM 1512, November 1993 [9]
Rykodisc RCD 10218/19, November 1993 *(US version)*

Disc One: 'Space Oddity' (5'14") *(3'31" on US edition)* / 'Changes' (3'33") / 'Starman' (4'13") / 'Ziggy

Stardust' (3'13") / 'Suffragette City' (3'25") / 'John, I'm Only Dancing' (2'46") / 'The Jean Genie' (4'06") / 'Drive In Saturday' (4'27") / 'Life On Mars?' (3'48") / 'Sorrow' (2'52") / 'Rebel Rebel' (4'28") / 'Rock'n'Roll Suicide' (2'58") *(UK only)* / 'Diamond Dogs' (6'03") / 'Knock On Wood' (3'02") *(UK only)* / 'Young Americans' (5'10") / 'Fame' (4'16") / 'Golden Years' (3'58") / 'TVC15' (3'43") / 'Sound And Vision' (3'00")

Disc Two: '"Heroes"' (3'35") / 'Beauty And The Beast' (3'33") / 'Boys Keep Swinging' (3'16") / 'DJ' (3'20") / 'Alabama Song' (3'50") *(UK only)* / 'Ashes To Ashes' (3'34") / 'Fashion' (3'23") / 'Scary Monsters (And Super Creeps)' (5'09") / 'Under Pressure' (3'58") *(4'01" on US edition)* / 'Wild Is The Wind' (5'59") *(UK only)* / 'Let's Dance' (4'07") / 'China Girl' (4'14") / 'Modern Love' (3'56") / 'Blue Jean' (3'09") / 'This Is Not America' (3'48") *(UK only)* / 'Dancing In The Street' (3'14") / 'Absolute Beginners' (5'36") / 'Day-In Day-Out' (4'14")

Additional tracks on US edition: 'Oh! You Pretty Things' (3'11") / 'Be My Wife' (2'55") / 'Look Back In Anger' (3'05") / 'Cat People (Putting Out Fire)' (6'43") / 'Loving The Alien' (4'39") / 'Never Let Me Down' (4'03") / 'Jump They Say' (3'54") / 'Peace On Earth/Little Drummer Boy' (4'23")

The title of this excellent compilation is actually a bit of a misnomer given that tracks like 'Ziggy Stardust' were never released as A-sides, but let's not be pedantic: until it was superseded by *Best Of Bowie* in 2002, *The Singles Collection* provided an invaluable starting point for the beginner, and for the fan it marked the CD debut of several rare 7" edits (though not all – 'Drive In Saturday', 'Fame', 'Golden Years' and 'Scary Monsters' are the full-length album versions). Collectors will prefer the US release (entitled *The Singles 1969 To 1993*) which, although substituting an inauthentic hacked-down 3'31" edit of 'Space Oddity' and omitting five tracks from the UK selection, includes two rarities: the full-length original version of 'Cat People (Putting Out Fire)' and, on a bonus CD with the first 40,000 pressings, 'Peace On Earth/Little Drummer Boy', complete with David and Bing's spoken preamble. The two releases feature different versions of 'Under Pressure', neither of which is the original 7" edit: the UK album has the slightly edited version previously found on *Queen Greatest Hits 2*, while the US album features the remix from *Classic Queen*.

THE GOSPEL ACCORDING TO DAVID BOWIE
Spectrum Music/Karusell 5500212, 1993

Another CD of Deram tracks.

ALL SAINTS
ALLSAINTS 1/2

'Warszawa' / 'Some Are' / 'Subterraneans' / 'Moss Garden' / 'Sense of Doubt' / 'Neuköln' / 'Art Decade' / 'The Mysteries' / 'Ian Fish, U.K. Heir' / 'Abdulmajid' / 'South Horizon' / 'Weeping Wall' / 'Pallas Athena' / 'A New Career In A New Town' / 'The Wedding' / 'V-2 Schneider' / 'Looking For Lester' / 'All Saints'

In 1993 Bowie compiled this exclusive double CD of instrumentals from *Low*, *"Heroes"*, *Black Tie White Noise*, *The Buddha Of Suburbia* and Philip Glass's *"Low" Symphony*, as a Christmas present for friends and colleagues. Limited to 150 pressings, privately distributed and never commercially available, the original *All Saints* has become a desirable and costly collector's item. A subsequent single-disc compilation, released in July 2001 and also called *All Saints*, featured a similar if condensed track-listing.

RARESTONEBOWIE
Trident Music International/Golden Years GY014, June 1995
Dolphin BLCK 86008, 1997

'All The Young Dudes' (4'10") / 'Queen Bitch' (3'15") / 'Sound And Vision' (3'24") / 'Time' (5'12") / 'Be My Wife' (2'44") / 'Footstompin'' (3'24") / 'Ziggy Stardust' (3'21") / 'My Death' (5'49") / 'I Feel Free' (5'20")

Although running to a paltry 36 minutes, MainMan's 1995 follow-up to *Santa Monica '72* is a minor treat. The highlight, despite its ropey sound quality, is the 1974 live recording of 'Footstompin''. Other attractions include the first proper release of Bowie's studio version of 'All The Young Dudes' and a 1973 radio commercial for *Pin Ups*, lurking on a hidden track at the beginning of the CD. The remainder of *RarestOneBowie* comprises live oddities from the 1970s, including a spunky 'Queen Bitch' recorded on 23 March 1976, and a brace of last-night rarities –

'Sound And Vision' and 'Be My Wife' – from Earls Court on 1 July 1978. Also on offer are *The 1980 Floor Show*'s version of 'Time' and a live rendition of 'My Death' from Carnegie Hall on 28 September 1972. On the desperate side are the gratuitous reappearance of the *Santa Monica '72* version of 'Ziggy Stardust' and an atrociously muffled recording of 'I Feel Free' from Kingston Polytechnic on 6 May 1972.

As with *Santa Monica '72*, the packaging features some pleasing archive photos and reproductions of MainMan memorabilia, including Mike Garson's receipt for the *Diamond Dogs* sessions and a deposit note for an Atlantic crossing by "Mr & Mrs Bowie (Jones) and child" on the *QEII*. A 1997 Japanese reissue was augmented by a further six tracks from *Santa Monica '72*.

LONDON BOY
Spectrum Music 5517062, 1996

Another repackage of Deram material, notable for its inclusion of the full 4'35" mix of the original 'Space Oddity' otherwise available only on the *Love You Till Tuesday* CD.

BBC SESSIONS 1969-1972 (SAMPLER)
NMC/BBC Worldwide Music NMCD 0072, July 1996

'Hang On To Yourself' (2'49") / 'Ziggy Stardust' (3'19") / 'Space Oddity' (4'13") / 'Andy Warhol' (2'54") / 'Waiting For The Man' (4'28") / 'Interview With Brian Mathew' (1'28") / 'Let Me Sleep Beside You (edited version)' (2'34")

As a taster for their proposed three-volume compilation of Bowie's BBC radio sessions (see Chapter 4), NMC and BBC Worldwide Music released this seven-track sampler. The project was shelved, leaving only this limited-edition CD which now exchanges hands for shockingly inflated sums. Despite offering slim pickings by comparison with EMI's subsequent double-disc set *Bowie At The Beeb*, it should be noted that this CD boasts a couple of otherwise unavailable cuts: 'Waiting For The Man' from the Hype session of 25 March 1970, and 'Andy Warhol' from the acoustic Bowie/Ronson session of 21 September 1971. All the other tracks reappear on *Bowie At The Beeb*.

THE DERAM ANTHOLOGY 1966-1968
Deram 8447842, June 1997

'Rubber Band (Single Version)' (2'05") / 'The London Boys' (3'20") / 'The Laughing Gnome' (3'01") / 'The Gospel According To Tony Day' (2'48") / 'Uncle Arthur' (2'07") / 'Sell Me A Coat' (2'58") / 'Rubber Band' (2'17") / 'Love You Till Tuesday' (3'09") / 'There Is A Happy Land' (3'11") / 'We Are Hungry Men' (2'58") / 'When I Live My Dream' (3'22") / 'Little Bombardier' (3'24") / 'Silly Boy Blue' (3'48") / 'Come And Buy My Toys' (2'07") / 'Join The Gang' (2'17") / 'She's Got Medals' (2'23") / 'Maid Of Bond Street' (1'43") / 'Please Mr Gravedigger' (2'35") / 'Love You Till Tuesday (Single Version)' (2'59") / 'Did You Ever Have A Dream' (2'06") / 'Karma Man' (3'03") / 'Let Me Sleep Beside You' (3'25") / 'In The Heat Of The Morning' (2'56") / 'Ching-a-Ling' (2'02") / 'Sell Me A Coat' (2'51") / 'When I Live My Dream' (3'49") / 'Space Oddity' (3'46")

After 30 years of repackages Decca finally released this valuable round-up of Bowie's Deram recordings, adding the independently recorded 'Ching-a-Ling' and 'Space Oddity' for good measure. With the exception of the second version of 'When I Live My Dream', which is bunched together with the material from the *Love You Till Tuesday* film, the compilation follows a chronological pattern. Tracks 5-18 comprise the *David Bowie* album in its original order, and are the compilation's only stereo tracks (the four *Love You Till Tuesday* soundtrack songs are mixed in the simulated stereo technique, which involves a fractional delay on one channel).

Decca had intended to include out-takes like 'Your Funny Smile', 'Bunny Thing' and 'Pussy Cat', but deferred to Bowie's wish that they remain unreleased. Also absent are the never-released first takes of 'Please Mr Gravedigger' and 'London Bye Ta Ta', the masters of which were lost back in the 1960s. A more annoying omission is 'When I'm Five', not actually recorded under the Decca contract but previously released on *Love You Till Tuesday*. 'Ching-a-Ling' and 'Space Oddity' are both the truncated edits used in the film rather than the full-length versions. These few gripes aside, this handsomely packaged CD is a must for the collector.

THE BEST OF DAVID BOWIE 1969/1974
EMI 7243 8 21849 2 8, October 1997 [13]

Bowie's 1997 re-sale of his back catalogue to EMI brought forth yet another hit compilation. 'John, I'm Only Dancing' is the 1973 "sax version", and other attractions are the stereo version of 1970's 'The Prettiest Star' single (previously on *Sound + Vision* in mono only, although the stereo mix later appeared on that compilation's 2003 reissue), and a cleaned-up remastering of Bowie's 'All The Young Dudes' which is superior to the one on *RarestOneBowie* (this would later resurface on the 2003 reissue of *Aladdin Sane*). The track-listing differed in some overseas versions.

EARTHLING IN THE CITY
AT&T/N2K 8116501, October 1997

Given away with the November 1997 American edition of *GQ* magazine, this six-track CD offers exclusive live versions of 'Little Wonder' (3'44") and 'The Hearts Filthy Lesson' (5'03") recorded at Bowie's fiftieth birthday concert. The remaining tracks were available on other formats of the *Earthling* singles.

THE BEST OF DAVID BOWIE 1974/1979
EMI 7243 4 94300 2 0, April 1998 [39]

EMI's sequel to *1969/1974* includes 'It's Hard To Be A Saint In The City', otherwise only available on *Sound + Vision*. 'Young Americans' is the 3'11" US single version (its first time on CD), while 'Golden Years', 'TVC15' and '"Heroes"' are also the single edits. The promo version substituted the 7" mixes of 'John, I'm Only Dancing (Again)' and 'D.J.' in place of the full-length ones.

I DIG EVERYTHING: THE 1966 PYE SINGLES
Essential ESM CD 712, June 1999
Essential ESM 10765, June 2000

Yet another repackage of Bowie's three Pye singles, this time in a beautiful boxed set of three individual CD singles, also appearing on 7" vinyl and, a year later, as a 10" EP. But why?

BOWIE AT THE BEEB
EMI 7243 5 28629 2 4 / 7243 5 28958 2 3, September 2000 [7]

Disc One: 'In The Heat Of The Morning' (3'01") / 'London Bye Ta Ta' (2'34") / 'Karma Man' (2'59") / 'Silly Boy Blue' (4'36") / 'Let Me Sleep Beside You' (3'16") / 'Janine' (3'01") / 'Amsterdam' (2'56") / 'God Knows I'm Good' (3'10") / 'The Width Of A Circle' (4'50") / 'Unwashed And Somewhat Slightly Dazed' (4'54") / 'Cygnet Committee' (8'16") / 'Memory Of A Free Festival' (3'17") / 'Wild Eyed Boy From Freecloud' (4'42") / 'Bombers' (2'53") / 'Looking For A Friend' (3'08") / 'Almost Grown' (2'16") / 'Kooks' (3'02") / 'It Ain't Easy' (2'51") *Disc Two:* 'The Supermen' (2'50") / 'Eight Line Poem' (2'52") / 'Hang On To Yourself' (2'48") / 'Ziggy Stardust' (3'23") / 'Queen Bitch' (2'57") / 'I'm Waiting For The Man' (5'22") / 'Five Years' (4'21") / 'White Light/White Heat' (3'46") / 'Moonage Daydream' (4'56") / 'Hang On To Yourself' (2'48") / 'Suffragette City' (3'25") / 'Ziggy Stardust' (3'22") / 'Starman' (4'03") / 'Space Oddity' (4'13") / 'Changes' (3'28") / 'Oh! You Pretty Things' (2'55") / 'Andy Warhol' (3'12") / 'Lady Stardust' (3'19") / 'Rock'n'Roll Suicide' (3'08") *Disc Three:* 'Wild Is The Wind' (6'21") / 'Ashes To Ashes' (5'03") / 'Seven' (4'12") / 'This Is Not America' (3'43") / 'Absolute Beginners' (6'31") / 'Always Crashing In The Same Car' (4'06") / 'Survive' (4'54") / 'Little Wonder' (3'48") / 'The Man Who Sold The World' (3'57") / 'Fame' (4'11") / 'Stay' (5'43") / 'Hallo Spaceboy' (5'21") / 'Cracked Actor' (4'09") / 'I'm Afraid Of Americans' (5'29") / 'Let's Dance' (6'20")

EMI's long-awaited compilation of highlights from Bowie's legendary BBC sessions materialized in September 2000, initially boxed with an exclusive fifteen-track bonus disc culled from Bowie's concert at the BBC Radio Theatre on 27 June that year. *Bowie At The Beeb* offers a rich feast of archival delights, unearthing several very obscure recordings including the elusive 'Memory Of A Free Festival' from the 1970 *Sunday Show* concert. The album's appeal was nevertheless mainstream, as demonstrated by its number 7 peak in the UK chart – the best showing for any Bowie compilation in a decade – and the reviews were universally ecstatic. Indeed, following David's triumphant homecoming at Glastonbury the previous

June, *Bowie At The Beeb* sealed his critical status as the undisputed elder statesman of popular music; in November 2000 a survey conducted among contemporary musicians in the *NME* voted Bowie the most influential artist of all time.

The breakdown of tracks is as follows: the first four tracks on Disc One hail from the *Top Gear* session recorded on 13 May 1968; the next two are from *The Dave Lee Travis Show* recorded on 20 October 1969; 'Amsterdam' to 'Memory Of A Free Festival' come from *The Sunday Show* recorded 5 February 1970; 'Wild Eyed Boy From Freecloud' is from Hype's *Sounds Of The 70s* set on 25 March 1970; and the remainder of Disc One is culled from *In Concert: John Peel* on 3 June 1971. Disc Two begins with a pair of tracks from the acoustic Bowie/Ronson session of 21 September 1971 (one of Bowie's finest BBC sessions, and sadly among the least well represented here), followed by the complete five-song *Sounds Of The 70s* session of 18 January 1972, and then the excellent five-song set from John Peel's *Sounds Of The 70s* show taped on 16 May. 'Starman' to 'Oh! You Pretty Things' comprises the entire *Johnnie Walker Lunchtime Show* set of 22 May 1972, and the last three cuts hail from Bowie's final BBC session of the decade, recorded for *Sounds Of The 70s* on 23 May 1972.

On the initial pressing, a mastering error resulted in tracks 4 and 12 on the second disc being identical: both were in fact the version of 'Ziggy Stardust' recorded on 16 May 1972. With admirable efficiency, EMI responded to this mistake by promptly issuing a one-track replacement CD of the missing track (BEE-BREP2) which was mailed to purchasers on request. Later pressings of the album corrected the error.

The attractive sleeve painting, based on a 1972 Mick Rock photo of David in the studio, was the work of *Diamond Dogs* veteran Guy Peellaert. "Guy works in a collage way," explained Bowie, "so what you see is a combination of photo and paint." The Japanese release (EMI TOCP 65631) included a deluxe 72-page booklet and an extra track in the form of 'Oh! You Pretty Things' from the acoustic session of 21 September 1971. Pre-publicity generated an array of promo and sampler CDs featuring tracks from the album, including free cover-mounts on various magazines and a very handsome eight-track sampler (BEEBPRO-6872) encased in a mock reel-to-reel tape box. EMI even issued a portable radio in the shape of an old-fashioned microphone, complete with a *Bowie At The Beeb* logo which lit up when the set was switched on.

The limited-edition bonus disc, entitled *BBC Radio Theatre, London, June 27, 2000*, offers a beautiful selection from Bowie's post-Glastonbury concert at Broadcasting House: there are joyous renditions of new material like 'Seven' and 'Survive', while fresh life is breathed into older numbers including a superb 'Always Crashing In The Same Car' and a truly exhilarating revamp of 'Let's Dance'. The curious decision to fade the audience sound to silence at the end of each track rather mars the overall atmosphere, but otherwise it's a splendid memento of the 2000 mini-tour – and arguably the best recorded of all Bowie's live albums.

ALL SAINTS: COLLECTED INSTRUMENTALS 1977-1999
EMI 7243 5 33045 2 2, July 2001

'A New Career In A New Town' / 'V-2 Schneider' / 'Abdulmajid' / 'Weeping Wall' / 'All Saints' / 'Art Decade' / 'Crystal Japan' / 'Brilliant Adventure' / 'Sense of Doubt' / 'Moss Garden' / 'Neuköln' / 'The Mysteries' / 'Ian Fish, U.K. Heir' / 'Subterraneans' / 'Warszawa' / 'Some Are'

This single-disc commercial reshuffle of Bowie's in-house 1993 compilation *All Saints* (see above) adds 'Crystal Japan' and 'Brilliant Adventure' to the original track-listing, but removes 'South Horizon' and all three *Black Tie White Noise* instrumentals. As on the first *All Saints*, 'Some Are' is Philip Glass's *"Low"* *Symphony* version; the others are the original Bowie cuts. The cover image of a blurred, negative-effect David with beard and shoulder-length hair was chosen by BowieNet members from a selection of eight pieces of artwork. It's hardly the most appealing of Bowie's album sleeves, but the compilation itself makes for an efficient and impressive summary of his more experimental work.

BEST OF BOWIE
EMI 7243 5 39821 2 6, November 2002 [11]
EMI/Virgin 72435-95692-0-8, November 2003
  (US/Canada reissue with bonus DVD)

Disc One (UK): 'Space Oddity' (5'14") / 'The Man Who Sold The World' (3'57") / 'Oh! You Pretty

Things' (3'13") / 'Changes' (3'34") / 'Life On Mars?' (3'50") / 'Starman' (4'13") / 'Ziggy Stardust' (3'13") / 'Suffragette City' (3'25") / 'John, I'm Only Dancing' (2'46") / 'The Jean Genie' (4'06") / 'Drive In Saturday' (4'30") / 'Sorrow' (2'55") / 'Diamond Dogs' (6'05") / 'Rebel Rebel' (4'30") / 'Young Americans' (3'15") / 'Fame' (4'17") / 'Golden Years' (3'29") / 'TVC15' (5'33") / 'Wild Is The Wind' (6'00")

Disc Two (UK): 'Sound And Vision' (3'05") / '"Heroes"' (3'36") / 'Boys Keep Swinging' (3'18") / 'Under Pressure' (3'57") / 'Ashes To Ashes' (3'37") / 'Fashion' (3'27") / 'Scary Monsters (And Super Creeps)' (3'34") / 'Let's Dance' (4'10") / 'China Girl' (4'18") / 'Modern Love' (3'58") / 'Blue Jean' (3'11") / 'This Is Not America' (3'53") / 'Loving The Alien' (4'45") / 'Dancing In The Street' (3'22") / 'Absolute Beginners' (5'38") / 'Jump They Say' (3'54") / 'Hallo Spaceboy (PSB remix)' (4'26") / 'Little Wonder' (3'43") / 'I'm Afraid Of Americans (V1)' (4'25") / 'Slow Burn (radio edit)' (3'57")

Bonus DVD with 2003 US reissue: 'Let's Dance (Club Bolly Mix Edit)' *(Video)* / 'Just For One Day (Heroes) (Edit)' *(Video)* / 'Black Tie White Noise (Live At Hollywood Center Studios, 8/5/93)' *(Video)* / 'Let's Dance (Club Bolly Extended Mix)' / 'Let's Dance (Bollyclub Mix)' / 'China Girl (Club Mix)' 'Just For One Day (Heroes) (Extended Version)' *(David Guetta vs Bowie)* / 'Loving The Alien (Scumfrog Remix)' *(The Scumfrog vs Bowie)* / 'Nite Flights (Moodswings Back To Basics Remix)'

Whether the world really needed yet another Bowie compilation by 2002 is a moot point, but the critical success of *Heathen*, alongside EMI/Virgin's retention of Bowie's back catalogue following his departure to Columbia, meant that it was more or less inevitable.

Released alongside the excellent DVD of the same title, *Best Of Bowie* superseded 1993's *The Singles Collection* and EMI's brace of 1997/1998 *Best Ofs* to become Bowie's standard greatest hits album. The UK version is a sturdy chronological trip through the classics, skimming through the post-*Let's Dance* 1980s and bypassing Tin Machine before resuming the story with 'Jump They Say' and a smattering of 1990s tracks.

However, the story doesn't end there. The elaborate gimmick used to promote *Best Of Bowie* was that its track-listing varied considerably from country to country, the better to reflect which songs had been popular in each territory. Accordingly, no fewer than 20 different versions of the album were released in October and November 2002; some countries released double-disc sets, others a single CD, while the US and Canada had both. Most releases are identifiable by the national flags reproduced in the hinge panel of the CD cases (the exceptions being the flagless UK, Eastern European and Argentinian/Mexican editions).

Most of the variant tracks on the different editions are readily available elsewhere, but collectors wishing to take advantage of the rarities on offer will be particularly interested in the New Zealand edition (EMI 7243 5 41925 2 4) which includes the first ever CD releases of the single mixes of 'Magic Dance' and 'Underground', the latter also appearing on the Chilean edition. Other minor rarities include the radio edit of 'Black Tie White Noise' (Denmark), the live version of 'Tonight' with Tina Turner (the Netherlands, where it was a number 1 hit in its day), and the US single version of 'Rebel Rebel' (Chile). In a solitary foray into the Tin Machine years, the US/Canada two-disc edition includes 'Under The God'. The UK, Greece and US/Canada editions feature the CD debut of the 7" edit of 'Scary Monsters', while several non-UK versions (USA/Canada, New Zealand, Greece, Netherlands, Denmark, Norway/Sweden, Chile, and Germany/Switzerland/Austria) carry the hard-to-find 7" edit of the original 'Cat People'. The last of these also includes the 1989 *Sound + Vision* remix of '"Helden"', while the last two feature the radio edit of 'When The Wind Blows'.

Some tracks ('Golden Years', '"Heroes"', 'Ashes To Ashes', 'China Girl', 'Modern Love', 'TVC15', 'Young Americans') vary between the album and single versions on different editions. Others are more consistent: notably, 'Slow Burn' is the previously hard-to-find radio edit.

Best Of Bowie's sleeve was a composite of David's face from different periods of his career, designed by '*hours...*' veteran Rex Ray; it also appeared on the accompanying DVD. Reviews of both were of the five-star variety and sales were healthy: while the DVD topped the UK music chart, the album peaked at number 11. Nearly a year after its release, the album was given a sales boost by the media coverage of *Reality*: in September 2003 *Best Of Bowie* leapt back up to number 25 in the UK chart, and by the following month it had spent no fewer than 45 weeks in the top 75.

In November 2003, the US/Canada single-disc version was reissued in a limited edition sleeve accompanied by a new bonus DVD consisting mainly of video and audio remixes from *Club Bowie*, while 2004's "Asian Tour Edition" (EMI 7243 5 7749 2 3), released to coincide with the Far East dates of A Reality Tour, combined the UK version with a bonus disc of *Club Bowie*.

CLUB BOWIE:
RARE AND UNRELEASED 12" MIXES
Virgin/EMI VTCD591, November 2003

'Loving The Alien' *(The Scumfrog vs David Bowie)* (8'21") / 'Let's Dance (Trifactor vs Deeper Substance Remix)' (11'02") / 'Just For One Day (Heroes) (Extended Version)' *(David Guetta vs Bowie)* (6'37") / 'This Is Not America' *(The Scumfrog vs David Bowie)* (9'12") / 'Shout (Original Mix)' *(Solaris vs Bowie)* (8'02") / 'China Girl (Riff & Vox Club Mix)' (7'08") / 'Magic Dance (Danny S Magic Party Remix)' (7'39") / 'Let's Dance (Club Bolly Extended Mix)' (7'56") / 'Let's Dance (Club Bolly Mix Video)' *(CD-ROM)*

The lurid day-glo orange packaging of this compilation, released at the height of the *Reality* boom, offers some indication of the eye-opening material within. Completists will value Virgin/EMI's collection of some of the more prominent club remixes of Bowie's work, but many of the unusual noises included on this CD will challenge even the most passionate collector. On the plus side are the Scumfrog remixes of 'Loving The Alien' and 'This Is Not America', both of which are likeable dance tracks, while the Asian remixes of 'Let's Dance' and 'China Girl' are certainly intriguing. However, the obscure repetitiveness of the remaining tracks will probably make sense only to the most chemically enhanced of hardcore clubbers – not exactly Bowie's natural fan constituency. The video of the 'Let's Dance (Club Bolly Mix)' is included in CD-ROM format.

The release threw up a number of variant formats, including a CDR promo which featured the otherwise unavailable 'Starman (Metrophonic Remix)' and the variant versions 'Just For One Day (Heroes) (Club Mix)', 'Shout (Amazon Dub)' and 'Magic Dance (Danny S Cut N Paste Remix)'.

MUSICAL STORYLAND
Worlds In Ink/Universal Music B0001073-02,
    April 2004

'Uncle Arthur' / 'Rubber Band' / 'There Is A Happy Land' / 'Did You Ever Have A Dream' / 'Sell Me A Coat' / 'Come And Buy My Toys' / 'Maid Of Bond Street' / 'Love You Till Tuesday' / 'When I Live My Dream' / 'Ching-a-Ling'

One of the most unusual Bowie-related projects yet undertaken, this charming book-and-CD release is the brainchild of California-based artist Jamilla Naji who, combining her love of Bowie's Deram recordings with her desire to publish a children's picture book, created an illustrated companion to ten of Bowie's late 1960s songs. Naji's acrylic paintings illustrate her interpretations of each song in an attractive and colourful style, poised somewhere between the naïve primitivism of Henri Rousseau and the dreamlike surrealism of Marc Chagall, while the accompanying CD allows children (and adults) to listen to the original recordings. *Musical Storyland* is available for shipping to US addresses via www.worldsinink.com.

OVERSEAS COMPILATION ALBUMS

A summary of variant compilations released outside the UK.

In The Beginning Volume Two
(1973 German Deram compilation)
David Bowie Coccinelle Variétés
(1973 French release of *The World Of David Bowie*, reissued 1983)
David Bowie Mille-Pattes Series
(1973 French release of *Images 1966-1967*)
El Rey Del Gay-Power
(1973 Spanish compilation of Deram tracks)
Disco De Ouro
(1974 Brazilian reissue of *The World Of David Bowie*)
Best Of David Bowie
(1974 Japanese double LP of tracks from *Space Oddity* to *Aladdin Sane*, reissued in 1976 as *David Bowie Special*)
David Bowie
(1976 Belgian reissue of *Images 1966-1967*, also issued as *David Bowie* in Argentina in 1978)
Starting Point
(1977 American Deram repackage)
Bowie Now
(1978 American promo-only compilation from *Low* and *"Heroes"*)
Collection Blanche
(1978 French reissue of *Images 1966-1967*)
20 Bowie Classics
(1979 Australian reissue of *Images 1966-1967*, minus 'Karma Man')
Profile
(1979 German Deram repackage)
Chameleon
(1979 Australian compilation from *Ziggy Stardust* to *Lodger*)
1980 All Clear
(1979 American promo-only compilation from *Space Oddity* to *Lodger*)
La Grande Storia Del Rock
(1979 Italian Deram package)
Rock Galaxy
(1981 German reissue of *Hunky Dory* and *Ziggy Stardust* as a double album)
David Bowie
(1981 Canadian reissue of Pye singles)

Historia De La Musica Rock
(1981 Spanish reissue of *Another Face*, reissued in 1982 as *Gigantes Del Pop Volume 28*)
Die Weisse Serie
(1982 German repackage of *Another Face*)
Bowie
(1982 Japanese reissue of *The World Of David Bowie*)
Superstar
(1982 Italian Deram repackage)
London Boys
(1982 Spanish compilation of 1966 Pye singles and other sixties Pye hopefuls)
Portrait Of A Star
(1982 French reissue of *Low*, *"Heroes"* and *Lodger* as a triple boxed set)
Die Weisse Serie Extra Ausgabe
(1983 German repackage of Deram tracks)
Ziggy '83
(1984 Canadian promo from the ABC broadcast of Bowie's Montreal concert in July 1983)
Early Bowie
(1984 Italian reissue of Pye singles)
30 Años De Musica Rock
(1984 Mexican reissue of *Another Face*)
David Bowie
(1985 Spanish reissue of Pye singles)
Early Years
(1987 French box set of *The Man Who Sold The World*, *Hunky Dory* and *Aladdin Sane*)
Starman
(1989 Russian compilation from *Space Oddity* to *Ziggy Stardust*)
David Bowie
(1990 Spanish Deram repackage)
The Laughing Gnome
(1996 German CD of UK *London Boy* compilation)
When I Live My Dream
(1997 German Deram compilation)
Rarest Live
(2000 Japanese compilation of tracks from *Santa Monica '72*)

(v) VARIOUS ARTISTS' COMPILATION ALBUMS

The only compilations listed are those which feature exclusive Bowie tracks, or the original release of tracks later made more widely available. The only tracks listed are those which are of particular interest to Bowie collectors.

GLASTONBURY FAYRE
Revelation REV 1/2/3, June 1972

'The Supermen' (2'41")

This now exceedingly rare triple album was an attempt to recoup the losses of the previous year's Glastonbury festival, at which David had performed. It saw the first release of Bowie's "alternative" studio version of 'The Supermen', later included as a bonus track on *Hunky Dory*. According to the sleeve notes, Bowie's "live tape recorded at Glastonbury will remain in our vaults until the revolution."

RUBY TRAX
Forty NME 40CD, September 1992

'Go Now' (4'30")

In addition to an exclusive live Tin Machine track, this three-CD charity release marketed by the *NME* and BBC Radio 1 in aid of the Spastics Society includes Tears For Fears' version of 'Ashes To Ashes', and a plethora of unlikely covers such as Billy Bragg's 'When Will I See You Again?' and EMF's 'Shaddap You Face'.

BEST OF GRUNGE ROCK
Priority P253708, 1993 *(US)*

'Baby Can Dance' (2'49")

BEYOND THE BEACH
Upstart CD012, October 1994 *(US)*

'Needles On The Beach' (4'32")

DAVID BOWIE SONGBOOK
Connoisseur VSOP CD236, 1997

'"Heroes"' *(Blondie)* / 'Space Oddity' *(The Flying Pickets)* / 'The Man Who Sold The World' *(Midge Ure)* / 'Kooks' *(Danny Wilson)* / 'Ziggy Stardust' *(Bauhaus)* / 'Rock'n'Roll Suicide' *(Tony Hadley)* / 'John, I'm Only Dancing' *(The Polecats)* / 'All The Young Dudes' *(Mott The Hoople)* / 'Watch That Man' *(Lulu)* / 'Rebel Rebel' *(Sigue Sigue Sputnik)* / 'Fame' *(Duran Duran)* / 'The Secret Life Of Arabia' *(Billy MacKenzie)* / 'Boys Keep Swinging' *(Susanna Hoffs)* / 'Ashes To Ashes' *(Tears For Fears)* / 'China Girl' *(Iggy Pop)* / 'Silver Treetop School For Boys' *(Beatstalkers)* / 'Over The Wall We Go' *(Oscar)*

This enjoyable compilation of Bowie cover versions by mainstream artists offers a selection of well-known recordings such as Lulu's 'Watch That Man', Bauhaus's 'Ziggy Stardust' and Blondie's live '"Heroes"', together with more obscure tracks including Billy MacKenzie's excellent 'The Secret Life Of Arabia', Susanna Hoffs's intriguing 'Boys Keep Swinging' and The Flying Pickets' indescribable 'Space Oddity'. Bowie collectors will be attracted by the two rare 1960s recordings: Oscar's 'Over The Wall We Go' (featuring guest vocals by David), and The Beatstalkers' 'Silver Treetop School For Boys'.

PHOENIX: THE ALBUM
BBC Worldwide/NMC PHNXCD1, 1997

'Hallo Spaceboy' (5'34")

LONG LIVE TIBET
EMI 7243 83314027, July 1997

'Planet Of Dreams' (4'37")

An added bonus for Bowie fans on this Tibet House Trust charity album is Terrorvision's cover of 'Moonage Daydream'.

THE BRIDGE SCHOOL CONCERTS VOL. 1
Reprise 946824-2, 1997 *(US)*

'"Heroes"' (6'34")

LIVE FROM 6A: GREAT MUSICAL PERFORMANCES FROM LATE NIGHT WITH CONAN O'BRIEN
Mercury Records 314536 3242, 1997 *(US)*

'Dead Man Walking'

99X LIVE XIV "HOME"
WNNX 5, 1998 *(US)*

'Dead Man Walking'

A limited run of this Atlanta WNNX Radio compilation came with a cover designed by Bowie.

RED HOT + RHAPSODY: THE GERSHWIN GROOVE
Antilles 314557788-2, October 1998 *(US)*

'A Foggy Day In London Town' (5'25")

WBCN: NAKED TOO
Wicked Disc WIC1009-2, November 1998 *(US)*

'Dead Man Walking'

SNL25: SATURDAY NIGHT LIVE – THE MUSICAL PERFORMANCES VOLUME 1
Dreamworks 0044-50205-2, September 1999 *(US)*

'Scary Monsters (And Super Creeps)'

VH1 STORYTELLERS
Interscope 0694905112, April 2000 *(US)*

'China Girl' (4'41")

SUBSTITUTE: THE SONGS OF THE WHO
edel/EAR ED183022, June 2001

'Pictures Of Lily' (4'59")

DIAMOND GODS: INTERPRETATIONS OF BOWIE
IHM/Ncompass IHCD 16, October 2001

'Loving The Alien' *(Iva Davies & Icehouse)* / 'Life On Mars?' *(En)* / 'Space Oddity' *(Brix Smith)* / '"Heroes"' *(Blondie)* / 'God Knows I'm Good' *(Bellatrix)* / 'The Man Who Sold The World' *(Tayce)* / 'I Can't Read' *(Tim Bowness & Samuel Smiles)* / 'The Laughing Gnome' *(Buster Bloodvessel)* / 'Panic In Detroit' *(The Aries Parallel)* / 'Rock'n'Roll Suicide' *(Hazel O'Connor)* / 'Real Cool World' *(Dead Eye Dolls)* / '"Heroes"' *(Nico)* / 'Loving The Alien' *(The Nine)* / 'Memory Of A Free Festival' *(David Fisher)*

Although less star-studded than *David Bowie Songbook* or the subsequent *Starman*, this useful compilation of cover versions includes, among other things, Hazel O'Connor's unsettling 'Rock'n'Roll Suicide', Iva Davies's beautiful acoustic 'Loving The Alien', Nico's excellent '"Heroes"', and Buster Bloodvessel's jaw-dropping techno interpretation of 'The Laughing Gnome'.

THE CONCERT FOR NEW YORK CITY
Columbia COL 5054452, November 2001

'America' (4'26") / '"Heroes"' (5'52")

STARMAN
UNCUT 2003 03, February 2003

'The Prettiest Star' *(Ian McCulloch)* / 'Starman' *(Culture Club)* / 'Fall In Love With Me' *(Guy Chadwick)* / 'The Gospel According To Tony Day' *(Edwyn Collins)* / 'Life On Mars?' *(The Divine Comedy)* / 'All The Young

Dudes' *(Alejandro Escovedo)* / 'The Man Who Sold The World' *(Midge Ure)* / 'Boys Keep Swinging' *(The Associates)* / 'Cracked Actor' *(Big Country)* / 'Funtime' *(Peter Murphy)* / 'John, I'm Only Dancing' *(The Polecats)* / '"Heroes"' *(Blondie)* / 'Rebel Rebel' *(Sigue Sigue Sputnik)* / 'Fame' *(Duran Duran)* / 'Ziggy Stardust' *(The Gourds)* / 'Space Oddity' *(The Langley Schools Music Project)* / 'Panic In Detroit' *(Christian Death)* / 'Rock'n'Roll Suicide' *(Black Box Recorder)*

The March 2003 edition of the UK's *Uncut* magazine was a Bowie special, including among its attractions this excellent free CD of cover versions. Two of the recordings (Ian McCulloch's 'The Prettiest Star' and Edwyn Collins's superb 'The Gospel According To Tony Day') were recorded exclusively for this release.

Other highlights include The Gourds' bonkers folk/reggae/Latino interpretation of 'Ziggy Stardust', Culture Club's atmospheric 'Starman', and Black Box Recorder's laid-back 'Rock'n'Roll Suicide'.

HOPE
London Recordings 50466 5846 2, April 2003

'Everyone Says 'Hi' (METRO Mix)' (3'42")

This charity compilation, in aid of War Child's campaign for the children of Iraq, included the rare 'METRO Mix' of 'Everyone Says 'Hi''. In Canada a double-disc variation entitled *Peace Songs* (Sony/BMG C2K91772) also featured the track.

3   LIVE

Naturally, documentation of Bowie's very earliest perform-
ances is at best sketchy, and we can never hope to draw up
definitive details of his repertoire and dates prior to the
1970s. Performances vary from night to night, and of
course not every song in the later tours' set-lists was per-
formed at every gig. Chapter 10 contains a comprehensive
chronology of individual dates and television appearances.

1947 – 1962: EARLY PERFORMANCES

Among the earliest musical influences that impressed
themselves on the imagination of the young David
Jones were Felix Mendelssohn and Danny Kaye.
"There was a piece of religious music that was always
played on the radio on Sunday called 'O For The
Wings Of A Dove'," Bowie told *Rolling Stone* in 2003.
"I must have been about six." This was undoubtedly
the famous 1927 recording of Mendelssohn's *Hear My*
Prayer, from which 'O For The Wings Of A Dove', sung
by the boy soprano Ernest Lough, became a staple of
religious broadcasting during the mid-twentieth century. "Not so far after that I heard 'Inchworm' by
Danny Kaye," David continued. "They are the first two
pieces of music that made any impression on me. And
they both have the same weight of sadness about
them. For some reason I really empathized with that."
In an interview for *Q* magazine in the same year he
went further: "'Inchworm' is my childhood. It wasn't a
happy one. Not that it was brutal, but mine were a certain type of British parent: quite cold emotionally and
not many hugs. I always craved affection cause of that.
'Inchworm' gave me comfort, and the person singing
it sounded like he'd been hurt too. And I'm into that,
the artist singing away his pain."

'Inchworm', written by Frank Loesser for the 1952
film musical *Hans Christian Andersen*, would go on to
exert a fundamental effect on Bowie's creative palette,
influencing compositions like 'Ashes To Ashes' and
'Thursday's Child' in later years. "I loved it as a kid,
and it's stayed with me forever," he told *Performing*
Songwriter in 2003. "You wouldn't believe the amount
of my songs that have sort of spun off that one song

… There's a child's nursery rhyme element in it, and
there's something so sad and mournful and poignant
about it. It kept bringing me back to the feelings of
those pure thoughts of sadness that you have as a
child, and how they're so identifiable even when
you're an adult. There's a connection that can be made
between being a somewhat lost five-year-old and feeling a little abandoned and having the same feeling
when you're in your twenties. And it was that song
that did that for me." So, too, did the unusual harmonic structures of *Hear My Prayer*; as he told Michael
Parkinson in 2002, these were "the pieces of music
that kind of broke my expectations. Holst's *Mars* was
another. Those notes were so weird. It didn't follow
anything that I knew, you know. And songs like that –
pieces of music where the notes didn't go the right
way – really got me."

David's introduction to rock and roll came not
long afterwards, and can largely be credited to his
half-brother Terry. Ten years David's senior, Terry was
one of two children born to Peggy Burns in the years
before she met David's father Haywood Stenton Jones
in 1946. "It was Terry who really started everything for
me," Bowie told his first biographer George Tremlett
many years later. "He was into all those different beat
writers, and listening to jazz musicians like John
Coltrane and Eric Dolphy … while I was still at
school, he would go up to town every Saturday
evening to listen to jazz in the different clubs … he
was growing his hair long, and rebelling in his own
way … it all had a big impact on me." In 1999 he
recalled that "Terry really opened up my mind. He
had an innate intelligence, an excitement about the
world and an appetite for knowledge. He taught me

how to learn things, how to go out of my way to discover things."

In 1953 the family had left David's birthplace at 40 Stansfield Road, Brixton, in favour of the leafy suburb of Bromley in Kent. There they changed addresses a couple of times before settling at 4 Plaistow Grove in June 1955. By now a new youth culture was emerging in force from America. "I saw a cousin of mine dance when I was very young," David later recalled. "She was dancing to Elvis's 'Hound Dog' and I had never seen her get up and be moved so much by anything. It really impressed me, the power of the music. I started getting records immediately after that. My mother bought me Fats Domino's 'Blueberry Hill' the next day. And then I fell in love with the Little Richard Band. I never heard anything that lived in such bright colours in the air. It really just painted the whole room for me."

Both 'Hound Dog' and 'Blueberry Hill' were UK hits late in 1956. A couple of years later, aged eleven, David began attending Bromley Technical High School, where he pursued a growing interest in rhythm and blues, skiffle and rock'n'roll. He had become the proud owner of a white plastic saxophone on which he taught himself Little Richard tunes, and had also begun to dabble in the ukulele and a home-made string bass made from a broom-handle and a plywood tea-chest. By 1958 he was a chorister at St Mary's Church, Bromley, alongside George Underwood and Geoffrey MacCormack, both of whom would remain friends for life. MacCormack, who first met David at the age of seven at Burnt Ash Primary School, would re-emerge as a backing vocalist and co-writer on several of Bowie's mid-1970s albums, and read a Psalm at David's wedding in 1992. David recalled in 1983 that MacCormack "had the big ska record collection, and it just wasn't worth competing with him, so I went straight into buying Chuck Berry, Little Richard and the blues stuff."

George Underwood would play in several of David's early R&B bands and later design some of his classic album sleeves. Apparently the two first met in 1957 at the 18th Bromley Scouts' Cub Pack. George owned an acoustic guitar, and it was this that provided the backing for David's first documented "rock" performance, at the Scouts' annual Summer Camp on the Isle of Wight in August 1958. The boys' set consisted of 'Cumberland Gap', 'Gamblin' Man' and 'Putting On The Style', three skiffle numbers which had featured on the A- and B-sides of Lonnie Donegan's chart-topping singles the previous summer.

For Christmas 1959, a fortnight short of his thirteenth birthday, David was given his first real saxophone by his mother. Soon afterwards he began taking weekly lessons from jazz saxophonist Ronnie Ross, who lived not far away in Orpington. Terry had recommended Ross after seeing him nominated as best jazz newcomer in *Downbeat* magazine. "I rung him up," David would remember many years later. "I said, 'Hi, my name is David Jones, and I'm twelve years old, and I want to play the saxophone. Can you give me lessons? He sounded like Keith Richards, and he said no. But I begged until he said, 'If you can get yourself over here Saturday morning, I'll have a look at you.' He was so cool."

"He had about eight lessons, one every two weeks and I charged him £2 a lesson," Ronnie Ross later recalled. "He stuck it out for that time and then disappeared." David would later enlist Ross to perform the famous sax solo on Lou Reed's 'Walk On The Wild Side'.

"For me the saxophone always embodied the West Coast beat generation," David recalled in 1983. "I was very entranced by that period of Americana. It became sort of a token, a symbol of freedom; a way of getting out of London that would lead me to America, which was an ambition at the time … Then when I started working with it, I found I didn't have a very good relationship with the sax and that lasted right the way through … I've always felt grossly uncomfortable playing it. I want it to do one thing and it wants me to do something else, and between us, we get something that comes and sounds peculiarly like my style of playing."

Another formative experience in David's musical education was a stint working at Vic Furlong's record shop in Bromley, where he was entranced by the sounds of James Brown, Ray Charles and Jackie Wilson, black musicians who were still very much on the periphery of the British market. In 1960, at the start of their third year at Bromley Tech, both David and George moved into the school's art stream where their creative predilections were encouraged by their progressive art master Owen Frampton, whose son Peter was also briefly a pupil at the school. Peter later recalled that he and David played Buddy Holly numbers like 'Every Day' and 'Peggy Sue' during school concerts. Over 25 years later, long after his own peak of fame as a rock musician, Peter Frampton would be reunited with David in the studio and on tour.

In 1962, around the time of the dissolution of George Underwood's short-lived band George And The Dragons (whose final performance at a school concert was apparently upstaged by the lost property lady's rendition of 'There's A Hole In My Bucket'), he and David approached another school band with a view to joining forces.

THE KON-RADS
June 1962 – September 1963

Musicians: David Jones/Dave Jay (*vocals, tenor saxophone*), George Underwood (*vocals*), Neville Wills (*guitar*), Alan Dodds (*guitar*), Dave Crook (*drums*), Dave Hadfield (*drums*), Rocky Shahan (*bass*), Roger Ferris (*vocals*), Christine Gill, Stella Gill (*backing vocals*)

Repertoire included: 'It's Only Make-Believe' / 'Quarter To Three (A Night With Daddy G)' / 'A Picture Of You' / 'Hey Baby' / 'In The Mood' / 'China Doll' / 'The Young Ones' / 'Sweet Little Sixteen' / 'Move It' / 'Lucille' / 'Good Golly Miss Molly' / 'Ginny Come Lately' / 'Let's Dance' / 'Hall Of The Mountain King' / 'I Never Dreamed'

Bromley Tech schoolboys Neville Wills, Alan Dodds and Dave Crook were already playing as a three-piece called The Kon-rads when George Underwood offered his services as lead singer. He promptly brought in David Jones to sing Joe Brown's 'A Picture Of You' ("he looked like Joe Brown in those days," remarked Underwood many years later), and to help out on vocals for a cover of Bruce Channel's 'Hey Baby'. David soon introduced his new tenor saxophone into the mix, and The Kon-rads were relaunched. According to legend the group's name had emerged when they supported Jess Conrad, who apparently introduced them as "my Conrads", but details of this particular tale are thin on the ground.

David's first documented date with the group was at a school fête on 16 June 1962. The *Kentish Times* reported a crowd of nearly 4000, although not all were watching when "a group of young instrumentalists called The Conrads [sic] played music on guitars, saxophone and drums."

"The Kon-rads did cover songs of anything that was in the charts," recalled David thirty years later. "We were one of the best cover bands in the area and

we worked a lot." By late 1962 George Underwood had left the band to be replaced by a new lead singer, Roger Ferris, while Dave Crook had been replaced on drums by Dave Hadfield and the ranks were swelled by new members Rocky Shahan and the Gill sisters. "I was originally in as a sax player," said David, "Then our singer, Roger Ferris, got beaten up by some greasers at the Civic, Orpington and I took over the vocals. I could only do Little Richard songs 'cos they were the only ones I really knew the words to." Thus it was that, following the customary show-opener 'In The Mood', the likes of 'Lucille' and 'Good Golly Miss Molly' were added to the repertoire. As David's confidence grew, other new additions included Brian Hyland's 'Ginny Come Lately' and Chris Montez's 'Let's Dance'.

The Kon-rads kept David busy into the spring of 1963, playing at youth clubs, church halls and dances. They did well enough to splash out on a band uniform ("I hated those suits," David later confessed, "They were brown corduroy"), while their restless young singer experimented with an array of extravagant hairstyles and, significantly, with his name: on the band's 1962 Christmas card it became "Dave Jay" (a change apparently inspired by the sax-heavy combo Peter Jay And The Jaywalkers), while drummer Dave Hadfield tells the Gillmans that David was already considering the name Bowie. He had also begun composing his own songs, some of which were added to the band's repertoire. According to Roger Ferris, David was already "getting into cutting up bits of paper with lines on them and throwing them in the air and seeing what came out. He was very avant-garde very early." Before long, however, The Kon-rads proved too restrictive an outfit for David's roving musical eye. "I wanted to move into rhythm and blues," he later said, "and they wouldn't. They wanted to stay with the Top 20. That's when I broke away."

Two crucial episodes occurred during David's time with the Kon-rads. The second, in August 1963, was his earliest known studio recording (see 'I Never Dreamed' in Chapter 1). The first happened earlier the same year, and in its own way had a more lasting effect. During a schoolyard quarrel over a girl, George Underwood punched David in the face, inadvertently inflicting what was diagnosed as traumatic mydriasis on David's left eye. "It was over this girl called Carol Goldsmith," Underwood revealed in 2001. "Obviously I didn't mean to hurt him as much as I did. I certainly didn't have a compass or a battery in my hand as people have claimed since. It was just a knuckle but it dislodged something and damaged part of his eye."

"It started bleeding and I was in hospital for months," David melodramatically claimed a few years later. In fact it wasn't quite that serious, but it did leave him with a susceptibility to migraines and impaired eyesight. "It's left me with a wonky sense of perspective," he said in 1999. "When I'm driving, for instance, cars don't come towards me, they just get bigger." Look closely at the oft-reproduced publicity shots of the Kon-rads, and you can see that David's eye is still bruised.

The most noticeable result of the punch was that the pupil of David's left eye remained permanently dilated. Contrary to popular legend the iris did not change colour, although his left eye often appears greenish-brown due to the paralysed pupil, while his right remains blue.

After David's departure the Kon-rads enjoyed a modicum of success, supporting The Rolling Stones on tour and even releasing a single, 'Baby It's Too Late Now', in 1965. Intriguingly, 2001 saw the discovery of another previously unknown Kon-rads single which some Bowiephiles, despite the absence of concrete proof, believe may date from David's time with the band (for more on the elusive 'I Didn't Know How Much', see 'I Never Dreamed' in Chapter 1).

THE HOOKER BROTHERS
July-September 1963

Musicians: David Jones *(vocals, tenor saxophone)*, George Underwood *(vocals, rhythm guitar, harmonica)*, Viv Andrews *(drums)*

Repertoire included: 'Tupelo Blues' / 'House Of The Rising Sun' / 'Blues In The Night (My Momma Done Told Me)'

In July 1963, aged 16, David left Bromley Tech to work as a junior "visualizer" at the American-owned advertising agency J Walter Thompson, "doing paste-up and initial design for things like raincoats," he recalled in 1993. "I hated it." In 2003 he recounted that "My immediate boss, Ian, a groovy modernist with Gerry Mulligan-style short crop haircut and Chelsea boots, was very encouraging about my passion for music, something he and I both shared, and

used to send me on errands to Dobell's Jazz record shop on Charing Cross Road, knowing I'd be there for most of the morning till well after lunch break. It was there, in the 'bins', that I found Bob Dylan's first album. Ian had sent me there to get him a John Lee Hooker release and advised me to pick up a copy for myself, as it was so wonderful. Within weeks my pal George Underwood and I had changed the name of our little R&B outfit to The Hooker Brothers and had included both Hooker's 'Tupelo' and Dylan's 'House Of The Rising Sun' in our set."

Substantial evidence of Bob Dylan's influence on David's songwriting lay some years ahead, but the naming of his new band betrayed a growing interest in the pioneering sounds of rhythm and blues and, as Bowie would later reflect, both Dylan and Hooker "became an integral part of what I tried to do eventually." The Hooker Brothers were a trio consisting of David, George Underwood and drummer Viv Andrews (later to play on The Pretty Things' first two hits, both covered by Bowie on *Pin Ups*). In the summer of 1963 they secured the first of David's many gigs at Peter Melkin's Bromel Club at the Bromley Court Hotel, and also played at the Ravensbourne College of Art, where George was now a pupil. "This was a group of sixteen and seventeen-year-olds playing blues," recalled Underwood. "Everything we did was copied, but not very well. Such songs as 'My Momma Done Told Me'."

The band also styled themselves The Bow Street Runners and Dave's Reds & Blues, the latter a coded reference to speed and barbiturate pills and, as Bowie recalled in 2000, "a sad and clumsy allusion to R&B." It appears that the band only performed a total of three or four times before Viv Andrews departed and the others moved on to form the group with whom David would cut his first ever disc.

DAVIE JONES AND THE KING BEES
April – June 1964

Musicians: Davie Jones *(vocals, tenor saxophone)*, George Underwood *(rhythm guitar, harmonica, vocals)*, Roger Bluck *(lead guitar)*, Dave "Frank" Howard *(bass)*, Bob Allen *(drums)*

Repertoire included: 'Liza Jane' / 'Got My Mojo Working' / 'Hoochie Coochie Man' / 'Louie, Louie Go Home' / 'Can I Get A Witness'

David was still working as a commercial artist when he and George Underwood formed The King Bees (occasionally hyphenated in publicity material of the time). The name derived from the Louisiana blues singer Slim Harpo's composition 'I'm A King Bee', then recently covered on The Rolling Stones' debut album. Legend has it that David met the three new members while waiting to have his hair cut. "Before you could say 'short back and sides', they decided to join forces," chirped the band's first press release. "I can't actually remember their names," David confessed in 1993. "They were from North London and were virtually professional. Quite scary." Nevertheless, he and George soon assumed control: "We inflicted our tastes on the others," Underwood later said.

In the spring of 1964 David made his first overtures to a potential manager. With a little help from his father, he wrote a letter to the wealthy washing-machine entrepreneur John Bloom to suggest that he might like to consider becoming the next Brian Epstein, with the King Bees his Beatles. Impressed by David's audacity but hardly knowledgeable about the music business, Bloom passed the letter on to his friend Leslie Conn, then manager of the Denmark Street publishing company Melcher Music. Conn secured The King Bees a gig at Bloom's wedding anniversary party at the Jack Of Clubs in Brewer Street, Soho, where the guests included Adam Faith and Lance Percival. It was not a success. "It was all a bit embarrassing," David recalled years later. "The party was very posh, with many guests in evening dress, and we all turned up in our T-shirts and jeans, ready to play rhythm & blues." Conn later said that "The noise was deafening ... people had their hands over their ears." Apparently the band got through two numbers before Bloom yelled, "Get 'em off! They're ruining my party!"

An audition with Decca was more successful and led soon afterwards to the recording of 'Liza Jane' (see Chapter 1). Another of Conn's contacts, the music publisher Dick James, was reportedly unimpressed by young Davie Jones but nonetheless agreed to publish 'Liza Jane'. At around the same time Conn introduced David to another of his protégés, Mark Feld – the future Marc Bolan. "We met each other firstly painting the wall of our then manager's office," David recalled in 1999. "'Hello, who are you?' 'I'm Mark, man.' 'Hi, what do you do?' 'I'm a singer.' 'Oh yeah? So am I. Are you a Mod?' 'Yeah, I'm King Mod. Your shoes are crap.' 'Well, you're short.' So we became really close friends."

It appears that David now shares Bolan's opinion of his sartorial tastes at the time. "I've always hated the way I looked when I was with the King Bees," he confessed in 2002. "It was that coalman's jacket I used to wear, the leather kind of waistcoaty affair. It was very long and it had no sleeves. It was what coalmen used to wear to put their sacks over their backs, but I thought it was an interesting fashion item! My hair was none too clever either."

With the release of 'Liza Jane' in June 1964, David somewhat precipitately left his job at the advertising agency, throwing his enthusiasm behind the Dick James Organisation's publicity campaign: "Davie's favourite vocalists are Little Richard, Bob Dylan and John Lee Hooker," proclaimed the press release. "He dislikes Adam's apples, and lists as his interests baseball, American football and collecting boots. A handsome six footer with a warm and engaging personality, Davie Jones has all it takes to get to the showbusiness heights, including talent." To promote the single, Conn secured The King Bees a succession of appearances at various London venues, notably clocking up David's first appearance at the Marquee Club, and also marking his first performances on television, playing 'Liza Jane' on *Ready, Steady, Go!* on 19 June and *The Beat Room* on 27 July. "We were a very typical Americanized London rhythm and blues outfit," David later recalled. "We were quite influenced by The Downliner Sect and we did a lot of pub work." However, the chart failure of 'Liza Jane' spelled the end of his involvement with the band. "The King Bees weren't very good, and we weren't going anywhere," admitted Underwood many years later. "We weren't blues people. We didn't want someone who could finger-pick like Chet Atkins; we wanted dirt and distortion." Without David, The King Bees released another unsuccessful single, 'You're Holding Me Down', before splitting.

Meanwhile, in August 1964, Leslie Conn introduced David to another act on his books: a six-piece Kentish band tipped to be at the vanguard of "the Medway Beat". Davie Jones had found his next band.

THE MANISH BOYS
August 1964 – March 1965

Musicians: Davie Jones *(vocals, saxophone)*, Johnny Flux *(lead guitar)*, Paul Rodriguez *(guitar, tenor saxophone, trumpet)*, Woolf Byrne *(baritone saxophone,* harmonica), Johnny Watson *(bass guitar, vocals)*, Bob Solly *(organ)*, Mick White *(drums)*

Repertoire included: 'Liza Jane' / 'I Pity The Fool' / 'Louie, Louie Go Home' / 'Take My Tip' / 'Last Night' / 'I Ain't Got You' / 'Duke Of Earl' / 'Love Is Strange' / 'Mary Ann' / 'Watermelon Man' / 'Hoochie Coochie Man' / 'Don't Try To Stop Me' / 'Little Egypt' / 'Night Train' / 'If You Don't Come Back' / 'Big Boss Man' / 'James Brown Medley' / 'Stupidity' / 'Can't Nobody Love You' / 'Hello Stranger' / 'You Can't Sit Down' / 'Believe To My Soul' / 'What'd I Say'

When David met them in August 1964, Maidstone's Manish Boys had already been together for four years and had undergone several changes of name (including Band Seven and The Jazz Gentlemen) before settling on a moniker derived from Muddy Waters's 1955 classic 'Mannish Boy'. Organist Bob Solly told *Record Collector* in 2000 that there was resistance within the band to the addition of David: "Initially we said no, but Conn said, 'He's got a recording contract, he's just made a record and he could be to your advantage.'" David met the band for rehearsals at saxophonist Paul Rodriguez's house at Coxheath. "He had a hell of a good voice and he was a very good sax player," Rodriguez later said. "He was a better musician than any of us." David rapidly assumed a governing role, steering the band towards R&B with his prized copy of James Brown's LP *Live at the Apollo*. The Manish Boys were quick to capitalize on the fact that David had already released a single, and on August 18 the *Chatham Standard* announced that "...other news from the boys is that they are now backing Decca recording star Davie Jones, whose group, the King-Bees, are no longer with him." The following day saw David's first gig with the band, at the famous Eel-Pie Island jazz club in Twickenham.

By the time of his association with The Manish Boys, David had begun dressing *à la mode*. "A popular thing was to go down to the back of Carnaby Street late at night and raid the dustbins," he later said. "You could pick up the most dynamite things down there!" Not only did David indulge his own love of clothes – something that has never deserted him – but he oversaw a sartorial makeover for the band. Within a month of his arrival, The Manish Boys were following David's example in clothes and hairstyles.

October 6 saw David's first studio session with the band, recording three unreleased demos at Regent Sound Studios (see 'Hello Stranger' in Chapter 1). A month later came David's first substantial television interview, although unlike his previous appearance on *Juke Box Jury*, it had little to do with his music. In a shameless attempt to court publicity David, whose thick blond hair now hung below his shoulders, claimed to have founded a society called The International League for the Preservation of Animal Filament, and it was in the guise of "president" that he found himself talking to novelist Leslie Thomas for the 2 November edition of the London *Evening News and Star*. Headlined "FOR THOSE BEYOND THE FRINGE", the item saw David claiming common ground with such hirsute greats as P J Proby, Screaming Lord Sutch, the Beatles and the Rolling Stones. The story was pounced upon by BBC Television's *Tonight*, which on 12 November featured the celebrated interview with David Jones, now spokesperson of the equally nonexistent Society for the Prevention of Cruelty to Long Haired Men. Flanked by the Manish Boys, David explained to Cliff Michelmore: "For the last two years we've had comments like "Darlin'" and "Can I carry your handbag?" thrown at us, and I think it's just had to stop now." Bass player John Watson added that the Society was contemplating CND-style protest marches, at which David quipped, "Baldermaston." This episode apparently netted David the princely sum of five guineas.

On 1 December 1964 The Manish Boys, now signed to the Arthur Howes Agency, began a six-date, two-shows-a-day tour of the north, playing support to Gene Pitney, The Kinks, Marianne Faithfull and Gerry & The Pacemakers. Although opening with the band composition 'Last Night' and adding David's single 'Liza Jane' to their repertoire, The Manish Boys' act leaned mainly on American-influenced blues and soul, including a James Brown medley and covers of Ray Charles, Solomon Burke, The Coasters and The Yardbirds. David's stage persona was developing noticeably camp mannerisms, which in addition to the band's notoriously long hair would lead a promoter in Cromer to tell them they were "obscene". They had to flee after a gig in Luton where, according to Rodriguez, "The general feeling of the audience appeared to be that the trumpet player was all right but the rest were a lot of fucking poofters." Bob Solly recalls that when, in late 1964, The Manish Boys auditioned at the BBC for a residency at Hamburg's Star-Club, David secured the job by assuring the German promoter that he was gay: "That was common in those days. People would say anything in order to get on." There is every indication, however, that David's alleged homosexuality during the period has been much exaggerated: it was at a Manish Boys gig that he first met fourteen-year-old Dana Gillespie, who became a girlfriend and remained in his circle into the 1970s. "My parents thought he was a girl," Gillespie later revealed. "He looked like Veronica Lake. His hair was much longer than The Beatles'. On stage, he wore these Sheriff of Nottingham type boots, a Russian peasant's shirt and a waistcoat. If you wore knee-length suede boots with long straight hair, you weren't the normal person on the street. He was always an outsider in that regard."

Not long afterwards The Manish Boys' recording career resumed in association with producer Shel Talmy, whose offer to take the group into the studio meant scrapping the Hamburg season. On 8 February 1965 they cut their Parlophone single 'I Pity The Fool', and when Leslie Conn secured a performance on BBC2's 8 March edition of *Gadzooks! It's All Happening*, David found himself involved in a second hair-orientated publicity stunt. The show's producer Barry Langford insisted that David cut his hair before the broadcast, which led to a preposterous demonstration involving the band's small coterie of fans picketing the BBC with placards reading "Be Fair to Long Hair". The *Daily Mirror* ran the story on 3 March with the headline "ROW OVER DAVY'S HAIR", and the following day's *Daily Mail* reported that the band had been dropped from the programme, quoting David saying "I wouldn't have my hair cut for the Prime Minister, let alone the BBC." The *Mirror* was back on the case on 6 March with the news that the band would be appearing after all, and would donate their fee to charity if viewers complained about David's locks. On the day of the show the *Evening News* published a photograph of the week's most publicized pop singer having his hair cut for the show after all. The *Mirror* wrapped up the saga the day after the TV show with an editorial lamenting that the existence of long-haired men was "nauseating", proof of "a sickness in the air".

Langford, of course, was a willing party to all this nonsense – certainly the publicity didn't do the programme any harm. Then again, it didn't do 'I Pity the Fool' much good, and within days of the broadcast David had parted company with the band after a dispute over billing. 'I Pity the Fool' had been credited simply to The Manish Boys, despite an earlier agreement that it was supposed to have been "Davie Jones and The Manish Boys". As early as April 1965 Paul Rodriguez would admit to the *Kent Messenger* that there had been "a furious row" over David's billing. In any event, the failure of the single put paid to any plans to record another. Bob Solly recalls meeting David in Shel Talmy's office in March: "We said to him, 'What about the next record?' And he said, 'What makes you think I wanna do another record with The Manish Boys?' … I think he was a nice fellow who sometimes had to be nasty in order to get on. He had no other thought in his head than success."

By April David was fronting his next group, The Lower Third, and the remaining Manish Boys disbanded not long afterwards. Guitarist Johnny Flux would later enjoy some unlikely successes under the name John Edward – he wrote and produced Renee & Renato's notorious 1982 smash 'Save Your Love', and designed, built and voiced the early 1980s ITV robot Metal Mickey. As a final footnote, Kenneth Pitt points out in his memoir that *Mirabelle* magazine's "Local Group Top Ten" voted The Manish Boys its sixth favourite band in the very same week that The Rats, a little-known Hull group who would later employ one Michael Ronson, were voted third.

THE LOWER THIRD
April 1965 – 29 January 1966

Musicians: Davy Jones/David Bowie *(vocals, guitar, saxophone)*, Denis "Tea-Cup" Taylor *(lead guitar)*, Graham Rivens *(bass)*, Les Mighall *(drums)*, Phil Lancaster *(drums)*

Repertoire included: 'You've Got A Habit Of Leaving' / 'Baby Loves That Way' / 'The London Boys' / 'Can't Help Thinking About Me' / 'Chim Chim Cheree' / 'Mars, The Bringer Of War' / 'Born Of The Night'

By April 1965 the Giaconda coffee bar in Denmark Street was David's regular haunt, as it was for so many young hopefuls on the fringes of London's music business, and it was here that David met his next band.

Originally a five-piece from Margate who had formed in 1963 as Oliver Twist and The Lower Third, the band had effectively split when three of its members decamped to London. In need of recruits, they promptly auditioned David at La Discothèque in

Soho. With David on sax and fellow auditionee Steve Marriott on vocals, the band ran through Little Richard's 'Rip It Up'. The result was adjudged a success, and while Marriott went off to form – almost immediately – The Small Faces, the other four joined forces as (the newly-spelt) Davy Jones and The Lower Third. Although hardly epic in length, this would be David's most significant stint with a band so far. During the same period he played the occasional gig with other bands, including The T-Bones and Sonny Boy Williamson.

"I guess it wanted to be a rhythm and blues band," David recalled in 1983. "We did a lot of stuff by John Lee Hooker, and we tried to adapt his stuff to the big beat – never terribly successfully. But that was the thing – everybody was picking a blues artist as their own … ours was Hooker."

Success was not immediate: the unsuccessful demo 'Born Of The Night' impressed nobody. On 20 May at R G Jones Studios, David and the band wrote and recorded two self-penned jingles for US radio, one for Youthquake Clothing and the other for an unidentified product called Puritan. Former Manish Boy Johnny Flux was now a DJ for pirate station Radio City, and he called in a favour by persuading David to record some further jingles for the Johnny Flux Show. It wasn't the most glorious of beginnings for a new outfit, and before The Lower Third had enjoyed any real success, drummer Les Mighall returned to Margate. He was replaced by Phil Lancaster, who had briefly played with the Dave Clark Five.

Despite the failure of 'I Pity The Fool', David's producer Shel Talmy successfully negotiated a Parlophone deal for The Lower Third and continued to supervise their session work. At around the time that the band recorded its first single 'You've Got A Habit Of Leaving', David quietly dumped Leslie Conn in favour of his first full-time manager: Ralph Horton was a Giaconda regular who worked as a booker at a Denmark Street agency. Previously a roadie for The Moody Blues but now assisting in the management of acts including Screaming Lord Sutch, Horton came on board after an audition at the Roebuck pub on Tottenham Court Road in early August. His first act as manager was to supervise a makeover of the long-haired teenagers; kitted out with hipster trousers and floral ties from Carnaby Street, they were frog-marched to Charles of Queensway for regulation Mod haircuts. Horton even encouraged the use of hair lacquer, which upset some of the band but not David,

who was already besotted by the dandified Mod image and its new cheerleaders, The Who.

Horton secured a series of summer engagements for The Lower Third, including a residency supporting The Who's regular Bournemouth Pavilion gigs. They also supported The Moody Blues at the Bromel Club, and Johnny Kidd & the Pirates and The Pretty Things during a Saturday residency at the Winter Gardens, Ventnor. A series of Saturday afternoon shows at the Marquee followed in September as part of "The Inecto Show", sponsored by Inecto Shampoo and taped for broadcast by pirate Radio London. It seems that The Lower Third's contribution was restricted to warm-up spots that were never actually broadcast.

"We were too loud on stage," David recollected. "We used feedback and sounds and didn't play any melodies. We just pulverized the sound, which was loosely based on Tamla-Motown. We had an ardent following of about a hundred Mods, but when we played out of London, we were booed right off the stage. We weren't very good." At David's instigation the band started behaving like The Who on stage – Denis Taylor thrashed his guitar and David smashed his microphone against the drumkit, breaking a cymbal on one occasion. "We were known as the second loudest group in London," Taylor said years later. "The Who were the first. A publisher … remarked that we sounded like a Lancaster Bomber flying through the studio." It's odd, then, to note David's apparent preference for well-behaved audiences: "We're not a 'scream' group," he declared in a Parlophone press release in August 1965. "We like our audiences to be quiet while we're performing a number, and then to give us a healthy response when we finish."

Ralph Horton did not prove to be The Lower Third's greatest asset, lacking both the tactics and the financial skills necessary for successful management. Nevertheless it was Horton who took the band from Shel Talmy to Tony Hatch, a producer whose style was arguably more suited to David's songs. And it was Horton who, under no illusions about his own limited cachet in the industry, opened a significant door in David's career when he elected to contact a more powerful manager.

On 15 September 1965 Horton telephoned Kenneth Pitt, manager of Manfred Mann and rising star Crispian St Peters – not to mention Bob Dylan during his English tours – to request assistance in furthering the prospects of The Lower Third. Pitt was busy with other clients and declined, but among the advice he offered was that the vocalist might consider changing his name to avoid confusion with the Davy Jones who was making waves as a versatile actor-singer and was about to find global fame with The Monkees. Horton passed on Pitt's advice, and on 17 September, The Lower Third were duly informed by their singer that he was now called David Bowie.

Denis Taylor thought the name ludicrous, remarking that it would "never catch on". Horton's flatmate Kenny Bell's first reaction was apparently to tell David that the new name was "fucking stupid". David would subsequently say that he chose the name because a Bowie knife is double-edged and "cuts both ways" – in fact a suggestion given to him much later by William Burroughs – and he also remarked that "I wanted a truism about cutting through the lies and all that." Incidentally, David has always, but always, pronounced the name to rhyme with "Chloë". It doesn't rhyme with "Howie", and nor is the correct pronunciation "Boo-ie" (this being the version favoured by many Americans including, almost certainly, the original Jim Bowie).

Shortly afterwards David Bowie and The Lower Third secured their deal with Pye Records and made their first recordings with Tony Hatch (see 'Can't Help Thinking About Me' in Chapter 1). On 2 November they failed an audition at the BBC, whose selection panel noted that they had "a singer devoid of personality." Later the same month Horton negotiated a miserable sponsorship contract with business entrepreneur Raymond Cook, who was assured 10 per cent of Bowie's earnings in exchange for limited financial investment. Kenneth Pitt later reproduced the text of this contract in his memoir *The Pitt Report*, rightly describing it as "an amazingly inept, do-it-yourself document".

New Year's Eve 1965 saw the group sharing the bill with Arthur Brown at the Golfe-Drouot Club in Paris, with further Parisian gigs following on 1 and 2 January. The release of 'Can't Help Thinking About Me' was imminent, but the preferential treatment given to David during the publicity push for the single was instrumental in driving a wedge between him and the rest of the band. Although a couple more live dates followed, the writing was on the wall for David Bowie and The Lower Third. Matters came to a head at the Bromel Club where, on 29 January, the band refused to play after being told by Horton that no wages were available for them that night. "David cried, but it made no difference," said Graham Rivens,

"We all had had enough."

"We realized that Dave wasn't backing us up," Phil Lancaster later recalled. "Looking back, it was absolutely right that we should split up ... David was the bloke with the songwriting ability and the individuality and the performing skills. It was absolute destiny that he was going to go off on his own." The Lower Third took their small place in the history books and Ralph Horton, already seriously in debt to Raymond Cook, was left with a potential solo artist on his hands.

THE BUZZ

10 February – 2 December 1966

Musicians: David Bowie *(vocals, guitar, saxophone)*, Derek Boyes *(keyboards)*, Derek Fearnley *(bass)*, John Eager *(drums)*, John Hutchinson *(lead guitar, February-June)*, Billy Gray *(lead guitar, July-November)*

Repertoire included: 'Can't Help Thinking About Me' / 'Do Anything You Say' / 'Good Morning Girl' / 'I Dig Everything' / 'I'm Not Losing Sleep' / 'You'll Never Walk Alone' / 'Breakout' / 'Take It With Soul' / 'Harlem Shuffle' / 'It's So Easy' / 'It's Getting Back' / 'Join The Gang' / 'The London Boys' / 'One More Heartache' / 'Dance, Dance, Dance' / 'Land Of A Thousand Dances' / 'See-Saw' / 'Come See About Me' / '(Please) Stay' / 'What Kind Of Fool Am I?' / 'It Doesn't Matter Anymore' / 'Shake' / 'Jenny Takes A Ride' / 'Hold On, I'm Coming' / 'Bunny Thing'

The disbanding of The Lower Third left David Bowie with a single to promote and no band to back him. From the 3-5 February 1966, auditions were held at the Marquee Club. Among the first to attend was drummer John Eager, followed by be-quiffed bassist Derek Fearnley, whose audition was rapidly followed by a compulsory haircut in Ralph Horton's bathroom. Guitarist John Hutchinson had just spent a year working in Sweden, and suspected that David was more impressed by his Scandinavian suede jacket and trousers than his musicianship. He in turn recommended an organist from Scarborough called Derek Boyes. This motley collection came together as The Buzz, apparently so named by Earl Richmond, a disc jockey from Radio London. David immediately assigned them with nicknames: John "Hutch" Hutchinson, Derek "Chow" Boyes, Derek "Dek"

Fearnley and John "Ego" Eager. The Buzz promptly went into rehearsal and a string of gigs began at Leicester University on 10 February.

On 4 March the band appeared on Associated Rediffusion TV's *Ready, Steady, Go!*, miming 'Can't Help Thinking About Me'. Three days later The Buzz recorded a new single, 'Do Anything You Say', which would be the first release credited simply to "David Bowie". There was to be none of the jockeying that had persisted in David's previous bands: "From day one," Eager told the Gillmans, "we knew this was David and a backing band."

Shortly before the release of 'Do Anything You Say', David's financial backer Raymond Cook tired of Ralph Horton's importunity and withdrew his assistance. On 31 March, the day before the single came out, Horton renewed his appeal to Kenneth Pitt.

On 17 April Pitt attended the second in a series of ten Sunday afternoon concerts at the Marquee, sponsored by Radio London and billed as "The Bowie Showboat" in recognition of David's modest but loyal following. "He sang songs from his Pye records, some R&B evergreens and several new songs of his own, all with intense conviction, as if each song was his ultimate masterpiece," Pitt wrote. "He oozed confidence and was in total command of himself, his band and his audience." At Horton's flat in Warwick Square a deal was struck the same evening: effectively Pitt now became Bowie's manager while Horton assumed the role of assistant and gigging scheduler. Pitt also assumed financial responsibility for the unpaid debts run up by Horton over the previous months, and set about disentangling David from a web of half-baked contractual agreements.

Pitt arranged extra gigs for The Buzz, including a spot supporting Crispian St Peters (who now had two of the year's biggest hits under his belt) at Blackpool's South Pier. June saw the band's first attempt to record 'I Dig Everything', adjourned when Tony Hatch decided to replace The Buzz with session musicians. With financial pressures still bearing heavily, "Hutch" resigned on 15 June and returned home to Yorkshire. His place was taken by 16-year-old Billy "Haggis" Gray from Kilmarnock, whose first gig was in Warrington on 2 July. He, too, was informed that he was very much a backing musician. "I had always been a little raver on stage," he recalled, "but Ralph came up to me and told me to calm it down as it detracted from David."

With the re-recorded 'I Dig Everything' due for release, Bowie led The Buzz through intensive rehearsals for a new stage act which was unveiled in Ramsgate on 26 August. The new show involved the use of pre-recorded backing tapes, the first David had used on stage, but the Ramsgate gig was bedevilled by technical problems and the tapes were scrapped after a similar disaster in Greenford the following night.

By September it had become clear that neither Tony Hatch nor Pye had their hearts in David's music, and it was without acrimony that Hatch released him from his contract. By now another season at the Marquee was under way; Radio London interviewed David at one of his concerts during September, when he revealed that he was working on a stage musical.

On 18 October David and The Buzz (minus Billy Gray but augmented by two session musicians) recorded the three studio tracks with which Pitt successfully won Bowie's Deram contract. However, by the time the *David Bowie* sessions got under way on 14 November, all was not well within The Buzz. David's songs were rapidly moving in a new, narrative direction, and although the band loved them his audience was unconvinced. The day before the first album session the band performed its last Marquee gig, a show that John Eager recorded in his diary as "pathetic". According to Dek Fearnley, tastes were changing: "The kids didn't want David's songs; they didn't understand them. The songs were too pretty for them and there were no guts in the music. All they wanted was soul." Although The Buzz retaliated by writing "WE HATE SOUL" on the side of their touring ambulance, subsequent evidence shows that by late 1966 they had been forced to capitulate to their audience. In 1999 Bowie posted a long-lost Buzz set-list on the Internet, remarking that "It's astonishing to me that 99% of our stage songs were soul and that I was writing in such a musical/vaudeville way." Alongside 'Join The Gang' and 'Can't Help Thinking About Me', The Buzz were now performing numbers like Marvin Gaye's 'One More Heartache' and The Supremes' 'Come See About Me'.

On 19 November, the same day that the tour ambulance broke down in Cromer, Billy Gray left the band and The Buzz continued as a trio. While Kenneth Pitt was out of the country, touring America and Australia with Crispian St Peters, financial matters came to a head once again. On 25 November Horton told The Buzz they would have to disband because of a lack of money. They offered to continue playing without payment but, according to Fearnley, "even with the band not being paid it couldn't survive. So we broke up."

Three engagements remained, and The Buzz officially ceased to exist after the Shrewsbury gig on 2 December 1966 – the very day that the 'Rubber Band' single was released. Bowie has since recalled that the band played The Velvet Underground's 'Waiting For The Man' at the final gig, although the date of Kenneth Pitt's return from America, bearing a pre-release test pressing of the Velvets' first album, casts doubt on this recollection. The musicians continued to contribute to the *David Bowie* sessions until February 1967.

THE RIOT SQUAD

March – May 1967

Musicians: David Bowie *(vocals, guitar, tenor saxophone)*, Rod Davies *(guitar)*, Croke Prebble *(bass)*, Bob Evans *(saxophone, flute)*, George Butcher *(keyboards)*, Derek Roll *(drums)*

Repertoire included: 'Waiting For The Man' / 'Dirty Old Man' / 'It Can't Happen Here' / 'Silly Boy Blue' / 'Little Toy Soldier' / 'Silver Treetop School For Boys'

Having completed the *David Bowie* album, David entered a period which lacked the continuity of previous band relationships. The first of many sporadic line-ups that flickered briefly between 1967 and 1972 was The Riot Squad, a band who already existed when David joined them for a run of about twenty gigs in the spring of 1967. David encouraged the band to wear extravagant, clownish face-paint and psychedelic accessories on stage. Kenneth Pitt recalls that they appeared at Oxford Street's Tiles club on 13 April with a flashing red police lamp, and that their live act included The Velvet Underground's 'Waiting For The Man' and The Fugs' 'Dirty Old Man'. Bowie later recalled that "I also made them cover Mothers of Invention songs. Not happily, I seem to remember, especially as my big favourite was 'It Can't Happen Here'. Frank's stuff was virtually unknown in Britain, and relistening to that song I can see why he wasn't on any playlists." Bowie's Velvets-styled out-take 'Little Toy Soldier' was cut with The Riot Squad at Decca Studios on 5 April, with Gus Dudgeon in the producer's chair. A tape exists of The Riot Squad rehearsing 'Little Toy Soldier', 'Silly Boy Blue' and 'Silver Treetop School For Boys' at the Swan in Tottenham.

1967 – 1968: STAGE BALL, FESTIVAL HALL AND CABARET

Musicians: David Bowie *(vocals, guitar)*

Cabaret Repertoire: 'Love You Till Tuesday' / 'The Day The Circus Left Town' / 'The Laughing Gnome' / 'When I'm Five' / 'When I'm Sixty-Four' / 'Yellow Submarine' / 'All You Need Is Love' / 'When I Live My Dream' / 'Even A Fool Learns To Love'

The Riot Squad had long since disbanded by November 1967, when David played two very different engagements. The first was in Amsterdam on November 10 when he performed 'Love You Till Tuesday' on the Dutch television show *Fanclub* – his first television appearance since March the previous year. The second was on 19 November, when he played a ten-minute live spot at London's Dorchester Hotel, this time accompanied by the Bill Saville Orchestra. The event was the Stage Ball on behalf of the British Heart Foundation, and Kenneth Pitt records that among those who enjoyed David's performance were Danny La Rue and Frazer Hines.

Outwardly, 1967 had seen the greatest advances yet in Bowie's career. His first album had garnered good reviews and the year ended with further acclaim for his part in Lindsay Kemp's *Pierrot In Turquoise* (see Chapter 6). Nevertheless, by now his finances were in a parlous state. *Pierrot In Turquoise* was arranged on a profit-share basis and, as any actor who has gone down that path will know, "profit-share" is a euphemism for "unpaid". Sales of *David Bowie* had not yet recouped David's original advance. After the excitement of the past twelve months, 1968 was to prove a year of frustrations.

Bowie's first live engagement of the year involved a trip to Hamburg to record three songs for ZDF television's *4-3-2-1 Musik Für Junge Leute* on 27 February. The show's producer Günther Schneider congratulated David on being "by far one of the most sensible and creative young artists I know." Not long afterwards, on a trip to London, Schneider would take David to see *Cabaret* at the Palace Theatre, and for this he deserves at least a footnote in the history of Bowie's theatrical influences.

Early March brought the second leg of *Pierrot In Turquoise* at London's Mercury Theatre, during which Bowie also returned to the Decca Studios with Tony Visconti to begin recording 'In The Heat Of The

Morning' and 'London Bye Ta Ta'. These were completed in April, and in the same month Bowie contributed backing vocals to The Beatstalkers' cover of his composition 'Everything Is You'. However, after nearly a year of rebuttals Decca's rejection of the proposed single 'In The Heat Of The Morning' proved the last straw, and by the end of April Bowie had left the label for good.

While Pitt busied himself trying to secure a new contract (being rejected by the Apple label among others), David recorded his second BBC radio session on 13 May. Next came a brief appearance in an eight-hour multiple-bill concert at Covent Garden's Middle Earth Club. This was in preparation for a twelve-minute spot on 3 June at the Royal Festival Hall, where David supported Tyrannosaurus Rex on a bill that also included Stefan Grossman and Roy Harper. The compère was John Peel, a newcomer to David's music who became a supportive ally in the years ahead.

David's brief spots at the Covent Garden and Festival Hall gigs consisted of a mime piece he had devised in the aftermath of *Pierrot In Turquoise*. Entitled *Yet-San And The Eagle*, it was performed against a specially prepared backing tape that incorporated 'Silly Boy Blue'. "He didn't sing at all but had a tape going," Marc Bolan later recalled, "and he'd act out a story about a Tibetan boy. It was quite good actually." Bowie later explained that the piece "told the story of how the Chinese had invaded Tibet and though the Tibetans may be struck down their spirit would fly for eternity." The piece culminated in the flying eagle mime that David would resurrect several years later for the Ziggy Stardust tour. According to Kenneth Pitt, "during the course of the [Festival Hall] performance an American voice suddenly shouted out, 'Stop the propaganda,' or words to that effect." More recently Bowie recalled that "Word had got around that I would be doing this spot of propaganda and all the Maoists turned up and heckled me, waving their little red books in the air. Marc Bolan was delighted and thought it an unmitigated success. I was trembling with anger and went home sulking." Nevertheless, *Yet-San And The Eagle* drew praise from the *International Times*, which noted that "David Bowie, although one or two drags were heckling him, received the longest and loudest applause of all the performers, and he deserved it. It was a pity that he didn't have a longer set."

David was continuing to audition for various film roles while working part-time at a Carey Street printing firm called Legastat. During the summer, financial pressures led to his reluctant decision to revive an idea originally proposed by Kenneth Pitt the previous December: that he should devise a one-man show specifically for the cabaret circuit. By late July he had begun rehearsing his act in earnest at Kenneth Pitt's flat, drawing up a repertoire (see above) which alternated his own compositions with several Beatles covers. His props included a glove-puppet "laughing gnome" and four home-made Beatle cut-outs, based on the *Yellow Submarine* figures which Pitt had borrowed from the film's production office. The pieces were linked by spoken interludes scripted by Pitt, and the variety-act ambience was sealed by the recitation of a poem: Roger McGough's 'At Lunchtime – A Story Of Love', later an influence on 'Five Years'.

Before the cabaret act was unveiled, David played a 25-minute spot at the Marquee on 1 August as support to Australian band The Groop, whose business affairs Pitt was managing during a British sojourn. Later the same month, David privately auditioned his 27-minute cabaret showcase twice in one day, firstly in Kenneth Pitt's office before the booking agent Sidney Rose, and later at the Astor Club for two more agents, Harry Dawson and Michael Black. The auditions met with no success and, as Pitt recounts, "I knew there and then that it was the end of the cabaret road." Pitt's recollection that Harry Dawson apologetically turned David down because he was "tremendous … marvellous … too good!" has been dutifully trotted out in many subsequent biographies, but in his 1988 book *Starmakers And Svengalis* Johnny Rogan finally tracked down Dawson, who told him, "I turned around to Ken and said, 'Let him have a good day job – he's never going to get anywhere'."

The abortive cabaret show has been held up as final proof of Pitt's inability to comprehend what he had in David Bowie, but while it was clearly a dreadful idea the episode has rebounded unfairly on Pitt's reputation. "Contrary to popular opinion," he told Christopher Sandford, "I *hated* cabaret. In the course of four years, I mentioned it to David once. That was when he was broke and unable to feed himself."

Within days of the ill-starred audition David had moved on once more, leaving Pitt's Manchester Street flat to live with his girlfriend Hermione Farthingale. By September the pair were performing in a new acoustic three-piece called Turquoise.

TURQUOISE/FEATHERS

14 September 1968 – 16 March 1969

Musicians: David Bowie *(vocals, guitar, mime)*, Hermione Farthingale *(vocals, mime)*, Tony Hill *(guitar, vocals (September-November))*, John Hutchinson *(guitar, vocals (November-March))*

Repertoire included: 'When I'm Five' / 'Lady Midnight' / 'One Hundred Years From Today' / 'Amsterdam' / 'Next' / 'Ching-a-Ling' / 'Life Is A Circus' / 'Space Oddity' / 'Sell Me A Coat'

In August 1968 David and Hermione Farthingale moved into a rented room in Clareville Grove, South Kensington, where they were to stay until their separation in early 1969. These were the "one hundred days" later lamented in 'An Occasional Dream'.

David's new venture synthesized his dabblings in Buddhism, mime and a new ingredient introduced to his creative palette by both Tony Visconti and Hermione: the acoustic American folk sound popularized by the hippy movement. Together with Tony Hill, formerly the guitarist with Misunderstood, they formed a "multimedia" trio called Turquoise, whose song-and-mime repertoire embraced David's more whimsical compositions (including a new one, 'Ching-a-Ling') and a selection of covers, including Bowie's first foray into the work of Jacques Brel.

Turquoise's first and last gig was a thirty-minute slot at London's Roundhouse on 14 September; from the following day's show at the Middle Earth Club, the group was re-named Feathers. After only a handful of dates Tony Hill left to join High Tide, and as of 17 November he was replaced by a former colleague from The Buzz, John "Hutch" Hutchinson. In addition to the songs, David now performed his mime 'The Mask', while the trio took it in turns to read poems between numbers. Feathers were not a great success, netting a total of three performances in November and December.

David had returned to Hamburg to record his second appearance on *4-3-2-1 Musik Für Junge Leute* on 19 September, and by early October plans were afoot to make the film eventually realized as *Love You Till Tuesday*. Feathers recorded 'Ching-a-Ling' on 24 October, while on 10 November, following his week's filming on *The Virgin Soldiers*, David was once again in Germany. This time the venue was Munich for an appearance on *Für Jeden Etwas Musik*, where he performed a mime routine and sang a song – which ones are uncertain, although given the timing 'The Mask' and 'Ching-a-Ling' seem likely contenders.

Over Christmas David played two solo dates at the Magician's Workshop in Falmouth, Cornwall, at the invitation of an acquaintance called Gerry Gill. He spent Christmas at Gill's house near Redruth, playing his two twenty-minute spots on Christmas Eve and Boxing Day, but was paid only expenses.

Feathers played another date at the Roundhouse on 4 January 1969 (where David was briefly introduced to his future wife Angela, although they wouldn't get to know each other until April). On 22 January David recorded his fabled Lyons Maid ice-cream commercial, and four days later shooting began on *Love You Till Tuesday*. By this time two major and not unrelated developments had occurred: David's relationship with Hermione was over, and he had written a new song called 'Space Oddity'.

On completion of the film Hermione left Feathers, and David and Hutch continued as a duo. In the short term, however, David embarked on six solo dates, performing his mime pieces *Yet-San And The Eagle* and *The Mask* as first support on a Tyrannosaurus Rex tour beginning in Birmingham on 15 February. Tony Visconti would later opine that this was a gesture of back-handed generosity on Bolan's part: "David was open to friendship but Marc was quite cruel about David's as yet unproven musical career," Visconti tells David Buckley. "I think it was with great sadistic delight that Marc hired David to open for Tyrannosaurus Rex, not as a musical act, but as a mime."

"I had no idea, from seeing him on the tour, that he had any musical aspirations at all," recalled Bolan's other support act, the sitar player Vytas Serelis. "I do remember thinking what an old woman he was, because he used to take hours to get his make-up on. He'd go on in a draggy costume with tights and everything, and do this fairly conventional Marcel Marceau-type act." John Peel, who compèred the tour, recorded in *Disc & Music Echo* that "David Bowie performs two of his mime things. It has been good to see the appreciation for what he does." Bowie would later credit Peel with persuading him to drop his mime act and concentrate on music.

When David and Hutch re-convened Feathers in early March, the mime and poetry were dropped and the pair concentrated instead on a more sophisticated folk sound based on their twin acoustic guitars and vocal harmonies. At the same time, now his *Virgin Soldiers* haircut had grown back sufficiently, David restyled himself with the straggly bubble-perm he continued to wear into 1970 ("not my greatest hairstyle," he ruefully observed twenty years later). With the arrival of the new look, many observed a new manner, as David began cultivating the fey, softly-spoken and effeminate persona which, with a few refinements, would remain his public image well into the 1970s.

All these developments came to a head on 11 March when Feathers played a Guildford Festival gig, not in Guildford itself but at the University of Surrey's London premises on Battersea Park Road. Kenneth Pitt described the performance as "a revelation", as a newly relaxed and confident Bowie carried the audience through the set with a stream of witty remarks and easy charm. Hutch later recalled that "The Battersea date was the first time I began to understand what David was doing. He never worked like that before and had never used such chat." To the Gillmans he added, "It was a sort of gay patter, with me as a quiet straight man ... I didn't know what to do except play guitar and sing, but it seemed to work." However, the financial rewards were insufficient for Hutch, and he left David's side to resume his former job as a draughtsman. "We could have become another Simon and Garfunkel," he later said. "That was another chance I missed."

Before Hutch's departure, he and David recorded a tape of acoustic demos which would prove instrumental in securing a new recording contract. By late June David was back in the studio, beginning work on his second album.

1969-1970: GROWTH, FREE FESTIVAL AND SOLO DATES

Musicians: David Bowie *(vocals, guitar)*, with *(selected dates only)*: Tim Renwick *(guitar)*, John Lodge *(bass)*, John Cambridge *(drums)*

Repertoire included: 'When I Live My Dream' / 'Space Oddity' / 'Let Me Sleep Beside You' / 'Amsterdam' / 'God Knows I'm Good' / 'Buzz The Fuzz' / 'Karma Man' / 'London Bye Ta Ta' / 'An Occasional Dream' / 'Janine' / 'Wild Eyed Boy From Freecloud' / 'Unwashed And Somewhat Slightly Dazed' / 'Fill Your Heart' / 'The Prettiest Star' / 'Cygnet Committee' / 'Threepenny Pierrot' / 'Columbine' / 'The Mirror' / 'Don't Think Twice, It's Alright' / 'She Belongs To Me'

Following the dissolution of Feathers, Bowie's live career followed its nose with a sporadic series of engagements during the run-up to the *Space Oddity* album. On 14 April he took up residence at the flat of his new friend Mary Finnegan in Foxgrove Road, Beckenham. Here, out of Kenneth Pitt's orbit, David and Mary established a folk club with the assistance of Calvin Mark Lee and Angela Barnett. Its inaugural meeting took place on Sunday 4 May in the function room of the Three Tuns pub on Beckenham High Street. Fifty people attended, and after a guest spot by Tim Hollier, Bowie performed an acoustic set against a projected psychedelic backdrop. "He was very together," recalled Finnegan later. "Barry Low brought his 'liquid whirl' and the people loved it."

The success of the first folk club meeting ensured a regular run of Sunday gatherings at the Three Tuns. The following week 90 people came, the week after 120, and thereafter the meetings spilled out into the pub's garden. "David was very idealistic in those days," said Mary, "and we began to get more of a community feeling. Love and Peace were moving out to the suburbs." As other creative types pitched in – poets, film students, even Mary Finnegan's children – the club developed into what was popularly called an "Arts Laboratory", and was renamed Growth. "There's a lot of talent in the green belt and there is a load of tripe in Drury Lane," David told *Melody Maker*. "I think the Arts Lab movement is extremely important." Among those who made guest appearances at meetings were Lionel Bart, Steve Harley, and Bowie's erstwhile mentor Chimi Youngdong Rimpoche. Of course, the reality of such a free-for-all fell short of the lofty idealism on which it was founded, as Bowie later admitted: "Very little happened at these 'happenings'. The idea was to let everyone take it over and do whatever they liked but, as is always the case with those situations, it ended up with three of us doing all the work and everyone else sitting on their arses."

Along with other early landmarks on Bowie's road to fame, the Three Tuns has since become something of a Mecca for fans. It was renamed the Rat and Parrot in the 1980s, but after a petition by the Beckenham Town Residents' Association in 2001, the Noble House Pub Company consented to revert its name to the Three Tuns. On 6 December 2001, a plaque was unveiled by Mary Finnegan and Steve Harley to commemorate the pub's key role in the development of Bowie's career, although two years later the plaque was removed as a change of ownership once again put the building's future in jeopardy.

In addition to the regular Arts Lab meetings at the Three Tuns, Bowie played various other gigs in the summer of 1969, most of which were one-man acoustic affairs. On 10 May David and Tony Visconti recorded an appearance with The Strawbs (miming to their number 'Poor Jimmy Wilson') for the BBC2 show *Colour Me Pop*, broadcast the following month.

On 24 July, by which time the *Space Oddity* sessions were under way, David flew with Kenneth Pitt to Valetta to take part in the Maltese Song Festival. From there they continued to Rome for a repeat performance at the Italian Song Festival, arranged by the same entrepreneur and with the same roster of artists. Pitt refutes the accusation made by some, notably Angela, that this sojourn was some sort of attempt to wrest control of David from his new coterie – "Our main reason for going to those Mediterranean countries was to get a free holiday in the sun … I made no demands, expected nothing," he insists. At the Maltese Festival David sang 'When I Live My Dream' to the backing of the house orchestra, and came second behind the winning Spanish entrant, Cristina. Before leaving for Italy he joined his fellow artists in an impromptu concert for the ship's company on board the aircraft carrier USS *Saratoga*. At the Italian Festival in Monsummano-Terme on 31 July he again performed 'When I Live My Dream', which received a "Best Produced Record" award.

Bowie and Pitt arrived home on 3 August to the awful news – not broken to David until after his gig at the Three Tuns that afternoon – that his father was seriously ill with pneumonia. David rushed to the bedside and is said to have pressed into his father's hands the trophy he had won at the festival. Haywood Jones died two days later.

While the *Space Oddity* sessions continued, 16 August saw the last hurrah of the Growth Arts Lab in the form of an open-air free festival held at Beckenham Recreation Ground. On the other side of the Atlantic, crowds were massing for the second day of the free-love generation's zenith, the three-day Woodstock festival. At Beckenham's rather more modest contribution to the global love-in, Bowie's headlining set was supported by performers including *Space Oddity* sessioners Tony Visconti and Keith Christmas, The Strawbs, Sun, Gas Works, Miscarriage,

Amory Kane, Bridget St John, Oswald K, Gun Hill, and Kamirah & Giles & Abdul. Also on offer were ceramic and jewellery stalls, puppetry and street theatre, a Tibetan shop, coconut shies and an assault course. The event was committed to legend in 'Memory Of A Free Festival', although the story famously goes that David's mood on the day was at odds with the nostalgic sentiments expressed in the song. Few have bothered to point out that he had buried his father only five days earlier.

On 25 August David was in Hilversum, Holland, recording a mimed performance of 'Space Oddity' for the Dutch television show *Doebidoe*. On 13 September he compèred another open-air concert, this time a smaller affair at Bromley's Library Gardens. On 2 October he recorded his first ever *Top Of The Pops* appearance and, as 'Space Oddity' began catching on, Kenneth Pitt arranged a twenty-minute support slot on a tour by Humble Pie, the band led by Steve Marriott and David's old schoolmate Peter Frampton. Their manager Andrew Oldham originally wanted Bowie to perform his mime routines, but acquiesced to his wish to play straight songs instead. The nine-date tour started in Coventry on 8 October, and later in the month David recorded a BBC radio session for *The Dave Lee Travis Show*.

It was during October that David and Angela moved to their celebrated home at Haddon Hall, a spacious Edwardian house converted into flats at 42 Southend Road, Beckenham. Bowie's apartment incorporated a grand central staircase leading to a stained-glass window and horseshoe-shaped landing whose connecting doors had been blocked off during the conversion, leaving what David and his friends dubbed the minstrels' gallery. Over the next few years Haddon Hall would become an unofficial demo studio, photo-shoot location, campaign office and all-purpose commune for the Bowie entourage, and was home at various times to such individuals as Tony Visconti and Mick Ronson. Its air of tattered Edwardian finery and its reputation as a haunted house (Bowie, Visconti and many others insist that they often saw the ghost of a young woman in the garden) made Haddon Hall the perfect setting for David's gradual rise to stardom.

Following the end of the Humble Pie tour, Bowie flew to Berlin – his first visit to a city that would later become pivotal to his music – to perform 'Space Oddity' on ZDF's *4-3-2-1 Musik Für Junge Leute*. November 2 saw another inaugural trip, this time to

Switzerland for *Hits A-Go-Go*.

Having played a couple of solo dates in England at the end of October, the following month saw Bowie begin a short tour of Scotland to coincide with the release of *Space Oddity*. Although three of the ten dates were cancelled this outing, on which David was backed by Junior's Eyes, can justifiably claim to be Bowie's first *bona fide* solo tour. Each show began with a Junior's Eyes support set, after which David replaced vocalist Graham Kelly to play a selection of numbers from *Space Oddity* peppered with a few covers. "It was quite a strange affair, a bit of a lash-up really," guitarist Tim Renwick later recalled. Bowie, whose previous gigging experience rested largely in the realm of loudly amplified R&B, was unprepared for the reception awaiting his new acoustic folk style: "I thought haughtily, 'I'll go out and sing my songs!', not knowing what audiences were like in those days. Sure enough, it was a revival of the Mod thing which had since turned into skinheads. They couldn't abide me. No way! The whole spitting, cigarette-flicking abuse thing by audiences started long before the punks of 1977 in my own frame of reference." Angela Bowie later recalled that the Gillingham audience was particularly hostile: "The crowd didn't want to hear David, they wanted to hear Buddy Holly. So I rounded up the support band and asked if any of them knew any Buddy Holly songs. They did, so David went out and played an entire set of Buddy Holly numbers and went down great! Then he came to the end and sang 'Space Oddity' and that was that. Everybody started throwing beer bottles and cigarette ends at him."

The most prestigious of the autumn gigs was David's headliner at the Royal Festival Hall's Purcell Room on 20 November. Kenneth Pitt had booked the concert a year earlier in the hope that David might have had some success by then, and his timing turned out to be immaculate. However, Pitt's dwindling influence and the ascendancy of David's new ally Calvin Mark Lee led to a dispute between the two over responsibility for promoting the gig, and each has since blamed the other for what ensued. The Purcell Room concert was a personal triumph for David, but was attended by so few journalists that its purpose – coverage in the national press – was confounded. Bowie was furious, and neither Pitt nor Lee would ever be fully trusted thereafter. "I have never seen him perform so well, either before or since," said Pitt many years later. "David Bowie happened that night. Had the press been there, everything that happened to him

in 1972 would have happened in November 1969."

Among the few who reviewed the show was Tony Palmer of the *Observer*, who commended the "sizzling concert" and the "spectacularly good" 'Space Oddity', but found some of David's "love reveries" – 'An Occasional Dream' and the like – "dreary, self-pitying and monotonous". *Music Now!* reported that "His performance was astounding. He had the audience bewitched with his words, his music, his voice and his professionalism. With simplicity and sincerity he sang his songs. He has his own style, but also great imagination and versatility."

On 30 November David performed 'Space Oddity' at Save Rave '69, an all-star charity show at the London Palladium in aid of the Invalid Children's Aid Association. The concert was attended by Princess Margaret, to whom David was presented. It was his final live show of the year and of the decade. On 8 January 1970, his twenty-third birthday, David performed at London's Speakeasy club after beginning work on the single version of 'The Prettiest Star' earlier the same day. This was the first of several one-off bookings organised through the NEMS agency. David played acoustic guitar, accompanied by Tony Visconti on bass and John Cambridge on drums. The gig was attended by Tim Hughes of *Jeremy* magazine, who recorded that Bowie sat "Perched precariously on two boxes – a luminous elfin face surrounded by an aureole of blond curls – he looks very vulnerable."

On 29 January David travelled to Aberdeen to record an appearance on Grampian TV's *Cairngorm Ski Night*. 'London Bye Ta Ta' was still being mooted as the forthcoming single and this was the song David performed, backed by a large studio orchestra. To make the trip financially worthwhile Pitt secured David an engagement at Aberdeen University the following night. When Lindsay Kemp, now based in Edinburgh, heard of David's forthcoming Scottish trip he contacted Pitt to offer David two days' work on a television adaptation of *Pierrot In Turquoise* (see *The Looking Glass Murders* in Chapter 6).

At the Marquee on 3 February Bowie was backed by a trio of *Space Oddity* veterans: Tony Visconti on bass, John Cambridge on drums and Tim Renwick on guitar. According to Kenneth Pitt it was at this Marquee gig that David was first introduced to Mick Ronson, a friend of Cambridge's from Hull who had been wooed down to London to meet Bowie at the drummer's insistence. This account is contradicted by Tony Visconti, who insists that Ronson had first entered the scene some months earlier (see 'Wild Eyed Boy From Freecloud' in Chapter 1). Whichever version is correct, within two days of the Marquee concert Bowie had hired Ronson as a full-time guitarist, and one of the cornerstones of his forthcoming success had been cemented into place.

HYPE

5 February – 16 May 1970

Musicians: David Bowie *(vocals, guitar)*, Mick Ronson *(guitar)*, Tony Visconti *(bass)*, John Cambridge *(drums)*

Repertoire included: 'Amsterdam' / 'God Knows I'm Good' / 'Buzz The Fuzz' / 'Karma Man' / 'London Bye Ta Ta' / 'An Occasional Dream' / 'The Width Of A Circle' / 'Janine' / 'Wild Eyed Boy From Freecloud' / 'Unwashed And Somewhat Slightly Dazed' / 'Fill Your Heart' / 'The Prettiest Star' / 'Cygnet Committee' / 'Madame George' / 'Memory Of A Free Festival' / 'Waiting For The Man'

The introduction of Mick Ronson to the Bowie camp in February 1970 was the latest in a succession of auspicious arrivals – Tony Visconti, Ken Scott, Angela Barnett – who would prove fundamental to David's commercial and artistic breakthrough. Ronson was Bowie's first true partner and collaborator, and many still believe that the level of his contribution to David's work has been underestimated. Ever a shy and self-effacing character, Ronson told a reporter many years later that "I was never really a writer, I was always more of a performer. David was a writer and a performer. What I'm good at is putting riffs to things, and hook-lines, making things up so songs sound more memorable." But there was more to Mick Ronson than that: his hard-boiled rock sensibility, combined with his multi-instrumental skill (Ronson's string arrangements and piano playing on albums like *Ziggy Stardust* are often criminally underrated) brought Bowie exactly the colleague he needed.

The chain of events by which Ronson entered Bowie's orbit is complicated and has often been misrepresented, so let us attempt an accurate – if potted – version. A classically trained pianist who turned during his teenage years to the violin, recorder and finally guitar, Mick Ronson hailed from Kingston-upon-Hull, where his early bands had included local pub outfits called The Mariners and The King Bees. The latter – no relation, of course, to Bowie's 1964 outfit – also featured future Steeleye Span bassist Rick Kemp, a connection that would pave the way for a Bowie collaboration many years later. After spells with The Crestas, The Voice and Wanted, in 1966 Ronson joined a three-year-old Hull band called The Rats, who had already cut a couple of flop singles (which pre-date Ronson and in which, contrary to widespread belief, he played no part). A band of ever-changing line-ups, The Rats were fronted at this stage by Benny Marshall, who would later play harmonica on 'Unwashed And Somewhat Slightly Dazed'. During the *Space Oddity* sessions Marshall was introduced to Bowie by drummer John Cambridge, another former Rat who had left to join Junior's Eyes in early 1969. Cambridge proceeded to recommend other members of The Rats to Bowie, in particular their talented guitarist. Meanwhile The Rats' replacement drummer was another Hull player, Mick "Woody" Woodmansey, who would soon displace John Cambridge once again.

At around the time that Benny Marshall was playing harmonica for Bowie, Ronson was making his vinyl debut, not with The Rats but as lead guitarist on Michael Chapman's *Fully Qualified Survivor*. This record was produced by Gus Dudgeon, hot on the heels of his work on 'Space Oddity', and indeed Dudgeon has claimed that it was this connection, and not John Cambridge, that brought about Ronson's first meeting with Bowie. If Tony Visconti's account is accurate, then it seems plausible that introductions might have taken place in London during the autumn of 1969. Whatever the case, by November Ronson was back in Hull with The Rats who, despite undertaking some studio sessions at around this time, were drifting into the doldrums. By January 1970, when John Cambridge travelled north to seek him out, Ronson was working as a municipal groundsman for Hull City Council, marking out the lines on a rugby pitch. Although on the point of abandoning music Ronson agreed to accompany Cambridge to London, where he was introduced (or else reintroduced) to Bowie at the Marquee on 3 February. "We just sat around in David's flat," Ronson recalled in 1984. "I picked up a guitar and jammed with him. He said, 'Hey, do you wanna come down to do this radio show and play with me?'" Sure enough, two days later Ronson was playing in Bowie's band.

The new four-piece received its baptism at the BBC's Paris Cinema Studio on 5 February 1970, in a live concert recorded for John Peel's *The Sunday Show* (see Chapter 4). "I didn't know anything, none of the material," Ronson later said. "I just sat and watched his fingers. I didn't really know what I was doing, but everybody seemed to like it. I don't know if it was treated as an audition or not, I never really thought of it like that. I was just playing, it was a normal thing for me."

After collecting a "Brightest Hope" award at *Disc & Music Echo*'s Valentine's Day Awards ceremony on 13 February, David withdrew to Haddon Hall, where the entire band was now living, to plan his next publicity offensive. The question of the new band's name was resolved during a telephone call to Kenneth Pitt. Bowie remarked to his manager that "the whole thing is just one big hype," to which Pitt responded, "Then why not call it The Hype?" In the event, *pace* Kenneth Pitt and nearly every subsequent piece of writing on the subject, the group was simply called "Hype" without the definite article, as evidenced by every surviving interview, poster and ticket. "I deliberately chose the name in favour of something that sounded perhaps heavy," David told *Melody Maker* the following month, "because now no-one can say they're being conned." It was his first significant embrace of the provocative artificiality that would inform his archetypal "plastic rock'n'roller" Ziggy Stardust.

The band made its concert debut on 22 February at an event called Implosion at London's Roundhouse, where they played alongside Caravan, The Groundhogs and Bach Denkel, bands who epitomized what Bowie later referred to as the "incredibly denim-y stage" of rock music that he and his peers would soon overthrow so spectacularly. It was an epoch-making moment for, after years of personal experimentation in costume and make-up, Bowie now coaxed his entire band to dress up with flamboyant theatricality. Hype arrived on the Roundhouse stage in outrageous costumes made by Angela Barnett and Liz Hartley, Tony Visconti's girlfriend. The outfits were apparently inspired by a night David and Angie had spent with the photographer Ray Stevenson, who had revealed a passion for comic-strip superheroes. Sure enough, each member of Hype assumed the persona of a gaudy cartoon character. Bowie himself became Rainbowman (in multi-coloured lurex tights, thigh boots and a billowing blue cape), Visconti was Hypeman (in a Superman-style outfit with a giant "H" on his chest), Ronson wore Bowie's 'Space Oddity' suit from *Love You Till Tuesday* to become Gangster-

man, while Cambridge, in a frilly shirt and outsized ten-gallon hat, was Cowboyman. A more incongruous mismatch with the other acts would be hard to imagine, and although the concert has been famously dubbed "the birth of glam rock", its reception on the night left a lot to be desired. "We died a death," Bowie admitted later. Among the denim-clad audience only Marc Bolan entered into the spirit of things, arriving dressed as a Roman legionary complete with a plastic breastplate from Woolworth's. For Tony Visconti the evening ended in humiliation: his clothes were stolen from the dressing room and he was forced to return home in his Hypeman costume.

All the same, Hype's Roundhouse concert deserves its place in history. The time was not yet right and some of the band were unconvinced, but for Bowie the die was cast. "I just stopped after that performance, because I knew it was right," he told the *NME* some years later. "I knew it was what I wanted to do and I knew it was what people would want eventually." In the meantime he put on a brave face, telling *Melody Maker* in March 1970 that "We've had these costumes made by various girlfriends which make us look like Dr Strange or the Incredible Hulk. I was a bit apprehensive about wearing them at the Roundhouse gig because I didn't know how the audience would react … but they seemed to accept it, which was nice."

Although Kenneth Pitt notes that David's and Angela's demands for a minimum fee of £150 per Hype show met with total failure, a handful of gigs followed during February and March, mainly at London Arts Lab venues already familiar to David. The night after the Roundhouse show, perhaps initially doubting its new name, the band played in Streatham under the moniker Harry The Butcher. At Hull University on 6 March (a gig arranged through The Rats' local connections) the band was joined on stage by Benny Marshall on harmonica. The following night's London gig was panned by *Disc & Music Echo*: "David Bowie, in ten-league boots and groovy gear, presented his new backing group line-up Hype. He needs an expert on sound balance … The show was a disaster. The volume on Mick Ronson's lead guitar was so high that not only did he block out David's singing but also completely over-powered John Cambridge's drums." Between Hype engagements, David played a few acoustic solo dates including a Mencap charity gig at the Albert Hall. "I want to retain Hype and myself as two separate working units whereby we can retain our own identities," he told *Melody Maker*.

On 11 March Hype played a second Roundhouse gig, this time supporting Country Joe McDonald along with Black Sabbath and Hawkwind among others. In 1998 some film footage of 'Waiting For The Man' from this second Roundhouse concert surfaced from a private collection, offering one of the very few moving picture records of David from the pre-Ziggy 1970s. Excerpts have since appeared in documentaries including VH1's *Legends* and A&E's *Sound & Vision*.

At 11.00am on 20 March, the day after a performance at the Three Tuns in Beckenham, David and Angela were married at Bromley Register Office in a low-key ceremony attended by a handful of Haddon Hall friends, including John Cambridge and Liz Hartley. Tony Visconti was unable to attend, being busy at a studio session with the Strawbs. An unexpected arrival was David's mother Peggy, who had got wind of the occasion the night before and alerted a couple of local papers, whose photographers were on hand to preserve the day for posterity. "Looks like *Hello!* Magazine were at this one too!" joked David in 1993 when *Q* magazine showed him a strip of shots from the *Kentish Times*. "Second biggest mistake of my life marrying that woman."

David's first marriage has generated a lot of overheated prose over the years. Claims and counter-claims continue about whether it was merely an excuse to resolve Angela's UK visitor status, a chance for David to get his hands on a green card, or a business contract whereby each agreed to promote the other's career in turn. The significance of Angela's role in David's rise to fame has been ludicrously overplayed in some quarters, but although her creative input is often exaggerated, her practical contribution as a fixer and all-round motivating force is beyond question. Speaking to *Rolling Stone* in 1993, Bowie made a rare comment on the subject: "The reason that we got married was for her to get a work permit to work in England, which really wasn't the basis for a good marriage. And it was very short, remember. I mean, by '74 we rarely saw each other. After that she would drop in or drop out for a weekend or so, but we were virtually living our separate lives. There was no real togetherness." The story did not end happily, and the aftermath has made for some poisonous literature – some of it by Angela herself – to which this book feels no inclination to add anything further.

On 25 March Hype recorded another BBC radio session, and five days later the band played its last gig, marking John Cambridge's final Bowie concert.

Following his studio work on the single version of 'Memory Of a Free Festival' early the following month, he returned to Hull, supplanted at Ronson's suggestion by Mick Woodmansey.

On 12 April, six days before sessions began for *The Man Who Sold The World*, Bowie played two half-hour solo spots alongside the Keef Hartley Band at Harrogate Theatre in Yorkshire. The engagement had come about following negotiations between Kenneth Pitt and the theatre's artistic director, Brian Howard, who was a fan of the *Space Oddity* album and wanted David to provide a musical and dramatic narration for the theatre's forthcoming adaptation of Sir Walter Scott's *The Fair Maid Of Perth* which was to combine, in Howard's words, "drama, music, folk and ballet as well as mobile sets and projections." David was initially keen on the idea but, like most of Pitt's 1970 projects, the plans were to run aground.

While the album sessions proceeded David played a few solo gigs, notably at the Ivor Novello Awards at London's Talk Of The Town on 10 May. 'Space Oddity' had won an award, and David performed the song to a large orchestral arrangement supervised by Paul Buckmaster and conducted by Les Reed in a live satellite broadcast to the US and the Continent. It was his first major American exposure, relayed to audiences at New York's Carnegie Hall and other locations throughout the US. Although not televised in Britain, the show was broadcast live on Radio 1, and video copies of this excellent performance have since leaked onto the bootleg circuit. Following the album sessions David's solo summer engagements included the May Ball at Jesus College, Cambridge.

Although the original Hype line-up had ceased to exist at the end of March, it's a little-known fact that the band forged ahead without David in the wake of the *Man Who Sold The World* sessions. The short-lived post-Bowie career of Hype and its successor Ronno, which introduced the name of Trevor Bolder into the history books, is discussed under *The Man Who Sold The World* in Chapter 2.

1971: SOLO DATES

Musicians: David Bowie *(vocals, guitar), with (selected dates only):* Mick Ronson *(guitar, piano),* Rick Wakeman *(piano),* Trevor Bolder *(bass),* Mick Woodmansey *(drums),* Tom Parker *(piano)*

Repertoire included: 'Holy Holy' / 'All The Madmen' / 'Queen Bitch' / 'Bombers' / 'The Supermen' / 'Looking For A Friend' / 'Almost Grown' / 'Kooks' / 'Song For Bob Dylan' / 'Andy Warhol' / 'It Ain't Easy' / 'Memory Of A Free Festival' / 'Oh! You Pretty Things' / 'Eight Line Poem' / 'Changes' / 'Amsterdam' / 'Waiting For The Man' / 'White Light/White Heat' / 'Fill Your Heart' / 'Buzz The Fuzz' / 'Space Oddity' / 'Round And Round'

In contrast to the non-stop gigging that would begin the following year, 1971 was one of Bowie's quietest periods in the live arena. On 20 January he made his only substantial television appearance of the year, performing his new single 'Holy Holy' on Granada TV. The following month he travelled to America on a short tour arranged by Mercury Records to promote *The Man Who Sold The World*. David Bowie's first trip to the land of his dreams began inauspiciously with a body-search at Washington's International Airport, where immigration officials were apparently alarmed at the spectacle of the long-haired, effeminate English musician.

Despite having acquired a green card when he married Angela, David was as yet unable to perform owing to the union stipulations of the American Federation of Musicians, and the promotion was restricted to interviews and personal appearances in Washington, New York, Chicago, Philadelphia, San Francisco and Los Angeles. Only in the exotic environment of a Hollywood party, thrown by Mercury promoter and LA scene-maker Rodney Bingenheimer, did David feel sufficiently liberated to don his Mr Fish dress. After watching Warhol's protégée Ultra Violet give a succession of interviews from a bath full of milk, he spent the evening strumming a selection of numbers from *The Man Who Sold The World*, perched cross-legged on a waterbed. Many years later, a snatch of 'All The Madmen' recorded at the party would appear on the 2004 soundtrack album of the Rodney Bingenheimer biopic *Mayor Of The Sunset Strip*.

While in America Bowie was interviewed by *Rolling Stone*'s John Mendelsohn, who inadvertently captured a crucial moment in the genesis of the coming superstar. David, whom Mendelsohn found "almost disconcertingly reminiscent of Lauren Bacall", announced that he was intending to "bring mime into a traditional Western setting, to focus the attention of the audience with a very stylized, a very Japanese style of movement." In the same interview Bowie made his

now famous pronouncement that rock music "should be tarted up, made into a prostitute, a parody of itself. It should be the clown, the Pierrot medium. The music is the mask the message wears – music is the Pierrot and I, the performer, am the message." In this convoluted conflation of Warhol, Marshall McLuhan and Lindsay Kemp, Bowie had set the template for Ziggy Stardust.

In May 1971, after months of intensive songwriting, demoing and toying with artificial group constructs like Arnold Corns and the Nick King All Stars, Bowie finally assembled a band to record his next album (see *Hunky Dory* in Chapter 2). He had played no substantial concerts for nearly a year, and his return to the live circuit in the summer of 1971 was not without its teething troubles. The first engagement was a concert session for BBC radio on 3 June (see Chapter 4). Bowie was unhappy with the results, and according to Bob Grace of Chrysalis he "freaked out" in the pub afterwards: "He thought his career was over, he thought he had blown it."

Thankfully he had not, and at the open-air Glastonbury Fayre festival in Somerset on 23 June, Bowie was warmly received despite some unusual circumstances. The previous night's schedule had overrun disastrously and David's slot was cancelled when the authorities insisted on a 10.30pm cessation. Undeterred, David began his set at dawn, just as the 8000 muddy festival-goers were stirring in their tents. The opening 'Oh! You Pretty Things' was interrupted by unsolicited contributions from a Swedish girl on an acid trip, while the second number was delayed as David removed a beetle from between the keys of his electric piano. According to Dana Gillespie, as he began singing 'Memory Of A Free Festival' "the sun came over the hill and lit him up and everyone warmed to him. He was a huge success." The following year's *Glastonbury Fayre* album, released to recoup the festival's losses, would feature David's studio re-recording of 'The Supermen'.

As the *Hunky Dory* sessions progressed David played a one-off acoustic set on 28 July at the Country Club in Hampstead, accompanied by Mick Ronson on guitar and Rick Wakeman on piano. The gig was attended by the cast of *Pork*, the controversial show that was about to open at the nearby Roundhouse, marking Bowie's first encounter with the future stars of the MainMan circus (see *Hunky Dory* in Chapter 2). Of the show itself, Wayne County later recalled that David "had on these baggy yellow pants, a floppy hat, long hippy hair. I hated the way he was dressed, although his songs were nice … 'Changes', 'Kooks', all those. He'd written 'Andy Warhol' by then, and when he played it Cherry [Vanilla] stood up and popped her tit out. The other 28 people in the audience all gasped."

On the completion of *Hunky Dory* in September, David returned to America with Angela, Tony Defries and Mick Ronson to sign his new contract with RCA. As on his earlier visit he was unable to perform, but the trip was memorable for a number of other reasons, not least seeing Elvis Presley in concert at Madison Square Garden. At the invitation of *Pork*'s Tony Zanetta, David met Andy Warhol at the Factory in Greenwich Village, while at the Ginger Man restaurant he was introduced by RCA's Dennis Katz to another hero, Lou Reed. "David was flirtatious and coy," Zanetta later recounted, "He was in his Lauren Bacall phase, with his Veronica Lake hairdo and eyeshadow. So he let Lou take the driver's seat conversationally." At an RCA reception at Max's Kansas City later the same evening, David had his first encounter with yet another pivotal figure in his career: Iggy Pop. After America, Bowie made a brief promotional tour of Belgium and the Netherlands, playing the occasional free show in bars and public houses.

Back in England, the *Ziggy Stardust* sessions now imminent, David and his band played at the Friars, Aylesbury on 25 September. Although in itself an inauspicious one-off, this date was of crucial importance as the first full concert by the band soon to be known as The Spiders From Mars. The show opened with Bowie and Ronson alone, performing acoustic versions of 'Fill Your Heart', 'Buzz The Fuzz', 'Space Oddity' (introduced by David as "one of my own that we get over with as soon as possible") and 'Amsterdam'. Trevor Bolder and Woody Woodmansey then joined in for 'The Supermen', and having played piano on 'Oh! You Pretty Things' and 'Eight Line Poem' David introduced Tom Parker, sometime organist with The Animals, to "take over the piano and play it properly for the rest of the evening." There followed four more *Hunky Dory* numbers, then 'Looking For A Friend', 'Round And Round' and a final encore of 'Waiting For The Man'.

Kris Needs, a local journalist who covered the gig, tells Dave Thompson that Bowie "was still going around with his long hair and floppy hats, but he was great to watch on stage. He had just got back from New York and was full of talk about the people he'd met there, Lou and Warhol, and he played 'Waiting For The Man' and 'White Light/White Heat', which was the first time I'd ever heard anybody acknowledge The Velvet Underground. The response to that gig was amazing. I still think that, more than any other show he played, it was that one which finally decided him that he could make a go of it in this country. After the show he was sitting there, very quietly, but very excitedly."

Busy in the studio, Bowie remained almost entirely absent from the stage until the end of January 1972, when he reappeared in Aylesbury with a rather different show. The quiet excitement detected by Needs had been justified. David Bowie's time had come.

THE ZIGGY STARDUST TOUR (UK)
29 January – 7 September 1972

Musicians: David Bowie *(vocals, guitar)*, Mick Ronson *(guitar)*, Trevor Bolder *(bass)*, Mick Woodmansey *(drums)*, Matthew Fisher *(keyboards, 20 April – 27 May)*, Robin Lumley *(keyboards, 2 June – 18 July)*, Nicky Graham *(keyboards, 19 August – 7 September)*

Repertoire: 'Hang On To Yourself' / 'Ziggy Stardust' / 'The Supermen' / 'Queen Bitch' / 'Song For Bob Dylan' / 'Changes' / 'Starman' / 'Five Years' / 'Space Oddity' / 'Andy Warhol' / 'Amsterdam' / 'I Feel Free' / 'Moonage Daydream' / 'White Light/White Heat' / 'You Got To Have A Job (If You Don't Work – You Don't Eat)' / 'Hot Pants' / 'Suffragette City' / 'Rock'n'Roll Suicide' / 'Waiting For The Man' / 'Life On Mars?' / 'Sweet Jane' / 'I Can't Explain' / 'John, I'm Only Dancing' / 'This Boy' / 'The Width Of A Circle' / 'Round And Round' / 'Lady Stardust' / 'My Death' / 'Wild Eyed Boy From Freecloud'

On 19 January 1972, three days before the "I'm gay" interview appeared in *Melody Maker*, journalist George Tremlett interviewed Bowie at the Royal Ballroom in Tottenham, where rehearsals were underway for the forthcoming tour. Tremlett was told that the staging would be "Quite outrageous, but very theatrical … it's going to be costumed and choreographed, quite different to anything anyone else has tried to do before … This is going to be something quite new."

Of course, the Ziggy Stardust stage show did not materialize in a vacuum. Ever since Little Richard's heyday, rock singers had worn mascara and flamboyant costumes, and to followers of Marc Bolan the glitter and spandex were nothing new. As recently as November 1971 Alice Cooper had wowed audiences at London's Rainbow Theatre with an outlandish show involving a live boa constrictor, a straitjacket and, finally, execution by electric chair. But Bowie was unimpressed by Cooper's theatrics, complaining to Michael Watts in the *Melody Maker* interview that "I think he's *trying* to be outrageous. You can see him, poor dear, with his red eyes sticking out and his temples straining. He tries so hard … I find him very demeaning. It's very premeditated, but quite fitting with our era. He's probably more successful than I am at present, but I've invented a new category of artist, with my chiffon and taff. They call it pantomime rock in the States." What was new about Bowie's offering was that he proposed not just to exhibit, but to inhabit the fantasy, to *become* Ziggy Stardust and play out his own rise and fall through the performance of the music itself.

Trevor Bolder later explained to the Gillmans that having completed work on the *Ziggy Stardust* album earlier in January, "we thought, This is the end of it, that's just the name of the album." But not long afterwards, "David started dragging us downstairs" to the basement flat of Haddon Hall, where a group of seamstresses overseen by Freddi Burretti began to work the musicians into "a band with costumes". As Bowie later put it, "I wanted the music to look like it sounded." With his encouragement the band grew their hair long and began to experiment in make-up. "I used to love getting into the eye-shadow and mascara stuff, loved it," Mick Ronson recalled, but the others were less enthusiastic. "To get the band into that stuff I had to tell them that the girls would really love it," Bowie said later. "Thank God it paid off … They never had so many women in their lives and so they got tartier and tartier."

The band's original costumes were based on those sported by the Droogs in Stanley Kubrick's 1971 film *A Clockwork Orange*. In addition to the deco-print two-piece he wore on the *Ziggy Stardust* sleeve photo, the early concerts saw David donning white satin trousers with a flock-patterned jacket ("My first and only stage costume change for those first few weeks," he later recalled), and the quilted rainbow jumpsuit later showcased on *Top Of The Pops*. Bowie had even considered wearing a bowler hat in the style of Malcolm McDowell's Alex in *A Clockwork Orange*, but in the end he settled for subverting the brutality of the film's

Droog uniforms. "I was determined that the music we were doing was the music for the *Clockwork Orange* generation," he said in 1993, "and I wanted to take the hardness and violence of those *Clockwork Orange* outfits – the trousers tucked into big boots and the codpiece things – and soften them up by using the most ridiculous fabrics. It was a Dada thing – this extreme ultraviolence in Liberty fabrics." *A Clockwork Orange* was Kubrick's first picture since *2001: A Space Odyssey*, and its impact on Bowie's work would be just as significant: David elected to open the Ziggy concerts with Walter Carlos's synthesized arrangement of *Ode To Joy* from Beethoven's ninth symphony, which accompanied the key scene of Alex's brainwashing. "Both of these films provoked one major theme: there was no linear line in the lives that we lead," David observed 30 years later. "We were not evolving, merely surviving. Moreover, the clothes were fab."

Bowie explained that The Spiders "played the part perfectly – they were a number one spacey punk-rock band, they were absolute archetypes, everyone was right out of a cartoon book." As the archive footage and photographs demonstrate, however, none of The Spiders ever quite succeeded in emulating their leader's androgynous chic. "Good old Trev," Bowie reminisced of his bassist in 1993, "he had a similar haircut but he insisted he kept his sideburns."

While David groomed the band, Tony Defries was grooming David for the trappings of stardom. A Hull acquaintance of Ronson's, a towering black Yorkshireman called Stuey George, was hired as Bowie's personal minder and bodyguard, and the pair were booked into top West End hotels for the occasional weekend in order to accustom themselves to the etiquette of being treated as VIPs. Publicists, secretaries and a full-time photographer, London Film School graduate Mick Rock (who would first encounter Bowie at the Birmingham Town Hall gig on 17 March), were added at RCA's expense to Defries's increasingly Colonel Parker-like empire.

Although not generally considered the first night of the tour itself, Bowie's new show was premiered at Aylesbury's Borough Assembly Hall on Saturday, 29 January 1972. The publicity billed David as "The Most Beautiful Person In The World": there was no reference to The Spiders, merely a pseudo-hippy message reading, "Homo Superiors … Bells … Feet … Worlds … Hello". Among the audience at the gig was Roger Taylor, already a fan, who had dragged Freddie Mercury along for the occasion: "We were blown away," Taylor recalled. "It was so fantastic, and like nothing else that was happening, and so far ahead of its time."

The Ziggy Stardust tour proper began on 10 February at the Toby Jug in Tolworth. "Oh, that's perfect!" Bowie laughed when reminded of the fact by Q's David Cavanagh in 1996. "Ziggy at the Toby. It was probably a pub. Things moved quite fast in those days, but Ziggy was a case of small beginnings. I remember when we had no more than twenty or thirty fans at the most. They'd be down the front and the rest of the audience would be indifferent. And it feels so special, because you and the audience kid yourselves that you're in on this big secret."

The earliest Ziggy Stardust concerts were based squarely on the new album, usually opening with 'Hang On To Yourself', and David's imploring "gimme your hands" routine was already being exploited as the final melodramatic flourish. There were a few numbers from earlier albums, and initially the warmest reception was usually given to his three-year-old hit 'Space Oddity'. Alongside the Velvet Underground and Jacques Brel covers were a couple of oddities which would soon disappear from the repertoire: Cream's 'I Feel Free' and the James Brown medley 'You Got To Have A Job' / 'Hot Pants'. The show lacked the theatrical excesses of the later Ziggy period, conforming instead to a tried-and-tested formula of a hard-rock electric opening, followed by a trio of stripped-down numbers (usually 'Space Oddity', 'Andy Warhol' and 'Amsterdam'), for which the rhythm section would sit back as Bowie and Ronson perched on stools downstage, armed only with their acoustic guitars. Then it would be back to the full electric assault, culminating in 'Suffragette City' and 'Rock'n'Roll Suicide'.

On 8 February The Spiders recorded their famous appearance on *The Old Grey Whistle Test*, performing 'Oh! You Pretty Things', 'Queen Bitch' and 'Five Years'. Only the latter two songs were originally broadcast, but full versions and out-takes from this excellent set have been widely aired ever since, eventually appearing on 2002's *Best Of Bowie* DVD. "I was very scared on that programme," Bowie remarked the following month, "cause they're all so serious about music!"

As February progressed, Bowie concentrated on sharpening the act on the basis of each night's experience. An early failure came at Imperial College when he attempted to step out across the audience's shoulders in the style of Iggy Pop – the crowd was too

sparse and he fell to the floor. He dyed his hair red for the first time later the same month, and during March the momentum grew. In Sunderland six fans arrived in wheelchairs, aping disablement until Bowie's entrance caused them to leap to their feet as if healed by their new Messiah. At another concert David was hoisted aloft by fans and carried around the auditorium in a lap of honour, a spontaneous act which so entranced Tony Defries that it was stage-managed for future gigs. Photos and posters were handed out free after the concerts, Defries reckoning that the surest way to cement Bowie in the minds of the nation's youth was to encourage them to stick him on their bedroom walls. RCA's marketing manager Geoff Hannington recalled watching the shows with "absolute amazement".

There was a month's break from late March, but with the release of 'Starman' and the resumption of live dates on 20 April, the campaign was stepped up and the show revamped. From April the band was augmented by a pianist, Procol Harum's Matthew Fisher. Defries invited a posse of journalists to the 6 May concert at Kingston Polytechnic, and a recording of the same gig was reputedly made for possible release as a live album. The only evidence of this that has ever come to light is a muffled audience bootleg, from which derives the version of 'I Feel Free' included on *RarestOneBowie*.

After the Kingston gig the stakes were raised, as greater press attention led to the booking of larger venues. On 14 May David entered Olympic Studios to record 'All The Young Dudes' with Mott The Hoople, and with The Spiders he taped no fewer than three BBC radio sessions later the same month. By now the Ziggy shows had begun to whip their audiences into a frenzy. In Worthing on 11 May Bowie climbed onto Mick Ronson's shoulders as he played and, still singing, was carried piggy-back into the crowd. In Newcastle the local paper described how "the audience welcomed every number with wild enthusiasm" and how Bowie, a "supreme showman", received a "genuine spontaneous standing ovation" at the end. Future star Neil Tennant was in the Newcastle audience and described the show many years later as the best gig of his life: "The venue was half-empty. He was electrifying. He dedicated a song to me and my friends, saying, 'This song is for the strange people in the audience'."

From the Newcastle show on 2 June pianist Robin Lumley replaced Matthew Fisher who, according to

Lumley, had "done a bunk ... for some unknown reason". With the release of *The Rise And Fall Of Ziggy Stardust And The Spiders From Mars* on 6 June the concert bookings rocketed. On 21 June The Spiders were seen performing 'Starman' on Granada TV's *Lift-Off With Ayshea*. In Croydon four days later, a thousand fans were turned away.

It was during this stage of the tour that another piece of the Ziggy mythology fell into place. At Oxford Town Hall on 17 June, photographer Mick Rock was on hand to capture forever the moment when David first knelt before Mick Ronson during his 'Suffragette City' solo and simulated fellatio on his guitar. Photographed again and again at subsequent concerts, the consummation of Bowie's provocative stage relationship with Ronson became one of the abiding images of rock, an outrage to rival Hendrix burning his guitar or Iggy Pop diving headlong into the crowd. According to Stuey George, it was a premeditated stunt calculated to cause "a stir" after Ronson had begun emulating Hendrix by playing his guitar with his teeth on stage. "David suggested taking it a stage further ... What you have to remember is that with David everything was choreographed." The original fellatio photograph was distributed to the press, and one of the most iconic images of Bowie was born. Once again Ziggy Stardust was undermining the assumed "masculinity" of rock performance, this time by subverting the implicitly heterosexual connotations of the guitar solo.

The stunt almost backfired when Mick Ronson learned that paint had been thrown over his parents' front door and daubed on the new car he had bought them, and that his sister was braving accusations in Hull that he was "a queer". According to some reports Ronson was only dissuaded from quitting the band by some fast talking from Bowie and Defries.

The Dunstable gig was filmed for posterity by Mick Rock, and a selection of clips later formed the video for the 1994 release of the live 'Ziggy Stardust' single from *Santa Monica '72*. This four-minute montage offers a valuable glimpse of The Spiders' early stage show, capturing David's remarkable elasticity, and catching Woody Woodmansey before his hair was cut short and dyed blond.

The turning-point came in early July, when The Spiders' famous *Top Of The Pops* performance of 'Starman' was followed three days later by a special "Save the Whale" gig on behalf of Friends Of The Earth at London's Royal Festival Hall. Support came from Marmalade and the JSD Band (Mott The Hoople had turned down the slot: "I knew what the bugger was up to," said Ian Hunter later, suggesting that Bowie had intended to give the band twenty minutes "with a lousy sound system", the better to reflect his own set), but there was no doubt about who the audience had come to see. Compère Kenny Everett introduced Bowie as "the second greatest thing next to God," and the press weren't far behind in their praise. "When a shooting star is heading for the peak, there is usually one concert at which it is possible to declare, 'That's it – he's made it,'" wrote Ray Coleman in *Melody Maker*. "Bowie is going to be an old-fashioned, charismatic idol, for his show is full of glitter, panache and pace. Dressed outrageously in the tightest multicoloured gear imaginable, Bowie is a flashback in many ways to the pop star theatrics of about ten years ago, carrying on a detached love affair with his audience, wooing them, yet never surrendering that vital aloofness that makes him slightly untouchable ... obviously revelling in stardom, strutting from mike to mike, slaying us all with a deadly mixture of fragility and desperate intensity." *Record Mirror* declared that "David Bowie will soon become the greatest entertainer that Britain has ever known ... His talent seems unlimited and he looks certain to become the most important person in pop music on both sides of the Atlantic." The *Guardian* found him "a remarkable performer", and even the *Times* hailed his music as "T S Eliot with a rock and roll beat."

The Festival Hall concert was notable for other reasons. After a standard set, the band was joined for the encores by Lou Reed, who had arrived from New York the previous day to begin work with Bowie on his new album *Transformer*. It was Reed's first appearance on the British stage, and although somewhat the worse for wear ("He was absolutely out of his head," an anonymous insider told the Gillmans, "I don't know if he was stoned or pissed or what"), he duetted with David on the Velvet Underground numbers 'White Light/White Heat', 'Waiting For The Man' and 'Sweet Jane'.

A week later on 16 July, Lou Reed and Iggy Pop (both fresh from solo performances at the King's Cross Cinema over the previous two days) were present at a Bowie press conference at the Dorchester Hotel, arranged for a group of American journalists who had been flown over by Defries to attend Bowie's Aylesbury gig the previous night. Following the press conference Defries began refusing interviews and access to David. It was the beginning of the next stage in his campaign to build up an aura of untouchable mystique around his star: the summer of 1972 also saw the hyping of Bowie's much-discussed dread of being shot on stage, and the exaggeration of his fear of flying (in reality a genuine but conquerable anxiety that had been exacerbated by an electrical storm while flying home from Cyprus with Angie in 1971) into a full-blown phobia necessitating heavily publicized and vastly inconvenient journeys by the Trans-Siberian Express and the *QEII*.

Defries's grasp on Bowie's affairs tightened at around the same time. In June 1972 he split from Laurence Myers, his partner at Gem Productions, who surrendered Gem's copyright control of Bowie's master recordings in return for $500,000 of Bowie's future earnings. Ignorant of this arrangement and still trusting Defries implicitly, David agreed to sign a new contract which allowed his manager a shocking 50 per cent of his future earnings. The contract was with a company Defries had purchased the previous year and which, on 30 June 1972, he registered under a new title: MainMan. It is a name now synonymous with the excess and exploitation towards which Bowie was irrevocably headed. "The problem is," Defries frankly told the Gillmans, "I don't think David could read or understood his own contracts."

After the Aylesbury gig of 15 July there was a month's break in Bowie's gigging schedule, as he concentrated instead on his studio commitments as co-producer of *Transformer* and *All The Young Dudes*. On 13 August he made a guest appearance for the encores of a Mott The Hoople concert in Guildford.

The UK tour was re-launched on 19 and 20 August with two high-profile performances at the Rainbow Theatre in Finsbury Park. Determined to raise his work to a suitably climactic new level, Bowie had summoned his old mime tutor Lindsay Kemp from Edinburgh to stage and choreograph the new shows. Under Kemp's direction, Bowie and The Spiders underwent two weeks' rehearsal at the Theatre Royal, Stratford East, simultaneously with the *Transformer* sessions. Kemp devised a series of avant-garde routines with his four dancers – Annie Stainer, Ian Oliver, Barbara Ella and Carling Patton – whom David dubbed the Astronettes, a name he would later recycle. The resulting gigs, billed as *The Ziggy Stardust Show*, were unveiled as a decadent multimedia spectacle, by far the most theatrical concerts Bowie had yet undertaken and arguably the most spectacular of the

entire Ziggy period. Ladders and catwalks framed the stage, giving David the opportunity to perform songs from different levels – a significant step towards the radical rock theatre he would attempt on later tours. The inspiration for this, he revealed, came from performances he had seen by the Living Theatre in London. The stage itself was covered with sawdust, an old Lindsay Kemp technique which, as David later explained, would allow dragged feet to "produce a trail indicating movement caught, so to speak, in the spotlight."

In another innovative move, the Rainbow shows were illuminated by slide projections against the backdrop: prior to Bowie's entrance, the screens displayed a montage of new images shot by Mick Rock at Trident during the *Transformer* sessions, juxtaposed with stills of rock icons like Elvis Presley and Little Richard. This, David explains in *Moonage Daydream*, was "to give a semblance of continuity to the Ziggy theme, as though he was already one of them. At other times, it was Warhol objects juxtaposed against their civilian counterparts. The Campbell's soup can, a packet of Kellogg's Corn Flakes, Andy's electric chair against a chair from Habitat, Marilyn and a girl from Orpington. And so on and so forth."

For the opening 'Lady Stardust' (added to the repertoire for the first time), a giant projection of Marc Bolan's face filled the backdrop while the dancers waltzed through dry-ice in identical Bowie masks. During 'Starman', Kemp dangled from the rafters dressed as an angel, while David added lines from the song's ancestor 'Over The Rainbow'. The newly-revived 'The Width Of A Circle' saw Bowie embarking on an elaborate mime sequence devised by Kemp which stayed in the show for the remainder of the Ziggy tour. Other new additions included 'Life On Mars?', 'I Can't Explain', 'Round And Round', the new single 'John, I'm Only Dancing', and 'Wild Eyed Boy From Freecloud' (a full-length rendition, unlike the medley version heard in later Ziggy concerts). 'Amsterdam' was replaced by another Jacques Brel cover, 'My Death', for the acoustic interlude. It was also at around this time that The Beatles' 'This Boy' was added to the repertoire as an occasional treat. The Rainbow shows heralded a third replacement keyboard player, Nicky Graham, who had accompanied some of The Spiders' BBC Radio sessions and now stayed with the band for the remainder of the UK tour.

There were new costumes too, including a selection of bomber-jackets chosen by Angela from

London boutiques, some spider-web leotards for the dancers which would reappear in the following year's *The 1980 Floor Show*, and, notably, Bowie's first Kansai Yamamoto costume: a tight-fitting red one-piece, later described by David as "the impossibly silly 'bunny' costume", which would remain a regular feature of Ziggy's live act thereafter. By introducing both Japanese costume and a mime element to Bowie's act, the Rainbow shows were instrumental in pushing him in the direction of kabuki theatre, a tradition he had so far plundered only for hairstyles and make-up. As 1972 progressed Bowie began using Japanese culture as another signifier for what was "alien" in his species of rock music. Kabuki literally means "song, dance, art", and its exotic make-up and physical expressionism, not to mention the fact that both male and female roles are played by men, gave it an obvious resonance for Bowie. The adoption of full-scale kabuki costumes the following year would alter his stage act forever.

A glimpse of the style of the Rainbow concerts survives in the form of the 'John, I'm Only Dancing' video, shot by Mick Rock during rehearsals on 18 August and featuring two of Kemp's dancers. Footage from the first Rainbow gig was later edited to accompany a live recording of 'Starman' made on the same night, but this remains unreleased.

Support at the Rainbow shows came from the latest glam sensation Roxy Music, whose debut single 'Virginia Plain' entered the chart the same week. Roxy had supported the tour in Croydon two months earlier, marking David's first encounter with his future collaborator Brian Eno. "The first time I met him I thought he looked more effeminate than I did," Bowie later recalled. "Really quite a shock."

Among those who attended the Rainbow concerts were Lou Reed, Mick Jagger, Alice Cooper, Rod Stewart, Andy Warhol and Elton John (who left before the end, announcing that Bowie had "blown it"). *Record Mirror* declared the show a "stunning production spectacle" with a "breathtaking finale", while the *NME*'s Charles Shaar Murray, soon to become one of David's foremost cheerleaders, found it "perhaps the most consciously theatrical rock show ever staged" and a "thoroughly convincing demonstration of his ascendancy over any other soloist in rock today". Lou Reed was overcome either by the show or by something else, and had to be carried out by Warhol and Kemp as he wept, "I have seen my music played and it was just beautiful!"

"Ironically enough, this would be the first and last time I would ever stage the Ziggy show on such a scale," Bowie later recalled. "We simply couldn't afford it." But it hardly mattered, because the essence of Ziggy, like the essence of kabuki, was not the scenery but the actor himself. "Although he was always called 'theatrical', Ziggy had very little stage show," Mick Rock pointed out in 2003. "Unlike Alice Cooper, who had this elaborate Grand Guignol set, Ziggy *was* the stage show – his costumes, his mime, his illusions, his dramatics. He did it all himself; he used himself. It was an amazing sleight of hand."

Such was the success of the Rainbow shows that a further ten UK gigs were booked for late August and early September, including another show at the Rainbow but otherwise staged mainly at venues run by the Top Rank organisation. By comparison with the Rainbow extravaganza these were toned-down affairs (the temporary loss of the costumes in transit even led to the band appearing in jeans and T-shirts at Manchester's Hard Rock Club), but by now David Bowie had conquered Britain. In Manchester on 3 September Defries dropped a new bombshell for the delighted entourage: RCA had consented to back an American tour which would begin later the same month.

THE ZIGGY STARDUST TOUR (US)
22 September – 2 December 1972

Musicians: David Bowie *(vocals, guitar)*, Mick Ronson *(guitar)*, Trevor Bolder *(bass)*, Mick Woodmansey *(drums)*, Mike Garson *(piano)*

Repertoire: 'Hang On To Yourself' / 'Ziggy Stardust' / 'The Supermen' / 'Queen Bitch' / 'Changes' / 'Life On Mars?' / 'Five Years' / 'Space Oddity' / 'Andy Warhol' / 'My Death' / 'The Width Of A Circle' / 'John, I'm Only Dancing' / 'Moonage Daydream' / 'Starman' / 'Waiting For The Man' / 'White Light/White Heat' / 'Suffragette City' / 'Rock'n'Roll Suicide' / 'Lady Stardust' / 'Round And Round' / 'The Jean Genie' / 'Drive In Saturday' / 'All The Young Dudes' *(29 November only)* / 'Honky Tonk Women' *(29 November only)*

With Bowie yet to score a chart hit in America, the US tour of autumn 1972 was a considerable financial gamble. RCA's American division remained uncertain of its level of commitment to its newest star, and Tony Defries instructed the entire Bowie entourage "to look and act like a million dollars", famously telling them in a pre-tour pep-talk that "so far as RCA in America is concerned, the man with the red hair at the end of the table is the biggest thing to have come out of England since the Beatles – and possibly before the Beatles." By contrast with the steady snowballing effect of the seven-month UK tour, the tactics of the American campaign were to arrive with all guns blazing.

Having broken Bowie in Britain, Defries now proposed to relocate his centre of operations to America. In August 1972 he established a MainMan office on New York's East 58th Street, and began populating it with staff chosen more for their outrageousness than their business acumen. Tony Zanetta, the *Pork* actor who had assisted Defries in his American dealings since returning to New York a year earlier, was now installed as MainMan's president, with fellow *Pork* veterans Leee Black Childers and Cherry Vanilla appointed vice-president and publicity officer respectively. "The most sensible thing to do was to hire actors to act the parts," claims Angela Bowie in her memoir, "so they wouldn't do anything in the stupid, old-fashioned dumb way it was always done … an actor playing a role is a lot better than some idiot doing it the way they've been doing it for thirty years because that's the way it's always been done. Fuck the way it's always been done, let's do it the way we want it to be done."

The original intention was to tour the full theatrical production staged at the Rainbow Theatre in August, but the idea was scrapped on grounds of cost. Nonetheless, outwardly the tour projected all the trappings of excess that Defries could coax from the cautious advances of the concert promoters. Expense accounts, hotel tabs, champagne and limousine bills were all forwarded to RCA. David and Angela arrived on board the *QEII* on 17 September, and were given a suite in Central Park's Plaza Hotel. The following day the band and entourage arrived at Kennedy Airport.

Bowie and Defries had agreed to open the US tour in Cleveland, Ohio, where local radio had been strong in its support of Bowie's last two albums and where a young devotee called Brian Kinchy had set up David's first US fan club, helping distribute cuttings and press releases around the country. In the late summer of 1972 Bowie had telephoned Kinchy from London to thank him for his support and, as Kinchy told the Gillmans, "When he said we may be starting in Cleveland I thought, Jesus!"

Only five days before the opening Cleveland gig, a fifth member of the band was recruited. Three temporary pianists had come and gone on the British tour, and the situation was once again vacant. At the suggestion of RCA's London executive Ken Glancey, Bowie and Ronson contacted Brooklyn jazz pianist Mike Garson, who had also been recommended by Annette Peacock, on whose album *I'm The One* he had recently played. At RCA's New York studios Ronson demonstrated the chords of 'Changes' and allowed Garson to repeat them. "I must have played for eight seconds," Garson later recalled, "and Mick said, 'You've got the gig.'" When asked by Defries to name his fee, Garson suggested what he thought was a realistic amount: "I reckoned that these guys must be on about $2000 a week so I'll only ask for $800," he told the Gillmans. "So I said $800 a week and he looked a little dazed but I couldn't tell what he was thinking. But he said, 'Fine,' and I thought, what an idiot I am, I should have asked for $1500." Not until much later would Garson discover that Defries was paying the other Spiders no more than £30 a week.

As the band entered last-minute rehearsals, 'Song For Bob Dylan' and 'Wild Eyed Boy From Freecloud' were dropped from the set-list. After the first handful of concerts 'Starman' and 'Round And Round' would also disappear; but there would soon be new additions, written on the road as the tour bus crossed America.

Bolstered by extensive publicity and wall-to-wall playing of the *Ziggy Stardust* album on local WMMS radio, the opening Cleveland Music Hall gig on 22 September, supported by Lindisfarne, was filled to its 3200-seat capacity. Fan club organizer Brian Kinchy sat next to Defries and recalled that it was "an amazing show. People were just going crazy. They were singing, they were clapping, they knew the words … I was in awe." After a ten-minute ovation the audience rushed the stage, and the *Cleveland Plain Dealer* dutifully reported that "a star has been born". WMMS broadcast a recording of the gig the following week.

The press response to the next concert, two days later in Memphis, Tennessee, was not so warm. The *Memphis Commercial Appeal* told its readers that Bowie "substituted noise for music, freaky stage gimmicks for talent, and covers it all up with volume". Even so, the 4335-strong capacity audience from Elvis Presley's home town "loved it. They screamed. They yelled. They danced on their seats and begged for more."

Four days later came the make-or-break concert of the tour, as the band returned to New York to play

Carnegie Hall. The *Pork* company had been promoting the concert for weeks in advance, distributing free tickets while simultaneously spreading rumours that they were unobtainable. MainMan reported 400 applications for the 100 RCA press passes on offer. "We peddled David's ass like Nathans sell hotdogs," Cherry Vanilla later told *Village Voice*. As the hype escalated, the concert became the showbusiness event of the season. Among the luminaries in the packed house were Andy Warhol, Truman Capote, Anthony Perkins, Alan Bates, Todd Rundgren and the New York Dolls. Despite a bad cold, Bowie rose to the occasion and gave one of his finest performances yet. According to *Melody Maker*, "A strobe was turned on, and the familiar tones of *Clockwork Orange* music cut the air, very loud, and quite suddenly, there was Bowie in New York City … trying every minute, and working like fury. And glory did it work. Mick Ronson was playing rock guitar like it should be played. No frills, just a quick wrist. The audience just loved him."

In the *New York Daily News* Lilian Roxon reported that David, "a great songwriter and lyricist as well as a great showman and entertainer", had won over a "skeptical, cynical audience." She concluded: "A star is born. I have always wanted to write that in a review and now I can." The *New York Times* hailed "a solidly competent stage performer who brings a strong sense of professionalism to every move he makes … He understands that theatricality has more to do with presence than with gimmickry, and that beautifully coordinated physical movements and well-planned music can reach an audience a lot quicker than aimless prancing and high-decibel electronics."

Newsday's Robert Christgau, on the other hand, complained that Bowie was "currently trying to ride a massive hype into superstardom" and questioned whether "songs about Andy Warhol written by an English fairy are enough for American audiences". Critics everywhere were drawing parallels with America's own war-painted sensation Alice Cooper, but Ellen Willis of the *New Yorker* dismissed the comparisons as "wilful incomprehension. There is nothing provocative, perverse or revolting about Bowie. He is all glitter, no grease, and his act is neither overtly nor implicitly violent." Willis also displayed a perceptiveness rare among her peers regarding the most controversial aspect of Britain's latest import: "As for his self-proclaimed bisexuality, it really isn't that big a deal. British rock musicians have always been less uptight than Americans about displaying, and even

flaunting, their 'feminine' side … Bowie's dyed red hair, make-up, legendary dresses, and on-stage flirtations with his guitarist just take this tradition one theatrical step further."

The Carnegie Hall concert was taped by RCA for a proposed live LP, although the only track yet to emerge on an official release is 'My Death' on *RarestOneBowie*.

The tour moved on to Washington and Boston (where the concert was also recorded, live tracks later appearing on *Sound + Vision Plus* and 2003's *Aladdin Sane* reissue). *Boston After Dark* dubbed David "the most important artist to have emerged in this decade". Returning to New York, the band entered RCA's studios to record David's new composition 'The Jean Genie', which received its live premiere in Chicago on 7 October. Detroit, St Louis and Kansas City followed, but by comparison with the rapturous receptions in the north, many southern venues seemed unwilling to accept this newly imported outrage. At Kansas only 250 people turned up, so David gathered them to the front and sat on the edge of the stage to give an intimate cabaret-style performance. According to Tony Zanetta's book *Stardust*, David reacted to the disappointment of small houses by drinking heavily: "He was so upset he got very drunk, and during the [Kansas] show he fell off the stage into the house. But he didn't miss a note." If this account is true, it marks the earliest substantial instance of David cushioning himself with intoxicants on stage, something that would become a serious problem two years later.

As the tour moved from city to city it gathered the inevitable stream of groupies and hangers-on, and by the time it arrived in Los Angeles for the Santa Monica concerts on 20 and 21 October, an entourage of 46 moved into the luxurious Beverly Hills Hotel at RCA's expense. The first date was recorded for American FM radio, and would receive an official release many years later as *Santa Monica '72*. On 27 and 28 October the video for 'The Jean Genie' was shot in San Francisco.

Although the tour had been due to end in California, Defries capitalized on its early success by adding new engagements. In Seattle there was another tiny audience to rival Kansas City, while some other planned dates were cancelled owing to poor sales. At Fort Lauderdale on 17 November Bowie unveiled another new composition, 'Drive In Saturday', and at around the same time he added another touch to Ziggy's increasingly alien visage: one night in Florida he shaved off his eyebrows, having persuaded Angela to do it first so that he could see what it looked like. He later claimed that the eyebrow-shaving was a drunken act of ill-temper spurred by Mott The Hoople's decision to turn down 'Drive In Saturday' as their next single.

The cool southern reception continued at Nashville, where Cherry Vanilla's lurid advance publicity about Bowie's homosexuality and her own Communist sympathies resulted in a right-wing demonstration outside the venue. The *Nashville Banner*, whose reporter stressed his aversion to "queers", described the 4500-strong audience as "subdued" and considered comparisons between Bowie and Presley ill-advised: "There is no similarity whatsoever, so far as talent is concerned."

Further north, the final few gigs did better business. Due to popular demand there were two sell-out performances back in Cleveland, this time at the larger Public Auditorium. On 29 November Bowie compèred a Mott The Hoople concert at the Tower Theatre, Philadelphia, joining the band to perform encores of 'All The Young Dudes' and 'Honky Tonk Women'. The following night saw the first of Bowie's three consecutive dates at the same venue, concluding the US tour. Philadelphia would become one of Bowie's foremost American strongholds, nurturing a loyal fan base and playing host to the recording of *David Live*, *Young Americans* and *Stage*.

By the end of 1972 Bowie could hardly be said to have cracked the States (as yet his best US chart performance was a feeble number 65 for 'Starman'), but the tour was a significant first step in a process that would take another three years to complete. In the short term its shocking expense would land MainMan in trouble with RCA. Everyone from Tony Defries downwards had lived far beyond their means; Tony Zanetta later estimated that the room service bill at the Beverly Hills Hotel alone came to $20,000. Ultimately RCA would recoup the costs of the tour from Bowie's own royalty share, while Defries retained his full 50 per cent. MainMan's wholesale milking of David Bowie had begun in earnest.

THE CHRISTMAS ZIGGY STARDUST TOUR
23 December 1972 – 9 January 1973

Musicians: David Bowie (*vocals, guitar*), Mick Ronson (*guitar*), Trevor Bolder (*bass*), Mick Woodmansey (*drums*), Mike Garson (*piano*)

Repertoire: 'Let's Spend The Night Together' / 'Hang On To Yourself' / 'Ziggy Stardust' / 'Changes' / 'The Supermen' / 'Life On Mars?' / 'Five Years' / 'The Width Of A Circle' / 'John, I'm Only Dancing' / 'Moonage Daydream' / 'The Jean Genie' / 'Suffragette City' / 'Rock'n'Roll Suicide' / 'Waiting For The Man' / 'Starman'

Bowie followed his first American tour with a short series of Christmas and New Year concerts in England and Scotland, beginning with two nights at the Rainbow Theatre supported by *Space Oddity* guitarist Tim Renwick's current band Quiver. The audiences were asked to bring children's toys to be distributed through Dr Barnardo's homes on Christmas Day ("I think we filled an entire truck with them," David recalled). With the *Aladdin Sane* sessions being fitted around the tour dates, the major innovation was the introduction of The Rolling Stones' 'Let's Spend The Night Together' as the opening number. David later described this phase of the Ziggy tour as "probably one of the best, highest energy jaunts of our short eighteen-month life."

THE 1973 ZIGGY STARDUST TOUR (aka THE ALADDIN SANE TOUR)
14 February – 3 July 1973

Musicians: David Bowie (*vocals, guitar, saxophone, harmonica*), Mick Ronson (*guitar, backing vocals*), Trevor Bolder (*bass*), Mick Woodmansey (*drums*), Mike Garson (*piano, mellotron, organ*), Ken Fordham (*alto, tenor and baritone saxophone*), John Hutchinson (*rhythm guitar, backing vocals*), Brian Wilshaw (*tenor saxophone, flute*), Geoffrey MacCormack (*backing vocals, percussion*)

Repertoire: 'Hang On To Yourself' / 'Ziggy Stardust' / 'Changes' / 'Soul Love' / 'John, I'm Only Dancing' / 'Moonage Daydream' / 'Five Years' / 'Space Oddity' / 'My Death' / 'Watch That Man' / 'Drive In Saturday' / 'Aladdin Sane' / 'Panic In Detroit' / 'Cracked Actor' / 'The Width Of A Circle' / 'Time' / 'The Prettiest Star' / 'Let's Spend The Night Together' / 'The Jean Genie' / 'Suffragette City' / 'Rock'n'Roll Suicide' / 'The Supermen' / 'Starman' / 'Round And Round' / 'Quicksand/Life On Mars?/Memory Of A Free Festival' / 'Wild Eyed Boy From Freecloud/All The Young Dudes/Oh! You Pretty Things' / 'White Light/White

Heat' / 'Love Me Do'

On 17 January 1973 David appeared with The Spiders on Granada TV's *Russell Harty Plus*, performing 'My Death' and 'Drive In Saturday'. Sharply dressed in a new Freddi Burretti outfit ("a parody of a suit and tie," he said) and a single enormous earring, David gave an entertaining interview, evidently delighting Harty with his saucy insinuations on subjects still considered taboo by television. On 24 January the *Aladdin Sane* sessions ended, and the following day he was stepping aboard the *QEII* in Southampton for another Atlantic crossing.

Unsurprisingly RCA had baulked at the cost of the 1972 junket, and Tony Defries had received a rap over the knuckles about expense accounts and hotel bills. As an economy measure the new US tour would play multiple dates in just seven cities, beginning with two nights in New York followed by a week's residency in Philadelphia. After America the show was due to travel to Japan, Britain and Europe, and then back to the States in the autumn, by which time it was hoped Bowie's American audience would be enormous. As history knows, the back-breaking 1973 leg of the Ziggy tour – generally referred to as the Aladdin Sane tour for obvious reasons – would in fact end under rather different circumstances.

David and Angela arrived in New York on 30 January 1973. As the finishing touches were put to *Aladdin Sane* at RCA Studios, it was revealed that Bowie's live band had been enlarged to include the album's two saxophonists, Ken Fordham and Brian Wilshaw, together with Geoffrey MacCormack on extra percussion and backing vocals. Another new arrival was David's old colleague from Feathers and The Buzz, John Hutchinson, recruited to provide rhythm guitar so that Bowie might concentrate on his increasingly acrobatic performances and costume changes.

Unsurprisingly the completion of *Aladdin Sane* heralded major changes to the set-list, which now incorporated every song from the new album bar 'Lady Grinning Soul'. Other songs were rearranged for a fuller band sound, including 'Space Oddity' which was now lifted from the acoustic set and transformed into a major production number. Another new arrival, albeit for the first couple of gigs only, was 'Soul Love', boasting a sax solo from David himself.

Also newly refined was Bowie's behaviour on stage. Perhaps responding to the meatier sound of his enlarged band and the rawer edge of the *Aladdin Sane* material, David's stage physicality became more assertively sexual, largely dropping the shy, fey quality he had projected to audiences the previous year. Whether this was the conscious adoption of a new "Aladdin Sane" character is in some doubt; to all intents and purposes he was still playing Ziggy Stardust, the name by which he had begun to introduce himself on stage. With the subtle change in demeanour came a new set of eye-opening costumes by the Japanese designer Kansai Yamamoto. "I like to keep my group well dressed, not like some other people I could mention," David told the press. "I'm out to bloody well entertain, not just get up on stage and knock out a few songs … I'm the last person to pretend I'm a radio. I'd rather go out and be a colour television set."

Embracing the conventions of kabuki theatre, in which changes of mask and costume denote changes of mood and personality, Bowie now began integrating his costumes into the "text" of the shows, conferring on the gaudy apparel an implied significance it had hitherto lacked. The portrayal of the schizoid character of Aladdin Sane was externalized by mime and masks (a point made explicit on the Diamond Dogs tour). In finest pantomime tradition Bowie now averaged between five and seven costume changes per show, and his new outfits included a quilted black PVC all-in-one with vast, rigid flares, which was torn away to reveal an embroidered white judo suit. In addition there were sharply stylized, ever-changing experiments in hair and make-up, largely at the behest of Pierre Laroche, who created the famous sleeve image for *Aladdin Sane* at around the same time. In early 1973 Bowie's shaggy mid-period Ziggy hairstyle was streamlined into a glossy leonine mane and dyed a darker red, and he began sporting silver lipstick, thick streaks of eyeliner and a gaudy white disc in the centre of his forehead.

Although there was still no stage scenery as such, the 1973 tour saw the addition of large banners on the backcloth, depicting a black zig-zag similar to *Aladdin Sane*'s trademark lightning-bolt. Intermittently lit by flashing strobes, the logo bore a passing resemblance to the Nazis' SS symbol, a fact largely unnoticed at the time but which, in retrospect, foreshadowed the more ominous stage settings of subsequent tours. "The flash on the original Ziggy set was taken from the 'high voltage' sign that was stuck on any box containing dangerous amounts of electricity,"

Bowie explained many years later. "I was not a little peeved when Kiss purloined it. Purloining, after all, was my job."

On 14 February the New York glitterati turned out for the opening concert at Radio City Music Hall. Andy Warhol, Truman Capote, Todd Rundgren, Bette Midler, Allen Ginsberg and Salvador Dali were in the audience to see David make an outrageous entrance, descending fifty feet to the stage in a metal cage. The show was a long one, 21 songs in all, and was rapturously received as Bowie and the audience goaded one another to ever-greater heights of theatrical frenzy. Mid-way through the final encore of 'Rock'n'Roll Suicide', the drama reached its peak when a man scrambled from the front row, grabbed Bowie and planted a kiss on his cheek, to which David responded by crumpling senseless to the floor. Members of the band initially assumed that David was simply going with the moment and ending the show on a note of high melodrama, but when he had to be carried offstage it became obvious that he had genuinely fainted. "It was pure nerves that caused that," Bowie recalled many years later. "I was absolutely terrified. Also I'd had some make-up done by Pierre Laroche … he did some brilliant things, but he used glitter on me for the first time, and it ran into my eyes. I did the whole show almost blind."

At both of the New York concerts, 'My Death' (now much enhanced by Garson's piano) was followed by a short intermission while a mind-expanding *2001*-style film of rushing stars and galaxies was projected onto the backdrop, accompanied by science-fiction sound effects. Thereafter this feature was dropped, as indeed was 'My Death' until the final shows at Hammersmith Odeon in July. Another epiphany in New York was David's first encounter with a young black dancer called Ava Cherry, later to become both backing singer and girlfriend.

Providing support for the third night and throughout the remainder of the US leg was Fumble, a British band David had seen on *The Old Grey Whistle Test* and whom he had used as support on the recent Manchester gig. Like the New York concerts, the seven shows at Philadelphia's Tower Theater were sell-outs. In Nashville and Memphis the homophobic element re-emerged – Bowie even received anonymous threats – but the *Press-Scimitar* reported that the "rapt" Memphis audience "exhibited a strange and somewhat puzzling attraction by Bowie", while the *Nashville Tennessean* gruffly admitted that "Bowie real-

ly is not a bad rock musician, if one can consider him such."

After the final concert at the Hollywood Palladium (also the last show to be supported by Fumble), Bowie boarded the SS *Oronsay* for the Pacific crossing to Japan. Arriving at Yokohama on 5 April, David was installed in Tokyo's Imperial Hotel. There he received a visit from Kansai Yamamoto, who had completed a further collection of stage costumes. Although the new designs included some tight-fitting jumpsuits of the kind hitherto favoured by Ziggy, Yamamoto also provided more flamboyant creations, including a flowing white robe decorated with Japanese characters reading "David Bowie", a silver leotard hung with a floor-length fringe of solid glass beads, a candy-striped spandex bodystocking, and a multi-coloured kimono that could be ripped away nightly to reveal only a red jockstrap (or, as David insisted on calling it, a Sumo wrestler's loincloth). "They were everything that I wanted them to be and more," David later wrote in *Moonage Daydream*. "Heavily inspired in equal parts by kabuki and samurai, they were outrageous, provocative, and unbelievably hot to wear under the stage lights." During the Japanese tour The Spiders joined David in going native, Trevor Bolder tying his long hair in a Samurai-style topknot to the delight of the crowds. Young Zowie, meanwhile, was making his debut appearance on tour; suitably decked out in a kimono, he attended his first ever Bowie concert in Tokyo.

David's singles had been doing well in Japan, and the scenes at the nine sell-out concerts were little short of frenzied. Lines of policemen monitored the activity of the front rows, routinely hurling stage-divers back into line. "It was accepted in Japan that people would dive onto the stage and they would get thrown off," recalled Hutch. Bowie later explained that "In Japan we were faced with an audience that we presumed didn't understand a word of what we were saying. Therefore I was more physically active than on any other tour I've ever done. Literally, I activated the whole thing with my hands and my body. I needn't have sung half the time." The *Japan Times* raved that Bowie was "the most exciting thing to have happened since the fragmentation of the Beatles. Theatrically he is perhaps the most interesting performer ever in the pop music genre."

The Japanese tour presented a stimulating change for David after the rock'n'roll excesses of his American jaunts; he visited moss gardens and kabuki and Noh theatre performances, learning new make-up techniques from Tamasaburo, the country's foremost kabuki actor. He had become fascinated by the life of Yukio Mishima, the homosexual novelist who had developed an obsession with the imperialist tradition of his Samurai family and committed ritual *seppuku* in 1970. These and other aspects of Japanese culture were to exert a powerful influence on Bowie's writing and lifestyle.

After visiting Nagoya, Hiroshima, Kobe and Osaka, on 20 April the Japanese tour ended where it had begun, in Tokyo. At the final gig an adoring crowd of fans stormed the stage, causing a bank of seating to collapse, fortunately without injury. While the entourage flew back to London, David embarked on the longest and most impractical yet of his non-flying escapades: after travelling 600 miles by boat to Vladivostok, he boarded the 6000-mile Trans-Siberian Express to Moscow. He was accompanied on the week-long train journey by Geoffrey MacCormack, Leee Black Childers and an American journalist called Bob Musel, who would later recall Bowie entertaining other passengers with an impromptu acoustic concert (which included 'Amsterdam' and 'Space Oddity') in his train compartment. David would later intimate that the culture-shock of travelling through checkpoints and witnessing the state systems of the Eastern bloc would have an impact on the paranoid themes of surveillance and totalitarianism that permeated *Diamond Dogs*.

Having made his rendezvous with Angela in Paris and spent an evening in the company of Jacques Brel, David arrived back in London on 4 May to find himself at the height of his popularity: *Aladdin Sane* was the number 1 album and 'Drive In Saturday' was peaking at number 3 in the singles chart. Several hundred fans and paparazzi congregated at Victoria Station to meet the boat train, only to be informed by loudspeaker that Mr Bowie would be arriving at Charing Cross instead. The scenes of mayhem that followed on the Underground were to be repeated throughout the forthcoming fifty-date UK tour, most of which had already sold out. In order to meet demand Defries would persuade the band to play two gigs per day at several of the pre-booked venues: at the height of the tour in late June the band would play 22 concerts in 16 days.

A week before the UK tour began, another chapter in Bowie history opened when the teenage magazine *Mirabelle* published the first instalment of David's

weekly "diary". This feature would run every week for the next two years, clocking up a total of 101 instalments until the final entry on 5 April 1975. The tone of wide-eyed innocence, the profusion of exclamation marks and the painstaking catalogue of Angela Bowie's social engagements make for immediately suspicious reading, and in 1998 David surprised nobody by admitting that the diary was actually written by MainMan's press officer Cherry Vanilla. Today the *Mirabelle* diaries offer a fascinatingly skewed account of the period between the final UK Ziggy tour and the release of *Young Americans*, revealing more about Cherry Vanilla's priorities and lifestyle than about those of a star who was becoming increasingly estranged from his management. The relentless plugging of other MainMan signings, the constant enthusing about "my incredible press lady, Cherry Vanilla", and the ruthless airbrushing of any mention of David's more controversial habits during the period, make for an often hilarious distortion of events.

On the eve of the UK tour David made the first step in patching up his differences with his former producer Tony Visconti, whom he hadn't seen since the completion of *The Man Who Sold The World* three years earlier. Visconti attended David's homecoming party at Haddon Hall on 5 May and was relieved to discover that "underneath all the make-up and stuff, it was really my old buddy David." Kenneth Pitt was similarly delighted to receive a surprise visit from David at his Manchester Street flat.

During rehearsals in early May there were several changes to the set. 'John, I'm Only Dancing' was dropped, as was 'Starman' after its brief return on the Japanese leg. In their place came a revamped 'White Light/White Heat' and a pair of beautifully constructed medleys: the first comprised excerpts from 'Quicksand', 'Life On Mars?' and 'Memory Of A Free Festival', while the second condensed 'Wild Eyed Boy From Freecloud', 'All The Young Dudes' and 'Oh! You Pretty Things'.

Despite the auspicious omens, the UK tour got off to a disastrous start. Defries had allowed grandiosity to overtake common sense by booking the 18,000-seat Earls Court Arena for the opening night on 12 May: the venue was twice the size of any David had previously played, but nonetheless the tickets had sold out within three hours. Today Earls Court is a customary venue for major concert tours, but in 1973 it had never played host to a rock concert of any kind. All did not go well. The acoustic was atrocious, the band's customary sound system totally inadequate, the seating insufficiently ranked, and the stage at floor level, meaning that few of the capacity audience could either see or hear what was going on. Before long there was a stampede near the front and altercations broke out among the crowd. By 'Space Oddity', halfway through the concert, there was chaos, and the band left the stage while order was restored. Kenneth Pitt judged it "a disaster". David was horrified and insisted that Defries cancel the tour's planned climax at Earls Court, replacing it with two nights in the more appropriate setting of Hammersmith Odeon.

One good thing emerged from the Earls Court debacle: during rehearsals, a nearby Ladbroke Grove studio became the venue for Mick Rock's classic video clip for 'Life On Mars?', which was released as a single in June and went top ten in the week the tour ended. And, despite a round of gleeful hatchet headlines ("Bowie Fiasco"; "Aladdin Distress"; "Drive-Out Saturday"), from the very next gig in Aberdeen four days later the remainder of the UK tour was a massive success. The *Sun* drooled that in Glasgow a couple had made love in the stalls to the strains of "the new god of pop'n'rock, back on the road with the freakiest show in Britain today." The *Daily Express* warned its readers about the dire new threat to the nation's morals: "26-year-old Bowie behaves more like a Soho stripper than a top pop star. He bumps, he grinds, he waggles his hips … His favourite [Spider] straddles the star on stage, who then simulates love with his strident guitar … David is a self-confessed bisexual. 'I'm not embarrassed about it. Are you?' he asks. The answer, inevitably, is 'Yes'." Bowie's fans thought differently, and at concert halls across the country there were riotous scenes of a kind seldom seen since the days of Beatlemania. Three limousines in succession were trashed by the nightly press of the crowd. The Brighton Dome banned Bowie from ever returning after an overexcited audience ripped up the venue's seats.

In Bournemouth on 25 May, BBC reporter Bernard Falk caught up with the tour and filed an 11-minute report for *Nationwide*, capturing backstage glimpses of The Spiders and frantic scenes of hysteria on the streets outside. Falk's barely concealed contempt for the "skinny lad with a pasty complexion" simmered throughout the item, and over some alarming shots of Bowie's getaway limo being mobbed by fans, Falk concluded: "When he dresses up and plasters his face, the kids of today see it as his way of flaunting [sic]

convention, and they respect him for it. It's worth wondering, though, what the beat age will spawn next, when someone like David Bowie isn't even freakish enough to shock us any more."

The tour ended with two dates at Hammersmith Odeon on 2 and 3 July. The final night, a star-studded affair attended by Mick Jagger, Lou Reed and Ringo Starr, was opened by a one-off support set from Mike Garson, who played a fifteen-minute instrumental medley of Bowie numbers on the piano. The concert itself was captured by the American filmmaker D A Pennebaker, best known for his Bob Dylan documentary *Don't Look Back* and his coverage of 1967's Monterey Pop festival. Pennebaker had been hired by RCA to shoot just half an hour of footage for an experimental new format called Selectavision: "This was a just-invented device for putting a video onto a record," the director explained to *Uncut* in 2003. "I never worked out exactly what it was, but it was years ahead of its time, which is maybe why it never survived. They wanted me to get a half-hour of his performance. But scouting the first show, I realized rapidly that we had to shoot the whole thing. There was a film to be made here." In his customarily grainy *vérité* style, Pennebaker filmed not only the concert itself, but caught fly-on-the-wall footage in David's dressing room and on the streets outside. After an edited screening on US television in 1974 and years of contractual wrangling, the film was finally released in 1983 as *Ziggy Stardust And The Spiders From Mars*, with a remixed DVD following in 2003.

Both band and audience were on an incandescent high which remains palpable even in Pennebaker's murky film. "There was a great last night tone," recalled Mick Ronson many years later, "there was a lot of energy there." Cut from both the film and live album was the guest appearance of Ronson's idol Jeff Beck, who joined the band to assist on encores of 'The Jean Genie' and 'Round And Round'. As Beck left the stage, Bowie stepped forward to speak. Having thanked the band and road crew, he paused before continuing, his announcement interrupted by repeated cheers: "Of all the shows on this tour this – this particular show will remain with us the longest, because not only is it – not only is it the last show of the tour, but it's the last show that we'll ever do. Thank you." Oblivious to the incredulous screams of "Noooo!" which all but drowned out his last two words, Bowie signalled to Hutch to begin the intro to 'Rock'n'Roll Suicide', and proceeded to play Ziggy

Stardust for the last time.

The reaction was monumental. "TEARS AS BOWIE BOWS OUT", declared the *Evening Standard*. "BOWIE QUITS", announced the *NME* on 7 July, quoting from a MainMan press release issued the day after the concert which stated that David "was leaving the concert stage for ever … The massive arenas of 80 US and Canadian cities will not now, or perhaps ever again, hold within their walls the magic essence of a live Aladdin Sane". The European sojourn and the proposed American tour, whose 38 confirmed shows were due to begin in Toronto on 1 September, had suddenly evaporated. "I don't want to do live concerts again for a long, long time," Bowie said on 4 July. "Not for two or three years at least." The fans were not alone in their surprise: famously, most of the band had known nothing about Bowie's decision either. "I couldn't hear it too well but he said something about retiring," Hutch later recalled. "Everybody in the band was looking at each other and saying, 'What?' Trevor and Woody seemed to take it worse because they felt double-crossed, they hadn't been told."

It was, of course, the only way to go. By catching the audience off its guard, Bowie had successfully fulfilled the self-immolation of Ziggy Stardust's apocalyptic narrative. That the Hammersmith speech remains probably the most discussed and dissected moment in Bowie's career is proof enough that it was a brilliant stroke of theatre. He is practically unique among rock performers in being able to point to one particular concert that still exerts this much mystique: that night in July 1973 has become one of Bowie's abiding works of art.

The romantic interpretation of Bowie/Ziggy's "retirement" remains the most attractive: that the artist, mentally besieged by the monster he had created, was driven to destroy him on stage before he himself was consumed, strangled by the mask like the character in David's 1969 mime routine. There's no shortage of fuel for this colourful thesis. Christopher Sandford's biography quotes fans who claim they met David in a deserted alley off Hammersmith Broadway only forty minutes before that final concert, finding him "on a razor's edge" and on the point of suffering "a Stephen Fry-like breakdown", desperately reluctant to perform at all. "Ziggy definitely affected him," said Mick Ronson many years later. "To do anything and to do it well, you have to become completely involved. He had to become what Ziggy was; he had to believe in him. Yes, Ziggy affected his personality. But he

affected Ziggy's personality. They lived off each other."

"I liked the ambiguity of not being able to separate the personas," Bowie himself has said. "It's the ominous enigma of the split personality, and which side is which…" Ever since the 1972 US tour, those close to David had noticed that his immersion in the rock-'n'roll lifestyle was making it harder for Ziggy to revert to plain old David Jones when he left the concert stage. "It was quite easy to become obsessed night and day with the character," he later admitted. "Everybody was convincing me that I was a Messiah, especially on that first American tour. I got hopelessly lost in the fantasy." On another occasion, he said, "My whole personality was affected … I thought I might as well take Ziggy to interviews as well. Why leave him on stage? Looking back it was completely absurd. It became very dangerous. I really did have doubts about my sanity … I think I put myself very dangerously near the line."

Without doubt there is truth in all this, but it should never be forgotten that David Bowie knows how to spin a good line. The man captured in Bernard Falk's news report and, briefly, in the backstage footage of Pennebaker's Hammersmith film, is not a demented rock god of the kind David himself would later send up in *Jazzin' For Blue Jean*, but a seasoned pro dragging on his cigarette as he prepares to meet his public. It is a lucid and level-headed David who explains to Falk that "I believe in my part all the way down the line … but I do *play* it for all it's worth, because that's the way I do my stage thing. That's part of what Bowie's supposedly all about. I'm an actor."

There are other, altogether more prosaic reasons which made Ziggy Stardust's final act of self-destruction remarkably convenient. What few outsiders realized at the time was that there were grave doubts over the viability of the projected third US tour. The original 1972 American jaunt had lost RCA something in excess of $300,000, and although MainMan had promised to pull in its horns, the Bowie roadshow continued to live far beyond its means in 1973. David's singles had yet to strike gold in America, and sales of his albums were no more than comfortable (by June *Ziggy Stardust*, the most successful, had only shifted 320,000 copies in a country where true success required seven-figure sales). The spring of 1973 had seen the rise of an American RCA executive called Mel Ilberman who proved more resistant than some of his colleagues to the blandishments of Tony Defries, and after a series of heated negotiations he pulled the plug on the third American tour, suggesting a smaller affair which Defries rejected. According to MainMan employee Jaime Andrews, the decision to "retire" Ziggy was made quite rationally as a face-saving measure: "It was a way to get press, and regroup and figure out what we were going to do."

Another compelling reason for the death of Ziggy was David's creative restlessness: at his best he has always been reluctant to stand still. "I had an awful lot of fun doing [Ziggy]," he explained soon afterwards, "…but my performance on stage reached a peak. I felt I couldn't go on stage in the same context again … if I'm tired with what I'm doing it wouldn't be long before the audience realized." And he was tired not only intellectually, but physically; by July the Ziggy Stardust tour had been running for eighteen months. "A good halfway through, nine or ten months into it, I knew it was over already," David told Michael Parkinson in 2002. "I just wanted to move somewhere else. There was a new kind of music I wanted to write, a different kind of theatricality I wanted to bring into it and all that. The last few months, I was really treading water. I couldn't wait to finish."

And in any case, by the time of Bowie's return to Britain in May, the charts were saturated with the vulgarized fallout of the groundwork he had laid down with Bolan and Roxy Music a year before. As early as December 1972, in the very week that 'The Jean Genie' entered the chart, the Strawbs had peaked at number 12 with 'Lay Down', a single whose B-side (or 'Backside' as it was entitled) was credited to "Ciggy Barlust and the Whales From Venus" which, if not exactly side-splitting, was an early indication that Bowie was already established enough to merit parody. In the week of Ziggy's retirement, the number 1 single was Slade's 'Skweeze Me Pleeze Me', while that summer's other regular chartbusters included Wizzard, Mud, Suzi Quatro, Sweet and Gary Glitter, whose kitsch classic 'I'm The Leader Of The Gang (I Am)' began its month-long residency at the top three weeks later. All these acts made hugely enjoyable records and never failed to raise a smile on Top Of The Pops, but in the process of colonizing glam rock, they had simultaneously emasculated it. Bowie later recalled that "it actually became a sense of embarrassment, iconically. I mean, in my feather boas and dresses, I certainly didn't wanna be associated with the likes of Gary Glitter, who was obviously a charlatan … we were very aware of it at the time and we were very miffed that people who had obviously never seen

Metropolis and had never heard of Christopher Isherwood were actually becoming glam rockers." For an artist who intended to keep one step ahead it was quite patently time to move on.

There can also be little doubt that drugs were beginning to play a part in Bowie's protean mentality. Although he was still some months away from the descent into serious addiction that would blight him during the remainder of the decade, by the summer of 1973 his outlook had already been affected by exposure to cocaine. Thirty years later he would recall that the making of the Ziggy Stardust album had been "drug-free apart from the occasional pill: amphetamines, speed … when we first started doing Ziggy we were really excited and drugs weren't necessary. The first eight months were real fun and then it soured for me. I went to America and got introduced to real drugs and it all went pear-shaped."

Finally there was the question of Bowie's deteriorating relationship with his band, born partly out of artistic frustrations and partly from MainMan's internecine politics. "I guess, at the time, [it] was a bit nasty," David admitted many years later, "…they wanted to remain doing what we were doing and I didn't. I was going somewhere else, and they didn't want to go. They were quite happy to play Jeff Beck covers." Personal differences had also begun to rear their heads during the second American tour. Mike Garson, then a committed Scientologist, had struck up a close friendship with Woody Woodmansey and Trevor Bolder, both of whom converted to the faith in 1973. Although Garson was to outlast all of the original Spiders, David admitted many years later that his pianist's proselytizing zeal "did cause us one or two problems. I was thinking of having him back in the band [in 1995] and the thing that really clinched it was hearing that he was no longer a Scientologist." Garson, who renounced Scientology in the early 1980s, later confessed that "I was probably too fanatical. I probably owe some people apologies from that viewpoint because I was a little pushy … I wanted to share what I knew and help people. But I'm not proud of that."

On the eve of the second US tour in February 1973, Woodmansey's friendship with the man they nicknamed "Garson The Parson" finally brought about the revelation of the enormous wage inequality among the band. It came as a shock to all concerned, and on arriving in New York Ronson, Bolder and Woodmansey confronted Tony Defries and demanded more money. Defries consented, but the damage was done. There were now other tensions within The Spiders. Bolder and Woodmansey were apparently offended by the addition of the extra musicians for the 1973 concerts, feeling that what had previously been presented as a coherent rock outfit was now being reduced to a solo star's backing group. Two years later Mick Ronson admitted that experiences in America "affected the band so badly. On whatever level you want to talk about. I'm talking about feeling within the band, about money, and the position of people in the band. It was a bad feeling." In a classic divide-and-conquer tactic, Defries had already promised Ronson a solo contract when, a fortnight in advance of Hammersmith, he forewarned him of Bowie's retirement. Ronson consented not to tell Bolder and Woodmansey, whom Angela Bowie believes had sealed their own fate from the moment of the pay revolt.

In the end, of course, MainMan's announcement that Bowie had quit the stage "for ever" proved to be wide of the mark; so too did David's declaration that he would not tour "for two or three years". Three months later, as a sop to American audiences deprived of the autumn tour, he would perform *The 1980 Floor Show* for NBC Television. By June 1974 he was on the road in America with the Diamond Dogs tour. The Hammersmith concert, it transpired, was merely Ziggy's last show.

The day after the final concert, MainMan hosted an extravagant wrap party at the Café Royal in Regent Street. The party, which has become known as "the Last Supper", was a star-studded event attended by every celebrity MainMan's telephonists could muster: Lou Reed, Mick and Bianca Jagger, Jeff Beck, Barbra Streisand, Ringo Starr, Paul and Linda McCartney, Cat Stevens, Lulu, Keith Moon, Elliott Gould, Tony Curtis, Britt Ekland, Ryan O'Neal, Sonny Bono, Spike Milligan, Peter Cook, Hywel Bennett and, magnificently, The Goodies. The musical entertainment was supplied by Dr John. It was at this party that Mick Rock snapped the famous photograph that purports to show David kissing Lou Reed – but which, on even the most rudimentary inspection, clearly shows nothing of the sort. "I'm not actually kissing him," David confirmed in 1993. "If you study it, I'm talking into his ear and he's talking into mine. I'm quite a way over. But it was near enough to a kiss for the press and they all printed it … No, I think Lou Reed is the last person in the world I'd want to kiss."

Also present at the party were Mick Ronson and Woody Woodmansey, but Trevor Bolder, disgusted by the previous night's unexpected climax, was nowhere to be seen. Although Bolder and Ronson would return on David's next album *Pin Ups*, Woodmansey would not. The Spiders never played together again.

In following the highs and lows of the eighteen-month tour that swept Bowie to stardom, a recurring feature has been the snowballing catalogue of celebrity doorsteppers attending the various openings and closings. But perhaps the most significant attendees were to be found not in the hospitality suite but in the audience, for there were unknown faces in the teenage crowds who would one day aspire to their own successes. Among the youngsters who attended the Ziggy Stardust concerts were Ian McCulloch, Pete Burns, George O'Dowd (who was among the fans who camped outside Haddon Hall in 1973 – he would later recall the day when "Angie opened the window and said, 'Why don't you all fuck off?' – we were thrilled!"), Holly Johnson, Marc Almond, Pete Shelley, Neil Tennant and Ian Curtis. The tour still regarded by many as Bowie's finest hour was also a potent breeding ground for the music of the future.

THE 1980 FLOOR SHOW

18 – 20 October 1973

Musicians: David Bowie *(vocals, guitar, tambourine, harmonica)*, Mick Ronson *(guitar, backing vocals)*, Trevor Bolder *(bass)*, Aynsley Dunbar *(drums)*, Mike Garson *(piano)*, Mark Carr Pritchard *(guitar)*, Ava Cherry, Jason Guess *(backing vocals)*, Geoffrey MacCormack *(backing vocals, percussion)*, Marianne Faithfull *(guest vocals)*

Repertoire: '1984/Dodo' / 'Sorrow' / 'Everything's Alright' / 'Space Oddity' / 'I Can't Explain' / 'Time' / 'The Jean Genie' / 'I Got You Babe' / 'Rock'n'Roll Suicide'

American audiences deprived of an autumn 1973 tour were appeased by a specially mounted "live" performance for NBC's rock show *The Midnight Special*. Directed and produced by Stan Harris, and recorded over three days before a 200-strong fan club audience at London's Marquee, *The 1980 Floor Show* captured a fascinating moment of transition between *Pin Ups* and *Diamond Dogs*.

In some ways the show's visual elements amounted to a short-lived resurrection of Ziggy Stardust, whom David was proposing to take to the West End stage at around the same time in a full-blown rock musical. Resplendent in his Ziggy hairstyle and backed by a troupe of dancers in cobweb outfits, David showcased a new parade of costumes designed by Freddi Burretti, Kansai Yamamoto and David's old colleague Natasha Kornilof. They included a red basque decked with ostrich plumes, a body-stocking decorated with leaping flames, and a curious half-leotard fronted by a keyhole motif. This last was inspired by a costume Bowie had seen in a picture from Tristan Tzara's 1923 production *La Coeur à Gaz*, inspired by the Zürich-based Cabaret Voltaire. "I have always loved Tristan Tzara's outrageous stage clobber," David wrote many years later in *Moonage Daydream*, "and eventually, in the late Seventies, staged three songs for *Saturday Night Live* based very heavily on his wonders." The most controversial of the new costumes was a fishnet body-stocking with a pair of gold lamé hands that clutched at David's chest as if from behind. A third hand, grasping his crotch, was removed at NBC's insistence, only for recording to be delayed when what remained of the outfit proceeded to reveal more than it should. Ken Scott recalls that Bowie, miffed by the costume alteration, "proceeded to do his best to mess up the re-takes. I think in the end they intercut between the two, but they did it really badly and it's noticeable on the final version." Bowie later remarked that the show was "shot abysmally".

In most respects, however, *The 1980 Floor Show* reflected new interests rather than past glories. The playlist derived mainly from *Pin Ups* and *Aladdin Sane*, but the most prominent feature was the new '1984/Dodo' medley, billed as a preview of Bowie's forthcoming adaptation of *Nineteen Eighty-Four*. Matt Mattox's elaborate choreography, including an opening sequence in which the dancers' whirling bodies coalesced into a series of tableaux spelling out the title of the show, indicated Bowie's growing stage-musical aspirations: Mick Ronson and the rest of the band were visually sidelined in favour of a theatrical presentation of Bowie the performer.

The musicians were drawn largely from *Pin Ups* personnel, with the addition of Arnold Corns guitarist Mark Carr Pritchard. Vocal backings were provided by The Astronettes, a three-piece group created by David as a showcase for his new girlfriend Ava Cherry. The two had first met in New York at the beginning of the year, and during the *Pin Ups* sessions had spent time together in Paris, where Ava was dancing in a ballet production. At the time of *The 1980 Floor Show* she was working with David on the ultimately abandoned Astronettes album and, for a while, co-habited with the Bowies in their new Oakley Street residence. She would become a familiar figure in David's circle over the next two years.

A surprise addition to the show was Marianne Faithfull, the 1960s starlet and sometime partner of both Brian Jones and Mick Jagger, who appeared in a backless nun's habit, wimple and all, to duet with David on a stunningly off-key cover of Sonny & Cher's 'I Got You Babe'. She also performed a couple of solo numbers, including her 1964 hit 'As Tears Go By'. Support for the 65-minute broadcast came from The Troggs and from Carmen, a Hispanic Los Angeles glam outfit whose debut album *Fandangos In Space* had been produced by Tony Visconti. He and his girlfriend Mary Hopkin were in attendance for the recording, as were Angela and Zowie, Lionel Bart, Dana Gillespie and ex-*Pork* drag queen Wayne County. Another new arrival was Amanda Lear, the cover star of Roxy Music's 1973 album *For Your Pleasure*, who was enlisted as MC for the event. She took the stage billed as "Dooshenka", presiding over the show in the style of a space-age Marlene Dietrich. Like Marianne Faithfull and Ava Cherry, she too became intimate with David at around the same time.

Recording began on 18 October with the solo sets by Carmen and Faithfull. The bulk of Bowie's contribution was shot on the following day, which was also when The Troggs performed their set. Each number was performed several times to allow the repositioning of the three-camera unit. The third and final day, on which the set was closed to the press and audience, was devoted to the title-sequence choreography, various pick-up shots and close-ups, and the elaborate staging of the current single 'Sorrow': as the dance troupe adopted frozen positions and the saxophone solo was mimed by a dancer in a silver top hat, David appeared in a two-piece suit and crooned the song to Amanda Lear.

NBC elected to censor more than Bowie's costumes. He had agreed to substitute the word "swanking" in the appropriate place in 'Time', while "goddamn" in the same number and "screw" in 'Dodo' were later blanked out for the broadcast. One song, 'Rock'n'Roll Suicide', was filmed in its entirety but cut from the finished show and has never seen the light of day.

The 1980 Floor Show saw David's final stage appearance with Mick Ronson and Trevor Bolder, the two Spiders who had survived the transition into the *Pin Ups* sessions. On the last night of shooting at the Marquee, Bowie and Ronson sat together in the dressing room. "We just nodded at each other, he looked over and grunted," recalled Ronson later. "Then he went back to doing his face. And that was the end of me and David." It wasn't quite, of course; Bowie went on to collaborate on Ronson's solo debut *Slaughter On 10th Avenue*, and many years later the pair would reunite in the studio and on stage.

Change was in the air. Ava Cherry, whom David was hyping as "the next Josephine Baker", was opening her eyes and ears to America's contemporary black music. Amanda Lear's interests in Continental art and cinema were also exerting an effect on David, who was already veering towards the decadent European trappings popularized by the previous year's smash hit film *Cabaret*. Although the stage productions of *Ziggy Stardust* and *Nineteen Eighty-Four* never materialized, the album and live show that took their place combined Orwell's vision with a potent combination of these new influences.

The 1980 Floor Show was premiered in America on 16 November 1973. Although NBC has subsequently screened both full-length and edited versions, the programme has still never been aired in Britain.

THE DIAMOND DOGS TOUR
14 June – 20 July 1974

Musicians: David Bowie *(vocals, guitar)*, Earl Slick *(guitar)*, Herbie Flowers *(bass)*, Tony Newman *(drums)*, Mike Garson *(piano, mellotron)*, Michael Kamen *(musical director, electric piano, moog, oboe)*, David Sanborn *(alto sax, flute)*, Richard Grando *(baritone sax, flute)*, Pablo Rosario *(percussion)*, Warren Peace, Gui Andrisano *(backing vocals)*

Repertoire: '1984' / 'Rebel Rebel' / 'Moonage Daydream' / 'Sweet Thing' / 'Candidate' / 'Changes' / 'Suffragette City' / 'Aladdin Sane' / 'All The Young Dudes' / 'Cracked Actor' / 'Rock'n Roll With Me' / 'Watch That Man' / 'Drive In Saturday' / 'Space Oddity' / 'Future Legend' / 'Diamond Dogs' / 'Panic In Detroit' / 'Big Brother' / 'Chant Of The Ever Circling Skeletal Family' / 'Time' / 'The Width Of A Circle' / 'The Jean Genie' / 'Rock'n'Roll Suicide' / 'Knock On Wood' / 'Here Today, Gone Tomorrow'

Even before completing work on *Diamond Dogs* in February 1974, Bowie was discussing plans to stage the album as a piece of spectacular rock theatre designed to take America by storm. "I must have the total image of a stage show," he had said the previous November. "It has to be total with me. I'm just not content writing songs, I want to make it three-dimensional."

Initially there was talk of expanding the stage concepts of *The 1980 Floor Show* and the abandoned *Ziggy Stardust* musical, but David's visions had already moved off in other directions. One of his latest idols was James Dean, pictures of whom adorned his Oakley Street house, and principal among his new creative influences was the company of Amanda Lear, who awakened his interest in Salvador Dali and, more significantly, took him to see Fritz Lang's seminal 1926 film *Metropolis* on his twenty-seventh birthday, 8 January 1974. The next day David trawled London's bookshops for every study of Lang he could find; his interest in the expressionist cinema of the German silents, in particular the New Realist school of Georg Pabst and the Nietzschean nightmares of *Metropolis* and Robert Wiene's 1919 classic *The Cabinet Of Doktor Caligari*, would prove central to the conception of his forthcoming stage show. German expressionism's collision of fairytale with freakshow, and its morbid obsession with dream-states, nightmares and comas within which the artist operates like a macabre puppeteer, would remain a crucial ingredient in Bowie's creative palette for the remainder of his career.

Choreographer Toni Basil was the first of several Americans summoned to Britain to discuss the tour with David. She had acted in *Easy Rider* and *Five Easy Pieces* and had choreographed George Lucas's *American Graffiti*. "We just clicked," Basil tells the Gillmans, "because neither of us felt that choreography was just steps. One number could have an acting premise, another could have a mime premise, another number had steps and another was more staged and choreographed. With somebody like him you don't have to be limited to one thing." Bowie already had ideas for the staging of individual numbers. "David had this idea about having ropes tied around the necks of some dancers," Toni Basil tells Jerry Hopkins. "When I told him he could do it if he was careful, he yelled at Corinne, 'The 'Diamond Dogs' number is back in!'"

Jules Fisher, a prominent lighting director whose credits included the first American tour of *Tommy* and the Broadway production of *Jesus Christ Superstar*, was also consulted by David. "For *Diamond Dogs*, he had an understanding of German expressionist art and film," Fisher later explained. "He wanted that image and I'd seen all of those films … He said, 'I see a town, like the one in *The Cabinet Of Doktor Caligari…*'" Fisher introduced Bowie to set designer Mark Ravitz, who recalled that "David gave me three clues: Power, Nuremberg, and Fritz Lang's *Metropolis*." Ravitz assembled a list of images suggested by his conversations with Bowie: "tanks, turbines, smokestacks … *ecce homo* drawings by George Grosz, grotesque decadence, flourescent tubing … state police, alleyways, cages, watchtowers, girders, beams, Albert Speer". Ravitz's original design, involving giant Nazi-style banners rising from the stage, was rejected by David in favour of a less literal interpretation of the three "clues".

Co-designed and constructed by Chris Langhart, the Diamond Dogs set was more elaborate than any previously attempted for a rock tour, and cost an unprecedented $250,000. Based on the expressionist designs of *The Cabinet Of Doktor Caligari*, a giant backdrop depicted the nightmarish Hunger City skyline, tilted in jagged perspective. To either side stood two massive aluminium skyscrapers, linked by a moving bridge which would rise and fall during the show. The specialist props, run by hydraulic mechanisms and early forms of computer control, were to be built from scratch.

On 11 April 1974 Bowie arrived in New York to preside over the publicity campaign for the imminent release of *Diamond Dogs* and to begin assembling musicians for the tour. Herbie Flowers, Mike Garson and Tony Newman were retained from the *Diamond Dogs* sessions. Having played lead guitar on the album himself David was without a soloist, and his first instinct was to reach back to a time before the arrival of Mick Ronson. In April he contacted *Space Oddity* guitarist Keith Christmas who, much to his surprise, was flown out to New York. There Christmas encountered a lifestyle he described to Christopher Sandford as "straight out of Fellini … David was doing amyl nitrate all of the time. He collapsed on the concrete stairs in one club. I grabbed him as he went down … A couple of nights later we were rehearsing alone in the studio. David took me into the loo, whipped out a double-sided razor and slashed into a huge chunk of coke. Some time around then it dawned on me I wasn't going to be on the tour." The two would briefly collaborate again a couple of years later, on the little-known out-take 'Both Guns Are Out There', but in the meantime Diamond Dogs was not for Christmas.

A potential replacement was quick to appear. "I've found a really incredible black guy called Carlos," David told pressmen at the post-show party of Todd Rundgren's Carnegie Hall gig. This was of course Carlos Alomar, soon to become one of Bowie's key collaborators. The two had met a few days earlier at RCA's 6th Avenue studios while recording Lulu's version of 'Can You Hear Me', and Bowie was immediately besotted. However, Alomar was already earning upwards of $800 a week in session fees and gigs with his band The Main Ingredient, and was unimpressed by Tony Defries's offer of $250 per week. Negotiations broke down and Alomar's place in Bowie history was deferred until later in the year.

After seeing a neo-classical ballet production based on the sculptor Auguste Rodin, David hired its composer, New York keyboardist Michael Kamen, as the tour's musical director. Kamen, who would later win fame as a film score composer and Pink Floyd arranger, introduced Bowie to saxophonist David Sanborn and a young guitarist called Earl Slick who played with Kamen's New York Rock Ensemble. Finally, backing vocalists Gui Andrisano and *Aladdin Sane* veteran Geoffrey MacCormack (now calling himself Warren Peace) were recruited to participate in Toni Basil's choreographed set-pieces, enacting the roles of the "Dogs" themselves who would shadow David's every move on stage.

Band and choreography rehearsals continued for four weeks in upstate New York. As the results were translated onto Mark Ravitz's elaborate set for dress rehearsals at Port Chester's Capitol Theater in early June, the vast technical demands of the show became apparent, not least during a serious incident on stage. "I've never met anyone who could think so fast on his feet," recalled Toni Basil. "The bridge broke when [Bowie] was on it. It was the first day of rehearsal with the set, a few days before the tour started. As the bridge was falling, he calculated precisely when it would hit, jumping into the air just before the crash to avoid the shock." Stage manager Nick Russiyan later told biographer Tony Zanetta that "The technical problems were never resolved before we left Port Chester. David was in great danger physically, and could have gotten electrocuted or killed."

The tension on set was compounded by other factors. With the exception of the two backing vocalists, the band were informed that they would spend most of the show concealed upstage behind black drapes, as the presence of eight musos together with their drumkits, keyboards and amplifiers would detract from the sci-fi spectacle of Hunger City. For their few appearances they were given tailor-made 1940s suits to wear, a move better received in some quarters than others: Earl Slick, whose long hair was shorn off at Bowie's behest to match the period feel, has recalled that drummer Tony Newman would regularly sabotage his costume and once even ripped it into tatters before the show. The band faced contractual fines if they ad-libbed or deviated from the rehearsed arrangements, but while some accounts have construed this as rock-star megalomania run wild, in truth it was grounded in sound technical considerations. With elaborate scenery flats and lethally heavy counter-weights flying hither and thither every evening, there could be no margin for error: an unscheduled extra couple of bars' worth of guitar solo could have created serious problems. In essence, the Diamond Dogs show had more in common with a stage musical than with a standard rock concert. This was its great fascination but also, perhaps, its fatal flaw.

There could be no doubting the sheer scale and spectacle of the show that opened at the Montreal Forum on 14 June. As the lights went down on Hunger City and a spotlight picked out David at the end of the first verse of '1984', the audience received the first major shock of the evening: Ziggy Stardust was well and truly dead. Devoid of war-paint, his auburn hair streaked strawberry blond and swept back James Dean-style, David wore a sharp blue two-piece suit, the first of a new set of costumes designed by Freddi Burretti. For American audiences packed with Ziggy clones who had been waiting a year to see their hero on stage, Bowie's transformation into Halloween Jack was their first taste of his propensity for change.

The music, too, had changed – not only from the proto-punk of The Spiders From Mars, but even from the raunchy garage and doom-laden synthesizers of the *Diamond Dogs* album itself. Rearranged to tap into the funky black sound David had begun to espouse, and yet dappled with an incongruous big-band feel emphasized by the saxophones, flutes and in particular Michael Kamen's plaintive oboe, the new band sounded more like a post-apocalyptic blues cabaret

than a rock group. Some numbers, notably 'The Jean Genie' and 'Rock'n'Roll Suicide', had been radically reconstructed as schmaltzy Vegas show-stoppers. If it was a shock, it was a magnificent one – but the real shock was the scenery.

A few numbers in, the amazing set began to perform. David sang 'Sweet Thing' from the raised catwalk in a voluminous trench coat, puffing on a Gitane beneath sodium street-lamps as he gazed down at the "Dogs" cavorting on the stage below. The skyscrapers dripped blood on cue. As Fisher later explained, "they were made of newsprint that could be torn apart, so Bowie actually climbed one of these towers and destroyed the building during the concert." For 'Aladdin Sane' David mimed with a kabuki stick-mask showing the character's trademark lightning-bolt, which also flashed from the skyscrapers above. He sang 'Cracked Actor' in sunglasses and Shakespearean doublet, caressing and French-kissing a skull while the Dogs cued him with a clapperboard, powdered his cheeks, photographed him and played spotlights across his face.

A hydraulic cherry-picker supported a chair set into an office window near the top of the stage-right skyscraper. Appearing in the chair, David sang 'Space Oddity' into a mike disguised as a telephone, and as the song reached "lift-off" the cherry-picker began to extend over the first six rows of the audience. As David later remembered, the chair "went out about forty foot over the audience's heads, and because of the beautiful lighting that we had, you didn't see the rest of the cherry-picker, you only saw the office chair suspended out there." 'Diamond Dogs' began with Bowie up on the catwalk, holding two trailing leashes to restrain the Dogs, who prowled the stage as the bridge descended to floor level. By the end of the song the Dogs themselves had taken over and tied Bowie up with the ropes. Then it was straight into 'Panic In Detroit' for which the ropes were unravelled to form a boxing ring in which David, now in red boxing gloves and fanned down by his bodyguard Stuey George, shadow-boxed an imaginary opponent and lost. For 'Big Brother' he sprawled atop a glittering ten-foot diamond while the Dogs savaged and scrabbled at it from beneath. The diamond rolled downstage before opening up to consume him; then the sides fell away revealing a giant jewelled hand, whose fingers unfurled to show David crouching in the palm, from where he sang 'Time'. 'The Width Of A Circle' revived the Ziggy show's familiar stuck-in-a-box mime routine, at the end of which David was dragged to his feet by the Dogs for a wrestling bout and street-fight to the strains of 'The Jean Genie', before singing a final, defeated 'Rock'n'Roll Suicide' alone on a chair.

There were more conventional moments between the set-pieces, including straightforward renditions of 'Watch That Man' and 'Moonage Daydream' (during which Earl Slick was allowed to take centre-stage for a guitar solo while David raced behind the set to position himself for 'Sweet Thing'), and a solo 'Drive In Saturday' in which David, alone on a bar stool, strummed an acoustic guitar while the Dogs sat to one side, eating popcorn. Otherwise the show was stage-managed down to the last note. After 'Rock'n'Roll Suicide' there were no encores, not even a bow. Instead the PA system announced that "David Bowie has already left the auditorium."

The reviews were ecstatic. A Toronto critic described the opening concert as "the most spectacular rock show I have ever seen", while the *Winnipeg Free Press* hailed it as "unique and brilliant". The *Owen Sound Sun-Times* hailed Bowie's "perfect, precision-honed showmanship", while *Melody Maker* reported to British readers that Bowie's "far-reaching imagination has created a combination of contemporary music and theatre that is several years ahead of its time … a completely new concept in rock theatre – the most original spectacle in rock I have ever seen."

However, the initial month of concerts took its toll. The technical demands were immense – for the opening night the scenery took 32 hours to erect, and thereafter the 15 roadies were supplemented by a 20-man union crew recruited at each venue. Nonetheless there were mechanical problems: the cherry-picker malfunctioned during one of the early concerts, leaving David with no option but to perform the next half-dozen numbers suspended in mid-air. On the way to Tampa, Florida, a bee flew into the cabin of one of the transport lorries and stung the driver, who swerved off the road and into a swamp. Crisis was transformed into triumph as the show's announcer declared, "Good evening, ladies and gentlemen. The concert you're going to see tonight is not the show we had planned for you. Due to an unfortunate road accident, half of our stage scenery, costumes, lighting equipment, is in a local swamp fifteen miles north of here. There was talk of cancelling tonight's performance, but David Bowie would not hear of it." The cheers that greeted the announcement heralded a terrific performance which ended in a twenty-minute standing ovation and the only encore of the tour.

The atmosphere backstage, however, was becoming overwrought. Members of the band noted that the collaborative and friendly atmosphere that had prevailed during rehearsals gradually evaporated on the road. A particular bone of contention was the band's resentment at being obscured behind the scenery. "They kept saying, 'We don't like playing behind these bleeding screens!'" David recounted two years later, "and I said, 'Well, you've got to, because I haven't got any parts for you – I don't want people to see you playing, because it doesn't look like a street if there's a bass amp stuck in the middle,' but it was very hard to convince them of that." Matters weren't helped by the two-tier boarding arrangements: while David, Defries and a select clique stayed in deluxe hotel suites, the remainder of the band was consigned to Holiday Inns. David's personal retinue, meanwhile, had been swelled by the arrival of Tony Mascia, a Bronx Italian and former sparring partner of Rocky Marciano, who backed up Stuey George's security duties and drove David's limousine. He would remain on the Bowie pay-roll long after the disintegration of MainMan.

In his *Melody Maker* review Chris Charlesworth remarked that Bowie's stage presence was far removed from the finely judged *simpatico* of the Ziggy concerts: "Not once does he address the audience or even allude to their presence, other than an odd grin," he wrote, adding that as a result Bowie seemed like "some kind of magical being", dripping with "almost total arrogance". Although this was a deliberate theatrical effect, it appears that it had begun to follow David offstage. Cocaine had wrought a major change in his disposition, as he himself has since averred. Ava Cherry told the Gillmans: "When I first met David, he didn't do drugs. When I first went to England, he would hardly smoke a joint. His personality was altogether different, he was sweet and kind and loving, I loved him so much. When we got to America people started coming on the tours and bringing lots of coke around and of course we were all doing it. But David has an extreme personality, so his capacity was much greater than anyone else's. He would start to change his personality sometimes. It didn't affect his music or how he created, but it would affect how he would react to people, those who really liked him and cared about him." According to Michael Kamen, "One minute he would be a wonderful sweet friend, somebody who was easy to talk to and fool around with. The next minute he was somebody who would burn through you with their eyes. It was a quite sudden switch." With the mood swings came the obvious physical evidence that David's habit was affecting him adversely. Cocaine suppresses appetite and dehydrates the body, and during the tour David's already slender frame became gaunt in the extreme.

According to Angela Bowie, who witnessed the tail-end of the tour, cocaine was also affecting David on stage. His performance, she wrote in her memoir, "was erratic. Sometimes, when the coke was working for him, he was brilliant ... Other times ... he missed cues and forgot moves and botched things up in all kinds of ways." Even so, she admits that "his voice stayed strong" and that "the show was a knockout".

Matters came to head when Herbie Flowers led a band revolt over payment for the *David Live* album. The band had not been informed of the plan to record any shows – according to Earl Slick, the first they knew of it was finding "extra mikes everywhere" at the Philadelphia soundcheck – and they turned to Flowers as their spokesman. "Probably David asked me to do the Diamond Dogs tour because he knew it was going to be a long, long tour and he needed somebody he could socialize with," Flowers told Jerry Hopkins, "And we got on very well for a while, until through seniority I became like the trade union representative for the musicians ... when we heard they were going to record a live album, I confronted David about it."

"Herbie went nuts," recalled Mike Garson. "'How can they do this without our permission? How come we're not getting paid? How come there's no contracts? We're not going on!' So we agreed that we weren't going on stage that night unless we got paid."

There was a confrontation in David's dressing room an hour before the first Philadelphia concert, at which Flowers rejected Tony Defries's proposal that the band members should each receive the union rate of $70 for the live album. Instead Flowers demanded $5000 apiece, a figure agreed beforehand among the disgruntled musicians. Tensions ran high; legend has it that David threw a chair at Flowers during the scene, but Stuey George has denied this: "He kicked the chair and it flew backwards," he told the Gillmans, "It wasn't directed at any person. David wouldn't actually get physical with anybody."

The musicians won the day, and Defries was compelled to sign an agreement that they would receive $5000 each – although, in classic MainMan style, they would not see it for two years, and then only after

launching legal proceedings. The Philadelphia concert began half an hour late and the atmosphere on stage was less than relaxed, but some considered the performance all the better for it: "When we went on stage," recalled Flowers, "the feeling of liberation in the band was glorious!"

Even before this debacle, Bowie's relations with Tony Defries were rapidly deteriorating. If David was suffering delusions of grandeur they were as nothing compared with the Colonel Parker wonderland now inhabited by his manager, who had become aloof and unavailable even to David, while opening Swiss bank accounts and moving into the gold and futures markets. David, meanwhile, had at last begun to discover the extent to which he had allowed himself to be exploited. He had always mistakenly believed that he owned a 50 per cent share of the company, but as the Diamond Dogs tour unwound he finally realized the true nature of the contracts he had signed with Defries: he owned no portion of MainMan, and while Defries pocketed a full 50 per cent of Bowie's income, David received what remained of his 50 per cent *after* all company expenditure was deducted. In practice this could mean almost anything Defries wanted it to. "Some of the concert promoters began talking to David, telling him how much he was making," recalled Ava Cherry. "David was amazed when he heard the figures. He had no idea at all." Bowie was all too aware that the tour was losing money hand over fist, costing more to mount each night than it could possibly take at the box office, and he was making up the shortfall out of his personal allowance. He had already abandoned plans to buy Richard Harris's London house in order to bail out the tour's running costs; now, as he became increasingly aware of the true nature of MainMan, the writing appeared on the wall for Defries.

By the time of the Philadelphia dates the show's tight script had already been sufficiently slackened to allow changes to the set: 'Knock On Wood' replaced 'Drive In Saturday', and there was room for an Ohio Players cover, 'Here Today, Gone Tomorrow'. All the same, David was rapidly tiring of the show's lack of spontaneity.

The Diamond Dogs tour never reached British shores, owing to the vast cost such an undertaking would have entailed. Tony Defries had initially attempted to sell the show to British promoters, and for a while a nine-day stint at the Wembley Empire Pool was mooted for autumn 1974, but to recoup the necessary costs the ticket prices would have had to begin at a prohibitive £7, unheard of at the time.

But despite its comparatively short run of 37 performances, the Diamond Dogs tour remains the stuff of legend. It was the first rock spectacle of its kind, redefining expectations of what was possible on the concert stage. Never before had a rock tour enlisted the services of a top theatrical designer, and many of the show's innovations – notably the cherry-picker and the hydraulic bridge – have since become commonplace. In 1976 Jules Fisher was hired to design a similarly ambitious set for The Rolling Stones ("They simply couldn't handle the kind of staging that Bowie had," he later recalled), while in the same year Mark Ravitz designed Kiss's Destroyer tour, which truly ushered in the age of pyrotechnic-fuelled stadium extravaganzas.

In its genre-defining theatricality the tour was a triumph on many levels. Angela Bowie later wrote that "I don't think there's ever been anything to match Diamond Dogs. Plenty of shows have been bigger, the expenditure of effort and funds more conspicuous by far, but none has been brighter. None has tried to mean as much or succeeded in communicating its meaning as effectively." Toni Basil believed that "it was the greatest set I have ever seen, it was the greatest rock show I have ever seen … The show was phenomenal, and David was absolutely brilliant." Tony Visconti has described the show as "one of the best things David has ever done on stage." The tour's coordinator Fran Pillersdorf told the Gillmans that Bowie "held the stage like Garland … He was the consummate showman. We were in an arena with thousands of screaming people, he was playing against a forty-five-foot set, and it was his show." For his part, Bowie recalled in 1993 that "It was quite an unbelievable, unbelievable headache, that tour – but it was spectacular. It was truly the first real rock and roll theatrical show that made any sense. A lot of people feel that it has never been bettered … it was something else, it really was."

Nonetheless, even on an aesthetic level the show had its drawbacks. The decision to hire a top-flight band of musicians resulted in a rather peculiar interpretation of the Diamond Dogs material. By any conventional definition it was probably the finest live band Bowie had yet employed, and in terms of sheer musicianship their performance is impossible to fault. But as Bowie recalled in 1997, "Some of my lines had sounded almost proto-punk because of my inabilities as a virtuoso. But by the time they took it on stage, they were playing it in a very musicianly style. Something was lost because of that. That album had a quality of obsession with what I wanted to get over. That's not there when I hear the gigs from that period … They play it too well and with too much fluidity. So to me, Diamond Dogs was never played well on stage, or at least never with the sensibility that the album had."

In its original form, the Diamond Dogs tour breathed its last over two nights at New York's Madison Square Garden – moved from the smaller Radio City Music Hall after increased demand – on 19 and 20 July. The Ringling Brothers Circus, which had a residency at the venue, was still in the process of vacating the loading area, and the presence of elephants and tigers made for an unusual atmosphere backstage. When the tour re-convened in September after a six-week break, during which David's relationship with his manager had deteriorated further, his cocaine habit had spun dangerously out of control, and he had retreated to Philadelphia to record most of the Young Americans album, it was immediately evident that things were going to be very different.

THE PHILLY DOGS TOUR

2 September – 1 December 1974

Musicians: David Bowie (vocals, guitar, harmonica), Earl Slick (guitar), Carlos Alomar (guitar), Mike Garson (piano, mellotron), David Sanborn (alto sax, flute), Richard Grando (baritone sax, flute), Pablo Rosario (percussion), Warren Peace, Anthony Hinton, Luther Vandross, Ava Cherry, Diane Sumler (backing vocals); plus, September only: Michael Kamen (musical director, electric piano, moog, oboe), Gui Andrisano (backing vocals), Doug Raunch (bass), Greg Enrico (drums); plus, October-December only: Emir Ksasan (bass), Dennis Davis (drums), Robin Clark (backing vocals)

Repertoire: '1984' / 'Rebel Rebel' / 'Moonage Daydream' / 'Sweet Thing' / 'Candidate' / 'Changes' / 'Suffragette City' / 'Aladdin Sane' / 'All The Young Dudes' / 'Cracked Actor' / 'Rock'n Roll With Me' / 'Knock On Wood' / 'Young Americans' / 'It's Gonna Be Me' / 'Space Oddity' / 'Future Legend' / 'Diamond Dogs' / 'Big Brother' / 'Time'/ 'The Jean Genie' / 'Rock'n'Roll Suicide' / 'John, I'm Only Dancing (Again)' / 'Sorrow' / 'Can You Hear Me' / 'Somebody

Up There Likes Me' / 'Footstompin'' / 'Panic In Detroit' / 'Win'

Also referred to as the "Soul tour", Bowie's autumn 1974 dates were officially a continuation of the Diamond Dogs show, but the staging, personnel and set-list were so altered as to become a different entity altogether. The resulting hybrid of the Diamond Dogs concerts with David's new Philadelphia-inspired sound has become known as the "Philly Dogs" tour.

Having recorded most of *Young Americans* at Sigma Sound in August 1974, David was impatient to perform the new work on stage. Although the elaborate Diamond Dogs stage effects were still in evidence for the opening shows at the Los Angeles Universal Amphitheater on 2-8 September, this was no more than an unwilling concession to Tony Defries, who had insisted that West Coast audiences be given a chance to witness the production. There was also the question of pulling out the stops for the BBC crew trailing David for Alan Yentob's documentary *Cracked Actor*, whose in-concert sequences were shot at the Los Angeles dates. Already, however, there were changes to the repertoire. The big production numbers remained intact, but gone were the more loosely choreographed 'Watch That Man', 'Drive In Saturday', 'The Width Of A Circle' and 'Panic In Detroit'. In their place came three of the new compositions recorded in Philadelphia: 'Young Americans', 'It's Gonna Be Me' and 'John, I'm Only Dancing (Again)'.

There were also line-up changes, brought about by the influx of new blood from the *Young Americans* sessions and the casualties of the Diamond Dogs tour. By the end of June, bass player Herbie Flowers had had his fill and returned to Britain. "If I'd have done the second half of the tour, I'd have died," he tells Jerry Hopkins. "I got home in one piece and my wife said, 'If you ever do that again, I'm leaving you.'" Tony Newman had left to work with George Harrison, and the pair were temporarily replaced by bassist Doug Raunch, on loan from Santana, and percussionist Greg Enrico, formerly of Sly & The Family Stone. *Young Americans* guitarist Carlos Alomar now made his live debut with Bowie, although Earl Slick and Michael Kamen, neither of whom had played at the Sigma sessions, returned to handle lead guitar and keyboards respectively. Swelling the ranks of backing singers were Anthony Hinton, Luther Vandross, Ava Cherry and Diane Sumler.

The Los Angeles concerts were a major showbiz draw, attended by Diana Ross, Bette Midler, Michael Jackson, Iggy Pop, Tatum O'Neal, Racquel Welch (then apparently considering a MainMan management offer which included plans to record an album produced by Dana Gillespie, which tragically never happened) and Elizabeth Taylor, who would befriend David during his Californian interlude. It was at Taylor's Beverly Hills house in September 1974 that David was first introduced to John Lennon, who would add his talents to the *Young Americans* album a few months later. Also present in Los Angeles was David's old friend Marc Bolan, his star already in the descendant.

The *Los Angeles Times* hailed the opening concert as "marvellously entertaining" and David himself as "stunning – a performer of immense style and ability". Following a week's residency at the Universal Amphitheater and a handful of concerts in San Diego, Tucson and Phoenix, there was a three-week break caused by a promoter's refusal to meet Tony Defries's financial demands (which by 1974 were often a staggering ninety-ten in MainMan's favour). David now leapt at the opportunity to refashion the show from top to bottom. The Diamond Dogs stage set was scrapped, given away to a school in Philadelphia to obviate storage costs, and at rehearsals in Los Angeles Bowie realigned the show as a straightforward stand-and-deliver performance with the band in full view. The only concession to theatricality was a white backcloth onto which simple patterns of light and colour were flashed. In the larger venues a live relay of the show itself was projected onto the backdrop. David, who now shouldered his acoustic guitar for a greater proportion of the numbers, performed on a sparkling stainless steel platform; the backing singers were confined to another. The clothes had changed too, as the Diamond Dog costumes developed into a succession of tapering zoot-suits and jodhpurs, again designed by Freddi Burretti and based on the combined wardrobes of James Dean and Frank Sinatra. The Philly Dogs stage outfits would mark Bowie's final collaboration with his friend Burretti, who sadly died in Paris in May 2001 at the early age of 49.

With the abandoning of the scenery came sweeping changes to the repertoire, as set-reliant numbers like 'Sweet Thing', 'Aladdin Sane', 'All The Young Dudes', 'Cracked Actor', 'Big Brother' and 'Time' were all dropped. 'Space Oddity' remained and 'Panic In Detroit' returned, both stripped of their elaborate routines. Among the new additions were 'Sorrow', 'Can

You Hear Me', 'Somebody Up There Likes Me', and an energetic cover of The Flare's 'Footstompin''. The still unfinished composition 'Win' would be added to the repertoire towards the end of the tour.

The reason for all the changes was twofold. In the first place the staging of the Diamond Dogs tour had placed an almost unbearable strain on all concerned, and David had come to regard the scenery as a financial as well as a creative albatross. Secondly and more compellingly, he was bored with *Diamond Dogs* and in love with his new music. "I was supposed to go all over America with it," he recalled in 1978, "and I only got to Los Angeles and I was bored stiff with it, and I threw the set away and came back with a completely different show … they were supposed to be selling the entire show on this spectacular set, and the kids would come and there was no set, no nothing, and there I was singing soul music!"

After filling in for the September dates, Doug Raunch and Greg Enrico had now departed, as had backing vocalist Gui Andrisano and keyboardist Michael Kamen, who was supplanted as musical director by Mike Garson. In their place came new blood: bassist Emir Ksasan from Carlos Alomar's band The Main Ingredient, *Young Americans* backing vocalist (and Alomar's wife) Robin Clark, and a figure who was to be a mainstay of Bowie's rhythm section for the remainder of the decade, New York drummer Dennis Davis. Considering that he would play on three tours and seven albums (including *Low*, renowned in rock history for its revolutionary percussion experiments), Davis remains one of the most under-appreciated of all Bowie's collaborators. "Dennis was so open," said David many years later. "He was almost orgiastic in his approach to trying out new stuff … I told him about a Charlie Mingus gig that I saw where the drummer had polythene tubes that would go into the drums, and he would suck and blow to change the pressure as he played. Dennis was out the next day buying that stuff. Dennis is crazy, an absolute loony man, but he had a lot of his own thoughts on things, and he would throw us all kinds of curve-balls."

The Mike Garson Band, as it was now called, opened each show with a series of soul numbers, with lead vocals supplied by the backing singers. The set included 'Love Train', 'You Keep Me Hangin' On', 'I'm In The Mood For Love' (sung by Ava Cherry), 'Funky Music (Is A Part Of Me)' (sung by Luther Vandross), 'Stormy Monday' (sung by Warren Peace perching on

Garson's piano), and finally a souled-up rendition of Bowie's own 'Memory Of A Free Festival'. The main set now usually began with either 'Rebel Rebel' or 'Space Oddity'.

The new show opened at the St Paul Civic Center on 5 October, moving through middle America for the next four weeks before descending on New York's Radio City Music Hall for seven dates. The first two were added by Defries at a late stage after the others had sold out, but unfortunately the extra concerts did poorly at the box office (another instance of MainMan's overweening self-belief: few artists could hope to sell out seven consecutive nights at Radio City). As a result Bowie was forced to open before the New York press in a half-empty house, and the critical reaction was frosty. The *New York Times* found David "self-consciously uncomfortable without routines to act out, and he was in hoarse voice". The *New York Post* likened the experience to a gaudy birthday cake "made out of cardboard, with a hollow centre", while *Zoo World* condemned the show as "a disaster … something like a bad night in Las Vegas … totally mediocre". In *Creem*, Lester Bangs epitomized American critics' attitude to Bowie during the 1970s, mistrusting the credentials of an artist who changes direction. Pleasantly referring to David as a "pasty-faced snaggletoothed little jitterbug", Bangs considered the show "a parody of a parody" which was "as full of ersatz sincerity as Jerry Lewis … Bowie has just changed his props: last tour it was boxing gloves, skulls and giant hands, this tour it's Black folk."

Even some of the band were unhappy with the new show. Earl Slick later complained that "David had gone completely in a direction I didn't like," while the ousted musical director Michael Kamen was in the audience for a show which he described to the Gillmans as "horrific – a sort of third-rate gospel revivalist meeting. The stage was full of large black people going 'Hallelujah' and shaking tambourines, and poor David was very thin and very white and completely out of his element."

Kamen's comment reveals one of the more disturbing aspects of the Philly Dogs phase. Bowie was now gravely debilitated by cocaine abuse, and his appearance by the end of 1974 was alarming. He looked emaciated, his voice was often hoarse and he required glasses of water lined up on Mike Garson's piano to re-hydrate himself during the shows. "When he grimaced his lips adhered to his gums," the Gillmans were told by David's cousin Kristina, who watched one of the New York concerts from the wings. "He would turn his back on the audience to run his finger around his mouth to free them." According to percussionist Pablo Rosario, "David was really wired. He was doing too much cocaine. He looked like a tiger in a cage going from side to side of the stage." Most distressing of all was the gold-topped walking cane that now became part of David's stage act. He gave the impression that it was nothing more than his latest prop, but the truth was that at times he couldn't keep himself upright without it. "Trust me, I prayed for him," Mike Garson said in 1999. "I was very concerned. He's very lucky he's alive, let's just put it that way."

At the same time, signs began to appear that David's imagination was expanding in ever more eccentric directions. It was during the Philly Dogs tour that he began peppering his interview patter with references to Kirlian photography, ghosts, UFOs, government conspiracy theories, the Kabbalah and, increasingly, Adolf Hitler. *Creem*'s Bruno Stein transcribed a post-show conversation in a Chicago hotel bar in which Bowie rambled disconcertingly about these and other topics, including the sinister agendas of advertising agencies and the "cultural manipulation" practised by the ancient Mayans. Looking back on the period twenty years later, Bowie observed that he was losing his grip on the division between his own personality and those of his stage characters: "As drugs started to take a more severe hold of my life, the ability within your conscious mind to actually deliver yourself into two separate parts disappear, and the lines blur, and it's only this one formless mutant that's left behind … it gets very messy in there…"

All things considered, one of the more incongruous sidelines of the period can be found in the unintentionally hilarious version of events still being peddled by Cherry Vanilla to readers of the teenage magazine *Mirabelle*. "I must admit that I'm getting rather attached to just getting anything I want from room service," reveals "David" in one entry, while another includes the innocent recollection that "Mick Jagger and Bette Midler arrived, and very soon I was in a relaxed state". "I've lost so much weight on this tour that I'm going to have to start getting back in shape," he reports cheerily on 4 January. "Angie is trying to fatten me up again with her home cooking!"

Indeed, while the Philly Dogs tour unwound MainMan continued to project a business-as-usual air to the outside world, despite massive debts on both sides of the Atlantic and further extravagances on the part of Tony Defries, whose dislike of Bowie's soul music was no secret and whose relationship with his errant client was now in terminal decline. Defries was attempting to groom Dana Gillespie and Wayne County for pop stardom (neither found it), and while David brought in the dollars MainMan announced that it was to produce a Broadway spectacular called *Fame*, written by *Pork* veteran Tony Ingrassia and based on the life of Marilyn Monroe. The show opened and closed on 18 November 1974 at a cost to MainMan of $250,000.

Despite the chaotic management situation, the physical self-destruction, the mental torment and an artistic direction many critics regarded as questionable, late 1974 represents one of the most fascinating and certainly one of the most poorly documented of all Bowie's live incarnations. Bootleg recordings which survive from the tour reveal a vital and gutsy show already transformed by the rhythm skills of Carlos Alomar and Dennis Davis into the prototype for what was coming next.

After a total of 46 concerts (nine more than the Diamond Dogs tour which preceded it), the Philly Dogs show closed in Atlanta on 1 December 1974 (a planned concert in Tuscaloosa the following day had been cancelled). Three days later, Dick Cavett's *Wide World Of Entertainment* screened an appearance that had been taped in New York on 2 November during the Radio City residency. There were excellent live performances of 'Young Americans', '1984' and 'Footstompin'', but David himself was looking terrible. At his most waxen and monosyllabic, he fended off Cavett's enquiries with hostile, almost inarticulate answers, sniffing obsessively and jabbing at the carpet with his walking-stick. "It was horrendous," he recalled twenty years later. "I had no idea where I was, I couldn't hear the questions. To this day, I don't know if I bothered answering them, I was so out of my gourd." As ever, the *Mirabelle* diary offered a different view to UK readers: "Dick Cavett and I got on very well," it claimed desperately, "and it was almost like sitting in my living room and talking to a friend." It was an inglorious conclusion to 1974, a year in which Bowie's increasingly fascinating musical transformations threatened to be eclipsed by his painfully visible physical and mental ones.

On 7 December *Disc & Music Echo* reported that the tour was to continue in Brazil in January 1975, after which Bowie would bring his soul show to mainland Europe and Britain. A fortnight later the *Mirabelle* diary stated that "Some of the dates for my European tour have been set. As it stands now, I'll be starting in the Scandinavian countries in March." By the New Year, however, plans for a European tour had evaporated amid the concluding sessions for *Young Americans* and the final meltdown of Bowie's relationship with his manager.

1975: SOUL TRAIN AND THE CHER SHOW

1975 was David Bowie's lost year, mired in drugs, alcohol and the ongoing legal dispute with MainMan. For the first time in three years David had no touring schedule, and between January and June he drifted between hotels and rented houses, first in New York and then in Los Angeles. The only substantial creative endeavours of the year came in its second six months, with the filming of *The Man Who Fell To Earth* and the recording of *Station To Station*.

A few isolated public appearances punctuated the year. At New York's Uris Theater on 1 March David presented Aretha Franklin with the "Best Female Soul Singer" gong at the Grammy Awards. Aretha ruffled a few feathers by exclaiming on national television that "I'm so happy I could even kiss David Bowie", but the occasion is best remembered for an oft-printed celebrity line-up of David flanked by Simon and Garfunkel, John Lennon and Yoko Ono. "Lennon and I were off our tree that night," Bowie later confessed, "and spent far too much time in a corner giggling like schoolboys and making snide remarks about everybody." On 8 September, fresh from completing *The Man Who Fell To Earth*, David played a couple of impromptu numbers with Bill Wyman and Ronnie Wood at Peter Sellers's birthday party in Los Angeles.

On 4 November, midway through the *Station To Station* sessions, ABC's black music show *Soul Train* featured David miming studio performances of 'Fame' and the brand new single 'Golden Years', marking only the second major appearance by a white artist on the programme (Elton John had beaten him to it by six months). Bowie's jittery, spaced-out interview between numbers marked a new low in coherency, and as he shamefacedly recalled in 1999, his attempt to mime 'Golden Years' was disastrous: "I hadn't bothered to learn it, and the MC of the show, who was a really charming guy, took me on one side after the third or fourth take, and he said, 'Do you know there

were kids lined up to do this show, who have fought their whole lives to try and get a record and come on here?'"

An appearance on CBS's *The Cher Show* followed on 23 November. Here Bowie performed 'Fame' and joined Cher on a lavish duet of 'Can You Hear Me', but the main attraction was a six-and-a-half-minute medley: beginning and ending with 'Young Americans', David and Cher shimmied their way through a succession of hoary US hits to the accompaniment of the studio orchestra: 'Song Sung Blue', 'One', 'Da Doo Ron Ron', 'Wedding Bell Blues', 'Maybe', 'Maybe Baby', 'Day Tripper', 'Blue Moon', 'Only You', 'Temptation', 'Ain't No Sunshine' and 'Youngblood'.

"Cher I adored, from what I remember," said David many years later, although recollections of his sartorial priorities are rather clearer: "I'd got this thing in my mind that I was through with theatrical clothes and I would only wear Sears & Roebuck, which on me looked more outlandish than anything I had made by Japanese designers. They were just like this middle America dogged provincialism. They were loud check jackets and check trousers. I looked very bad. And very ill." On another occasion he recalled that Cher was initially frosty, but "warmed up when we sang together ... I was probably this crazed anorexic figure walking in, and I'm sure she didn't know what to make of me."

Five days after *The Cher Show*, British television viewers were treated to a live satellite interview with a pie-eyed David on ITV's *Russell Harty Plus*. The Spanish government had requested emergency use of the satellite to announce the death of General Franco, but David declined to relinquish his spot, confirming to Harty that he was looking forward to "coming home in May to play shows, look at you and be English again."

THE STATION TO STATION TOUR
2 February – 18 May 1976

Musicians: David Bowie (*vocals, saxophone*), Stacey Heydon (*guitar*), Carlos Alomar (*guitar*), George Murray (*bass*), Tony Kaye (*keyboards*), Dennis Davis (*percussion*)

Repertoire: 'Station To Station' / 'Suffragette City' / 'Waiting For The Man' / 'Stay' / 'Sister Midnight' /

'Word On A Wing' / 'TVC15' / 'Life On Mars?' / 'Five Years' / 'Panic In Detroit' / 'Changes' / 'Fame' / 'The Jean Genie' / 'Rebel Rebel' / 'Diamond Dogs' / 'Queen Bitch' / 'Golden Years'

Also referred to as the "Thin White Duke" and the "White Light" tour, Bowie's 1976 roadshow signalled the end of his mid-1970s sabbatical in America and the beginning of his relocation to Europe. It was to prove one of the most controversial periods of his career, but also produced one of the finest shows he has ever toured.

Rehearsals began in December 1975 at Keith Richards's studio in Ocho Rios, Jamaica. Bowie's relationship with his new manager Michael Lippman had disintegrated during the *Station To Station* sessions, and David finally sacked him at the beginning of 1976, issuing a lawsuit on 27 January in an attempt to recover earnings he claimed Lippman had withheld. The suit was destined to drag on until the autumn, providing an unwelcome distraction during the *Low* sessions; Lippman eventually won and disappeared from Bowie's story, later to become George Michael's manager. During the *Station To Station* sessions Lippman had taken Earl Slick onto his books and won him a solo contract with Capitol Records, driving a wedge between Bowie and his guitarist. Slick, who recalled that his "relationship with David just vaporized", attributes the falling-out to a misunderstanding with Bowie's management team. In Slick's place Bowie hired an unknown 21-year-old Canadian called Stacey Heydon. Roy Bittan was also unavailable, so former Yes keyboardist Tony Kaye joined the otherwise intact *Station To Station* band.

Occasionally introduced by David as "Raw Moon", the five-piece group was his smallest live band since the early days of The Spiders, and the standard of musicianship has rarely been bettered. The band whipped up a visceral, driven sound for the new songs and oldies like 'Five Years' and 'Panic In Detroit', the latter extended by an epic-length drum solo from Dennis Davis. Of the chosen set-list, Bowie told reporters that "I think 'Jean Genie' is a gas, I still like that one. I still love 'Changes'. All the songs I still do I still like, but I'm not doing 'Golden Years' or 'Space Oddity'. I've really been radical for this show and I won't do any hits for the sake of doing hits." In fact 'Golden Years' did make one or two appearances during the early concerts, but was dropped when David had difficulty reproducing its somersaulting vocal

range. Perhaps the most interesting addition to the set (again for a few American dates only) was 'Sister Midnight', a new song which would be recorded for Iggy Pop's *The Idiot* later in the year. Iggy had spent much of 1975 in Los Angeles in an even worse condition than David, and had recently discharged himself from a psychiatric institute he had voluntarily entered to wean himself off heroin. Now David's constant companion, he became a permanent member of the Station To Station entourage.

There were other changes in the air. David had already made the decision to sever his connections with Los Angeles, and as rehearsals continued Angela Bowie was busy house-hunting in Switzerland, where she had helped to negotiate residency. The house she found, a chalet near Lausanne called Clos des Mésanges, became David's official residence as of mid-1976, although it would seldom be his home over the next few years.

On 3 January, by which time rehearsals had moved to New York, the band appeared on *The Dinah Shore Show*, performing superb versions of 'Stay' (its first outing, a fortnight ahead of the album's release) and 'Five Years'. The show offered little indication of the forthcoming tour's presentation, owing more to the style of his Philly Dogs concerts: while the band wore rhinestone-encrusted Vegas outfits, David danced exuberantly in a dark blue shirt and voluminous flares.

By contrast the staging of the tour itself, when it opened in Vancouver on 2 February, seemed almost a reaction against the excesses of 1974. This time no attempt was made to disguise the paraphernalia of speaker cables, amps and lighting rigs. After pre-show tapes of Kraftwerk's *Radio-Activity* (Bowie had apparently considered asking the group to play as support), the show began with a projected film sequence from the 1928 Luis Buñuel/Salvador Dali silent *Un Chien Andalou*, showing a razor-blade cutting into an eyeball. Thereafter the visual element was provided entirely by banks of white light against black backdrops, capturing the stark spectacle of David Bowie in his latest incarnation. During the first few dates David experimented with costumes for his new character, and early gigs saw him take to the stage in tight turned-up jeans, laced boots and Bob Dylan cap (an ensemble not entirely unlike the earliest Ziggy costumes), and also in a softer outfit dominated by a pair of enormous yellow flares. However, within the first few days a far more forbidding image had crystallized and would remain unchanged for the duration of the tour. The Thin White Duke stalked the stage in pleated black trousers, black waistcoat and white shirt, his hair slicked tightly back like a Weimar cabaret singer straight out of Isherwood's Berlin. David told *Melody Maker* that the new show was "more theatrical than Diamond Dogs ever was … it's by suggestion rather than over-propping. It relies on modern, twentieth-century theatre concepts of lighting and I think it comes over as very theatrical."

From Vancouver the tour travelled down the West Coast (coinciding with David's final departure from California – he emptied his house during the three-night residency in Los Angeles) before zig-zagging across America for two months. Reviewing the second night, the *Seattle Times* revealed that "Bowie came on like a suave French boulevardier" and when not singing "would either walk off or dance in a sort of angular, jumpy way, with lots of squats and stiff-legged stretches." There were teething troubles, however: David was "drenched in big spots and banks of fluorescent lights that caused a buzz in the sound-system", and in the critic's opinion his saxophone playing in 'TVC15' left something to be desired: "I hope he meant to contrast with the band, because he did – he sounded like he was playing another tune." By the time the tour had moved into America's heartlands the praise was less reserved and the showbiz glamour of 1974 was back with a vengeance: guests at the Los Angeles concerts included Elton John, Rod Stewart, Britt Ekland, Patti Smith, Christopher Isherwood, David Hockney, Ray Bradbury, Alice Cooper, Carly Simon, Ringo Starr and even the President's son Steve Ford. The *Los Angeles Times* found David "happier, more confident, and relaxed", while six weeks later the *New York Times* considered the closing US date at Madison Square Garden the best Bowie show yet, noting the impressive effect of David's "cool, hostile distancing".

The Nassau Coliseum gig on 23 March was recorded by RCA and a selection broadcast on *The King Biscuit Flower Hour*. Two tracks from this excellent recording, 'Word On A Wing' and 'Stay', were later included on the 1991 reissue of *Station To Station*, and high-quality bootlegs of the radio broadcast make this one of the finest live Bowie recordings in circulation.

Three days earlier, on 20 March, had come the first of two inflammatory episodes. After the Rochester concert Bowie's hotel room was raided by police and, with Iggy Pop and two companions, he was arrested on suspicion of marijuana possession. The case never

came to trial, and in retrospect it's remarkable that this was the nearest Bowie ever came to a drugs bust. But by the time the case was dropped it had been overshadowed by a far larger controversy, which was to blight the remainder of the tour.

From 7 April the show began its European leg – Bowie's first concerts outside America since 1973 and his first ever major dates on mainland Europe. Back in February, David had explained that the show's blinding searchlights and follow-spots were inspired by German expressionist cinema and the photography of Man Ray. Now, as the tour moved into Europe, journalists who had been listening to his recent political pronouncements had different ideas. "It might have been staged by Speer," wrote one reviewer.

It was during the latter half of the Station To Station tour that Bowie's deluded fixation with the origins and symbols of Fascism landed him in serious trouble with the media, who were just as disposed to exploit controversy as Bowie was to court it. The lure of a good meaty scandal has prompted many historians to misrepresent the story: certainly Bowie was partly to blame, but the pulse-quickening tales of Nazi salutes and dictatorial ambitions have been greatly distorted to the detriment of our understanding of a very significant episode.

Much – too much – has been made of David's alleged far-right sympathies during the 1970s, not least by the National Front, who years after the controversy were still trying to claim David for their own in risible newsletter articles: "It was Bowie who horrified the music establishment in the mid seventies with his favourable comments about the NF … Bowie who, on the album *Hunky Dory*, started the anti-Communist musical tradition which we now see flourishing amidst the new wave of Futurist bands", claimed the National Front's youth paper *Bulldog* in 1981. In fact Bowie had never said anything remotely favourable about the National Front. What he *had* said, mostly a year earlier during his darkest Los Angeles days, was nonetheless naïve and irresponsible. In August 1975 he had told the *NME* that "There will be a political figure in the not too distant future who'll sweep this part of the world like early rock and roll did … the best thing that can happen is for an extreme right government to come. It'll do something positive at least, to cause commotion in people and they'll either accept the dictatorship or get rid of it."

Bowie had long been interested in the life of Adolf Hitler, and had expressed genuine admiration for his media-manipulation and stagecraft. "Look at some of his films and see how he moved," he told Cameron Crowe in 1975. "When he hit that stage, he worked an audience. Good God! He was no politician. He was a media artist ... he would march into a room to speak and music and lights would come on at strategic moments. It was rather like a rock'n'roll concert. The kids would get very excited – girls got hot and sweaty, and guys wished it was them up there. That, for me, is the rock'n'roll experience."

There was nothing in that particular disquisition, perceptively analytical as it was, that could be construed by anyone with half a brain as genuinely sinister. In many ways it was no more than a restatement of ideas which had informed dozens of his songs: 'Cygnet Committee', 'Saviour Machine', 'Star', 'Big Brother', 'Somebody Up There Likes Me' and countless others had long encouraged their audience to consider the razor's edge between glamour and oppression. As early as December 1969 Bowie had told *Music Now!* that "This country is crying out for a leader. God knows what it is looking for, but if it's not careful it's going to end up with a Hitler." Sadly, things took a turn for the worse as the Station To Station tour began. In February 1976 *Rolling Stone* quoted David as saying, "I think I might have been a bloody good Hitler. I'd be an excellent dictator. Very eccentric and quite mad." This, like several other pronouncements published in *Rolling Stone* and *Playboy* during 1976, derived from David's coke-infested interviews with Cameron Crowe the previous year. The *Playboy* article reveals a harsh and unsympathetic figure, dismissing peers and predecessors with arrogant put-downs and holding forth on the virtues of "fast" drugs, but between the provocative quotes there are flashes of ironic self-ridicule which have long since been forgotten. At the end of the interview Crowe asked Bowie if he stood by everything he had said, to which David replied, "Everything but the inflammatory remarks." Crowe himself was under no illusions: Bowie, he asserted, was "fully aware that he is a sensational quote machine. The more shocking his revelation, from his homosexual encounters to his Fascist leanings, the wider his grin ... The truth is probably inconsequential." However, then as now, few readers were interested in context. The damage had been done.

When the tour reached Berlin, the rumour spread that David had been photographed outside Hitler's bunker. Then, during a short mid-tour vacation with Iggy Pop, David's possessions were searched on a train at the Russian-Finnish border, and books about Albert Speer and Josef Goebbels were confiscated by Soviet guards. Bowie said they were research material for a musical he was writing about Goebbels. By now the accumulation of incidents was encouraging journalists to pursue the "Nazi" angle. At a press conference in Sweden David was reported as saying, "As I see it, I am the only alternative for the premier in England. I think Britain could benefit from a Fascist leader. I mean, Fascist in its true sense, not Nazi. After all, Fascism is really nationalism. In a sense, it is a very pure form of communism."

On 2 May the tour finally reached London where, in a well-staged publicity stunt, David arrived at Victoria Station in an open-topped Mercedes. He stood up in the car to acknowledge the crowds of fans who had gathered to welcome him back to Britain, and what happened next has been hotly contested ever since. Myth would have it that in front of the assembled posse of photographers Bowie snapped up his right arm in a Nazi salute. Photographs flooded the newspapers and at last the proof seemed overwhelming.

David was quick to react. He furiously denied that he had made a salute, saying that the photographers had caught his arm in mid-wave. Looking at the photos today, it is patently clear that this is exactly what happened. It's his left hand that is waving, and furthermore it looks nothing like a salute. "I don't think I'd have done anything as daft as that," he said in 1993. "They were waiting for me to do something like a Nazi salute and a wave did it for them." The whole episode has, in any case, been puffed up in retrospect: contrary to popular assumption, the text beneath the *NME*'s famous "Heil and Farewell" photograph (in which David's arm isn't even *raised*) made no mention of a salute.

His stay in Britain was only to last a week – the six sold-out shows at the Wembley Empire Pool were the only UK dates of the entire tour – and he agreed to meet just one journalist, Jean Rook of the *Daily Express*. She asked him, of course, about the alleged comment concerning Fascist rule in Britain. Bowie implied that the remarks had been an ironic response to provocative questioning: "If I said it – and I've a terrible feeling I did say something like it to a Stockholm journalist, who kept asking me political questions – I'm astounded anyone could believe it. I have to keep reading it to believe it myself. I'm not sinister ... I don't stand up in cars waving to people because I think I'm Hitler. I stand up in cars waving to fans – I don't write the captions under the picture." Rook pointed out that it was all good publicity, and asked if it mattered. Bowie replied, "Yes, it does. It upsets me. Strong I may be. Arrogant I may be. Sinister I'm not … What I'm doing is theatre, and only theatre. All this business about me being able to raise 7000 of my troops at the Empire Pool by raising one hand is a load of rubbish … What you see on stage isn't sinister. It's pure clown. I'm using my face as a canvas and trying to paint the truth of our time on it. The white face, the baggy pants – they're Pierrot, the eternal clown putting over the great sadness of 1976."

As ever, Bowie's argument was that he was holding up a mirror, performing a symbolic character in his ongoing dramatization of the *zeitgeist*, a concept to which Fleet Street was unlikely to listen. His articulate rebuttals of the "Nazi" allegations were sidelined in favour of the juicy quotes, and it took Bowie a long time to live down the controversy. Reviewers arrived at the Wembley concerts in May 1976 primed by the events of the previous few days. *Sounds* commented on the show's "stormtrooper vibe", *The Guardian* considered it "more Nazi than futuristic", and *Melody Maker* noted that it "raised echoes of his recent controversial comments about Fascist rule for Britain."

The Wembley concerts were, however, well reviewed. *Melody Maker* went on to describe the show as "undoubtedly funky" while the visuals were "inspired … a brilliant glare of black and white expressionism that emphasised the harshness of the music and reflected upon his image as a white-shirted, black-suited creature of Herr Ishyvoo's cabaret. It was, I think, the most imaginative lighting of a rock concert I have ever seen." At the end of the first Wembley gig, Bowie was so overcome by the ovation that he left the stage in tears.

The tour ended in Paris on 18 May. By the autumn Bowie had moved to Berlin, and to the intellectual titans of the tabloid press this was proof enough of where his sympathies lay. He was entranced by the social and sexual freedoms of Isherwood's city, but appalled to discover that his own name had already been annexed by Nazi fanatics, some of whom beat a path to his door; he is even said to have seen his name daubed on the Berlin Wall, the last two letters twisted into a swastika. In 1977, Britain's Rock Against Racism movement printed a leaflet called "Love Music – Hate Racism", which printed an image of Bowie's silhouette next to those of Enoch Powell and Adolf Hitler.

Bowie's reaction to this groundswell was to manifest itself in a demonstrable swing to the left and a torrent of angry songs. In 1978 he told an American interviewer that "There's a very negative aspect in England at the moment which has reared its ugly head … there's now a party there called the National Front which is the fourth strongest party in the country … I don't think it is an answer to anything at all. It's an answer to an idiot's dream." He added pointedly that "I used the Thin White Duke at one time, which unfortunately backfired a bit in England, but I tried to theatrically show what could happen."

Today Bowie blames the entire episode on a combination of his own naivety and the media's inability to resist a feeding frenzy. In 1993 he told the *NME* that his interest in the mythological aspects of Nazism was entirely abstract, and that the Victoria incident shook him into reality: "My interest in them was the fact that they supposedly came to England before the war to find the Holy Grail at Glastonbury and this whole Arthurian thought was running through my mind … The idea that it was about putting Jews in concentration camps and the complete oppression of different races completely evaded my extraordinarily fucked-up nature at that particular time. But, of course, it came home to me very clearly and crystalline when I came back to England."

Amid the inevitable streamlining of the facts since 1976, one of the greatest casualties has been the truth of what the Station To Station show was actually like. History has it that Bowie cut a glacial, arrogant figure on stage, a permanently smouldering Gitane clamped between his sneering lips as he glided from one slab of industrial rock into another. At best this is only half the story. The Thin White Duke may well have been, in Bowie's words, "a very nasty character indeed", but the shows were exuberant and joyous. David entered in character at the opening of each concert, but as the show progressed he would play the sax, execute all his usual dance steps and tell jokes between songs. He sweated profusely and would often peel off his waistcoat and shirt to perform the latter numbers topless, and in Evansville he even stood on top of the piano to sing 'Golden Years'. On the Diamond Dogs tour David had seldom if ever spoken to the audience; this time around it was difficult to get him to shut up. On more than one occasion, following the band introductions, he told Tony Kaye to stop playing the intro to 'Changes' so that he could chat at length with the crowd. His garrulousness owed partly to the fact that he was now weaning himself off cocaine and had turned instead to brandy, and bootlegs reveal that his rambling speeches were often completely incoherent. 1976 wasn't a very happy year for David Bowie, but that doesn't mean that the tour was some sort of robotic nightmare. Paul Gambaccini described the show as "the finest performance by a white artist I had ever seen", while Bob Geldof, who met Bowie backstage in Brussels, recalled the performance as "just staggeringly brilliant ... one of the best shows I've ever seen." These are by no means isolated opinions; the Station To Station show achieved a peak of musical excellence that would arguably not be matched by another Bowie tour for nearly twenty years.

THE 1977 IGGY POP "THE IDIOT" TOUR

1 March – 16 April 1977

Musicians: Iggy Pop *(vocals)*, David Bowie *(keyboards)*, Ricky Gardiner *(guitar)*, Tony Sales *(bass)*, Hunt Sales *(percussion)*

Repertoire: 'Raw Power' / 'TV Eye' / 'Dirt' / '1969' / 'Turn Blue' / 'Funtime' / 'Gimme Danger' / 'No Fun' / 'Sister Midnight' / 'I Need Somebody' / 'Search And Destroy' / 'I Wanna Be Your Dog' / 'Tonight' / 'Some Weird Sin' / 'China Girl' / '96 Tears' / 'Gloria'

While *Low* raced up the UK chart Bowie opted for anonymity in the spring of 1977 by playing keyboards on Iggy Pop's first tour since the demise of The Stooges. The set-list comprised a package of old Stooges favourites boosted by material from *The Idiot* and three new songs which would later appear on *Lust For Life*. In Britain Iggy was being widely hailed as the founding father of punk, and the *Evening Standard* soberly informed readers of his "bizarre stage appearances that have included antics like vomiting over a member of the audience, smashing his teeth out with a microphone and smashing a broken glass against his chest."

The band was completed by *Low*'s guitarist Ricky Gardiner and two new arrivals. The Sales brothers, drummer Hunt and bassist Tony, were the sons of Texan stand-up comedian and Sinatra Rat-Pack acolyte Soupy Sales. Former members of Todd Rundgren's band, they would go on to play on *Lust For Life* and, a decade later, would feature in a more notorious attempt by David to seek anonymity within a democratic band structure.

"It was the first time I'd ever really put myself into a band since The Spiders," Bowie later said. "It was great not having the pressure of being the singer up front ... Iggy would be preening himself before he went on and I'd be sitting there reading a book." Bowie was punctilious about not diverting press attention away from Iggy: as *Sounds* reported, "If you wanted David, you also got the band." On stage, he stayed behind his keyboard and barely looked at the audience. It was a generous and at the same time a canny manoeuvre; Bowie's presence undoubtedly helped Iggy to sell tickets, but at the same time it removed him from centre-stage at a time when any remotely mainstream artist was in danger of being rubbished by the cheerleaders of punk.

The tour opened at the Friars, Aylesbury, where Bowie had played some of the early Ziggy Stardust gigs five years earlier. After six British dates came an Atlantic crossing, on a schedule that left David no alternative but to conquer his fear of flying. Some of the American concerts were supported by up-and-coming new wave act Blondie. On 15 April, the penultimate night of the tour, the band appeared on *The Dinah Shore Show* to perform 'Sister Midnight' and 'Funtime'. Contrary to popular myth, however, at no point did David ever duet with Iggy on Otis Redding's 'That's How Strong My Love Is' or his own 'Fame' (both songs were featured on Iggy's subsequent Bowie-less Lust For Life tour, and the inaccurate claims of generations of bootleggers later gave rise to the misconception that David was involved).

Although both David and Iggy had come a long way since the self-destructive excesses of their last stay in America, the wolf was still at the door: "There were too many drugs around at the time," said Bowie in 1993. "I was going through these really ambivalent things because I kept wanting to leave the tour to keep off drugs. The drug use was *unbelievable* and I knew it was killing me, so that was the difficult side of it. But the playing was fun."

Iggy Pop resumed touring in the autumn of 1977 after completing work on *Lust For Life*. On this second tour the Sales brothers were accompanied by Stacey Heydon (formerly of Bowie's Station To Station tour band), while ex-Stooges keyboard player Scott Thurston took the place of David, who was now immersed in promotional duties for *"Heroes"*. Iggy's live albums *TV Eye* and *Suck On This!* both feature recordings from the 1977 tour.

THE STAGE TOUR

29 March – 12 December 1978

Musicians: David Bowie *(vocals, keyboards)*, Carlos Alomar *(guitar)*, Adrian Belew *(guitar)*, Dennis Davis *(percussion)*, George Murray *(bass)*, Simon House *(violin)*, Sean Mayes *(piano)*, Roger Powell *(keyboards)*, Dennis Garcia *(keyboards, 11-14 November only)*

Repertoire: 'Warszawa' / '"Heroes"' / 'What In The World' / 'Be My Wife' / 'The Jean Genie' / 'Blackout' / 'Sense Of Doubt" / 'Speed Of Life' / 'Breaking Glass' / 'Beauty And The Beast' / 'Fame' / 'Five Years' / 'Soul Love' / 'Star' / 'Hang On To Yourself' / 'Ziggy Stardust' / 'Suffragette City' / 'Rock'n'Roll Suicide' / 'Art Decade' / 'Station To Station' / 'Stay' / 'TVC15' / 'Rebel Rebel' / 'Alabama Song' / 'Sound And Vision'

In February 1978, fresh from filming *Just A Gigolo* in Berlin, Bowie took his son Joe on a safari holiday in Kenya. Then he flew to Dallas where, on 16 March, he joined rehearsals for what was to be his biggest concert tour so far, visiting the US, Canada, Europe, Japan and, for the first time, Australia. Rehearsals had begun several days earlier under the musical direction of Carlos Alomar who, with Dennis Davis and George Murray, made up Bowie's now familiar rhythm section. The bulk of the show was to comprise material from *Low* and *"Heroes"*, but as neither Robert Fripp nor Brian Eno cared for touring, David recruited four newcomers: Sean Mayes on piano, Adrian Belew on lead guitar, Roger Powell on synthesizers and, by way of innovation, Simon House on violin. Mayes, who had accompanied Bowie's *Top Of The Pops* performance the previous October, was a member of the band Fumble who had supported David's 1973 US tour. His posthumously published diary *We Can Be Heroes* provides a fascinating insight into the Stage tour and the *Lodger* sessions.

Eno had recommended Roger Powell, formerly of Todd Rundgren's Utopia and fresh from working on Meat Loaf's *Bat Out Of Hell*, while Simon House, who had recently been playing with Hawkwind, was an old schoolmate of David's who had neither seen nor heard from him in 15 years. Adrian Belew was a 28-year-old Kentuckian who had been discovered in a Nashville bar by Frank Zappa, with whom he was touring when he met Bowie in Berlin. "I had exactly a week between gigs," Belew told a journalist at the time. "During it, Bowie taught me thirty or forty of his

songs. He works fast." Belew later recalled that his decision to work with Bowie caused some friction with Frank Zappa, who had been hoping to retain his services – when the three met in a Berlin restaurant, Zappa "was very unfriendly to David", whom he insisted on calling "Captain Tom".

"I'm going out as myself this time," David said in a pre-tour interview. "No more costumes, no more masks. This time it's the real thing. Bowie Bowie." Certainly the Stage tour (no more than a semi-official title, after the album it spawned), was Bowie's least extravagant live show for many years, although his stage persona was as flamboyant as ever and the broad visual strokes were calculated to impress in the increasingly large venues he was now playing. The Diamond Dogs tour had played to halls with an average capacity of 7500; for the Philly Dogs shows this had risen to 10,000, while for the Station To Station tour the mean was around 14,000 in America and 7000 in Europe. (Of course, none of these averages reveal the highs and lows: Madison Square Garden and Washington Captal Center, both visited in 1974 and 1976, held over 19,000, Bowie's biggest audiences so far. Conversely, some venues on the 1976 European tour were mere 3000-seaters.) The statistics for the new tour were broadly similar to the Station To Station outing, although the greater number of European dates meant an increase in the total audience, while a clutch of giant open-air venues on the final Pacific leg would set new attendance records: 20,000 each in Adelaide and Sydney, and 40,000 apiece in Melbourne and Auckland.

To make an impression in these arenas, David elected to develop the stark approach of the 1976 staging. The ceiling of fluorescent tubes which had formed part of the Station To Station tour's lighting rig was expanded to create enormous panels of striped light, hanging like prison bars at the back and sides of the stage, which would pulse moodily during the slow instrumental pieces and flash frantically during rock numbers like 'Rebel Rebel' and 'Suffragette City'.

Despite Bowie's promise of "no more costumes", the Stage tour in fact saw a new wardrobe unrivalled in variety since the days of Ziggy Stardust. The outfits were designed by Natasha Kornilof, who had worked with Bowie in the days of Lindsay Kemp's *Pierrot In Turquoise* and again on his 1972 Rainbow Theatre concerts and *The 1980 Floor Show*. "We had torn bits out of magazines and we did small drawings and we had lots of ideas," recalled Kornilof. The resulting new-look Bowie, resplendent in a succession of tight shirts, snakeskin jackets, matelot caps and ballooning pleated trousers which fleetingly became known in fashion circles as "Bowie pants", offered a softer, more approachable image than any he had presented since the days of 'Space Oddity'. The band, meanwhile, were given unusually free rein in their choice of attire: after flirting with the idea of going on stage in a spacesuit, Adrian Belew settled for a succession of Hawaiian shirts and casual slacks; George Murray alternated between a black and white kimono and a cowboy outfit (the silhouette of the latter can be seen on the cover of *Stage*); Simon House plumped for leather jackets and jeans; and Sean Mayes and Carlos Alomar experimented in the latest punk styles.

The show opened in San Diego on 29 March. After a pre-show tape compiled from tracks by Lou Reed, Iggy Pop and The Rutles, the concert began to the funereal atmospherics of 'Warszawa', which remained the opening number throughout the tour. With the only movement coming from Carlos Alomar's conductor's baton, 'Warszawa' presented a bravely static tableau which was, in its way, just as theatrical as Bowie's past curtain-raisers: the show then gathered momentum with the second number, '"Heroes"'. As well as the Berlin material, a smattering of mid-1970s numbers and the later addition 'Alabama Song', the big surprise of the Stage tour was the revival of seven songs from the *Ziggy Stardust* album, rearranged for Bowie's new, synthesizer-heavy futurist sound. David sprung the idea on the band halfway through rehearsals, arriving one day to announce, "Let's do the whole of the *Ziggy* album, that'll surprise them!" Sean Mayes records that the final *Ziggy* selection was made "only after learning the whole lot".

The *Ziggy* songs were usually played *en bloc* immediately after the ten-minute interval, causing a minor sensation during the tour's early dates. The idea of the famous 'Ziggy Stardust' riff rendered on violin might sound unlikely, but the critical response was warm. "As he went through such provocative, new-age rock tunes as 'Five Years', 'Suffragette City' and 'Rock'n'Roll Suicide', it was easy to see how deep Bowie's impact on rock has been," wrote Robert Hilburn in the *Los Angeles Times*. "The first great rock star to emerge in the 70s, Bowie didn't turn out the most hits, write the largest batch of noteworthy songs or necessarily draw the biggest crowds, but he shook the rock'n'roll epicentre more than any other single figure in that period … he remains a towering figure in rock, one whose

side steps are more interesting than most lesser artists' biggest leaps forward." Others agreed. "A superb live show," said the *New York Times*, "and the enthusiasm at the end of Monday night's concert … was a genuine attestation of excellence." *Variety* noted that "Bowie is uncanny in his ability to pick musicians," describing Adrian Belew's guitar as "a riveting and pivotal force".

After the opening night, the band played an impromptu set in the bar of their San Diego hotel. Despite the party atmosphere that prevailed throughout the tour, relations within the band were not without their tensions; Alomar and Belew have admitted to a certain mutual friction, while Bowie himself was moving through a fragile stage in his post-addiction recovery, often unwell and prone to drinking bouts. Several of the band, including Mayes in his diary, recall Bowie as a friendly but often distant figure on the tour, sometimes unapproachable even by his colleagues due to the protective ministrations of Coco Schwab.

The ninth concert, in Dallas on 10 April, was filmed for a six-song US television broadcast entitled *David Bowie On Stage*. The shows in Philadelphia, Providence and Boston were recorded for the live album *Stage*, and at around the same time 'Rock'n'Roll Suicide' was dropped from the set to be replaced by 'Alabama Song'.

The two Detroit concerts in late April were marked by riotous crowds, causing David to stop in the middle of 'Ziggy Stardust' on the first night to berate the over-zealous bouncers, and necessitating an unscheduled break in 'Beauty And The Beast' on the second while the stage was cleared of a mountain of flowers, frisbees, scarves, toilet rolls and other projectiles (earlier the same night David had altered the words of 'The Jean Genie' to "smiles like a toilet roll" as yet another one sailed past his head). In Toronto David was reunited with Lindsay Kemp, who was in town performing *Salome*. In Boston police officers removed two girls who had interpreted Bowie's injunction to "let yourself go" as a cue to strip topless during 'The Jean Genie'. At the same gig someone had smuggled in a pair of giant beach balls which were inflated and bounced around the audience during the concert; when they reached the stage David gamely punched them back into the crowd, doubtless making a mental note to incorporate the idea into a future live show.

The American leg ended at Madison Square Garden and, as ever, David Bowie in New York was a major event: Andy Warhol noted in his diary that "only two tickets came for the Bowie concert and everyone wanted to go." Among those in the audience at the Garden (where, just as in 1974, the presence of the Ringling Brothers Circus made for a surreal atmosphere backstage) were Robert Fripp, Earl Slick, Brian Eno, Dustin Hoffman and members of Talking Heads. Also present was a 14-year-old boy called Sterling Campbell, who had been invited along by his new neighbour Dennis Davis. "I told him I play drums and he invited me to the show," Campbell recalled many years later. "That show was my first introduction to David's music and to the brilliance of Dennis Davis. And I knew what I wanted to do with my life!" Campbell soon became Davis's student, and many years later was to take over as Bowie's principal drummer.

The end of the US tour was celebrated with parties at two of New York's hippest venues, Hurrah's and Studio 54. Thereafter the show moved to Europe, opening in Frankfurt on 14 May after a short break in which Bowie had flown to Paris to overdub some dialogue for *Just a Gigolo*. In Berlin (where, before the show, Alan Yentob interviewed him for *Arena*), David broke off in the middle of 'Station To Station' to remonstrate in German with a over-zealous bouncer who was manhandling a fan, earning him massive respect from the local press. After the Vienna concert on 22 May the band gathered in a hotel room to listen to a cassette of the *Stage* album. "They loved it and jumped out of their seats," Tony Visconti later recalled – although Adrian Belew contradicts this, telling David Buckley that he "hated" the LP with its "thin and awful" sound. The Marseilles gig on 27 May was interrupted by a powercut – just after 'Blackout', appropriately – and a female fan took advantage of the darkness to jump on stage and kiss David. "I didn't know where she came from and I didn't have time to ask her name," he later joked. There was an enforced interval of over an hour before the performance could continue, this time without the neon lighting rig. In the interim the band had been driven back to their hotel to protect them from the crowd.

On 30 May the band recorded a special mini-concert in Bremen before a 150-strong studio audience for Germany's ZDF show *Musikladen Extra*. Sean Mayes wrote that "our only problem was adjusting to such a small and self-possessed audience. One girl, who was close enough to reach out and touch David's leg, sat with her back to the stage for the entire performance. Eat your hearts out Bowie fanatics!" The

show was broadcast on 4 August, and has since been repeated by MTV and other music stations. A planned video and CD release in 1996 was stalled by copyright problems.

Like all Bowie's major tours, the 1978 shows were heavily bootlegged. Four tracks from one such recording, 'Soul Love', 'The Jean Genie', 'Fame' and '"Heroes"', taped in Gothenburg on 4 June, were later included on a semi-legal 1993 Japanese compilation album called *David Bowie Best Selection*.

Having travelled through Germany, Austria, France and Scandinavia, the tour arrived in Britain. On 13 June, the day before the first UK concert, David attended an Iggy Pop gig at The Music Machine in Camden. Also in attendance was Johnny Rotten, and the three met for drinks after the show; Iggy joined the Bowie entourage for the next week. At Newcastle City Hall, a venue on Bowie's 1973 tour, the backstage visitors included Trevor Bolder and David's former bodyguard Stuey George. The UK tour ended with three shows at the 18,000-seater Earls Court Arena. The disaster of 1973 was happily not repeated, and the concerts were a triumph. On the last night, which was recorded by RCA, 'Sound And Vision' was hastily dredged from the rehearsal repertoire and added as a final encore on the spur of the moment. Together with 'Be My Wife' from the same concert, this recording later appeared on *RarestOneBowie*.

The critics were delighted, remarking on the contrast with the controversy that had attended Bowie's last London concerts. The *Financial Times* found a "confident, happy Bowie, finished with excess and quite content to sing though his songbook to his very faithful fans" in an atmosphere "more exciting than for Bob Dylan a fortnight earlier". The *Times* reported that "Predictably, the audience went wild. Less predictable was the warmth, even affection Bowie showed for them. A change for him, for us and, one might add, for the better." The *Evening News* called him "a totally controlled performer," adding that "It would be foolish to dismiss him solely as a rock star. He is an interesting painter, an innovative lighting expert, an actor and an artist." The Earls Court shows were filmed by David Hemmings, but although extracts were previewed on *The London Weekend Show* the film was never released, apparently because Bowie's opinion of the result tallied pretty much with his opinion of *Just A Gigolo*. "Dave came down to Spain to see my cut," said Hemmings later. "He decided at the end of the day that he didn't want to release it." Another factor may have been Bowie's reluctance to see profits from the film go to RCA, with whom he had a serious spat at around this time (see *Stage* in Chapter 2). In 2001 Bowie recalled of the film that "I simply didn't like the way it had been shot. Now, of course, it looks pretty good, and I would suspect that it would make it out some time in the future." The Earls Court film would prove to be Bowie's last collaboration with David Hemmings who, after scoring a considerable acting comeback in movies like *Gladiator* and *Last Orders*, sadly died in December 2003.

On 2 July, the day after the final Earls Court show, the band convened at Tony Visconti's Good Earth Studio to record 'Alabama Song'. There followed an interval of four months, during which David took the band to Montreux to begin work on *Lodger*. *Stage*, meanwhile, was released on 25 September.

After a week's rehearsal in Sydney, the Pacific leg opened at Adelaide's Oval Cricket Ground on 11 November. Not only was it Bowie's first Australian concert, it was also the first open-air gig of the tour and, indeed, David's first ever large-scale outdoor concert. The repertoire remained almost identical to the previous leg of the tour, although 'Speed Of Life' had now been dropped. For the first two dates of the Australian tour, local keyboardist Dennis Garcia deputized for Roger Powell, who was working on a delayed project with Utopia.

At the 40,000-capacity Melbourne Cricket Ground on 18 November the audience was soaked by torrential rain, but the band played on. Sean Mayes's account paints a graphic picture of the mayhem: "the bedraggled fans had a punk look with their ruined hair and streaky make-up. But the mood was fantastic – when you're soaked you don't give a damn! David loved the rain but the shiny black stage was like wet ice, and once he slipped and nearly went arse-over-tit into the front row … David wiped the soles of his shoes between numbers. Simon dried his violin bow every now and then … During the encores, a few fireworks went off and one or two rockets soared up onto the canopy."

From Australia the tour moved to New Zealand, where the 41,000-strong crowd at Auckland's Western Springs broke the country's previous attendance records. Next the band flew north for Bowie's first Japanese concerts since 1973. The opening gig in Osaka was broadcast on Japanese FM radio, while the final show of the entire tour, at Tokyo's NHK Hall on 12 December, was filmed for *The Young Music Show*.

Japanese translations of the song titles and lyrics were flashed across the screen in the edited broadcast, during which Dennis Davis, who had already donned warpaint and taken to bashing two giant gongs during the Japanese gigs until David confiscated them, can be seen wearing a gorilla mask for a couple of numbers.

After the gig, RCA hosted a 1920s-themed "Gigolo Party" to mark the end of the tour and the forthcoming release of *Just A Gigolo*. David stayed in Japan, spending Christmas in Kyoto with Coco Schwab. As early as October 1977 he had told the *NME* that he intended to spend time there: "I want something very serene around me for a few months to see if that produces anything," he said, adding enigmatically that "It is also important to my private life that I go to Kyoto."

Although perhaps not as exciting as some of Bowie's previous live outings, the Stage tour was a huge commercial and critical success. The cool reception of some historians and the comparatively sterile listening experience of the heavily mixed *Stage* album have conspired to enshrine the tour in the collective imagination as a bit of a bore, but this is a little unfair. By incorporating the synthesizer instrumentals from the Berlin albums between the big hits, the show may not have replicated the visceral excitement of past glories (David himself later admitted that the live rendition of 'Warszawa' was "a bit yawn-making"), but the band was one of the most proficient he had ever assembled: "each musician is full of dazzling musical personality," said Tony Visconti later, and it only takes a couple of minutes in the company of *Stage* to confirm that opinion. More than any other Bowie tour of the 1970s, it was a critically fêted sell-out wherever it went. And, as ever, it was hugely influential. Within a matter of months *Top Of The Pops* would be swamped by synthesizer acts whose chilly glares and neon-lit, dry-ice-billowing, jumpsuit-wearing visuals were directly descended from the Stage tour.

1979 – 1980: TELEVISION SPECIALS

Following the end of the Stage tour in December 1978, Bowie entered the longest period he had yet spent away from the live arena. Over the next five years he would make only a handful of live appearances, most of them on television.

First came a little-documented appearance in March 1979, when David appeared on stage at New York's Carnegie Hall to play viola alongside Philip

Glass, Steve Reich and John Cale in a performance of the latter's 'Sabotage'. The following month saw David's appearance on *The Kenny Everett Video Show*, miming to 'Boys Keep Swinging' in a performance which marked the beginning of a long and fruitful working relationship with the show's director, David Mallet.

On 15 December 1979 David recorded a trio of songs for NBC's *Saturday Night Live* (not an accurate title on this occasion, as the sequence was broadcast nearly a month later on 5 January). He was joined by Carlos Alomar, Dennis Davis and George Murray, together with Hall & Oates guitarist G E Smith (later to appear in the 'Fashion' video), Blondie keyboardist Jimmy Destri, and a pair of extraordinary backing singers in draggy make-up and three-quarter-length dresses. One was the cult German artist Klaus Nomi, making his first mainstream appearance after being "discovered" by David posing as a human mannequin in the window of New York boutique Fiorucci's. His fellow vocalist was Joey Arias, another Fiorucci acolyte, but it was Nomi whose career subsequently took off. He secured a recording deal with RCA who released his extraordinary debut album in 1981. He died only two years later, one of the first celebrity victims of AIDS.

Now firmly entrenched in the avant-garde new wave posture of his *Scary Monsters/Elephant Man* period (he first saw the Broadway production of the latter during the same trip to New York), Bowie had devised a striking sequence of routines for *Saturday Night Live*. For 'The Man Who Sold The World' he was carried downstage by the backing singers in a rigid wasp-waisted morning suit which left only his head and forearms free, and having completed the number he was duly carried away. The costume, he later revealed, was inspired by the Edwardian cabaret artist Hugo Ball, who would be carried on stage in a tube at Zürich's Cabaret Voltaire. "I combined the tube device with another Dada costume, that of a highly stylised men's evening dress with huge shoulders and bow tie," he explained in 1999. For 'TVC15' he reappeared in a blue jacket, pencil skirt, stockings and high heels, resembling a cross between an airline stewardess and Rosa Klebb, while a toy dog sat at his feet with a television screen in its mouth. Finally, 'Boys Keep Swinging' saw David's head superimposed over a dancing rod-puppet body which he operated himself (even producing a cheeky *membrum virile* at the song's climax), the whole overlaid by chromakey onto the

background shot of the band. This was based on an act he had seen in German fairgrounds: "the performer, dressed in black, would attach a small body puppet ... below his chin. This gave the effect of a human-headed marionette." The *Saturday Night Live* set remains one of Bowie's finest television appearances, the excellent renditions of the songs themselves in no way subordinate to the brilliantly eccentric staging. 'The Man Who Sold The World' and 'TVC15' have arguably never been bettered live.

On 31 December 1979 both *Kenny Everett's New Year's Eve Show* and, in America, *Dick Clark's Salute To The Seventies*, featured mimed studio performances of Bowie's new acoustic version of 'Space Oddity'. The *Kenny Everett* performance, again directed by David Mallet, is of particular interest in that it used images later developed for the following year's 'Ashes To Ashes' video. It was also the scene of an unhappy incident according to Gary Numan, a Bowie fan who had followed his career with something akin to hero-worship since the mid-1970s (speaking many years later, Numan admitted that during the Station To Station tour "I dyed my hair orange with gold sprayed in the front and wore a waistcoat with Gitanes cigarettes in my pocket, even though I didn't smoke. I don't think I looked very cool. When I managed to get to the front, I was holding one of those glowing green sticks that you used to get at gigs. I lobbed it at Bowie during 'The Jean Genie' and caught him in the chest – probably the greatest moment of my life at that point"). In the wake of Numan's success in 1979, Bowie had made disparaging remarks about an artist regarded by many as little more than a tribute act, describing him as a "clone" in *Record Mirror* and adding that Numan had "not only copied me, he's clever and he's got all my influences in too." Numan claims that he had already recorded his own performance for the same Kenny Everett special when, spotted across the floor by Bowie during the taping of the 'Space Oddity' sequence, he was taken to one side by David Mallet and asked to leave the studio. A few days later Numan was informed that his own segment would not be used in the show after all, a turn of events he attributes to Mallet's need to appease his most lucrative promo client. In 2000 Bowie described this story as "apocryphal", telling Q that "If he were asked not to come onto the set, it would have been during rehearsals. I do remember having told the studio people that he was welcome to come in for the actual shoot. He never appeared."

David returned to American TV on 3 September 1980 – in between his own performances of *The Elephant Man* in Chicago – to perform superb versions of 'Life On Mars?' and 'Ashes To Ashes' with members of the *Scary Monsters* band (plus *Saturday Night Live* veteran G E Smith and The Rumour's drummer Stephen Goulding) on an edition of NBC's *The Tonight Show With Johnny Carson*. It was Bowie's only major promotional appearance for *Scary Monsters* and indeed his last live performance until 1983. After the closing night of *The Elephant Man* on 3 January 1981, his only other appearance of note before retreating from the public eye came on 24 February when he attended the *Daily Mirror*'s Rock And Pop Awards ceremony in London, collecting the "Best Male Singer" award from Lulu.

THE SERIOUS MOONLIGHT TOUR

18 May – 8 December 1983

Musicians: David Bowie (*vocals, guitar, saxophone*), Earl Slick (*guitar*), Carlos Alomar (*guitar*), Tony Thompson (*percussion*), Carmine Rojas (*bass*), David LeBolt (*keyboards*), Steve Elson, Lenny Pickett, Stan Harrison (*saxophones*), Frank Simms, George Simms (*backing vocals*)

Repertoire: 'Star' / '"Heroes"' / 'What In The World' / 'Look Back In Anger' / 'Joe The Lion' / 'Wild Is The Wind' / 'Golden Years' / 'Fashion' / 'Let's Dance' / 'Red Sails' / 'Breaking Glass' / 'Life On Mars?' / 'Sorrow' / 'Cat People (Putting Out Fire)' / 'China Girl' / 'Scary Monsters (And Super Creeps)' / 'Rebel Rebel' / 'I Can't Explain' / 'White Light/White Heat' / 'Station To Station' / 'Cracked Actor' / 'Ashes To Ashes' / 'Space Oddity' / 'Young Americans' / 'Soul Love' / 'Hang On To Yourself' / 'Fame' / 'TVC15' / 'Stay' / 'The Jean Genie' / 'Modern Love' / 'Imagine'

By 1983 Bowie had been absent from the touring circuit for an unprecedented five years, and the pre-release publicity for *Let's Dance* promised a spectacular new show. Like the album itself, the Serious Moonlight tour was consciously designed to "normalize" Bowie for a mass audience. "I was getting really pissed off for being regarded as just a freak," he said in 1983. "I won't be trying to put on any pose or stance. You won't see Mr Iceman Cometh or weird Ziggy or whatever. I was just gonna be me, having a

good time, as best I can … That was my premise for this tour: to re-represent myself."

As ever, strong visuals would be central to Bowie's latest self-reinvention. The set was originally entrusted to Derek Boshier, creator of the *Let's Dance* album artwork, but his elaborate designs were rejected as too costly. Instead Bowie contacted Diamond Dogs tour veteran Mark Ravitz, who created a stage environment more elaborate than any since 1974, yet bold and simple enough to work in multi-thousand-seater venues. Four enormous fluted columns of translucent polythene dominated the stage, while giant neoclassical lintels hovered above them, suggesting a cross between a Palladian temple and *Star Trek*. "It's kind of like some sort of new architecture," said Bowie, "combining classicism and modernism." To stage right was a giant hand, pointing upwards after the fashion of Michelangelo's *Creation of Adam* (famously pastiched by the *E.T.* film poster just a few months earlier), towards a glittering crescent moon hanging stage left. At some of the major venues, like Milton Keynes Bowl and Madison Square Garden, a larger inflatable moon would hang over the audience, breaking open to shower the crowd with silver and gold balloons at the end of each show.

However, the main visual cues derived from the previous two tours, relying not on props but on a truly spectacular light show. Bowie's keynote was the same as it had been for years: "He said he wanted German expressionism," said lighting designer Allen Branton, "and I went and bought all the books." Branton based his plot around 40 Vari-lites, computer-controlled lamps capable of panning, tilting, rotating and switching between any of 60 colour gels. Today Vari-lites are standard in every television quiz-show, but Branton's use of them in 1983 was a spectacular innovation for the rock stage. "Every show thus far, including mine, has generally hung them in the same horizontal plane, on the overhead light grid," he explained. "I wanted them on different planes. Turned on 90 degrees. Stretching their physical parameters." Adding conventional washes and internal lighting for the giant columns, Branton created set-piece landscapes: stark blue backlight for 'Cat People', sultry reds and yellows for 'Red Sails', flickering strobes and harsh green cross-beams and searchlights for 'Scary Monsters'. "Fellini, Ziegfeld and Steven Spielberg would all be proud of us," remarked Branton.

The initial fortnight's rehearsals in a Manhattan studio were overseen by musical director Carlos

Alomar, back on board after his absence from *Let's Dance*. In April David joined the band in rehearsal at Las Calinas, near Dallas. Alongside the *Let's Dance* personnel the new faces included sometime Village People and Billy Joel keyboardist David LeBolt, and saxophonist Lenny Pickett, whose arrival brought together the sax trio who would be dubbed The Borneo Horns in the tour brochure. The ten-piece band was Bowie's biggest since 1974, and in another throwback to the year of the Diamond Dogs it included two choreographed backing vocalists, Frank and George Simms.

Serious Moonlight remains Alomar's favourite of the six Bowie tours he has played to date – "it was the first tour where we did all of the hits," he tells David Buckley, adding that he particularly enjoyed creating "all these fabulous horn arrangements so that every song sounded as if it had just been recorded." During the tour Bowie confirmed that Alomar's rearrangements were crucial to the show's identity: "Before, I've had up to three synthesizers onstage. The music had sort of industrial, mechanized-sounding connotations to it. That's another aspect that I wanted to lighten up on … The choice of musicians has helped, because they're not familiar with my music. So they've interpreted it more from a soul-based background. Inherently, there's a lighter-hearted characteristic coming through the music, than if I had used my original musicians who had it in their minds, 'Oh yeah, I know Bowie, he wants doom and gloom in here.'"

Towards the end of the Dallas rehearsals, as the band worked with choreographer Chris Dunbar in advance of their departure for a final week of preparation at the Vorst Nationaal in Brussels, a crisis arose with the eleventh-hour sacking of lead guitarist Stevie Ray Vaughan. The problem had nothing to do with Vaughan's ability: on the contrary, as rehearsal bootlegs reveal, his unique contribution to the band's sound was striking. Bowie later remarked that "Stevie was pulling notes out of the air that no-one could have dreamed would have worked with my songs." Unfortunately drugs and management problems were afflicting Vaughan, who was apparently at loggerheads with Bowie over impositions of choreography and costume, strictures against drug-taking on tour, and in particular the fee he was receiving. Vaughan claimed that Bowie's management had also reneged on a verbal promise that his group Double Trouble would support some of the British and American dates. Bowie, who had already departed for Europe to under-

take promotional duties when the crisis arose, would later say that he was "almost blackmailed" by Vaughan's "cartoon of a manager", explaining that half an hour before the coach was due to leave for the airport to take the band to Brussels, Vaughan's manager "demanded to renegotiate Stevie's fee, there and then, giving him a higher salary than any other musician on the tour, otherwise he would pull Stevie from the tour. As I was thousands of miles away in Belgium and with twenty minutes to go, our promoter took it upon himself to make a decision which would change the entire sound of the show."

Thus, with less than a week to go until opening night, Vaughan was dismissed. "When the rest of the party arrived in Belgium," Bowie later recalled, "Carmine Rojas, my bass player, told me that it was one of the most heartbreaking moments he had ever witnessed on the road, Stevie left standing on the sidewalk with his bags surrounding him. Carmine was convinced that Stevie had no idea that his manager was going to pull such a scam or, if he did, that this guy had convinced Stevie that he could pull it off." The rest of the band rallied against any controversy, Alomar telling journalists that "David has never made any money before, and on this tour there are a lot of people making sure that he's going to make some money. As far as our money situation, come on, that's just fine. Everybody's making over four figures [per week]." Despite the stance of Vaughan's manager, this was evidently no re-run of the *David Live* pay mutiny. (Vaughan, who was later reconciled with Bowie, tragically died in a plane crash in 1990.)

Ironically, Vaughan was replaced by a guitarist whose last contribution to the Bowie story had also involved pulling out of a tour at the last minute. Earl Slick, who had toured with David in 1974 and played on *Station To Station* before parting company on frosty terms, was hastily contracted and flown out to Brussels on 14 May. "Everything was straightened out," Slick said of his former quarrel with David. "There was communication, a lot of joking and fooling around. In the old days I'd show up at the theatre and literally not see him except for the stage part. Now it's back to normal. Business as usual." Carlos Alomar put in frantic extra rehearsal time with Slick, who spent four days locked in a hotel room "with coffee pot after coffee pot", learning the 31 songs on the setlist.

Bowie had laid down the law to his band about drug-taking, and his personal regimen on the Serious

Moonlight tour was a far cry from the coke-bombed madness of the mid-1970s. He began each day with two hours of aerobics and shadow-boxing. "This is a long tour and I want to be in shape," he told reporters. "I don't want it to be like the old days, when I felt it was almost my duty to end up a wreck. I thought that was what you had to do to be a substantial artist." He had also conquered his much-vaunted fear of flying: along with the new lifestyle came the ultimate touring accessory, a private 707 jet.

Although the show was more tightly choreographed than the 1976 or 1978 tours, Bowie had avoided intricate stagecraft in favour of broad strokes which, like the set and lighting, were well conceived for giant venues. There was a revival of 1974's skull-and-shades routine for 'Cracked Actor'. The four giant columns filled with smoke during 'Station To Station', and Bowie sang 'Ashes To Ashes' inside one of them as it rolled downstage. In the same number, the Simms brothers played ball with a giant inflatable globe, which then sat in a spotlight for 'Space Oddity' before being kicked out across the audience during 'Young Americans'. For other numbers there were stunningly frenetic light shows, while 'Life On Mars?', 'Wild Is The Wind' and 'Space Oddity' were delivered from points of stillness in a solitary spotlight. There was rudimentary choreography for 'Fashion' (Bowie and the Simms boys acting as catwalk models), while 'Let's Dance' was the cue for David to perform some shadow-boxing. For 'Red Sails' he mimed climbing a mountain, while Lenny Pickett executed what Bowie called a "whirling dervish" dance suggested by the saxophonist during rehearsals. But these were the exceptions: most of the numbers were performed in a straight stand-and-deliver style, with David the unchallenged centre of attention.

Bowie devised his two-piece pastel suits with wardrobe designer Peter Hall, whose work he had admired in recent New York productions of La Bohème and Zoot Suit. For most concerts David would begin in a powder-blue suit and striped schoolboy tie, changing during the 15-minute interval (usually between 'White Light/White Heat' and 'Station To Station') into a peach two-piece with a polka-dot bowtie slung around the collar. Other outfits included a lime-green suit and a white naval jacket with gold piping. His handsome thirtysomething features were highlighted by a candyfloss mop of peroxide hair, teased into the lacquered 1950s meringue already seen in the 'Let's Dance' video. Hall also designed the band costumes,

which Bowie described as "a slight parody on all the New Romantics ... I thought it might be nice to make it look a bit like Singapore in the fifties." Hall cast each musician against a different cultural backdrop. "He saw Carlos as the Ghandi type, or actually more of a prince," said Bowie. The Simms brothers wore striped blazers and fedoras, Carmine Rojas a sailor's cap and sarong, and David LeBolt a coolie hat. The three-man sax section were dressed as a Cossack, an Alpine mountaineer and a safari hunter. Only late-comer Earl Slick appeared to escape Hall's attentions, sporting a standard rock-guitarist T-shirt and a Knopfler-style headband.

More than any previous Bowie tour, the set-list was unashamedly a greatest hits package aimed at acquainting the new mass audience with Bowie's back catalogue. With only four tracks from Let's Dance included, the sense that Bowie was touring a new album was slight. As usual, those fortunate enough to attend the earlier dates were rewarded with the fullest sets. 'Joe The Lion' and 'Soul Love' didn't make it past Brussels, 'Wild Is The Wind' and 'Hang On To Yourself' were scrapped over the next few days, and lost before the end of the tour were 'TVC15', 'I Can't Explain' and 'Red Sails'. Halfway through the US leg the set-list was reshuffled, promoting 'Look Back In Anger' to curtain-raiser while the opening 'Jean Genie/Star' medley was relegated to the encores. Looking back on the tour in 1987, David said that "I was really pushing it, trying to do all those Ziggy things ... it was fine for the first few weeks, then I thought, God, I wish I'd dipped into more stuff from Lodger and maybe some of the "Heroes" things, Low even. I'm not doing 'Star' again. That was quite hard."

Bowie was in superb voice, although during his five-year touring break a lifetime of smoking had finally caught up with his higher register, necessitating the re-pitching of melodies like 'Life On Mars?' and 'Golden Years'. He picked up his acoustic guitar for 'Space Oddity' and 'Young Americans', and occasionally played saxophone for the final encore 'Modern Love'. The instrumental arrangements were a mixed bag: Earl Slick's recreation of 'Station To Station' and his hard-edged solo in 'White Light/White Heat' were magnificent, but elsewhere the overpowering sax section threatened to outstay its welcome. Nobody could fault the appropriate and lovely sax interludes in 'Sorrow' and 'Young Americans', but the use of saxophones to replace the edgy guitar intro of 'Breaking Glass' or the bassline of 'Scary Monsters' made for an uncomfortable listening experience. Bowie's flirtation with that bane of 1980s pop, the over-produced horn section, would continue to bedevil his next couple of albums.

After Bowie's flying visit to Cannes to promote *Merry Christmas Mr Lawrence*, The Serious Moonlight tour opened in Brussels on 18 May. The *NME*'s Charles Shaar Murray raved about "the best-staged and best-lit concert I can remember", remarking that "every moment of the way, Bowie's staging supports, enhances, underlines and comments upon the music … the arrangements for the tour demonstrate that Bowie is at least as interested in revitalising his music as he is in simply reproducing it, as he did on the Stage tour." Murray concluded that "Not on the basis of his legend or his publicity, but on the strength of this show, Bowie is the finest white pop performer alive."

From Brussels the show moved through a handful of dates in Germany and France before flying to Los Angeles to headline the third and final day of the US Festival in San Bernardino, where the 150,000-strong audience was by far the biggest Bowie had ever played. Also on the bill were Van Halen, Men At Work, Stevie Nicks, The Clash, U2 and The Pretenders. Bowie's widely reported $1.5m booking for the festival broke industry records for the highest flat fee paid to a solo performer for a single concert, and was instrumental in brokering the Serious Moonlight tour in general: "That opened up some places to play, especially in the Far East," David revealed, adding that it also "paid for a second set to get built," enabling the road crew to leapfrog ahead. Although good for Bowie, the US Festival was a disaster for its organisers, who were faced with untold losses and the consequences of a serious riot on the hard-rock-oriented second day, resulting in two deaths and 145 arrests.

Bowie returned to Europe for three nights at Wembley Stadium which had sold out within 24 hours, followed by further dates in Britain and the Continent. By now the tour was a massive success, but that didn't stop the British music press crying foul (in fact, it probably encouraged them). "This new, very visible Bowie says much to us about the rewards of mediocrity that maintain rock's motion," said the previously enthusiastic *NME*, while *Sounds* dismissed David's new act as "the thinking man's Frankie Vaughan … musical fish and chips". *Melody Maker* explained that "The concerts confirmed what those singles with Queen and Bing Crosby should already

have told us. The man who sold the world can now be safely filed away under family entertainment. And all the family is buying." The tabloids were more accommodating, the *Sun* perceiving in Bowie "the mystique of Bob Dylan" and "the sheer animal excitement of Mick Jagger", while the *Daily Express* commended the show's "utmost style", noting that "For the first time in his thirteen-year career, Bowie played Bowie straight." The UK concerts were so over-subscribed that further dates were added in Edinburgh and Milton Keynes, a story repeated throughout the tour. Booking agent Wayne Forte later explained that regional promoters had initially underestimated Bowie's popularity: "It was a hard sell in Europe, especially outdoor dates. Promoters felt David wasn't an outdoor act and was a reserved-seat act for an older, well-dressed audience … And then things went crazy. The promoters went wild. They wanted the biggest stadiums."

While in Britain Bowie visited Madame Tussaud's, who had just unveiled his waxwork – at the time he was the only rock singer other than Presley and The Beatles to be so commemorated. Press coverage focused on the peculiar demands of selecting not one but two different matching eyeballs, while David declared himself "really pleased" to be positioned next to George Orwell.

Providing support during various legs of the tour were UB40, Icehouse, The Beat, The Tubes and Peter Gabriel. The Paris gig on 8 June – attended by 'China Girl' star Jee Ling among others – was marked by a rather silly incident in which the famously outspoken Kevin Rowland of Dexys Midnight Runners announced during the band's support set that "David Bowie is full of shit!", dubbing him "a bad Bryan Ferry". Not surprisingly the band was booed off. Rowland told reporters, "We only agreed to the show because France is an important market for us, not because I have any respect for Bowie." He later went on to record the theme to the BBC sitcom *Brush Strokes*.

June 30 saw a special gig in aid of the Brixton Neighbourhood Community Association, held in the presence of Princess Michael of Kent at by far the smallest and most evocative venue of the entire tour: the 2800-capacity Hammersmith Odeon, where Ziggy Stardust had announced his retirement ten years earlier almost to the day. Tickets for the show, which at a steep £25 and £50 included a compulsory donation, sold out immediately, raising an eventual total of

£93,000 for the charity. Wild reports that the gig would see the rebirth of Ziggy and The Spiders were unfounded; the show proved to be a standard but intimate Serious Moonlight set, stripped of the scenery that simply wouldn't have fitted in the venue. Members of the support band Amazulu joined David for the final encore of 'Modern Love'.

The Hammersmith gig did see another reunion of sorts. Tony Visconti, who had been passed over as producer of Let's Dance, had been invited to the Edinburgh gig two days earlier with a view to correcting the sound balance after reviews had criticized the acoustic quality of the concerts. "My immediate response was 'Why don't you get Nile Rodgers to do it?'" admitted Visconti later, "But I got off my act and flew up to Edinburgh. I stomped around in the field and made a few notes … and I confirmed their worst fears about the sound – it was appalling. They said, 'Okay, will you come to the benefit concert at Hammersmith Odeon and put it right?' I went to the rehearsals and they just literally let me have the board so I did the sound that afternoon … David jumped from the stage and I asked him what he thought of it. 'Sounds great,' he said, and 'Will you do the rest of the tour with me?' … but the answer was basically 'No,' I just couldn't drop all my plans for the year." This was to be the beginning of a long professional estrangement between David and arguably his most talented and empathic producer, a break which many consider crucial to an understanding of Bowie's creative unsteadiness over the next decade. After Hammersmith the two lost contact, apparently because of Visconti's willingness to talk to journalists about subjects David considered private. The air was finally cleared in 1998 when, to the rejoicing of many fans, they began working together again.

The mammoth American leg followed from July to October in a wave of unprecedented Bowiemania. The New York Post considered the show "flawless", while the New York Times found Bowie "subtler, more ferocious, more moving and more dazzling – intellectually and sensually – than anything the art world's most celebrated performance artists have come up with." Week after week the ticket grosses topped Billboard's box office statistics. David was on the cover of Time magazine, and post-show parties were the toast of the celebrity circuit, attracting names like Michael Jackson, Cher, Raquel Welch, Barbra Streisand, Bette Midler, Prince, Tina Turner, Susan Sarandon, Sissy Spacek, Henry Winkler, Irene Cara, Donald Suther-land, Tom Conti, sundry Rolling Stones, Joe Jackson, Nile Rodgers, Ian Hunter, David Byrne, Richard Gere, Paul Newman, John McEnroe, Dustin Hoffman, Grace Jones, Bryan Ferry, Elton John and Yoko Ono (at the last of the three Madison Square Garden shows David dedicated 'Space Oddity' to "a little boy called Sean," the late Mr Lennon's youngest).

The Montreal Forum show on 13 July was broadcast on American radio, and 'Modern Love' from the same gig was later released as a B-side. The accompanying video was shot in Philadelphia on 20 July, the same night that a girl invaded the stage during the band introductions, grabbed hold of David and inadvertently smashed his acoustic guitar before being escorted off. "I want to apologize for my mother," Bowie deadpanned to the crowd. Two months later on 11 and 12 September, the full-length Serious Moonlight video was shot by David Mallet at the 11,000-seater PNE Grandstand in Vancouver. There were plans to release a live album mixed by Let's Dance engineer Bob Clearmountain from the various recordings, but the idea was dropped.

Those lucky enough to see the show on 4 September, the second of two nights in Toronto, received the biggest treat of the tour. "We have got a very exceptional surprise for you at the end of this evening, and I'm not going to tell you anything about it," teased David while introducing the band. After the first couple of encores he announced, "I was walking through a corridor in Toronto last night, and I ran into somebody I haven't met for eight years, and I said, what are you doing tonight? … I'd like to introduce one of the original Spiders From Mars – Mick Ronson!" Relations between Bowie and his legendary guitarist had been nonexistent since 1975, when Ronson had spoken out in disparaging terms about Bowie's wayward lifestyle in Los Angeles. Now based in Toronto, Ronson had decided that a reconciliation was due: "When I heard the show was on in Toronto, I called up Corinne and asked for some tickets," he recalled. "I saw David, and the first thing he asked was if I wanted to play. I told him I couldn't … But by the next evening I just thought, sod it, why not? So I went down to the Grandstand and we did 'Jean Genie' and it was great. Earl Slick lent me his guitar, and I'd heard him playing solos all night so I thought, 'Right, no solos, I'll go out there and thrash.' So I did, I really thrashed that guitar, swinging it around my head and banging into it, and afterwards David told me it was Earl's prize guitar and all the while I'd been playing he'd been petrified! Poor Slick, I didn't know."

In October the tour moved to Japan (where Nagisa Oshima attended the first night), in November to Australia and New Zealand (where the Toarangtira Maoris honoured David with a tribal ceremony), and ended with four December dates in the Far East, taking in Singapore, Bangkok and Hong Kong. These last four concerts weren't officially part of the Serious Moonlight tour, which had its last night proper in Auckland on 26 November, where the 74,480-strong audience was the largest ever recorded for an Australasian concert and was believed to be the greatest single gathering of people in New Zealand's history: one in 50 of the country's population was at the Bowie gig. During the encores Bowie was joined on stage by James Malcolm, the boy who had played his brother in *Merry Christmas Mr Lawrence*. The nuclear arms race was dominating the world's headlines, and Bowie ended the Auckland concert with an impassioned oration ("I wish our world leaders would stop their insane inability to recognize that we wish to live peacefully!"), and, with Malcolm, released two white doves into the sky before the final encore.

The so-called "Bungle In The Jungle" tour that followed was a last-minute addition born of David's enthusiasm to play the Far East – the carrot after the Western tour's stick, as he himself termed it – and was reckoned as a financial loss from the outset. The majority of the road crew were dispensed with and the set, costumes and Vari-lites were abandoned, but nevertheless the pared-down show was seen by 70,000 people over the four nights. Bowie's Far Eastern travels were commemorated by Gerry Troyna's fly-on-the-wall film *Ricochet*. In Singapore both 'China Girl' and 'Modern Love' had been banned from radio play as potentially subversive, and the police imposed a 60-foot gap between stage and audience at the concert. The Bangkok gig coincided with the King of Thailand's birthday, marked by fireworks at the end of the show and a dedication delivered by George Simms, a formidable linguist who had previously added to Bowie's German and Japanese addresses by announcing shows in French, Swedish and Dutch.

The final Hong Kong date, 8 December 1983, was the third anniversary of John Lennon's death. Earl Slick, who had played lead guitar not only on 'Fame' but on Lennon's 1980 comeback *Double Fantasy*, suggested marking the occasion with a one-off rendition of 'Across the Universe', to which Bowie replied, "Well, if we're going to do it, we might as well do 'Imagine'." The rapidly rehearsed one-off performance of Lennon's classic was introduced before the encores and, needless to say, was ecstatically received.

In every conventional sense the Serious Moonlight tour was a massive success, consolidating Bowie's new mainstream audience and generating the sort of revenue that can only be boggled at – David is said to have referred to the tour in private as his "pension plan". The 97 concerts were attended by over 2.6 million people, reflecting not only the success of *Let's Dance* but also the fact that Bowie was, for the first time, appealing to a generation of fans equipped with nostalgia and disposable incomes. It was by far the biggest rock tour of 1983, breaking house attendance records wherever it went. Bowie became the first artist to sell out four consecutive nights at the Philadelphia Spectrum, while massive sales at the 16,500-capacity LA Forum prompted the California Angels baseball team to threaten a lawsuit over "disruption" of their ticket sales at the Anaheim Stadium, which was four times larger and which, as the *coup de grâce*, Bowie proceeded to fill a month later. Japanese hair salons were besieged by demands for the peroxided "Bowie Cut", while in Europe wholesalers were mystified by a rush on the sales of women's red shoes to wear – and fling – at the concerts.

But in the long term the tour was a mixed blessing. In the very act of propelling Bowie to living-legend status, it created a millstone around his neck. "I was something I never wanted to be," he later admitted. "I was a well-accepted artist. I had started appealing to people who bought Phil Collins albums. I like Phil Collins as a bloke, believe me, but he's not on my turntable twenty-four hours a day. I suddenly didn't know my audience and, worse, I didn't care about them." In recent years Bowie has tended to overplay the notion that he was a cult artist before 1983 (not strictly true, as demonstrated by his top ten hits, record-breaking album sales and sell-out concerts at Madison Square Garden and Earls Court a decade earlier), but there can be no doubt that the Serious Moonlight tour brought him an unthinkably massive audience of a kind unlike any he'd had before. In making the mistake of trying to give this audience what he thought it wanted, Bowie would soon falter badly. Contrary to popular belief not everything he did during the remainder of the 1980s was useless, but it would be a long time before he returned to his natural habitat on the creative fringe.

1985: TINA TURNER AND LIVE AID

Musicians (Live Aid): David Bowie *(vocals)*, Kevin Armstrong *(guitar)*, Matthew Seligman *(bass)*, Neil Conti *(drums)*, Pedro Ortiz *(percussion)*, Clare Hurst *(saxophone)*, Thomas Dolby *(keyboards)*, Tessa Niles, Helena Springs *(backing vocals)*

Repertoire (Live Aid): 'TVC15' / 'Rebel Rebel' / 'Modern Love' / '"Heroes"' / 'Let It Be' / 'Do They Know It's Christmas?'

On 23 March 1985 Bowie made a surprise appearance during the encores of a show on Tina Turner's Private Dancer tour at the Birmingham NEC. David Mallet filmed the concert, which has since been aired on television and released on video. Sporting a white jacket, wing collar, black trousers and one of his less successful hairstyles, Bowie joined Tina in a duet of 'Tonight' and a medley combining Chris Montez's 'Let's Dance' with his own hit of the same name. The performance – not one of David's greatest moments – appeared on various Tina Turner compilations, including 1988's *Live In Europe*, the 1992 CD single 'I Want You Near Me', and the 1994 CD & Video double pack *Tina Live – Private Dancer Tour*.

During the 'Absolute Beginners' sessions at Abbey Road three months later, Bowie informed his group that "I've got this little gig – can you do it?" Ever since Bob Geldof had confirmed plans for a concert on 13 July in aid of Ethiopian famine relief, Bowie had been high on his wish list. Plans for a transatlantic satellite link-up with Mick Jagger were abandoned and in its place came the recording of 'Dancing In The Street' (see Chapter 1). Thereafter, augmented by keyboard wizard Thomas Dolby and saxophonist Clare Hurst, the band rehearsed a shortlist of seven songs on three consecutive Sundays at Bray and Elstree Studios. The final rehearsal was recorded and each band member given a tape.

Bowie's technical preparations for Live Aid were among the most meticulous of the day. According to the compère Andy Peebles, "his army took over" from the Live Aid crew for the duration of his set. At midnight on 12 July Bowie was still backstage at Wembley, examining blueprints and discussing the stadium's dead spots. Allegedly he even scripted Peebles's introduction.

In a double-breasted grey suit and gravity-defying blow-dry (provided the previous day by Freddie Mercury's partner Jim Hutton), Bowie at Live Aid cut a figure somewhere between his Serious Moonlight and Diamond Dogs personae. Early in the day he spent an hour in the royal box with the Prince and Princess of Wales. His set began at 7.20pm with a rollicking 'TVC15', followed by smooth, sax-driven versions of 'Rebel Rebel' and 'Modern Love', and finally the undisputed highlight, a splendid '"Heroes"' which Bowie dedicated "to my son, to all our children, and to the children of the world."

The general consensus is that Queen stole the show at Live Aid, but with his uniquely evocative '"Heroes"' Bowie came an honourable second. He was originally to have played another number, 'Five Years', but at the last minute he sacrificed the remainder of his allotted time to introduce a film compiled from newsreel footage of the Ethiopian famine. Bob Geldof later recalled showing David the video backstage: "Bowie was sobbing … he says, I want to drop a song and introduce this." Sure enough, as the band left the stage David announced, "Let us not forget why we are here. People are still starving." The film, backed by The Cars' 'Drive', remains one of the abiding images of Live Aid. "That tape was the turn-around moment in the entire event," said Geldof. More money was pledged immediately after its transmission than at any other time during the concert.

Bowie's contribution to Live Aid didn't end with his set: in addition to the screenings of 'Dancing In The Street', he joined the all-star backing group who helped Paul McCartney through a technically hampered 'Let It Be', and sang the opening line of 'Do They Know It's Christmas?' for the final encore. "We should make it an annual event," he enthused afterwards. For many years the Live Aid recordings remained unreleased, but at the time of writing a DVD is scheduled for Christmas 2004.

In the twenty months following Live Aid Bowie made only two concert appearances. The first came on 19 November 1985 when he took to the stage at New York's China Club for an impromptu jam on 'China Girl' and other numbers with a band including Iggy Pop, Stevie Winwood, Carlos Alomar, Carmine Rojas and Ron Wood (the occasion was the birthday of *Labyrinth* drummer Steve Ferrone, who also played). The second was his live performance of 'Dancing In The Street' with Mick Jagger at the Prince's Trust Concert at Wembley Arena on 20 June 1986. A little under a year later, with a new album under his belt, Bowie was back on the road.

THE GLASS SPIDER TOUR
30 May – 28 November 1987

Musicians: David Bowie *(vocals, guitar)*, Peter Frampton *(guitar)*, Carlos Alomar *(guitar)*, Carmine Rojas *(bass)*, Alan Childs *(drums)*, Erdal Kizilcay *(keyboards, trumpet, congas, violin)*, Richard Cottle *(keyboards, saxophone)*, Melissa Hurley, Constance Marie, Viktor Manoei, Stephen Nichols, Craig Allen Rothwell aka "Spazz Attack" *(dancers)*

Repertoire: 'Up The Hill Backwards' / 'Glass Spider' / 'Day-In Day-Out' / 'Bang Bang' / 'Absolute Beginners' / 'Loving The Alien' / 'China Girl' / 'Rebel Rebel' / 'Fashion' / 'Scary Monsters (And Super Creeps)' / 'All The Madmen' / 'Never Let Me Down' / 'Big Brother' / 'Chant Of the Ever Circling Skeletal Family' / "87 And Cry' / '"Heroes"' / 'Sons Of The Silent Age' / 'Time Will Crawl' / 'Young Americans' / 'Beat Of Your Drum' / 'New York's In Love' / 'The Jean Genie' / 'Dancing With The Big Boys' / 'Zeroes' / 'Let's Dance' / 'Time' / 'Fame' / 'Blue Jean' / 'I Wanna Be Your Dog' / 'White Light/White Heat' / 'Modern Love'

In March 1987 Bowie took a five-piece backing group to press conferences in Toronto, New York, London, Paris, Madrid, Rome, Munich, Stockholm and Amsterdam, previewing his forthcoming world tour with performances of 'Day-In Day-Out', 'Bang Bang' and "87 And Cry'. He promised that the tour itself would be "overflowing with make-up, costumes and theatrical sets" (sadly not "theatrical sex", as one of the British tabloids excitedly reported).

The fact that the press conferences were mini-concerts in themselves is an indication of the commercial scale of Bowie's new undertaking. Glass Spider was to be his most extravagant rock-theatre spectacular since the Diamond Dogs show – but now the venues were massive stadiums and the budgets and expectations were far higher. In the spring of 1987 Bowie negotiated a sponsorship deal with Pepsi, for whom he filmed a commercial with Tina Turner (see *Creation* in Chapter 6). There was a feeling of betrayal in some quarters that rock's great outsider, whose anti-American anger was still manifest in 'Day-In Day-Out', should be linking arms with one of the quintessential symbols of corporate business. Bowie freely admitted that the motive was to raise capital for a massively expensive tour. "I could have afforded to tour on my own, but I couldn't have afforded to tour

in quite such an elaborate way," he told *i-D* magazine.

The key creative personnel were all veterans of past extravaganzas. Lighting design was in the hands of Serious Moonlight's Allen Branton, while Mark Ravitz once again designed the stage set, but perhaps most significant was the return of Diamond Dogs choreographer Toni Basil. Since last working with David, she had choreographed Talking Heads and scored a hit of her own, 1982's transatlantic smash 'Mickey'. In collaboration with New York's avant-garde ISO Dance Theater, Basil devised a series of *outré* routines and recruited five professional dancers to develop them with David, who attested to collecting "lots of bruises" during rehearsal. To allow the necessary freedom of movement, for the first time he elected to use headset mikes of the kind pioneered by Kate Bush on her 1979 Tour Of Life.

In early April the promotional band, now augmented by the addition of Erdal Kizilcay, began an eight-week rehearsal period in New York. Work shifted the following month to Rotterdam's Ahoy Hall and Feyenoord Stadium, where Ravitz's breathtakingly preposterous "Spider Environment" had been constructed: a network of scaffolding and catwalks reminiscent of his original Hunger City set, dwarfed by a fifty-foot-high spider whose glowing body and illuminated legs framed the split-level stage. Bowie told reporters that the show, like the song it was named after, was "based on that part of a child's life when he realizes he can't rely on his parents forever." He promised "a lot of elements, movement, dialogue, fragments of film, projected images. Ultra-theatrical … The show has a slight narrative form that's tenuous to say the least; it's almost what I believe a modern musical should look like. It has a lot to do with the audience and how they perceive rock music and all those clichés and stereotypes." Promotional billboards displayed a chaotic collage of rehearsal shots, tigers, spiders, horses and circus clowns.

The show that opened in Rotterdam on 30 May was nothing if not spectacular, beginning with a protracted rock-star entrance which ensured that the audience had already worked itself into a frenzy by the time David appeared. After a pre-show tape of The Kronos Quartet's classical arrangement of 'Purple Haze', Carlos Alomar appeared alone on stage, thrashing up a storm of Hendrix-style guitar reminiscent of Robert Fripp's performance on 'It's No Game'. True to the original he was cut off in his prime by a disembodied but familiar scream of "Shut up!", eliciting an outbreak of mass hysteria from the crowd. Suddenly the stage was alive with activity as four of the dancers abseiled to the stage from the belly of the giant spider. Garishly attired like the extras in the 'Ashes To Ashes' and 'Fashion' videos – leathers, tutus, New Romantic make-up and *Rocky Horror* drag – the dancers mimed to the first of several pre-recorded dialogue interludes, a cut-up of images of urban brutality, before moving into the first verse of 'Up The Hill Backwards'. Finally the music segued into the opening chords of 'Glass Spider', and as Bowie's voice was heard intoning the spoken narration, he emerged at last from the spider's mandibles, descending to the stage in a chair and speaking into a telephone in the style of 1974's 'Space Oddity' routine. From then on all hell broke loose as Peter Frampton burst from the shadows to deliver the first of many guitar solos, the dancers enacted frantic spidery movements, and Bowie, in a refulgent red suit and spats, danced downstage to meet his public.

The remainder of the show was a non-stop blitzkrieg of crazed routines. At the beginning of 'Bang Bang' David hurled himself at the audience, Iggy Pop-style, only to be pulled back by the dancers who then dragged a screaming fan from the front row and thrust her towards him. When David started to fondle her he received a slap in the face and was dragged into a raunchy *pas de deux* as the girl, Melissa Hurley, dropped her screaming fan act and revealed herself to be the fifth member of the dance team, planted in the front row in a lampoon of the transparent fakery of Bruce Springsteen's 'Dancing In The Dark' video (not to mention Bono's real-life re-enactment of it at Live Aid).

After some more barely comprehensible dialogue during the intro to 'Absolute Beginners' ("We can't have rock stars cross-breeding with normal people!"), Bowie embarked on a long and elaborate vogue routine with dancer Viktor Manoei, while the others unravelled Melissa Hurley's dress to create a new backdrop. 'Loving The Alien' offered an elaborate dumb-show in which Bowie and the dancers became blind-folded "believers". 'Scary Monsters' found David prowling the catwalks way above the stage. 'Fashion' heralded a staggering piece of choreography marrying the 1974 boxing mime with a new sequence in which the dancers physically hurled Bowie about the set. For 'Never Let Me Down' he knelt downstage, wilting between verses only to be revived by Melissa Hurley's oxygen mask. "87 And Cry' adapted another Diamond Dogs routine as David, now in a futuristic

jumpsuit, was tied up with ropes by helmeted astro-nauts. In 'Sons Of The Silent Age' Peter Frampton took over the chorus while Bowie acted as puppeteer to Constance Marie's remarkable contortionist act. For 'Let's Dance', Hurley and Nichols performed a body-popping duet while the others' giant silhouettes were projected against the backdrop.

Most extravagant of all was 'Time': head to foot in gold lamé, Bowie perched atop the giant spider, sporting a pair of angel's wings which unfurled on cue. During the first chorus he descended into the body of the spider and abseiled back to the stage, in the process incorporating a meticulous recreation of "The Hanged Man" of the Tarot, his outstretched arms and crossed-leg posture hailing specifically from the 1942 Thoth Tarot deck designed by none other than Aleister Crowley: this transmogrification from angel to Crowley's Hanged Man was one of several echoes of darker times incorporated into the show, most of which were entirely lost on the audience.

During an extended 'Fame' the dancers assembled a Sputnik-like sculpture out of drums, music stands and guitar fretboards, winched it aloft and joined David in a body-thrashing dance. The final 'Modern Love' was choreographed as an extended walk-down and bow. Throughout it all, Allen Branton's massive light show surpassed even his Serious Moonlight achievements. The spider changed colour from blue to pink to gold to green, while the barrage of Vari-lites set into its belly created landscapes of colour and light that changed with each song: twinkling blue stars for 'Glass Spider', banks of yellow squares forming a city skyline for 'China Girl', and madly flashing spotlights for 'Rebel Rebel'.

In short, the show was outrageous and utterly unprecedented. Stadium bands like Kiss and Queen had staged pyrotechnic spectaculars before, but no rock show had ever approached Glass Spider's mind-boggling circus of light, sound and contemporary dance. As theatre, it was spellbinding – if you were close enough to see what was going on. What suffered, inevitably, was the music.

Bowie himself was garlanded with praise. *Smash Hits* dubbed him "a living legend" whose singing was "excellent" and who looked "barely older than he did 15 years ago as Ziggy Stardust." The *Los Angeles Times* gushed about his "radiant, sexy superstar aura that may not have been equalled in pop-rock since Presley," while the *Independent* paid homage to "the visage of the rock idol with the polish of the Vegas crooner." But of the show itself, reservations abounded. "The star was there," continued the *Independent*, "what was in alarmingly short supply was taste … Bowie has built a career on making hollowness inspirational so it's surprising that such a past master should have lost the knack of structuring a spectacle." *Smash Hits* complained that the frantic stage activity was impossible to follow, branding the dialogue interludes "completely unintelligible" and adding that "if it wasn't for his bright red suit, you'd be hard pressed to say which scurrying, ant-like figure was David Bowie." *Melody Maker* found a "paucity of ideas" and *Sounds* dismissed the show as "frenzied schlock and half-baked goofing". There were even unkind comments about the latest hairstyle: fifteen years earlier it had looked exotic and striking when framing the visage of Aladdin Sane, but by 1987 it had become known as the "mullet" and was irredeemably uncool, associated with an endless parade of Euro-soft-rockers and celebrity footballers.

Despite the reviews, the tour did phenomenal business, progressing through 86 performances in 15 countries. The opening night in Rotterdam was the sixteenth birthday of Bowie's son, who was introduced to the audience for a 60,000-strong singalong of 'Happy Birthday'. On 6 June David held a press conference at Berlin's Hansa By The Wall, in the very room where he had recorded *"Heroes"* ten years earlier. On the same evening he headlined the last night of a three-day festival in the Platz der Republik, and thousands of East German fans gathered on the opposite side of the Berlin Wall to hear the concert. Border police eventually dispersed the gathering with tear gas, and the ugly scenes were later described by *Bild* as "a defining moment" in the pro-unification climate that would bring down the Wall two years later. "I'll never forget that," Bowie recalled in 2003. "It was one of the most emotional performances I've ever done. I was in tears. They'd backed up the stage to the wall itself so that the wall was acting as our backdrop. We kind of heard that a few of the East Berliners might actually get the chance to hear the thing, but we didn't realize in what numbers they would. And there were thousands on the other side that had come close to the wall. So it was like a double concert where the wall was the division. And we could hear them cheering and singing along from the other side. God, even now I get choked up. It was breaking my heart. I'd never done anything like that in my life, and I guess I never will again. When we did '"Heroes"' it really felt

anthemic, almost like a prayer. However well we do it these days, it's almost like walking through it compared to that night, because it meant so much more. That's the town where it was written, and that's the particular situation that it was written about."

In Florence, tragically, a lighting engineer was killed when he fell from the scaffolding. But foremost among the tabloid tattle that followed the tour were the events of 9 October, when a woman called Wanda Lee Nichols alleged that Bowie had assaulted her "in a Dracula-like fashion" in a Dallas hotel room. When the case eventually came to court it was dismissed within two hours, but in the meantime Pepsi made the precipitate decision to withdraw their television commercial.

Although it was certainly derided in some quarters from the very outset, the Glass Spider tour's notoriety has since snowballed out of all proportion. It's customarily likened to the worst excesses of *Spinal Tap*, and of course it was always going to be anathema to those who think rock stars should stand downstage with only a guitar and a mike-stand for company. All such criticisms might be dismissed if only the music itself had shone through as it should, but sadly it was this, and nothing to do with the dance routines, that was Glass Spider's biggest pitfall. In many ways it was a beautifully full and professional sound, but what it lacked was the necessary bite, its ever-present spangles of synthesizer smoothing away the native edginess of songs like 'The Jean Genie' and 'Time'. Tellingly, the numbers that really succeeded were often those unfettered by choreography: as *Rolling Stone* noted of the East Rutherford show, "When Bowie cast off the frills and ripped through 'Rebel Rebel' and 'China Girl', he displayed all the authority for which his shows are renowned … Unfortunately, they only served to make the excesses more apparent."

Just as he had during the Diamond Dogs tour, Bowie rapidly grew tired of playing to a script. Several of the *Never Let Me Down* numbers were dropped mid-tour ('New York's In Love' didn't make it past the first seven dates), while 'The Jean Genie' and 'Young Americans' were drafted in as crowd-pleasers. By the time the *Glass Spider* video was recorded during the eight-show residency at the Sydney Entertainment Centre, Bowie's sense of relief during the unadorned straight-to-audience numbers was palpable. He was visibly invigorated by the chance to bring a tougher guitar sound to the show in a duet with guest guitarist Charlie Sexton (the first time in many moons, incidentally, that Bowie had picked up an electric guitar on stage). The last of four shows in Melbourne the following week saw much of the spider set and production numbers abandoned due to high winds and heavy rain. Five days later, on 28 November, the tour closed in Auckland. "It was so great to burn the spider in New Zealand at the end of the tour," David remarked later. "We just put the thing in a field and set light to it. That was such a relief!"

In later years Bowie would look back on the tour with diminishing affection. The first major interview with Tin Machine, in Q magazine's June 1989 issue, saw Bowie's new colleagues launch an attack on the Glass Spider show that appeared to take David somewhat by surprise. "To come to its defence, I liked the video of it," he said. "But I overstretched … It was so big and so unwieldy and everybody had a problem all the time, every day, and I was under so much *pressure* … I just had to grit my teeth and get through it which is not a great way of working."

Even so, Bowie has leapt to the show's defence on more than one occasion, pointing out in 1997 that it was considerably more successful when it played smaller, indoor venues: "I'd designed it to be an all-enveloping kind of spectacular, inasmuch as it was a bit three-ring circus, there were always three or four events happening at the same time on stage … Individually there were some incredibly good ideas on that stage, and in a small environment it really worked well … but when you're a thousand rows back it just becomes this huge mass of confusion. None of it makes any sense, and that was a really bad mistake." As the Wembley audiences discovered to their cost, the mistake was compounded when bad weather scuppered not only Bowie's flying angel routine but also the overall acoustics; 1987 was a poor summer and many of the European concerts were blighted by wind and rain, while daylight conditions negated many of the lighting effects that make such an impression on the video version.

But the Glass Spider tour was by no means the bloated disaster of repute, and even Bowie has now written it off a little too zealously. For one thing, the show was unavoidably a victim of bad timing. In the post-Live Aid atmosphere there was a general feeling that rock's aristocracy was due for a drubbing, and Bowie was not alone in attracting ridicule in 1987. Veteran journalist Chris Roberts, then with *Melody Maker*, enjoyed the show but found himself under "overwhelming peer group pressure not to like it."

For another thing, although it has come to be regarded as the epitome of overblown stadium excess, Glass Spider was hugely influential. The cutting-edge ensemble choreography which soon became *de rigueur* among stadium superstars like Prince, Madonna and Jacksons Michael and Janet (not to mention the relentless parade of synchro-dancing boy bands), owes a tremendous debt to Glass Spider. Paula Abdul's group abseiled onto the stage at the 1990 Grammy Awards. The Rolling Stones' 1989/90 Steel Wheels tour borrowed freely from the show, while U2, the Pet Shop Boys and indeed Bowie himself recycled the multimedia aspects to develop future live concepts. The immaculate 'Absolute Beginners' routine brought vogue-dancing out of New York's gay clubs and into mainstream pop a full three years before Madonna's hit single, and provided a springboard for the visuals of Bowie's own 1990 tour.

And when the set-list strayed away from *Never Let Me Down* and the obligatory golden oldies, it was positively thrilling. The emphasis on *Scary Monsters (And Super Creeps)* is revealing, particularly when it emerges that 'Scream Like A Baby' and 'Because You're Young' were still being rehearsed in Rotterdam mere days before the tour opened. Sadly they were abandoned before the first show (as was the less enticing 'Shining Star'), but other rarities made the final selection: no other Bowie tour has offered 'Up The Hill Backwards', 'All The Madmen' or 'Sons Of The Silent Age'. The unexpected revival of 'Big Brother', complete with a blockbusting Latin drum solo, was a huge treat. Better still, as the video reveals, when the songs really gelled they were terrific. The surprisingly hard-rocking renditions of 'China Girl', 'Blue Jean', 'I Wanna Be Your Dog' and 'White Light/White Heat' give the lie to accusations of sludgy, middle-of-the-road performances, and the combination of tight guitar work and Richard Cottle's superb saxophone breaks in 'Sons Of The Silent Age' and 'Young Americans' is positively blissful.

The Glass Spider tour wrought two other major developments in Bowie's life. Firstly, he entered into a relationship with dancer Melissa Hurley: "We fell in love after the tour was over, while having a holiday in Australia," said Bowie later. The couple became engaged and rumours of an imminent marriage persisted until, three years later, they quietly parted. Another three years passed before Bowie spoke of the relationship, recalling Melissa as "such a wonderful, lovely, vibrant girl … I guess it became one of those older men, younger girl situations where I had the joy of taking her around the world and showing her things. But it became obvious to me that it just wasn't going to work out as a relationship – and for that she would thank me one of these days. So I broke off the engagement."

The second by-product of the Glass Spider tour was another relationship, this time a creative one. In November 1987 Bowie was given a cassette by Sarah Gabrels, a PA on the tour. It was a tape of guitar demos by her husband Reeves, and within a matter of days it had set Bowie in a new direction – one which he would later acknowledge as the path to his salvation as an artist.

INTRUDERS AT THE PALACE / WRAP AROUND THE WORLD
1 July 1988 / 10 September 1988

Musicians: David Bowie *(vocals, guitar)*, Reeves Gabrels *(guitar)*, Kevin Armstrong *(guitar)*, Erdal Kizilcay *(bass)*

Repertoire: 'Look Back In Anger'

1988 was the first year for two decades in which not a single new Bowie record was released, and David's only major public endeavour was a one-off performance at London's Dominion Theatre as part of "Intruders At The Palace", a benefit concert in aid of the Institute for Contemporary Arts. Bowie elected to present a suitably avant-garde interpretation of one of his songs in collaboration with Edouard Lock, principal designer and choreographer for the Montreal-based dance group La La La Human Steps, whom he had originally approached in 1987 with a view to working on the Glass Spider tour. Bowie later described the group as operating "where punk and ballet clash"; their experimental dance works, with titles like *Human Sex*, *New Demons* and *Businessman In The Process Of Becoming An Angel*, combined extreme, almost violently gymnastic choreography with spectacular mixed-media visuals to produce works of chaotic energy. "It's not mime, it's not dance," said Bowie. "It's something else."

For the ICA show Bowie and Lock devised a cutting-edge routine with the group's principal dancer Louise LeCavalier. The eight-minute performance of 'Look Back In Anger' that emerged was a fascinating moment of transition between Glass Spider and Tin Machine, distilling the best of both without the unpalatable excesses of either. The gutsy, acrobatic dancing was an obvious progression from the previous tour, and Lock's pre-recorded big-screen projections of Bowie and LeCavalier, mimicking the paces they were simultaneously enacting on stage, was a refinement of Glass Spider's '"Heroes"' sequence. Meanwhile Bowie's plain charcoal suit and the aggressive, metallic guitar sound emanating from his backing group provided a taste of things to come. It was captivating, and to many observers it delivered more in eight minutes than Bowie had achieved in the preceding five years. Chris Roberts raved in *Melody Maker* that "It wasn't a relative of pop. It was purely fantastical … They slap one another across the face, tickle the chin, hurl, whirl and assault. The flickering video shows Bowie and LeCavalier, monochrome icons freezing with fear and lust…"

For Bowie, the ICA gig was to have far-reaching consequences. Lock's interactive video-projection techniques and LeCavalier's body-thrashing dance style would later form the touchstone of the Sound + Vision tour. More significantly, the ICA gig marked Bowie's first collaboration with Reeves Gabrels (see *Tin Machine* in Chapter 2), who played guitar alongside Live Aid's Kevin Armstrong and Glass Spider's Erdal Kizilcay. For the first and only time in Bowie's live career, the percussion was provided solely by a drum-machine. The group also recorded a studio version of the revamped 'Look Back In Anger', which later appeared as a bonus track on the 1991 reissue of *Lodger*.

On 10 September 1988, the 'Look Back In Anger' performance was reprised as part of an ambitious live global television link-up called *Wrap Around The World*. Masterminded from PBS's New York studios by the Korean video artist Nam June Paik, the event involved broadcasts from New York, Tokyo, Seoul, Jerusalem and Rio de Janeiro, which were beamed to participating countries across the world including Japan, South Korea, China, the Soviet Union, the US, Germany, Israel and Brazil. Bowie was at the WNET Studios in New York where, in addition to presenting the 'Look Back In Anger' performance, he held a conversation via satellite with his sometime movie co-star Ryuichi Sakamoto, who performed live from Tokyo.

THE 1989 TIN MACHINE TOUR
14 June – 3 July 1989 (plus 4 November 1989)

Musicians: David Bowie *(vocals, guitar)*, Reeves Gabrels *(guitar)*, Tony Sales *(bass)*, Hunt Sales *(drums, vocals)*, Kevin Armstrong *(guitar)*

Repertoire: 'Amazing' / 'Heaven's In Here' / 'Sacrifice Yourself' / 'Working Class Hero' / 'Prisoner Of Love' / 'Sorry' / 'Now' / 'Bus Stop' / 'Run' / 'Tin Machine' / 'Maggie's Farm' / 'I Can't Read' / 'Shakin' All Over' / 'Baby Can Dance' / 'Pretty Thing' / 'Crack City' / 'Under The God' / 'You've Been Around'

Tin Machine's first live performance was a secret warm-up gig in the spring of 1989 at a club in Nassau, while the album sessions were still in progress. "We weren't announced," said Reeves Gabrels. "We just walked up on stage and you could hear all these voices whispering, That's David Bowie! No, it can't be David Bowie, he's got a beard!" Following this low-key baptism and an appearance performing 'Heaven's In Here' at the International Music Awards in New York on 31 May (after which Tina Turner's mother told a reporter that "I liked it better when David was singing songs!"), rehearsals continued in Manhattan for a small-scale inaugural tour. There were to be only twelve shows in all – three in America, four on mainland Europe and five in Britain – and all in venues with a capacity of no more than 2000. It was an intense reaction against the expansiveness of the Glass Spider circus. "Non-theatrical, definitely," Bowie declared. "Just a six-piece horn section and a trapeze artist!"

Joined on stage by their often overlooked fifth member Kevin Armstrong, the 1989 incarnation of Tin Machine cut a straightforward, monochrome dash in black trousers, white shirts and – at the beginning of the evening at least – jackets and ties. Otherwise the visuals were restricted to a few stark lighting effects. It was a studiously stripped-down garage aesthetic, but it was inevitably rendered theatrical by the very fact that the bearded, perspiring, chain-smoking vocalist within a fingertip's reach of the audience was a global superstar who had seldom played venues this small since 1973 – indeed one of them, St George's Hall in Bradford, was a veteran of the Ziggy Stardust tour.

The set-list, too, was entirely uncompromising. Bowie had made it clear that his current enthusiasms began and ended with Tin Machine, but nobody had seriously imagined he wouldn't throw in the occasional oldie – a hard-boiled 'Scary Monsters' perhaps, or a guitar-heavy 'Suffragette City'. But it was not to be. Tin Machine stuck to their own songbook: the whole of the first album save 'Video Crime', bolstered by a trio of new compositions and a couple of hoary 1960s covers. The absence of Bowie's back catalogue was a source of disappointment to some, but without a doubt it was the decisive factor in cementing Tin Machine's genuine band identity. In a move that was to develop further on the second tour, Bowie even surrendered centre stage to Hunt Sales for one number, a prototype of the *Tin Machine II* track 'Sorry'. This and other try-outs were indicative of the wholesale rejection of the scripted shows that had peaked with Glass Spider. "Thirty per cent of every night was improvisation," Gabrels tells David Buckley, "and the Sales brothers were rooted in that."

In Amsterdam on 24 June, video screens were erected outside the 1500-seater venue to mollify the 25,000-strong crowd that had gathered in the hope of getting tickets. At this gig the little-seen 'Maggie's Farm' video was shot, while the accompanying single and sundry live B-sides were recorded the following night at La Cigale in Paris. Excerpts from the same show were broadcast on Westwood One FM radio.

As might have been predicted from the album, the amplified cacophony that issued from the speakers was not for the faint-hearted. The show was sweaty, unpolished, bowel-shatteringly loud, and quite unlike anything Bowie had done since his days fronting The Lower Third. For the devotee it was exhilarating, for others something of a challenge, but it had its admirers among the press. "Mr Bowie couldn't completely give up theatricality any more than Johnny Cash could give up wearing black," wrote Jon Pareles in the *New York Times*. "The lighting, while not too fancy, provided more variation than the average club setup – white-and-shadow effects designed to emphasize how stark the setting was. And Mr Bowie has retained his easy grace onstage." Such praise was thin on the ground, however. Most critics would have preferred to hear 'Let's Dance' and slammed the shows accordingly. Still smarting from the poor reception accorded to Glass Spider, Bowie's resolve hardened and he all but quoted the self-pitying lyrics of 'I Can't Read' to one reporter: "I can't get anything right. I can't go big. I can't go small. Whichever way I go is wrong."

The tour ended on 3 July, and a few days later Bowie opened the £1m Brixton Community Centre, partially funded by his charity concert at Hammersmith Odeon in 1983. He then took a holiday in Indonesia while Reeves Gabrels played guitar for The Mission's forthcoming album *Carved In Sand*. Later in the year Tin Machine reconvened in Australia to begin work on their second album, playing a one-off gig at Moby Dick's in Sydney on 4 November. Recording continued on and off until January 1990, when the project was temporarily suspended as Bowie unexpectedly announced his return to the stadium arena for his biggest solo tour yet.

THE SOUND + VISION TOUR

4 March – 29 September 1990

Musicians: David Bowie *(vocals, guitar, saxophone)*, Adrian Belew *(guitar)*, Erdal Kizilcay *(bass)*, Michael Hodges *(drums)*, Rick Fox *(keyboards)*

Repertoire: 'Space Oddity' / 'Changes' / 'TVC15' / 'Rebel Rebel' / 'Golden Years' / 'Be My Wife' / 'Ashes To Ashes' / 'John, I'm Only Dancing' / 'Queen Bitch' / 'Starman' / 'Fashion' / 'Life On Mars?' / 'Blue Jean' / 'Let's Dance' / 'Stay' / 'China Girl' / 'Ziggy Stardust' / 'Sound And Vision' / 'Station To Station' / 'Alabama Song' / 'Young Americans' / 'Panic In Detroit' / 'Suffragette City' / 'Fame' / '"Heroes"' / 'The Jean Genie' / 'Gloria' / 'Pretty Pink Rose' / 'Modern Love' / 'Rock'n'Roll Suicide' / 'White Light/White Heat' / 'Waiting For The Man'

Barely six months after touring Tin Machine's hard-rock repertoire around a handful of club venues, a newly beardless David appeared at press conferences in New York and London to unveil a massive seven-month solo tour whose statistics would surpass even Serious Moonlight and Glass Spider: 106 performances in 24 countries, including his first forays into eastern Europe and South America, the latter marking the first Argentinian concert by a British artist since the Falklands War.

Uniquely, the tour had no new album to promote. The impetus came from EMI in conjunction with the Massachusetts-based label Rykodisc, who in 1989 had begun remastering and reissuing Bowie's former RCA catalogue, beginning with the lavish box set *Sound + Vision*. While David immersed himself in Tin Machine, Ryko had been pressing him to promote the reissue programme with a "greatest hits" tour. "It's

been thrown at me for some years," he told reporters, "Both from audiences and from producers of rock shows, who've said, Why don't you just go all the way and do all the songs that they know? You've never done it and it'd be great. I'd go, Oh, I don't want to; it's corny, no. Then I gave in last year when Ryko said it would be great if you would help support this thing."

To quash suggestions that a greatest hits tour smacked of a sell-out, Bowie had hatched a couple of gimmicks guaranteed to generate a *frisson* among the faithful and mass publicity everywhere else. Firstly, it was announced that the set-list for the tour would be partially determined by the most popular titles logged in an international telephone poll. Secondly, and far more shockingly, Bowie nonchalantly declared that the price of his agreeing to the tour was that thereafter he would never perform his greatest hits again.

It was a master stroke of publicity. Bowie explained the reasons behind the decision: "I went away and thought, Well, I've never done it before, I'm sure by the end I'll never want to do it again, so what about if I do these songs for the last time – just do them on this tour and never do them again? That would give me a motivation for the entire tour, knowing each night that I do them, I get that much closer to never singing 'Ground Control to Major Tom…' again." Elsewhere he admitted, "I know I'll miss them desperately. They're very fine songs to work with and I love singing most of them, but I don't want to feel that I can always fall back on them." The press thrilled to the idea, and pre-tour sales were phenomenal. In Britain, two dates at the 12,000-seater Docklands Arena sold out immediately, and when a third concert was added the tickets went in eight minutes flat. Bowie's initial resolve to avoid playing open-air venues went out of the window as demand escalated. Extra UK dates were added for later in the summer at Manchester's Maine Road stadium and the 65,000-capacity Milton Keynes Bowl.

The presentation of the tour took its cue from a combination of the Glass Spider and Tin Machine shows. Bowie assembled a pared-down backing group of four musicians – other than Tin Machine, his smallest live band since the early Ziggy concerts in 1972. "I've noted that there's been a great emphasis on the older bands and older artists to go out with very large contingents," he told MTV, "so I thought, okay, just do the opposite then … Stripped-down, I think is the word, so that it does become a keyboards, bass, drums, lead guitar interpretation of the songs that I've done over the years."

The only familiar face from recent times was Glass Spider veteran Erdal Kizilcay, now promoted to bass guitar. Bowie initially asked Reeves Gabrels to play lead guitar, but Gabrels declined the offer on the grounds that it would invalidate the Tin Machine project: "We were trying to make the band point," Gabrels explained later, "and if I'd done the tour, the Sales brothers would have been pissed off and it would have confused the issue a whole lot more." Instead Bowie appointed Adrian Belew, last heard on *Lodger* and the Stage tour, as musical director and lead guitarist. In the years since working with Bowie, Belew had pursued a solo career as well as playing with Paul Simon, Tom Tom Club, Talking Heads and Robert Fripp's resurrected King Crimson.

"I wanted the band to sound very plain and unadorned," Belew told *International Musician*. "I also wanted them to go from sounding like an orchestra for 'Life On Mars?' to sounding like a garage band for 'Panic In Detroit'." In January 1990 Bowie contributed two songs to Belew's solo album *Young Lions*, as a result of which he recruited Belew's keyboardist Rick Fox and drummer Michael Hodges. When asked why, for the first time since 1974, he was embarking on a solo tour without his trusty sideman Carlos Alomar, David explained: "Carlos is a wonderful guitar player with whom I'm sure I'll work again, but the fact that he is so familiar with the songs is the reason I didn't choose him for this tour. It needed the air of unfamiliarity." He also suggested that despite the show's retrospective nature he was approaching the material in a new context: "I didn't have to think myself back to rediscover what I was on about in any of those songs. I'm approaching it strictly from now."

With the predictable results of the telephone poll tweaked by some less obvious additions from David himself, the set list was whittled down to the obvious curtain-raiser 'Space Oddity' followed by two or three songs per album from *Hunky Dory* up to *Let's Dance*, with the balance marginally in favour of those perennial standard-bearers *Station To Station* (four songs) and *Ziggy Stardust* (five, plus 'John, I'm Only Dancing'). Curiously, the only album from this period other than *Pin Ups* to go entirely unrepresented was *Lodger* – the one featuring Adrian Belew – although the contemporaneous cover 'Alabama Song' was revived. Less surprisingly, the only post-1983 oldie to make the list was 'Blue Jean'. Held in New York in January 1990, initial rehearsals took only two weeks. Marrying the music with Bowie's latest visual concept took rather longer.

After the Glass Spider debacle, all eyes were on the staging of Sound + Vision, and here was where the tour moved into top gear. At the January press conference Bowie told reporters that the show would be "nowhere near as ambitious as Glass Spider in size, but qualitatively, in essence, I think it's as theatrical." To MTV he explained that "I want to keep the stage as minimalist as possible, I really wanted it to have the feel of an opera or ballet stage where it was just one large dark space that could be lit in a theatrical fashion." Against this setting the Canadian designer and choreographer Edouard Lock, with whom Bowie had collaborated on 1988's ICA benefit, was entrusted with realizing a spectacular new interactive concept. Central to the staging of the show was a gigantic gauze screen that would rise and fall at various times for the projection of pre-recorded video images and live relays, while the lighting phased the results through different levels of transparency. "We're using a real opera screen," explained Bowie. "It's the largest use of video ever: forty-foot by fifty-foot high video images through state-of-the-art projection systems built for it." He described the final effect as "like an enormous Javanese shadow puppet show."

The concept was grounded in Bowie's ongoing fascination with the distance between the perception of stardom and the reality, and thus was conceived the idea that he would interact on stage with projected images of himself. Scenographers Luc Dussault and Lyn Lefevre worked with Edouard Lock to devise the means of computer-controlling the screen projections, which were set in motion by a signal activated on Rick Fox's keyboard at the start of each song. The pre-recorded sequences, some of which were also used in the 'Fame 90' video, were directed by up-and-coming filmmaker Gus Van Sant, whose *Drugstore Cowboy* had wowed art-house critics the previous year. These comprised mainly black-and-white shots of Bowie playing his guitar and dancing with Louise LeCavalier, who had performed with David at the 1988 ICA gig. LeCavalier told the *Montreal Gazette* that she was very impressed by Bowie's "quality of movement ... He can be many things when he moves – both aristocratic and funky."

However, there was to be no return to the cluttered, over-busy dance routines of the Glass Spider show. "What I wanted to avoid was the usual pitfalls," explained Lock. "You can amplify sound to reach large areas; the problem is that the technology hasn't extended itself to visuals. You can still go to the stadium and see a pea on stage. You can't see anything of the performer's face … I don't think people come to stadiums for the music. They can listen to records if they want that. They come to the stadium to meet the artist … I wanted to build an architecture based around the person as opposed to the set."

Accordingly, the Sound + Vision set was black and bare by comparison with its predecessors. The only architectural detail was a gold-painted frieze of cherubs and gargoyles (laughing gnomes?) along the apron stage; otherwise the rigging was supplemented only by two gargantuan cloths hung on either side of the proscenium, presenting the audience with two titanic silhouettes: on the left, the shock-haired, thrashing figure of Louise LeCavalier, and on the right, the narcissistic, posing-into-the-microphone profile of Bowie himself.

The tour opened at La Colisée in Quebec on 4 March. During the pre-show music the gauze descended, blank and unlit, to cover the entire stage. As the music peaked, the two gigantic silhouettes on either side burst their moorings and billowed to the ground. Behind each, a bank of white light slammed up as the opening chords of 'Space Oddity' rang out. A fifty-foot high projection of Bowie's face faded into view and gazed down at the stage in profile, while through the gauze a spotlight picked out the tiny figure of David himself, strumming his guitar and singing the opening lines. The giant face rotated to survey the audience and its lips articulated Major Tom's countdown. "The crowd are amazed," wrote Steve Sutherland in *Melody Maker*, "No one has ever seen anything like this before." As entrances go, it was ten times simpler than Glass Spider and immeasurably more effective: at once epic and intimate, its visual impact was guaranteed even from the back row of the biggest stadium. Three weeks later, beginning at the Edinburgh show on 23 March, the drama of the opening sequence would be enhanced by a further plundering of Bowie history, as the regular pre-set music became the synthesized *Clockwork Orange* version of Beethoven's *Ode To Joy* – the same classical-futurist tape that had opened the Ziggy Stardust concerts.

The rest of the show was equally stunning. During 'Rebel Rebel' Bowie picked up a video camera and filmed the crowd, whose ecstatic faces were relayed onto the projection screen, fulfilling the breakdown of the artist/spectator confrontation long ago proposed in 'Andy Warhol': "put you all inside my show". For 'Life On Mars?' Bowie was dwarfed by his former self as the screen played the song's original 1973 video to devastatingly emotive effect. 'Let's Dance' and 'China Girl' were accompanied by wild, erotic dance duets between Bowie and LeCavalier. 'Fame' resurrected the vogue-dancing clip and flickering flames from the 1990 video.

Not every song was swamped by video effects: elsewhere the architecture was created by bold washes of light. 'Panic In Detroit' featured rotating red police lamps. 'Station To Station' saw Bowie looming over the footlights, lit eerily from beneath. For 'Ziggy Stardust' he played guitar, bathed in blood-red light and relishing the chance to ham up the never-again angle; at the end of the song he would slowly disentangle himself from his guitar, put it down on the stage and walk away, head in hands. There was room, too, for innovation in the form of a vigorous rendition of David's gift to Adrian Belew, 'Pretty Pink Rose', while 'Fame' segued into a disorientating recreation of the recently-released 'Fame 90 House Mix'. After the customary ritenuto on the line "break down and cry", 'Young Americans' developed into a sprawling blues workout incorporating a selection of old standards.

At the opening handful of Canadian concerts, Bowie was briefly joined on stage by Louise LeCavalier and Donald Weikert of La La La Human Steps, who performed a body-slamming dance during 'Suffragette City'; Bowie pulled Edouard Lock on stage for applause before the final encores.

Visually, then, the concerts were sensational. Bowie himself, trim in a charcoal Tin Machine suit and, after the short interval, foppishly remodelled as a latter-day Thin White Duke in swashbuckling lace-trimmed blouse and waistcoat, was on fine form. He played more guitar than on any tour since 1973, and added some freestyle saxophone to 'TVC15'. Reservations abounded, however, regarding the musical arrangements. The band produced an often weedy, thin little sound that rang hollowly around the cavernous arenas and outdoor stadiums. Adrian Belew has admitted that a four-piece band was unequal to the task: "a saxophone is vital on 'Young Americans', and I always felt that you couldn't fill that role with the guitar … it would have been nice to augment a few things here and there." Belew also claims that the backstage atmosphere was not always wonderful; he alone was permitted to join David in front of the screen for guitar duets and solos, while the rest of the band were all but concealed among the upstage flats. Belew reveals that his colleagues were "gravely disappointed" and that Rick Fox "nearly quit the tour several times", while an incident in which Erdal Kizilcay misinterpreted an ad-libbed gesture from David as an invitation to join him downstage resulted in an ugly scene.

Reviews were quick to criticize the instrumental shortcomings, although most had nothing but praise for the overall spectacle. The *Times* declared that Bowie's "presence was little short of majestic". *Melody Maker*, meanwhile, adored the visual concepts but laid into the band in no uncertain terms: "The turgid tub-thumpers are thankfully hidden behind columns, but the terminally pratty Adrian Belew, with his ghastly tie and ponytail, bounces about nauseatingly and labours under the delusion that weird guitar noises are automatically art."

It's always been customary for Bowie to shuffle his set-lists and drop a few numbers as a show develops, but seldom has there been such a drastic cull as on the Sound + Vision tour. In March Bowie was forced to truncate the set at his last two London gigs due to strain on his throat. His voice continued to suffer on the lengthy American leg, and during the summer a whole clutch of songs was struck off the playlist. Sadly but predictably, most of the casualties were among the more obscure and enticing numbers – those selected by Bowie rather than by the telephone poll. 'Queen Bitch' was relegated to a mid-song break in 'Fashion', and then dropped altogether. 'Be My Wife', 'Golden Years', 'TVC15', 'John, I'm Only Dancing', 'Alabama Song' and even 'Rock'n'Roll Suicide' bit the dust, while 'Starman' was only ever performed at a handful of gigs. The extended 'Young Americans' soul-jam was scrapped in favour of a mid-song jump into 'Suffragette City' after a piece of outrageous mummery in which Bowie really did "break down and cry", collapsing to the stage for anything up to two minutes (David's future collaborator Moby, who saw the show at Giants Stadium, later described this routine as "the coolest thing I've ever seen a musician do on stage", prompting Bowie to recall that "I just stayed there … just seeing how far I could take it"). But as Radio 1's live transmission of the superb Milton Keynes show on 5 August bore witness, there was still plenty to enjoy – including a new segue from 'The Jean Genie' into Van Morrison's 'Gloria'. This had its origins in the Cleveland show of 20 June, when U2's Bono had

joined Bowie on stage to duet on the number. A wide array of other covers would be incorporated into 'The Jean Genie' during the tour, including several that had a wider significance for Bowie, among them 'Tonight', 'I Wanna Be Your Dog' and 'Try Some, Buy Some'.

In Brussels on 21 April David unexpectedly embarked on the opening lines of 'Amsterdam' during the band introductions, but rapidly ground to a halt when it became clear he'd forgotten the words. Other unscheduled appearances during the tour were made by the old standard 'You And I And George' and the *West Side Story* number 'Maria'. The Tokyo concert on 16 May, which fell before the reshuffle and included many of the tour's rarer items, was broadcast on Japanese television. Also captured for TV were the Lisbon gig of 14 September and the tour's final night, before a 100,000-strong crowd in Buenos Aires on 29 September. Reports circulated that an official video shot in Paris was scheduled for a September 1991 release, but this never emerged.

The Sound + Vision tour may not have been the greatest musical showcase of Bowie's live career but, as its name suggested, the sound was only one half of the equation. As a piece of *son et lumière* the show was stunning, and at their best the ravishing visuals bristled with emotive power, as the always rapturous response to 'Life On Mars?' bore witness. And what of the much-vaunted pledge that this was the last ever outing for Bowie's back catalogue? "I have the same freedom as all of us – that is, to change my mind!" he laughed in 1999. He explained that what he'd really meant was that he would never again systematically tour his greatest hits and, give or take Glastonbury 2000, he has been true to his word. For the record, his first transgression of the pledge came in 1992 when he sang '"Heroes"' at the Freddie Mercury tribute concert, and over the ensuing years the vast majority of the Sound + Vision songs have gradually reappeared in the repertoire, alongside altogether more obscure and exciting revivals.

Thirteen years later, when promoting *Reality* and its accompanying world tour, Bowie told more than one interviewer that the main reason for Sound + Vision's most talked-about gimmick had been a lack of self-confidence in his new material: "It was such turmoil for me at that point," he admitted in 2003. "I didn't know if my songs were any good. I'd spread myself very thin and I didn't want to be intimidated by my own catalogue, so I thought I would really have to begin again. For myself, I would have to start anew, build a new catalogue and see where it takes me. What will I be like as a writer? Let's do it and find out. And as the nineties progressed I felt my writing was getting stronger and stronger … I now feel very confident about touring and putting new songs against old songs. I don't feel intimidated, it's as simple as that."

Following hard on the heels of the sense of closure afforded by the Sound + Vision tour, Bowie's personal life coincidentally took a major turn. During the tour his engagement to Melissa Hurley had come to an end, and at a dinner party on 14 October, only a fortnight after the last show, he was introduced to his future wife.

THE TIN MACHINE "IT'S MY LIFE" TOUR
5 October 1991 – 17 February 1992

Musicians: David Bowie *(vocals, guitar, saxophone)*, Reeves Gabrels *(guitar, vocals)*, Tony Sales *(bass, vocals)*, Hunt Sales *(drums, vocals)*, Eric Schermerhorn *(rhythm guitar, vocals)*

Repertoire: 'Bus Stop' / 'Sacrifice Yourself' / 'Goodbye Mr. Ed' / 'Amazing' / 'I Can't Read' / 'You Can't Talk' / 'Sorry' / 'One Shot' / 'Go Now' / 'Stateside' / 'Betty Wrong' / 'I've Been Waiting For You' / 'Under The God' / 'You Belong In Rock N'Roll' / 'Amlapura' / 'Baby Universal' / 'Debaser' / 'If There Is Something' / 'Heaven's In Here' / 'Shakin' All Over' / 'Shopping For Girls' / 'A Big Hurt' / 'Crack City' / 'Pretty Thing' / 'Tin Machine' / 'Baby Can Dance' / 'Waiting For The Man'

Bowie's first live appearance of 1991 was during the encores at a Morrissey concert in Los Angeles on 6 February, when the two performed a duet of Marc Bolan's 'Cosmic Dancer'. They had first been introduced backstage at David's Manchester gig the previous August, marking the first in a series of encounters over the next five years.

Later in 1991, the release of *Tin Machine II* heralded an outing far larger than the band's low-key 1989 tour. This time the itinerary took in 12 countries and 69 performances after a protracted period of warm-up gigs and press shows. Rehearsals began in July in St-Malo, France, and continued the following month at the Factory Studios in Dublin. After brief jaunts to London to appear on BBC1's *Paramount City* and *Wogan*, and to record a live BBC radio session on 13 August, the band returned to Dublin to play secret warm-up gigs at the Baggot Inn and the Waterfront Rock Café. "We're still only about halfway through rehearsals but it's coming together," Bowie told the *Irish Times*, "Hence the reason for doing these gigs. It's a chance to try out new material and count the mistakes." The *Sunday Tribune* reported that the band "crashed out heavy metal guitar solos and riotous drum rolls over Bowie's thin, nasal vocals." According to the *Irish Times*, "There were times at The Baggot and The Waterfront when the music's sense of primal release harkened back to the days when Mick Ronson was bending the frets as Bowie's chief Spider From Mars."

Tin Machine then departed for America to play a gimmicky press show on 25 August at Rockit Cargo LAX, an end-of-runway unit at Los Angeles Airport. The gig was later broadcast by ABC Television, and footage of the event, complete with aeroplanes whizzing overhead, was used in the 'Baby Universal' video. There followed a launch party for *Tin Machine II* on 27 August, at which Bowie fulfilled a lifetime's ambition when he met his earliest rock hero, Little Richard. "What I'd never realized," David later recounted, "is that he had an eye just like mine." After playing three more trade-only shows in America, Tin Machine flew to Milan for the tour's first night proper on 5 October.

Dubbed "It's My Life" after the publicity material's prominent use of the tattoo across Hunt Sales's shoulders, the tour was essentially a continuation of the band's previous no-frills staging. The lighting was a little more stagey, featuring a psychedelic lava-lamp swirl for 'You Belong In Rock N'Roll' and some ghostly footlighting for 'I Can't Read', but the biggest visual difference was Bowie himself. The bearded, middle-aged rocker of the 1989 tour was replaced by a clean-shaven and heavily tanned frontman who, for the first time since 1976, would often respond to the sweltering club temperatures by stripping off his shirt halfway through the set and continuing topless. Even when fully dressed, the band's attire was considerably less formal than the sombre charcoal suits of the previous tour: they now sported a summery selection of Hawaiian shirts and brightly-coloured jackets designed by Thierry Mugler, David's favourite designer of the time. Less endearingly, it was not uncommon for both Bowie and Hunt Sales to arrive on stage sporting T-shirts proclaiming "Fuck You, I'm In Tin Machine". One wonders whose idea that was.

In addition to most of *Tin Machine* and all of *Tin Machine II*, the set-list included Pixies' 'Debaser', Neil Young's 'I've Been Waiting For You', for which Reeves Gabrels took lead vocal, and The Moody Blues' 'Go Now', fronted by Tony Sales. Hunt, meanwhile, seized the limelight for 'Stateside' and 'Sorry'. In addition to his guitar work, Bowie was now playing a great deal of saxophone, while Kevin Armstrong's place on rhythm guitar was taken by newcomer Eric Schermerhorn, later to play on Iggy Pop's *American Caesar*.

Aside from the predictable complaints from those who wanted to hear Bowie's golden oldies, the critical response was far from bad. According to the *Manchester Evening News*, "Bowie booted into touch the critics who have tried to squeeze the life out of Tin Machine's so far brief career." *Melody Maker* described David as "lean, newly tanned and unusually relaxed," adding that "this year's Bowie is a very different proposition from the neurotically nervy character who shuffled a trifle uneasily through his farewell-then-greatest-hits tour."

The most significant event of the tour came in Paris at the end of October when David proposed to his new love. The Somalian-born model and actress Iman Abdulmajid was best known during the 1980s as the face of the Tia Maria commercials, and was now setting up her own cosmetics company and carving out an acting career in films such as *No Way Out* and *Star Trek VI*. Something of a Bowie fan, Iman had seen several of David's concerts before the two were introduced at a friend's dinner party in October 1990. "I make no bones about it," David later said, "I was naming the children the night we met. I knew that she was for me, it was absolutely immediate." In the ensuing year Iman had made a cameo appearance in *The Linguini Incident* and joined David on a six-week Italian holiday, and now the couple were travelling together on the It's My Life tour. Chartering a boat on the Seine as the setting for his proposal, David arranged for a musician to serenade Iman with Doris Day's 'April In Paris', and as the boat passed under the Pont Neuf he dropped to his knees, sang 'October In Paris' and proposed marriage. "I knew I had to sing to express how I felt in the best way I can," he said. "Luckily, it worked … it was not something we had discussed at any length and she was not expecting it. She was shocked, but she didn't hesitate for a second." News of the engagement broke in early November.

Meanwhile the tour pressed on. The Hamburg gig on 24 October was filmed for the video *Oy Vey, Baby: Tin Machine Live At The Docks*. A performance of 'Baby Can Dance' from the same gig, not included on the video, later appeared on the compilation album *Best Of Grunge Rock*. By the time the tour reached Britain a new tradition had been established whereby fans would throw packs of Marlboro cigarettes, Bowie's preferred brand, on stage. On 11 November at the Brixton Academy (only a couple of minutes' walk from David's birthplace on Stansfield Road), a flying Marlboro packet struck him in the eye, necessitating a brief cessation and Bowie's first appearance in an eye-patch since the days of 'Rebel Rebel'.

Brixton Academy was the final European venue for the tour, which recommenced four days later at Bowie's beloved Philadelphia Tower Theater. While in America there were performances on *Saturday Night Live* and *The Arsenio Hall Show*, and all proceeds from the Chicago gig on 7 December were donated to the city's Children's Memorial Hospital. Marking the final Vancouver concert with a one-off revival of 'Waiting For The Man', Tin Machine went their separate ways over Christmas, reconvening for a final 13-date Japanese tour that began in Kyoto on 29 January and ended – as did Tin Machine's career – in Tokyo on 17 February.

Over a year later Bowie was still talking about Tin Machine as a going concern, claiming that the band intended to reconvene for a new album at the end of 1993. In reality, when the tour ended it was all over bar the live album. A string of concerts in Chicago, Boston, New York, Sapporo and Tokyo had been recorded for *Oy Vey, Baby* which, like the Hamburg video, accurately commemorated the It's My Life tour as a loud, confrontational exorcism of Bowie's fast-evaporating creative crisis.

Subsequent reports have revealed that Hunt Sales's recreational habits were a major catalyst in the band's demise. In the wake of David Buckley's *Strange Fascination* Bowie confirmed the rumours: "I guess it's now out because somebody's written about it in a book," he said in 2000, "but one of our members had a serious drugs problem … and that really destroyed the band more than anything else. It got to a situation where it was just intolerable. You didn't know if the guy was gonna be dead in the morning … we just couldn't cope." He added that the tour was "a nightmare" as a result.

In any case, it seems more than likely that larger issues were at play. Tin Machine had, in Reeves Gabrels's words, fallen "on the grenade of *Let's*

Dance", muffling Bowie's 1980s explosion and clearing the creative decks for a man now obviously itching to resume his solo career. "Once I had done Tin Machine, nobody could see me any more," David said some years later. "They didn't know who the hell I was, which was the best thing that ever happened, because I was back using all the artistic pieces that I needed to survive and I was imbuing myself with the passion that I had in the late seventies." Bowie's artistic renaissance didn't happen overnight, but by 1992 the light at the end of the tunnel was shining brightly.

THE FREDDIE MERCURY TRIBUTE CONCERT
20 April 1992

Musicians: David Bowie *(vocals, saxophone)*, Annie Lennox *(vocals)*, Ian Hunter *(vocals, guitar)*, Mick Ronson *(guitar, vocals)*, Brian May *(guitar)*, John Deacon *(bass)*, Roger Taylor *(drums)*, Tony Iommi *(guitar)*, Joe Elliott, Phil Collen *(backing vocals)*

Repertoire: 'Under Pressure' / 'All The Young Dudes' / '"Heroes"'

Freddie Mercury lost his struggle against AIDS-related symptoms on 23 November 1991. Collecting a posthumous Brit Award on his behalf in February 1992, the remaining members of Queen announced a special concert at Wembley Stadium to raise awareness of the disease. The Freddie Mercury Tribute Concert, also referred to as the "Concert For Life", rapidly snowballed into the most talked-about charity gala since Live Aid, and the 72,000 tickets sold out in under two hours. Rehearsals took place at Bray Studios over the two days immediately prior to the big night. Bowie's presence at the concert had never been in doubt and there was, of course, no mystery about which Queen song he would be singing. It was revealed that Freddie's part would be taken by Annie Lennox, formerly of Eurythmics but now launching her solo career with her soon-to-be number 1 album *Diva*.

The Bowie/Lennox spot came near the end of the evening, after performances by the likes of Def Leppard, Extreme, Metallica, Guns N'Roses, Robert Plant, Paul Young, Seal and Lisa Stansfield. Annie Lennox sported a silver blouse, a voluminous tutu and a swathe of black make-up across her eyes, while Bowie appeared in his familiar *Tin Machine II* guise:

healthy tan, swept-back hair, lime-green Thierry Mugler suit, shirt and tie. The pair launched into a vigorous 'Under Pressure' during which Annie threw herself at David and pawed his face during the final chorus, leaving the stage to tumultuous applause. David next introduced his old colleagues Ian Hunter and Mick Ronson. It was the latter's first appearance with Bowie since their one-off reunion at a Serious Moonlight gig in Toronto nine years earlier, and would lead to his forthcoming contribution to *Black Tie White Noise*. Backed by Queen, the trio launched into a nostalgic 'All The Young Dudes', with Hunter on lead vocal and Bowie playing sax. Hunter then left the stage (unexpectedly by the look of it, muttering something in Bowie's ear that seemed to take him by surprise), but Ronson remained to deliver a superb guitar line on a blistering and impassioned '"Heroes"'. Just as it seemed that Bowie would exit in a blaze of brilliance, he cut short the final "just for one day" and launched into an oration about the victims of "…this relentless disease. I'd particularly like to extend my wishes to friend Craig," he said, turning to look directly into the TV camera, "I know you're watching, Craig – and I'd like to offer something in a very simple fashion, but it's the most direct way that I can think of doing it." Then, before an estimated audience of a billion people, he dropped to his knees and hoarsely recited The Lord's Prayer.

Bowie later said that it was an entirely spontaneous act and that he was "the most surprised man in Wembley" when it happened. Craig, he explained, was a playwright friend from New York in the last stages of an AIDS-related illness; he died two days later. "My friend Craig was not a Christian, but I thought that prayer the most appropriate," David said the following year. "For me, it's a universal prayer." It was clearly meant in all sincerity, but unfortunately the Lord's Prayer incident looked clumsy and mawkish, opening the floodgates for pitiless ridicule from those who had been waiting for a chance to take a pop at his first post-Tin Machine performance. "In hindsight, as it was so alien a gesture within the context of rock, it remains a favourite personal rock 'moment' for me," said Bowie in 2000. "It was astounding to find that I could complete the prayer in front of so many thousands of people without hearing a pin drop … there's an aspect of my personality which continually asks my audience, 'How long will you tolerate this?'"

After the show Bowie hosted a party graced by

most of the concert's glitterati, including Liza Minnelli and Elizabeth Taylor, whose sixtieth birthday party he had attended the previous February. Two days later David and Iman flew to Lausanne to be married.

The concert was released on video in November 1992, while the performance of 'All The Young Dudes' was included on Mick Ronson's posthumous 1994 album *Heaven And Hull*. Footage of Bowie and Annie Lennox rehearsing 'Under Pressure' at Bray Studios (and superior to the concert version it is, too) later appeared in the 1995 television documentary *The Queen Phenomenon: In The Lap of the Gods*. Both rehearsal and performance footage were reused in the video for 1999's 'Rah Mix', while in May 2002 the concert was released on DVD, complete with an updated version of the documentary and full rehearsal footage of 'Under Pressure'.

1993: BLACK TIE WHITE NOISE

Although Bowie elected not to tour *Black Tie White Noise*, he made a couple of appearances on American television to promote the album in May 1993, performing tracks with the help of Al B Sure! on *The Arsenio Hall Show* and *The Tonight Show With Jay Leno*. Later in the year, on 1 December, David compered the Concert of Hope, a World AIDS day benefit at Wembley Arena attended by the Princess of Wales, where the acts included George Michael, Mick Hucknall and kd lang.

THE OUTSIDE TOUR

14 September 1995 – 20 February 1996

Musicians: David Bowie *(vocals, saxophone)*, Peter Schwartz *(musical director, keyboards)*, Reeves Gabrels *(guitar)*, Gail Ann Dorsey *(bass, vocals)*, Zachary Alford *(drums)*, Carlos Alomar *(guitar)*, Mike Garson *(keyboards)*, George Simms *(keyboards, backing vocals)*

Repertoire: 'Scary Monsters (And Super Creeps)' / 'Hallo Spaceboy' / 'Look Back In Anger' / 'The Voyeur Of Utter Destruction (As Beauty)' / 'The Hearts Filthy Lesson' / 'Breaking Glass' / 'I'm Deranged' / 'A Small Plot Of Land' / 'Joe The Lion' / 'I Have Not Been To Oxford Town' / 'Outside' / 'We Prick You' / 'Jump They Say' / 'Andy Warhol' / 'The Man Who Sold The World' / 'Teenage Wildlife' / 'My Death' / 'Nite Flights' / 'Under Pressure' / 'What In The World' / 'Strangers When We Meet' / 'Thru' These Architects Eyes' / 'The Motel' / 'Boys Keep Swinging' / 'D.J.' / 'Moonage Daydream' / 'Diamond Dogs' / 'Subterraneans' / 'Warszawa' / 'Reptile' / 'Hurt'

By 1995 Bowie had been absent from the concert stage for three years, and early in the year he declared that he felt no inclination to tour again. Nevertheless, by September he had embarked on what would snowball into his most intensive period of touring for 20 years.

Pressed by his new label Virgin, David initially agreed to promote *1.Outside* in America with "no more than six dates". In August, rehearsals began in New York with a seven-piece backing band. Joining *1.Outside* personnel Gabrels, Alomar and Garson were Serious Moonlight veteran George Simms and musical director Peter Schwartz, who had previously appeared in the *Black Tie White Noise* video. Drummer Zachary Alford, whose previous employers included Bruce Springsteen, Billy Joel and the B52's (he appears in the 'Love Shack' video), was recommended to Bowie by *1.Outside* percussionist Sterling Campbell. "Zach is Sterling's best pal," explained David. "Sterling got a great offer from Soul Asylum to become an integral part of the band, and quite rightly he said, 'Look guys, I'd love to do the tour, but this is a real opportunity for me to join a group proper. But you might like this kid.'" Alford would become a crucial contributor to Bowie's music, as would the final newcomer, bassist Gail Ann Dorsey. A solo artist with two albums to her name, Dorsey had played with Gang Of Four and The The, and was recording with Roland Orzabal's one-man version of Tears For Fears when the call came from Bowie.

By early September David had been persuaded to extend the American leg to 25 dates and make preparations for a European tour. As the itinerary grew to become Bowie's largest since Sound + Vision, he began issuing pre-emptive warnings that this was to be no greatest hits extravaganza. The set-list drew heavily from the new album, otherwise sticking to the more obscure corners of his back catalogue, in particular *Low* and *Lodger*. 'Scary Monsters', 'Breaking Glass' and 'Jump They Say' were the only vintage A-sides in the original repertoire, while choices like 'Joe The Lion', 'Teenage Wildlife' and 'My Death' were guaranteed to delight hardcore fans and bewilder everyone else. 'The Man Who Sold The World', enjoying new-found fame in the wake of Nirvana's 1993 *Unplugged* performance, was drastically reworked in a trip-hop arrangement, while 'Andy Warhol' was realigned as an electric bass number.

Opening for Bowie on some dates of the US tour was Reeves Gabrels, playing numbers from his new solo album *The Sacred Squall Of Now*. The main support act was Nine Inch Nails, the Californian hardcore outfit whose 1994 album *The Downward Spiral* (featuring Bowie sideman Adrian Belew on one track) had gone top ten in Britain and America. Vocalist Trent Reznor was among several cutting-edge American rockers who had joined Kurt Cobain in acknowledging a debt to Bowie, revealing that he had listened to *Low* every day during the *Downward Spiral* sessions. At the American shows David would make his first appearance during Nine Inch Nails' set, joining the group to perform 'Subterraneans' (which remained exclusive to the Nine Inch Nails gigs), together with 'Scary Monsters', 'Hallo Spaceboy' and two numbers from *The Downward Spiral*, 'Reptile' and 'Hurt'.

By aligning himself with Nine Inch Nails in America Bowie risked scorn, but undoubtedly achieved exposure and credibility of the kind that his timely chumminess with Suede's Brett Anderson had created in Britain at the time of *Black Tie White Noise*. With artists like Reznor and the Smashing Pumpkins' Billy Corgan talking about Bowie in interviews – not to mention the rise of Marilyn Manson, scandalizing middle America with his Alice Cooper-meets-Ziggy Stardust freakshow – the time was ripe for Bowie to reclaim the US market.

The Outside tour opened in Hartford, Connecticut on 14 September, on a stage set recalling the cluttered artist's studio from the 'Hearts Filthy Lesson' video. Ripped, billowing drapes hung to the rear. A paint-strewn table and chair and a handful of stiff-limbed mannequins were dotted about the stage. Dangling overhead were surreal sculptures: a body in a sack, a crouched figure trapped in an armillary sphere, a set of rotating fluorescent tubes like animated sunbeds which descended to menace Bowie during 'Nite Flights' and 'Andy Warhol', and a metallic mobile spelling out a cryptic legend that would change from one night to another: usually it was the 'All The Madmen' refrain of "Ouvrez Le Chien", but on some of the early dates the variations included "Strange KO", "Noise Angel" and "Man Made". For some numbers Bowie would sprawl across the table and chair; for others he danced like a puppet beneath the stark white lights. In 'A Small Plot Of Land' he scurried across the rear of the set, reshaping the scenery by releasing a series of banners. The overall effect, very much in keeping with the set-list itself, was evocative of the avant-garde posture Bowie had adopted during his *Lodger/Elephant Man/Scary Monsters* period. His costumes favoured the same late-1970s aura of artist's-garret chic: usually he would appear in a paint-streaked jumpsuit, peeled away and tied at the waist to reveal a T-shirt or vest. Occasionally he displayed a few days' growth of stubble, and for the first time in many years his make-up was extravagant, expressionistic and there to be seen.

The opening Hartford show preceded the release of *1.Outside* by ten days, and like several of the early concerts it left its audience bemused. A New York concert a fortnight later was reviewed for *Mojo* by Cliff Jones (later lead singer of Gay Dad), who reported that Bowie was pelted with bottles and pretzels by the nonplussed crowd: "Bewilderingly random solos and strange sinewy scales battle against a pounding techno backing while inhuman piano runs tumble from the speakers. Extremely unsettling but strangely thrilling, as though someone has randomly rewired the Rock Machine … in some indefinable way, Bowie remains a curious pioneer – and pioneers, as they say, get all the arrows."

During the US tour there were live performances on *The Late Show With David Letterman* and *The Tonight Show With Jay Leno*, while on 18 September Bowie and Mike Garson attended a private charity function in a New York hotel to perform superb piano-and-voice versions of 'A Small Plot of Land' and 'My Death'. Added to the repertoire at the New York gigs a few days later were 'Look Back In Anger' and 'Under Pressure', for which Gail Ann Dorsey lent her considerable vocal talents to the Freddie Mercury role. 'Joe The Lion', 'What In The World' and 'Thru' These Architects Eyes' were all dropped before the end of the American leg, which closed in Los Angeles on 31 October; Bowie hosted a Hallowe'en wrap party where the guests included Brad Pitt and John Lydon. Thereafter the tour moved to Britain, where six days of rehearsal at Elwood Studios near Watford yielded four new additions to the set: 'The Motel' (which now became the usual opener), 'Boys Keep Swinging', 'D.J.' and 'Moonage Daydream'. On 7 November, during the rehearsal week, Bowie and Brian Eno attended Q magazine's awards ceremony to receive an Inspiration Award from Jarvis Cocker, who introduced them as

"Mr Hunting Knife" and "Mr Liver Salts". Three days later the band performed 'Strangers When We Meet' live on *Top Of The Pops*.

The UK tour opened at Wembley Arena, where Bowie's backstage visitors included Bill Wyman, Bob Geldof, Glen Matlock, Tony Blair and his 73-year-old former manager Kenneth Pitt. The support slot was filled by Morrissey, now promoting his album *Southpaw Grammar*. British critics were distinctly underwhelmed, the *Times* branding the show "an uphill slog", while the *NME* declared that "It is thunderous, but sadly not thunderously good," going on to admit that "a sweetly mysterious 'My Death' displays grace and subtlety" but dismissing the show overall as a "grinding, grime-laced farrago."

A common complaint was that Bowie was short-changing his fans by avoiding the greatest hits, a criticism he dismissed out of hand: "If they didn't know that I wasn't going to be [playing the hits], they must have been living under a rock." Later he told *Q*, "I know what happens when I play the classics. I know the outcome. So why would I want to do it again? Other than for financial remuneration, which frankly I don't need ... In ten years' time, when I'm playing to halls with no audience whatsoever, my contemporaries can turn round and say, 'Well that's the reason we didn't do what you did.' But we'll see." This, surely, was the point. The Outside tour wasn't a greatest hits package for corporate hospitality outings; it was a new show for audiences interested in Bowie's progress as an artist.

Six numbers from the final Wembley gig were later broadcast on Radio 1. From London the tour moved to Birmingham and Dublin, before the band flew to Paris to play 'The Man Who Sold The World' at MTV's European Music Awards. There had been plans to perform the song as a duet with Polly Harvey, but according to Bowie the collaboration "didn't work out ... we both had different ideas on what the arrangement should be. It ended friendly enough but I doubt that we will get back together again."

After Paris the UK tour resumed. There was a minor sensation when Morrissey, whose support sets had been uncharacteristically lacklustre and occasionally ill-tempered (a sulky aside to the Wembley audience – "Don't worry, David will be on soon" – only succeeded in raising a mass cheer), disappeared before the Aberdeen gig and never returned. The support slot was filled on later dates by a variety of local bands. Five years later, Morrissey hinted at a falling-out with David, remarking that "I left the tour because he put me under a lot of pressure and I found it too exhausting. He wouldn't even phone his mother without considering the impact on his career status. Bowie is principally a business. He surrounds himself with very strong people and that's the secret of his power – that everything he does will be seen in a certain light." Not exactly renowned for his readiness to forget a grudge, Morrissey's bitterness over the episode appears to have increased rather than dwindled over the years. In Channel 4's 2003 documentary *The Importance Of Being Morrissey* he claimed that he had left the tour because he objected to Bowie's suggestion that his support set end with a crossover duet (as the Nine Inch Nails set had done on the American leg), adding that "You have to worship at the temple of David when you become involved. He was a fascinating artist in 1970, '71, '72, but not now." In March 2004, as he prepared to follow Bowie's footsteps as curator of the Meltdown Festival, Morrissey told *GQ* magazine that David was "not the person he was. He is no longer David Bowie at all. Now he gives people what he thinks will make them happy, and they're yawning their heads off. And by doing that, he is not relevant. He was only relevant by accident." Morrissey's opinions on pots and kettles are not recorded.

On 2 December came the first in a string of television appearances with a performance on BBC2's *Later... With Jools Holland*. Bowie's muted demeanour during his interview with Holland may be put down to a hastily covered-up incident that had occurred during rehearsals. Sharing the show's billing were Oasis, whose vocalist Liam Gallagher was absent due to what the BBC described as a "sore throat". In fact what had happened was that Gallagher, in one of his tiresome attempts at rock'n'roll outrage, had declared Bowie to be "a washed-up old fart" and attempted to throw a punch at him. He was escorted from Television Centre and lead vocals were taken over by his brother.

The 13 December gig at the Birmingham NEC was billed as the "Big Twix Mix Show", a bumper event also featuring the Lightning Seeds and Alanis Morissette. 'Hallo Spaceboy' was performed twice during the evening for the benefit of a film crew shooting the promo for the forthcoming single; this footage was later scrapped when the decision was taken to release the Pet Shop Boys remix. Excerpts from the Birmingham show were televised by the BBC, while recordings of 'Under Pressure' and 'Moonage

Daydream' from the gig were released as B-sides.

On 14 December the band performed a live set for Channel 4's *The White Room*. In the New Year the tour moved to the Continent, where 'Diamond Dogs' was added to the repertoire during rehearsals in Helsinki. Over the course of the 23 European dates, the band performed live sets for Swedish, Dutch and French television; on Dutch TV's *Karel* Mike Garson gave a one-off rendition of 'Warszawa'.

The European dates concluded in Paris on 20 February. The previous night had seen the most prominent of the many television appearances that propped up the tour, as the band flew to London for the Brit Awards at Earls Court. The evening was dominated by the legendary Michael Jackson/Jarvis Cocker incident, but final billing was given to Bowie, who arrived on stage in a black suit, stiletto heels and a giant "SEX" earring to collect an Outstanding Contribution award from opposition leader Tony Blair. Amusingly the future people's Prime Minister arrived at the podium to the strains of 'Fashion' ("turn to the left, turn to the right"), and in a fulsome introduction hailed Bowie as "an innovator – he's pushed the frontiers back, he's a man not afraid to go up the hill backwards." Bowie, whose chief motive was to perform his latest single ("I'm not big on the award bit at all," he said later, "I think it's rubbish"), was mercifully less grandiloquent: "Thank you Tony, thank you everyone else. I think I'll go and sing at you." Having performed 'Hallo Spaceboy' with the Pet Shop Boys and a medley of 'Moonage Daydream' and 'Under Pressure' with the tour band, he was back in Paris the same night.

Setting aside those critics who felt cheated by the absence of familiarity (which would doubtless have bred only their contempt), the Outside shows saw a vigorous, vital Bowie throwing himself into music which he genuinely believed in. Brian Eno's diary records several telephone calls during the tour in which David was "full of excitement about his concerts" and had "the enthusiasm of a teenager." The band was arguably Bowie's strongest since 1976, with Zachary Alford and Gail Ann Dorsey in particular investing the *1.Outside* material with renewed guts and power. Obscure oldies like 'Teenage Wildlife', 'D.J.' and the re-orchestrated 'My Death' were real highlights, evincing a perfect thematic sympathy with the new material. Hang the critics: the Outside tour was Bowie's finest in twenty years.

THE 1996 SUMMER FESTIVALS AND EAST COAST BALLROOM TOURS

4 June – 21 July 1996
6 September – 14 September 1996

Musicians: David Bowie *(vocals, saxophone)*, Reeves Gabrels *(guitar)*, Gail Ann Dorsey *(bass, vocals)*, Zachary Alford *(drums)*, Mike Garson *(keyboards)*

Repertoire: 'The Motel' / 'Look Back In Anger' / 'The Hearts Filthy Lesson' / 'Scary Monsters (And Super Creeps)' / 'Outside' / 'Aladdin Sane' / 'Andy Warhol' / 'The Voyeur Of Utter Destruction (As Beauty)' / 'The Man Who Sold The World' / 'A Small Plot Of Land' / 'Strangers When We Meet' / 'I Have Not Been To Oxford Town' / 'Teenage Wildlife' / 'Diamond Dogs' / 'Hallo Spaceboy' / 'Breaking Glass' / 'We Prick You' / 'Jump They Say' / 'Lust For Life' / 'Under Pressure' / '"Heroes"' / 'My Death' / 'White Light/White Heat' / 'Moonage Daydream' / 'All The Young Dudes' / 'Baby Universal' / 'Telling Lies' / 'Little Wonder' / 'Seven Years In Tibet'

Following its final Paris gig the Outside tour disbanded until June 1996, when a slimmed-down group reconvened for dates in Japan, Russia and Iceland, followed by a string of Summer festivals in Europe. Although still officially billed as the Outside tour, the changes in line-up and repertoire effectively rendered it a separate entity, which has come to be known as the 1996 Summer Festivals tour. Gone were George Simms, Peter Schwartz and Carlos Alomar (who later confessed that he hadn't enjoyed the Outside tour at all, finding times changed and Bowie inaccessible). What remained was a more rock-oriented core band who would remain in place for the subsequent recording of *Earthling*. The set-list had also undergone changes, losing 'I'm Deranged', 'D.J.' and 'Boys Keep Swinging', while 'Oxford Town' and 'Teenage Wildlife' were dropped after the first date on 4 June. In their place came new attractions, including 'Aladdin Sane', 'White Light/White Heat', 'Lust For Life' (a first for Bowie, roped in following its exposure in *Trainspotting*) and, most surprisingly, Tin Machine's 'Baby Universal'. There was also a hint of the future: unveiled in Nagoya on 7 June was an all-new composition called 'Telling Lies' which David had written during the break in touring.

Gone, too, were the more elaborate elements of the Outside tour's stage set. Bowie, now resplendent in a spiky shock of carrot-coloured hair reminiscent of his Ziggy days, had taken to wearing black leather trousers, lace-edged blouses and a distressed Union Jack frock-coat co-designed with Alexander McQueen: not only the *Earthling* songs but the *Earthling* look were beginning to emerge.

In Tokyo on 5 June Bowie was joined for 'All The Young Dudes' by Japanese singer Tomoyasu Hotei. Two weeks later Russian television broadcast a 50-minute compilation from the Kremlin Palace show in Moscow, where the Russian David Bowie fan club presented their hero with an antique balalaika at the end of the evening. Other TV coverage included an epic 106-minute German broadcast of the Loreley Festival gig on 22 June, ITV extracts from the Phoenix Festival on 18 July, and MTV reports from shows in Belgium and Iceland. The Tel Aviv and Ballingen gigs were broadcast on FM radio in their respective countries, while a six-song selection from the Phoenix Festival was aired live on Radio 1.

The tour wrapped in Switzerland in late July, and almost immediately Bowie took his band to New York's Looking Glass Studios to begin work on *Earthling*. In early September, while sessions were still in progress, the band played four low-key ballroom gigs in Philadelphia, Washington, Boston and New York, premiering two new compositions, 'Little Wonder' and 'Seven Years In Tibet'.

THE BRIDGE SCHOOL CONCERTS
19-20 October 1996

Musicians: David Bowie *(vocals, guitar)*, Reeves Gabrels *(guitar)*, Gail Ann Dorsey *(bass, vocals)*

Repertoire: 'Aladdin Sane' / 'The Jean Genie' / 'I'm A Hog For You Baby' / 'I Can't Read' / 'The Man Who Sold The World' / '"Heroes"' / 'You And I And George' / 'Let's Dance' / 'China Girl' / 'White Light/White Heat'

Since 1986 Neil Young has organized an annual charity event in aid of the Bridge School for the disabled in Hillsborough, California. In 1996 Bowie joined the bill at Mountain View's Shoreline Amphitheater, alongside Billy Idol, Patti Smith, Pearl Jam, Pete Townshend and Young himself.

Traditionally the Bridge School benefit is a semi-acoustic affair, and Bowie accordingly played acoustic guitar while his two backing musicians, Reeves Gabrels and Gail Ann Dorsey, were plugged in. On the first evening David made humorous reference to Pete Townshend's earlier set by launching into a brief snatch of The Who's 'Anyway, Anyhow, Anywhere', and in a similarly playful mood he attempted to teach Gabrels the Coasters' chestnut 'I'm A Hog For You Baby', replacing the line "love you all night long" with something rather ruder. On the second night he busked the sentimental ditty 'You And I And George', which he had formerly played at a couple of Sound + Vision gigs.

The Bridge School concerts saw Bowie's first revival since 1990 of 'The Jean Genie' and the reappearance of 'I Can't Read', which had just been re-recorded during the *Earthling* sessions, but the real surprises were the jokey acoustic revivals of 'Let's Dance' and 'China Girl'. A recording of '"Heroes"' from the second night later appeared on the US compilation album *The Bridge School Concerts Vol. 1*.

Four days later, Bowie was back with his full *Earthling* band to perform 'Little Wonder' and 'Fashion' (another new revival) at the VH1 Fashion Awards at Madison Square Garden.

DAVID BOWIE AND FRIENDS – THE FIFTIETH BIRTHDAY CONCERT
9 January 1997

Musicians: David Bowie *(vocals, guitar, saxophone)*, Reeves Gabrels *(guitar)*, Gail Ann Dorsey *(bass, keyboards, vocals)*, Zachary Alford *(drums)*, Mike Garson *(keyboards)*, plus guests as below

Repertoire: 'Little Wonder' / 'The Hearts Filthy Lesson' / 'Scary Monsters (And Super Creeps)' & 'Fashion' *(with Frank Black)* / 'Telling Lies' / 'Hallo Spaceboy' *(with Foo Fighters)* / 'Seven Years In Tibet' *(with David Grohl)* / 'The Man Who Sold The World' / 'The Last Thing You Should Do' & 'Quicksand' *(with Robert Smith)* / 'Battle For Britain (The Letter)' / 'The Voyeur Of Utter Destruction (As Beauty)' / 'I'm Afraid Of Americans' *(with Sonic Youth)* / 'Looking For Satellites' / 'Under Pressure' / '"Heroes"' / 'Queen Bitch' & 'Waiting For The Man' & 'Dirty Blvd.' & 'White Light/White Heat' *(with Lou Reed)* / 'Moonage Daydream' / 'Happy Birthday' / 'All The Young Dudes' & 'The Jean Genie' *(with Billy Corgan)* / 'Space Oddity'

"An ageing rock star doesn't have to opt out of life," Bowie told Jean Rook in 1979. "When I'm fifty, I'll prove it." And, eighteen years later, he did, launching his new album *Earthling* in a star-studded charity concert at Madison Square Garden.

The decision to stage the show in New York was, Bowie explained, a logistical one. "All my crew are American," he told the BBC apologetically. "Economically, it was more feasible to do it in the States than take all the caboodle back to Europe." The venue was also a convenient one for the roster of predominantly American artists booked as special guests: the Smashing Pumpkins' Billy Corgan, David Grohl and his Foo Fighters, Frank Black (long admired by David, who had been citing the influence of Pixies on his work for nearly a decade), and best of all Lou Reed, introduced by David as "the king of New York". There were British guests too; as support Bowie had chosen rising Anglo-Canadian stars Placebo, and in a long overdue collaboration he secured the services of Robert Smith, The Cure's brilliant singer-guitarist who had attested to Bowie's influence on his work for many years. "Smith and Jones together at last!" joked David. "He doesn't seem fifty," said Smith later, "He seems about 15 and 100 at the same time." Following the gig, Smith (whose tongue-in-cheek birthday present for David was a fossilized chameleon) enlisted Reeves Gabrels and Mark Plati to guest on The Cure's 1997 single 'Wrong Number'. Gabrels, who would go on to play live dates with The Cure at the end of the year, later revealed that Madonna was also among the concert's mooted guests until late in the day.

With *Earthling* not due on the shelves for another month and only 'Telling Lies', 'Little Wonder' and 'Seven Years In Tibet' thus far unveiled on stage, the show boasted several brand new songs. All but two of the *Earthling* tracks were performed, as were a couple from *1.Outside*, while most of the obvious crowd-pleasers were held back until late into the evening. Brilliantly, the new songs threatened to steal the show: 'Seven Years In Tibet' and 'Battle For Britain' were delivered with devastating energy and conviction, while 'Hallo Spaceboy', augmented by no fewer than three drummers courtesy of the Foo Fighters, was a riot. Even so, the concert achieved an appropriate air of nostalgia with the unexpected revivals of 'Quicksand', 'Queen Bitch' and 'Space Oddity'.

The staging was an intriguing combination of old and new. The Outside tour set was augmented by the reappearance of Sound + Vision's gauze screen and accompanying projections: 'Moonage Daydream' was now backed by images from the 'Life On Mars?' video while 'Battle For Britain' featured the 'Fame 90' vogue routine. 'Telling Lies' harked back to Serious Moonlight's bouncing globe, as David unleashed a horde of giant inflatable eyeballs on the unsuspecting crowd. But the most remarkable visual aspect was the incorporation of Tony Oursler's unsettling "Media Sculptures", as featured in the 'Little Wonder' video. Pre-filmed shots of Bowie's face were projected onto the blank heads of the malformed figures dotted about the set: during 'Looking For Satellites' the stage came alive with distorted Bowie-faces chanting the backing vocals.

Dressed in a lace-edged black shirt and a succession of foppish jackets, including his Union Jack coat and a preposterous *Labyrinth*-style rococo number for the encores, David was in fine voice and appeared to enjoy himself immensely. His duet with Robert Smith was a particular joy – two of British rock's great suburban poets side by side, picking out 'Quicksand' on their acoustic guitars, was a sight to cherish – but the highlight, surely, was Lou Reed's guest spot. Seldom has Reed let slip such a broad grin as the one that spread across his face when he and David launched into the opening bars of 'Queen Bitch'. The inclusion of Reed's 'Dirty Blvd.' was a masterstroke, and Gail Ann Dorsey later said that "looking over to see David and Lou Reed together was the greatest thrill for a little girl from Philadelphia."

A less certain note was struck by Billy Corgan's rather self-serving contributions to 'All The Young Dudes' and 'The Jean Genie', but by that stage in the evening it mattered little. The party mood was sealed by the presentation of a birthday cake while Gail Ann Dorsey led the audience in 'Happy Birthday', and David's closing performance of 'Space Oddity', again accompanied by the Sound + Vision projections, was the perfect encore. "I don't know where I'm going from here," he told the crowd, "But I promise I won't bore you."

There were criticisms in some quarters that Bowie didn't use the occasion to reconvene old line-ups and turn the gig into a nostalgia trip, but this is surely missing the point: that's exactly what David Bowie doesn't do, and for once the critics were firmly on his side. "More than most performers his age, Mr Bowie has repeatedly staked his career on the new," said the *New York Times*. "In the new songs Mr Bowie sang, he uses jungle as an overlay of double-time energy and implacable noise, revitalising what might have been stately arena anthems." The *New York Daily News* noted that the concert "kept one eye firmly on the future. Instead of serving up dewy-eyed rehashes of sounds from eras dead and gone, Bowie … shook classic numbers to their core. He also devoted roughly one-third of the show to recent and brand new material." According to the *Boston Globe*, "The startling triumph of this set was that Bowie's new material is his strongest in years … both edgy and immediately accessible."

The pay-per-view broadcast on American TV (directed, incidentally, by 'Time Will Crawl' veteran and Robert Smith acolyte Tim Pope) included bonus performances of 'I Can't Read' and 'Repetition', recorded backstage at Madison Square Garden.

THE EARTHLING TOUR

7 June – 7 November 1997

Musicians: David Bowie *(vocals, guitar, saxophone)*, Reeves Gabrels *(guitar)*, Gail Ann Dorsey *(bass, keyboards, vocals)*, Zachary Alford *(drums)*, Mike Garson *(keyboards)*

Repertoire: 'Quicksand' / 'I'm Deranged' / 'Pallas Athena' / 'V-2 Schneider' / 'Fun' / 'Is It Any Wonder' / 'O Superman' / 'The Last Thing You Should Do' / 'Telling Lies' / 'Stay' / 'Battle For Britain (The Letter)' / 'Hallo Spaceboy' / 'Fashion' / 'Under Pressure' / 'Little Wonder' / 'The Motel' / '"Heroes"' / 'Scary Monsters (And Super Creeps)' / 'Outside' / 'Looking For Satellites' / 'The Man Who Sold The World' / 'Strangers When We Meet' / 'I'm Afraid Of Americans' / 'Seven Years In Tibet' / 'The Jean Genie' / 'The Voyeur Of Utter Destruction (As Beauty)' / 'White Light/White Heat' / 'Queen Bitch' / 'Waiting For The Man' / 'All The Young Dudes' / 'Dead Man Walking' / 'Fame' / 'The Hearts Filthy Lesson' / 'Look Back In Anger' / 'Panic In Detroit' / 'Always Crashing In The Same Car' / 'Moonage Daydream' / 'I Can't Read' / 'The Supermen' / 'My Death'

Following a month's sabbatical after his fiftieth birthday concert, Bowie and his four-piece band remained on call from February through to April 1997 with a string of television and radio appearances (see Chapter 10) to promote the release of *Earthling*. Bowie's 8 February performance of 'Scary Monsters'

for NBC later appeared on the compilation *Saturday Night Live – 25 Years*. On 12 February, CNN and MTV were on hand to record David unveiling his star on Hollywood's Walk Of Fame. On 14 March he was in Toronto to film the video for the forthcoming single 'Dead Man Walking', a song that would become the focal point of public appearances over the next month: three different performances, recorded on 8 and 10 April, would later appear on the US compilations *Live From 6A*, *Live I IV* and *WBCN: Naked Too*.

In mid-April the band crossed the Atlantic to begin rehearsals for their next major tour. Like the Outside jaunt it would last six months, by the end of which Bowie had been touring, on and off, for well over two years. "Honestly, it would be a sin not playing live when I've got a band like this," he told *Q*. "They're the best group I've had in twenty years, right up there with The Spiders in terms of cohesive musicianship and attitude."

Rehearsals began on 20 April at the Factory Studios in Dublin, previously the rehearsal venue for Tin Machine's It's My Life tour. The set-list drew on the repertoire established during 1996 and at the birthday concert, and among the influx of *Earthling* tracks (all of them save 'Law (Earthlings On Fire)') came additions like 'V-2 Schneider', 'Fame' and 'Pallas Athena'. Certainly the most startling new arrival was a nine-minute reworking of Laurie Anderson's 'O Superman' on which Gail Ann Dorsey sang lead vocal. In addition to her bass guitar and vocal chores Dorsey was now playing keyboards, while some of the more techno-oriented numbers were enhanced by pre-recorded DAT backings (questions were raised about quite how much of the show depended on programmed samples, but if nothing else it demonstrated that Bowie had indeed moved into the techno-dance realm).

During rehearsals the band visited London to play 'Dead Man Walking' on *Top Of The Pops*. After a secret show at Dublin's Factory on 17 May, rehearsals moved to the Brixton Academy in preparation for two warm-up gigs at London's 720-capacity Hanover Grand. It was the first time since 1972 that Bowie had kicked off a tour in his home country.

The Hanover Grand shows on 2 and 3 June were billed respectively as "Famous Fame" and "Little Wonderworld". The announcement that each would be split into two parts – a conventional round of songs followed by a "dance" set – attracted a great deal of interest from the British press, who were busy filling column inches with barbs about why a 50-year-old rock star who had just floated his back catalogue on the stock exchange felt the need to embark on a tour of sweaty little clubs. On this occasion, in the presence of the likes of Noel Gallagher, Gary Oldman and Goldie (for whose album *Saturnzreturn* David had recorded his contribution a few days earlier), Bowie successfully seduced many critics. The *Mirror* raved about "one of the most astonishing concerts I've ever seen," describing the sound as "awesome", the band "easily his best since The Spiders" and the overall package "a blistering answer to those who say he's lost the plot". But not all went according to plan on the opening night, as the *Guardian*'s Caroline Sullivan reported: "At the end [of the first set] he confirmed that his 'little drum'n'bass set' would follow the interval – and the audience voted with its feet." As far as Sullivan was concerned, there was a happy ending: "Those who left missed something fearfully loud, sweaty and hypnotic. Bowie, honking away on his saxophone, looked more like one of his new jungle buddies than like David Bowie Plc. Which is the way it should be."

The "dance set" turned out to consist of hard-hitting and radical reworkings of the likes of 'Pallas Athena', 'I'm Deranged', 'Dead Man Walking' and 'The Last Thing You Should Do'. The most unusual feature was an extended revision of 'Fame' based around a sample of the line "Is it any wonder?", which would later be restructured in the studio as 'Fun'.

Prompted by the first night's exodus, Bowie switched the sets for the following evening to perform the drum'n'bass numbers first. Barbara Ellen of the *Observer* was mightily displeased: "exhaustingly tedious ... we all have to stand around for an aeon, listening to what sounds like the cast of *Star Wars* falling down a fire escape. During 'Little Wonder' from the *Earthling* album, the bass vibrations got so unpleasantly deep and loud, I could feel my internal organs changing position. If I start urinating out of my nipples, I will know who to blame ... For God's sake man, you're a living legend. In future, play the old stuff, and stop trying so hard." The *Mail On Sunday*'s Giles Smith was more interested in the present, confessing that although he enjoyed the post-interval oldies, "a small, perverse part of me would have been interested to see him keep the faith – thundering on in the first mode until the last fan was either entirely won over or had left the building under a white flag."

Melody Maker gave the show an unmitigated slating, describing the new material as "more dishearteningly wretched than you could ever imagine." The *NME* was similarly dismissive of the *Earthling* songs but remained cautiously happy about the show in general, commending 'V-2 Schneider' as "surely the funkiest he's sounded in 20 years", 'White Light/White Heat' as "breathtaking", and finding 'Fame' and 'Fashion' "both kicked up the arse by more nostril-terrifying bass."

A further warm-up gig followed in Hamburg before the Earthling tour's official opening night at Lubeck on 7 June. A string of club dates followed before the "dance" numbers were either abandoned or incorporated into the main set. The favoured warm-up acts were now techno DJs rather than support bands. Just as the new music was more gutsy and instinctive than the 1.*Outside* material, so the band's performances had become less regimented. David himself, his red-dyed hair fading to blond during the course of the summer, had taken to wearing baggy slacks, polo-necks, T-shirts and even jogging bottoms, although an element of theatre remained in the loose-fitting white Nehru suit and the outrageous brocaded Indian ensemble he sported at some of the festival dates.

Although the show was less stagey than its predecessor, Bowie's penchant for set-dressing was still in evidence: the stage was dotted with abstract *objets*, including the inflatable eyeballs that had appeared at the fiftieth birthday gig. The lightshow was stunning, tapping into the club ambience with a furious stroboscopic assault on the senses, but the main visual element was provided by a series of disorientating back-projections: a psychedelic whirlpool for 'Little Wonder', a flashing chessboard of squares for 'Stay', a trip down a *2001* time-tunnel for 'V-2 Schneider', expanding stars and stripes for 'I'm Afraid Of Americans', and what the *Glasgow Herald* described as "a porno vid that would make Madonna blush" for 'Fashion'. Although deferring to his band during the solos Bowie remained an animated focal point, dropping into little mime routines throughout the show – plucking imaginary arrows from his body, Saint Sebastian-style, was a new favourite. Most of the time, however, he was busy playing either acoustic guitar or saxophone.

The previously sceptical *NME* described Bowie's headliner at the Phoenix Festival on 20 July as "almost too marvellous for words", going so far as to pronounce 'Little Wonder' "an ace Bowie tune". The previous night the band had appeared in the festival's

Radio 1 Tent to play a drum'n'bass set as "Tao Jones Index", the pseudonym under which a limited-edition 12" single of 'V-2 Schneider' and 'Pallas Athena', recorded in Amsterdam on 10 June, appeared the following month.

After the final European show in Budapest on 14 August, there was a three-week break before the tour reconvened in Vancouver. Rehearsals for the American leg saw some changes to the set – 'Outside' and 'I'm Deranged' were performed only a couple more times, while '"Heroes"' and 'Pallas Athena' were dropped altogether. In their place came several new additions, notably 'Panic In Detroit', 'The Supermen', and the concert debut of the *Low* classic 'Always Crashing In The Same Car'. The last two numbers made several appearances in a series of two-man acoustic guitar sessions recorded by Bowie and Gabrels for various radio stations during the American leg, alongside 'I Can't Read', 'Scary Monsters' and 'Dead Man Walking' (see Chapter 10).

The tour zig-zagged across America for the next two months. The Boston gig on 1 October became the first Bowie concert to be webcast live on the Internet. Five days later, David found time to film the video of 'I'm Afraid Of Americans' in New York with Trent Reznor. The 14 October concert at Port Chester's Capitol Theater (the scene, many years earlier, of technical rehearsals for the Diamond Dogs tour) was added at short notice for broadcast on MTV's *Live At The 10 Spot* after a last-minute cancellation by The Rolling Stones; Bowie warmed up with three untransmitted numbers before playing an excellent 50-minute set for the broadcast. The following day's gig at Radio City Music Hall was for the GQ Awards, from which a four-song set was broadcast on VH1 the following month.

In late October, by which time David had cultivated an alarming new Mohican hairstyle, the tour moved into Central and Southern America for its final six dates. The last, in Buenos Aires on 7 November, was broadcast in two instalments on Argentine television. Noting that this was where the Sound + Vision tour had wrapped seven years earlier, Bowie delighted the press by declaring, "It's my new tradition to finish my tours in Argentina!" In fact there were brief reprises of the tour in early December, when Bowie played a couple of dates in California, and on 29 January 1998, when he guested at *Howard Stern's Birthday Show*, later broadcast on E!TV. There were rumours of a duet with Radiohead at the 1998 Grammy Awards

(at which Bowie had two nominations, for *Earthling* and 'Dead Man Walking'), but this came to nothing.

If the Earthling tour lacked a little of its predecessor's sense of total theatre, then it substituted a raw energy and excitement not always evident in the Outside shows. The reworking of old favourites was for the most part scintillating: 'Quicksand' became a triumphant opening number, Bowie beginning alone on acoustic guitar while the band assembled behind him to strike up for the second chorus. 'The Jean Genie' gathered speed after a slow blues intro adapted from the 1974 version. 'Fame' was transformed by sinister keyboard effects and deafening blasts of bass. Crucially, such revivals remained vital and coherent within the context of Bowie's latest musical enthusiasms: the techno-styled 'V-2 Schneider' and the excellent rendering of 'O Superman' were entirely of a piece with the *Earthling* manifesto. Moreover, just as on the Outside tour, the new numbers held their own with admirable aplomb.

Soon afterwards Bowie spoke of releasing *Earthling Live*, an album culled from recordings of the European tour. He mixed the album in 1998 with Reeves Gabrels and Mark Plati, but Virgin pulled the release from their schedules. Later the same year, tracks from the project were made available to BowieNet subscribers in downloadable form, and in 2000 the live CD was distributed exclusively to BowieNet members as *liveandwell.com*.

THE 'HOURS...' TOUR
23 August – 12 December 1999

Musicians: David Bowie *(vocals, guitar)*, Page Hamilton *(guitar, September onwards)*, Reeves Gabrels *(guitar, August only)*, Mike Garson *(keyboards)*, Gail Ann Dorsey *(bass)*, Mark Plati *(acoustic guitar)*, Sterling Campbell *(drums)*, Holly Palmer *(backing vocals)*, Lani Groves *(backing vocals, August only)*, Emm Gryner *(backing vocals, September onwards)*

Repertoire: 'Life On Mars?' / 'Thursday's Child' / 'Can't Help Thinking About Me' / 'Seven' / 'China Girl' / 'Rebel Rebel' / 'Survive' / 'Word On A Wing' / 'Drive In Saturday' / 'I Can't Read' / 'Always Crashing In The Same Car' / 'If I'm Dreaming My Life' / 'The Pretty Things Are Going To Hell' / 'Repetition' / 'Changes' / 'Something In The Air' / 'Stay' / 'Cracked Actor' / 'Ashes To Ashes' / 'I'm Afraid Of Americans'

Bowie's first live appearance of 1999 came at the Brit Awards on 16 February, when he joined Placebo for a duet of Marc Bolan's '20th Century Boy'. The performance was reprised at a Placebo gig in New York a month later, when David also joined the band for 'Without You I'm Nothing'. On 8 May he appeared at the Hynes Convention Center in Boston to receive an honorary degree from Berklee College of Music, from which Reeves Gabrels had graduated in 1981.

Three months later, on 23 August, Bowie performed his first full-length set since the end of the Earthling tour, in an exclusive session at Manhattan Center Studios for VH1's *Storytellers*. First broadcast in edited form on 18 October, the show provided a taster for the forthcoming album *'hours…'*. David was joined by co-producer Mark Plati and most of the *Earthling* band – the only absentee was Zachary Alford, replaced by *1.Outside* and *'hours…'* drummer Sterling Campbell. In hooded top and trainers, his hair now longer than at any time since 1971, David unveiled a handful of new numbers and some jaw-dropping archive selections. Alongside unexpectedly mainstream revivals like 'China Girl' and 'Rebel Rebel', there were rare treats in the form of 'Word On A Wing' and 'Drive In Saturday', not performed since 1976 and 1974 respectively. But the biggest surprise was the resuscitation of the 1966 single 'Can't Help Thinking About Me': unheard for 33 years, its revival marked the first time since 1970 that David had performed any of his pre-*Space Oddity* material. The performance of 'China Girl' later appeared on the *VH1 Storytellers* album. During rehearsals for the show, the band also taped 'Thursday's Child', 'Survive' and 'The Pretty Things Are Going To Hell' for the BBC's *Top Of The Pops* and *TOTP2*.

It had been announced the previous spring that Bowie was to headline a massive "Millennium Concert" at Gisborne in New Zealand, becoming the first singer to perform as the sun rose on the year 2000. In August, however, the Gisborne concert was cancelled owing to poor sales. Instead, on the heels of the *Storytellers* performance, Bowie announced an autumn promotional tour to accompany the release of *'hours…'*. Although there would be only eight concerts, there would also be studio performances for well over a dozen television shows in the USA, Canada and Europe.

In September Bowie announced that "Page Hamilton, ex-Helmet founder member, will stand in on lead guitar for Reeves Gabrels on these shows.

Reeves will finish off two projects that have impending deadlines in October." Rumours of a tiff with Reeves Gabrels were rapidly denied. "We didn't have a falling out," Gabrels informed fans over the Internet on the same day as Bowie's announcement. "It was obvious to me that I needed to get on with my own thing. My album [*Ulysses (della notte)*] will be out in mid-October and I'm really into that … It is all amicable and we plan on reuniting for the next studio project." A few months later the story appeared to have changed, as the guitarist admitted that he and Bowie had "drifted apart." In an interview for *Guitar World* in 2001, Gabrels confessed that the parting of the ways had been his own fault. "Over time, I started thinking of David as the singer in *my* band – how twisted is that?" he laughed. "That was why I was getting frustrated with him near the end; I wanted the music to go one way and he wanted it to go another way. And when push came to shove, I had to remember whose name was on those albums, and I didn't. I lost perspective." To date, the VH1 *Storytellers* show remains the guitarist's final work with Bowie.

Late September saw the beginning of an intensive round of television spots to promote *'hours…'* (see Chapter 10). By the time Bowie appeared on *The Late Show With David Letterman* on 4 October, he was looking somewhat peaky. The following day, an acoustic set at New York's Virgin Megastore and an appearance on *The Howard Stern Show* were both cancelled when he succumbed to a bout of gastro-enteritis. Having flown to Britain on 8 October, a fully recovered and ebullient David gave a hysterical interview to Chris Evans on Channel 4's *TFI Friday*.

The following night saw Bowie's six-song set at the all-star NetAid concert at Wembley Stadium. Coordinated by U2's Bono, NetAid was a major initiative to raise awareness of global poverty and launch a website to pool charity resources. Other artists at Wembley included The Corrs, Eurythmics, George Michael, Stereophonics, Catatonia and Robbie Williams, while the linked events in Geneva and New Jersey featured Bono, Pete Townshend, Bryan Ferry, Texas, Puff Daddy and Jimmy Page. By the standards of previous charity extravaganzas NetAid was not a resounding success (post-mortems spoke of a lack of clear charity goals translating into a half-empty stadium in New Jersey), but nonetheless the event raised $12 million.

On 10 October Bowie played an invitation-only gig at the Dublin HQ, sponsored by Guinness, who had staged promotional competitions to win tickets. It was the first full-length show since the *Storytellers* gig, with a broadly similar set-list bolstered by more shock resurrections in the shape of 'Changes' and 'Repetition'. Thereafter the tour moved to the Continent, where 'Something In The Air' was added to the set at the 1000-seater Elysée Montmartre in Paris. This gig expanded to almost twice its scheduled length when Bowie opted for an extended encore. "I was only supposed to play 45 minutes," he told the delighted crowd, "but Paris is a special city for me. It's here that I got engaged." Three live tracks from the concert later appeared on the CD single of 'Survive'. While in Paris, Bowie was presented with the prestigious order of Chevalier des Arts et Lettres by the French cultural minister Catherine Trautman.

The Vienna gig on 17 October included a rare performance of 'If I'm Dreaming My Life', otherwise included only in the *Storytellers* set but cut from its transmission. This show, which coincided with the launching of BowieNet Europe, was available as a live webcast. In between the full-length gigs October saw a host of television appearances on the Continent. Back in London on 25 October Bowie played a live session for Radio 1's *Mark Radcliffe Show*, before returning to America – his departure from Heathrow later appeared on BBC1's docusoap *Airport*.

In Las Vegas on 28 October, Bowie received the inaugural "Legend" award at Warner Brothers' first WB Radio Music Awards. November 16 saw 'Thursday's Child' and another new revival, 'Cracked Actor', performed on *Late Night With Conan O'Brien*, plus a humorous version of 'What's Really Happening?' with lyrics submitted by the host. The first full-scale gig for a month was at New York's Kit Kat Club on 19 November, where 'Stay', 'Ashes To Ashes' and 'I'm Afraid of Americans' were added to the set. The show was broadcast on the SFX radio network and given a live webcast by the American Express *Blue Concert* series; tracks from the gig would later be included on formats of the 'Seven' single. Three days later Bowie played a ten-song session for the Canadian TV station Musique Plus, before once again crossing the Atlantic. Back in London he recorded a set for BBC2's *Later… With Jools Holland*, gave an interview to a clearly besotted Jeremy Paxman on *Newsnight*, and played a gig at the London Astoria. "We were all so nervous because there was all these famous people in the audience," Mike Garson later recalled. "Mick Jagger was there and Pete Townshend and they all went backstage. David

was great in that show."

The final two gigs followed the same week in Milan and Copenhagen, where backing vocalists Emm Gryner and Holly Palmer performed a last-night ditty called 'Shrink That Sweater' inspired by an incident earlier in the week when one of the crew had accidentally shrunk Bowie's purple pullover. David entered into the party spirit with a self-parodying announcement that "Not only is it the last show of the tour, but it's the last show – of the millennium!" The Danish newspaper *Ekstra Bladet* described the gig as "possibly the greatest music event on Danish soil ever," and an hour-long compilation was shown on Danish television the following May.

The day after the Copenhagen gig the band travelled to Gothenburg to record appearances on Swedish television. Bowie's final public appearance of 1999 was on the 30 December edition of Channel 4's *The Big Breakfast*, in which he gamely swapped places with the boom operator, donned an apron to help out in the kitchen, and played baseball with a collection of Christmas toys. It was the parting shot in a hectic promotional tour which had found David apparently happier and more relaxed than ever before. His breathlessly anecdotal interview style was pure stand-up, exemplified by the deliriously rambling account on *TFI Friday* of his Indonesian holiday in 1983. Better still was the music itself, sparklingly performed by a superb band. Bowie was in his finest voice for many years and, perhaps inspired by Mike Garson's sumptuous makeover of 'Life On Mars?', he was effortlessly rediscovering high notes long presumed dead. The potentially alarming revival of stadium crowd-pleaser 'China Girl' turned out to be a triumph, retooling the number with the darkness and attack of Iggy Pop's original, and even 'Rebel Rebel' successfully shed the predictability of its 1980s appearances. 'Can't Help Thinking About Me' proved a positive revelation rather than a comic novelty, while 'Drive In Saturday' and 'Word On A Wing' were simply majestic. Best of all, the *'hours…'* material was delivered with grace, conviction and flair. Once again, the new songs stole the show – which, for David Bowie, is exactly how things should be.

2000: NEW YORK AND GLASTONBURY

16 June – 24 July 2000

Musicians: David Bowie *(vocals, guitar)*, Earl Slick

(guitar), Mike Garson *(keyboards)*, Gail Ann Dorsey *(bass, guitar, clarinet, vocals)*, Mark Plati *(guitar, bass)*, Sterling Campbell *(drums)*, Holly Palmer *(backing vocals, percussion)*, Emm Gryner *(backing vocals, keyboards, clarinet)*

Repertoire: 'Wild Is The Wind' / 'Life On Mars?' / 'Golden Years' / 'Changes' / 'Stay' / 'China Girl' / 'Survive' / 'Absolute Beginners' / 'Ashes To Ashes' / 'Rebel Rebel' / 'Fame' / 'This Is Not America' / 'All The Young Dudes' / 'Starman' / 'The Man Who Sold The World' / 'Under Pressure' / 'Station To Station' / 'Seven' / 'Thursday's Child' / 'The Pretty Things Are Going To Hell' / 'Hallo Spaceboy' / 'Ziggy Stardust' / '"Heroes"' / 'Let's Dance' / 'I'm Afraid Of Americans' / 'The Jean Genie' / 'Cracked Actor' / 'Little Wonder' / 'I Dig Everything' / 'The London Boys' / 'Always Crashing In The Same Car'

On 13 February 2000 the world's press bubbled with the happy news that Mr and Mrs Bowie were expecting a new addition to the family. David was said to be "utterly overjoyed" and told the press that "It's been a long and patient wait for our baby, but both Iman and I wanted the circumstances to be absolutely right, and didn't want to find ourselves working flat out during the first couple of years of the baby's life."

With the baby due in August, David revealed that his return to the concert stage for a handful of summer engagements would be his last for some time: "That's it for about 18 months," he told the *Mirror*, "I'm becoming a recluse now!"

In late March, after an absence of 17 years from the Bowie camp, guitarist Earl Slick joined members of the *'hours…'* tour band for rehearsals in New York. "Playing with Bowie is like coming home," said Slick, whose presence ensured the addition of three further *Station To Station* numbers to the previous year's repertoire. Among the other surprises were revivals of 'Starman', 'Ziggy Stardust', 'Let's Dance' and even 'Absolute Beginners', together with the live premiere of another mid-1980s hit, 'This Is Not America'. Following the resurrection of 'Can't Help Thinking About Me', the appearance of 'I Dig Everything' and 'The London Boys' fuelled speculation that David was planing to cut a new album of his 1960s songs.

The band played two warm-up gigs on 16 and 19 June at New York's Roseland Ballroom, the second of which was free and exclusive to BowieNet subscribers. A third show on 17 June was called off at two hours'

notice when David found he was unable to sing, having contracted a mild dose of laryngitis and strained his voice on the first night; it was the first time in his career that he had been forced to cancel a concert for vocal reasons. Apparently David had suffered several minor ailments in recent weeks, as his body adjusted to his decision to quit smoking in anticipation of the arrival of Iman's baby (a resolution that wasn't to last; he was back on the Marlboro Lights by October). The BowieNet show was attended by Iman, Duncan, Susan Sarandon and various members of The Cure. The band was joined for the encores by Thomas Dolby, and also in attendance was David's veteran drummer Dennis Davis.

On 23 June the band appeared on Channel 4's *TFI Friday*, taping four songs of which only the first two, 'Wild Is The Wind' and 'Starman', were transmitted. Two days later came Bowie's headlining set at the Glastonbury Festival, his first appearance at the event since 1971. Glastonbury coordinator Michael Eavis could scarcely contain his delight, describing Bowie's set as "absolutely fantastic. He promised me the show of a lifetime and he delivered it." The critics, too, were in raptures: "a masterclass in superstardom," declared the *Mirror*, reporting that "Other big-name acts watched open-mouthed." The *NME* raved about "the breadth and intent of this fantastic performance," while the *Times* believed that "it will be remembered as the occasion at which Bowie won new respect."

On 27 June a more intimate concert was taped at London's BBC Radio Theatre for broadcast later in the year. The star-studded audience included Boy George, Simon Le Bon, Lulu, Bob Geldof, Russell Crowe, Meg Ryan and Richard E Grant. Mike Garson, who had provided appropriate curtain-up music for each gig on the tour ('I'll Take Manhattan' in New York; 'Greensleeves' at Glastonbury) played Gershwin's 'A Foggy Day In London Town' as the band took to the stage. David was still being dogged by throat problems, and during the encores was forced to call an adjournment while he downed a glass of water. The band played an instrumental jam based on 'The Jean Genie' until Bowie returned to the fray, refreshed and apparently cured, and once again happy to banter with the audience.

An excellent hour-long selection from the concert was screened on BBC2 on 24 September, the day before the release of *Bowie At The Beeb*, whose initial pressings also included a bonus live disc with fifteen tracks from the gig, bearing witness to a charged, proficient performance radiating enthusiasm and warmth. Indeed, despite his illness David's bonhomie was if anything even more pronounced than in the previous year. For the 2000 dates he had taken to wearing a succession of flamboyant three-quarter-length coats, and with his luxuriant hair now teased into soft waves, he resembled nothing so much as his *Man Who Sold The World* persona of thirty years earlier. His vocal problems barely affected the standard of the performances, which were spectacular. Numbers like 'Life On Mars?' and the superb 'Wild Is The Wind' (a pair of songs which David reprised at the Yahoo! Internet Life Online Music Awards in New York on 24 July, where he was nominated Online Pioneer of 2000) showcased a dramatic, full-bodied Bowie, evidently relishing his reunion with one of his finest guitarists, and bowing out of live performance – for the time being at least – in magnificent form.

2001 – 2002: THE TIBET HOUSE BENEFITS AND THE CONCERT FOR NEW YORK CITY

Musicians (Tibet House Benefit Concerts): David Bowie *(vocals, guitar, harmonica)*, Philip Glass *(piano)*, Tony Visconti *(bass)*, Sterling Campbell *(drums)*, Martha Mooke, Gregor Kitzis, Meg Okura, Mary Wotten *(Scorchio Quartet)*, Moby *(guitar – 2001 concert only)*, Adam Yauch *(bass – 2002 concert only)*, David Harrington, John Sherba, Hank Dutt, Jennifer Culp *(Kronos Quartet – 2002 concert only)*

Musicians (The Concert For New York City): David Bowie *(vocals, Omnichord)*, Mark Plati *(guitar)*, Gail Ann Dorsey *(bass)*, Paul Shaffer *(keyboards)*, Sid McGinnis *(guitar)*, Will Lee *(bass)*, Anton Fig *(drums)*, Felicia Collins *(guitar, percussion)*, Tom Malone *(horns)*, Bruce Kapler *(horns)*, Al Chez *(horns)*, Nikki Richards *(backing vocals)*, Elaine Caswell *(backing vocals)*, Curtis King *(backing vocals)*

Repertoire: '"Heroes"' / 'Silly Boy Blue' / 'People Have The Power' / 'America' / 'I Would Be Your Slave' / 'Space Oddity'

Following his appearance at the Yahoo! awards on 24 July 2000, Bowie retreated from the limelight to work on *Toy* and to devote time to his domestic life. His only high-profile appearance for the remainder of the year was at the VH1 Fashion Awards at Madison Square Garden on 20 October, where he presented Stella McCartney with the "Fashion Designer Of The Year" award.

In January 2001, news began to filter through that Bowie was to perform at the Tibet House Benefit concert at New York's Carnegie Hall, marking his first appearance at the famous venue since the 1970s. "I'll be doing a couple of songs with both Moby and Philip Glass," David revealed, whetting fans' appetites for the renewal of two of his more stimulating collaborative relationships. Before becoming the darling of the chill-out club scene with the global success of his album *Play*, Moby had remixed Bowie's 1997 single 'Dead Man Walking', while David's previous work with Philip Glass encompassed not only the *Low* and *"Heroes"* symphonies but also a live appearance at Carnegie Hall way back in 1979.

The concert on 26 February, in aid of the Tibet House Trust which had previously benefited from such projects as the 1997 album *Long Live Tibet*, was a far more cutting-edge affair than the average charity bash, and was adjudged a great success by critics and fans alike. "It has a low profile," David noted approvingly in an interview for *Newsday*. "Given the nature of the artists, it sells out, but it's not a trumpet-blowing thing. It's a very comfortable situation." Performers included Patti Smith, Emmylou Harris, Natalie Merchant, Dave Matthews, and Pakistan's qawwali master Rahat Nusrat Fateh Ali Khan. Bowie's brief two-song set came a little over an hour into the proceedings, his reunion with Moby and Glass rendered even more exciting by the appearance of Tony Visconti on bass – the first time he had shared a stage with David since the days of Hype over thirty years earlier. With additional string backing by the Scorchio Quartet, Bowie's set consisted of his customary benefit-gig classic '"Heroes"' and, by way of acknowledging both the Tibetan theme of the evening and his recent studio sessions, an extraordinarily beautiful revival of his 1966 number 'Silly Boy Blue'. At the song's climax a troupe of monks from the Drepung Gomang Buddhist Monastic University swelled the sound with chants and percussion, in what *Rolling Stone* later described as "the most moving moment of the evening". The concert ended with Patti Smith leading the assembled company in an energetic performance of her 1988 song 'People Have The Power', during which she pulled David over to her microphone for a spirited duet.

Bowie had announced beforehand that this would be his only live date of 2001, but events were to dictate otherwise. In the wake of the 11 September terrorist attacks on New York and Washington, David was characteristically quick to rally his Internet community. "Life here will continue," he told BowieNet members on 12 September. "New Yorkers are a resilient and fast thinking people. In this way they really do resemble my own Londoners. They came together quickly in massive community support and silent determination." When it was announced that Madison Square Garden would play host to a major benefit concert, the presence of rock music's foremost New Yorkers was a foregone conclusion. Sure enough the show, which took place on 20 October 2001 before an audience consisting mainly of FDNY officers and other rescue workers, was a star-studded affair featuring Jon Bon Jovi, Eric Clapton, The Who, Macy Gray, Janet Jackson, Mick Jagger, Keith Richards, Billy Joel, Elton John, Paul McCartney, and a host of Hollywood stars. There was even a sequence of short films celebrating the spirit of New York, donated by the likes of Woody Allen, Spike Lee and Martin Scorsese. David undertook the challenge of opening the concert, which he chose to do in unexpected but charming style with a pared-down interpretation of Simon and Garfunkel's 'America', which he performed sitting cross-legged in a pool of light, accompanying himself on a low-tech 1980s Omnichord keyboard. Thereafter the lights came up for an inevitable but wonderfully impressive '"Heroes"', for which David was joined by Mark Plati on guitar, Gail Ann Dorsey on bass, and the concert's eleven-piece house band, billed as "The Orchestra For New York City" (trivia buffs will note that they included *Never Let Me Down* guitarist Sid McGinnis and *Tonight/Black Tie White Noise* backing vocalist Curtis King). For the first time in many moons Bowie was backed on stage by a full horn section, and on this occasion the results were undeniably superb. The Concert For New York City was broadcast live on America's VH1, with edited highlights later screened by CBS and other stations. A double CD of the concert appeared the next month, with a DVD following in 2002.

On 22 February 2002 Bowie performed once again at the Tibet House Benefit concert at Carnegie Hall, this time sharing the bill with Ray Davies, Beastie Boy Adam Yauch, and newcomers Chocolate Genius, who opened the show with an acoustic rendition of 'Soul Love'. Bowie began his own set with a dramatic premiere of the *Heathen* composition 'I Would Be Your Slave', again accompanied by Tony Visconti, Sterling

Campbell and the Scorchio Quartet. Then came an unexpected and sumptuous orchestration of 'Space Oddity' (David's first performance of the number since his fiftieth birthday concert five years previously), for which Philip Glass played piano and Adam Yauch took over on bass, while Visconti conducted the assembled strings of the Scorchio and Kronos Quartets. *Rolling Stone* described the result as "stunning". Once again, Bowie and his band joined Patti Smith at the end of the evening for a final encore of 'People Have The Power'.

MELTDOWN 2002 AND THE HEATHEN TOUR
10 May – 23 October 2002

Musicians: David Bowie (*vocals, guitar, keyboards, saxophone, Stylophone, harmonica*), Earl Slick (*guitar*), Gerry Leonard (*guitar*), Mark Plati (*guitar, keyboards*), Gail Ann Dorsey (*bass, vocals*), Mike Garson (*keyboards*), Sterling Campbell (*drums, keyboards*), Catherine Russell (*backing vocals, keyboards*)

Repertoire: 'Speed Of Life' / 'Breaking Glass' / 'What In The World' / 'Sound And Vision' / 'Always Crashing In The Same Car' / 'Be My Wife' / 'A New Career In A New Town' / 'Warszawa' / 'Art Decade' / 'Weeping Wall' / 'Subterraneans' / 'Sunday' / 'Cactus' / 'Slip Away' / 'Slow Burn' / 'Afraid' / 'I've Been Waiting For You' / 'I Would Be Your Slave' / 'I Took A Trip On A Gemini Spaceship' / '5.15 The Angels Have Gone' / 'Everyone Says 'Hi'' / 'A Better Future' / 'Heathen (The Rays)' / 'China Girl' / 'Let's Dance' / 'I'm Afraid Of Americans' / 'Ashes To Ashes' / 'Fame' / 'Hallo Spaceboy' / 'Absolute Beginners' / 'Fashion' / 'Changes' / 'Starman' / 'Ziggy Stardust' / '"Heroes"' / 'White Light/White Heat' / 'Stay' / 'Life On Mars?' / 'Space Oddity' / 'I Feel So Bad' / 'One Night' / 'Look Back In Anger' / 'Survive' / 'Alabama Song' / 'Rebel Rebel' / 'Moonage Daydream' / 'The Bewlay Brothers'

On 11 February 2002, two weeks before his performance at the Tibet House Benefit concert, it was announced that David Bowie had accepted the post of Artistic Director at Meltdown, the annual music and arts festival hosted by London's South Bank complex. Each of the nine previous Meltdown Festivals had been curated by a guest director hailing from the avant-garde end of the musical spectrum: George Benjamin, Louis Andriessen, Elvis Costello, Magnus

Lindberg, Laurie Anderson, John Peel, Nick Cave, Scott Walker and, most recently, Robert Wyatt. Each Meltdown director is given free rein to assemble his or her fantasy festival, creating an eclectic programme of rock, classical and contemporary music, film, theatre and exhibitions, reflecting their own personal passions and interests. Previous Meltdowns had yielded memorable performances from a host of artists both mainstream and obscure: among the veterans were Nina Simone, Ryuichi Sakamoto, Lou Reed, Radiohead, Deborah Harry, Sonic Youth, Blur, Tricky and Kylie Minogue.

David Bowie's Meltdown 2002 (as the event was officially entitled) ran from 13-30 June, the main focus of attention being a non-stop schedule of concerts in the Royal Festival Hall and its smaller adjoining venue, the Queen Elizabeth Hall. For Bowie fans, the event was given an added frisson by the fact that the South Bank had played host to some crucial dates in David's early career: the Purcell Room had been the scene of his showcase concert on 20 November 1969, while the Royal Festival Hall itself had played host to a mime performance in 1968 and, more memorably, to the breakthrough Ziggy Stardust gig on 8 July 1972, at which David had been joined on stage by Lou Reed.

Bowie announced that he was excited by the opportunity to curate Meltdown: "I was very disappointed two years ago when I had to decline Scott Walker's invitation to perform, so I am thrilled that I get a second chance to contribute in whatever way I can." Glenn Manx, the South Bank's Producer of Contemporary Culture, pronounced himself "thrilled and honoured" by Bowie's acceptance of the post, describing David as "the quintessential Meltdown Director. His way of thinking makes an eclectic festival like Meltdown possible."

The main line-up for Bowie's Meltdown was announced in April 2002, with extra attractions added over the following month. Among the artists performing on the Royal Festival Hall's main stage were The Divine Comedy (17 June), Coldplay with guest Pete Yorn (22 June), Suede (23 June), Mercury Rev (27 June) and Supergrass with guest Bobby Conn (28 June). The Queen Elizabeth Hall, meanwhile, played host to some rather more idiosyncratic artists, including an eye-opening double bill comprising cult singer-songwriter Daniel Johnston and Bowie's old favourite the Legendary Stardust Cowboy (15 June), stand-up comedian Harry Hill (17 June), Television with guests Luke Haines and Stew (19-20 June), Kimmo

Pohjonen Kluster and the Lonesome Organist (18 June), and Asian Dub Foundation playing their live score to Mathieu Kassovitz's film La Haine (21-22 June). More mainstream offerings in the Queen Elizabeth Hall included an acoustic set by The Waterboys (16 June) and two nights with Badly Drawn Boy (26-27 June), while a more unusual choice was Matt Johnson's relaunched The The (25 June). A late cancellation by Gorillaz and Terry Hall, who had been scheduled to perform at the Festival Hall on 21 June, made way for the last-minute addition of rising New York "electro-clash" exponents Fischerspooner.

There were initial mutterings from some quarters that Bowie's Meltdown programme was more conservative and mainstream than those of previous years (indeed, in May Bowie was even moved to publish a defence of his Meltdown line-up in the Times after journalist Stuart Maconie had accused him of pandering to the masses), but on close inspection Bowie had in fact gone farther into the left field than many of his predecessors. Nobody who attended the frankly indescribable Daniel Johnston/Legendary Stardust Cowboy evening could possibly accuse Bowie of making concessions to popular taste, and for every Coldplay or Supergrass there was a Baby Zizanie, a Peaches, a Polyphonic Spree or a Bollywood Brass Band. "My choice of billing reflects both my populist and fringe tastes in music," declared Bowie, and nowhere was this clearer than in the series of free concerts sponsored by BBC Radio 3 on the Festival Hall Ballroom stage: they included such unlikely acts as Swedish punk-funk outfit (International) Noise Conspiracy, Teutonic obscurantist Uwe Schmidt (here adopting the name Senor Coconut to play a series of salsa reworkings of Kraftwerk songs), and Terry Edwards And The Scapegoats, who played a set of ska interpretations of Bowie numbers, including 'Speed Of Life', 'Sorrow', 'Cat People', 'TVC15', 'Rebel Rebel' and 'Boys Keep Swinging'.

Even more unusual were Lonesome Organist Jeremy Jacobson, a one-man band of bizarre homemade instruments, and Finnish duo Kimmo Pohjonen Kluster who, on the evening before their Queen Elizabeth Hall performance, played an extraordinary Ballroom set of reinterpreted Bowie classics including 'Abdulmajid', 'Warszawa', 'Sense of Doubt', 'We Prick You' and 'Life on Mars?'. Pohjonen's part-vocal, part-accordion music is played live over pre-treated samples made by percussionist Samuli Kosminen. "My music is obscure, psychedelic and sometimes beautiful," said Pohjonen, "like Finnish weather." Another notable coup was the revival of the Langley Schools Music Project, the 1970s brainchild of music teacher Hans Fenger, whose legendary recordings of Canadian schoolchildren singing pop classics like 'God Only Knows' and 'Space Oddity' were released on CD in 2002 as *Innocence And Despair*. Invited by Bowie to relaunch the project, Fenger collaborated with children from eight Lambeth schools for their free Ballroom performance on 21 June, which duly culminated in 'Space Oddity'.

These Bowie covers were not the only tributes to Meltdown's curator: The Divine Comedy included an excellent cover of 'Ashes To Ashes' in their set, while Television's Tom Verlaine, whose 'Kingdom Come' had been covered by David on *Scary Monsters* back in 1980, returned the compliment with an encore version of 'Psychotic Reaction' in which he sang snatches of Bowie lyrics over an ethereal backing.

In addition to the programme of concerts, David Bowie's Meltdown included *Sound And Vision* (see Chapter 7), an exhibition of work by young artists selected from the Bowieart website, and *Digital Cinema*, an eclectic choice of films created in the digital medium which were screened throughout June at the neighbouring National Film Theatre. "I can guarantee that if you've not seen digi-film before, you are in for an astonishing few hours," said David, whose selections included mainstream titles like *The Pillow Book* and *24 Hour Party People* alongside obscurities such as Oshii Mamoru's Japanese virtual-reality fantasy *Avalon* and Zacharias Kunuk's Inuit epic *Atanarjuat: The Fast Runner*.

The Meltdown programme began and ended with the festival's only fundamentally Bowie-oriented evenings: on 13 June the London Sinfonietta, conducted by Marin Aslop, performed Philip Glass's *Low* and *"Heroes"* symphonies at the Royal Festival Hall, while the closing date of 29 June, billed as "The New Heathens Night", was to be a headlining concert by the man himself. For Bowie, however, Meltdown was only part of an ongoing package of gigs to promote the release of *Heathen*. Preceded by a handful of live appearances in New York, the Heathen tour proper would begin at Meltdown before embarking on a series of summer festival dates.

Rehearsals began in New York in early May. Assembling a band consisting mainly of veterans of the 2000 tour together with *Heathen* newcomers Catherine Russell and Gerry Leonard, Bowie intimated that the greatest hits package of two years earlier was not about to be repeated: "I capitulate every now and again and give them what they want," he said, "but I get mad at myself because that's not really what I do, or what I like. I'm very selfish about what I want to do, and as I get older I get more selfish." Nevertheless, the first public preview leaned heavily on mainstream oldies: in a five-song set for MTV's Tribeca Film Festival at New York City's Battery Park on 10 May, the band played 'China Girl', 'Slow Burn', 'Afraid', 'Let's Dance' and 'I'm Afraid Of Americans'.

On 30 May David reprised the solo performance of 'America' he had given at the previous year's Concert For New York City. This time the occasion was a charity auction at Manhattan's Javits Center, organized by the Robin Hood Foundation who had coordinated much of the city's post-11 September fundraising activities. "It's an amazing charity," said David. "It is run and paid for by the wealthy of New York, therefore there are no expenses whatsoever. Every single penny made goes to charity. They are the biggest funder of schools in New York's poorest neighbourhoods. They've also made it possible for, so far, over 700,000 uninsured kids to get access to health care. Since 1988, they've raised literally millions and millions of dollars and started more programmes than I can remember." The Foundation asked David to sing 'America' as a curtain-raiser for the auction, which was hosted by Mike Myers and Diane Sawyer. "I went over straight after my own rehearsals and did the song for them, then went home for dinner," said David. "They raised – wait for it – $14,000,000 in one night."

On 2 June came the first in a series of television recordings, as the band taped a set of nine songs at New York's Kaufman Studios for use by the BBC's *Top Of The Pops* and *TOTP2*. Before a small audience of BowieNet members, the band played four numbers from *Heathen* ('Slow Burn', 'Cactus', 'Gemini Spaceship' and 'Everyone Says 'Hi''), four fresh oldies ('Sound And Vision', 'Ashes To Ashes', 'Fame' and 'Absolute Beginners'), and a second performance of 'Slow Burn' for use as a generic promotional clip. 'Slow Burn' duly appeared on *Top Of The Pops* on 7 June, with other songs popping up in subsequent editions of *TOTP2*. Further TV performances would follow on *The Late Show With David Letterman* on 10 June ('Slow Burn') and *Late Night With Conan O'Brien* on 19 June ('Slow Burn' and 'Cactus').

The first full-length show of the tour was a warm-up gig at New York's Roseland Ballroom on 11 June. Access was exclusive to BowieNet members, who were rewarded by a remarkable departure from Bowie's usual style of set-list. David had already told a couple of interviewers that he was intending to perform both *Low* and *Heathen* in their entirety, and this is exactly what he did. "The two albums kind of feel like cousins to each other," he explained later. "They've got a certain sonic similarity." For the opening *Low* section David wore a Thin White Duke-style waistcoat and trousers with white shirt with black tie, an outfit created, as were most of the suits he wore on stage during 2002, by the New York-based designer Hedi Slimane. During the *Low* performance David played keyboards on 'Warszawa' and 'Art Decade', harmonica on 'A New Career In A New Town', and saxophone for the closing 'Subterraneans'. After a 10-minute interval the band returned, David now clad in the three-piece Burberry tweed suit that appeared in the *Heathen* publicity photos, to play his new album from start to finish. He then changed into a scarlet frock-coat and black silk trousers for encores of 'Hallo Spaceboy', 'Ashes To Ashes', 'Fashion' and 'I'm Afraid Of Americans'. It was a highly unusual experiment (making *Low* and *Heathen* the first Bowie albums other than *Tin Machine II* to be performed in their entirety on a single tour, and the first ever to be played in uninterrupted album order at a single gig), and was adjudged an unqualified triumph by those lucky enough to attend.

On 14 June the band played four songs at New York's Rockefeller Plaza for NBC's *The Today Show* (while, during the soundcheck, Bowie even busked an impromptu rendition of 'Rock'n'Roll Suicide'). The following day saw a 13-song concert on the A&E channel's interactive TV show *Live By Request*, which allows viewers to request numbers by telephone or email. Unsurprisingly, more oldies were added to the set-list for the occasion, with 'Changes', 'Starman', 'Ziggy Stardust' and '"Heroes"' returning from the 2000 repertoire. In the UK, a re-edited version of *Live By Request* would be screened on ITV in December, cutting the telephone calls but adding two extra songs ('I've Been Waiting For You' and 'Cactus') which were not shown by A&E.

On 26 June Bowie arrived in Southampton after a leisurely five-day crossing on the *QEII*. The following evening was spent at BBC Television Centre recording an interview special with Jonathan Ross, during which the band played 'Fashion', 'Slip Away', 'Be My Wife',

'Everyone Says 'Hi'' and 'Ziggy Stardust'. Edited to 45 minutes ('Be My Wife' was among the excisions), the show was transmitted the following week as *Friday Night With Ross And Bowie*. In the meantime, 29 June found compère and performer reunited for Bowie's long-awaited Meltdown concert at the Royal Festival Hall. Providing excellent support on the "New Heathens Night" were the Portland-based Dandy Warhols, while the festivities continued after the gig with a DJ set hosted by Jonathan Ross, on whose Radio 2 show David had appeared earlier in the day. Bowie was delighted by his choice of support act, whose work he had been championing for some time: "The Dandy Warhols are a terrific band both on stage and on record," he had said the previous November. "Their writing seems to get better with every album." The admiration was mutual: in September 2000 The Dandy Warhols' lead singer Courtney Taylor-Taylor had told the *NME* that Bowie was "a superhero because he always did it better and farther than everybody else … and today he's just as unbelievable and irresistibly beautiful as ever."

The London show attracted a star-studded audience including Robert Smith, Brian Eno, Siouxsie Sioux, Toyah Willcox, Kylie Minogue, Bono, Stephen Duffy, Tracey Emin, Janet Street-Porter, and members of Duran Duran and Supergrass. Bowie's set again consisted of complete performances of *Low* and *Heathen*, although this time *Low* was re-ordered to divide the long instrumental tracks: entering to the strains of 'Weeping Wall', David joined the band for 'Warszawa' before returning to the beginning of the album. 'Art Decade' was inserted after 'Sound And Vision', and the set again ended with 'Subterraneans'. During the ten-minute interval Bowie changed from his Thin White Duke outfit into a white silk suit for the superb performance of *Heathen* which followed. Although the length of the set and the Festival Hall's curfew regulations forced David to be a little less chatty between numbers than usual, he found the time to ask who had seen The Legendary Stardust Cowboy's Meltdown concert ("What a professional!" he laughed on relating the trouser-dropping antics with which The Ledge had concluded his set), and dedicated '5.15 The Angels Have Gone' to John Entwistle, whose death had been announced the previous day.

Returning to the stage in the scarlet coat he had worn at Roseland, Bowie was joined for the first encore by The Dandy Warhols, bringing a total of six guitars to the stage for a magnificent rendition of

'White Light/White Heat', a new addition to the repertoire. The encores continued with 'Fame', 'Ziggy Stardust', 'Hallo Spaceboy' and 'I'm Afraid Of Americans'.

The Roseland and Meltdown concerts set a template for the unadorned performance style that would prevail throughout the Heathen tour: besides David's costume changes and the customary state-of-the-art lighting (including, at most gigs other than Meltdown, a backdrop spelling "BOWIE" in multiple lightbulbs), the only real concession to theatricality came in the form of a spot of play-acting in the early stages of 'Sunday', during which David and Gail Ann Dorsey indulged in some synchronized hand-movements, and in 'Heathen (The Rays)', at the climax of which Bowie would bow his head and place a hand on Dorsey's shoulder, allowing her to guide him off stage as though he were blind. It was an effective theatrical construct, evocative not only of the blind-eyed *Heathen* sleeve image but also of the choreography that had accompanied 'Loving The Alien' – another song of faith and heathenism – on the Glass Spider tour many years earlier. 'Heathen (The Rays)' would remain the usual closing number of the tour's pre-encore set, Bowie's "blind" exit ending the main part of the show on a suitably understated flourish.

"I can't remember a time when I was received so warmly," David told reporters backstage after the Meltdown concert. "It was fantastic." Sure enough, the press reaction was unanimous. "If there is one area in which Bowie excels it is in creating a sense of occasion, and he didn't disappoint," reported the *Times* in a five-star review, hailing Bowie's appearance at the Festival Hall as "a resplendent vision of lithe, ageless cool ... whatever changes Bowie has weathered, he remains a natural performer and a supremely gifted musician." The *Sun* remarked that "a nonchalant Bowie was strutting on the stage like a cocky teenager ... at 55 the Thin White Duke still looks great and sounds great." Another five-star review in the *Guardian* declared the concert "an extraordinary event", remarking that Bowie "seems so ageless, flashing a toothy grin as he snakes his lithe, angular body about the stage. His vocals are as spine-shivering as ever." The *Daily Telegraph* announced that "this has to be up there with the best. He was alive, animated, focused, evidently having the time of his life, and he was backed by a singularly awesome band ... Sensational, and unforgettable."

As the tour moved from London to a string of festival dates in France, Norway, Denmark and Belgium, it became apparent that the rigid structure of the Meltdown repertoire was by no means the be-all and end-all of Bowie's 2002 repertoire. Although most of the *Low* and *Heathen* material would be retained (including further near-complete performances of *Low* in Cologne, Montreux and Berlin), some numbers were dropped altogether. Neither 'A Better Future' nor, surprisingly, 'Slow Burn' resurfaced after Meltdown, while 'Gemini Spaceship' enjoyed only one further trip as the set-list rapidly transformed into a more eclectic and crowd-pleasing selection from Bowie's recent and distant past. The Paris show on 1 July (recorded by ARTE television and transmitted on 12 September) saw the addition of 'Stay' as the show opener, while an ecstatically brilliant 'Life On Mars?' opened the batting in Norway and thereafter remained the usual curtain-raiser, beginning with Mike Garson on solo piano and building into a breathtaking full-band orchestration during the second verse. More unexpected was a one-off performance of 'Space Oddity' at the Horsens Festival in Denmark (David would later tease some audiences with a brief snippet of 'Space Oddity' on his Stylophone after 'Slip Away', while Cologne was subjected to a Stylophonic snatch of 'Do-Re-Mi').

Back in the UK, David and Iman attended the Serpentine Gallery's annual party in Hyde Park on 9 July, and the following day the tour resumed at Manchester's Move Festival, where Meltdown signings Suede and The Divine Comedy played in torrential rain before the clouds parted for Bowie's headlining set. Rumours of a duet with Suede proved unfounded, but Bowie's performance received breathless notices. "As the hits kept coming, there was an overwhelming sense that Bowie is now more relaxed than he has been for years," reported the *Manchester Evening News*. "The voice, of course, was as glorious and theatrical as ever." The *Daily Star* considered the show "pitch perfect ... the crowd went wild. If Bowie ever gets bored with belting it out after all these years in the business, he certainly hides it well." The *Daily Telegraph* raved about "Bowie's incredible rebirth as a performer. He is clearly having the time of his life on this tour, aided by an astonishingly tight, virtuoso band ... it's hard to describe how awesome was the impact ... Such is Bowie's aura, that undeniable sense of otherness that makes even those who gave up on him in the 1980s flock back to him like space cadets to the commander."

From Manchester the tour headed back to the

Continent. Cologne's mammoth 30-song set included the first *Low* performance since Meltdown – now minus 'Weeping Wall', as would remain the case for the rest of the tour – and two performances of 'Everyone Says "Hi"' for the benefit of the cameras which were filming the song's little-seen live video. Next came Nimes, Lucca, and a headlining set at the prestigious Montreux Jazz Festival. Returning to America on the *QEII*, Bowie next linked up with Moby's twelve-date Area: 2 Festival tour of the United States and Canada, during which he performed alongside acts including Busta Rhymes, Ash, Blue Man Group and Moby himself. Busy promoting his new and conspicuously Bowie-influenced album *18*, Moby had already described David as "my favourite musician of the 20th century" and "an amazing live performer". David had struck up a close friendship with Moby in recent months, inviting him to remix 'Sunday', participating in several joint interviews to promote *Heathen* and *18*, and even giving Moby the hat he wore in *The Man Who Fell To Earth* as a Christmas present. Posting on his website immediately after the opening Area: 2 date in Bristow on 28 July, Moby gushed about his star guest: "David Bowie was beyond great. I can't believe that I stood at the side of the stage watching David Bowie perform at my festival. Oh my goodness. He was so good. The new songs from *Heathen* sounded wonderful … the song about Oogie and Uncle Floyd has such a heartbreaking, elegiac quality to it. I'm a very happy little festival organizer."

The press concurred: "It may be Moby's tour, but through outstanding songs and sheer animal magnetism, David Bowie owns Area: 2," reported the *Washington Times*. The *Toronto Star* announced that Bowie "proved the one real uniting force of the day … Curiously, too, it wasn't the Bowie classics that went over best, although a closing run at 'Ziggy' certainly left the throng on a high note. Rather, it was later material – the electro-shocked 'I'm Afraid Of Americans' and 'Hallo Spaceboy', the '80s standard 'Let's Dance', a massive cover of Neil Young's 'I've Been Waiting For You' and the brooding title track from his excellent new *Heathen* disc – that kept most of the crowd on its feet." The *Courier Post* reported that "the performance was enhanced by some of the best live vocal work Bowie has delivered in years. He seems to have found his way back to slightly higher registers; the icy edge that informed his earlier style was frequently employed to great effect." The *Rocky Mountain News* reported that the Denver show "left the crowd

breathless and stunned", while the *Orange County Register* hailed Bowie's Los Angeles set as "one of the great performances of the year." The *Times Dispatch* went so far as to say that "Although Moby closed the concert, the majority of the audience came to see the man who should have headlined the night, Mr Thin White Duke himself." For his part, David seemed unfazed by taking second billing for the first time in living memory: "I'm taking full advantage of second spot on the show and getting in the car afterwards and driving home to New York every night," he explained, "so that I can be there when Lexi wakes up in the morning." Commuting also allowed the band to record an appearance on NBC's *Last Call With Carson Daly* on 1 August, playing 'Cactus' and 'Everyone Says 'Hi''. The same two songs featured on *The Tonight Show With Jay Leno* on 12 August, during which Moby played percussion on 'Everyone Says 'Hi'', and provided guitar and vocals on 'Cactus'.

Given the multiple bill, Bowie's Area: 2 sets were markedly shorter than the other 2002 dates, averaging around 16 numbers each. The Jones Beach set on 2 August was cut short by an electrical storm: songs like 'I'm Afraid Of Americans' and '"Heroes"' were rendered particularly dramatic in torrential rain punctuated by rolls of thunder and flashes of lightning, but conditions finally became too dangerous and the set was curtailed after a mere 12 numbers. The longest Area: 2 set was reserved for the final date, at the dramatic Gorge Amphitheater outside Seattle. The concert fell on the 25th anniversary of Elvis Presley's death, and Bowie elected to mark the occasion by swelling his encores with the inclusion of what he described as "hasty but enthusiastic" covers of the Presley classics 'I Feel So Bad' and 'One Night'. "The Gorge was just the most splendid location for a finale," David remarked afterwards, "and, because of its majesty, put me in mind of the mountain Shokan location where it all began last year with the recording for *Heathen*."

Midway through the Area: 2 tour it emerged that Bowie would be returning to Europe to play six more concerts in September and October. Before the gigs got under way, David appeared at London's Natural History Museum on 3 September to collect an Outstanding Achievement prize from Stella McCartney at *GQ*'s Men of the Year Awards. There followed a handful of TV spots to promote the European release of the 'Everyone Says 'Hi'' single, including performances on Swedish TV's *Bingolotto* and Bowie's first ever appearance on BBC1's flagship chat show *Parkinson*, for which he gave a lengthy interview and followed 'Everyone Says 'Hi'' with a pared-down 'Life On Mars?', accompanied only by Mike Garson. The show was considered a great success, and Bowie would be back on *Parkinson* little more than a year later.

On 18 September, the day before *Parkinson* was recorded, the band played an excellent ten-song live session in front of a small audience at the BBC's Maida Vale Studios. Broadcast on Radio 2 a fortnight later, this show featured five further additions to the repertoire in the form of 'Look Back In Anger', 'Survive', 'Alabama Song', a heavily restructured 'Rebel Rebel' with a new low-key guitar intro, and finally the undisputed highlight: David's first ever live performance of 'The Bewlay Brothers'. For many fans, the long-awaited live debut of this most legendary and enigmatic of songs was the talking point of 2002; 'The Bewlay Brothers' would reappear only twice more, in the following month's concerts in Hammersmith and Brooklyn. September 20 saw Bowie back at the BBC for the third time in as many days, this time to record an appearance on BBC2's *Later... With Jools Holland*. In addition to a short interview (during which David commandeered Holland's piano to perform a snatch of The Legendary Stardust Cowboy's 'Paralyzed'), the band played 'Rebel Rebel', 'Look Back In Anger', '5.15 The Angels Have Gone', 'Heathen (The Rays)' and 'Ashes To Ashes', although only 'Rebel Rebel' and the two *Heathen* numbers were included in the show's transmission a month later.

The European concert dates began on 22 September with an epic 31-song gig in Berlin, which included another near-complete performance of *Low* and the introduction of 'Moonage Daydream' to the repertoire. The show was widely considered to be one of the year's finest concerts, reaching a peak with an emotive performance of '"Heroes"'. "There's no other city I can do that song in now that comes close to how it's received," David reflected the following year. Recalling the remarkable events of the Glass Spider tour's Berlin Wall concert in June 1987, he remarked that "This time, what was so fantastic is that the audience – it was the Max Schmelling Hall, which holds about 10-15,000 – half the audience had been in East Berlin that time way before. So now I was face to face with the people I had been singing it to all those years ago. And we were all singing it together. Again, it was powerful. Things like that really give you a sense of what performance can do. They happen so rarely at

that kind of magnitude." The Berlin concert was filmed, and reports circulated for a while that a DVD release would be forthcoming. It wasn't, but a 13-song selection was broadcast on German television the following February.

The European tour continued with dates in Paris, Bonn and Munich, before reaching what was arguably its pinnacle on 2 October when, for the first time since 1983, Bowie returned to the legendary London venue where he had famously killed off Ziggy Stardust some 29 years earlier: although now trading under the ungainly name of the Carling Apollo Hammersmith, to many it will forever remain the Hammersmith Odeon. The celebrity-studded audience included erstwhile Bowie stalwarts Brian Eno, George Underwood and John Cambridge. Incorporating an array of classics old and new, including the first full-blown concert outing for 'The Bewlay Brothers', the Hammersmith gig ended the European dates on a dazzling high.

In the days after Hammersmith there followed a couple of TV appearances, on Germany's *Wetten Dass...?* and Italy's *Quelli Che Il Calcio*, before the band returned to New York. The original intention had been to end the tour in Hammersmith but, as David would later recall, "we had a number of New York TV commitments at hand, so I needed to keep the band together for another couple of weeks before they drifted off to family and friends for the winter." The solution was to line up a series of concerts following the route of the New York Marathon, and thus was born the five-date extension to the Heathen tour that came to be known unofficially as the "New York Marathon" or the "Five Boroughs tour". The dates were swelled to eight with the addition of a performance of 'Rebel Rebel' and 'Cactus' at Radio City Music Hall for VH1's Fashion Awards on 15 October, and two final shows at another pair of venues steeped in Bowie history: Philadelphia's Tower Theater and Boston's Orpheum. The accompanying TV spots included a performance of 'Afraid' and 'I've Been Waiting For You' on *Late Night With Conan O'Brien*, which would later undergo an unusual transformation: when the show was repeated by NBC the following May the visuals, including Bowie's performance, were rendered entirely in clay-mation animation.

The "New York Marathon" dates were trailed by photographer Myriam Santos-Kayda, whose excellent book *David Bowie: Live In New York* commemorated the concerts in rehearsal and performance. Bowie's foreword to the book summed up the successful conclusion of the Marathon dates at Manhattan's Beacon Theater: "When Gail Ann and I slow danced through 'Absolute Beginners' that night, we both felt just that. It didn't seem like the end of a long and gruelling year, but a new time with a horizon that went on forever. As we left the stage that night to the sound of Gerry's last guitar hurrah, we hugged in the wings and felt sad for maybe the first time all year."

It had indeed been a golden year for David Bowie: the widespread acclaim accorded to *Heathen* was compounded by the success of the tour, while the thirtieth anniversary reissue of *Ziggy Stardust* and November's *Best Of Bowie* cemented the impression of 2002 as something of an *annus mirabilis*. October brought the agreeable news that David had finished a very respectable 29th place in the BBC's much-publicized *Great Britons*, an enjoyably absurd jamboree in which the public was invited to vote for the "greatest" figure in the nation's history while watching endless television shows in which celebrities promoted their favourite candidates. Bowie was the third highest musician in the poll (Lennon and McCartney both made the top 20), which exclusively revealed that he was greater than Charles Dickens, George Stephenson and Sir Walter Raleigh, but less great than William Shakespeare, Charles Darwin and Michael Crawford. So now you know.

Despite the fact that 2002 had been Bowie's most high-profile year for quite some time, his family commitments had ruled out the possibility of a major world tour: instead, the Heathen tour amounted to some 36 concert dates, punctuated by several leisurely breaks. "Touring has become harder and harder for me," David had admitted in the summer of 2002. "This new set of shows that I'm doing this year are actually not too many to cope with really. I'm doing about a dozen in Europe and a little more than a dozen in the States, which means I'll be able to get home." Nevertheless, the 2002 concerts – in particular the string of triumphant autumn engagements that were added some time after that statement – proved to be of immense significance in reinvigorating David's appetite for large-scale touring. Following the universally applauded success of the Heathen tour, 2003 would see Bowie's full-scale return to the world stage.

More so than the uncompromising set-lists of the mid-1990s or the mainstream package of Glastonbury 2000, the Heathen tour succeeded in being all things to all men, allowing David to delight the faithful with superb performances of *Low* and *Heathen*, while at the same time pulling more crowd-pleasing material out of the hat when the occasion required. David was delighted with his new band: "I now have the feeling we are one of the strongest bands I've ever worked with," he enthused in June 2002, "and it's very exciting to be on stage with them." Nobody who saw the concerts could disagree: the addition of the immensely talented Gerry Leonard on second lead guitar lent an extra textural depth to a band which, grounded in Gail Ann Dorsey's spectacular bass, Mark Plati's dextrous rhythm work and Earl Slick's searing solos, now offered one of the most guitar-heavy line-ups of Bowie's live career. The sound, although full, remained beautifully clear and atmospheric, with Sterling Campbell's percussion and the excellent keyboard work of Mike Garson and Catherine Russell underpinning the arrangements to perfection. Bowie's own contributions on guitar, saxophone, keyboards and harmonica (not to mention Stylophone on the truly spectacular 'Slip Away') bore witness to a more hands-on role in the band's sound than of late, and his voice was on stunning form. In short, the Heathen tour offered further evidence that the quality of David Bowie's live performances seems only to increase with every passing year.

TIBET HOUSE BENEFIT 2003
28 February 2003

Musicians: David Bowie *(vocals)*, Gerry Leonard *(guitar)*, Tony Visconti *(bass)*, Martha Mooke, Gregor Kitzis, Meg Okura, Mary Wotten *(Scorchio Quartet)*

Repertoire: 'Loving The Alien' / 'Heathen (The Rays)' / 'Waterloo Sunset' / 'Get Up, Stand Up'

On 28 February 2003 Bowie took a break from the *Reality* sessions to make his third annual appearance at the Tibet House Benefit concert at Carnegie Hall, alongside such artists as Laurie Anderson, Ziggy Marley, Rufus Wainwright and Ray Davies. In keeping with previous years his choice of songs was both unusual and revealing, opening with a delicate acoustic rendering of 'Loving The Alien' for which he was backed only by Gerry Leonard on guitar. It was the first time he had performed the number since 1987's Glass Spider tour and, given the mood of the western world in February 2003, it was a timely and provocative revival. This was followed by a similarly pared-down acoustic reading of 'Heathen (The Rays)', supported by a beautiful string arrangement orchestrated by Tony Visconti and played by the Scorchio Quartet, with support from Leonard on acoustic guitar and Visconti on bass. There followed Bowie's duet with the legendary Ray Davies on The Kinks' classic 'Waterloo Sunset', for which the pair were backed by Lenny Kay and members of the Patti Smith Band, and at the end of the concert Bowie joined in a mass rendition of Bob Marley's 'Get Up, Stand Up'.

A REALITY TOUR

19 August 2003 – 21 July 2004

Musicians: David Bowie *(vocals, guitar, Stylophone, harmonica)*, Gerry Leonard *(guitar, vocals)*, Earl Slick *(guitar)*, Gail Ann Dorsey *(bass, vocals)*, Mike Garson *(keyboards)*, Sterling Campbell *(drums, vocals)*, Catherine Russell *(guitar, keyboards, vocals, percussion, mandolin)*

Repertoire: 'New Killer Star' / 'Pablo Picasso' / 'Never Get Old' / 'The Loneliest Guy' / 'Looking For Water' / 'She'll Drive The Big Car' / 'Days' / 'Fall Dog Bombs The Moon' / 'Try Some, Buy Some' / 'Reality' / 'Bring Me The Disco King' / 'Modern Love' / 'Cactus' / 'Battle For Britain (The Letter)' / 'Afraid' / 'Sister Midnight' / 'I'm Afraid Of Americans' / 'Suffragette City' / 'Fantastic Voyage' / 'The Man Who Sold The World' / 'Rebel Rebel' / 'Hang On To Yourself' / 'Heathen (The Rays)' / 'A New Career In A New Town' / 'Hallo Spaceboy' / 'Fame' / 'Breaking Glass' / 'Changes' / 'Under Pressure' / 'Sunday' / 'Ashes To Ashes' / '"Heroes"' / 'Slip Away' / 'Let's Dance' / 'Ziggy Stardust' / 'Loving The Alien' / 'China Girl' / 'White Light/White Heat' / 'The Motel' / '5.15 The Angels Have Gone' / 'The Jean Genie' / 'Fashion' / 'All The Young Dudes' / 'I've Been Waiting For You' / 'Sound And Vision' / 'Be My Wife' / 'Always Crashing In The Same Car' / 'Five Years' / 'Life On Mars?' / 'Starman' / 'Panic In Detroit' / 'Blue Jean' / 'Quicksand' / 'The Supermen'

During the Area: 2 tour in the summer of 2002, Bowie had let slip to journalist Dean Kuipers that he was contemplating the possibility of not undertaking any more solo tours. Whether this was an idle fancy, a momentary declaration of solidarity with the mixed-bill festival circuit, or a deliberate piece of mischief remains uncertain, but there is no doubt that by the end of the year the story was very different. The success of October 2002's landmark Hammersmith gig and the subsequent "New York Marathon" dates had replenished Bowie's appetite for touring to a degree that surpassed even the enthusiasm he had displayed during the *Earthling* period. "I was very, very happy with how we were on stage and what we sounded like, and how we were able to interpret the material," he said in 2003 of the Heathen tour. "And I really wanted to go back out this year, so I was highly motivated to have an album that represented the band." The result would be reflected not only in *Reality*, written and recorded with a specific view to its live potential, but also in the staggering scale of the ensuing tour. Originally touted as Bowie's most extensive live outing since the mid-1990s, A Reality Tour would soon eclipse any such comparison, outstripping even Sound + Vision, Glass Spider and Serious Moonlight to become, in terms of individual dates, the longest tour of his career.

Officially announced on 16 June 2003, the new show was dubbed "A Reality Tour", the indefinite article emphasizing the album's dalliance with the notion that there can be no absolute definition of reality. "Last year's shows were such a tremendous high and the audiences so responsive," Bowie told *Billboard*. "My band is playing at the top of its form right now, and it would be foolish not to play a tour this year while we're in such good spirits about the live-show aspects of our work." Initial bookings were spectacularly healthy (the first night at Dublin sold out in five minutes), leading to the swift addition of second dates at many of the European venues, including Paris, Dublin, Birmingham and London. Ever the innovator, Bowie endorsed a "Virtual Ticket" scheme designed to attract custom to BowieNet, whereby every ticket sold for A Reality Tour contained an access code entitling the ticket holder to follow the tour online via snippets of exclusive audio and video footage.

Rehearsals began in New York in July 2003. The band was identical to that of the Heathen tour but for the absence of Mark Plati, who had departed after the *Reality* sessions to become musical director of Robbie Williams's "Weekends Of Mass Distraction" tour, playing at the star's sold-out Knebworth concerts among others. In his absence, Gerry Leonard was promoted to the role of bandleader. "The songs on this album are fantastic live," Bowie enthused. "I was so excited about how they feel. They were the first things that we learned when we went into rehearsals, and they are truly going to be great stage songs."

August 19 saw the first live date, a low-key warm-up gig for BowieNet members at the 500-capacity Chance Theater, a former picture house in the upstate New York town of Poughkeepsie. The short set gave a tantalizing indication of the delights to come on the tour: in addition to six *Reality* songs and a smattering of *Heathen* numbers, the set-list included the live debut of 'Fantastic Voyage', the surprise resurrection of 'Sister Midnight' for the first time at a Bowie gig since 1976, and a pair of *Ziggy Stardust* numbers – 'Hang On To Yourself' and 'Suffragette City' – that hadn't been heard in many years. Neither had 'Modern Love', which became the last of the trio of *Let's Dance* hits to find its way back into Bowie's post-Sound + Vision repertoire.

September saw the pre-tour publicity machine swing into action as *Reality*'s release date approached. On 1 September Bowie appeared on the German radio station EINS, selecting an hour's worth of his favourite records, while September 4 found him recording a two-hour TV special for the France 2 channel, featuring interviews and a seven-song performance which included a duet of 'Fashion' with Blur's Damon Albarn. Bowie had already spent much of 2003 praising Blur in general and their latest album *Think Tank* in particular; during tour rehearsals in July, David and members of his band had attended a Blur gig at New York's Hammerstein Ballroom, and he related how "back at the studio the next day we tried to fit 'Song 2' onto everything we played" – a running gag that would continue to resurface during A Reality Tour. Other guests on the France 2 show included French artists Air and Françoise Hardy (who delighted David by revealing that *1.Outside* was her favourite Bowie album), while there were satellite contributions from Moby, Mick Rock and The Dandy Warhols, who were once again preparing to support Bowie on tour. Since their appearances together in 2002 David had continued to champion The Dandy Warhols, whose May 2003 album *Welcome To The Monkey House* had been co-produced by Tony Visconti and featured Nile Rodgers among its guest musicians. "We were approaching it as if it was a Bowie collection," guitarist Pete Holmström would later say of the album's recording process. One track, 'I Am A Scientist', used a sample from 'Fashion', while drummer Brent DeBoer pointed out that 'I Am Sound' was heavily influenced by 'Ashes To Ashes': "It has that great, pumping

bassline – when Bowie heard it he said, 'That's one of mine!'" Bowie had even expressed a wish to play saxophone on the T Rex-style 'Hit Rock Bottom', but his 2002 touring commitments had made it impossible. Following The Dandy Warhols' support on the initial European leg of A Reality Tour, the slot would be filled by Macy Gray on the first US leg, various local artists in the Pacific countries, and, on Bowie's return to America in the spring of 2004, by The Polyphonic Spree and Stereophonics.

The biggest pre-tour publicity event came on September 8, when the band performed before an intimate audience of BowieNet members and celebrities at London's Riverside Studios in an unusual and highly publicized stunt designed to launch both album and tour. Billed as "the world's first live and interactive music event", the performance was beamed live to 86 cinemas in 22 countries worldwide, including Brazil, Italy, Germany, Sweden, Poland, Denmark, France, Norway, Canada, Australia, America and Britain, reaching an audience totalling some 50,000. Owing to time delays, Asia, Japan and Australia received the show the following day, while the US, Canada and South America held cinema screenings a week later on 15 September. It wasn't actually the first live cinema syndication of a rock concert (Korn, for one, had staged a similar event across America in 2002), but it was by far the largest and most elaborate yet attempted, the first to be broadcast in 5.1 surround sound, and the first to boast an "interactive" element with the participating cinemas.

Prior to the satellite link-up Bowie treated the Riverside Studios audience to a warm-up consisting of 'A New Career In A New Town' and snatches of Blur's 'Song 2' and Link Wray's 'Rumble'. As the concert went live to cinemas around the world, the band launched into a spirited rendition of the entire *Reality* album. Tony Visconti was on hand at Riverside to mix the performance in DTS 5.1 sound, although apparently not every receiving cinema technician proved equal to the challenge, and a few began screening the show minus the lead singer's audio input. "I was disheartened to read that some cinema attendees could not hear David's voice clearly or not at all, in some cases," Visconti remarked the following day. "I can assure you that the sound in the recording truck was amazing as we were monitoring in 5.1 surround sound the entire time." After the performance of *Reality*, there followed a question-and-answer session hosted by Jonathan Ross, during which various pre-selected cinemagoers were invited to pose questions to David via satellite. Despite a few technical hitches the event was considered a great success, and the evening concluded with an encore of six oldies and a final rerun of 'New Killer Star'. The main *Reality* segment was later included as a bonus DVD with the so-called 'Tour Edition' of the album released in November 2003.

The roster of pre-tour appearances continued with a return visit to BBC1's *Friday Night With Jonathan Ross*, recorded on 11 September and transmitted the following day. The band performed 'New Killer Star', 'Modern Love' and 'Never Get Old', although only the first two were broadcast. September 18 found Bowie performing the same three songs at New York's Rockefeller Plaza for the 2003 Toyota Summer Concert series on NBC's *The Today Show*, while a day earlier he taped 'New Killer Star', 'Never Get Old' and 'Hang On To Yourself' for *Last Call With Carson Daly*. 'New Killer Star' popped up again for CBS's *The Late Show With David Letterman* on 22 September. The following day saw David and the band recording a five-song session for AOL online; for a week from 10 October, AOL's Broadband subscribers could access the exclusive performance of 'New Killer Star', 'I'm Afraid Of Americans', 'Rebel Rebel', 'Days' and an unusual acoustic version of 'Fall Dog Bombs The Moon'. Thereafter, the songs were offered via AOL Music one at a time for six months, 'New Killer Star' later appearing for sale at Apple's iTunes Music Store.

Following the extensive round of publicity appearances and TV shows, the band moved to Brussels at the end of September for a final week of production rehearsals on the tour set, which had been conceived by Bowie in collaboration with designer Therese Deprez and visual director Laura Frank. "I'm not really very keen to put on much of a theatrical show, in terms of big sets and elephants and fireworks and things like that," he remarked in 2003. "Of course, it doesn't mean that I won't go back on my word, because that's part and parcel of what I do for you – part of my entertaining factor is lying to you!" A year earlier he had told *Billboard* that "I got pretty sick with touring in the 1980s", describing shows like Serious Moonlight and Glass Spider as "major, major undertakings" which were "huge and unwieldy".

Even so, the tour that opened in Copenhagen on 7 October would prove to be Bowie's most visually arresting endeavour since Sound + Vision, and in some respects it was even more theatrical. The stage was dominated by the backdrop of a giant LED screen,

raised several feet above stage level, at the base of which a raised catwalk ran the width of the stage before debouching into two platforms thrusting out into the audience on either side of the playing area. Staircases led down from the rear catwalk to the stage, while hanging above the platforms were a series of huge, bleached white tree branches, dangling gracefully to either side of the stage. High above the downstage area loomed another bank of LED screens, faceted in a giant semi-circle to convey the on-stage action to the farthest reaches of each venue.

The countdown to curtain-up began as the piped pre-show music moved into the *Reality* bonus track 'Queen Of All The Tarts (Overture)', followed by a bluesy work-out as the lights slowly began to dim. After 25 seconds or so the music petered to a halt, whereupon Bowie's amplified voice was heard saying "No, let's keep that going, that was good – Gerry, pick that up again!" Naturally this caused great excitement among the crowd, and as the music struck up once again the lights dimmed to blackout and the giant screens began showing a garish cartoon of the band in rehearsal, fronted by Bowie on harmonica. Echoing the comic-strip-versus-real-life imagery of the *Reality* packaging, the cartoon image on the screen was slowly wiped across by a genuine piece of film of the band in rehearsal, whereupon the musicians began to appear on the rear catwalk, silhouetted against the giant projections as they walked down the stairs to take their places (a tricky business for some: in November the UK *Mirror* published a tour diary by Gail Ann Dorsey, in which she confessed to suffering from vertigo on the raised platforms). Bowie himself was the last to arrive, surreptitiously taking his place centre-stage in the dark while all eyes were on the screen, ensuring a moment of real impact as he was revealed in a blaze of spotlights amid the opening strains of 'New Killer Star'. It was one of the most theatrically effective of all Bowie's stage entrances, its teasing step-by-step nature recalling the elaborate preamble of the Glass Spider show while deftly avoiding its bombast.

As in his pre-tour appearances, Bowie adhered to an adaptable but instantly recognizable visual image for A Reality Tour. In the place of the shiny suits and silk shirts of the 2002 concerts came a collection of artfully thrown-together outfits that suggested a raggle-taggle image of post-punk chic: tattered black jeans, baseball boots and pumps, tight-fitting T-shirts and waistcoats, neckerchiefs and scarves, and a succession of denim jackets and distressed tail-coats which were usually discarded after the first couple of numbers.

The staging of individual songs was very simple, although the lighting and screen effects ensured that the show remained big, broad and theatrically effective. Bowie delivered most numbers in a straightforward centre-stage style, although there were a few choreographed moments, including an athletic rendering of 'Hallo Spaceboy' in which he ran the length of the rear catwalk, framed by psychedelic pulses of light, careering out onto the stage-left platform to loom over the audience and falling to his hands and knees as he stretched out to the crowd imploringly. 'Bring Me The Disco King', which opened many of the encores during the initial leg of the tour, found him sitting on the upstage catwalk beside Mike Garson's piano before prowling onto the stage-right platform, picking his way between the dangling branches before finally reaching the audience.

Many songs, like 'Sunday' and 'Reality', were backed by abstract animated swirls and patterns on the giant screens, mixed with live footage of the band relayed from on-stage cameras; others were accompanied by pre-filmed material. 'The Motel' was played against a slowly shifting backdrop of quasi-Hitchcockian images of suburban America, gradually giving way to flames and explosions as the song reached its climax. 'The Loneliest Guy' saw Bowie's face gliding mournfully among the trees in a wintry forest. Perhaps most strikingly of all, 'I'm Afraid Of Americans' was accompanied by a disturbing high-energy animation in which a couple's physical interaction moved from dancing to violence to sex and back again, while all around them images of American capitalism – big cars, cola bottles and a suspiciously familiar-looking cartoon mouse – danced, vibrated and spun angrily.

A real show-stopper was 'Slip Away', which began with a clip of Oogie and Uncle Floyd from *The Uncle Floyd Show* beamed onto the screens, while the chorus featured a "follow the bouncing ball" sequence as Oogie's head, against a backdrop of stars, bobbed along the scrolling lyrics, prompting the audience into a mass singalong (on the opening night in Copenhagen there was a short-lived speaker failure during 'Slip Away', and what might have been disastrous during another song became a positive triumph as the crowd carried the number until the sound was restored). 'Sunday', which often came midway

through the main set, was augmented by a lengthy guitar solo from Earl Slick while David left the stage for a breather and a change of shirt. 'Heathen (The Rays)' ended the main set on many of the early dates, allowing David and Gail Ann Dorsey to reprise the "blind" exit routine they had perfected on the previous tour; in later shows the song was often moved elsewhere in the set as '"Heroes"' became a more common choice to conclude the main section.

Bowie's ease and confidence on stage was palpable from the opening moments of the show, and although the video and lighting effects were certainly impressive, the real theatricality resided in its star performer. "The more confident I get, the less and less I use on stage," David declared in 2003. "These days I'm just wearing a suit, and that's about it. That's my full theatricality and I'm really enjoying it, especially as an interpreter of songs. I tell you, the thing that's been inspiring for me getting older is that it feels and seems my writing is staying buoyant. It feels strong and the songs have a real resonance, and it makes me very confident now about plunging back and doing old stuff as well. I really steered away from that during the early nineties, because I wasn't at all confident about what I was writing then and I just didn't know if it stood up to the old stuff. So, I kind of cleared the decks just to get back on my feet as a writer and to not feel too much comparison being thrown at myself, even if it was self-inflicted. Now, however, I can take anything from the past and put it alongside what I'm currently doing, and I feel, 'Hey, this is a really good chronological show.' It dips into every period and I feel that everything is as strong as the one that it's played against."

The growing sense that Bowie no longer felt intimidated by his own back catalogue was certainly borne out by the set-lists for A Reality Tour, which continued the Heathen shows' policy of relaxing David's formerly guarded attitude to the more populist numbers, in the process finding a happy medium midway between the confrontational no-hits policy of the Outside tour and the predictable golden oldies package of Sound + Vision. The result was a repertoire that laid appropriate and justified emphasis on Bowie's recent material, but also paid considerably more than lip-service to his classics and even revived some obscure nuggets, managing to please both the hardcore fan and the casual concert-goer. Thus the chilly atmospherics of 'The Motel' and 'The Loneliest Guy' rubbed shoulders with crowd-pleasers as mainstream as 'Rebel Rebel', a glut of *Ziggy Stardust* numbers, and even the three *Let's Dance* singles (although 'Modern Love', a frequent choice during the preliminary TV appearances, disappeared from the tour after just two outings and didn't resurface again until the Toronto gig in April 2004).

The most interesting choices not only delighted the faithful but also appeared to suggest a pleasingly subversive agenda: alongside the bleak pessimism of much of the *Heathen* material and the cloaked political anger of 'Fall Dog Bombs The Moon' came a succession of revivals which combined to suggest a calculated stance regarding the unhappy state of affairs on the world stage at the time of the tour: making its first ever live outing was 1979's anti-war parable 'Fantastic Voyage', while a delicate acoustic reworking of 'Loving The Alien' laid bare the song's implicit plea for communication and tolerance between faiths. When, during the week of George W Bush's behind-closed-doors "state visit" to the UK in November 2003, Bowie dedicated a particularly blistering rendition of 'I'm Afraid Of Americans' to "our visitor this week", he won a hearty response from the Birmingham NEC audience.

In pre-tour interviews David revealed that the band had rehearsed fifty different songs, enabling him to alter the set-lists radically over time and serve up different treats in venues where he was due to perform more than one show. He was true to his word: although the average length of each show hung around 25 or 26 songs, by the beginning of 2004 the band had performed more than fifty different numbers during the tour, and while previous years had tended to see an initially varied repertoire gradually whittled down to an increasingly predictable set, A Reality Tour found Bowie chopping and changing throughout, dropping some numbers for weeks on end before unexpectedly reinstating them, introducing surprise new additions, moving encores into the main set and vice versa. Each night's set-list was drawn up at the soundcheck, but such was the band's proficiency that Bowie was even able to make changes mid-show: "I leave gaps in the set-list where I can just call out for a song," he explained, "depending how the audience is reacting." It was a far cry from the days of Glass Spider or Sound + Vision when, barring the occasional encore, the repertoire was more or less pre-ordained months in advance.

As well as delighting the audiences, this arrangement did much to obviate the perennial problem of Bowie himself getting bored on tour. "See, some songs are great, but if you play them over and over again they don't have that much in them," he told one interviewer. "It just becomes singalong time, and it's not much fun for us as musicians. Like 'Starman' – it's a nice song, and we'll do that occasionally, but to do that every night, it really doesn't draw upon your prowess. I can't do a full evening's worth of those because I'll go barmy. You really become a karaoke machine. It's great to be able to do 'The Motel' and '5.15 The Angels Have Gone' and things like that, because they really push you as a performer and a musician."

Even the all-important opening number was open to experimentation. For the first seven shows the night began with 'New Killer Star', but this was demoted to second place at Frankfurt in favour of 'The Jean Genie' ("That was the catalyst for an unexpectedly brilliant show," wrote Gail Ann Dorsey in her *Mirror* diary). From Milan onwards 'Rebel Rebel' became the customary curtain-raiser and would remain so for the rest of the tour, although there was still room for manoeuvre: unusually, the Amneville set opened with 'The Loneliest Guy' and 'Days' before resuming a more familiar playing order, while one show in Las Vegas opened with 'Hang On To Yourself'. By contrast, the final song of the set remained 'Ziggy Stardust' throughout the tour, the screens flashing a giant "BOWIE" over the final chord.

'Sister Midnight' was among the rarer treats; after its appearance at the Poughkeepsie warm-up gig it didn't surface again until Munich, and only rarely thereafter. Of the *Reality* songs, by far the rarest was 'Try Some, But Some' which, like 'Days' and 'Looking For Water', made few appearances on the initial European dates before becoming rather more familiar during 2004. One of the most exciting late additions was 'Five Years', which appeared towards the end of an epic-length concert at Berlin's Max Schmelling Halle and remained a strong contender in the increasingly Ziggy-dominated encores thereafter. Its addition had been instigated by Sterling Campbell busking the opening drumbeat during the Vienna soundcheck a few days earlier, prompting David to revive the number for the first time in 25 years.

The fluid approach to the repertoire undoubtedly paid off. "I'm having a ball," Bowie told an Australian interviewer in February 2004. "We're five months into it and I'm not even vaguely bored. I'm having just a super time. Judging by the audience reaction to this tour, I think I've done the right thing. I think I've chosen quite accurately how far I can go with quite new and obscure things, and how much I should balance that with pieces everybody knows." In addition to the ever-changing set-lists, David was in his usual playful mood between songs; as well as regular bursts of Blur's 'Song 2' and the occasional foray into Link Wray's 'Rumble', the gigs brought other unexpected interludes. In Vienna David played a snippet of Frank Zappa's 'It Can't Happen Here', while at several concerts he teased the crowd after 'Slip Away' by launching into a snatch of 'Space Oddity' on his Stylophone. There were other unscheduled excursions into songs as diverse as 'Golden Years', 'Do You Know The Way To San José?', 'YMCA' and 'Get It On'. In Cologne on 31 October David marked Hallowe'en by acting out scenes from The Birds between numbers, culminating in Catherine Russell and Gail Ann Dorsey launching into the spooky song sung by the children in the Hitchcock movie. "I suppose you would have to be a big fan of The Birds to get it," Dorsey wrote in her diary. "It went right over the audience's heads."

During the first couple of years of the new century Bowie had, for perhaps the first time ever, begun to carry a little extra weight, but by the time of A Reality Tour he looked leaner and fitter than he had in a decade. He sparred regularly in the boxing ring and was accompanied on tour by a personal trainer. "I'm a fairly disciplined man," he said in 2003. "I don't cut corners. And I can see that it really pays dividends to have put in a fair amount of training before going on tour. I mean, at 56 it's not as easy as when you're twentysomething." Bowie's physical fitness was apparent not only in the remarkable athleticism with which he threw himself around the stage, but also in the magnificent condition of his voice. The touring schedule made concessions to his family life too, as Iman and Alexandria accompanied him on several of the legs: "What we tend to do is get a house somewhere in the vicinity of the area that we are working," David explained, "and then I kind of fly back there each night."

On 15 October, while Bowie played Rotterdam, a pre-recorded live performance was beamed to the Royal Albert Hall during an event called Fashion Rocks For The Prince's Trust. Billed as "the largest fashion-music performance ever staged", the evening involved a host of the world's leading designers showing elements of their autumn and winter collections to the live accompaniment of various bands and singers, all in aid of The Prince's Trust. Those per-

forming at the Albert Hall included Robbie Williams, Bryan Ferry and Elton John, while Bowie's live performance of (naturally) 'Fashion' was beamed onto a giant screen behind the stage during the finale. The show was transmitted on Channel 4 on 19 October, although Bowie's segment was largely obscured by the closing credits and edited highlights of the evening. October 17 saw David pay a return visit to German TV's Die Harald Schmidt Show to play 'Never Get Old' and 'New Killer Star'. Also during the European leg, David and Iman found time to undertake a photo session for Tommy Hilfiger; shot in Amsterdam's Amstel Hotel, the pictures received widespread exposure during the designer's spring 2004 campaign.

Having played some remarkably long sets during the European leg, David's voice began to suffer in mid-November. Throat problems forced the Nice gig to be curtailed to an unusually short 20 numbers, and when David's condition was officially diagnosed as laryngitis, the Toulouse concert scheduled for 12 November was cancelled, marking only the second such incident in Bowie's live career (the first had been the cancellation of a BowieNet gig in June 2000). Happily he bounced back again in Marseille two days later, even adding the notoriously challenging 'Life On Mars?' to the repertoire for the first time, seemingly in defiance of his throat problems. As ever the song was rapturously received, and it remained a pillar of the set-list thereafter.

In Birmingham on 20 November, David followed 'Under Pressure' with an impromptu performance of 'Happy Birthday' for Gail Ann Dorsey. The two Dublin shows, of which the second broke the tour's records with a mammoth 35 numbers, were filmed for a planned DVD release in 2004. 'Starman' was added to the set at the second of two shows at Wembley Arena, where the celebrity concert-goers included Paul Merton, Eddie Izzard, Phil Manzanera, Brian Eno, Jack Dee, Beverley Knight and Ricky Gervais, whose award-winning comedy series The Office had made mischief with perceptions of "Reality TV" in a style not dissimilar to Bowie's own interest in the area ("I've turned on so many Americans to that series," David said in 2003. "They don't get it immediately, you know – they're not sure if this is supposed to be like the 'reality' thing or whatever, but once they do – the whole band love it now"). Meanwhile, at a BowieNet aftershow party on 25 November, fans were treated to a live set by Heathen veteran and Bowie collaborator Kristeen Young, with soundboard duties being taken by Tony Visconti, who was in London to produce Tim and Neil Finn's new album.

On 27 November David recorded his second appearance in a little over a year on BBC1's *Parkinson*, playing 'Ziggy Stardust' and 'The Loneliest Guy'. As the initial European leg concluded in Glasgow the following night, reports began to emerge that the tour would be extended into the summer of 2004. Bowie informed the delighted Glasgow crowd that the band would be returning to Scotland for the T In The Park festival in July, and a clutch of other European summer festival dates were announced shortly afterwards.

Meanwhile, the first North American leg of the tour got off to a difficult start when David was unexpectedly beset by further health problems. The laryngitis that had afflicted him a month earlier paled by comparison with the bout of influenza that laid him low for several days in early December, and no fewer than five gigs in the US and Canada were cancelled and hastily rescheduled for 2004 before the North American leg got off to a belated start in Montreal on 13 December. This left only two more shows in the tour itinerary before the Christmas break, although there was a further concert at Paradise Island in the Bahamas on 20 December. This one-off show was not billed as part of A Reality Tour proper, tickets being available only via a series of promotions and competitions. A 90-minute segment of the Bahamas gig was broadcast live by a number of US radio stations.

December 21 saw Bowie's name linked to a story that caused a sensation in the British press for a few days, when the *Sunday Times* published a secret list of celebrities who had turned down civil honours at various times in the past. The story had been kick-started some weeks earlier when the poet Benjamin Zephaniah broke with the customary protocol of polite silence and went public with the fact that he had refused an honour on ethical grounds. The *Sunday Times*'s subsequent acquisition of a leaked list of "refuseniks" proved to be a major embarrassment to the establishment, sparking a media debate about the relevance of the 700-year-old honours system. It was revealed that among the famous names who had turned down honours in recent years were Albert Finney, Vanessa Redgrave, Alan Bennett, John Cleese, Helen Mirren, Honor Blackman and George Melly. David Bowie, it transpired, had turned down a CBE in 2000 – hardly a surprising revelation given Tony Blair's solicitousness towards him in the 1990s. Asked some months earlier to comment on Mick Jagger's

acceptance of a knighthood, David had told the *Sun* that "I would never have any intention of accepting anything like that. I seriously don't know what it's for. It's not what I spent my life working for. It's not my place to make a judgment on Jagger, it's his decision, but it's just not for me." Pressed on a similar question by Jonathan Ross a year earlier, David had wryly remarked, "I would suggest that they give it to somebody who would give a damn ... I'm not sure what I'd do with it. I'd lose it or break it, or put it in a drawer and lose the key."

Following the Christmas break, the US tour resumed on 7 January 2004 in the traditional Bowie stronghold of Cleveland. Two days later a lengthy gig in the Motor City saw the appropriate addition of 'Panic In Detroit', which remained a regular feature of the set-list during the US leg. A more unusual new arrival was 'Blue Jean', which made an unexpected appearance during the last of three shows at Chicago's Rosemont Theatre.

The first leg of the US tour concluded in Los Angeles on 7 February, whereafter the band flew to the Southern hemisphere for Bowie's first Australasian concerts since the Glass Spider tour seventeen years earlier. The Pacific leg began in Wellington, New Zealand on 14 February at the open-air Westpac Stadium. Heavy rain necessitated the abandoning of the thrust platforms, and Bowie even donned a hooded top and anorak as the downpour continued. From New Zealand the tour moved to Australia, where the second of two concerts at the Sydney Entertainment Centre saw the surprise addition of 'Quicksand' to the repertoire. The Adelaide show a couple of days later heralded an unexpected change of outfit, as for the first time on the tour David abandoned the denim look in favour of a grey zoot-suit and trilby reminiscent of his Serious Moonlight image. "No reason for the change," he remarked afterwards, "just felt like it." On 24 February the band played 'The Man Who Sold The World' and 'New Killer Star' on the Australian TV chat-show *Rove Live*.

From Australia the tour moved to Singapore, Japan and Hong Kong before returning for a mammoth second leg in the US and Canada which lasted from late March to early June. In Kelowna on 11 April, the band included a medley of Broadway numbers towards the end of the show, while in Berkeley five days later Bowie added 'The Supermen' to the set-list. During the encores at the same show he was joined on stage by The Polyphonic Spree for 'Slip Away', an innovation which resurfaced on subsequent dates. Thereafter the band returned to Europe to play the summer festival circuit, headlining alongside acts such as The Strokes, The Darkness, the re-formed Pixies, Suzanne Vega and The Charlatans at a variety of fixtures, including Bowie's debut appearance at the UK's Isle Of Wight Festival.

Wherever A Reality Tour went, the press reaction was seldom short of ecstatic; review after review remarked not only upon the band and the staging, but on the unprecedented strength and beauty of Bowie's vocal performance. The *Manchester Evening News* remarked on how the opening UK show served up "gem after gem" and declared it "genius", while the *Times* considered the show "breathtaking" and "sublime", noting that "Bowie performed with complete authority but also a strange kind of charm – as if the battles with his myth and the baggage of his past were now resolved." The extent to which the *Reality* material wowed the critics can be summed up by the *Guardian*'s comment that "The swaggering 'New Killer Star' has the indescribable but unmistakable feel of a Bowie classic. In fact, there aren't nearly enough new songs aired. 'Changes', 'Under Pressure' and the rest are delivered to perfection." The *Birmingham Post* observed that "Bowie himself looked remarkably fresh faced, far younger and healthier than anyone with his past dare hope for. A decorative stage set and excellent lighting set the scene, but with the singer in top form vocally, little was needed in the way of props."

Reviewing the first Dublin show, the *Irish Independent* opined that "the Thin White Duke can still lay claim to the title of Rock'n'Roll's greatest showman. And what a show ... The accompanying light and visual spectacle was a sight to behold, but never threatened to outshine the real star of the show ... Bowie still manages to project more charisma during one song than most modern-day stars manage in a career." The *Sun* judged the Glasgow gig "stunning ... Bowie at his best", while the *Scotsman* announced that "Now is a good time to be David Bowie, and a good time to be a fan of David Bowie. The Thin White Duke looked more dazzling than ever, his voice is in supple shape and, thanks to his wonderful intuitive band, everything else sounds great too ... In 2003, this ultra-cool 50-something has wired back into the spirit, the strut and the stance that makes him peerless still."

Le Monde reported that Bowie was "in fantastic

vocal form. Moving from arrogant glamour to affectedness, one minute a haughty crooner, the next a vulnerable troubadour, his music surpasses that of all the rockers of his generation." The *Hamburger Morgenpost* hailed "a fabulous show, that took your breath away and left you drained of emotion ... It can't get much better than this."

In America the news was just as good. "Never has Bowie seemed as comfortable in his own skin as he does now," reported *Billboard*. "At a sold out Madison Square Garden in New York, he confidently held court in his adopted home like he had nothing to prove, as sure of the strength of his latest material as he was of his versatile backing band. Fit and laid-back, the constantly grinning Bowie looked as giddy as a school kid, belying his nearly sixty years. His voice also sounded as unique and powerful as ever ... new songs like 'New Killer Star' and 'Reality' revealed how vibrant a songwriter and performer Bowie remains ... Don't call it a comeback, since Bowie never went away. But artists new and old could stand to learn from Bowie's smiling, hip-swiveling, gregarious example, even if few could match his energy and enthusiasm."

The topical content of the show was not lost on the critics; in Chicago the *Daily Herald* remarked that "The most relevant coupling – 'I'm Afraid of Americans' and '"Heroes"' – did not need explaining. When the grinding guitars, paranoid chorus and Christ-like postures of the first met the swooning optimism of the second, Bowie expressed more about the state of world affairs over the past few years than most political pundits ever could."

Quite besides the thrilling proficiency of one of the finest live bands he has ever assembled, the sheer verve with which Bowie attacked the often epic-length concerts was both exciting and touching to behold. Seldom, if ever, had he displayed such constant and infectious enthusiasm on stage. And, as both David and the critics agreed, the new material more than matched up to the golden oldies: songs like 'New Killer Star', 'The Loneliest Guy', 'Never Get Old', 'Slip Away' and 'Bring Me The Disco King' were integral and immensely popular ingredients in the show, drawing as much respect and admiration as the classics. All of which meant that A Reality Tour was not only the longest of Bowie's career, but also, beyond doubt, one of the greatest.

4   tHE BBC raDIO sessions

Bowie's many studio performances for radio and television are covered elsewhere in this book, but one particular series of recordings merits closer inspection. Between 1967 and 2002 Bowie recorded sixteen major sessions for BBC radio. In 1996, following their successful Beatles release Live At The BBC, BBC Worldwide Music announced plans for a compilation of Bowie's radio sessions, even going so far as to release the now rare BBC Sessions 1969-1972 sampler. That project was shelved owing to clearance problems, giving way to the release in September 2000 of EMI's long-awaited double CD Bowie At The Beeb, featuring a rich selection of recordings from Bowie's classic 1968-1972 sessions.

Owing to the often repetitive set-lists and the common practice of splitting up individual tracks for repeat broadcasts, accurate documentation of the BBC sessions has become something of a minefield over the years. Latter-day compilations, including two archive broadcasts in 1987 and 1993 (quite separate but both, confusingly enough, also called Bowie At The Beeb), have improved the availability of the recordings but have sometimes attributed individual tracks inaccurately. Pick-and-mix bootlegs confuse matters even further for those seeking to complete a collection. This chapter aims to disentangle the web.

Unless otherwise noted, all sessions were originally transmitted on BBC Radio 1.

TOP GEAR
• Recorded: 18/12/1967 • Broadcast: 24/12/1967 • Repeat: 28/1/1968 • Venue: Piccadilly Studio 1 • Producer: Bernie Andrews

'Love You Till Tuesday' / 'Little Bombardier' / 'In The Heat Of The Morning' / 'Silly Boy Blue' / 'When I Live My Dream'

Bowie's first BBC session came about when Kenneth Pitt discovered that Bernie Andrews, producer of John Peel's Sunday afternoon show Top Gear, was an admirer of the David Bowie album. David received ten guineas for the recording, which was backed by the seven-piece Arthur Greenslade Orchestra in arrangements which remained faithful to Bowie's studio recordings. 'Love You Till Tuesday' closely followed the single version, right down to the 'Hearts And Flowers' coda, while 'When I Live My Dream' replicated the 'Version 2' recording. Bowie apparently agreed to include 'Little Bombardier' only after repeated requests by Bernie Andrews. The show was broadcast on Christmas Eve, Bowie sharing the bill with Jimi Hendrix, Traffic, Family and Ice.

It appears that the mysterious 'Something I Would

Like To Be', which The Pitt Report claims was recorded for the session, is no more than a myth; it did not appear in the broadcast and has never been referred to by any other source. Kenneth Pitt is equally adamant that 'In The Heat Of The Morning' was not played at the session, although it definitely was. It's therefore to be conjectured that 'Something I Would Like To Be' might exist in Pitt's notes as a working title for 'In The Heat Of The Morning', a new song at the time whose official Decca recording lay three months in the future, appearing in this session with a very different arrangement and lyrics.

TOP GEAR
• Recorded: 13/5/1968 • Broadcast: 26/5/1968 • Repeat: 20/6/1968 • Venue: Piccadilly Studio 1 • Producer: Bernie Andrews

'London Bye Ta Ta' / 'In The Heat Of The Morning' / 'Karma Man' / 'When I'm Five' / 'Silly Boy Blue' (not broadcast until repeat)

For Bowie's second Top Gear set, this time sharing a bill with The Animals, Family, Alan Bown and Mike

Stewart, David enlisted the arranging skills of his new producer, and the extravagant fourteen-piece band was duly billed as the Tony Visconti Orchestra. They included John McLaughlin on guitar, Herbie Flowers on bass (pre-dating his work on 'Space Oddity' by over a year), a pre-Blue Mink Barry Morgan on drums, and Alan Hawkshaw on keyboards. Tyrannosaurus Rex's Steve Peregrine Took joined Tony Visconti on backing vocals.

'Silly Boy Blue' was only aired in the repeat broadcast; it was standard BBC practice at the time to hold back a track or two for the repeat. 'When I'm Five' from this session is the only full studio recording David ever made of the song, and it was this version that later appeared in the *Love You Till Tuesday* film and on its accompanying soundtrack album. With the master tapes remaining in the hands of Bowie and Tony Visconti the remainder of this session has never leaked onto the bootleg circuit, and as a result the appearance of every track bar 'When I'm Five' on *Bowie At The Beeb* was greeted with considerable excitement. The majestic arrangement of 'Silly Boy Blue' is of particular note.

THE DAVE LEE TRAVIS SHOW

• *Recorded:* 20/10/1969 • *Broadcast:* 26/10/1969 • *Venue:* Aeolian Hall Studio 2 • *Producer:* Paul Williams

'Unwashed And Somewhat Slightly Dazed' / 'Let Me Sleep Beside You' *(not broadcast)* / 'Janine' *(not broadcast)*

For this short but excellent session David was backed by *Space Oddity* band Junior's Eyes: Mick Wayne (guitar), John "Honk" Lodge (bass), Tim Renwick (guitar) and John Cambridge (drums). BBC records reveal that Junior's Eyes lead singer Graham Kelly was also present, although it's uncertain whether he contributed to the session.

Only 'Unwashed And Somewhat Slightly Dazed' was broadcast, alongside the then-current 'Space Oddity' single and a short interview with Brian Mathew recorded the same day. An excerpt from the interview, plus 'Let Me Sleep Beside You' from this session (a superb rendition, perhaps Bowie's definitive recording of the number), appeared on the *BBC Sessions 1969-1972* sampler, while both of these tracks plus 'Janine' were included on *Bowie At The Beeb*.

THE SUNDAY SHOW

• *Recorded:* 5/2/1970 • *Broadcast:* 8/2/1970 • *Venue:* Paris Cinema Studio • *Producer:* Jeff Griffin

'Amsterdam' / 'God Knows I'm Good' / 'Buzz The Fuzz' / 'Karma Man' / 'London Bye Ta Ta' / 'An Occasional Dream' / 'The Width Of A Circle' / 'Janine' / 'Wild Eyed Boy From Freecloud' / 'Unwashed And Somewhat Slightly Dazed' / 'Fill Your Heart' / 'The Prettiest Star' / 'Cygnet Committee' / 'Memory Of A Free Festival' / 'Waiting For The Man' *(not broadcast)*

Although they would not call themselves "Hype" until a fortnight later, Bowie's new backing band (referred to as "The Tony Visconti Trio" in BBC documentation) made its debut at this hour-long concert, the sixth programme in a new series of shows compered by John Peel and recorded before a live audience.

For the first four numbers David accompanied himself alone on acoustic guitar, before being joined by Tony Visconti (bass) and John Cambridge (drums) for a couple of songs, with Mick Ronson adding his guitar skills from 'The Width Of A Circle' onwards. It was Bowie's first live performance with Ronson: "I met him for the first time about two days ago, through John the drummer" David remarks at one point between numbers. As well as marking the first appearance of a prototype version of 'The Width Of A Circle', the session offers a brace of Biff Rose covers, one of which would later be recorded for *Hunky Dory*. The other, 'Buzz The Fuzz', is more of a rarity. Live recordings of 'An Occasional Dream', 'God Knows I'm Good', 'Cygnet Committee' and 'Memory Of A Free Festival' are also exclusive to this session. The latter was edited down from its original 6'40" length to just over three minutes when the concert overran its allotted hour; for the same reason, a five-and-a-half minute version of 'Waiting For The Man' was cut before the broadcast and has never seen the light of day.

For many years this session was available only in the form of a decidedly ropey off-air recording available on various bootlegs. *Bowie At The Beeb* changed all that, including 'Amsterdam', 'God Knows I'm Good', 'The Width Of A Circle', 'Unwashed And Somewhat Slightly Dazed', 'Cygnet Committee' and 'Memory Of A Free Festival' from this historically fascinating concert.

SOUNDS OF THE 70s: ANDY FERRIS
• *Recorded:* 25/3/1970 • *Broadcast:* 6/4/1970 •
Repeat: 11/5/1970 • *Venue:* Playhouse Theatre Studios
• *Producer:* Bernie Andrews

'The Supermen' / 'Waiting For The Man' / 'The
Width Of A Circle' / 'Wild Eyed Boy From Freecloud'
(not broadcast until repeat)

The first three songs from this Hype session were
broadcast on the April 6 edition of the new *Sounds Of
The 70s* series, hosted by Andy Ferris, and all four were
aired by David Symonds on 11 May. They are easily
distinguished from later BBC versions by Hype's guitar-heavy, almost prog-rock sound. Kenneth Pitt
records in his memoir that it was during this session
that he first experienced the uncomfortable atmosphere that presaged his fall from grace; he would cease
to be David's manager a few weeks later. 'Waiting For
The Man' from this session appears on the *BBC
Sessions 1969-1972* sampler, while the excellent 'Wild
Eyed Boy From Freecloud' is its sole representative on
Bowie At The Beeb.

IN CONCERT: JOHN PEEL
• *Recorded:* 3/6/1971 • *Broadcast:* 20/6/1971 • *Venue:*
Paris Cinema Studio • *Producer:* Jeff Griffin

'Queen Bitch' / 'Bombers' / 'The Supermen' /
'Looking For A Friend' / 'Almost Grown' / 'Kooks' /
'Song For Bob Dylan' / 'Andy Warhol' / 'It Ain't Easy'
/ 'Oh! You Pretty Things' *(not broadcast)*

Bowie's second live concert session saw him sharing
the bill with Mike Heron, formerly of the Incredible
String Band, in John Peel's *In Concert* series. Living out
his Warholian Factory fantasies in the weeks leading
up to the *Hunky Dory* sessions, David invited a selection of friends and colleagues to make guest appearances during the session. "This is going to be incredibly complicated," began compere John Peel, and he
wasn't wrong: in addition to the core band of Mick
Ronson, Woody Woodmansey and Trevor Bolder,
David had brought along vocalists Dana Gillespie
(who sang 'Andy Warhol'), George Underwood (who
sang 'Song For Bob Dylan' and the third verse of 'It
Ain't Easy'), Geoffrey Alexander (who sang the second
verse of 'It Ain't Easy' and backing vocals on 'Almost
Grown') and Mark Carr Pritchard (who sang 'Looking

For A Friend'). Peel introduced Pritchard as being
"with a group called Arnold Corns who have a single
called 'Moonage Daydream', which nobody on the
BBC has played at all, which is a great pity." Bowie's
sidemen were referred to as "members of a group
called Ronno" who were apparently "gonna be making an LP fairly soon."

Many years later, Trevor Bolder would recall that
this concert was the first time he had ever seen David
in his Mr Fish dress: "I'd seen him in jeans and T-shirt,
and all of a sudden this guy comes out wearing a
bloody dress, covered in make-up, and I was like:
what the hell's this? Cos I'd not seen him, I didn't
know he was gonna come out with that sort of thing.
I just thought he was going to come out like anybody
else would play, nicely dressed or whatever. And it was
a radio show with a small audience, so no one was
gonna see him!"

Despite David's own reservations it was an entertaining set, and marked several significant firsts. Most
of the songs were new to the repertoire, and with four
very different early versions of forthcoming *Hunky
Dory* tracks (including 'Kooks', composed only days
earlier), two songs that were later scrapped ('Looking
For A Friend' and 'Bombers', the latter with David on
piano), a complete one-off ('Almost Grown'), and a
free-for-all finale of 'It Ain't Easy' pre-dating the
release of *Ziggy Stardust* by an entire year, the recording is of immense historical interest. Sadly time con-
straints resulted in the cutting of 'Oh! You Pretty
Things' before broadcast, and this number is now lost.

The date of this session has been widely misquot-
ed as 5 June, but BBC records and *Bowie At The Beeb*
confirm that 3 June is correct. 'Bombers', 'Looking For
A Friend', 'Almost Grown', 'Kooks' and 'It Ain't Easy'
are included on *Bowie At The Beeb*.

SOUNDS OF THE 70s: BOB HARRIS
• *Recorded:* 21/9/1971 • *Broadcast:* 4/10/1971 •
Repeat: 1/11/1971 • *Venue:* Kensington House Studio
T1 • *Producer:* John Muir

'The Supermen' / 'Oh! You Pretty Things' / 'Eight
Line Poem' / 'Kooks' / 'Fill Your Heart' *(not broadcast
until repeat)* / 'Amsterdam' *(not broadcast)* / 'Andy
Warhol' *(not broadcast)*

Again for *Sounds Of The 70s* but this time presented by
"Whispering" Bob Harris, this session is unique in

that David was joined only by Mick Ronson for a pared-down and largely acoustic set which is also notable as the only session of the 1960s and 1970s to be recorded in stereo. Both Bowie and Ronson contributed guitar, piano and vocals to a selection of songs recently recorded during the *Hunky Dory* sessions. According to engineer Bill Aitken, "It was a strange session: two voices, two acoustic guitars or, on some numbers, two electric guitars. The electric guitars sounded very strange as neither Bowie or Ronson had brought in amplifiers; consequently the guitars were direct injected. The fact that they DI'd led me to think they weren't taking the session too seriously. However, it's worth a listen."

"My own feeling then was that Mick Ronson's contribution to Bowie's sound and style was something he was never given enough credit for," said Bob Harris later. "I like to think that duo session was a rare moment of Bowie, in effect, acknowledging that Ronson was not just a sideman, but an integral part of his sound."

As in the previous session, 'The Supermen' followed the "alternative" arrangement as subsequently recorded during the *Ziggy Stardust* sessions. 'Andy Warhol', one of the two tracks never broadcast, was included on the *BBC Sessions 1969-1972* sampler, while 'The Supermen' and 'Eight Line Poem' represent the session – arguably one of Bowie's best – on *Bowie At The Beeb*.

SOUNDS OF THE 70s: JOHN PEEL
• *Recorded:* 11/1/1972 • *Broadcast:* 28/1/1972 • *Repeat:* 31/3/1972 • *Venue:* Kensington House Studio T1 • *Producer:* John Muir

'Hang On To Yourself' / 'Ziggy Stardust' / 'Queen Bitch' / 'Waiting For The Man' / 'Lady Stardust' *(not broadcast until repeat)*

As *Ziggy Stardust* loomed on the horizon, the Spiders recorded a succession of very similar sets for BBC radio, often confused over the years as bootleggers have combined and incorrectly labelled the results. However, most of the sets can be accurately identified by minor variations in Bowie's rendition of the lyrics.

The confusion gets off to a flying start with this very elusive session which, presented by John Peel, saw the first major unveiling of *Ziggy Stardust* material. The *BBC Sessions 1969-1972* sampler CD claims to

include 'Hang On To Yourself' from this session, but in fact it features the version from the next *Sounds Of The 70s* session, recorded a week later. Furthermore, the CD's liner notes state that 'Hang On To Yourself' is the only surviving track from this session. This is incorrect – on the contrary, every song from this session *except* 'Hang On To Yourself' has appeared on bootlegs, usually in considerably inferior quality to the other 1972 sessions. Notably, this is the only session from the 1970s to be omitted entirely from *Bowie At The Beeb*.

Identifying lyrics for this session: 'Queen Bitch' begins "Well, I'm up on the eleventh floor". 'Waiting For The Man' contains "dark grey building, up three flights of stairs".

SOUNDS OF THE 70s: BOB HARRIS
• *Recorded:* 18/1/1972 • *Broadcast:* 7/2/1972 • *Venue:* Maida Vale Studio 5 • *Producer:* Jeff Griffin

'Queen Bitch' / 'Five Years' / 'Hang On To Yourself' / 'Ziggy Stardust' / 'Waiting For The Man' *(not broadcast)*

This tight electric session was recorded by the Spiders only a week after its predecessor, this time for an edition of *Sounds Of The 70s* presented by Bob Harris. It's worth noting that the two January 1972 sessions coincided with the recording of the last few tracks of the *Ziggy Stardust* album itself at Trident: while laying down these BBC tracks, the Spiders were simultaneously working on the original versions of 'Suffragette City', 'Starman' and 'Rock'n'Roll Suicide'.

'Hang On To Yourself' from this session appeared on the *BBC Sessions 1969-1972* sampler CD, wrongly labelled as coming from the previous *Sounds Of The 70s* set. The entire set is included on *Bowie At The Beeb*, although the album's initial pressing accidentally substituted the recording of 'Ziggy Stardust' from the 16 May 1972 session.

Identifying lyrics for this session: Bowie's vocal for 'Queen Bitch' begins with a whispered "Oh yeah!" before "Mmm, I'm up on the eleventh floor", and after the first line David says "Louder"; 'Five Years' is unique to this session, and has "I had to cram so much, everything in there"; 'Hang On To Yourself' has "she'll come to the show tonight, praying to the light *machines*"; 'Ziggy Stardust' has "played it left hand, but *played* it too far"; 'Waiting For The Man' has "grey dirty building, up three flights of stairs".

SOUNDS OF THE 70s: JOHN PEEL

• *Recorded:* 16/5/1972 • *Broadcast:* 23/5/1972 •
Repeat: 25/7/1972 • *Venue:* Maida Vale Studio 4 •
Producer: Pete Ritzema

'Hang On To Yourself' / 'Ziggy Stardust' / 'White Light/White Heat' / 'Suffragette City' / 'Moonage Daydream' (*not broadcast until repeat*)

On the eve of *Ziggy Stardust*'s release the Spiders recorded three further sessions. The first was for a Tuesday night John Peel show incorrectly billed in some documentation as *John Peel With Top Gear, Sounds Of The 70s*, a title which has done nothing to ease the confusion of historians. For this recording Ronson, Bolder and Woodmansey were joined by pianist Nicky Graham, whose frenetic dexterity on tracks like 'Suffragette City' and 'White Light/White Heat' help to make this tight, exuberant set arguably the best of the 1972 sessions.

The revised repeat featured 'Moonage Daydream' for the first time, but omitted 'Hang On To Yourself' and 'Ziggy Stardust'. The latter appears on the *BBC Sessions 1969-1972* sampler, while the entire set is included on *Bowie At The Beeb*.

This session is more easily identifiable than its immediate predecessors, not least because it features two songs ('Suffragette City' and 'Moonage Daydream') that were included in no other BBC set. Identifying lyrics for the others: 'Hang On To Yourself' has "*Comes* to the show tonight, praying to the light *machine*"; 'Ziggy Stardust' has "*Well, he* played it left hand, but *made* it too far"; 'White Light, White Heat' has the ad-lib "White light make me sound like Lou Reed".

THE JOHNNIE WALKER LUNCHTIME SHOW

• *Recorded:* 22/5/1972 • *Broadcast:* 5-9/6/1972 •
Venue: Aeolian Hall Studio 2 • *Producer:* Roger Pusey

'Starman' (*broadcast 6-9/6/1972*) / 'Space Oddity' (*not broadcast*) / 'Changes' (*not broadcast*) / 'Oh! You Pretty Things' (*broadcast (5/6/1972*)

For this session the Spiders were joined once again by pianist Nicky Graham, something of an unsung hero of Bowie's 1972 tour whose work is showcased well on the faithful recreations of 'Changes' and 'Oh! You Pretty Things' included here. Unusually, the recording

of 'Starman' incorporated a remixed backing tape of the string arrangements from the Trident original, but the remainder of the performance is entirely new. Rather than showcasing the whole session, Johnny Walker networked one song per show for five days in a row: 'Oh! You Pretty Things' on 5 June, followed by 'Starman' on four consecutive days. 'Changes' and 'Space Oddity' were not broadcast, but the latter was included on the *BBC Sessions 1969-1972* sampler, while the complete session appears on *Bowie At The Beeb*.

Identifying lyrics for this session: 'Space Oddity' includes the ad-lib "I'm just a rocket man", while the full-band rendition of 'Oh! You Pretty Things' is easily differentiated from the stripped-down acoustic version recorded the previous year. 'Starman' and 'Changes' are unique to this session.

SOUNDS OF THE 70s: BOB HARRIS

• *Recorded:* 23/5/1972 • *Broadcast:* 19/6/1972 •
Venue: Maida Vale Studio 4 • *Producer:* Jeff Griffin

'Andy Warhol' / 'Lady Stardust' / 'White Light/White Heat' / 'Rock'n'Roll Suicide'

Recorded only a day after its predecessor, Bowie's final BBC session of the 1970s was for Bob Harris's *Sounds Of The 70s* and once again saw pianist Nicky Graham joining the Spiders in the studio. All but 'White Light/White Heat' were later included on *Bowie At The Beeb*.

Identifying lyrics for this session: 'Andy Warhol' ends with David ad-libbing a camp impersonation of Warhol, concluding with "Well, I only look at the pictures myself"; 'Lady Stardust' ends with him saying "Wrong song"; 'White Light, White Heat' begins with "White light gonna take me outta my brain". In 'Rock'n'Roll Suicide', which is unique to this session, Bowie mutters "I'm gonna lift this mike up a bit" over the opening bars.

MARK GOODIER'S EVENING SESSION

• *Recorded/Broadcast:* 13/8/1991 • *Venue:* Maida Vale Studio 5 • *Producer:* Jeff Smith

'A Big Hurt' / 'Baby Universal' / 'Stateside' / 'If There Is Something' / 'Heaven's In Here'

After a break of nineteen years, Bowie returned to the

BBC in August 1991 to record a set with Tin Machine, broadcast live on *Mark Goodier's Evening Session*. The five tracks were later released on various formats of Tin Machine's 'Baby Universal' single.

CHANGESNOWBOWIE
• *Recorded:* 1/1997 • *Broadcast:* 8/1/1997 • *Producer:* Mark Plati

'The Man Who Sold The World' / 'The Supermen' / 'Andy Warhol' / 'Repetition' / 'Lady Stardust' / 'White Light, White Heat' / 'Shopping For Girls' / 'Quicksand' / 'Aladdin Sane'

During rehearsals in New York for his fiftieth birthday concert, Bowie recorded nine songs exclusively for Radio 1's retrospective *ChangesNowBowie*. Interspersed with an interview by Mary Anne Hobbs, the often surprising selection offered a revealing insight into David's own perception of his career as he reached his half-century. For the mainly acoustic set, David was accompanied by Reeves Gabrels (guitar), Gail Ann Dorsey (bass and vocals), Mike Garson (piano) and Zachary Alford (drums). The session was produced by Mark Plati, who later recalled that "We did most of the songs in a day, just David, Reeves and Gail together live. I added some strings and keys after the fact. David did six lead vocal tracks in two hours."

MARK RADCLIFFE
• *Recorded/Broadcast:* 25/10/1999 • *Venue:* Maida Vale Studio 4 • *Producer:* Will Saunders

'Survive' / 'Drive In Saturday' / 'Something In The Air' / 'Can't Help Thinking About Me' / 'Repetition'

During the *'hours…'* promotional tour Bowie and his band performed a live session before a studio audience for Radio 1's *Mark Radcliffe* show. Only four songs had been planned, but 'Repetition' was squeezed in at the last moment.

THE SATURDAY MUSIC SHOW
• *Recorded:* 25/10/1999 • *Broadcast:* 6/11/1999 • *Venue:* Maida Vale Studio 4 • *Producer:* Chris Whatmough

'Survive' / 'China Girl' / 'Survive' / 'Changes'

Back-to-back with the previous *Mark Radcliffe* session, Bowie recorded a further two tracks for Billy Bragg's Radio 2 *Saturday Music Show*, followed by two more for broadcast on Chris Evans's *Breakfast Team* on Virgin Radio.

DAVID BOWIE – LIVE AND EXCLUSIVE
• *Recorded:* 18/9/2002 • *Broadcast:* 5/10/2002 • *Venue:* Maida Vale Studio 4 • *Producer:* Sarah Gaston

'Sunday' / 'Look Back In Anger' / 'Cactus' / 'Survive' / '5.15 The Angels Have Gone' / 'Alabama Song' / 'Everyone Says 'Hi'' / 'Rebel Rebel' / 'The Bewlay Brothers' / 'Heathen (The Rays)'

On the eve of his autumn 2002 European dates, Bowie and the Heathen tour band recorded this superb live session before a studio audience. It was broadcast on Radio 2 a fortnight later as a one-off show entitled *David Bowie – Live And Exclusive*. In addition to showcasing several *Heathen* songs (including the new single 'Everyone Says 'Hi'', released two days before the recording), the set also saw the unveiling of several numbers new to the 2002 repertoire, notably the debut of the reworked 'Rebel Rebel' and, to the delight of Bowie fans the world over, the first ever live performance of 'The Bewlay Brothers'.

FURTHER NOTES ON THE BBC SESSIONS

On 8 February 1972 Bowie and the Spiders performed 'Queen Bitch', 'Five Years' and 'Oh! You Pretty Things' for BBC2's *Old Grey Whistle Test*. Although not a BBC session proper, these three tracks have also made their way onto bootlegs, muddling matters still further. Similarly, Bowie's *Top Of The Pops* 'Starman' appearance on 5 July 1972 is not to be confused with the radio sessions.

A BBC radio broadcast dated 21/9/1972, featuring 'John, I'm Only Dancing', 'Star' and 'Lady Stardust', has been widely bootlegged and is often cited as another of Bowie's radio sessions. It isn't; the songs are merely adulterated versions of the original album tracks.

In addition to the studio sessions, Radio 1 has made several live broadcasts from Bowie's concerts. On 13 July 1983 a Serious Moonlight gig from the Montreal Forum was taped for radio; on 30 August 1987 a Glass Spider show was broadcast from

Montreal's Olympic Stadium; on 5 August 1990 a Sound + Vision concert was broadcast from the Milton Keynes Bowl; a half-hour Outside tour selection was recorded at Wembley Arena on 18 November 1995; the last six songs from the Phoenix Festival on 18 July 1996 were broadcast live; and the NetAid concert on 9 October 1999 was also relayed live, together with a backstage interview.

BBC Radio has also produced several excellent Bowie documentaries over the years. Recommended are Radio 1's four-part *The David Bowie Story* (May 1976, updated in six parts in May 1993), and Radio 2's three-part *Golden Years* (March 2000). Finally, Bowie himself narrated Radio 2's excellent two-part history of London's Marquee Club (the scene of many of his own early concerts including the 1966 *Bowie Showboat* gigs and 1973's *1980 Floor Show*), broadcast in July 2001.

5   the videos

David Bowie is justly renowned as one of the pioneers of rock video: with typical perversity, he had a full-length film of promos under his belt before he'd recorded his first hit single. Love You Till Tuesday *was followed by Mick Rock's evocative series of Ziggy-era clips, of which Lester Bangs later identified 'John, I'm Only Dancing' as "the very moment the modern idea of a video was born" – certainly it preceded Queen's 'Bohemian Rhapsody', ubiquitously lauded as the first rock video, by a full three years. Perfunctory clips for 'Be My Wife' and '"Heroes"' appeared in 1977, but it seems likely that the sheer potential of video was brought home to Bowie in the same year by the work of the unsigned futurist band Devo, who had shot polished "conceptual" videos in the place of conventional demos. In 1978 Bowie described Devo as "fantastic" and announced that he was to produce their first album, although in the*

end that task was undertaken by Brian Eno. In 1979, by which time American artists as diverse as Blondie, Village People and Michael Jackson were using the visual medium as an integral part of the process of making hits, Bowie emerged at the vanguard of the video age. His trio of brilliant clips for 'Boys Keep Swinging', 'D.J.' and 'Look Back In Anger' were the most influential videos of their day, and 1980's classic 'Ashes To Ashes' defined the parameters of the new art form. Subsequent creations like 'China Girl', 'Jump They Say', 'Little Wonder' and 'New Killer Star' have ensured that Bowie remains at the frontier of rock video.

Individual videos are covered under the appropriate entries in Chapter 1. What follows is a guide to Bowie's official releases, and other shows and films of particular interest.

LOVE YOU TILL TUESDAY

• 1969/1984 (28 mins) • Kenneth Pitt Ltd/Polygram SUPC 00022 • *Director:* Malcolm J. Thomson

'Love You Till Tuesday' / 'Sell Me A Coat' / 'When I'm Five' / 'Rubber Band' / 'The Mask (A Mime)' / 'Let Me Sleep Beside You' / 'Ching-a-Ling' / 'Space Oddity' / 'When I Live My Dream'

In September 1968, when Bowie made his second appearance on the Hamburg-based ZDF pop show *4-3-2-1 Musik Für Junge Leute*, its producer Günther Schneider suggested to Kenneth Pitt the possibility of making a half-hour special for the channel. Pitt was unhappy with "the way in which the Germans were handling colour television, then in its infancy," but he took the idea back to London and in early October he and David met with Malcolm Thomson, a former assistant of Pitt's now involved in the film industry. A script was drawn up comprising five of Bowie's Deram songs and the recent compositions 'When I'm Five' and 'Ching-a-Ling', together with David's mime rou-

tine 'The Mask'. The film was to include supporting appearances by his Feathers cohorts Hermione Farthingale and John Hutchinson, billed simply as "Hermione" and "Hutch", who joined David on vocals for 'Ching-a-Ling' and the remixed version of 'Sell Me A Coat'.

When outside funding was not forthcoming Pitt elected to finance the project himself, intending to recoup costs by selling the film to television companies at home and abroad. Pitt regarded ZDF as a key target, and in an attempt to improve his chances in that quarter he enlisted Schneider's production assistant Lisa Busch to provide German translations of 'Love You Till Tuesday', 'When I Live My Dream' and 'Let Me Sleep Beside You', together with a German voiceover for 'The Mask'.

In January 1969 David took refresher classes at the Dance Centre, visited the dentist for cosmetic work on his teeth, and attended appointments for the fitting and styling of a wig to cover his lingering *Virgin Soldiers* short back and sides. The fact that Bowie wears a wig throughout *Love You Till Tuesday* is seldom acknowledged, but once pointed out it becomes alarmingly obvious. Late January saw the filming of his Lyons Maid ice cream commercial and, rather more significantly, the composition of a new song. Pitt had urged him to produce "a very special piece of material that would dramatically demonstrate David's remarkable inventiveness and would probably be the high spot of the production." David wrote 'Space Oddity'.

Shooting began on 26 January with silent location sequences of David, Hermione and Hutch on Hampstead Heath for 'When I Live My Dream'. Three days later David recorded his German vocals at Trident. Filming resumed at Clarence Studios in Greenwich on 1 February, when the shooting of 'Ching-a-Ling' and 'Sell Me A Coat' marked Hermione's final appearance in the film and, it seems, in David's life. Pitt recalls hearing a quarrel emanating from the dressing room that day, and has since opined that Hermione only agreed to appear in the film as a parting gesture.

The following day saw the first audio recording of 'Space Oddity' at Morgan Studios in Willesden. On 3 February David was back in Clarence Studios, shooting 'Rubber Band' and 'Love You Till Tuesday', followed the next day by 'Let Me Sleep Beside You' and the studio sections of 'When I Live My Dream'. February 5 was devoted to 'The Mask', and the day after saw filming begin on the 'Space Oddity' sequence. Apparently Thomson, whose ambitions lay in the direction of soft porn, wanted the star-maidens in 'Space Oddity' (played by production assistant Suzanne Mercer and glamour model Samantha Bond – not to be confused with the actress now best known as 007's Miss Moneypenny, who was all of seven years old at the time) to be considerably more explicit, "but the climate of the times was against it," he told the Gillmans. "Besides, I didn't think Ken Pitt would approve." Finally, 7 February saw the completion of 'Space Oddity' and the filming of 'When I'm Five'.

Costs escalated during post-production, and the narration originally intended to link the songs was scrapped. Although Kenneth Pitt arranged the occasional private screening, no television station or film distributor expressed an interest. He was dismayed to discover that Günther Schneider had now left ZDF, while the BBC's only suggestion was that Pitt should consider making a similar film with Tom Jones. *Love You Till Tuesday* remained unreleased until May 1984, when Pitt finally recovered his costs by issuing it on home video in partnership with Polygram. Although Bowie took no part in promoting or approving the release, he is understood to have adored the result and encouraged his friends to see it.

Love You Till Tuesday may be cheap and unintentionally amusing in places, but as a record of David Bowie before fame beckoned its survival can only be welcomed. One could hardly wish to capture a more fascinating moment in his creative development, for the film witnesses the precise point at which he began grasping his identity as a solo performer and staging his music in a genuinely theatrical environment. Most revealing, not to say prophetic, is 'The Mask'. A boy steals a mask which makes his friends and family laugh, and he wins fame and fortune through the abjectly trivial act of putting it on in public. As his reputation spreads he becomes arrogant and disdainful of the common herd until finally, making love with his ego before a packed house at the London Palladium, he finds he cannot remove the mask and dies of suffocation on stage. "The papers made a big thing out of it," concludes the voiceover as the lights dim on his lifeless body. "Funny though – they didn't mention anything about a mask." Those who believe Bowie had no game-plan in the 1960s need look no further than this film.

ZIGGY STARDUST AND THE SPIDERS FROM MARS

• 1973/1983/2002 (86 mins) • Miramax/MainMan/ Warner Video PES 38022 *(VHS)* • EMI DVD 7243 4 92987 9 8 *(DVD)* • *Director:* D A Pennebaker

'Hang On To Yourself' / 'Ziggy Stardust' / 'Watch That Man' / 'Wild Eyed Boy From Freecloud/All The Young Dudes/Oh! You Pretty Things' / 'Moonage Daydream' / 'Changes' / 'Space Oddity' / 'My Death' / 'Cracked Actor' / 'Time' / 'The Width Of A Circle' / 'Let's Spend The Night Together' / 'Suffragette City' / 'White Light/White Heat' / 'Rock'n'Roll Suicide'

Don Pennebaker's film of the final Ziggy Stardust concert, shot at Hammersmith Odeon on 3 July 1973, was intended for theatrical release as early as Christmas of the same year under the title *The Last Concert*. An hour-long version was screened on US television in October 1974 and this, along with an unlicensed broadcast on an Italian pirate station, was notable for including the Jeff Beck encores absent from the later release. The raw sound of the 1974 version (mixed by Bowie with Mike Moran) was also a very different affair, with the guitar and bass drowning out nearly everything else, including the drums and occasionally Bowie's vocals.

The American broadcast was followed by nearly a decade of disputatious wrangling between the film's financiers, its executive producer Tony Defries, and latterly Jeff Beck himself. It was finally granted a release in October 1983 under the title *Ziggy Stardust And The Spiders From Mars*. "I dragged it out last year and had a look," Bowie explained, "and I thought, 'This is a *funny* film! This boy used to dress like that for a living? ... Wait till my son sees this!" *Ziggy Stardust And The Spiders From Mars* arrived minus the Beck encores, and with a soundtrack newly remixed by Bowie, Tony Visconti and Bruce Tergeson. "I don't know what I was on when I did it the first time," confessed David. The accompanying live album, *Ziggy Stardust: The Motion Picture*, featured slightly different mixes by the same team.

Although a priceless record of a pivotal occasion, Pennebaker's film is not without its shortcomings. The dark, grainy images and the director's penchant for hand-held, focus-pulling *cinéma-vérité*, which had been employed to such great advantage in his Bob Dylan film *Don't Look Back*, do little justice to the extraordinary costumes and strutting theatricality of the show. On the few occasions when David is in focus and not masking his face with a guitar or hand, he is often little more than a head and shoulders picked out in a blob of red light.

Nonetheless, the intensity of the performance and the hysteria of the crowd make this a far more exciting glimpse of a live performance than any of Bowie's later, glossier concert videos, offering first-hand evidence of his celebrated physical rapport with both Mick Ronson and the audience. Also worthy of note are the underrated excellence of Trevor Bolder's Jack Bruce-influenced bass style and Woody Woodmansey's primal drumming. Nowhere is this clearer than in the hypnotic prog-punk section of 'The Width Of A Circle', in which Bowie leaves the stage to change costumes while the Spiders lock horns in a ferocious wall of noise that appears to wreak an almost hallucinatory effect on the delirious crowd, who are captured trance-like in the flickering strobe lights.

In addition to the concert footage itself there are backstage scenes of David, looking every bit as tired as might be expected of a rock star at the end of an eighteen-month tour, submitting to the caresses of Pierre Laroche's make-up brush and executing hectic costume changes while the band holds sway on stage. Most revealing of all are the fleeting revelations about Tony Defries's business practices ("It's all in code," David mutters as he studies a mysterious telex sent to his manager from MainMan's New York offices, "I didn't know he did business in code – can't understand a word of this!") and the uncomfortable evidence of the Bowies' deteriorating marriage. Angela is seen signing autographs for the fans massing beneath the Hammersmith flyover, before arriving in the dressing room to David's manifestly feigned delight. "If, as I did recently, you watch the backstage scenes where David and I are talking," Angela later wrote in her autobiography, "you can see what I didn't want to: David's smiling face when it's turned towards me is a mask." Bowie seems far happier on stage where, in this historic film, he and his band are never less than spectacular.

A DVD release of the 1983 version appeared in some territories in 2000, but this was rapidly superseded by Tony Visconti's stunning Dolby Digital 5.1 remix, which was premiered at New York City's Film Forum on 10 July 2002 and released on DVD in March 2003 under the elongated title *Ziggy Stardust And The Spiders From Mars: The Motion Picture*. The absence of any extra surviving footage meant that, unlike the accompanying CD remix, there were no new additions to the film; but the sound is a revelation, and the additional attraction of a commentary by both Tony Visconti and Don Pennebaker makes this DVD one of the Bowie fan's essential purchases.

CRACKED ACTOR
• 1974 (60 mins) • BBC Television • *Director:* Alan Yentob

Although neither an official Bowie product nor an available video release, Alan Yentob's 1974 film deserves mention as arguably the finest documentary made about David Bowie. Filmed in and around Philadelphia and Los Angeles during August and September 1974, the show was produced for the BBC's *Omnibus* and was provisionally entitled *The Collector*, after a comment David had made in a Russell Harty interview the previous year.

We have many reasons to be grateful for Yentob's

film. First and foremost, *Cracked Actor* boasts footage of the astonishing Diamond Dogs stage show, and although the dimly-lit images and confused close-ups are only a marginal improvement on the 1973 Hammersmith film, these are priceless glimpses of a legendary chapter in Bowie history. Were it not for the presence of Yentob's crew David would already have scrapped the Diamond Dogs set, and already the *Young Americans* influence is making itself felt: after a glimpse of David rehearsing 'Right' with Ava Cherry, Luther Vandross and Robin Clark at Sigma Sound, the film concludes on the live rendition of 'John, I'm Only Dancing (Again)' with which Bowie closed the Los Angeles gigs.

Cracked Actor also offers an uncomfortable fly-on-the-wall insight into one of the darker periods of Bowie's life and career. There are notorious shots of an emaciated David slumped in the back of a MainMan limousine as the nighted streets of Hollywood flick past the windows. "Hope we're not stopped," he mutters as a police siren sounds, banishing any doubt concerning the source of his anxiety with the classic coke addict's overstated sniff. "*Cracked Actor* is extremely painful for me to watch," David said in 1997, "because I know what my interior life was like and I was unbelievably screwed up. I can't tell you how bad life was for me."

Even more telling is a moment of hostile body-language between David and Tony Defries, who is glimpsed in a backstage shot of the band preparing to take the stage. Also of note is an early sighting of Corinne Schwab, sharing the back of David's limo as Tony Mascia drives through the desert. Other highlights include shots of David undergoing torture by plaster of Paris for his Aladdin Sane kabuki mask, and the host of fabulous American fans interviewed by Yentob. "I'm just the space cadet, he's the commander," coos one girl, while a rather scary boy from Arizona tells Yentob that David is "from his own universe." When pressed on the question of what universe that might be, the glazed-over boy elucidates, "The Bowie universe."

Perhaps the most valuable aspect of *Cracked Actor*, however, is the deflating effect it has on the mythology surrounding Bowie's mid-1970s exile in America. There is little question that the man we meet in Yentob's film is unwell and maybe even a mite unhinged, but he is also articulate, funny and clever, communicating the mixed emotions of a sensitive and perceptive soul trapped in a vulgar rock'n'roll setting.

A member of the BBC crew later described David as "charming … like the only sober person in a roomful of drunks", and this is how he emerges from *Cracked Actor*. Bowie later told Yentob that he had watched the film "again and again", because "it told the truth".

Yentob's shots of a solemn, silent Bowie viewing footage of his 1973 farewell concert in a darkened room fired the imagination of Nicolas Roeg, who saw *Cracked Actor*'s first UK broadcast on 26 January 1975 and wasted little time in contacting David to discuss *The Man Who Fell To Earth*.

DAVID BOWIE VIDEO EP
• 1983 (12 mins) • PMI MVT 9900042 • *Directors:* David Mallet, Jim Yukich

'Let's Dance' / 'China Girl' / 'Modern Love'

Released with a 15 certificate, this three-track 1983 compilation remains the only official source of the uncut 'China Girl' video.

SERIOUS MOONLIGHT
• 1984 (90 mins) • Warner Music Vision 4509 968393 • *Director:* David Mallet

'Look Back In Anger' / '"Heroes"' / 'What In The World' / 'Golden Years' / 'Fashion' / 'Let's Dance' / 'Breaking Glass' / 'Life On Mars?' / 'Sorrow' / 'Cat People (Putting Out Fire)' / 'China Girl' / 'Scary Monsters (And Super Creeps)' / 'Rebel Rebel' / 'White Light/White Heat' / 'Station To Station' / 'Cracked Actor' / 'Ashes To Ashes' / 'Space Oddity' / 'Young Americans' / 'Fame'

Serious Moonlight was recorded on 11 and 12 September 1983 at the 11,000-seater Pacific National Exhibition Coliseum in Vancouver. The video was expected to do big business and director David Mallet left little to chance: local DJ Terry Mulligan took the stage before the show and drilled the audience on how to respond to the cameras, while Mallet's assistants scoured the audience to select 50 attractive young women who were given seats on the front row.

Mallet lets the songs and stage visuals speak for themselves, although there are occasional moments of directorial flash. The opening sequence depicts Bowie wandering through a Vancouver market. He makes his first entrance on stage surrounded by a halo of after-images, and during 'Ashes To Ashes' the picture turns paintbox-negative to emulate Mallet's original video. Each new number is introduced by a video caption giving the title and year ('Space Oddity' hails from 1972, apparently), accompanied by a photo of David from the appropriate period.

Absent are 'Red Sails' and the encores of 'Star', 'Stay', 'The Jean Genie' and 'Modern Love', all of which were performed at the Vancouver concerts. Otherwise the performances are more or less intact, although the extended intro of 'Station To Station' is missing while vocal overdubs were added to '"Heroes"' and, as is painfully obvious at one point, 'Ashes To Ashes'. But for the most part this is a smart, honest document, recording everything from Earl Slick's spectacular guitar solos to the Simms boys' occasionally irksome choreography. There's the chance to enjoy the 'Cracked Actor' skull routine, admire the spectacle of Bowie booting a giant inflatable globe around the auditorium, and marvel at his timing as it bounces back on stage and he heaves it onto his shoulders in an impromptu Atlas routine. It's neither as historically weighty as *Ziggy Stardust And The Spiders From Mars* nor as outrageously spectacular as *Glass Spider*, but as live videos go it's probably more solid and entertaining than either.

The UK release originally came on two separate tapes: *David Bowie: Serious Moonlight* ran from 'Look Back In Anger' to 'China Girl', while *David Bowie: Live* featured 'Scary Monsters' onwards. The subsequent 90-minute compilation gave better value for money despite losing the interview footage included on the originals.

RICOCHET

• 1984 (59 mins) • Vision Video VVD 084 • *Script:* Martin Stellman • *Director:* Gerry Troyna

Gerry Troyna's film is a curious document of the Serious Moonlight tour's Far Eastern dates in December 1983. *Ricochet* affects to be a fly-on-the-wall glimpse of David Bowie at work and play in Hong Kong, Singapore and Bangkok (in that order, despite the fact that Hong Kong actually came last), but parts of the film are blatantly scripted. Bowie is portrayed as an outsider, slipping away from the pressures of his schedule to wander abroad and soak up the exotic cultures of the three cities. Notwithstanding

the bright and breezy image of the 1983 package, one is reminded here of his Berlin period, a feeling pushed home by the use of two instrumentals from *"Heroes"* as incidental music.

Among the Hong Kong highlights are a glimpse of a copycat band rehearsing 'Ziggy Stardust', and footage from a press conference where Bowie traces his interest in the East back to his days with Lindsay Kemp. Over dinner he discusses China's takeover of the colony, still 14 years into the future. In Singapore he has his fortune told in a temple, visits the Raffles Hotel and is disappointed that he can't watch an opera rehearsal. In Bangkok he goes to a seedy club, takes a night trip in a canoe to the strains of 'Moss Garden', and finally visits a Buddhist shrine and listens to a Thai band. Interpolated between these vignettes is a rather irritating sub-plot about a young fan trying to get hold of a ticket; more rewarding is the concert footage of 'Look Back In Anger', '"Heroes"' and 'Fame' (but despite what it says on the sleeve blurb, not 'Ricochet', which was never performed on this or any other tour). Although dark, grainy and shot with none of the high-gloss technique of David Mallet's *Serious Moonlight* video, these live cuts are excellent, intense versions which often have the edge on the Vancouver recordings.

JAZZIN' FOR BLUE JEAN

• 1984 (21 mins) • Nitrate/PMI MVS 9900274 (*reissue: EMI PM0017*) • *Starring:* David Bowie, Louise Scott, Chris Sullivan, Graham Rogers, Kenny Andrews, Eve Ferret, Mark Long • *Script:* David Bowie, Julien Temple, Terry Johnson • *Director:* Julien Temple

In 1983 Michael Jackson famously pushed back the boundaries of rock video with his extravagant *Thriller* promo, and it wasn't long before David Bowie got in on the act. The result was the 21-minute feature *Jazzin' For Blue Jean*, directed by Bowie newcomer Julien Temple, the *enfant terrible* of British film who had trailed The Sex Pistols during the late 1970s and made his professional break with *The Great Rock'n'Roll Swindle*. Temple's early pop promos included Culture Club's 'Do You Really Want To Hurt Me' and ABC's 'Poison Arrow', while in 1983 he had directed The Rolling Stones' *Undercover* trilogy, thrilling the press by claiming he had nearly turned down the job because he didn't consider Jagger and company radical enough for him. The tit-for-tat poaching game between Bowie and the Stones showed no signs of abating in 1984, and while Mick Jagger secured the services of Nile Rodgers for his solo album *She's The Boss*, Bowie contacted Julien Temple. Together they developed a storyline from Bowie's plot, and playwright Terry Johnson was hired to polish the dialogue. Bowie's role remained hands-on throughout the production. "I get a lot of input from him," said Temple. "Which is very different from the Stones, who always want you to do everything yourself."

Jazzin' For Blue Jean was shot at Shepperton Studios and Kensington's Rainbow Room in August 1984 (not, as often claimed, at Soho's Wag Club, which is where Temple directed the MTV Awards 'Blue Jean' promo a few days later). "This is going to be like the old-style fifties short," said Bowie. "The song definitely takes second place to the plot and the characters. There's quite a lot of dialogue and different parts of the song crop up in different places. It's about a boy, a girl and a rock star." *Jazzin' For Blue Jean* is an amusingly resonant comedy in which Bowie takes two contrasting roles: Vic, the odd-job man with his eye on a girl, and Screamin' Lord Byron, the flamboyant rock star whose forthcoming gig provides Vic with the perfect date. Bowie's transformation into Byron, which saw him plastered in slap for the first time since 'Ashes To Ashes', would be his last full-blown characterization for many a year. His *Arabian Nights* costume, complete with turban and ballooning trousers, was designed by Alison Chitty.

Bowie lookalike Ian Ellis was pressed into action for the scenes in which Vic meets Byron. In a segment cut from the finished film, Bowie as Vic runs up to the catwalk during 'Blue Jean' and shouts to his alter ego, "We're at a table in the corner! I think you're doing really great, they really like ya!" – at which point Byron's boot stamps down on his hand. The three musicians hired to mime as the backing group came from real bands, although none had yet enjoyed chart success: the drummer was Physique's Paul Ridgeley, the guitarist Daryl Humphries from The Blondini Brothers, and the bassist was none other than Richard Fairbrass, then playing with Ian Flesh but later to find fame as the lead singer of Right Said Fred. The band's movements, like Bowie's, were choreographed by David Toguri. "Bowie moves like a wave," he said. "There is a weight behind his movements, a real authority. And he makes every move his own ... His concentration is extraordinary."

"Bowie is just getting better and better as an actor," said Julien Temple during the shoot. "And the guy is so acute and precise about what he wants ... I've never seen a video crew get so involved with a performer. It's extraordinary in the music field to have someone who understands film like Bowie because film and music don't often mix."

"I've had so much fun on this thing with Julien," said Bowie. "I can't wait to see it ... it's nothing particularly revolutionary in story terms, it's pretty lightweight, it's comedy material ... I think one thing that it does do is serve as demythification of the rock star, I hope. I do a very campy type of rock star and a very Ernie type of character, which is fun."

Jazzin' For Blue Jean is an unqualified triumph: the choreographed 'Blue Jean' section itself is spectacular, but above all the film is a superb showcase for Bowie's genuine comic talent. His instinct for physical comedy is beautifully precise, as evidenced by the running gag about the ill-fitting shoe Vic has borrowed for the date, and his timing throughout is marvellous. As Vic, Elastoplast on nose, he comes on like a junior Tony Hancock, painting himself into corners with increasingly tall tales ("David Hockney introduced us ... I write his lyrics," he blusters at one point, while the "Whoosh-Oleander" scene achieves an almost Woody Allen level of comic pain). As Screamin' Lord Byron he's a ridiculous, powder-puffed, pill-guzzling old luvvie. In public the star maintains an arrogant, flouncing swagger, and the adulation of the audience who ape his every move is almost sinister; but backstage he is a paranoid child, arriving in an oxygen mask, whining petulantly and surrounded by sycophants and bodyguards. Vic's desperate patter to the bouncer might almost be a review of the Serious Moonlight show ("I caught that tour in Berlin – I thought they hung the music up on too much light and trickery, bit OTT, don't you agree?"), and his final diatribe at the rock star ("You conniving randy bogus Oriental old queen! Your record sleeves are better than your songs!") is hysterically close to the bone. There's even room for a dig at "Frankie Say" T-shirts, *the* fashion accessory of the summer of '84. "God, I hate those damn things, I really hate them!" laughed Bowie at the time.

The comic unravelling of the rock star's mystique is framed by a series of cinematic jokes: in the opening scene Vic is pasting up a poster of Screamin' Lord Byron when he spots the girl and, imagining he is in a film, describes in voiceover exactly what we see

("Dead trendy, a long-shot down the street from a high POV, 'cause I was on me ladder"). At the end the fiction is self-consciously exploded: the last shot is a slow pull-out to reveal the film crew as Vic becomes Bowie, squabbling with the director: "Look, it's my song, my concept, my neck! I told you before, Julien, if she gets into the car with the rock star it's far too obvious…" until finally Temple shouts "Cut!"

Jazzin' For Blue Jean won cinema distribution supporting *The Company Of Wolves*, and received a late-night screening on Channel 4. The film was subsequently released on home video, and later appeared as a concealed "Easter Egg" on 2002's *Best Of Bowie* DVD. The extract featuring 'Blue Jean' itself has been widely shown and features in *The Video Collection* and *Best Of Bowie*.

DAY-IN DAY-OUT

• 1987 (18 mins) • PMI MVR 9900682 • *Directors:* Julien Temple, David Bowie, David Mallet

'Day-In Day-Out' / 'Loving The Alien' / 'Day In Day Out (Extended Dance Version)'

When 'Day-In Day-Out' was censored by broadcasters in Britain and America, PMI released a video EP of the single edit and the 'Extended Dance Version', with 'Loving The Alien' as an added bonus. With an 18 certificate, this remains the only release of the uncut 'Day-In Day-Out'.

GLASS SPIDER

• 1988 (107 mins) • Video Collection VC 4043/ VC 4044 • Image Entertainment 6198 • *Director:* David Mallet

'Up The Hill Backwards' / 'Glass Spider' / 'Day-In Day-Out' / 'Bang Bang' / 'Absolute Beginners' / 'Loving The Alien' / 'China Girl' / 'Rebel Rebel' / 'Fashion' / 'Never Let Me Down' / '"Heroes"' / 'Sons Of The Silent Age' / 'Young Americans' / 'The Jean Genie' / 'Let's Dance' / 'Time' / 'Fame' / 'Blue Jean' / 'I Wanna Be Your Dog' / 'White Light/White Heat' / 'Modern Love'

Recorded over eight shows at Sydney Entertainment Centre in November 1987 (although the bulk comes from the concert on 6 November), David Mallet's video captures the staggering enormity of the Glass Spider tour in its closing weeks. Like *Serious Moonlight* it was originally released in two separate instalments (with the break coming after '"Heroes"'), but these were superseded by a 1990 compilation of the two. In some Far East territories a DVD release followed in 1999.

Despite the critical drubbing the tour received, this is actually a hugely enjoyable record of a show best observed at close quarters. Sadly several of the tour's more enticing rarities are absent (no 'Big Brother', no 'All The Madmen'), and although David turns in a fine performance his end-of-tour voice is a little husky at times. There are nevertheless some splendid numbers, including a sublime 'Sons Of The Silent Age', a tip-top 'Young Americans', a surprisingly rocked-up 'Blue Jean' and a six-minute reworking of 'The Jean Genie'. Love them or loathe them, the technical routines and in particular the dancers are truly astonishing; and there's also the chance to boggle at Carlos Alomar's spiky hair and hologram shades, and shout at the hugely irritating girl in the front row who knows all the words and has devised her own hand-jive routines.

Glass Spider gets a rough deal, but until the day that either the Diamond Dogs or Sound + Vision shows are made available on video, this release leads the field for those wishing to see David Bowie delivering a rock-theatre spectacular.

TIN MACHINE

• 1989 (13 mins) • *Director:* Julien Temple

'Pretty Thing' / 'Tin Machine' / 'Prisoner Of Love' / 'Crack City' / 'Bus Stop' / 'Video Crime' / 'I Can't Read' / 'Working Class Hero' / 'Under The God'

Filmed at the New York Ritz, Julien Temple's 13-minute *Tin Machine* film is a medley of performance-style clips from the 1989 album. Each song segues headlong into the next ('Bus Stop' only gets as far as its first verse, for example, before the band slips into 'Video Crime'), until the film culminates in the full-length 'Under The God' promo. Clips were aired on television at the time but the film was rarely screened in its entirety, although it did enjoy brief distribution as a supporting feature in UK cinemas. *Tin Machine* has yet to appear on video, despite the fact that in 1999 Bowie cited it as his all-time favourite of his own music videos.

OY VEY, BABY – TIN MACHINE
LIVE AT THE DOCKS
• 1992 (88 mins) • Polygram 0853203 • *Directors:*
Rudi Dolezal, Hannes Rossacher

'Bus Stop' / 'Sacrifice Yourself' / 'Goodbye Mr. Ed' / 'I
Can't Read' / 'Baby Universal' / 'You Can't Talk' / 'Go
Now' / 'Under The God' / 'Betty Wrong' / 'Stateside' /
'I've Been Waiting For You' / 'You Belong In Rock
N'Roll' / 'One Shot' / 'If There Is Something' /
'Heaven's In Here' / 'Amlapura' / 'Crack City'

To film the second Tin Machine tour Bowie turned to
German directors Rudi Dolezal and Hannes
Rossacher, the so-called "Torpedo Twins" who had
earned their spurs with the 1986 video for Falco's
'Rock Me Amadeus' before going on to direct a string
of increasingly brilliant promos for Queen. Shot at
The Docks, Hamburg on 24 October 1991, *Oy Vey,*
Baby does a reasonable job of capturing the live Tin
Machine experience, generally offering more palatable
fare than the album whose name it shares. Interspers-
ing the performance with backstage glimpses and the
obligatory scenes of queuing fans, the directors alternate rock-steady tripod shots with fashionably shaky
hand-held close-ups, darting between monochrome
film and colour VT in a manner that's *de rigueur* nowadays but seemed quite radical in 1991. With sound
mixed and produced by Tim Palmer, the performance
itself showcases the best and worst of Tin Machine's
live act. The highlights include raw, exciting renditions
of 'Under The God' and 'Goodbye Mr. Ed' and a truly
affecting deconstruction of 'I Can't Read', but the prevailing tone is more accurately characterized by an
interminable 'Stateside' and a horribly self-indulgent
nine-minute assault on 'Heaven's In Here', including a
preposterous middle passage in which Reeves Gabrels
unplugs his guitar and passes the buzzing flex into the
crowd. 'Baby Universal' is just the studio version
dubbed onto the live visuals, but a heavily reworked
'Betty Wrong', with slow saxophone interludes, is
more worthy of attention. There's a chance to see each
member of the band take lead vocals: in addition to
the horrible 'Stateside', we have Tony Sales performing
'Go Now' and Reeves Gabrels singing 'I've Been
Waiting For You'. A valuable document, but in truth an
item for completists only.

BLACK TIE WHITE NOISE
• 1993 (63 mins) • BMG 74321 166223 • EMI
72434 90634 9 5 • *Directors:* David Mallet, Mark
Romanek, Matthew Rolston

Interview / 'You've Been Around' / 'Nite Flights' /
'Miracle Goodnight' / 'Black Tie White Noise' / 'I Feel
Free' / 'I Know It's Gonna Happen Someday' /
'Miracle Goodnight' *(clip)* / 'Jump They Say' *(clip)* /
'Black Tie White Noise' *(clip)*

Rather than tour *Black Tie White Noise* Bowie elected
to promote the album with David Mallet's hour-long
video, which combined interview footage with
behind-the-scenes shots of the album sessions, and six
mimed performances shot at Hollywood Center
Studios on 8 May 1993 (an additional mimed performance of 'Don't Let Me Down & Down' was
filmed, but failed to make the final cut). The result is
a useful companion to the album, offering glimpses
of Mick Ronson at work on 'I Feel Free' and David
rehearsing the vocal of 'I Know It's Gonna Happen
Someday', although Mallet's new "videos" are distinctly cut-price and unimaginative. According to Q,
"it could have been done cheaper, but not very much,"
and certainly these drab clips aren't a patch on the
three official *Black Tie White Noise* videos included at
the end of the tape which, together with the delightful
coda of out-takes from 'Miracle Goodnight', are worth
the price of admission in themselves. In 2001 a DVD
version was released in some Far East territories, while
in 2003 a remastered DVD was included with EMI's
10th Anniversary CD reissue of *Black Tie White Noise*.

THE VIDEO COLLECTION
• 1993 (105 mins) • PMI PM 807 • *Directors:* Mick
Rock, Stanley Dorfman, Nick Ferguson, David Mallet,
David Bowie, Jim Yukich, Julien Temple, Steve Barron,
Tim Pope, Jean Baptiste-Mondino, Gus Van Sant

'Space Oddity' / 'John, I'm Only Dancing' / 'The Jean
Genie' / 'Life On Mars?' / 'Be My Wife' / '"Heroes"' /
'Boys Keep Swinging' / 'Look Back In Anger' / 'D.J.' /
'Ashes To Ashes' / 'Fashion' / 'Wild Is The Wind' /
'Let's Dance' / 'China Girl' / 'Modern Love' / 'Blue
Jean' / 'Loving The Alien' / 'Dancing In The Street' /
'Absolute Beginners' / 'Underground' / 'As The World
Falls Down' / 'Day-In Day-Out' / 'Time Will Crawl' /
'Never Let Me Down' / 'Fame 90'

Released to tie in with *The Singles Collection* (and in almost identical packaging), this efficient round-up of most of Bowie's official promos from 1972 to 1990 was the only major compilation of Bowie videos until the arrival of 2002's *Best Of Bowie* DVD. The video skips any mention of Tin Machine and leaves the *Black Tie White Noise* promos to the documentary released only a month earlier.

The Video Collection was enthusiastically hailed at the time (*Q* went so far as to nominate it "the greatest video collection ever seen"), but even so, there are a number of gripes that even the casual fan might feel justified in raising. In the first place, the quality of the mastering is ropey in places – far better prints of 'The Jean Genie' have been aired over the years, and even the 1980s videos look rather mushy on this tape. Secondly, stereo sound has been dubbed onto the early videos, doubtless with the best of intentions but often completely out of synch with the pictures. Thirdly, despite a PG rating, 'China Girl' and 'Day-In Day-Out' are the bowdlerized versions favoured by *Top Of The Pops* and MTV. And finally, several videos are missing – obscure ones to be sure, but that would make their inclusion all the more pleasing: 'The Drowned Girl' and 'When The Wind Blows' are conspicuous by their absence, as are the less essential clips for 'Under Pressure' and 'This Is Not America'. It would have been nice, too, to see the mid-1970s TV appearances commonly used as promos, such as the Dutch TV 'Rebel Rebel', the *Soul Train* clip of 'Golden Years' and *The Cher Show* performance of 'Fame' (since the latter appears halfway down the right-hand side of the 'Fame 90' video, there presumably isn't a clearance problem). As it stands, *The Video Collection* suffers from a gaping chasm between 1973 and 1977.

But omissions and edits aside, there is much to admire in this brilliant collection. Alongside the classic clips are less familiar pleasures like 'Look Back In Anger' and 'Wild Is The Wind', little-seen rarities like 'Be My Wife' and 'Never Let Me Down', and even the previously unseen video for 'As The World Falls Down', scheduled for a Christmas 1986 release but shelved at the last minute.

BEST OF BOWIE

• 2002 (252 mins) • EMI 72349010390 • *Directors:* Mick Rock, D A Pennebaker, Stanley Dorfman, Nick Ferguson, David Mallet, David Bowie, Jim Yukich, Julien Temple, Steve Barron, Tim Pope, Jean Baptiste-Mondino, Gus Van Sant, Mark Romanek, Matthew Rolston, Roger Michell, Sam Bayer, Floria Sigismondi, Rudi Dolezal, Hannes Rossacher, Dom & Nick, Walter Stern

'Oh! You Pretty Things' (from *The Old Grey Whistle Test*) / 'Queen Bitch' (from *The Old Grey Whistle Test*) / 'Five Years' (from *The Old Grey Whistle Test*) / 'Starman' (from *Top Of The Pops*) / 'John, I'm Only Dancing' / 'The Jean Genie' / 'Space Oddity' / 'Drive In Saturday' (from *Russell Harty Plus Pop*) / 'Life On Mars?' / 'Ziggy Stardust' (from *The Motion Picture*) / 'Rebel Rebel' (from *Top Pop*) / 'Young Americans' (from *The Dick Cavett Show*) / 'Be My Wife' / '"Heroes"' / 'Boys Keep Swinging' / 'D.J.' / 'Look Back In Anger' / 'Ashes To Ashes' / 'Fashion' / 'Wild Is The Wind' / 'Let's Dance' / 'China Girl' / 'Modern Love' / 'Cat People (Putting Out Fire)' (from the Serious Moonlight tour) / 'Blue Jean' / 'Loving The Alien' / 'Dancing In The Street' / 'Absolute Beginners' / 'Underground' / 'As The World Falls Down' / 'Day-In Day-Out' / 'Time Will Crawl' / 'Never Let Me Down' / 'Fame 90' / 'Jump They Say' / 'Black Tie White Noise' / 'Miracle Goodnight' / 'Buddha Of Suburbia' / 'The Hearts Filthy Lesson' / 'Strangers When We Meet' / 'Hallo Spaceboy' / 'Little Wonder' / 'Dead Man Walking' / 'Seven Years In Tibet' / 'I'm Afraid Of Americans' / 'Thursday's Child' / 'Survive'

"Easter Eggs": 'Oh! You Pretty Things' (alternative take from *The Old Grey Whistle Test*) / Russell Harty interview, January 1973 / *Ziggy Stardust* DVD advert / Full-length *Jazzin' For Blue Jean* film / 'Blue Jean' (alternative Wag Club video) / 'Day-In Day-Out' (alternative dance mix) / 'Miracle Goodnight' (alternative mix) / 'Seven Years In Tibet' (Mandarin language version) / 'Survive' (live in Paris 1999)

Issued alongside the *Best Of Bowie* CD in November 2002, EMI's lavish two-disc DVD set superseded all previous compilations to become the most extensive collection of Bowie videos yet released. Both sound and vision were restored and remastered for the release by Abbey Road Interactive: "'The Jean Genie' track took a day to restore," the project's business developer Alex Reid later revealed. "The whole project took about a week and a half."

In addition to updating the run of official clips previously included on *The Video Collection*, this excellent set goes considerably further, adding such pleasures as the *Old Grey Whistle Test* session from 1972, the same year's seminal performance of 'Starman' from *Top Of The Pops*, the Dutch TV clip of 'Rebel Rebel' and, perhaps most excitingly, the *Russell Harty Plus* performance of 'Drive In Saturday' and the *Dick Cavett* rendition of 'Young Americans'. Sidestepping any mention of Tin Machine, *Best Of Bowie* moves on to scale new heights with the onset of Bowie's frequently brilliant 1990s videos.

The 50 minutes' worth of concealed "Easter Eggs" are also highly impressive, including an excerpt from David's 1973 interview with Russell Harty, the rare MTV Awards promo for 'Blue Jean', and the full-length *Jazzin' For Blue Jean* film. Also available are another *Whistle Test* take of 'Oh! You Pretty Things', the Mandarin language version of 'Seven Years In Tibet', a couple of superfluous remixes, and a splendid live 'Survive' from the 1999 tour.

The remastered soundtrack and prints are generally excellent. Some of the TV archive material is of variable quality, but that's to be expected; otherwise, the majority of this DVD looks and sounds simply stunning. Even the menus, each backed by a different Bowie instrumental, are beautiful.

However, nothing is perfect, and sadly there are a few lapses even on this marvellous release. As on *The Video Collection*, both 'Day-In Day-Out' and 'China Girl' are the expurgated versions re-edited for TV exposure, and although 'The Hearts Filthy Lesson' is considerably more complete than the version originally shown by MTV, it's still a few edits short of the real thing. Despite the remastering, a few of the clips – notably the *Lodger* songs and 'Buddha Of Suburbia' – appear to have been sourced from NTSC copies and are of decidedly inferior quality to the rest. It's a pity that the TV performances of 'Fame' and 'Golden Years' could not have been featured alongside 'Rebel Rebel' and 'Young Americans' (indeed, given that the latter was licensed from the Dick Cavett performance, it's a

shame that 'Footstompin'' wasn't included too), and a few *bona fide* videos are still missing ('The Drowned Girl', 'Under Pressure', 'This Is Not America', 'When The Wind Blows', and of course everything by Tin Machine). The liner notes are none too reliable either, among other things resurrecting the inaccurate old chestnut about the *Top Of The Pops* 'Starman' appearance dating from April 1972 (it was in fact recorded on 5 July and transmitted the following day).

But in the final analysis these are all minor quibbles: for all its flaws *Best Of Bowie* is still one of the most beautifully compiled and consistently brilliant music DVDs on the market. It comes as no surprise that it entered the UK music chart at number 1 and remained in the top ten for several weeks.

SOUND & VISION

• 2003 (90 mins) • Stax/Prometheus/Foxstar STX 2074 • *Director:* Rick Hull

This 90-minute Bowie biography was originally screened by America's A&E network on 4 November 2002, appearing on DVD a year later. Despite a few gaps and inexactitudes it's a good solid account of Bowie's career, featuring interviews with figures as diverse as Iman, Brian Eno, Tony Visconti, Iggy Pop, George Underwood, Geoffrey MacCormack, Mick Rock, Toni Basil, Carlos Alomar and Nile Rodgers. The wealth of rare archive material includes an array of childhood photographs, the celebrated "Society for the Prevention of Cruelty to Long-Haired Men" clip from the *Tonight* show in 1964, performance excerpts from *The Image* and *The Elephant Man*, film of Hype performing 'Waiting For The Man' in 1970, and even footage from David and Iman's wedding. Dedicated fans won't learn anything new, but it's a handsome enough stocking-filler.

I'LL GIVE YOU TELEVISION...

No subsequent Bowie documentary has ever matched 1974's *Cracked Actor* for sheer historical value, but a few individual broadcasts are worthy of mention. Alan Yentob caught up with David in two subsequent BBC interviews, firstly for *Arena* in 1978 and then for the 1997 special *Changes – Bowie At Fifty*. In the same month ITV chipped in with *An Earthling At 50*, while France's Canal + offered an excellent documentary called *A Part Ça … David Bowie*, which included a feast of rare clips (David at the 1975 Grammy Awards, live footage from the Station To Station tour, the 1980 Crystal Jun Rock commercial, David's wedding to Iman), and several rare interviewees speaking about David (John Lennon, Philip Glass, Cherry Vanilla, Guy Peellaert, Amanda Lear).

In May 1989 BBC2's *Def II* screened an excellent half-hour documentary following Tin Machine through tour rehearsals in New York. Hugh Thomson's 1996 BBC/WGBH co-production *Dancing In The Street – A Rock And Roll History* devoted an episode called 'Hang On To Yourself' to the more American-oriented aspects of the Bowie/Iggy/Reed/Alice Cooper axis, containing interviews with Bowie

and Mick Ronson together with monochrome footage of a long-haired David meeting Andy Warhol in 1971, and even a brief extract of the future MainMan crew hamming it up in *Pork*. Michael Apted's 1997 documentary film *Inspirations* includes an interview with Bowie during preparations for his fiftieth birthday concert, while Matthew Collings's Channel 4 series *Hello Culture*, screened in 2001, devoted much of its final episode to Bowie's attainment, exploitation and subversion of fame. Another documentary worth hunting down is VH1's *Legends*, first transmitted in September 1998, which not only unearthed seldom-seen live footage from the Philly Dogs and Sound + Vision tours, but even boasted a clip of Hype performing live in 1970. This last gem was among the clips that later turned up in A&E's *Sound & Vision*, released on DVD in 2003 (see above). On a less elevated note, the BBC's dumbed-down and opportunistic *Liquid Assets: Bowie's Millions*, premiered in March 2003, is a vulgar and intrusive disgrace to journalism, of interest only for a couple of rare interviewees including Calvin Mark Lee and Angela Bowie at her most revisionist.

OTHER ARTISTS' VIDEO RELEASES

BING CROSBY'S MERRIE OLDE CHRISTMAS

(Bing Crosby)
• 1977 (52 mins) • ITC 4401 • *Director:* Dwight Hemion

Reissued on home video in the 1990s, Bing's 1977 Christmas spectacular includes his duet with David on 'Peace On Earth/Little Drummer Boy', plus an exclusive rendition of '"Heroes"' and a host of terrifying guest appearances by Ron Moody, Stanley Baxter, Twiggy, the Trinity Boys' Choir and the Crosby family themselves.

BOX OF FLIX *(Queen)*
• 1991 (160 mins) • PMI MVB 9913243 • *Directors:* Various

This double video of Queen's complete works includes David Mallet's video for 'Under Pressure',

also available on *Greatest Flix II*, a solo-tape release of the second half of the set.

THE FREDDIE MERCURY TRIBUTE CONCERT

(Various Artists)
• 1992 (200 mins) • PMI MVB 4910623 • *Director:* David Mallet

This double-tape VHS compilation of the April 1992 tribute concert includes Bowie's three-song set, but has long been deleted and is in any case superseded by the superior 2002 DVD release.

TINA LIVE – PRIVATE DANCER TOUR
(Tina Turner)
• 1994 (55 mins) • PMI 72434 9130838 • *Director:* David Mallet

This release includes Bowie's guest appearance at Tina's Birmingham NEC concert on 23 March 1985. An excerpt was later included on the 2000 DVD release *The Best Of Tina Turner – Celebrate!*

CLOSURE *(Nine Inch Nails)*
• 1997 (74 mins) • Acme Filmworks Inc • *Director:* Jonathan Rach

This US compilation includes Bowie performing 'Hurt' with Nine Inch Nails on the US leg of the Outside tour, plus backstage footage of David with Trent Reznor.

THE CONCERT FOR NEW YORK CITY
(Various Artists)
• 2002 (296 mins) • Columbia/SMV Enterprises 54205 9 • *Director:* Louis J Horvitz

This mammoth double DVD compilation of the star-studded post-September 11 benefit concert, recorded at Madison Square Garden on 20 October 2001, opens with Bowie's excellent performances of 'America' and '"Heroes"'.

THE FREDDIE MERCURY TRIBUTE CONCERT
(Various Artists)
• 2002 (200 mins) • Parlophone 7243 4928699 3 • *Directors:* David Mallet, Rudi Dolezal, Hannes Rossacher

The original VHS release of 1992's Freddie Mercury Tribute Concert was made redundant by this double DVD, released in May 2002 to mark the tenth anniversary of the event (and to tie in with the London opening in the same month of Queen's stage musical *We Will Rock You*). The first disc features highlights from the marathon concert, during which Queen's surviving members backed a parade of celebrity guests. Bowie's appearance – Lord's Prayer and all – is included in its entirety, and there's a valuable bonus in the form of a complete rehearsal of 'Under Pressure' (with George Michael mouthing the words from the sidelines), shot at Bray Studios. The second disc features an updated version of the Torpedo Twins' 1995 documentary *The Queen Phenomenon: In The Lap of the Gods*, which includes interview footage of Bowie and is now rather prosaically called *The Freddie Mercury Tribute Concert Documentary*. With superbly remixed sound and skilfully re-edited footage favouring close-ups of the performers rather than endless long shots of Wembley Stadium, the concert itself is a huge improvement on the original broadcast: we get to see more of Mick Ronson, and there's even a new glimpse of Bowie's flummoxed expression as he turns away from the audience after the Lord's Prayer, suggesting that he was just as surprised by it as everyone else was.

JESUS? .. THIS IS IGGY *(Iggy Pop)*
• 2002 (52 mins) • Quantum Leap /Arte Video QLDVD 0341 • *Directors:* Gilles Nadeau, Gérald Guignot

This DVD is a re-titled release of a 1998 French TV documentary originally called *La Rage de Vivre* ("Lust For Life"), with added English narration. It's a brisk but useful summary of Iggy Pop's career and boasts a wealth of archive clips, including footage of Iggy and Bowie performing 'Funtime' on *The Dinah Shore Show* in 1977. There are also a couple of archive interviews with David, and a very brief snippet from Mick Rock's seldom seen 1972 'Ziggy Stardust' promo film.

GREATEST VIDEO HITS 2 *(Queen)*
• 2003 (240 mins) • Parlophone 4909839 • *Directors:* Various

This remastered DVD includes David Mallet's video for 'Under Pressure', and bonus footage of Bowie and members of Queen discussing the song.

6   the actor

Overviews of Bowie's career have often given short shrift to his acting, but with nearly 20 feature films, a number of television plays and a celebrated Broadway run to his credit Bowie the actor is all too easily dismissed. He has always been philosophical and self-critical about his film career, describing it on one occasion as "splashing in the kids' pool", but his cinematic aspirations remain an integral part of his identity as an artist. True to form, he has generally been attracted to idiosyncratic art-house directors whose work is far removed from the Hollywood mainstream. "I have, on the whole, avoided Hollywood like the plague," he commented in 2000. "One cameo for Scorsese to me brings so much more satisfaction than, say, a James Bond."

This chapter sets out, in chronological order, Bowie's work in film, television and theatre, and concludes with a breakdown of cancelled projects, rumours and apocrypha.

THE IMAGE

• GB, Border Films, 1967 • *Director/Writer:* Michael Armstrong • *Starring:* Michael Byrne, David Bowie

In September 1967 Bowie made his first film, a fourteen-minute black and white short written and directed by young actor-turned-filmmaker Michael Armstrong, who had previously offered Bowie the lead in his abortive feature project *A Floral Tale* three months earlier. *The Image* was an altogether less ambitious piece of work, a two-hander about an artist (Byrne) and a boy (Bowie). Armstrong described it as "a study of the illusionary reality world within the schizophrenic mind of the artist at his point of creativity." Looking back in 1983, Bowie described it as "an underground black and white avant-garde thing done by some guy. He wanted to make a film about a painter doing a portrait of a guy in his teens, and the portrait comes to life and, in fact, turns out to be the corpse of some bloke. I can't really remember all the plot, but it was a fourteen-minute short and it was awful."

The three-day shoot, for which Bowie netted £30, commenced on 13 September when David was required to stand in the rain outside a window, looking in to where the artist painted his portrait. The "rain" was provided by a hose, and by the time the shots were completed David was soaking. According to Kenneth Pitt, "He was then brought inside where willing hands stripped him of his clothes and an exul-tant Michael Armstrong pounced on him with a large white bath towel and proceeded to rub warmth back into his shivering body."

Given an X certificate, *The Image* was released the same year and sank into obscurity until the spring of 1973, when an attempt to cash in on Bowie's celebrity won it a handful of screenings sandwiched between porn movies at the Jacey Cinema off Trafalgar Square. In 1984, at the height of Bowie's marketability, *The Image* received a low-circulation video release. "Gasp with horror as your hero gets murdered," remarked the *NME*, "not once, not twice but five times. Gasp with astonishment as he gets up entirely unharmed. Wonder with puzzlement how his acting career ever survived the carnage."

PIERROT IN TURQUOISE

• 28 December 1967 – 30 March 1968 • Playhouse Theatre, Oxford • Rosehill Theatre, Whitehaven • Mercury Theatre, London • Intimate Theatre, London • *Director:* Lindsay Kemp • *Writers/Devisers:* Lindsay Kemp, Craig San Roque • *Starring:* Lindsay Kemp, David Bowie, Jack Birkett, Annie Stainer

In the autumn of 1967, while Decca's selection board grew ever more intransigent in their dealings with David's recordings, he learned that the 29-year-old actor and mime Lindsay Kemp had been so impressed by the *David Bowie* album that he was using it as interval music during his shows. Suitably flattered, David attended one of Kemp's performances and was immediately entranced by the potential of mime. "Anything I had seen before owed most everything to Marceau and that classical school of cute or terminal whimsy, walking against the wind and suchlike," Bowie wrote in *Moonage Daydream* many years later. "Kemp, on the other hand, was sawing away at Genet and reinterpreting episodes from *The Maids* and *Salome*." Immediately impressed, David began attending Kemp's classes in dance and movement (but not in mime itself, contrary to popular belief) at the Dance Centre in Floral Street. "He was considerably more inhibited than he is now, and considerably less confident," Kemp tells the Gillmans, whose biography not only credits him with tutoring David in stage movement and make-up, but makes no bones about the fact that the teacher-pupil relationship blossomed into something rather deeper. However, the more excitable elements of the story must be treated with caution: several years after these revelations, Kemp admitted that "the rather theatrical versions I invented … were not intended to be *deliberately* untruthful, you understand, simply more impressive."

It was also during late 1967 that David's interest in Tibetan Buddhism, encouraged by his new friend Tony Visconti, reached its height. Biographers and contemporary sources differ over the extent of David's devotion to the cause, although most agree that his later assertion that "I was within a month of having my head shaved, taking my vows and becoming a monk" might be erring on the side of exaggeration. Nevertheless, having befriended the Tibetan refugee Chimi Youngdong Rimpoche in September 1967 at the Tibet Society's headquarters in Hampstead, Bowie and Visconti paid a visit to the Samye Ling Tibetan Centre at Eskdalemuir in Scotland. David, however, would choose to assimilate what he had learned into his own belief system: "I was actually studying mime with Lindsay Kemp by then," he told George Tremlett, "and he was so earthly that I learned from him that people are much more important to me than ideas."

Before long Kemp had cast David in his forthcoming mime production, a devised piece called *Pierrot In Turquoise*. The title was a combination of Kemp's previous work, *The Strange World Of Pierrot Flour*, and an idea from Bowie himself. "David suggested 'Turquoise' as it was the Buddhist symbol of everlastingness," recalled Kemp. "He was very into Buddhism at the time and he had these beautiful Tibetan boots, I

remember." Like the earlier pieces, *Pierrot In Turquoise* dealt with the eternal triangle between Pierrot (Kemp), Columbine (Stainer) and Harlequin (Birkett), the threat to Pierrot's romantic prospects. One of Kemp's new routines involved offering Columbine a flower which, when he was rejected, he exchanged for a hangman's rope, while in another he opened up his insides, threw away his heart and used his intestines as a skipping rope.

Kemp described David's role of Cloud as "a kind of protean narrator-figure" whose constant changes deceived and tricked the hapless hero. Plastered in clown-white and dressed in a pink-and-purple spotted blouse, knee-breeches and Elizabethan ruff, David cut a figure startlingly similar to the sad-faced clown he would play in the 'Ashes To Ashes' video thirteen years later.

During the show Bowie performed 'When I Live My Dream' and 'Sell Me A Coat', together with three specially written compositions, 'Threepenny Pierrot', 'Columbine' and 'The Mirror', all accompanied on piano by Michael Garrett. The overwrought programme notes reflected David's Buddhist leanings: "Resurrected on Tibet with the strange blue flying god in his mind, David Bowie sings. An echo of bronze gongs and music hall angel … music by David Bowie, nineteen years old climbing the turquoise ice Himalayas." (Amid the flower-power hyperbole, the reporting of David's age was becoming increasingly wide of the mark. He was already 20 at the time the *David Bowie* sleeve-notes had claimed he was 19, and he turned 21 during the run of *Pierrot In Turquoise*.)

The production opened on 28 December 1967 with a one-off performance at the Oxford Playhouse. *The Stage* commended Bowie as an "inventive composer" who "makes several striking appearances as Cloud, a multi-guised character", while the *Oxford Mail* said "David Bowie has composed some haunting songs, which he sings in a superb, dreamlike voice," but nonetheless found that the show itself "only hints at universal truths Marcel Marceau somehow manages to express." The *Financial Times* declared that "Mr Bowie is a young pop-singer whose songs tend to follow ambition beyond the boundaries of his talent."

From Oxford *Pierrot In Turquoise* moved north to Whitehaven's Rosehill Theatre from 3-5 January. The lavish little theatre was the creation of a wealthy silk manufacturer, Sir Nicholas Sekers, and was a port of call for many internationally renowned acts. "I was in heaven," Kemp tells the Gillmans. "I had sponsorship

that I had never had before. I had a new show opening. I was in love with an angel who loved me. I had
everything – or so I thought." In fact, as Kemp soon
discovered, David was having an affair with the costume designer Natasha Kornilof, who would return
many years later to design Bowie's 1978 stage outfits,
most memorably, his 'Ashes To Ashes' costume. As
Pierrot In Turquoise reached Whitehaven, the discovery
that the show harboured its own backstage love-trian-
gle resulted in a particularly melodramatic performance, on a day when both Kemp and Kornilof apparently staged half-hearted suicide attempts.

After two months' break *Pierrot In Turquoise* recon-
vened in London, first at the Mercury Theatre (5-16
March) and finally at the Intimate Theatre in Palmers
Green (26-30 March).

Reports that Bowie spent two years in a mime
troupe are greatly exaggerated: *Pierrot In Turquoise*
would later be reworked without David, but during
his involvement the show notched up no more than
21 performances. Nonetheless the impact on his creative imagination was tremendous. Kemp, he later
said, was "very fundamental in teaching me quite a bit
about stagecraft, how lighting worked, how you could
use your body on stage to make a dramatic statement.
I hopefully could do any of the shows that I have done
without any of the scenery or props that I've used,
because a lot of it was body-work."

"I was desperately keen on mime at the time," he
recalled in 1993. "I thought it was the greatest thing –
the way in which you could transform an open space
and create things by suggestion. But I got over it pretty quick. I decided that I'd have to incorporate it in
presenting music. I knew at the time that I wanted to
present music in a very theatrical fashion but I wasn't
sure exactly how … Eventually it all solidified itself
with Ziggy." On another occasion he described the
experience of *Pierrot In Turquoise* as "wonderful,
incredible. It's a great experience living with this sort
of rancid, Cocteau-ish theatre group in these bizarre
rooms that were decorated and hand-painted with
elaborate things. The whole thing was so excessively
French, with Left Bank existentialism, reading Genet
and listening to R&B. The perfect bohemian life."

Bowie's interest in mime resurfaced in his 1968
piece *Yet-San And The Eagle*, and again in his multimedia trio Feathers. 'The Mask', the short piece performed in 1969's *Love You Till Tuesday*, would form the
bedrock of many of his stage routines during the
1970s, and mime remains an element in his visual

repertoire. His working relationship with Lindsay
Kemp resumed briefly in 1970 with *The Looking Glass
Murders*, and again in 1972 when Kemp directed the
Ziggy Stardust shows at the Rainbow Theatre.

Another consequence of Bowie's association with
Lindsay Kemp, who once joked that David would
manage "three press-ups and he's off to the coffee bar
to chat up the birds," was his introduction to a Dance
Centre student called Hermione Farthingale (real
name Hermione Dennis). She would soon join him
on stage and, after a short but intense relationship,
leave an indelible mark on his songwriting.

THE PISTOL SHOT

• BBC Television, 20 May 1968 (repeated 24
December) • *Director:* John Gibson • *Writer:*
Nicholas Bethell • *Starring:* Ann Bell, Peter Jeffrey,
John Ronane, Ilona Rogers

On 30 January 1968, David and his new girlfriend
Hermione Farthingale filmed their appearance in *The
Pistol Shot*, a BBC2 drama based on the life of
Alexander Pushkin (not a Chekhov play, as Bowie
sources often claim). Both had been recruited from
Lindsay Kemp's classes at the Dance Centre. Wearing
satin breeches and a powdered wig, David's brief
appearance involved dancing a minuet with Hermione.

THE VIRGIN SOLDIERS

• GB, Columbia Pictures/Carl Foreman, 1969 •
Director: John Dexter • *Writer:* John Hopkins (*Novel:*
Leslie Thomas) • *Starring:* Hywel Bennett, Nigel
Patrick, Lynn Redgrave, Nigel Davenport, Rachel
Kempson

Less than a week after the recording of 'Ching-a-Ling'
in October 1968, David found work as a walk-on in
the film adaptation of Leslie Thomas's army memoir
set in Singapore. "I'm in it for about twenty seconds as
an extra," he recalled in 1983. "I don't know how it
developed into a thing I've done as an *actor*. I've never
seen *The Virgin Soldiers* either so I'm not sure if I'm
actually even in it still. I know that I was thrown over
a bar in it." More recently, he has begun denying he
was ever in the movie. "People are always saying, if
you look very closely you can see David Bowie," he
said in 1993. "But I was never actually in it. I didn't get
the part … got me hair cut off for nothing. I think I

kept the clothes. Nicked 'em. It was some consolation."

Quite how he could have nicked the clothes from a film he was never in is a mystery, but of course David is notorious for rewriting his past as the fancy takes him. What seems to have happened is that in July 1968 he had failed a screen test for a *speaking* part in the film, but Kenneth Pitt's persistence led to the offer of a walk-on role in the recreation hall scene. Pitt records that David's six days of shooting began on 29 October, when he received his short back and sides haircut. The extant photographs of Bowie in his smuggled-out costume were taken by Pitt at David's Clareville Grove house, and one of them appeared in the following year's edition of the actors' directory *Spotlight*. So yes, David Bowie does appear in *The Virgin Soldiers*, albeit for no more than the blink of an eye. A little over 35 minutes into the film, just after Hywel Bennett has said "I've had six Drambuies" and Roy Holder corrects the number to "Eight", a pie-eyed but instantly recognizable David is carried past in the background by the barman.

LUV

On 22 January 1969, a few days before shooting commenced on *Love You Till Tuesday* (see Chapter 5) and in the very same week that he wrote 'Space Oddity', Bowie appeared in a thirty-second television commercial for a Lyons Maid ice cream called *Luv*, directed by none other than Ridley Scott. The commercial featured David and several other young actors scampering up and down the stairs of a London bus as they mimed to the jingle: "Luv, luv luv / Let me give it all to you / Let me know that someday you'll do the same for me / Luv, luv, luv!"

Kenneth Pitt reports that David earned himself 25 guineas plus residuals and did his best to keep his costume as a souvenir, until a panicky telephone call from the production company put paid to that idea. In 1998 the BBC's *Before They Were Famous* dredged up a brief clip from this forgotten masterpiece.

THE LOOKING GLASS MURDERS
• Scottish Television, 8 July 1970 • *Director/Deviser:* Lindsay Kemp • *Starring:* Lindsay Kemp, David Bowie

In late January 1970, Bowie was in Aberdeen to record an appearance on Grampian TV and play a gig at the town's university. A few days earlier Lindsay Kemp, now based in his home town of Edinburgh, got wind of David's sojourn north of the border and contacted Kenneth Pitt to offer two days' work on a new television adaptation of *Pierrot In Turquoise*. David agreed to reprise his role as Cloud, and after rehearsals on 31 January the show, initially called *Another World* but retitled *The Looking Glass Murders* for transmission, was recorded at Edinburgh's Gateway Theatre on 1 February. It was a curious throwback for David who, by the time of the programme's transmission in July, had completed work on *The Man Who Sold The World*.

THE MAN WHO FELL TO EARTH
• GB, British Lion, 1976 • *Director:* Nicolas Roeg • *Writer:* Paul Mayersberg (*Novel:* Walter Tevis) • *Starring:* David Bowie, Rip Torn, Candy Clark, Buck Henry, Bernie Casey, Jackson D Kane

In January 1975 the avant-garde British film director Nicolas Roeg, whose previous credits included *Performance*, *Walkabout* and *Don't Look Now*, was preparing to shoot his adaptation of Walter Tevis's novel *The Man Who Fell To Earth*. Peter O'Toole had already turned down the lead role when Roeg, who believed in "odd omens", chanced to see the BBC screening of Alan Yentob's *Cracked Actor* on 26 January. Within minutes he had telephoned screenwriter Paul Mayersberg to tell him to switch on. "Watching that film," Roeg said years later, "he was my film's character, Mr Newton. My reaction was, 'That's him all right, all wrapped up and done.'"

Without further ado Roeg contacted Bowie, who was then in the process of extricating himself from Tony Defries in the aftermath of the *Young Americans* sessions. A meeting was arranged a fortnight hence at Bowie's New York apartment. "He arrived on time and I was out," David later recalled. "After eight hours or so, I remembered our appointment. I turned up nine hours late, thinking, of course, that he'd gone. He was sitting in the kitchen." Despite this inauspicious start, the meeting was a success: David accepted the role.

Shooting was postponed, however, when Columbia Pictures withdrew from the project. Roeg's avowedly uncommercial work had long been regarded with suspicion and even downright hostility in Hollywood, and he sought alternative backing from British Lion. Finding himself at liberty David moved in the meantime to Los Angeles, where he now approached the darkest days of his cocaine period. There was a brief, abortive attempt to record some new material with Iggy Pop in May (see 'Moving On' in chapter 1), but otherwise David's day-to-day life was a blur. "I was zonked out of my mind most of the time," he later admitted. "In Los Angeles I was surrounded by people who indulged my ego, who treated me as Ziggy Stardust or one of my other characters, never realizing that David Jones might be behind it." He maintained that his drug abuse was not recreational, but to stimulate him and keep him awake and working. "You can do good things with drugs, but then comes the long decline. I was skeletal. I was destroying my body."

Things improved a little in June, when the eleven-week shoot finally began in and around Albuquerque and Lake Fenton, New Mexico. Later in the year the *Station To Station* sessions would push David to his personal nadir, but for the meantime he successfully weaned himself off the worst excesses of substance abuse, and was encouraged to build up his emaciated frame on a diet of ice cream; his rapid fluctuations in weight would cause continuity problems for the film crew.

David, who spent up to five hours being made up for the sequences featuring his alien form, won universal praise from the crew for his patience and professionalism. Mayersberg recalled that he was "word perfect. I don't remember seeing a fluff. It was unnerving in some ways." When Bowie was called upon to catch a bottle knocked over by Candy Clark, who played his human girlfriend, Mayersberg noted that he "did that three or four times and every time he caught it in exactly the same way. Hard things to do – but he was absolutely immaculate."

"My one snapshot memory of that film is not having to act," Bowie said in 1993. "Just being me as I was was perfectly adequate for the role. I wasn't of this earth at that particular time." Of his co-star Candy Clark his memories were less than fond. "I didn't get along at all well with that girl Candy," he recalled. "She was so histrionic and she had one of those voices that could peel paint off the wall."

David had parted with his girlfriend Ava Cherry in Los Angeles, and was accompanied on the shoot by Coco Schwab, Tony Mascia and Geoffrey Mac-Cormack. Between shooting he explored the countryside, scanning the skies for UFOs and visiting the bat-infested Carlsberg Caverns where he declared he would like to stage a concert, "with thousands of vam-pire bats descending on the audience's heads." Most of his spare time, however, was spent in his trailer or at the ramshackle and snake-infested *pied-à-terre* found by Schwab, reading voraciously ("I took four hundred books down to that film shoot," he later recalled), painting in a makeshift studio, and working on a volume of short stories called *The Return Of The Thin White Duke* which he described as "partly auto-biographical, mostly fiction, with a deal of magic in it." His growing interest in the occult would later spill out on *Station To Station*, and in the meantime it began to dominate his public utterances. Of Nicolas Roeg he said, "He is an old warlock … something magical happens on every film that he does." Years later, and in better health, David spoke glowingly of his director. "It didn't take long for me to realise the man was a genius. He's at a level of understanding of art that tremendously overshadows me. I was, and still am, in awe of Roeg. Total awe."

Visually, *The Man Who Fell To Earth* is sublime. The barren, heat-hazed New Mexico locations are captured with a breathtaking sensitivity charged, like all of Roeg's pictures, with a sense of man's relationship with an isolating landscape. The story, which is slight but charged with implication, sees Thomas Jerome Newton (Bowie) arriving in Middle America and founding a prosperous business empire by establishing patents on several remarkable inventions. In reality he is a visitor from a drought-stricken planet, the inventions are based on alien technology, and his plan is to fund a space programme that will return him home in time to save his family. In the original novel Newton's mission is explicitly to find water to rescue his dying world, but Roeg consciously downplays this strand, preferring to foreground the character's defeat at our hands, his loss of identity and the frustration of his hopes. He is corrupted by human weaknesses – alcohol, television and an inadequate affair – and is at last kidnapped by a mysterious government department, experimented upon, unwittingly blinded, and released a broken man. The final scene sees Newton a ruined, alcoholic recluse, wondering whether his wife will ever hear the song he has recorded as a message to her (radio waves, travelling through space, may eventually reach his doomed planet; he has no other way left to contact her).

The film is oblique and relentlessly parablaic, saturated by suggestive images of Bowie as Howard Hughes, Icarus, Adam, and Christ, the quintessential man who fell to Earth; Newton suffers a Judas-like betrayal at the hands of Rip Torn's character. His fall is both the Fall of Man, and a surrender to the forces of gravity whose laws were discovered by his namesake. Closer to home are the tantalizing links with Bowie's own experiences of American assimilation: Roeg would later explain that he had been eager to cast "someone who was inside society but awkward in it," while Bowie admitted that "the character in the original book had strong resemblances to the kind of isolationist characters that I'd been producing, so it was a fairly accurate piece of casting." The famous sequence of Newton slumped before a bank of chattering television screens, indiscriminately absorbing the Babel of modern America, resonates with Bowie's own cultural osmosis: like Newton, in 1975 he was displaced from his home and apparently weakened, diluted and corrupted by an alien environment. He later admitted to "being Newton for six months" after finishing work on the film, while Roeg recalled that "During the making of the film David got more than into the character of Mr Newton … towards the end I realized a big change had happened in his life." Bowie added that "The thing I objectively remember taking with me was the wardrobe. I literally walked off with the clothes, and I used the same clothes on the Station To Station tour." He also retained Newton's slicked-back, blond-streaked red hair, a style which became synonymous with the Thin White Duke.

Of the film itself David once said that "I didn't enjoy it as a movie to watch. It's very tight. Like a spring that's going to uncoil, it's got these terrific tensions … these very inhibited feelings in it." On another occasion he added that "Nic does revolting stuff that creates such challenging vignettes! Nic's love scenes must be some of the most perverse ever filmed. There's a quality to them that is so cruel. There's something about Nic's films which is awfully worrying but I think the magnetism of his movies is the wariness and worry they create." Roeg himself was characteristically oblique about the film: "There is a lot of drinking. It's all about drinking, actually. It is a love story and it is a science fiction movie and it is about drinking. One of the great lines in it is 'Why not?' It is about people who say, 'Have a drink,' and people who reply, 'Why not?'" This isn't quite as obtuse as it might seem; part of the film's enduring power is its anxiety about the ease with which we succumb to failure and forgetfulness. "I wanted it to have a very real sense of America, although it is certainly not about any one place," continued Roeg. "It's just a look at the human

condition which could be anywhere. It is a science fiction film without the hardware. We haven't got a dial in it. No dials! There are certain sci-fi-type shots in it, but not done with a great deal of final expertise because the actuality doesn't matter. Audiences are sophisticated today. They've seen the most perfect model shots after 2001. We paid attention to another kind of detail."

The Man Who Fell To Earth received its British premiere in Leicester Square on 18 March 1976. Ironically, while most of the American cast were present, the British star was on tour in the States; Angela, now all but estranged, represented him at the screening. In Europe the film was released as Roeg had intended, but in America the print was heavily edited by the distributor. "I was floored when it came out over here," David told an American interviewer a few years later, "and twenty minutes cut out of it – hacked out of it. It brought the thing to its knees; a bad thing to do to Nic's movie."

Reviews were cautiously polite, usually singling out Bowie as the film's strongest card. "Pallid and gaunt and required to give a low-key performance, David Bowie makes a convincing alien life form whose loneliness is beyond human experience," said Screen International, adding that "the inherent pathos of the character gives heart and soul to the technical wizardry." The Guardian observed that the "story spreads itself into the realms of political and moral allegory, and much else besides since it is also a romance as much about the mystery of love as of the universe." The Financial Times claimed there were "enough ideas for six films", noting that "with his enamelled, bony features and his soft feminine voice, Bowie is ingeniously right as the alien, a still centre around which the more flamboyant supporting performances and Roeg's own pyrotechnic direction can whirl and spark to often thrilling effect."

Not all the critics were convinced, however: "Once you have pierced through its glittering veneer, you find only another glittering veneer underneath", wrote Michael Billington in the Illustrated London News. The Daily Express found "more holes than a string vest", while the Daily Telegraph complained of "a succession of often stunning pictures, rather precariously related to rock music, or by overrunning dialogue, but in themselves contributing more to our mystification than understanding" (not unlike the syntax favoured by Daily Telegraph critics, then). "There is a punch line, but it takes forever, and great expectations slump away," said Charles Champlin of the *LA News*. In the *Times*, David Robinson was even less charitable: "You feel finally that all that has been achieved has been to impose an aura of mystery and enigma where essentially there is none". The *Spectator* was more succinct: "one of the best bad movies I have ever seen."

The Man Who Fell To Earth has aged well and confounded those who considered it merely fashionable. It is a long film and in many ways a difficult one, perhaps increasingly so as our attention-spans are chipped away by today's diet of stultifying blockbusters. But it handsomely repays the courtesy of a committed viewing, and remains Bowie's most significant work as a film actor.

JUST A GIGOLO

• West Germany, Leguan, 1979 • *Director:* David Hemmings • *Writers:* Ennio de Concini, Joshua Sinclair • *Starring:* David Bowie, Sydne Rome, Kim Novak, Marlene Dietrich, David Hemmings, Maria Schell, Curt Jurgens

Following his round of interviews and television appearances to promote *"Heroes"* in the autumn of 1977, Bowie spent some time in Japan and Thailand before returning to Switzerland for Christmas. There he was visited by David Hemmings, the actor-turned-director best known for his role in Antonioni's 1966 pop-art classic *Blow Up*. Hemmings wanted Bowie to appear in his forthcoming movie *Gigolo*, already being touted as the biggest and most expensive German film since the end of the War, with a budget of DM 12 million.

David was initially no more enthusiastic about the project than about any of the numerous scripts he was being sent (at the time he was said to be considering a film of *The Threepenny Opera* and another on the life of Egon Schiele). However, he was intrigued by the idea of working with Hemmings, whom he described as "a real actor's director", and the idea of a movie set in pre-Holocaust Berlin appealed to his long-standing interest in Christopher Isherwood's city. The deciding factor was that the film's German producer, Rolf Thiele, had persuaded Marlene Dietrich to come out of her 17-year retirement to appear in the picture. Bowie was entranced by the idea of co-starring with such an icon ("Marlene Dietrich was dangled in front of me," he later admitted), and signed up.

Just A Gigolo, as it was now called, began shooting

in Berlin in January 1978. Bowie was playing the central character Paul, a young Prussian who returns from the Great War to find his world changed forever. Lofty aspirations are dashed by intrigue and embroilment in the Berlin underworld, and he becomes a gigolo in the employ of Baroness von Semering (Dietrich). Finally he is killed by a stray bullet in a street brawl between Nazis and Communists, who squabble over his body until the Nazis finally carry him off and bury him, a hero to a cause he did not support.

"I've tackled a subject I'm fascinated with," said Bowie at the time. "That of gigolos, male escorts and male hookers for women. I've known various individuals in those professions, yet I've found they're rather inscrutable and difficult to get to know – therefore, the role was that much more of a challenge." He added: "It also allows me to display a more sensual, sexual side of myself that was totally lacking in *The Man Who Fell To Earth*, where I didn't even have any genitals."

"David has a very special quality," said Hemmings later. "The camera adores him. You can't shoot him and lessen his attractiveness. The nature of the character he played demanded that I shy away from this. We took him into the worst shop in order to find the filthiest clothes and the real down-and-out look that was necessary for the character, and everything that David put on, it looked as if he'd just created a new fashion. It was absolutely extraordinary, and very funny … If I put on heavy wellies and old cords and a sweater and a cloth cap, I'd look like a gardener. David looked like he'd just been asked by *Vogue* to do a cover."

Although Bowie would later recall such enjoyable experiences as dancing the samba with his co-star Kim Novak, the shoot was not without its tensions. The film crew was recruited from both England and Germany, leading to interminable language and union problems. There were frictions among the cast. The biggest question mark of all hung over Marlene Dietrich's involvement. Although she had agreed to appear she now refused to leave her Paris apartment, where she was apparently busy writing her memoirs. With the exception of Rolf Thiele, nobody – not even Hemmings – had even met her. Hemmings was eventually compelled to reschedule his shoot and move one of the sets to Paris to accommodate Miss Dietrich, by which time Bowie had shot all of his scenes and departed for a Kenyan holiday with his son, and thence to rehearsals for the Stage tour. He never met Dietrich, although shots were spliced together to imply otherwise.

Admirably loyal to the production, Bowie suggested to reporters at the time that Dietrich's isolation had its good side. "I think it's quite nice in the context of the film, because she's forever the observer, really," he claimed manfully in 1979, "and knowing that, it makes her even more of the observer – mystical, wonderful Cocteau character that she is." In reality, however, his disappointment at not meeting Marlene Dietrich was compounded by bitter disappointment with the finished movie. "The film was a cack, a real cack," he told the NME's Angus McKinnon two years later. "Everybody who was involved in that film, when they meet each other now, they look away! Yes, it was one of those. Well, we've all got to do one and hopefully I've done mine now … the first year or so after I'd made the thing I was furious, mainly with myself. I mean, oh God, I really should have known better. Every real, legitimate actor that I've ever met has told me never to even approach a film unless you know the script is good." In the same interview, he famously dubbed Just A Gigolo "my 32 Elvis Presley movies contained in one."

The press was in complete agreement. Hemmings insisted that the film was intended as a black comedy, "lightly ironic, tongue in cheek", which concerned itself with "exploding the myth of Germanic organization"; but critics attending the Cannes Festival preview set it up as a new Cabaret and then slated it for failing to meet their expectations. It was turned down by every major British distributor before finding a home with the inexperienced independent Tedderwick. Hemmings began re-editing the picture to suit his new distributors, but finance ran out. "I walked off the picture three-quarters of the way through the process," he later said. "Someone else finished the cut and butchered it. The music by Manhattan Transfer was cut to ribbons. Women in the film who gossiped all the way through the picture to provide a narrative sense were cut out for the most part. In all, twenty minutes of the film was removed, including all the humour and irony." In this form the movie was premiered to a hostile reaction in Berlin on 16 November, while Bowie was absent on the Australian leg of the Stage tour. Hemmings successfully negotiated the right to re-edit Just A Gigolo yet again in time for its UK release. The long-awaited British premiere was at the Prince Charles Cinema in Leicester Square on 14 February 1979, where David arrived on the arm of actress Viv Lynn. Both wore kimonos and wooden clogs; one wag suggested that they should have worn suits of armour.

The Financial Times said that the cast "fall like ninepins before the hamhanded staging and the choppy, frenetic, try-anything editing", while the Sunday Mirror considered the film "all show and no substance", adding that Bowie was "completely miscast". Much of the vitriol was reserved for David in particular. The Daily Telegraph led the assault: "The dramatic ability Bowie possesses is less enshrined as a living fact, than embalmed as a dead talent. Bowie's anaesthetized features worked well enough in his first film, The Man Who Fell To Earth. But then he played a man from outer space. Now he's supposed to be one of us; an occasional inflection of face or voice would have helped the illusion." According to the Morning Star, Bowie "exudes about as much warmth as a fridge", while the NME said that his "dramatic ambitions obviously far outweigh his abilities. Bowie might look the part as a foppish Prussian gentleman turned gigolo traipsing through 1920s Berlin, but he can't play it. An illusion is burnt to a crisp every time he opens his mouth or tries to convey any depth or detail of character. Bowie's efforts throughout are comically inept."

There were a few kinder notices; Variety claimed that the film "delivers a lot of bitter-sweet entertainment and is never less than engrossing," while "Bowie goes through his tumbleweed paces with engaging appeal". Films & Filming commended "an original and often deeply moving movie" in which David's "essentially filmic features are convincingly Aryan and his little-boy-lost air admirably conveys Paul's naïveté and inborn idealism." But the general response was summed up by Time Out: "It often goes for laughs it hasn't a hope of getting; sometimes it aspires to tragic dignity and looks truly inept. It would be kinder to yourself and to everybody involved to overlook it."

Just A Gigolo spawned one of the more obscure Bowie recordings, 'Revolutionary Song', which appeared on the soundtrack album and was released as a single in Japan.

It was, incidentally, during the shooting of Just A Gigolo that David filed for divorce, following Angela's explosive conduct over Christmas 1977 that had culminated in her much-publicized (mainly by herself) suicide attempt on Bowie's thirty-first birthday. January 1978 saw the first of Angela's many kiss-and-tell exposés to the tabloid press, in this case the Sunday Mirror.

THE ELEPHANT MAN

- 29 July 1980 – 3 January 1981 • Centre of Performing Arts, Denver • Blackstone Theater, Chicago • Booth Theater, New York • *Director:* Jack Hofsiss • *Writer:* Bernard Pomerance • *Starring:* David Bowie, Donal Donnelly, Patricia Elliott, Richard Clarke, Jeffrey Jones, Judith Barcroft, Dennis Creaghan

In December 1979, while in New York to record his appearance on *Saturday Night Live*, Bowie saw the Broadway production of Bernard Pomerance's play *The Elephant Man*. The show had first been produced in 1977 at London's Hampstead Theatre where, despite being a flop, it had attracted the attention of the American producer Richard Crinkley, who subsequently opened it in New York to great acclaim. By the time Bowie saw the play it was already a major success, having collected a clutch of awards for its author, director and cast.

The Elephant Man was, of course, based on the true story of Joseph "John" Merrick, the pitifully deformed man who was rescued from a circus sideshow in 1884 by the surgeon Frederick Treves, and went on to become the toast of fashionable society and a touchstone for the conscience of Victorian England. Pre-dating David Lynch's famous 1981 film, the play was at best a loose adaptation of Merrick's life and its popular success owed much to the fine line it trod between moral symbolism and sentimentality; at one point Merrick exclaims "Sometimes I think my head is so big because it is so full of dreams," while another character observes of the Elephant Man that "We polish him so that he may better reflect ourselves." When Bowie saw the play, Merrick was being played by the British actor Philip Anglim who, in accordance with the script directions, portrayed the character without recourse to prosthetic make-up or visual trickery of any kind, instead conveying Merrick's condition by the expressive distortion of his speech and semi-naked body. When Merrick was first revealed in a spotlight during a lecture by Treves, the actor was required to crumple his body in a series of moves as each successive deformity was described, and thereafter retain the same physicality for the duration of the play. Bowie later remarked that he "liked it as a piece of writing, and for myself I thought I would have loved to have the part if it had ever been offered to me – but it hadn't been, and that was the last I thought about it."

In February 1980, while Bowie was recording *Scary Monsters* at New York's Power Station, he was approached by the play's 29-year-old director Jack Hofsiss, who was preparing to recast the Broadway production while the original company went on tour. "He'd seen the play and we talked about it," recalled Hofsiss later. "His perceptions were right on the money. I began to think about David Bowie filling the role when Philip Anglim went into the road company. I wanted someone who would generate more interest in the play. I also wanted someone I'd find interesting. I saw *The Man Who Fell To Earth* and I knew of his stage presence, his sense of theatre in rock. He saw the larger elements of rock songs. The isolation he experienced in *The Man Who Fell To Earth* was similar to *The Elephant Man*."

Hofsiss, however, made no immediate offer. While Anglim went on the road with *The Elephant Man* and other actors took over on Broadway, Bowie returned to London to complete work on his album, visiting Iggy Pop in Berlin in April and shooting the 'Ashes To Ashes' video in May. The following month David was back in New York, where Hofsiss now approached him with an offer to take over the role of Merrick, apparently giving David only 24 hours to make up his mind. "I think that Hofsiss knew that if I'd had time to think about it I would have dropped out," said David later. "He was very clever psychologically in forcing me to face an issue like that."

With only a day to consider the offer of a six-month contract (including a month's rehearsal and no get-out clause), David readily accepted. The role, of course, was right up his street. "I always look for parts with an emotional or physical limp," he said, "And I always seem to get them. I kind of like characters with some kind of impediment. It's just an interesting thing to play around with, and I've never gone overboard with the idea of myself as any kind of romantic lead." He took his new role seriously, flying back to Britain to examine Merrick's skeleton, together with the other relics still kept at the London Hospital: photographs, body casts, clothing, and the paper model of a church constructed by Merrick. P G Nunn, the assistant curator of the hospital museum, later recalled that "David asked pertinent questions. He wanted to know how Merrick walked, how he spoke. I told him he could not have run, because he had no hips. And there was a great distortion of the mouth, because the tongue was thick and pushed to one side." Medical opinions still differ about the precise nature of the condition (or combination of conditions) suffered by

Merrick, but the usual diagnoses are neurofibromatosis and the so-called Proteus Syndrome, both incurable conditions which progressively distort bone and tissue.

"I felt the clue to playing the role successfully was to avoid pathos," said Hofsiss. "David felt Merrick's street savvy would have kept him from buying into hospital sympathy. Up to that time, replacement actors had done variations on the original actor's interpretations … David came up with an original view." Hofsiss asked Bowie to replace Philip Anglim on the provincial tour, allowing him to break in the role over a week in Denver and a further month in Chicago, before going on to open in the full critical glare of Broadway. No free tickets were released for the Denver shows and the national press was actively discouraged from attending. As the show's Broadway press agent Josh Ellis explained, "I don't think it's fair to put any scrutiny on David without giving him a chance to work his way into the role. If he's marvellous in Denver, he'll be marvellous in Chicago. And if he's not, well, why should we risk exposing him?"

After a fortnight's rehearsals in New York Bowie flew to San Francisco to watch Anglim's final performance, and then joined the road company for further rehearsals in Denver. Concetta Tomei, who played Mrs Kendal in the touring cast, told *Rolling Stone*: "Bowie has the technique of magnetising people, and that is something you just can't learn in a school or out of books. The guy is an actor and you can't really water it down. He's not a rock performer going into acting, he's an actor." By all accounts Bowie's commitment and conduct in rehearsal was meticulous; on the one occasion he was late he apologized individually to each member of the company.

"In order to play the role, you have to master the physical life and the vocal life of the character very quickly," said Hofsiss. "It has to become second nature to you." Bowie had resumed his mime training in preparation, and Hofsiss engaged a chiropractor to teach David a series of exercises essential to assuming Merrick's physicality: "I had to use the pre-imposed exercises before and after performances to get myself into and out of it," Bowie explained. "One's spine can be damaged very badly. I had one night of excruciating pain when I didn't do the exercises."

Bowie's opening night in *The Elephant Man*, on 29 July at the Denver Centre for Performing Arts, attracted instant praise from the local press. "When he pounded his hands on the bathtub and repeated phrases over and over, he brought magic and music to

the play's language," reported *Trouser Press*. "And, after a powerful final scene, when he came out for bows nattily attired in cravat and formal suit and shirt, graciously holding hands with the rest of the cast, he seemed the perfect incarnation of a stage matinee idol. The Denver audience may not have known it, but they were applauding one of the most courageous and broadening moves yet taken by a rock star." *Variety* was equally impressed: "Drawing on an early mime background and the resourceful staging of his rock shows, Bowie displays the ability to project a complex character … In scene after scene he builds poignantly, crying for the chance to become civilized, though he knows he will always be a freak; pleading for a home, though he knows his presence disturbs; and questioning the rules of society, though his well-being depends on their acceptance. Judging from his sensitive projection of this part, Bowie has the chance to achieve legit stardom."

During the opening week in Denver, Bowie's new single 'Ashes To Ashes' was released to widespread acclaim, and with a double whammy of critical approval under his belt the subsequent four weeks at Chicago's Blackstone Theater saw him courting publicity more readily; it was here that he gave a renowned and lengthy interview to Angus MacKinnon of the *NME*. By the time *The Elephant Man* reached Broadway's Booth Theater, expectations were high and there was, as Jack Hofsiss recalled, "an intense curiosity about whether David could pull it off."

On Broadway Bowie was performing with an entirely new cast, necessitating further rehearsals. At the same time he was promoting *Scary Monsters (And Super Creeps)*, even rushing from rehearsals to perform 'Ashes To Ashes' and 'Life On Mars?' on Johnny Carson's *The Tonight Show* on 5 September, where he also discussed the play and Merrick's illness. The opening night on 23 September was a major event, attended by Andy Warhol, David Hockney, Christopher Isherwood, Oona Chaplin, Elizabeth Taylor, Brian Eno, Aaron Copland and William Burroughs. Bowie's mother, and his ever-loyal early manager Kenneth Pitt, both flew in from London. "David was stunningly good," Pitt later said. "It was particularly gratifying for me, because so much of it seemed to flow from his mime training around the time of *Love You Till Tuesday*." Bowie's Montreux neighbour Oona Chaplin was similarly impressed, judging David "breathtakingly good at expressing physical agony."

The notices were ecstatic. "Bowie Blazing on Broadway!" trumpeted the *New York Post*, who described his performance as "simply electrifying". The city's press fell over themselves to praise the show and its new star. "When it was announced that David Bowie would play the title role in *The Elephant Man*, it was not unnatural to think he had been cast simply for the use of his name," began the *New York Times*. "Dismiss the thought now. Yes, more young people in designer jeans and leather now show up at the Booth Theater than before, and yes, they probably show up because Mr Bowie is a celebrated rock star. Fortunately, he is a good deal more than that, and as John Merrick, the Elephant Man, he is splendid." *Theater* magazine said that Bowie had "the exquisite stillness that the best actors have … the physical precision of his acting is really something to see." New York's *Daily News* praised Bowie's "piercing and haunted" portrayal of "restrained, tortured eloquence" and commended his ability to judge "the difference between having an act and acting". *Back Stage* magazine said he "acquitted himself magnificently." The *Village Voice* found Bowie "breathing new life into *The Elephant Man*", his interpretation "not so vulnerable as Philip Anglim and less ironic (he lacks Anglim's boyish beauty), but his portrait is more precise, more colourful, and much funnier." There was a lone voice of dissent: John Simon of *New York* magazine claimed that David's "reedy voice, when distorted as the part demands, becomes a falsetto sawing that slices intelligibility in half, and his androgynously pretty face and street-wise punk-rock sexiness finish off what pathos his acting left intact". But the few doubters were submerged by the avalanche of praise for a performance described by the *Times* as "one of the events of New York's theatrical season."

The Broadway show's weekly box office take rose from a September low of $61,000 to a record $119,000 for David's third week in the role. Even in Britain the interest was high, and on 10 October the BBC's *Friday Night And Saturday Morning* featured excerpts from the play and an interview with David conducted by Tim Rice.

As the Broadway run progressed David found time to pursue other projects in his daytime hours, shooting his appearance in *Christiane F.* and the video for 'Fashion' in quick succession in early October. Staying at the Carlyle Hotel, he frequented Japanese restaurants and happily told interviewers that he enjoyed the anonymity of the New York lifestyle. "The most you get is 'Hi Dave, how's it going?', it's a very neighbourly characteristic," he told a reporter for the *Times*. "They don't get as excited at meeting you as in London, which is still a bit star-conscious. Here you see Al Pacino walking around or Joel Grey jogging. It's quite easy to do that. It's great."

However, two weeks after this interview was published, New York was the scene of rock music's darkest day. On 8 December 1980 John Lennon was shot dead by an obsessive fan outside his apartment, and for David as for many others, things would never be quite the same again. Over the next few days it was reported that Mick Jagger, Rod Stewart, Paul McCartney and many others were tightening their personal security and withdrawing from the public glare. In New York, Bowie reportedly panicked when he first heard the news but held firm to his stage commitments. Jack Hofsiss later recalled: "The day after John was shot, I offered to re-stage the show so that David could leave the stage periodically when he wasn't needed, to keep his time on stage at a minimum. He absolutely refused. We increased the security at the theatre, but he made no demands." It later emerged that Lennon's killer Mark Chapman had seen *The Elephant Man* and had even photographed Bowie at the stage door; among the items found in his hotel room was a programme in which David's name had been circled in black. Chapman later bragged to a girlfriend that he could have shot either star. It would be prurient to speculate on Bowie's feelings in the aftermath of the tragedy, but two things are known to be true: he elected not to renew his contract for *The Elephant Man*, which expired with the final performance on 3 January (the cast presented him with the play's backcloth as a souvenir); and, connection or no, he cancelled plans for a 1981 tour to promote *Scary Monsters*. Instead he withdrew to his home in Switzerland and began the most concertedly reclusive year of his career so far.

Over 20 years later, in March 2002, *The Elephant Man* returned to Broadway in a new production directed by Sean Mathias. Billy Crudup played Merrick opposite Rupert Graves as Treves, with incidental music provided by Bowie's sometime collaborator Philip Glass. In June 2002 Bowie revealed that he had been offered the role of Treves.

CRYSTAL JUN ROCK

See 'Crystal Japan' in Chapter 1.

CHRISTIANE F. WIR KINDER VOM BAHNHOF ZOO

• West Germany, Maran Film/Popular Film/Hans H. Kaden/TCF, 1981 • *Director:* Ulrich Edel • *Writer:* Hermann Weigel • *Starring:* Natja Brunckhorst, Thomas Haustein, Jens Kuphal, Rainer Wölk, Jan Georg Effler, Christiane Reichelt, Daniela Jaeger, Kerstin Richter, David Bowie

This bleak German picture about a teenage girl's descent into drug addiction and prostitution was sold to audiences as a true-life biopic, although it was later exposed as a plausible fiction. It features a soundtrack of Bowie's late 1970s music, and David appears in the biggest set piece, a heroin-trip scene supposedly set at one of his concerts but in reality filmed at New York's Hurrah club in October 1980. In a red jacket and black jeans similar to those he had worn on *The Tonight Show With Johnny Carson* a month previously, David lip-synched to the *Stage* version of 'Station to Station' on the redressed Berlin nightclub set; as he was appearing nightly on Broadway at the time, director Ulrich Edel had no option but to shoot the sequence in New York. The same set was then used for the shooting of David's 'Fashion' video.

BAAL

• BBC Television, 2 February 1982 • *Director:* Alan Clarke • *Writer:* Bertolt Brecht (*Translation:* John Willett; *TV Adaptation:* John Willett, Alan Clarke) • *Starring:* David Bowie, Jonathan Kent, Juliet Hammond-Hill, Zoe Wanamaker, Tracey Childs, Robert Austin, Russell Wootton, Julian Wadham, Paola Dionisotti, Polly James, Leon Lissek

Shortly after recording 'Under Pressure' with Queen in July 1981, Bowie travelled to London to play the title role in the BBC's production of Bertolt Brecht's *Baal*, whose producer Louis Marks had flown to Montreux with director Alan Clarke to woo him for the role. Bowie was impressed by Clarke's previous work and was in any case immediately attracted to the project. *Baal* was Brecht's earliest play, written in 1918 as a student diatribe against Hanns Johst's expressionist piece *The Lonely One*. Satirising Johst's tale of an unacknowledged artist who redeems his dissolute lifestyle and dies at peace with God and the world, Brecht created in Baal a monster of sensuality and self-gratification, a ribald, drunken strolling player named after a

bestial pagan deity. Despite his repulsive appearance and egocentric amorality Baal is irresistible to women, which makes him envied, admired and despised by men. He seduces every girl who comes his way before abandoning them to pregnancy or suicide, and finally murders his best friend, goes on the run, and dies alone in a woodcutter's cottage. Throughout the action Baal's character and aspirations are established by 'Baal's Hymn', which traces his progress from his mother's womb to the cold womb of the earth. The lingering motif is Baal's perception of the sky above him, an expressionist metaphor for his shifting moods and experiences. It is large and pale at his birth, lilac for his drunken nights, apricot for his repentant mornings, and a rainbow of other colours throughout the play, but ever-present, a canopy of infinity encompassing transient human life.

By comparison with Brecht's later work *Baal* is at best an unbalanced experiment, a despairing portrayal of chauvinism and excess in the years leading up to the Great War; Brecht would later admit that he considered the play lacking in wisdom. It is by no means as accomplished or as popular as the playwright's greatest work, and when it is performed at all, the revised 1922 version is usually the preferred text. Louis Marks and Alan Clarke went back to basics, using an adaptation of the 1918 original.

The death of John Lennon was still a recent memory and Bowie had hitherto spent a reclusive 1981 in Switzerland. "He wanted a car and a bodyguard," recalled Marks later. "He wanted to be assured of his privacy and security. Of course, we provided him with what he needed. Otherwise, I might add, he was given no more than any other actor. He worked for the standard BBC fee."

Rehearsals lasted a month, and recording for the studio-bound production took place at Television Centre over five days in the hot August of 1981. Bowie's co-stars included Jonathan Kent as Baal's doomed friend Eckart, Zoe Wanamaker as the lover he abandons pregnant by the roadside, and *Secret Army* star Juliet Hammond-Hill as his upper-class mistress. "He was an actor in the company of actors," said Marks. "He was there on time. He worked the full period required. There were no problems. He was utterly exhausted when we finished. The studio was typically overheated and Alan was a perfectionist, so there were at least five or six takes for every scene. The last of the five shooting days we recorded the songs and halfway through the morning, someone in the basement of the BBC started up a pneumatic drill. We lost the entire morning. We started over in the afternoon. David was wearing these tight-fitting boots and he was drenched in sweat at the end of the day, but never a word of complaint." As Baal, Bowie was given the most convincingly unflattering makeover of his professional career, a vision in ragged clothes, unkempt beard and rotten teeth.

During the play Bowie performs five songs in all, accompanying himself on the banjo. *Baal* was written before Brecht's famous partnership with Kurt Weill, and all but one of the songs were set to new arrangements by Dominic Muldowney (the exception was 'The Drowned Girl', which used Weill's setting from *The Berlin Requiem*). Bowie, who described Baal himself as "super-punk", likened the numbers to medieval plainsong. After shooting finished, David relocated to Hansa Studios in September and re-recorded the *Baal* numbers with Muldowney and Tony Visconti, eliminating the dialogue interjections in 'The Dirty Song' and 'The Ballad Of The Adventurers', and knitting the episodic 'Baal's Hymn' into one long number. The fruits of these sessions, markedly different from the televised versions of the songs, were released by RCA in February 1982 to coincide with the play's transmission.

"Baal is someone who lives his life to the full," Louis Marks told the *Radio Times*. "He's rather like a rock star of today. We realised that we needed someone who was a star in his own right, someone to mirror the person himself. Bowie was ideal … He's a natural for the part. For one thing, he certainly knows his Brecht. He's very well read and particularly interested in pre-First World War German drama and art. Working with him, it was apparent that he did have an instinctive understanding of the character."

Baal is an uncompromising production, made at a time when television drama was allowed to appeal to the intellect as well as to the senses, and it's a Brecht production first and a star vehicle second. Certainly it's a curious piece of television whose stylistic decisions make for occasionally indigestible viewing, but the conviction of its execution together with the deeply thoughtful playing invest the whole with an authority rarely seen on today's small screen. The camerawork and blocking are genuinely Brechtian, distancing and alienating the viewer by keeping nearly every scene in long-shot with an absolute minimum of close-ups. The lighting is wilfully theatrical (at one point a character opens a curtain and the studio lights bounce up, quite deliberately, a full second

later) and the episodic progression of scenes is framed by carefully stilted captions such as "Two years later Baal discovers a (to him) new kind of love", and "In the years 1907-1910 we find Baal and Eckart tramping across South Germany". These appear on the right-hand side of a split screen, while on the left Bowie introduces each vignette with another verse of 'Baal's Hymn'. True to Brecht, the production concerns itself not with spectacle and certainly not with naturalism, but with its own self-conscious theatricality. The scenes of Baal and Eckart "tramping across South Germany", for example, are achieved on an entirely blank set on which Bowie and Jonathan Kent perform their dialogue while repeatedly walking towards the camera, cutting back to the start of an identical shot each time they reach it. Bowie's performance, too, is authentically Brechtian; some reviewers chose to dismiss his curious vibrato delivery as straightforward bad acting, but the mannered chant in which he delivers his lines is firmly in the tradition of the distanced, dispassionate recordings of Lotte Lenya and of Brecht himself. *Baal* addresses the artist's conflicting impulses of detached observation and intense sensory experience, or what translator John Willett referred to as the desire "to live his own writing and write his own living". Baal is not a realistic "character". He is an aggregation of poetry and symbols, and Bowie plays him accordingly.

None of this, of course, made *Baal* particularly easy viewing, and matters weren't helped by the BBC's quixotic decision to schedule the play on 2 March 1982 opposite Thames Television's justly garlanded production of John Mortimer's *A Voyage Round My Father*, starring Laurence Olivier. "It seems daft to say we had a contest between Lord Olivier, our greatest living actor, and David Bowie, professional weirdo, rock idol and actor on TV last night," declared Hilary Kingsley in the *Daily Mirror*, who went on to dub *Baal* "…a total flop. I cannot believe even the most besotted of David Bowie's fans could have tolerated more than a few moments of it. The hero, a tramp-poet haunting German high society in 1912, was rotten in every sense – a drunk, a slob, a know-all, a seducer, a murderer, who apparently decomposed before our eyes. That the BBC could spend a small fortune on this repulsive and rightly ignored tableau is a cause for top level concern." The repulsed Ms Kingsley wasn't alone in drawing unfavourable parallels between the two TV plays on offer that night: "only those observing strict, medieval, Lenten penitential rites would have denied themselves the pleasure of watching Laurence Olivier as Mortimer senior to boggle at this baleful piece of Brecht," said the *Times*, noting nevertheless that Bowie "did as good a job as possible of playing this amoral, anti-social poet". Other reviewers agreed in praising Bowie but damning the production. "*David Bowie in Baal* the BBC calls it," said the *Sunday Times* incorrectly, "as if the actor were more interesting than the play, and for once Aunty's right." The *Daily Telegraph* considered it "perverse" to cast Bowie "then subdue him in an emotionless production", while the *Daily Express* opined that "The grim Bertolt Brecht play with music is hardly the best vehicle to project the spectacular Bowie style and Mr Bowie's acting talents are swamped in the general angst." *Melody Maker* found "none of the dramatic dominance which made *The Elephant Man* so memorable". The *Sun* caught the general mood when it said that Bowie "confirmed that he is a creditable actor. But what an unspeakable play in which to prove it!"

Baal was never repeated, although it received a screening 20 years later during a retrospective of Alan Clarke's work at the National Film Theatre in March 2002. Ultimately the production is less than satisfying, but it remains one of the key roles in Bowie's acting career and one of which he can be justly proud. His slack-jawed, cynical screen presence and virtuoso death scene (scrabbling across the floor in deafening silence for one last glimpse of the sky) are deserving of real praise.

THE HUNGER

• US, MGM/UA, 1983 • *Director:* Tony Scott • *Writers:* Ivan Davis, Michael Thomas (*Novel:* Whitley Strieber) • *Starring:* Catherine Deneuve, Susan Sarandon, David Bowie, Cliff de Young

After completing work on the *Baal* EP and shooting videos for 'The Drowned Girl' and 'Wild Is The Wind', Bowie took a prolonged holiday. He began 1982 by accepting another acting role, this time for the British director Tony Scott, whose brother Ridley had made his name a couple of years earlier with *Alien* and was now consolidating his success by putting the finishing touches to his sci-fi epic *Blade Runner*. By contrast, *The Hunger* was to be Tony Scott's first feature film, following a string of highly praised television commercials. He later recalled his own nervousness, and said that Bowie "tried to put me at ease right away and was

very friendly".

The Hunger was based on a story by the Texan horror novelist Whitley Strieber, and by comparison with *The Elephant Man* or *Baal* it was distinctly lowbrow stuff. Bowie plays John Blaylock, an eighteenth-century vampire still alive in present-day New York, where he haunts Manhattan's discotheques with his 6000-year-old lover Miriam, played by Catherine Deneuve. When not on the prowl for blood donors, they teach classical music to students in their beautiful house, which has a crematorium in the basement for the disposal of unwanted remains. In the film's set piece Bowie's character suddenly ages 200 years in a matter of minutes, and as he retreats to his coffin, Miriam starts a new affair with a doctor, played by Susan Sarandon.

Shooting began in London on 1 March 1982 (the day before the BBC screened *Baal*), and continued on and off until July. Locations included a house in Mayfair, the gay nightclub Heaven (where Bauhaus performed 'Bela Lugosi's Dead' for one of the key sequences), Luton Hoo in Bedfordshire, and the obligatory *Dracula* location of Whitby in North Yorkshire. It was Bowie's most protracted stay in Britain for some years, and although he was occasionally seen in London's trendier clubs he generally kept a low profile. By all accounts he was as committed as ever to his role: "There was a scene in which he had to play the cello," recalled scriptwriter Michael Thomas. "Most actors would have faked it, appearing only in indirect or long shots, using a professional musician for the close-ups. Not David. He fucking learned how to play the cello! He worked like a bastard until he could play a decent Bach cantata!" (One doubts whether even Bowie, though he *is* a professional musician, would be capable of persuading a cello to sing a cantata; but let that pass.)

As the shoot neared completion, a series of unpleasantly sensational reports appeared in the British papers following David's visit to his half-brother Terry, still a patient at Cane Hill Hospital in south London, where he had recently attempted suicide. There were those, primarily one of David's aunts, who spoke to the tabloids about his alleged lack of financial support, and with characteristic sensitivity the *Sun* weighed in with an item culled from second-hand clippings headlined "I'M TERRIFIED OF GOING MAD, SAYS BOWIE." Not surprisingly David left London shortly afterwards, bound for the South Pacific and his next film project.

He was on his Serious Moonlight tour by the time *The Hunger* was released in 1983 in a blaze of hype. "*The Hunger* is a mood, a look, an ambience created by Tony Scott. It is the lighting of Stephen Goldblatt, it is the production design of Brian Morris, it is the clothes created by Milena Canonero", waxed one of the tag lines, while another attempted an equally doomed stab at minimalism with "Bowie & Deneuve together. Shock. Horror." Critics and filmgoers alike were less than impressed. There was praise for the three principals and for the amazing make-up during Bowie's ageing sequence, but the general consensus was that the movie was hamstrung by its restless pop-video editing and its rapid degeneration into little more than softcore lesbian porn. Film historian Peter Nicholls described *The Hunger* as an "attempt to sell vampirism through chic imagery, as if it were soap, and blood is just another colour to highlight a pastel décor … It is a slick film, not entirely hollow, but its ambitions though discernible remain unrealized." *The Observer* concluded that it was "One of the most incoherent and foolish pictures of recent months". Frankly, it would be hard to disagree. *The Hunger* is a handsomely mounted film but not a particularly good one; it's an archetypal triumph of style over content, and after the art-house integrity of Bowie's previous acting credits it represents something of a comedown. When asked about the film later, Bowie remained quietly diplomatic: "I felt very uncomfortable with that role," he said in 1987, "although I loved being involved in a Tony Scott movie."

MERRY CHRISTMAS MR LAWRENCE
• GB, Recorded Picture/Cineventure/Oshima, 1983 •
Director: Nagisa Oshima • *Writers:* Nagisa Oshima, Paul Mayersberg (*Novel:* Laurens van der Post) •
Starring: David Bowie, Tom Conti, Ryuichi Sakamoto, Takeshi, Jack Thompson, Johnny Okura

As early as 1980, while still performing in *The Elephant Man* on Broadway, Bowie was approached by the renowned Japanese director Nagisa Oshima with a view to starring in his next movie. Bowie was immediately attracted to the idea of working with Oshima, whose early credits included *Boy* and *The Ceremony*, and whose award-winning masterpiece *Ai No Corrida* (*In The Realm Of The Senses*) had sparked a famous Japanese obscenity trial in 1976. Oshima's new project was an adaptation of Laurens van der Post's 1963

short-story trilogy *The Seed And The Sower*. "He asked me if I had read the book and I hadn't," said Bowie, "But I had certainly seen a few of his movies and I immediately agreed to do it without seeing the script, mainly because it was such an opportunity, a once-in-a-lifetime experience to work with someone like Oshima." The screenplay was co-written by Oshima and *The Man Who Fell To Earth*'s Paul Mayersberg, who now tailored the role for Bowie. "I wrote the lines thinking of David saying them and I semi-consciously changed things to suit him," said Mayersberg, who found Bowie a different man from the one he had known in 1975: "He doesn't seem quite as tense or hyper … He has become more physical rather than mental – health rather than disease has become interesting to him."

Just as *Ai No Corrida* had been rejected by Japanese backers and eventually produced with French money, so *Merry Christmas Mr Lawrence*, with its homosexual subtext and unflattering portrayal of Japanese wartime atrocities, was forced into postponement while Oshima found finance in England and New Zealand. When he was ready to begin shooting on Rarotonga in the Cook Islands in the summer of 1982, Oshima contacted Bowie with only three weeks' notice. "I'd just finished *The Hunger* and the last thing I wanted to do was make a movie!" recalled Bowie. "I just wanted to have a holiday. So I took advantage of the situation and took my holiday in the South Pacific. I got to know the islands pretty well before Oshima got there with the crew, so by the time everyone arrived I felt pretty much as if I'd been on the island for some time, which, in fact, I was supposed to have been in my role."

In *Merry Christmas Mr Lawrence* Bowie plays Jack Celliers, a Major in the Allied forces who emerges from a jungle commando mission to Java and surrenders to the Japanese army. Interned in a prisoner-of-war camp he attracts the attention of the commandant Captain Yonoi (Ryuichi Sakamoto), a self-despising misfit tormented by his repressed homosexuality. The friendship between the maverick Celliers and the gentle humanist Lawrence (Tom Conti) sustains them through a series of brutal experiences, until Celliers confesses to Lawrence that his life is consumed by guilt over his failure to protect his handicapped brother through a childhood of humiliation. Celliers finds redemption when he saves a British officer from death by intervening in the execution to kiss the besotted Yonoi before the entire camp; as punishment he is buried up to his neck in sand and dies of exposure and thirst, while his comrades survive.

"In the film I embrace the idea of war because of my guilt about my dealings with my family, specifically my younger brother, who was a hunchback from birth," explained Bowie. "I disown all responsibility for looking after him to an extent that leads him into terrible social situations, but I just stand there in the wings … without ever running to his defence. All this starts to work on me over the years, and comes to a point where my life becomes meaningless because of the dishonourable way I've treated my brother, so when the war comes, I throw myself into it, looking for salvation, but really, it's that now I can die, can die honourably doing something." One of the most poignant aspects of the film is the parallel between Celliers' emotional history and that of David himself, as he admitted to a reporter at the Cannes Film Festival. "I found in Celliers all too many areas of guilt and shortcomings that are part of me," he said. "I feel tremendous guilt because I grew so apart from my family. I hardly ever see my mother and I have a step-brother [sic] I don't see any more. It was my fault we grew apart and it is painful – but somehow there's no going back."

Like Bowie, Ryuichi Sakamoto was a well-known rock artist in his own country; his Yellow Magic Orchestra had pioneered electronic music in much the same way that Bowie's Berlin albums had in the west. Shortly before filming commenced Sakamoto had released 'Bamboo Houses', the first of several collaborations with David Sylvian, a Bowie admirer who for many years seemed to base his image on David's 1974 look. Sakamoto later wrote the excellent incidental score for *Merry Christmas Mr Lawrence*, although the accompanying Sylvian collaboration 'Forbidden Colours', a top 20 hit in 1983, does not actually feature in the film. Oshima explained that he had cast both Bowie and Sakamoto not just for their box office potential, but for their ability to galvanize the supporting cast: "I like working with non-professionals," he later said. "It has an interesting effect on the professional actors in the cast. When they are confronted by the non-professionals, they become more honest and truthful in their performances."

Shooting in the Cook Islands and later New Zealand (for the flashback scenes of Bowie's childhood with his brother) was completed in seven weeks. David later described it as "my first experience of movie-making that wasn't incredibly boring. I've spent more time making movies just sitting on my arse, waiting for my call, then doing ten takes of something and going away for two or three hours while they change the lighting set-up. Oshima cancelled that out for me. Two takes and it was done … It was shot in sequence, the majority of it, and edited in the camera. And for the first time, I was caught up in the momentum of making a film." When Bowie asked Oshima if he could do a re-take, "he said, 'If you like. But my editor very old man. So tired these days. No point in taking more. He only look at first one anyway.' It was a bit like making old rock and roll records, when James Brown and his band would do it just once." At the end of shooting in November, David staged a ribald revue for the cast and crew, before returning to New York to begin work on *Let's Dance*.

The Serious Moonlight tour was in full swing by the time *Merry Christmas Mr Lawrence* was released in 1983. Reviews were mixed (the *Sunday Times* said the film "always seems like a cocktail of saleable ingredients rather than genuine cinema"), although Bowie himself was generally praised. The *Sunday Telegraph* found him "superb", the *Guardian* "formidable", *Variety* "remarkable", *Playboy* "electric" and the *New York Times* "mercurial and arresting". *Village Voice* considered David "a movie star's movie star".

Today *Merry Christmas Mr Lawrence* remains cautiously well-regarded. Some have claimed that it offers little more than a retread of territory already covered by *The Bridge On The River Kwai*, but in place of that movie's *Boy's Own* heroes and villains Oshima achieves something disturbingly intangible: a genuine examination of the clash of two incompatible cultures and a meditation on the nature of evil, guilt, friendship and redemption. Bowie's performance is at times truly haunting, and the tension between his character and Sakamoto's – both remarkable in the film for their striking, unsettling beauty as well as for their performances – is quite electric. But although Bowie gets first billing, the film really belongs to the excellent Tom Conti, who as Lawrence himself occupies the greater screen time and gives the film its moral and narrative heart. *Merry Christmas Mr Lawrence* occupies a worthy place alongside *The Elephant Man* and *The Man Who Fell To Earth* as one of the substantial achievements of Bowie's acting career.

YELLOWBEARD

• US, Orion/Seagoat, 1983 • *Director:* Mel Damski • *Writers:* Peter Cook, Graham Chapman, Bernard McKenna • *Starring:* Graham Chapman, Cheech and Chong, Peter Cook, Marty Feldman, Michael Hordern, Eric Idle, Madeline Kahn, James Mason, John Cleese, Spike Milligan, Susannah York, Beryl Reid

Despite a strong cast of *Monty Python* veterans and other cult comedians (it was Marty Feldman's last movie), Mel Damski's knockabout pirate spoof is a lacklustre attempt at an all-star comedy, a genre undergoing a mini-renaissance at the time. Holidaying in Mexico after the completion of *Let's Dance* at the end of 1982, David chanced to meet his old friends Graham Chapman and Eric Idle on an Acapulco beach and agreed to make a one-shot cameo as a character called Henson, whose sole *raison d'être* is a rather lame visual gag about a shark – as he turns to exit, we see a rubber fin protruding from his back. Though not without its moments, the film was a flop. "The atrocious script and haphazard direction elicit generally embarrassing performances from all concerned," sizzled Kim Newman in *MFB*. Bowie also appears in *Group Madness*, a 50-minute behind-the-scenes feature – more an anarchic romp than a documentary – shot during the filming of *Yellowbeard*.

THE SNOWMAN

• UK, Channel 4, 1983 • *Director:* Dianne Jackson • *Writer:* Raymond Briggs • *Starring:* Raymond Briggs, Peter Auty

In a cosy woolly jumper, and surrounded by childhood memorabilia, Bowie filmed a 30-second introduction to the celebrated BAFTA-winning animation based on the book by Raymond Briggs. The film has since become a Channel 4 Christmas tradition, although Bowie's introduction has usually been omitted from subsequent screenings.

INTO THE NIGHT

• US, Universal, 1985 • *Director:* John Landis • *Writer:* Ron Koslow • *Starring:* Jeff Goldblum, Michelle Pfeiffer, Richard Farnsworth, Irene Papas, Paul Mazursky, Roger Vadim

Into The Night is an old-fashioned attempt at a Cary Grant-style caper movie, in which the everyman hero's chance encounter with a mysterious girl leads to an unwilling adventure with emerald smugglers. Although Bowie's role is a tiny walk-on, it remains one of his personal favourites. "*Into The Night* was a gas," he recalled later. "It's nice to do cameos." He plays a ham-fisted hit-man called Colin, and won praise for his comic delivery despite the film's lukewarm reception.

ABSOLUTE BEGINNERS

• GB, Virgin/Goldcrest/Palace, 1986 • *Director:* Julien Temple • *Writers:* Richard Burridge, Christopher Wicking, Don MacPerson (*Novel:* Colin MacInnes) • *Starring:* Eddie O'Connell, Patsy Kensit, David Bowie, Ray Davies, James Fox, Lionel Blair, Steven Berkoff, Mandy Rice Davies

Colin MacInnes's 1959 novel *Absolute Beginners* was never a mass seller, but it was a cult almost from the day it went on sale. It's a valuable document of the moment in the late 1950s when London was changed forever by the socio-economic empowerment of the teenager: "we'd loot to spend at last, and our world was to be our world, the one we wanted…" No longer tied back by post-war austerity, a new generation began gathering in the espresso bars of Soho to plan for the day they would inherit the earth. Among them, of course, was David Jones.

Julien Temple discovered the novel in 1981 while researching a television programme on 1950s style, and immediately purchased the film rights. Over the next three years he developed a script, and it was while shooting *Jazzin' For Blue Jean* in 1984 that Bowie learned of the project, telling the *NME* that it "should do a lot for young British film-making. It feels essentially *London*, but London not in a passé way. The excitement of London, which has never been featured properly. I mean, there are so many stories of young America and young New York … For instance, he deals with the fifties black riots in Notting Hill, and that's an area which has never been treated on film. That's an extraordinary thing to have even dug up; so few people remember that it even happened. He's got a very good chance of carrying it off. I'd love to do a feature with him."

Bowie's wish came true when Temple approached him to provide a theme song for the movie, and David asked whether there might be a role for him too. In early 1985 it was announced that he was to appear in *Absolute Beginners*, now in pre-production with finance from Virgin and Goldcrest, the London-based company that had just scored a major success with *The Killing Fields*. Press releases promised an old-fashioned musical on a lavish scale, and as further cast names were announced, media gossip about the movie started generating a snowball effect. Since the international success of the Oscar-laden *Chariots Of Fire* and *Gandhi* a few years earlier, each new home-grown movie of any stature was subjected to intense scrutiny by the British press. The tabloids began talking about *Absolute Beginners* as the great white hope for the beleaguered British film industry. This, of course, was fatal.

In June 1985, Bowie recorded his three soundtrack songs at Abbey Road. Filming continued through the summer at Shepperton Studios, where elaborate sets had been constructed to represent the Soho, Notting Hill and Pimlico of 1958. The mock-up street scenes were intended to achieve the slightly unreal Technicolor quality of 1950s film musicals, and also to allow freedom of camera movement and obviate the costs of using genuine London locations. Even so, the budget soon began to rocket. Filming was blighted by non-stop rain, and a sound stage caught fire after an electrical accident. Two members of the cast caught pneumonia while others, including Bowie, were laid low by a cold epidemic. Temple's determination not to compromise on his vision led to re-shoots, and as production costs mounted the press started to smell a sensation. *Vanity Fair* claimed that the budget had risen to over $11 million, and although this was small beer by Hollywood standards, Goldcrest's *Revolution* had just bombed catastrophically and all but wiped the company out. All of a sudden *Absolute Beginners* was being portrayed not as British film's brightest hope, but its last chance. The papers ran gleeful stories about how many jobs depended on its success at the box office. Finding himself saddled with an unwanted responsibility, Julien Temple took the uncomfortable step of running an advertisement in the trade papers to suggest that people should lower their expectations of the film's ability to be an industry cure-all. This, of course, was interpreted by the popular press as an admission that *Absolute Beginners* was going to be rubbish. Someone fabricated a rumour that the picture was so bad that it might never be released. ITV's *Spitting Image* laid into the

film, in the process unveiling a Bowie puppet who would appear intermittently on the show over the next few years (usually characterized as a grating salt-of-the-earth cockney singing 'Maybe It's Because I'm A Londoner'). In *Time Out* Julie Burchill concocted "Ten reasons why nobody should bother going to see *Absolute Beginners*." And all before anyone had seen a frame of it.

Temple and his cast stood shoulder-to-shoulder and braved out the barrage of pre-release ridicule, and the early omens were good: released in March 1986, Bowie's excellent title song was a big hit. "Musicals are going to make an enormous comeback," he told *Today*, the new British daily that was vying with *Absolute Beginners* and Sigue Sigue Sputnik as the media hype of the season. "*Absolute Beginners* is very interesting, the nearest thing I can think of to it is *Guys And Dolls*. It's really quite extraordinary, it's very stylized … a fifties *Singin' In The Rain* feel." He spoke also of the background of anti-immigration unrest that underpinned the movie's comedy sheen: "I remember the riots. I remember mainly the prison sentences they handed out afterwards. It was unbelievable how they stopped the thing overnight. They put these guys in jail for ten years, incredible sentences and all of a sudden there weren't any white thugs wanting to go down to Notting Hill Gate to cause trouble."

On 1 March Channel 4 screened *A Beginner's Guide To Absolute Beginners*, featuring behind-the-scenes footage and interviews with the stars. Bowie told presenter Paul Gambaccini that Julien Temple was "one of the most interesting directors around, terrific to work with," and explained that his role as the rapacious advertising executive Vendice Partners was a chance to revenge himself on an industry he had disliked ever since his stint as a commercial artist in the early 1960s: "I worked in advertising when I first left school, and I loathed it." Temple paid tribute to Bowie's contribution to the film: "The character he plays really represents the whole change of Britain in the fifties – the frozen food, the cars with fins. David knew just how to get the right mid-Atlantic accent for an adman trying to be so slick and American but every so often slipping back into cockney." Bowie explained that the voice came straight from his superiors at the advertising agency: "There was this continual fluctuation, which I thought was a good way to play Vendice. And I enjoyed playing him. He's such a bastard."

Absolute Beginners went on general release after a royal premiere on 2 April 1986. It performed respectably at the British box office, and in America it made $300,000 in its first seven weeks, a perfectly decent showing for a British movie at the time. But there was no way it was ever going to achieve the impossible targets set by over-excited journalists; because it didn't single-handedly resuscitate the British film industry, the picture was branded an unqualified disaster. It's still regarded today as some sort of grand folly, often by people who've never seen it.

The reality is less extreme than the myth. *Absolute Beginners* is no masterpiece, but neither is it the awful mess its reputation suggests. Several reviews at the time were positively glowing: "No doubt about it," proclaimed the *Sun*, "THE film of 1986," while the *Daily Mail* called it "a riot of colour and action." Others commended individual set pieces but bemoaned the lack of overall focus, a view with which it would be hard to disagree. "All that noise, all that energy, so little governing thought," said *Time Out*, while *Melody Maker* qualified its praise of Bowie by wondering what he was actually doing in the film: "His lavish set piece, 'That's Motivation', is worth watching, and Bowie's role hints at comic potential as well as displaying his increasing confidence as an actor. But the over-riding impression is that the part has been tacked on as a vehicle for the great man, and never properly integrated into the ever-shifting crazy paving of the plot."

There's plenty to admire in *Absolute Beginners*; in fact, it's an exasperating movie for the very reason that *some* of it is so wonderful. The cinematography is magnificent, the tone set early on by a mind-bogglingly complex travelling shot through the teeming Soho street set that recalls the famous opening scene of *Touch Of Evil*. The sets are amazing and the choreography, by *Jazzin' For Blue Jean*'s David Toguri, is superb, lending a stylized quality to the crowd scenes as well as to the dance numbers. Although the picture would undoubtedly benefit from a tighter structure, the individual set pieces are frequently stunning, from Patsy Kensit's orgiastic dance routine with a troupe of bare-chested satyrs to Ray Davies's big number 'Quiet Life', performed against a fusillade of sight-gags in a life-sized, three-storey doll's house set. In between there are unexpected delights like Steven Berkoff's apoplectic cameo at a Mosley-style fascist rally, and Lionel Blair's seedy pop promoter with unsavoury designs on his latest protégé. As the narrator-hero Colin, the excellent Eddie O'Connell both looks and sounds uncannily like the callow young Bowie of *Love*

You Till Tuesday. Bowie himself, although only on screen for about 20 minutes, gives great value as the cynical salesman who talks in a stream of marketing clichés: offering a cigarette to Colin, he says "You're never alone with a Strand," a 1950s slogan famous for backfiring when consumers identified the brand with lonely, friendless individuals. "David had a very good memory for all that kind of thing," said Temple. "Like knowing the jackets he wore shouldn't be padded. And E-type Jaguars were an important part of the period for him."

But the film lacks focus, and nowhere more so than in the soundtrack. With songwriters as diverse as Ray Davies, Sade, Paul Weller and Jerry Dammers, the major difference between *Absolute Beginners* and an old-fashioned film musical is its sheer lack of cohesion. Moreover, several of the songs simply aren't good enough. Bowie's big number 'That's Motivation' exemplifies the problem, squandering a huge cinematic effort on a duff piece of music. It aspires to be a grandiose Busby Berkeley routine (David dances on a giant typewriter, climbs Mount Everest, tap-dances in the clouds, flies on a Kirby wire and finally appears as a ringmaster, cracking his whip at the centre of a nightmarish miasma of commercialization), but the song itself is such a dreadful stiff that a scene which should have been a show-stopper is almost painful to watch.

Nevertheless, Temple's overarching vision is convincingly cinematic. The romantic storyline and the racial powder keg both gather momentum under a relentlessly baking sun ("It's been building with the heat all summer, right in front of my eyes," says Colin as the urban tensions reach breaking point near the end), and both find their apotheosis in a final thunder-cracking downpour. This metaphysical meteorology is a touch of directorial license: the summer of 1958 was not a particularly hot one, and Temple explained that he was superimposing the sweltering heatwave of punk's *annus mirabilis*, 1976. "London in long spells of hot weather becomes quite different … almost magical," he said, recalling the summer he had spent following the Sex Pistols with a film camera. Temple's nostalgic punk sensibility is fundamental to *Absolute Beginners* which is, after all, a film about a disaffected youth culture battling to maintain its idealism against the predations of marketing men. The swift fate of punk is a further referential layer to add to a movie whose ancestry in musical cinema can be traced in directions as diverse as *Guys And Dolls*,

Cabaret, West Side Story and A Clockwork Orange. The eclecticism is both a strength and a weakness: one of the problems with Absolute Beginners is that the entire film seems to be in inverted commas. It's not a musical about the 1950s so much as a pastiche of a 1950s musical. A decade earlier Absolute Beginners might have made more sense to audiences, but in 1986 it was out of step with the mood of cinema, then firmly entrenched either in gritty realism or out-and-out fantasy, but rarely a mixture of both. For many, the spectacle of a violent knife-fight developing into a Grease-style dance routine was just too confusing to cope with.

Absolute Beginners is certainly a flawed picture, but it's also a unique and valuable one, which undeservedly became a casualty of circumstances beyond its control. Oscars are dished out to far worse films than this.

LABYRINTH

• US, Tri-Star, 1986 • Director: Jim Henson • Writer: Terry Jones • Starring: David Bowie, Jennifer Connelly, Toby Froud, Brian Henson, Ron Mueck, David Shaughnessy, Michael Hordern, Percy Edwards

During the US leg of the Serious Moonlight tour in 1983, Jim Henson, creator and mastermind of the Muppets, offered Bowie the lead role in his forthcoming picture Labyrinth. "Way back when we first started working on the story, we came up with this idea of a Goblin King," explained Henson later, "And then we thought, 'Wouldn't it be wonderful to have music and someone who can sing?' David was our first choice from the very beginning, and he liked the idea. So the whole thing was really written with him in mind." By the time Bowie and Henson made their respective cameos in the John Landis comedy Into The Night, the project was already in pre-production.

With the backing of executive producer George Lucas and a budget of $20 million (twice that of Absolute Beginners), Labyrinth was a major undertaking in children's cinema. In 1982 Henson had scored a minor hit with the cult favourite The Dark Crystal, and his new project was a further incursion into the fantasy vogue exemplified by films like Krull, Legend and The Neverending Story, subscribing to the tried-and-tested formula of the classic fairytale quest.

Sarah (Jennifer Connelly), a daydreaming teenager forced to babysit for her brother, idly wishes the child

spirited away by goblins. Enter Jareth, the Goblin King (Bowie), who abducts the child to a grotesque fantasy world and gives Sarah thirteen hours to rescue him before he is irrevocably turned into a goblin. Needless to say, Sarah must face untold perils and enlist all manner of eccentric comrades in her mission. Her uneasy alliance with the cowardly dwarf Hoggle teaches them both about the virtues of friendship and courage, while Jareth's seductive magnetism threatens to engulf Sarah's innocence as the clock ticks away.

"Jim gave me the script, which I found very amusing," Bowie explained at the time. "It's by Terry Jones, of Monty Python, and it has that kind of slightly inane insanity running through it. When I read the script and saw that Jim wanted to put music to it, it just felt as though it could be a really nice, funny thing to do." Of his role as Jareth, he suggested that "one feels that he's rather reluctantly inherited the position of being Goblin King, as though he would really like to be, I don't know, down in Soho or something." Henson elaborated: "His role is similar to being the leader of a gang. Everyone in the kingdom does what he says until Sarah comes along – and she defies him. The goblins David controls are like members of his gang. He treats them terribly but they do anything he says."

Decked out in a preposterous Tina Turner fright-wig and a succession of fantastically foppish outfits, Bowie began work on Labyrinth at Elstree Studios in late 1985. "Early on, his first couple of scenes were with Hoggle, and David kept wanting to look off-stage to where the voice was coming from," said Henson later. "It took him a little while to get used to that." Another hurdle involved the filming of Jareth's spectacular conjuring tricks with crystal balls, a running motif throughout the film. These were accomplished by the illusionist Michael Moschen, who would crouch behind Bowie's cloak and thrust his hands through the sleeves to replace Bowie's arms; the process was far from easy and led to multiple re-takes. During shooting David enthused about his 14-year-old co-star: "Jennifer was absolutely right for the part of Sarah. She's extremely pretty, with looks rather like those of the teenage Elizabeth Taylor – she's also a damn good actress." Sarah's baby brother was played by Toby Froud, son of the film's conceptual designer Brian Froud, while the film's choreographer was Cheryl "Gates" McFadden, later to find fame as Star Trek's Dr Beverly Crusher.

Bowie wrote and recorded five songs for the film, and in Britain the soundtrack album appeared some six months before the movie itself. *Labyrinth* finally hit UK cinemas in December 1986, but on both sides of the Atlantic the critics were unimpressed. *Variety* called the film "a crashing bore", complaining that there was "no real charm or texture to capture the imagination." Bowie's involvement was similarly ridiculed, the *Star* demanding to know, "Where have we failed, that this papery old queen is a hero to our kids?" More recently, Bowie himself has given the impression that he is none too proud of the movie. Asked by an interviewer in 2002 to nominate the "most Spinal Tap moment" of his career, he responded: "Oh God! I thought *Labyrinth* got pretty damn near it," adding, rather mysteriously, "but I was made to do that."

Predictably, the same sort of folk who go cross-eyed with embarrassment at 'The Laughing Gnome' would prefer it if *Labyrinth* didn't exist, but some recent Bowie biographers have rightly begun to concede that it deserves greater recognition. For anyone with an ounce of childhood still in them *Labyrinth* is a terrific movie and, deservedly, it was a box office hit of Christmas 1986. It has the humanity, warmth, moral progress and heroic sentiment one associates with the best children's cinema, from *Chitty Chitty Bang Bang* and *The Jungle Book* right back to *The Wizard Of Oz*, from which Henson and Jones take many of their cues. Sarah's Dorothy-like progress draws on a whole tapestry of other sources including *Alice In Wonderland*, Cocteau's *La Belle Et La Bête*, C S Lewis's Narnia books, Raymond Briggs's *Fungus The Bogeyman*, Maurice Sendak's *Where The Wild Things Are* and even Neil Jordan's *The Company Of Wolves*. In fact, the improving morality lessons are hung on a framework of references straight from Angela Carter's feminist fairytales, and Sarah's struggle to rescue the child operates as a metaphor for the preservation of her own innocence on the eve of adulthood. Jim Henson confirmed that the film was "about a person at the point of changing from being a child to a woman. Times of transition are always magic … The world that Sarah enters exists in her imagination. The film starts out in her bedroom and you see all the books she's read growing up – *The Wizard Of Oz*, *Alice In Wonderland*, the works of Maurice Sendak. And the world she enters shows elements of all these stories that fascinated her as a girl."

Bowie's Jareth, a strikingly erotic figure for a children's movie, tempts Sarah to put away childish things in a succession of positively Freudian confrontations. At her first rejection of him he flings a snake at her. Later he follows the example of *Snow White*'s wicked queen and tricks Sarah into eating a poisoned fruit, triggering a hallucinatory sequence in which, *Cinderella*-like, she enters a decadent Venetian masked ball, an adult world both alluring and repugnant. In another scene the nightmarish Junk Lady hands Sarah a tube of lipstick and urges, "Go on, dear, make yourself up!" But with the help of the Muppet characters (who, in an obvious nod to *The Wizard Of Oz*, are animated fantasies of the toys we see in her bedroom at the beginning), Sarah resists all attempts to corrupt her, rescues the child and abolishes Jareth by defying his last ultimatum. Back at home she begins to put away her childhood toys, but then relents and admits that she needs them, whereupon her bedroom explodes into a riotous Muppet party and the camera pulls outside to where the banished Jareth watches in the guise of an owl. Innocence prevails and adulthood can wait for another day: it's *exactly* the same as Bowie's 1966 composition 'There Is A Happy Land' ("It's a secret place, and adults aren't allowed there, Mr Grownup…").

Being a Terry Jones script, there are great jokes as well. Fairytale conventions are systematically subverted: ominous rock faces break off their doom-laden warnings to converse in camp Yorkshire accents, pretty gossamer fairies turn out to be vicious pests to be dispatched with fly-spray, and there's a milk bottle at the door of the forbidding goblin castle.

Labyrinth is also a visual feast. The art direction is stunning throughout, particularly in the *Cinderella* pastiche and in the majestic final confrontation on an optical-illusion set inspired by M C Escher's *Relativity*. Bowie's songs, too, have been much maligned. The irritating 'Chilly Down' we could do without, but the theme song and 'As The World Falls Down' are among his strongest work of the period. Given the melodramatic Muppet mayhem all around him he's in danger of underplaying the villainous moments, but Bowie comes into his own in the quieter, seductive scenes. His final slow-motion grimace when he knows he's been defeated is among the most beguiling moments he's ever committed to celluloid. For those sufficiently grown-up to admit the inner child, *Labyrinth* is ready for a major re-evaluation.

"CREATION"

In the spring of 1987 Bowie raised funds for the forth-coming Glass Spider tour by signing a sponsorship deal with soft drinks giant Pepsi, for whom he filmed a high-profile television commercial with Tina Turner. "Money is the only reason anyone would want to do a commercial, don't you think so?" he admitted during filming, which took place in an Amsterdam TV studio.

Entitled *Creation*, the 60-second advert was a pastiche of *Frankenstein* via *Metropolis*, set to a new recording of 'Modern Love' with lyrics reworked to fit Pepsi's motto of the time, "The Choice For A New Generation". David appears as a mad professor in bow tie, spectacles, white lab coat and slicked-down hair, plotting to create the perfect woman in his ramshackle laboratory. He takes a sip from his Pepsi bottle before accidentally spilling the contents into the works. Cue a big explosion and a driving wind which blows off his glasses, transforms his clothes and miraculously re-styles his hair, while his creation – Tina Turner, of course – emerges in a cloud of smoke from an incongruous red telephone box (*Ziggy Stardust* parallels no doubt intended). They gallivant off to an American diner and dance around a Pepsi machine to the suitably re-worded lyrics. Absolutely dreadful, and an absolute hoot.

The commercial was destined to be another casualty in Pepsi's troubled history of pop-star product endorsements. On 9 October 1987, David was accused of assaulting a female fan in Dallas. The case was later dismissed, but at the first whiff of controversy the courageous multinational withdrew the Bowie/Turner commercial from the airwaves. As a result it was only ever screened a handful of times.

THE LAST TEMPTATION OF CHRIST
• US/Canada, Universal, 1988 • *Director:* Martin Scorsese • *Writer:* Paul Schrader (*Novel:* Nikos Kazantzakis) • *Starring:* Willem Dafoe, Harvey Keitel, Barbara Hershey, Harry Dean Stanton, André Gregory, David Bowie

In 1984, during the shooting of *Jazzin' For Blue Jean*, Bowie told the *NME* that Martin Scorsese and Paul Schrader were planning to film Nikos Kazantzakis's novel in which Jesus is tempted by the fantasy of escaping the Cross to die an old man. "They've got Harvey Keitel to play Pontius Pilate," said David, "and

I think at one point it was supposed to be De Niro as Jesus, but now I think they're going for an unknown. Strangely enough, they can't raise a cent of finance for it in America."

In fact Scorsese had begun working on the project as early as 1980, but the studio dropped the project following threats from Christian pressure-groups. When the film eventually appeared in 1988, Jesus was played by Willem Dafoe and Judas by Harvey Keitel. Sting, who had earlier been cast as Pontius Pilate, was now unavailable, and the role was offered to Bowie. Fresh from the Glass Spider tour, David flew to Morocco in December 1987 to shoot his cameo. It's the briefest of appearances – a three-minute interrogation scene for which David spent only two days on set – but it's a key sequence and Bowie acquits himself well with a thoughtful, unshowy performance. The film caused an uproar in America, where members of the religious right decided that it would be more Christian to burn effigies of Scorsese than to find out what his complex, elegiac and brilliant film was actually about.

DREAM ON
• US, HBO, 1991 • *Director:* John Landis • *Writer:* David Crane, Marta Kauffman • *Starring:* Brian Benben, Chris Demetral, Denny Dillon, Wendie Malick

Bowie's guest appearance in HBO's comedy series was recorded in 1991 shortly after he had finished work on *The Linguini Incident* (see below), although *Dream On* was the first of the two to be aired. *Dream On* was a weekly sitcom written by the duo who would later create *Friends*; revolving around the misadventures of hapless publisher Martin and his ex-wife Judith, its central gimmick was Martin's habit of reflecting on his experiences through appropriate flashbacks from old movies and TV shows. Bowie, who was attracted to the show by the involvement of his old friend John Landis, appeared in the first two episodes of the second season, a two-parter entitled *The Second Greatest Story Ever Told* which began transmission on 7 July 1991. He played Sir Roland Moorcock, the larger-than-life director of a biopic about Judith's new husband. In one of his lesser-known excursions into acting, Bowie acquits himself well with a fine comic performance.

THE LINGUINI INCIDENT

• US, Rank/Isolar, 1992 • *Director:* Richard Shepard • *Writers:* Richard Shepard, Tamar Brott • *Starring:* Rosanna Arquette, David Bowie, Eszter Balint, André Gregory, Buck Henry

Originally entitled *Linguini* and co-funded by Bowie's management company Isolar, this harmless but negligible comedy was shot in late 1990 following the end of the Sound + Vision tour. David's future wife Iman, whom he had met in October, makes a cameo appearance, while supporting actor André Gregory had previously played John the Baptist in *The Last Temptation Of Christ*. Bowie plays a love-lorn bartender who teams up with a waitress and wannabe escapologist (Arquette) to steal Harry Houdini's ring from an antique shop, paving the way for possibly the most laboured tag-line in movie history: "He wants to be tied down. She wants to be tied up. It's not what you think!" It's a trivial film that was panned by the few papers who noticed it at all; *Variety* observed that "energetic actors can't overcome the uninspired, poverty-row production values". The final ignominy came in January 2000 when the picture was reissued on DVD with the appalling new title *Shag-O-Rama*, complete with psychedelic packaging blatantly attempting to cash in on the *Austin Powers* franchise.

TWIN PEAKS: FIRE WALK WITH ME

• US, Guild/Twin Peaks, 1992 • *Director:* David Lynch • *Writers:* David Lynch, Robert Engels • *Starring:* Sheryl Lee, Ray Wise, Kyle MacLachlan, Harry Dean Stanton, Kiefer Sutherland, David Bowie

Bowie filmed his two-minute cameo in David Lynch's prequel to the cult television serial in the summer of 1991, prior to commencing publicity duties for *Tin Machine II*. Devotees of *Twin Peaks*'s mannered obfuscation will find rich pickings in Bowie's appearance as Agent Phillip Jeffries, a tormented witness to diabolical goings-on who briefly materializes as if from a different dimension. Looking every inch the *Tin Machine II*-period Bowie (white suit, Hawaiian shirt and all), he affects a creditable Southern States drawl and is gone before there's any chance of the viewer deducing what's supposed to be going on. Which is undoubtedly the whole idea. The Region 1 DVD release includes deleted sequences featuring Bowie.

FULL STRETCH

• ITV (Meridian), 5 January 1993 • *Director:* Antonia Bird • *Writers:* Dick Clement, Ian La Frenais • *Starring:* Kevin McNally, Reece Dinsdale, Sue Johnston

Largely forgotten among Bowie's acting work is his cameo in the first episode of this short-lived comedy drama about a down-at-heel limousine company, written by the creators of *Porridge*, *The Likely Lads* and *Auf Wiedersehen, Pet*. Bowie appears as himself, snoozing in the back of a stretch Mercedes and blithely unaware of the comic mishaps besetting chauffeur Reece Dinsdale in his attempts to cross Central London to get the star to his gig. The scenes were shot around Pall Mall, Piccadilly Circus and St James's on a Sunday afternoon in 1992. "We chose Sunday because we thought it would be a quiet day," Reece Dinsdale said later, "but it was absolutely choc-a-bloc with cars and tourists, and we just could not get the shots in." On meeting Bowie, Dinsdale confessed to being "completely tongue-tied, but he was very charming and lovely. And when it came to doing the scene, he knew his lines and was very professional. He did it in one with no messing about."

BASQUIAT

• US, Guild/Eleventh Street/Miramax, 1996 • *Director/Writer:* Julian Schnabel • *Starring:* Jeffrey Wright, David Bowie, Dennis Hopper, Gary Oldman, Michael Wincott, Willem Dafoe, Benicio Del Toro, Christopher Walken, Courtney Love

Julian Schnabel's biopic of Jean-Michel Basquiat, the young graffiti artist who briefly became the darling of the New York art world before his drug-related death in 1988, began filming under the working title *Build A Fort, Set It On Fire* in June 1995. Bowie was full of enthusiasm for the project: "The first film about an American painter, and it's a *black* painter," he pointed out to *Ikon*. "Not Pollock, or Johns, or de Kooning – although John Malkovich as Pollock would've been stunning." Having recently visited the Africa 95 exhibition in Johannesburg, he explained that African artists "look on Basquiat as their Picasso, who made it in a white world. I'm not even sure Julian realizes the reverberations of his own movie. It's an informal, poignant story of a tragic life. How, by tacit agreement, an artist and society endeavour to demolish the artist himself." Some years later, Bowie would contribute an essay on Basquiat to the book *Writers On Artists*, an anthology of monographs published in 2001.

As Bowie indicated, *Basquiat* isn't merely a biography; its strength lies in the portrayal of the fickle, irresponsible environment of high-powered art cliques, in which a nobody can be promoted to a celebrity on the whim of a dealer anxious to discover the next big thing. It's a quiet, admirably restrained piece of filmmaking, and in the plum role of his own sometime muse Andy Warhol, Bowie all but steals the picture. By turns funny and tragic, he displays a sense of timing and attention to detail that transcends the caricature he could easily have plumped for. David's scenes were shot in the space of ten days. "I only had 7000 words," he revealed at the time, "and once I got them in the right order, it was a doddle. I mean, a most challenging role." He wore Warhol's genuine clothes and wig for the part. "They still smelt of him," he said. "I even had his little handbag – a very sad little bag with all kinds of devices to make you better." An overlooked jewel, this is without doubt one of Bowie's finest screen performances.

Trivia buffs take note: before fame beckoned, Jean-Michel Basquiat appeared as the DJ in Blondie's 'Rapture' video.

EVERYBODY LOVES SUNSHINE
(aka B.U.S.T.E.D.)
• GB, IAC/Isle Of Man Film Commission/Bozie Films, 1999 • *Director/Writer:* Andrew Goth • *Starring:* Goldie, Andrew Goth, David Bowie, Rachel Shelley, Clint Dyer

Bowie's role in writer/director Andrew Goth's debut came about through his friendship with the film's star, drum'n'bass artist Goldie, on whose album *Saturnzreturn* David had already guested. Trailed as "a hard-hitting gangland drama", the film concerns warring triads operating against the backdrop of Manchester's club scene, with a suitably hardcore soundtrack also provided by Goldie. A bespectacled Bowie plays Bernie, fixer for the gang headed by Terry (Goldie) and Ray (Goth), two cousins who are released from prison as the film begins. Bernie attempts to mediate between Ray, who now wants to go straight, and the psychotic Terry, whose determination to wreak his revenge on a rival gang spirals out of

control with disastrous results.

Shooting commenced on 21 February 1998 on the Isle of Man, later moving to Liverpool for five weeks. Distribution of the low-budget independent was sporadic: it played to a few festivals and Japanese cinemas before going straight to television, receiving its British premiere on Sky TV in on 16 June 1999. Although filmed and premiered as *Everybody Loves Sunshine*, the picture was retitled *B.U.S.T.E.D.* for its initial video and DVD release in January 2000, before reverting to the original title on later reissues.

Bowie's scenes are spread thinly and amount to no more than 15 minutes in all, but his effortlessly cool presence as the world-weary Bernie, an old-time gangster in the Kray mould, outclasses everyone and everything connected with this otherwise desperate piece of filmmaking, whose juvenile fantasies of masculinity and risible "gangsta" pretensions couldn't possibly be taken seriously by anyone who's seen Ali G – or indeed by anyone who's seen *Brighton Rock*, which was made 50 years earlier, has exactly the same plot, and is cooler, tougher and superior in every conceivable respect.

IL MIO WEST
• Italy, 1999 • *Director/Writer:* Giovanni Veronesi (*Novel:* Vincenzo Pardini) • *Starring:* Harvey Keitel, Leonardo Pieraccioni, David Bowie, Sandrine Holt

With Bowie's scenes shot in Garfagnana, Tuscany over two weeks in June 1998, this serio-comic spaghetti Western was released across Italy the following December. David plays Jack Sikora, a psychopathic, gun-toting pistolero in cowboy hat and shades, who rides into town in pursuit of his arch-enemy Johnny (Harvey Keitel). Bowie explained that he had been attracted by the script's uniquely European translation of American archetypes: his character, for example, drags a photographer everywhere he goes in order to capture his acts of violence and death.

MR RICE'S SECRET
• Canada, New City Productions, 2000 • *Director:* Nicholas Kendall • *Writer:* Joel Wyner • *Starring:* David Bowie, Bill Switzer, Teryl Rothery, Garwin Sanford

Filmed as *Exhuming Mr Rice* but re-titled with the children's market in mind, this TV movie was shot in Vancouver in the summer of 1998. Told in flashback, the story begins with the funeral of Mr Rice (Bowie), whose young neighbour, Owen, suffers from Hodgkin's disease. Pursuing a series of cryptic clues left to him by the old man, the boy embarks on a search for an elixir which, it transpires, had kept Mr Rice alive for 400 years. But the expected outcome of this fantastical device is neatly overturned, affirming the film's themes of positive thinking and the banishment of fear, as summed up by Bowie's key line: "It's what you do in life that's important, not how much time you have or what you wish you'd done."

Bowie explained that he had been attracted to the project by the script: "I thought it was charming – a very touching, compassionate piece of work, very well written." Of his portrayal of Mr Rice, whom he described as an embodiment of "the better qualities in all of us", he revealed that "I keep getting images of my dad."

Being a mainstream family film about a boy coming to terms with a terminal illness, *Mr Rice's Secret* is inevitably a little saccharine in places, but for the most part it skilfully avoids sentimentality and offers an honest, unflinching account of a child's emotional turmoil. Bowie's young co-star Bill Switzer is excellent, and David's own carefully understated performance as the boy's mentor, while not exactly requiring him to flex his acting muscles, is very nicely judged. The *Hollywood Reporter*, which found the film "uplifting, enchanting and outstanding", announced that "Bowie has never been better."

Originally intended for a straight-to-TV premiere, *Mr Rice's Secret* was previewed at the Griffoni Film Festival in July 1999 and was then showered with awards at various European film festivals before its screening on The Family Channel. A US theatrical premiere followed in December 2000. The subsequent DVD release includes extensive behind-the-scenes footage of Bowie and Switzer filming one of their scenes.

THE HUNGER

• Showtime Television, 1998-1999

In 1998 American networks began screening *The Hunger*, a Canadian-made horror anthology series based loosely on the concepts created in the film of the same name in which Bowie had starred back in 1982. In November it was announced that David would be taking over from Terence Stamp as the "host" for the show's second series. He began recording his spoken introductions in Montreal in late 1998, appearing in the episodes *Soul Snatcher*, *Bump In The Night* and *Smoke, Mirrors And Paranoia*. In addition, Bowie acted in an instalment called *Sanctuary*, filmed in March 1999 and transmitted the following September. He played Julian Priest, an artist obsessed with the macabre, and according to the *Los Angeles Weekly* his "I'm still-a-good-looking-actor vibe and relaxed delivery are, apart of course from the customary gratuitous nudity, the best thing about the show." The series received its first British screening on the Sci-Fi Channel from March 2000.

ZOOLANDER

• US, Paramount, 2001 • *Director:* Ben Stiller • *Writers:* Ben Stiller, Drake Stather, John Hamburg • *Starring:* Ben Stiller, Owen Wilson, Christine Taylor, Will Ferrell, Milla Jovovich

Ben Stiller's enjoyably camp comedy, which inserts a *Manchurian Candidate*-style assassination thriller into the narcissistic world of the fashion industry, grew from a character he had originally created in a short film for the 1996 VH1 Fashion Awards, at which Bowie also performed. After producing a follow-up film for the 1997 ceremony, Stiller resolved to launch his brain-dead supermodel Derek Zoolander in a full-length movie. *Zoolander* boasts an array of cameo appearances by celebrities such as Claudia Schiffer, Billy Zane, Sandra Bernhard and Donald Trump, many of them shot ad-lib at the VH1 Fashion Awards on 20 October 2000. Bowie's guest appearance, willingly sending up the media's image of him as the ultimate arbiter of cool, is rather more integral to the plot. "The script is hilarious," David revealed before filming in September 2000. "There is a *Fight Club* style 'walk-off' between the two star models, and I act as the referee." Having made an over-the-top entrance accompanied by a freeze-frame, an on-screen caption and a snatch of 'Let's Dance', Bowie proceeds to milk his two-minute scene for all it's worth. "It was just too funny a script to walk past," he confessed later. "An absolute hoot!" He was right: *Zoolander* is thoroughly daft and highly recommended.

RUTLES 2: CAN'T BUY ME LUNCH

• US, Warner Bros *(unreleased at time of writing)* • *Director:* Eric Idle • *Writer:* Eric Idle • *Starring:* Eric Idle, Neil Innes, Ricky Fataar, John Halsey

In October 2000, Bowie revealed that his old friend Eric Idle had asked him to film a spoof interview for a new documentary about Idle's fictional band The Rutles, originally created for the 1978 classic *All You Need Is Cash*. "I obviously have said yes," Bowie enthused. "This should be an absolute laugh." His interview segment was duly shot in Los Angeles in February 2001. Unreleased at the time of writing, *Can't Buy Me Lunch* also features contributions from the likes of Billy Connolly, Carrie Fisher, Tom Hanks and even Salman Rushdie.

MAYOR OF THE SUNSET STRIP

• US, First Look Media, 2004 • *Director/Writer:* George Hickenlooper

In the wake of hits like *Bowling For Columbine* and *Touching The Void*, the vogue for big-screen documentaries meant that Bowie's contribution to George Hickenlooper's film, although not an acting role as such, was seen on cinema screens worldwide. *Mayor Of The Sunset Strip* charts the career of the famed Hollywood club promoter Rodney Bingenheimer, who was pivotal in introducing David to American audiences in the early 1970s. Previously known for the 1991 *Apocalypse Now* documentary *Hearts Of Darkness*, Hickenlooper attracted a host of stars to the film, including David Bowie, Mick Jagger, Paul McCartney, Alice Cooper, Cher, Deborah Harry and Rodney Bingenheimer himself. The accompanying soundtrack album included an obscure rarity in the shape of a poor-quality snippet of David singing 'All The Madmen' at a Hollywood party in February 1971.

HOOKED TO THE SILVER SCREEN...

Like his music, Bowie's acting career has turned up numerous speculative and unfulfilled projects. Ever since the mid-1970s he has also spoken of a desire to write and direct for the cinema, ambitions which remain unrealized. He has acted as executive producer to a couple of little-known foreign films: Büvös vadász (1994), a fantasy by the Hungarian filmmaker Ildikó Enyedi, and Passaggio Per Il Paradiso (1996), an Italian romantic comedy directed by Antonio Baiocco.

What follows is a summary of some of the film and television jobs that never materialized. Some are well documented; others, inevitably, remain the stuff of rumour and hearsay.

1960s

In August 1966 Bowie was invited to contribute lyrics to a short film musical composed by the then unknown Carl Davis. Kenneth Pitt sent David's demo tape and lyric sheets to the producers in March 1967, but nothing more was heard of the project.

In 1967 David auditioned for the role of David Copperfield in *The Touchables*, while in June of the same year he was approached by a young actor called Michael Armstrong, who was planning a low-budget film of his high-camp adaptation of *Orpheus In The Underworld* entitled *A Floral Tale*. David was offered the role of Orpheus – prophetically, a pop singer who is torn to pieces by his fans – but the film was abandoned when the script was thrown out by the BBFC, whose powers were wider then than now, on the grounds that it featured explicit homosexuality. Bowie, who is said to have written and possibly demoed seven pieces of music for the project, would appear in Armstrong's short *The Image* later in the year.

Late in 1967 Bowie attempted to write a television play entitled *The Champion Flower Grower*. It centred around a Yorkshire gardener called Haywood "Woody" Kettlewell (Haywood, interestingly enough, being the Christian name of David's father), whose success in a local flower show wins him a weekend in London. There he meets a group of flower-power hippies, with hilarious consequences: "A handful of weirdies who wouldn't know one end of a bullock from t'other," declares Woody, whom David envisaged being played by Hywel Bennett, while proposing himself in the role of a backward boy called Sammy Slap. Kenneth Pitt submitted the script, with a copy of the *David Bowie* album, to Sydney Newman, BBC Television's Head of Drama. A Script Unit subordinate returned the following reply: "To be quite brief, Mr Bowie has really not yet begun to consider what a play *is* and this total lack of dramatic development just rules the script out for us. With regrets I return the manuscript and, what my secretary assures me, is a splendid LP."

In 1968 Bowie tried for film roles in *Oh! What A Lovely War* and *Alain*, and reached the second auditions for the London production of *Hair*. Noted song-and-dance man Lionel Blair has also recalled auditioning the young Bowie for a stage musical in 1968. In the autumn, Lindsay Kemp invited David and Hermione Farthingale to join him in Scotland for a Christmas production of *Puss In Boots*; tragically, they turned him down. Also in 1968 Michael Armstrong reappeared on the scene to offer Bowie a role in his feature-length horror film *The Dark*. The part was eventually taken by Julian Barnes and the film appeared in 1969, re-titled *The Haunted House Of Horror* and starring Dennis Price and Frankie Avalon. Armstrong's final unsuccessful attempt to employ Bowie was for a theatrical revue in March 1969 which, according to a note David wrote to Kenneth Pitt, could "do nobody in the cast anything but harm. It stinks."

In November 1969, when 'Space Oddity' was on its way down the UK chart, Bowie auditioned for the role eventually played by Murray Head in John Schlesinger's *Sunday, Bloody Sunday*, which appeared in 1971 and was showered with awards and nominations. Journalist and filmmaker Tony Palmer met Bowie in December 1969 to discuss the possibility of working on a film of *Groupie Girl*.

1970s

In January 1970 Kenneth Pitt was contacted by Brian Howard, artistic director of Harrogate Theatre in North Yorkshire, a repertory house renowned to this day for its excellent pantomimes. Howard's attempt to involve Bowie in a production of *The Fair Maid Of Perth*, which led to two solo gigs at the theatre on 12 April, is discussed under "Hype" in Chapter 3.

February 1970 saw Bowie exploring possible musical involvement in the films *Silver Lady* and *Perspective*. The following month, midway through Hype's live career, Kenneth Pitt recalls being asked by an impecunious David to arrange more work in television commercials. Having procured Bowie a day's engagement on an advert for Wall's sausages, Pitt was apparently rebuffed by an angry David snapping, "I don't want to do television commercials!"

On 14 April 1970, the very day that he was recording the single version of 'Memory Of A Free Festival', David attended an unsuccessful audition for Frank Nesbitt's bucolic melodrama *Dulcima*, which appeared in 1971 with a cast headed by John Mills. A more upsetting loss in the same month was the shelving of a proposal by Tony Palmer, who had reviewed David glowingly in the Observer the previous year, to make a fly-on-the-wall documentary which would have followed the *Man Who Sold The World* sessions and life at Haddon Hall.

With the departure of Kenneth Pitt from Bowie's career in 1970, the auditions and acting projects dried up until 1973, when the MainMan publicity machine began circulating the first of many rumours. Around the time of the second US Ziggy tour it was reported that Bowie was to play the lead role in a film of Robert Heinlein's *Stranger In A Strange Land*, about a Martian visitor to Earth. In fact the story was invented by Tony Defries, and with David's connivance at press conferences it became assimilated into established fact.

As discussed elsewhere in this book, in November 1973 David spoke of staging *Ziggy Stardust* as a rock musical; his fullest account of the planned show can be found in the *Rolling Stone* interview reproduced in *The Bowie Companion*. At the same time his fabled adaptation of George Orwell's *Nineteen Eighty-Four* was being mooted, as were plans to launch Amanda Lear in *Oktobriana: The Movie*, with music written and produced by David. This project was still being discussed as late as May 1974; for further details on all three, see *Diamond Dogs* in Chapter 2.

Elizabeth Taylor, who befriended David in 1974, invited him to appear with her in George Cukor's remake of the 1940 Shirley Temple fairytale *The Blue Bird*. Gossip columnists announced in November that Bowie was indeed to co-star, but in fact he dismissed the script as "a very dry, high French fairytale with nothing to say," telling an interviewer later that it was "a rotten part" and "a rotten film" – an opinion echoed by many critics when the movie appeared in 1976. Nevertheless the episode was a significant one, being the first instance that Bowie's name had been bandied around Hollywood circles in connection with a major film; *The Man Who Fell To Earth* followed soon afterwards.

In late 1974 rumours flew that Bowie was to star in a biopic about Frank Sinatra. When David took Ava Cherry to see Sinatra perform in Las Vegas, he sent a note backstage. Word came back that Ol' Blue Eyes was too busy to meet people and that he didn't want "some faggot" playing him on screen. Many years later, Bowie revealed that it was apparently Sinatra's daughter Nancy who had "stupidly suggested that I play him in a movie. God, he hated that. 'I don't want a fag playing me!' He was absolutely terrified that I might be taken seriously. He hated long hair, hated anything limey!"

In 1975 David made plans to write, direct and star in a film version of *Diamond Dogs*. "I'm finally going to make the film I've been wanting to do for so long," his ghostwritten diary informed *Mirabelle* readers in January 1975. "It's going to have a *Diamond Dogs* theme and I start right away!" Probably revealing more about the aspirations of the true diarist than the reality of Bowie's intentions, "David" also revealed that the film would star MainMan regulars Tony Zanetta, Wayne County and Cyrinda Foxe, along with Iggy Pop and Terence Stamp.

Five years later Bowie revealed that *Diamond Dogs* had progressed as far as silent black and white test footage he had shot in his suite at New York's Pierre Hotel. "I built three or four-foot high buildings out of clay on tables. Some were standing up, others were crumbling and I took the camera and put a micro-lens on it, zooming down the streets in between the tables." Tony Visconti recalls filming electronic inlays of Bowie walking through the model sets. "I wanted to make a film of *Diamond Dogs* so passionately," said David. "I really wanted to do that. I had the whole roller-skating thing in there. We had no more cars because of fuel problems – which was super stuff to look back on and say yes, I thought that then – and these characters with enormous, rusty, sort of organic-looking roller skates with squeaking wheels that they couldn't handle very well. Also I had groups of these cyborg people wandering around looking so punky..." Bowie made these comments in 1980,

when he announced his intention to release the *Diamond Dogs* footage with a new musical accompaniment. The idea was dropped, but David was still mindful of the film as recently as 1996: a flying saucer from the test footage was used in the sleeve artwork of *Earthling*, and at the same time he recalled that John Lennon was present for some of the test footage: "Every now and then the camera catches sight of him in the background, sitting there with his guitar playing hits of the day and saying, 'What the bloody hell are you doing, Bowie? It's so negative, all your shit, all this *Diamond Dogs* mutant crap!'"

David announced in 1975 that he intended to follow *The Man Who Fell To Earth* with a stint of writing and directing for the cinema; there were rumours of a film based somehow on the *Young Americans* album, and in August he told the *NME* that "I've done nine screenplays over the past year ... I'll probably do the one I wrote for myself and Iggy Pop and Joan Stanton. I haven't even got a title for it yet and I don't really want to go into the story. But it's very violent and depressing, it's not gonna be a happy film." In late 1975 Bowie screen-tested for a role in *The Eagle Has Landed*.

One of the forgotten near-misses of the Thin White Duke period was the announcement in 1976 that Ken Russell was to direct *Bowie*, a three-and-a-half-hour biopic scripted by William Burroughs in which David would portray himself. "The script is meaningless," he told the *Sunday Times*, "but the clothes are nice." It remains unclear whether the story was a wind-up, but it certainly never happened.

There were rumours that Bowie was offered a part in Ingmar Bergman's 1977 film *The Serpent's Egg*, while in late 1977 it was reported that he was to star in *Wally*, a biopic about the German expressionist painter Egon Schiele which was due to shoot in Vienna in 1978. Bowie confirmed his involvement, but the film was never made. Another non-starter in 1978 was a German film of *The Threepenny Opera* in which Bowie was said to be starring.

1980s – 2000s

In 1982 it emerged that David had turned down the role of Satan in Richard Loncraine's film remake of Dennis Potter's banned television play *Brimstone And Treacle*; the part went instead to Sting. In 1983 Bowie was invited to play the disfigured villain Sharaz Jek in Peter Davison's final *Doctor Who* adventure: the show's director, Graeme Harper, was later quoted as saying that he wanted David "because he'd studied mime and used it quite extensively during the early years of his career. Bowie also had the kind of cocksure eloquence that Jek needed." The part eventually went to ballet principal Christopher Gable.

1984 saw rumours that David was to appear in *The French Orpheus* and *Benja The King*, and would be playing the lead in an American TV production about the Pied Piper. In the same year his name was mentioned in connection with *Burton And Speke*, eventually released in 1989 as *Mountains Of The Moon* with Iain Glen in the role.

Bowie was approached regarding the soundtrack for Roger Deakins's *1984*, starring Richard Burton and John Hurt. "No, I'm not doing that," he told *NME*. "There was talk of me doing that at one time, but I don't have enough time. I've seen bits of it and I think it's a fabulous movie. Really, really good." The film was eventually scored by Eurythmics, together with *Baal* composer Dominic Muldowney.

At around the same time, director Derek Jarman approached Bowie with a view to starring in a film called *Neutron*, but the project was shelved. The director would later claim that he believed Bowie had pulled out because he mistakenly believed Jarman to be a disciple of the Elizabethan magician Dr John Dee, whose magical system formed part of Aleister Crowley's Golden Dawn teachings. Dee had featured as a character in Jarman's earlier film *Jubilee*, and supposedly Bowie, in a flashback to his mid-1970s obsessions, had taken fright on seeing the Dee memorabilia residing in Jarman's flat. However, this colourful anecdote remains entirely unconfirmed by anyone other than the late director.

Early publicity for 1985's James Bond outing *A View To A Kill* announced that Bowie was lined up to play the psychopathic villain Max Zorin. A spokesman for Albert Broccoli went on record as saying that "David would make the perfect villain. We plan to exploit his unique physical oddity – his different-coloured and different-sized eyes", but by September 1984 Bowie was already quashing the story: "Absolutely out of the question. Yes, I was offered that … I think for an actor it's probably an interesting thing to do, but I think that for somebody from rock it's more of a clown performance. And I didn't want to spend five months watching my double fall off mountains." Subsequently turned down by Sting, the role eventually went to Christopher Walken (not, as often claimed, Grace Jones, who played Zorin's sidekick). Speaking many years later, Bowie explained that "it simply was a terrible script and I saw little reason for spending so long on something that bad, that workmanlike. And I told them so. I don't think anyone had turned down a major role in a Bond before. It really didn't go down too well at all. They were very tetchy about it."

In 2000, Bowie revealed that "The only Hollywood movie I regret having passed on was a piece that Ridley Scott wanted me very much to do. He even determined that if I didn't do it he wouldn't make it. Unfortunately I was touring at that time so it became an impossibility. He never did make it, so at least I know that I don't have to kick myself too hard."

In June 1989 it was reported that Bowie was to be the musical director of *The Delinquents*, a romantic teen drama that saw Kylie Minogue's first attempt to market herself as a sex-kitten; he withdrew from the project later in the year. Rumours of Bowie as a *Doctor Who* villain resurfaced in 1993 when the BBC planned a one-off anniversary special called 'The Dark Dimension', but the show was never made. And it has even been whispered in some quarters that Bowie makes an uncredited appearance in *Star Wars: Episode 1 – The Phantom Menace*.

In September 2000 the BBC announced that Bowie had turned down yet another *Doctor Who* role, this time for a webcast radio episode called 'Death Comes To Time'. In February 2001 various newspapers reported that Bowie had come to the financial rescue of Kate Winslet's dream project *Thérèse Raquin*, but by 2002 the film had been shelved. In the summer of 2001 rumours once again circulated that David had been asked to play Frank Sinatra in a new biopic, but he was quick to quash the story. At around the same time a rumour emerged that David was to take on the role of Count Dracula in an Italian TV mini-series. It remains unclear whether Bowie was ever genuinely offered the part, which was eventually played by Patrick Bergin. And finally, media gossip in 2003 that Jude Law was set to play David Bowie in a forthcoming biopic was utterly unfounded.

7   tHE artiSt anD tHE wriTEr

Like many a creative soul who dabbles in more than one medium, David Bowie has weathered his share of ridicule for having the audacity to be a painter as well as a rock singer. He remains unconcerned by the pigeon-holing instincts of critics: "I'm determined that if I want to paint, do installations or design costumes, I'll do it," he said in 1996. "If I want to write about something, I'll write about it."

Bowie's enthusiasm for the world of fine art infiltrated his lyrics as early as 1969, with a reference to Braque in 'Unwashed And Somewhat Slightly Dazed'. His penchant for antiques and paintings has been noted ever since Tony Visconti and Kenneth Pitt observed him blowing substantial amounts of his earliest 'Space Oddity' royalties on *objets d'art* for Haddon Hall. Today Bowie's private collection includes pieces by Rubens, Auerbach, Gilbert and George, Bomberg, Hirst and Tintoretto but, as is so often the case, the extent of his acquisitions has been wildly exaggerated. "Last week I was approached by a magazine about doing an interview on my 'Surrealist and Pre-Raphaelite' collection," he revealed in March 2003. "This was news to me. I'm sure there are many a wonderful Dali or Burne-Jones up for grabs, but there are none in my collection … Yes, I do have a (too frequently remarked upon) Tintoretto and a small Rubens … But the majority of what I have are British 20th century and not terribly big names. I've gone for what seemed to be an important or interesting departure at a certain time, or something that typified the atmosphere of a certain decade, rather than go for Hockneys or Freuds or whatever. To many people, this would seem to make my collection kind of boring as it is not loaded with front-page items. But I like it."

It was in Los Angeles in 1975 that David began painting in earnest, reaching his first peak of activity in Berlin two years later. He has always found painting not only a stimulus but also a challenge: "I don't think you have to love something to be able to produce something which is creative out of it," he said in 1983 when discussing his tribulations as a saxophonist. "I have the same relationship with paint. It's a struggle and we hate each other, but it doesn't have to mean you can't eventually get something onto a canvas that has a lot of spikiness to it."

It was not until the mid-1990s that he felt sufficiently confident to begin exhibiting his work formally. Around the time of the *1.Outside* sessions he became a familiar figure in the contemporary art scenes of various European capitals. In 1994 he purchased Peter Howson's Bosnian war painting *Croatian and Muslim* for £18,000 after the Imperial War Museum refused to hang it. In the same year he became a member of the editorial board of *Modern Painters*, a publication for which he would go on to interview the likes of Balthus, Roy Lichtenstein, Jeff Koons, Tracey Emin and Damien Hirst. "I love it," he said in 1999. "For me it's far preferable being on that end of it. I'm interested in how artists work. The process. How they got where they got, why they're like they are, how they do what they do. Those three things are what you want to find out about a person you admire."

Bowie's public dialogues with contemporary artists continue to crop up in the popular press. He later said of his time interviewing for *Modern Painters* that "I just enjoyed the heck out of it, knocking on some famous painter's door and saying, 'Hello, I'm your interviewer!' I did the last interview with Lichtenstein, about two weeks before he died. That was an extraordinary experience. But for me, the most rewarding one that I did was Balthus. I just talked with him for about four hours, and the magazine was so excited because nobody had seen him in twenty years. It was the most extensive interview done with him in forty years, and I see it quoted now in quite academic things. 'From the Bowie interview…' Whoa, that's me! That was a joy to do, because he was such a gentleman and so mysterious and knew he was pulling you along into his myth. There were so many secrets about him … The total reversal of that was Jeff Koons, who is absolutely what you see is what you get. I put Jeff in the same position that Warhol had during his lifetime. I think Jeff is among the greatest of American artists, and it's taken a long time for people to actually start thinking about him like that. Nobody could take him seriously. The big porcelain sculpture of Michael Jackson. Why would you want to do that? It's absurdism. But in a way, there's something incredibly poignant and immediate about his works, which you felt with Warhol. There's a naivety about both of them, but you can't help suspecting that there must be something else going on."

At around the time that he began contributing to *Modern Painters*, Bowie's own work was becoming increasingly prolific. In September 1994 he contributed a series of boxed prints called *We Saw A Minotaur* to an all-star auction arranged by Brian Eno in aid of the War Child charity. The exhibition, entitled *Little Pieces From Big Stars*, was held at the Flowers East Gallery in London and included contributions from Iggy Pop, Kate Bush, Neil Tennant, Robert Fripp, Pete Townshend, Bryan Ferry, Paul McCartney and many others. In keeping with the *1.Outside* album then in production, *We Saw A Minotaur* was a multimedia concoction in which computer-enhanced Minotaur pictures accompanied a narrative about a fictional playwright called Joni Ve Sadd who, in association with Ira Benno (as anagrams go, these are not tricky), devises a post-millennial stage-play in the year 2003. Following the auction, at which Bowie's pieces raised over £10,000, the work was included in the *Minotaur Myths And Legends* exhibition at London's Berkeley Square Gallery in November and December. Here David, who also designed the exhibition's poster, found his work on show alongside that of Picasso, Francis Bacon, Elizabeth Frink and Michael Ayrton.

Also in 1994 he famously designed a wallpaper pattern for Laura Ashley, a move that invited widespread derision. "Well, it's not very original," he commented. "Robert Gober and a number of others, even Andy Warhol, did them. It's just part of a tradition."

April 1995 saw Bowie's first one-man exhibition, a retrospective at London's Cork Street Gallery entitled *New Afro/Pagan And Work 1975-1995*. It included oil portraits of himself and Iggy Pop from Berlin, charcoal portraits of his *1.Outside* colleagues, computer-generated Minotaur images, and a silver mask cast from his face. Two pieces were inspired by a recent journey to South Africa, where David and Iman had attended the Johannesburg Biennale, conducted a photo shoot for *Vogue* and met President Mandela: *Dry Heads* was a large canvas depicting a black man and a white woman sharing a shower, while *Ancestor* was based on David's discovery that "One of the stories prevalent in Africa is that the ghosts of one's ancestors are white … so I just took that and did a series of ancestor figures with kind of Ziggy Stardust haircuts."

Bowie's friendships with Andy Warhol and Julian Schnabel made him the ideal choice to portray the former in the latter's 1996 film *Basquiat* (see Chapter 6). David contributed a design to War Child's fashion show Pagan Fun Wear, designed the poster for the 1995 Montreux Jazz Festival (quite an honour: previous designers include Hockney and Haring), and was present at the opening of the Tate's new gallery in St Ives. In 1995 his friendship with Damien Hirst produced a joint work entitled *Beautiful Hallo Space-boy Painting*. Bowie revealed that Hirst shared his fascination with the Minotaur, and that plans were afoot to create the ultimate piece of conceptual art by grafting a bull's head onto the body of an anonymous human donor and housing it in a purpose-built labyrinth on a Greek island. Perhaps thankfully, this particular piece of art remained genuinely conceptual.

In 1996 David remixed 'A Small Plot Of Land' as the theme music for the BBC series *A History Of British Art*, and sponsored an "Outside" International Art Competition whose panel of judges he joined on the closing day of the Outside tour. In the same year his installations with Tony Oursler (whose unique visual concepts were showcased in Bowie's 'Little Wonder' video and on the Earthling tour) were exhibited at the Florence Biennale. David's work with Oursler was also examined in a segment of the 1997 documentary *Inspirations*, a 100-minute film in which director Michael Apted discussed aspects of the creative process with a variety of artists working in different media (they also included Bowie's Sound + Vision collaborators Edouard Lock and Louise LeCavalier). Visiting David during preparations for his fiftieth birthday concert, Apted even filmed an exclusive in the form of a brief improvised song called 'Dead Men Don't Talk (But They Do)'.

In 1997 Bowie launched 21, his own fine arts publishing company, whose first title was *Blimey! From Bohemia to Britpop: The London Art World from Francis Bacon to Damien Hirst* by the artist and commentator Matthew Collings. April 1998 saw one of the more eccentric episodes in David's relationship with the art world when he was revealed as one of the perpetrators of an elaborate hoax: William Boyd's monograph on the life of Nat Tate, an obscure artist who had committed suicide in 1960, was published by 21 in a handsome edition with forewords by noted names in modern art. At an official launch several respected art critics made fools of themselves by sounding off about Nat Tate's life and work, but it didn't take long for someone to notice that the artist's name was blatantly concocted from "National" and "Tate", London's two biggest art galleries. Nat Tate was not merely an April Fool joke but a cutting exposure of the fragile web of reputation and credibility that holds the art world together.

At around this time Bowie's magazine articles had begun leading him towards a blossoming sideline as a writer of monographs, forewords and sleeve-notes with an artistic and pop-cultural bent: back in 1985 he had written liner notes for *Too Many Fish In The Sea*, an album by Carlos Alomar's wife Robin Clark, and by the turn of the century such commissions were becoming commonplace. Bowie's short preface in the Nat Tate book was followed by an essay on Jean-Michel Basquiat in the 2001 anthology *Writers On Artists*, and he wrote forewords for Jo Levin's 2000 publication *GQ Cool*, Mick Rock's 2001 photography portfolio *Blood And Glitter*, and Q magazine's 2002 special *The 100 Greatest Rock'n'Roll Photographs*. His substantial contribution to Genesis Publications' lavish 2002 book *Moonage Daydream* amounted to a full-scale memoir of the Ziggy Stardust years. Also in 2002 David provided thoughtful and revealing liner notes for the posthumous release of erstwhile collaborator Stevie Ray Vaughan's *Live At Montreux 1982-85*, while the following year he contributed sleeve notes to The Spinners' compilation *The Chrome Collection*. He even contributed the testimonial "Funny, fast, witty and brutal" to the cover blurb of *truecrime*, a 2003 novel by Jake Arnott ("Whenever he's got a new book out I drop everything," Bowie said elsewhere, "knowing that the next couple of hours are going to be pure gangland bliss").

David's paintings have occasionally been used as album artwork, the most obvious instance being the self-portrait *Head Of DB* which adorns the sleeve of *1.Outside*. Universal/Polygram's 1997 reissues of The Walker Brothers' albums *Portrait, Images* and *Take It Easy With The Walker Brothers* included a portrait of the band painted by David, who also donated a piece entitled *Costume For The Unborn Minotaur* for use as the sleeve design of Swiss artist Sandro Sursock's 1998 album *Zero Heroes*. The album's back cover featured a portrait of David with Iggy Pop, Coco Schwab, Sursock and Charuvan Suchi (both of whom, incidentally, had provided backing vocals on 'Zeroes' during the *Never Let Me Down* sessions in Montreux), sitting on a Max Ernst statue of the Minotaur.

The 1998 British International Motor Show at the Birmingham NEC included a display of customized Austin Minis designed by celebrities: Bowie came up with a mirror-festooned creation. In the same year his ten-foot painting *The Death Of Mama Wati*, made in collaboration with South Africa's Beezy Bailey, was exhibited at the Gallery New York in Brugg, Switzerland. In November 1998 the Museum Ludwig in Cologne opened its *I Love New York* exhibition, which included a conceptual work entitled *Line* – ten pairs of drawings made by David Bowie and Laurie Anderson while on the telephone to each other. January 1999 saw New York's Rupert Goldsworthy Gallery holding a successful Bowie show, and the following summer Antwerp's Studio Propaganda exhibited a collection of his paintings. He has contributed various items to the New York Academy of Art's *Take Home A Nude* charity auctions, including in 1999 a black canvas studded with the word "nipples" in Braille, and in 2001 a set of three prints depicting cut-up collages of photographic and painted nudes of both genders.

In December 1999 Bowie lent seven of his old costumes to the New York Metropolitan Museum's *Rock Style* exhibition. The collection, which moved in 2000 to Cleveland's Rock and Roll Hall of Fame and London's Barbican Centre, included David's 'Ashes To Ashes' and Thin White Duke outfits, his *Earthling* jacket, three Ziggy creations and the Glass Spider 'Time' costume. Also featured in the exhibition was some rare live footage from the Station To Station tour.

Bowie renewed his collaboration with Tony Oursler for the release in July 2000 of *Fantastic Prayers*, an interactive CD-ROM "installation" created by Oursler with performance artist Constance De Jong and composer Stephen Vitiello. Among its virtual environments is a graveyard in which an accidental click of the mouse reveals David making a cameo appearance as the "flower director".

In October 2000 David donated a self-portrait entitled *Dhead LXIII* to the ArtAid exhibition at London's Vinopolis Gallery in support of the HIV charity Crusaid, and in the same month he gave two portrait prints of his wife Iman to the Berklee College of Music for auction. In November he contributed a photograph called *East Side Other* to *Life's Ups And Downs*, a photo-book in aid of charities for the homeless which also featured pictures by the likes of George Michael, Kylie Minogue, Elvis Costello and Brian Eno. Also in November 2000, David contributed two pieces to the Royal College of Art's *Secret* auction, for which several hundred artists from Damien Hirst to Terry Gilliam created over 1500 postcard-sized pieces of work, the idea being that buyers would be unaware of the artist's identity – famous or otherwise – until they had purchased their postcard and turned it over to read the signature. When the project was repeated the following year, Bowie donated three more pieces.

In February 2001 David helped to launch Sotheby's "Art Against Addiction" auction, and later the same year he donated another piece to the Crusaid charity – this time a study of his baby daughter Alexandria's hand – to be used in a series of 2001 Christmas cards. Bowie again exhibited at New York's Rupert Goldsworthy Gallery in November 2001. Opening in the same month at London's Tate Modern was an Andy Warhol retrospective, which included rare film footage of a *Hunky Dory*-era Bowie performing mime for Warhol during the pair's famous first meeting at the Factory in 1971. November 2002 saw the opening of an exhibition called *Why Are You Creative?* at Frankfurt's Museum of Communication, which included artwork by figures as diverse as David Bowie and the Dalai Lama, and in the same month another of David's paintings was sold at ArtAid's annual Crusaid auction.

David's interest in art history has extended to providing voiceovers for various art documentaries, notably *Resurrecting Stanley*, an excellent edition of *Omnibus* devoted to the life and career of Stanley Spencer, transmitted on BBC2 on 3 March 2001. On a less highbrow level, he narrated a two-hour US documentary called *Hollywood Rocks The Movies: The 1970s*, premiered on the AMC channel on 30 August 2002.

Bowie has also become the subject of several paintings, not least Paul McCartney's canvas *Bowie Spewing* which appears in his retrospective collection *Paul McCartney: Paintings*, published in 2000. When asked if he minded the title, Bowie laughed, "Of course not – but what a coincidence, I'm currently working on a song that's called 'McCartney Shits'." October 2000 saw the opening of *Painting The Century*, a major exhibition at London's National Portrait Gallery which sought to hang one portrait per year in a cultural *tour d'horizon* of the twentieth century. A portrait of David and Iman by Stephen Finer took its place alongside paintings by the likes of Picasso, Munch, Bacon and Freud. The exhibition ran until February 2001. A more permanent exhibit in the National Portrait Gallery is another oil portrait of David by Stephen Finer, painted in 1994.

In November 2000 the American multimedia artist T J Wilcox used images of Bowie in his short film *The Little Elephants*, a surrealistic narrative blending *Babar* with *The Elephant Man* in the tale of an ugly duckling who travels from the jungle to the big city, transforms into David Bowie, and lives happily ever after. From June to September 2002, the Museum of Television and Radio in Los Angeles and New York hosted a *David Bowie: Sound + Vision* exhibition devoted to Bowie's career in the various creative media. Meanwhile, from August to September 2002 San Francisco's Gallery 16 hosted *Fascination*, an exhibition by artists whose work was influenced by Bowie, including erstwhile collaborators Rex Ray and Myriam Santos-Kayda. A similar venture was the February 2003 exhibition at Amsterdam's Stip Gallery called *Up The Hill Backwards! The Golden Years Of David Bowie*, in which 18 Dutch artists showed work inspired by David. In an entirely different sphere, artist Jamilla Naji's 2004 children's book *Musical Storyland* (see 'David Bowie Compilation Albums' in Chapter 2) is a collection of paintings illustrating ten of Bowie's 1960s compositions. In February-March 2004 photographer Denis O'Regan, who trailed Bowie for many years and was the official photographer on the Serious Moonlight and Glass Spider tours, held a *Bowie 78-90* exhibition at Camden's Proud Gallery.

Critical reaction to Bowie's art has been mixed. In a "blind" critique of the work of various celebrity artists for the *Daily Mirror* in September 2000, the notoriously outspoken critic Brian Sewell described Bowie's 1995 painting *Zenzi* as "ghastly" and "messy": "It simply doesn't work. The hand which drew it is clumsy." In 2001 Matthew Collings, who was rather more accommodating towards one of David's paintings in a similar feature for *Q* magazine, devoted much of the last episode of his Channel 4 series *Hello Culture* to the subject of Bowie's status as a pop-cultural icon, painting an entertaining but sympathetic portrait of the artist-celebrity. Bowie's 1995 Cork Street exhibition was widely praised, and he remains one of the few rock-musician painters whose work is accommodated and even admired within the art establishment.

Having reached a peak of activity in the mid-1990s, the frequency of Bowie's dabblings in the world of fine art went into decline alongside the increasing momentum of his reinvigorated recording career; by the time of *Heathen* and *Reality*, he was spending less time on extra-curricular projects and was painting only rarely. "I've been so taken with the music side of my life over the last couple of years that I've done nothing I'm particularly excited about," he told the *New York Post* in 2003. "But I've always found painting or sculpting has helped the progress of my music, especially in the early nineties." When asked what had brought about this change, he explained that "I've gotten much more confident about my writing. My need to work things out in another art form has diminished."

A selection of Bowie's paintings, prints and sculptures can be viewed (and purchased) at his art website www.bowieart.com, which also runs a showcase for art school students to enable them, as David explains, "to show and sell their work without having to go through a dealer. Therefore, they really make the money they deserve for their paintings." In 2001 Bowieart launched the Window Pain Project, a series of exhibitions in the windows of busy London streets, again dedicated to the work of artists embarking on their careers. A group of young artists selected from Bowieart dominated the *Sound And Vision* exhibition assembled by David for Meltdown 2002. Displayed in the Royal Festival Hall foyer throughout the Meltdown programme in June 2002, *Sound And Vision* offered a showcase for current and recent graduates from British colleges whose work was linked by the common thread of appealing to stimuli other than the purely visual. According to the Meltdown publicity, the works were "concerned with the intensities of musical or popular pleasures, employing contemporary culture as their language or sound as their source."

8   Interactive

"I don't think we've even seen the tip of the iceberg," Bowie told Newsnight's *Jeremy Paxman in December 1999. "I think the potential of what the Internet is going to do to* society – both good and bad – is unimaginable. I think we're actually on the cusp of something exhilarating and terrifying."

The Internet has become one of the most significant galvanizing influences in Bowie's creative landscape. Ever enthusiastic about new technologies, David was involved in the electronic media before most of us knew they existed: "We had electronic mail in '83," he revealed at NetAid, "and by '87, '88, I had the first artist newsgroup up ... so I've been fooling around with the Internet for a really long time." In September 1996 'Telling Lies' became the first Internet release by a mainstream artist, and websites dedicated to Bowie began proliferating at around the same time. The launch of David's own ISP, BowieNet, on 1 September 1998 was the next logical step.

Along with the usual Internet privileges, subscribers to BowieNet receive access to online chats with David and his collaborators, news, downloadable exclusives, sales of David's art, and of course the chance to see Bowie's name alongside one's own (yourname@davidbowie.com). In 1999 Bowie's online activities expanded into the field of financial services: BowieBanc.com offers savings accounts, credit cards and cheque-books adorned with David's image, in what it assures customers is a "complete look/feel experience designed around Bowie's music, art, and lifestyle". Less than a year after its foundation BowieNet was being valued at £300 million, and profiles of David had begun to appear in industry write-ups about the Internet's prime movers and shakers. In July 2000, BowieNet won the Best Artist Site award at the Yahoo! Internet Life Online Music Awards.

Unlike many Internet moguls Bowie is a keen user himself, revelling in the delights of chat-rooms and the Web's more trivial sideshows. "I am the first one to pop off to the 'slap a Spice Girl' site and the 'punch a Hanson'," he told *The Big Issue* in 1998. "And I real-ly like the site called 'Virtual Autopsy'. You get to take an entire body apart." He is entirely tolerant of the numerous Bowie fan sites, even when they advocate the trading of unofficial recordings: "I am absolutely not into shutting them down. In fact, quite the reverse. I like the idea of a network community. If I was 19 again, I'd bypass music and go straight to the Internet. When I was 19, music was still the dangerous communicative future force, and that was what drew me into it, but it doesn't have that cachet any more. It's been replaced by the Internet which has the same sound of revolution to it."

Among the most significant BowieNet projects so far is the "virtual CD" *liveandwell.com*, launched in 1998 to replace the abandoned *Earthling Live* album. Downloadable recordings from the 1997 tour were released through BowieNet, before being issued in 2000 on the *liveandwell.com* CD, an exclusive gift for BowieNet subscribers. Another high-profile project was the "cyber-song contest" to complete the lyrics of the *'hours...'* track 'What's Really Happening?'. In July 2000, BowieNet members were invited to choose their favourite mix of one of the live tracks for use on the *Bowie At The Beeb* bonus disc, and in 2001 they selected the cover artwork for the *All Saints* compilation. April 2001 saw the launch of BowieRadio, a BowieNet subsidiary which allows users to listen to an online "radio" station (playing Bowie tracks, naturally, alongside others chosen by David) while surfing the Net. Such events marked the first step in what Bowie calls "a new demystification process going on between the artist and the audience ... the interplay between the user and the provider will be so in simpatico it's going to crush our ideas about what mediums are all about."

In common with many artists, Bowie's CD singles from 1999 onwards have often included PC-playable video material. In the same year 'hours…' became the first album by a mainstream artist to be made available on the Internet in downloadable form, while July 2000 saw EMI reissuing 20 studio albums (*Space Oddity* to *Tin Machine*, and *1.Outside* to 'hours…') for commercial download. The same month saw Bowie's cameo appearance in artist Tony Oursler's interactive CD-ROM *Fantastic Prayers* (see Chapter 7). In November 2003, Sony UK released 'Never Get Old' as a download single, while two months earlier the little-heard 'Your Turn To Drive' had seen limited release as a promotional download for those who purchased *Reality* online from HMV. In April 2004 Sony launched an online remix competition in association with Audi of America, inviting contestants to compete for the prize of an Audi car by creating "mash-ups" from pre-selected Bowie clips using downloadable software.

Three other interactive projects merit special mention…

JUMP: THE DAVID BOWIE INTERACTIVE CD-ROM

MPC/Ion 76896-40004-2, 1994

Bowie's earliest commercial venture into PC technology was this pioneering but now antiquated CD-ROM. Released in 1994, *Jump* invited users to "Enter Bowie's Creative Universe" by manipulating video footage from 'Jump They Say' and viewing extracts from the *Black Tie White Noise* documentary. *Jump* has inevitably dated but its amusing details, which include hidden animations and sound triggers together with a background 'Lift Music' version of 'Jump They Say', are not without charm.

OMIKRON: THE NOMAD SOUL

In 1999 Bowie and Reeves Gabrels provided eight songs for the computer game *Omikron: The Nomad Soul*, created by Quantic Dream and Eidos Interactive, best known as the company behind *Tomb Raider*. The game, which spent two years in development, boasts over 400 different environments in its four virtual city locations, 150 characters in "3D real time", four hours of dialogue and over 1200 different responses. It seems likely that Bowie was attracted by *Omikron*'s Buddhist overtones: when a character dies, he or she is reincarnated in the body of whoever happens to be nearest. David appears in the game as "Boz", leader of "The Awakened", and with Gabrels and Gail Ann Dorsey he can be encountered performing in the bars and streets of Omikron City. "You never know where you'll see us," Bowie explained. "It's fascinating and advanced. It won't be long, I think, before video games have the same appeal as the cinema, once they begin involving more screenwriters, people who work with story and character." David's wife Iman also appears in the game as a bodyguard for hire.

"I moved right away from the stereotypical industrial game music sound," revealed David. "My priority in writing music for *Omikron* was to give it an emotional subtext. It feels to me as though Reeves and I have achieved that." *Omikron* features variant versions of every track from 'hours…' except 'If I'm Dreaming My Life', 'Brilliant Adventure' and 'What's Really Happening?', plus the B-side 'We All Go Through' and four otherwise unavailable instrumentals, 'Awaken 2', 'Jangir', 'Qualisar' and 'Thrust'.

AMPLITUDE

In May 2003, nearly a decade after *Jump: The David Bowie Interactive CD-ROM*, Sony PlayStation 2 released its music-mixing game *Amplitude* – effectively, a far more sophisticated variation on the same idea. Among the songs that could be manipulated and remixed "within more than 20 immersive levels" (whatever that means) was an interactive version of the METRO remix of 'Everyone Says 'Hi''. Other artists whose recordings featured in the game included Garbage, Pink, Weezer and Blink 182.

apocrypha

Tales of uncredited recordings by David Bowie are legion, although most of them are nonsense. There are rumours, for example, that the Deram-era Bowie was responsible for the anonymous versions of the Beatles' 'Penny Lane' and the Monkees' 'A Little Bit Me A Little Bit You' included on the 1967 covers compilation *Hits 67*. Other anonymous covers of the era sometimes attributed to a cash-strapped Bowie include versions of Donovan's 'Hurdy Gurdy Man' and Don Partridge's 'Rosie'. The uncredited singer sounds not unlike David in his Anthony Newley phase, but there is no corroboration of the story and it seems highly unlikely that the recordings would have gone unmentioned in Kenneth Pitt's otherwise painstaking *The Pitt Report*.

David is often incorrectly said to feature on various singles released by his early bands after he had left them, notably The King Bees' 'You're Holding Me Down' and The Kon-rads' 'Baby It's Too Late Now', both of which are unquestionably after his time. The rare US/Canadian Kon-rads single 'I Didn't Know How Much', discovered in 2001, is a trickier proposition, but proof of David's presence on the recording has yet to emerge – and, and in the light of the 1965 Kon-rads studio tape which emerged a year later, it seems highly unlikely.

Contrary to the extravagant claims made by the liner notes of 1989's *Radio One* album, Bowie did not provide backing vocals on Jimi Hendrix's BBC session recording of 'Day Tripper', which was performed for *Top Gear* on 15 December 1967. David was indeed in the studio for the same show, but the idea that he sang on the Hendrix session is, in his own words, "Rubbish. Wish it were true though."

Famously, Bowie is rumoured to provide backing vocals and saxophone on 'Oh Baby'/'Universal Love', a 1970 single credited to Dib Cochran & The Earwigs. The rumour is without foundation: the group was in fact fronted by Tony Visconti and backed by a collection of his 1970 collaborators: Marc Bolan, John Cambridge, Tim Renwick and Rick Wakeman. Mick Ronson was present for the recording and may have added a guitar line, but contrary to rumour neither Bowie nor Bolan's bongo player Mickey Finn appear on the recording.

Bolan aficionados have also suggested that Bowie provided handclaps on the 1968 Tyrannosaurus Rex hit 'Debora', and later sax and backing vocals on 'New York City', 'Dreamy Lady', 'London Boys' and 'I Love To Boogie', all of which were released as singles between July 1975 and June 1976. Tony Visconti insists that this is untrue: "It's hearsay, it's what fans would love to believe," he told Barney Hoskyns. "If David Bowie had appeared on any of his records, believe me, Marc would have been the first to talk about it."

Bowie is rumoured to appear on The Rolling Stones' 1974 album *It's Only Rock'n'Roll*, and also on Ron Wood's solo debut *I've Got My Own Album To Do* from the same year. He was certainly present for some of the Stones sessions in Hilversum, where he was putting the finishing touches to *Diamond Dogs*, and Wood certainly played on his 1973 cover of 'Growin' Up', but Bowie's presence on either album remains unsubstantiated. The actor Christopher Lee recalls being summoned at around the same time to discuss a duet with Bowie, but apparently the pair were unable to agree on a suitable song.

One of several rumours from Bowie's lost year in Los Angeles is an alleged contribution to Keith Moon's 1975 solo album *Two Sides Of The Moon*. Along with Ringo Starr, Ron Wood (again) and Klaus Voorman, Bowie is said to have played on the outtakes 'Do Me Good', 'Real Emotion' and 'Naked Man', later included on some reissues. Again, there is no proof of Bowie's involvement. Even less likely is the suggestion that he appears on an alleged studio duet with John Lennon, again supposedly from 1975, performing 'Let's Twist Again'. The track has appeared on bootlegs but fails to convince, and Lennon's girlfriend May Pang, later Tony Visconti's wife, has confirmed that the two *Young Americans* tracks were Lennon's only recordings with Bowie.

Yet another alleged 1975 session, this time with Nina Simone, is said to have taken place at RCA's West Coast Studios in Los Angeles. It is known that David met Simone during this period and was a great admirer of her work – his recording of 'Wild Is The Wind' was made in her honour – but there is no evidence of a collaboration.

Bowie is unreliably rumoured to play saxophone on the Mekons' album *The Mekons*. Similarly dubious is a trio of bootleg instrumentals entitled 'Low', 'Lodger 1' and 'Lodger 2', which purport to hail from unspecified Bowie/Eno sessions during the late 1970s.

There is no doubt about David's presence on the 1979 John Cale demos 'Velvet Couch' and 'Pianola', but there is no proof whatsoever of his alleged involvement in a further series of Cale demos, some of which later resurfaced among his solo work: titles vary from bootleg to bootleg, but the dodgy demos include 'I've Nothing More To Destroy', 'Honi Soit', 'Cry Like A Pony' (aka 'Ride The Pony'), 'Baby Candy', 'Wednesday', 'Mandela Tribute', 'Looking For A Friend', 'Where Have You Been, My Only Love' and 'Augusto Pinochet'.

DON'T THINK YOU KNEW YOU WERE IN THIS SONG...

Among the songs rumoured to be *about* David Bowie are Brian Eno's 'Spider And I' (from 1977's *Before And After Science*), Bauhaus's 'King Volcano' (from 1983's *Burning From The Inside*), and the 1973 Rolling Stones tracks 'Angie' and 'Dancing With Mr D' (both from *Goat's Head Soup*). Isabelle Adjani's eponymous 1983 album includes a song with the punning title 'Beau Oui Comme Bowie' ("Handsome, yes, like Bowie"). Bongwater offered the track 'David Bowie Wants Ideas' on 1991's *Double Bummer*, while Phish recorded a song called 'David Bowie' on 1992's *Junta*. Dutch artist Gyllene Tider's eponymous 1990 album included a song called 'Åh Ziggy Stardust (Var Blev Du Av?)' ('Ah Ziggy Stardust, what became of you?'). Veruca Salt's 1997 album *Eight Arms To Hold You* includes a track called 'With David Bowie', although contrary to rumours David made no contribution to the recording.

Straightforward Bowie parodies include the HeeBeeGeeBees' seminal 1981 track 'Quite Ahead Of My Time' and Liam Lynch's 2003 offering 'Fake Bowie Song: Eclipse Me'. Less than hilariously, The Strawbs' 1972 track 'Backside' was credited to "Ciggy Barlust and the Whales From Venus".

Rather more uplifting is a song called 'Magical' which appears on Gail Ann Dorsey's 2003 album *I Used To Be...* Bowie's long-time bassist wrote the song as a paean to David in 1998, at a time when she was in low spirits and uncertain whether she would work with him again (as subsequent tours have demonstrated, she need not have worried).

There are lyrical references to Bowie in songs by the Clash ('Clash City Rockers'), Kraftwerk ('Trans-Europe Express'), the Undertones ('Mars Bars'), Joni Mitchell ('The Hissing Of Summer Lawns'), Bon Jovi ('Captain Crash And The Beauty Queen From Mars'), Dave Stewart ('Chelsea Lovers'), Bush ('Everything Zen'), Marilyn Manson ('Apple Of Sodom'), Boy George ('Who Killed Rock'n'Roll'), Tori Amos ('Riot Poof'), Kathi McDonald ('Bogart To Bowie'), Reunion ('Life Is A Rock But The Radio Rolled Me'), Nina Hagen ('New York New York'), The Wild Ones ('Bowie Man'), Yellow Magic Orchestra ('Tighten Up'), Tom Petty and the Heartbreakers ('The Same Old You'), Robyn Hitchcock ('1974'), Red Hot Chili Peppers ('Californication'), Snake Rock ('No More Glamour Boys'), Bubbi Morthens ('Blindsker'), Danny Boy ('Castro Boys'), Adam And The Ants ('Friends'), Peter Schilling (his 1984 single 'Major Tom (Coming Home)' is a sequel to 'Space Oddity'), Panic On The Titanic ('Major Tom'), Def Leppard (their 1987 song 'Rocket' mentions Major Tom), Robbie Williams (his 2000 hit 'Rock DJ' mentions 'Ground Control'), The Smiths ('Sheila Take A Bow' borrows from 'Kooks'), Jeffrey Gaines ('Somewhat Slightly Dazed'), the Subhumans ('No More Gigs'), the Beastie Boys ('Car Thief'), Funkadelic ('White Funk'), Parliament ('P. Funk'), Crash Pad ('TS/TV'), The Bloodhound Gang ('Legend In My Spare Time'), Dr Hook ('Everybody's Making It Big But Me'), Crash Pad ('TSTV'), The Angry Samoans ('Get Off The Air'), Brian Jonestown Massacre ('Since I Was Six (David Bowie I Love You)'), Black Randy & the Metrosquad ('Pass The Dust, I Think I'm Bowie'), Saucer ('Knick-Knacks For David Bowie'), The Treatment ("The Rise & Fall Of David

Bowie And The Glamrockers From Hammersmith'), Lockwood McCay ('T Rex And The Thin White Duke'), The Clean ('David Bowie'), The Batfish Boys ('The Birth Of Rock And Roll'), Tracy Bonham ('One Hit Wonder') and Patricia Kaas ('Hotel Normandy'). No Doubt's 2004 single 'It's My Life' included a mix named, for no readily apparent reason, the 'Thin White Duke Remix'. *The Man Who Fell To Earth* cops a mention in Big Audio Dynamite's 'E=MC^2', and there's even a mention of "David Bowie LPs" in John Sullivan's closing music for the long-running BBC1 sitcom *Only Fools And Horses.*

Music videos are by no means immune to Bowie references either. Marc Almond dresses as a host of pop icons including a Ziggy-era Bowie in the video of his 1995 single 'Adored And Explored' (and on the sleeve of its follow-up single 'The Idol'), while Spice Girl Mel C dons a replica of David's 'Rebel Rebel' pirate outfit during a fantasy sequence in 1997's cinematic triumph *Spiceworld The Movie*. 2003's no less cerebral masterpiece *Charlie's Angels: Full Throttle* finds Drew Barrymore fighting in full Aladdin Sane make-up to the strains of 'Rebel Rebel'. Depeche Mode's Martin Gore dressed as Aladdin Sane for a back-projection film used on the band's 1998 tour, while in October 2001 Boy George performed 'Starman' in full Bowie make-up for his winning turn in ITV's *Popstars In Their Eyes* celebrity contest. In May of the same year, regular contestant Tony Perry had reached the *Stars In Their Eyes* final with his performance of 'Ashes To Ashes', dressed as Bowie in his 1996 Brit Awards outfit. In December 2002, a follow-up celebrity special saw Boy George repeat his victory, this time singing 'Sorrow' in Aladdin Sane make-up. In the same month the ubiquitous Bowie acolyte Jonathan Ross followed suit, dressing as Ziggy for BBC1's *They Think It's All Over* Christmas special. The video of Pulp's 2002 single 'Bad Cover Version' lampooned Band Aid's 'Do They Know It's Christmas?', assembling a studio full of lookalikes including a Bowie double who not only bears an uncanny physical resemblance to David but also pulls off a creditable vocal impersonation. The sleeve of 'Bad Cover Version' was a parody of the *Ziggy Stardust* album cover, right down to the typeface and the tinted colours. A similar trick was attempted by the Baltimore-based artist CEX, whose 2003 album *Being Ridden* features a recreation of the *"Heroes"* album cover pose.

The *Aladdin Sane* sleeve, another of rock's classic images, has been aped and parodied by all and sundry. In 2001 it was appropriated by an advertising campaign for Absolut vodka, while in 2002 a cartoon version by Matt Groening, featuring Homer Simpson as Aladdin Sane, was among a series of album cover parodies featured in *Rolling Stone.*

Several bands have named themselves after Bowie songs or lyrics, among them Simple Minds (from 'The Jean Genie'), King Volcano (from 'Velvet Goldmine'), Belfast punk outfit Rudi (from 'Star') and Saviour Machine. One of U2's early names was The Hype, while Joy Division were at one time called Warsaw (and also recorded a song of the same name) in honour of 'Warszawa'. Nick Lowe responded to *Low* by calling a 1977 EP 'Bowi', while the Pink Fairies' album *Kings Of Oblivion* takes its name from 'The Bewlay Brothers'. Suede's 1994 epic *Dog Man Star* is named after three pivotal early Bowie albums (*Diamond Dogs, The Man Who Sold The World* and *Ziggy Stardust*).

Bowie's work has even inspired various works of fiction, including the titles of novels such as Kate Muir's *Suffragette City* (1999) and Alan Watt's *Diamond Dogs* (2000). Philip K Dick's 1981 novel *Valis* features a series of characters and scenarios inspired directly by the author's fascination with Bowie and in particular *The Man Who Fell To Earth*. The protagonist of Eric Idle's 1999 comic novel *The Road To Mars* is a "4.5 Bowie Artificial Intelligence Robot", doubtless named in honour of Idle's long friendship with David. Harland Miller's 2000 novel *Slow Down Arthur, Stick To Thirty* charts the adventures of a Bowie impersonator in Yorkshire in the early 1980s. "I kind of quite like the idea," David remarked after reading the book, "though I'm not sure he's a very good writer." Similar territory is covered by *This Little Ziggy*, a comic memoir by Martin Newell published in 2001. Dave Thompson's 2002 epistolary novel *To Major Tom: The Bowie Letters* tells the narrator's story via a series of fan letters written to Bowie over the years.

HOW THE OTHERS MUST SEE THE FAKER...

Bowie has been portrayed, lampooned and parodied in countless send-ups like ITV's *Spitting Image* and Channel 4's *The Comedy Lab*, but without doubt the funniest and best is BBC2's cult classic *Stella Street* (1997-present) in which John Sessions and Phil Cornwell impersonate a pantheon of unlikely celebrities who inhabit a leafy suburb of London. Cornwell's affectionate rendering of Bowie as a maladroit loser, given to ineffectual karate moves, extempore compositions ("There's a man in the moon, and 'e plays on the spoons, 'e goes golfing in Troon"), failed acting auditions, and unexpected mid-sentence bursts of his histrionic vocal technique, is savage but brilliant. Those not yet initiated in the delights of *Stella Street*, whose central character Mrs Huggett is one of the unsung heroines of modern Britain, are strongly advised to seek out the videos and DVDs.

August 2000 saw the London debut of a Bowie-related fringe play entitled *From Ibiza To The Norfolk Broads*, which ran for a month at the Camden People's Theatre. Written and directed by Adrian Berry, the play dealt with anorexic teenager Martin's obsession with Bowie. From his hospital bed, Martin indulges in *Kiss of the Spiderwoman*-style dream sequences in which he communicates with Bowie (voiced for the production by comedian Rob Newman) while various songs from 'Little Wonder' to 'Rock'n'Roll Suicide' reflect his predicament. The production, hailed by *Time Out* as "one of those rare things: a fringe play which exceeds all expectations", was revived in August 2001 at the Edinburgh Fringe Festival, where Bowie fans could also see Des de Moor and Russell Churney performing a critically acclaimed cabaret show based on David's songs called *Darkness And Disgrace*, which had opened at London's Rosemary Branch Theatre in April 2000 before touring the Home Counties. *Darkness And Disgrace*, which interspersed an eclectic selection of Bowie numbers with literary excerpts throwing light on his work (Orwell, Heinlein and so on) was revived at London's Pentameters Theatre in February 2003, and the same year saw the release of a CD recording of songs from the show. Not to be outdone, in March 2001 director David Hollywood unveiled a "conceptual theatre piece" called *Life On Mars* at the Wentworth Falls School of Arts in Australia. According to press releases the production tackled "themes of suburban life, alienation, fame and self-destruction" as told through the story of two brothers from the Bewlay family whose parents are a couple of kooks. Oh dear. The show transferred to Sydney's Newton Theatre the following November.

Cameron Crowe's 2000 film *Almost Famous*, inspired by the director's experiences as a teenage rock reporter on the US tour circuit in the mid-1970s (he famously interviewed Bowie at the height of his Los Angeles exile), features what is perhaps the cinema's first "fictional" portrayal of Bowie, in a scene in which a mob of fans crowd around a briefly-glimpsed Ziggy lookalike in a hotel lobby. David, who described *Almost Famous* as "a terrific film", had of course already appeared as himself in 1981's *Christiane F.*, and later reprised the role in Ben Stiller's 2001 comedy *Zoolander*.

Still the most prominent Bowie take-off in recent years is American writer/director Todd Haynes's 1998 glam fantasia *Velvet Goldmine* which, despite its creator's half-hearted denials ("No, it's not Bowie and Iggy Pop," he claimed in a pre-release interview), is a sustained exercise in obscure and parodic re-enactments of Bowie's 1970s career. In addition to Bowie ("Brian Slade") and Iggy Pop ("Curt Wild"), there are blatant approximations of Kenneth Pitt, Tony Defries, Angela Bowie, Coco Schwab, Ava Cherry, Marc Bolan and Freddi Burretti. There's even a cameo by Bowie's one-time guru Lindsay Kemp as a pantomime dame. Whether or not the cast are aware of it, Haynes devotes much of his film to the painstaking re-enactment of mythical moments from the Ziggy period: there is a re-staging of Bowie and Ronson's guitar-fellatio routine, for example, and a shot-for-shot recreation of Don Pennebaker's backstage footage from Hammersmith. Brian Slade's dialogue is peppered with quotations from Bowie interviews.

Bowie was originally invited to cooperate on *Velvet Goldmine* which is, of course, named after one of his songs. His music was central to Haynes's conception: 'All The Young Dudes', 'Velvet Goldmine', 'Lady Stardust', 'Moonage Daydream', 'Sweet Thing', 'Lady Grinning Soul' and Bowie's 'Let's Spend The Night Together' were all in the original storyboards. "I read the script thoroughly and I made sure that I saw all of Todd Haynes's movies to see what kind of a filmmaker he was," said Bowie in 1999, "and then I said no!" In the end, the nearest the film gets to a Bowie contribution is a snatch of Lou Reed's 'Satellite Of Love'.

Velvet Goldmine is splendidly performed and ravishingly photographed, and the pastiches of concert footage and promo films are delightful – although the cutting-edge New Romantic chic of the visuals has no period sensibility whatsoever. The real problem is that the film takes itself far too seriously. Moreover, it pretends to be a fiction while simultaneously sucking on the lives of real people, with the result that it leaves a rather bitter taste in the mouth. "I really hope Bowie can see in the film the affection and respect I have for him," said Haynes in 1998. Frankly, I wouldn't count on it. It's not remotely surprising that Bowie dissociated himself from the movie, because the portrayal of "Brian Slade" is wholly unsympathetic and often openly offensive.

In any case, *Velvet Goldmine* ultimately tells us more about Todd Haynes than it does about David Bowie. For Haynes, glam rock clearly represents the triumphant enfranchisement of clandestine, guilt-ridden gay youth, and of course that was one of its most positive achievements. But in reducing the whole story to a series of baroque sexual fantasies bolstered by every iconic gay utterance of Bowie's career, Haynes misappropriates glam and does it few favours. "I think *Velvet Goldmine* was grossly inaccurate about those times," declared Tony Visconti in 1998. "I think it was unfair to borrow from Bowie's life and distort it so much, and create the illusion that it was Bowie, and not some fictional character. Basically, I thought it was a gay porn film disguised as a musical." Mick Rock concurred, believing that the film "had nothing to do with that period … Make-up was nothing to do with being gay." Even Angela Bowie has weighed in against *Velvet Goldmine*, telling an interviewer in 2000 that she considered the film "muddled around in glam rock masturbatory narcissism."

To reject an exclusively gay reading of glam is to admit the more complex reality. Of course David Bowie made life better for a lot of gay kids and we mustn't underestimate that achievement, but his weapons were those of the aesthete: artifice, intelligence and imagination. *Velvet Goldmine* is big on Oscar Wilde (whom Haynes appears to consider a gay man first and a mildly influential writer second), but makes no investment in glam's genuine Wildean connection, which is surely its essential bookishness. Glam, like Wilde, thrived on intellectual dilettantism and the flaunting of a mannered, middle-class ennui. Where "Brian Slade" truly differs from his *alter ego* is

that he's a leaden, inarticulate yobbo who wouldn't know Jack Kerouac, Tibetan Buddhism or German expressionism if they bit him on the backside.

Bowie has by and large kept his counsel about *Velvet Goldmine*, although he did remark in one interview that "The film didn't understand how innocent everyone was then, about what they were getting into. Also, there was a lot more shopping." In 2002 he offered the less guarded opinion that "I thought the sex scenes were good, but I thought the rest of it was utter garbage." Haynes seems unwilling to accept that glam was never anything more than what Oscar Wilde called "a delicate bubble of fancy", built on hype and rejoicing in its own flimsiness. At the end of the picture he gets all sulky about the idea that his hero has sold out and betrayed some sort of authentic ideal. This in the end makes *Velvet Goldmine* a rather silly and spiteful film.

A more intelligent, creative and rewarding exploration of Bowie's native territory is to be found in John Cameron Mitchell's remarkable rock theatre creation *Hedwig And The Angry Inch*, which began life as a fringe theatre project in 1994 before becoming an Off-Broadway success in 1998, and was finally adapted into a film, directed by and starring Mitchell, in 2001. Bowie, who was among many celebrities drawn to the New York run when the show began receiving rave reviews and critics' awards, was sufficiently impressed to co-produce the Los Angeles transfer in October 1999. "*Hedwig* is the most wholly rounded piece of rock theatre that we've seen in years," he said at the time.

Framed by the tragicomic anecdotes of a German "song-stylist" who has undergone a botched sex-change operation in order to escape East Berlin, *Hedwig And The Angry Inch* tells of a picaresque quest for love, fulfilment and identity, offering both the division of Berlin and the tradition of stage transvestism as metaphors for the Aristophanic androgynes whose quest for their missing halves is described in Plato's *Symposium*. Stephen Trask's excellent glam-punk songs pursue the theme in a style clearly indebted to the likes of Lou Reed, Iggy Pop and David Bowie, influences freely acknowledged in the dialogue: of particular interest are the stomping *Transformer*-style number 'Wig In A Box' and the final cathartic 'Midnight Radio', musically and lyrically a close cousin of 'Rock'n'Roll Suicide', culminating in a reiterated entreaty to "Lift up your hands!" The film offers plenty of nods to Bowie's influence (a guitar fellatio scene, Hansel's Thin White Duke hairstyle, and a blatant 'Starman' arm-round-the-guitarist's-shoulder moment in the final number), but while many critics drew obvious parallels with Bowie's Berlin period and his androgynous Ziggy persona, *Hedwig* is ultimately very much Mitchell's own creation, its sharp, intelligent themes transcending mere pastiche. As *Variety Entertainment* observed of the Los Angeles theatre transfer, "David Bowie has signed on as a producer for this open-ended LA run, and the match is ideal. Hedwig's unparalleled identity crisis and effortless charisma capture the essence of glam-rock in a way that the film *Velvet Goldmine* never touched, and take it into a political and global context." By the time of the film's release in 2001 (complete with publicity photographs by – who else? – Mick Rock), *Hedwig* had deservedly become a cult of *Rocky Horror Show* proportions.

10

DATELINE

RECORDING & RELEASES	STAGE	TV & FILM
1958	**1958**	**1958**
	August ? Isle of Wight *(David Jones and George Underwood perform at 18th Bromley Scouts summer camp)*	
1962	**1962**	**1962**
	June 16 Bromley Technical High School *(this and all dates to May 1963 as The Kon-rads)* Month Unknown ? Bromley, Church Hall *(rehearsals)* ? Chislehurst Caves, Kent November 17 Cudham, Village Hall	
1963	**1963**	**1963**
August 30 The Kon-rads record 'I Never Dreamed' at Decca Studios	Month Unknown ? Orpington, Civic ? West Wickham, Wickham Hall May 18 Biggin Hill, Hillsiders Youth Club 25 Bromley Technical High School *(2 shows)* ? West Wickham, Ravensbourne College of Art July ? Bromley, Bromel Club *(this and next 3 dates as The Hooker Brothers)* ? West Wickham, Ravensbourne College of Art August ? Bromley, Bromel Club September ? Bromley, Bromel Club	
1964	**1964**	**1964**
June 5 Single release: 'Liza Jane'	April 14 London, Jack Of Clubs *(this and next 5 dates as Davie Jones and the King Bees)* May 15 London, Marquee 17 London, Café des Artistes 21 London, Roundhouse June 7 London, Bedsitter, Holland Park Avenue	June 6 'Liza Jane' features on BBC's *Juke Box Jury*. 19 'Liza Jane' performed on

RECORDING & RELEASES	STAGE	TV & FILM
	Month Unknown ? London, Bricklayer's Arms, Old Kent Road	Associated Rediffusion's *Ready, Steady, Go!* July 27 'Liza Jane' performed on BBC2's *The Beat Room*
	August 19 London, Eel-Pie Island *(this and all dates to 20 March 1965 as The Manish Boys)* 30 Ipswich September 2 London, Eel-Pie Island 9 Braintree ? Luton ? Chislehurst Caves 19 London, The Scene 21 Chatham, Invicta Ballroom 23 Medway County Youth Club 26 London, Acton Town Hall 27 London, Flamingo Club 29 Isleworth	
October 6 'Hello Stranger', 'Love Is Strange' and 'Duke Of Earl' recorded at Regent Sound Studios	October 2 Borehamwood, Lynx Club 7 London, Eel-Pie Island 9 London, Finchley 10 Newmarket 13 London, Putney 17 Leigh-on-Solent, Tower Ballroom 25 Leigh-on-Solent 31 Bromley November 6 London, Marquee 7 Bedford 8 London, Eel-Pie Island 13 Hastings, Witchdoctor 14 Maidstone, Agricultural Hall 20 Bromley, Justin Hall December 1 Wigan, ABC Cinema *(2 shows)* 2 Hull, ABC Cinema *(2 shows)* 3 Edinburgh, ABC Cinema, Lothian Road *(2 shows)* 4 Stockton, Globe Cinema *(2 shows)* 5 Newcastle *(2 shows)* 6 Scarborough *(2 shows)* 13 Bedford	November 12 David gives his first TV interview on BBC's *Tonight*, as spokesman for "The Society For The Prevention Of Cruelty to Long-Haired Men"
1965	**1965**	**1965**
February 8 'I Pity The Fool' and 'Take My Tip' recorded at IBC Studios	February 1 Maidstone, Star Ballroom March 4 Bournemouth 10 Bromley, Bromel Club 20 Cromer, Olympia Ballrooms April ? London, La Discothèque *(David auditions for The Lower Third)*	March 8 'I Pity The Fool' on BBC2's *Gadzooks! It's All Happening*

RECORDING & RELEASES	STAGE	TV & FILM
May 'Born Of The Night' demoed at Central Sound Studios 20 The Lower Third record radio jingles at R G Jones Studios	8 Minster, Working Men's Club *(this and all dates to September 1965 as Davie Jones and The Lower Third)* 10 Sheerness, Sheerness & District MCC Conservative Club 11 Minster, Working Men's Club May 17 Littlestone, Grand Hotel 28 Bournemouth, Pavilion 30 Bournemouth, Pavilion June 4 Bournemouth, Pavilion 5 Queensborough, Borough Hall 11 Brighton, Starlight Rooms 12 Manchester, King's Head 13 London, Roebuck Pub *(The Lower Third audition for Ralph Horton)* 14 Leeds, White Bear Tavern 19 Edgbaston, Happy Towers Ballroom 23 Tadcaster, Fairlight Gardens 25 Bournemouth, Pavilion 26 Bromley, Bromel Club 27 Bournemouth, Pavilion July 2 Bournemouth, Pavilion 3 Isle of Wight, Ventnor Winter Gardens 4 Bournemouth, Pavilion 10 Isle of Wight, Ventnor Winter Gardens 17 Isle of Wight, Ventnor Winter Gardens 24 Isle of Wight, Ventnor Winter Gardens 25 Sheerness, Sheerness & District MCC Conservative Club 31 Isle of Wight, Ventnor Winter Gardens	
August 20 Single release: 'You've Got A Habit Of Leaving'	August 7 Isle of Wight, Ventnor Winter Gardens 14 Isle of Wight, Ventnor Winter Gardens 19 London, 100 Club 21 Isle of Wight, Ventnor Winter Gardens 26 London, 100 Club 28 Isle of Wight, Ventnor Winter Gardens September 4 London, Marquee 7 London, 100 Club 11 London, Marquee 14 London, 100 Club 18 London, Marquee 21 London, 100 Club 25 London, Marquee	

RECORDING & RELEASES	STAGE	TV & FILM
	28 London, 100 Club October 8 London, Marquee (this and all dates to 29 Jan 1966 as David Bowie and the Lower Third) November 5 London, Marquee 19 London, Marquee December 10 London, Marquee 24 London, La Discothèque 31 Paris, Golfe-Drouot Club	
November 2 The Lower Third audition for the BBC		December 31 Clip of Paris concert is thought to have been shown on French TV
1966	**1966**	**1966**
January 14 Single release: 'Can't Help Thinking About Me'	January 1 Paris, Montmartre Bus Palladium 2 Paris, Golfe-Drouot Club 6 London, Victoria Tavern (launch party for 'Can't Help Thinking About Me') 7 London, Marquee 12 Newmarket, Community Hall 15 Harrow, Alexander Tavern 17 Carlisle, Holly Bush 19 Birmingham, Cedar Club 28 Stevenage, Town Hall 29 London, Marquee (matinee); Bromley, Bromel Club (cancelled) February 3-5 London, Marquee (The Buzz auditions) 10 Leicester, Mecca Ballroom (this and all remaining 1966 dates as David Bowie and The Buzz) 11 London, Marquee 26 Chelmsford, Corn Exchange 28 Eastbourne, Club Continental	
March 7 'Do Anything You Say' and 'Good Morning Girl' recorded at Pye Studios	March 5 Birmingham, Cranes Record Shop ? Crawley ? Bournemouth 12 Brighton, Club 101 ? Southampton 18 High Wycombe, Target Club ? Nottingham ? Peterborough ? Newmarket 25 Harrow, Alexander Tavern	March 4 'Can't Help Thinking About Me' on Associated Rediffusion's Ready, Steady, Go!
April 1 Single Release: 'Do Anything You Say'	April 2 Carlisle, Holly Bush 3 Edinburgh (cancelled) 4 Dundee, College 5 Glasgow, Green's Playhouse 6 Hawick 9 Thetford, Guildhall (2 shows) 10 London, Marquee (first of the "Bowie Showboat" gigs sponsored by	

RECORDING & RELEASES	STAGE	TV & FILM
	Radio London)	
	17 London, Marquee	
	24 London, Marquee	
	25 Chester	
	May	
	1 London, Marquee	
	8 London, Marquee	
	15 London, Marquee	
	18 Thetford, Guildhall	
	22 London, Marquee	
	29 London, Marquee *(matinee);* Blackpool, South Pier	
	30 Bishop's Stortford, Rhodes Centre	
June	June	
6 'I Dig Everything' demoed at Pye Studios	5 London, Marquee	
	12 London, Marquee	
	13 Ramsgate, Coronation Ballroom	
	14 Cambridge, Corn Exchange	
	17 Catford	
	18 Thetford, Guildhall	
	19 Brands Hatch, Racing Track	
	22 Bognor Regis, Shoreline Club	
	23 Lowestoft	
	24 Dunstable, California Ballroom	
	27 Great Yarmouth, Britannia Theatre	
July	July	
	2 Warrington, White Lion Hotel	
5 'I Dig Everything' recorded at Pye Studios	3 London, Marquee	
	15 Loughton, Youth Centre	
	30 Bishop's Stortford, Rhodes Centre	
August	August	
	12 Leicester, Latin Quarter	
	13 Boston, Gliderdrome	
19 Single release: 'I Dig Everything'	21 London, Marquee	
	26 Ramsgate, Coronation Ballroom	
	27 Greenford, Starlite Ballroom	
	28 London, Marquee	
	September	
	4 London, Marquee	
	11 London, Marquee	
	18 London, Marquee	
	23 London, Marquee	
	25 London, Marquee	
October	October	
	2 London, Marquee	
	9 London, Marquee	
18 'The London Boys', 'Rubber Band' and 'Please Mr Gravedigger' recorded at R G Jones Studios	16 London, Marquee	
	23 London, Marquee	
	29 Bognor Regis, Shoreline Club	
	30 London, Marquee	
November	November	
	6 London, Marquee	
14 *David Bowie* sessions begin at Decca Studios	13 London, Marquee	
	19 Cromer, Olympia Ballrooms	
	26 Gosport, Community Centre	
	27 King's Lynn, Maid's Head	
December	December	
2 Single release: 'Rubber Band'	2 Shrewsbury, Severn Club	

RECORDING & RELEASES	STAGE	TV & FILM
1967	**1967**	**1967**
February 25 *David Bowie* sessions end April 14 Single release: 'The Laughing Gnome' June 1 Album release: *David Bowie* 3 'Love You Till Tuesday' version 2 and 'When I Live My Dream' version 2 recorded at Decca Studios July 14 Single release: 'Love You Till Tuesday' September 1 'Let Me Sleep Beside You' and 'Karma Man' recorded at Advision Studios December 18 BBC radio session for *Top Gear* recorded at BBC Piccadilly Studios	March 13 Tottenham, The Swan *(rehearsals with The Riot Squad)* April 13 London, Tiles Club *(David Bowie and The Riot Squad)* 14 London, Marquee *(solo date)* November 19 London, Dorchester Hotel *(solo date)* December 28 Oxford, Playhouse *(first performance of Pierrot In Turquoise)*	 September 13 Begins filming *The Image* November 10 'Love You Till Tuesday' performed on Dutch TV's *Fanclub*
1968	**1968**	**1968**
    February Demo sessions for *Ernie Johnson* and 'Even A Fool Learns To Love' March 12 'In The Heat Of The Morning' and 'London Bye Ta Ta' begin recording at Decca Studios May 13 BBC radio session for *Top Gear* recorded at BBC Piccadilly Studios	January 3-5 Whitehaven, Rose Hill Theatre *(3 performances of Pierrot In Turquoise)* March 5-16 London, Mercury Theatre *(12 performances of Pierrot In Turquoise)* 25 London, Intimate Theatre *(rehearsals)* 26-30 London, Intimate Theatre *(5 performances of Pierrot In Turquoise)* May 19 Covent Garden, Middle Earth Club *(solo mime date)* June 3 London, Royal Festival Hall *(solo mime date)* August 1 London, Marquee *(solo date)*	January 30 Bowie and Hermione Farthingale film their minuet for BBC2 play *The Pistol Shot* February 27 'Love You Till Tuesday', 'Did You Ever Have A Dream' and 'Please Mr Gravedigger', filmed in Hamburg for German ZDF TV's *4-3-2-1 Musik Für Junge Leute* March 16 *4-3-2-1 Musik Für Junge Leute* broadcast May 20 *The Pistol Shot* shown on BBC2

RECORDING & RELEASES	STAGE	TV & FILM
	? London, Astor Club *(audition for cabaret act)* September 14 London, Roundhouse *(this date as Turquoise)* 15 Covent Garden, Middle Earth Club *(this and next 6 dates as Feathers)* 16 London, Wigmore Hall	September 19 Appears on German ZDF TV show *4-3-2-1 Musik Für Junge Leute*
October 24 'Ching-a-Ling' and 'Back To Where You've Never Been' recorded at Trident Studios		October 29 Begins filming for *The Virgin Soldiers*
	November 17 London, Hampstead Country Club December ? Birmingham, Arts Lab *(cancelled)* 6 London, Drury Lane Arts Lab 7 Brighton, Sussex University 14 Birmingham, Arts Lab *(cancelled)* 24 Falmouth, Magician's Workshop *(solo date)* 26 Falmouth, Magician's Workshop *(solo date)*	November 11 Appears on German TV show *Für Jeden Etwas Musik* December 24 *The Pistol Shot* repeated on BBC2
1969	**1969**	**1969**
January 29 German vocals for 'Lieb' Dich Bis Dienstag' and 'Mit Mir In Deinem Traum' recorded at Trident Studios February 1 Original version of 'Space Oddity' recorded at Morgan Studios	January 4 London, Roundhouse *(as Feathers)* February 11 Brighton, Sussex University *(as Feathers – David and Hutch only)* 15 Birmingham, Town Hall *(solo mime date. This and remaining dates to 8 March are as support on T.Rex tour)* 17 Croydon, Fairfield Halls 22 Manchester, Free Trade Hall 23 Bristol, Colston Hall March 1 Liverpool, Philharmonic Hall 8 Brighton, Dome 11 London, University of Surrey *(this and next two dates as Feathers – David and Hutch only)* 14 Guildford, Town Hall 16 Lincoln, Assembly Rooms April 29 Ealing, College of Technology May 4 Beckenham, Three Tuns 6 Hampstead, Three Horseshoes 9 Hampstead, Three Horseshoes 11 Beckenham, Three Tuns	January 22 Films commercial for Luv ice cream 26 Filming begins on *Love You Till Tuesday* February 7 Filming ends on *Love You Till Tuesday* May 10 Records appearance with The Strawbs on BBC2's *Colour Me Pop*

RECORDING & RELEASES	STAGE	TV & FILM
	18 Beckenham, Three Tuns	
	22 London, Wigmore Hall	
	25 Beckenham, Three Tuns	
June	June	June
	5 Beckenham, Three Tuns	
	15 London, Marquee	14 *Colour Me Pop* shown on BBC2
20 'Space Oddity' and 'Wild Eyed Boy From Freecloud' (B-side version) recorded at Trident Studios		
July	July	
11 Single release: 'Space Oddity'	15 Hounslow, White Bear	
16 Remaining *Space Oddity* sessions begin at Trident Studios	18 Beckenham, Three Tuns	
	24 Valetta, Hilton Hotel *(Maltese Song Festival)*	
	? USS *Saratoga (David gives impromptu performance for ship's crew while in Valetta)*	
	31 Pistoia, Monsummano-Terme *(Italian Song Festival)*	
	August	August
	3 Beckenham, Three Tuns	
	16 Beckenham Recreational Ground *(The "Growth" free festival)*	
	22 Wolverhampton, Catacombs Club	25 Records performance of 'Space Oddity' in Holland for TV show *Doebidoe*
		30 *Doebidoe* shown on Dutch TV
	September	
	13 Bromley, Library Gardens	
October	October	October
	1 Downham, Folk Club	2 Records 'Space Oddity' appearance for BBC1's *Top Of The Pops*
	8 Coventry, Coventry Theatre *(this and all dates to 26 October supporting Humble Pie, except where stated)*	
	9 Leeds, Town Hall	9 *Top Of The Pops* features 'Space Oddity'
	10 Birmingham, Town Hall	
	11 Brighton, Dome	
	12 Beckenham, Three Tuns *(not as support)*	
	13 Bristol, Colston Hall	
	16 London, All Saints' Church Hall, Powis Gardens *(not as support)*	16 'Space Oddity' performance repeated on *Top Of The Pops*
	17 Exeter, Tiffany's *(not as support)*	
	19 Birmingham, Rebecca's Club *(not as support)*	
20 BBC radio session for *The Dave Lee Travis Show* recorded at BBC Aeolian Hall Studios	21 London, Queen Elizabeth Hall	
	23 Edinburgh, Usher Hall	
	25 Manchester, Odeon Theatre	
	26 Liverpool, Empire Theatre	
	30 Gravesend, General Gordon *(2 shows)*	29 Films 'Space Oddity' performance in Berlin for *4-3-2-1 Musik Für Junge Leute*
	31 Gillingham, Aurora Hotel *(2 shows)*	
November	November	November
	7 Perth, Salutation Hotel *(first date of Scottish tour, backed by Junior's Eyes)*	2 Swiss SRG TV show *Hits A-Go-Go* features 'Space Oddity'
	8 Kilmarnock, Grand Hall	
	9 Dunfermline, Kinema Ballroom	
	10 Glasgow, Electric Garden	
	11 Stirling, Albert Hall *(cancelled)*	

RECORDING & RELEASES	STAGE	TV & FILM
14 Album release: *David Bowie* (later re-titled *Space Oddity*)	12 Aberdeen, Music Hall *(cancelled)* 13 Hamilton, Town Hall *(cancelled)* 14 Kirkcaldy, Adam Smith Hall *(matinee)*; Edinburgh, Frisco's *(evening)* 15 Dundee, Caird Hall 18 Croydon, Arts Lab 19 Brighton, Dome 20 London, Royal Festival Hall Purcell Room 21 Devizes, Poperama 30 London, Palladium *("Save Rave '69")*	 22 German ZDF TV show *4-3-2-1 Musik Für Junge Leute* features 'Space Oddity' (filmed on October 29) December 5 Appears on RTE television show *Like Now*
1970	**1970**	**1970**
January 8,13,15 'The Prettiest Star' (single version) and 'London Bye Ta Ta' (second version) recorded at Trident Studios February 5 BBC radio session for *The Sunday Show* recorded at Paris Cinema Studio March 25 BBC radio session for *Sounds Of The 70s* recorded at Playhouse Theatre Studios April 3,14-15 'Memory Of A Free Festival' single recorded at Advision Studios 18 *The Man Who Sold The World* sessions begin at Trident Studios May 10 Ivor Novello Awards broadcast on BBC Radio 1 22 *The Man Who Sold The World* sessions conclude at Advision Studios	January 8 London, Speakeasy 14 Lewisham, Old Tiger's Head 18 Beckenham, Three Tuns 30 Aberdeen, Johnston Hall February 1 Edinburgh, Gateway Theatre *(performs in The Looking Glass Murders)* 3 London, Marquee 22 London, Roundhouse *(first appearance as Hype; all remaining February/March shows with Hype except where stated)* 23 London, Streatham Arms *(as Harry The Butcher)* 28 Basildon, Arts Centre March 1 Beckenham, Three Tuns *(solo)* 3 Hounslow, White Bear 5 Beckenham, Three Tuns *(solo)* 6 Hull, University 7 London, Regent Street Polytechnic 11 London, Roundhouse 12 London, Royal Albert Hall *(solo charity show)* 13 Sunderland, Locarno Ballroom 14 Guildford, University of Surrey *(solo)* 19 Beckenham, Three Tuns *(solo)* 30 Croydon, Star Hotel April 12 Harrogate, Harrogate Theatre *(2 shows)* 27 Stockport, Poco-a-Poco Club May 10 London, Talk Of The Town *(performs 'Space Oddity' at the Ivor Novello Awards)* 21 Scarborough, The Penthouse	January 29 Performs 'London Bye Ta Ta' for Grampian TV's *Cairngorm Ski Night* February 1 Scottish Television films *The Looking Glass Murders* at Gateway Theatre, Edinburgh 27 *Cairngorm Ski Night* shown on Grampian TV May 10 'Space Oddity' featured on live screening of Ivor Novello Awards to US and the Continent

RECORDING & RELEASES	STAGE	TV & FILM
	June 16 Cambridge, Jesus College July 4 Bromley, Queens Mead Recreation Ground 5 London, Round House 17 Southend, Cricketers Inn August 1 Southend, Eastwoodbury Lane November ? Stockport, Poco-a-Poco Club	July 8 *The Looking Glass Murders* shown on Scottish Television
1971	**1971**	**1971**
April Album release: *The Man Who Sold The World* June *Hunky Dory* sessions begin at Trident Studios, continuing until August 3 BBC radio session for *John Peel's Sunday Concert* recorded at Paris Cinema Studio July 9 'It Ain't Easy' recorded at Trident Studios September 21 BBC radio session for *Sounds Of The 70s* recorded at Kensington House Studios November 8 Main *Ziggy Stardust* sessions commence at Trident Studios with 'Star' and 'Hang On To Yourself' 11 'Star', 'Ziggy Stardust', 'Velvet Goldmine' and 'Sweet Head' completed 12 'Moonage Daydream', 'Soul Love', 'Lady Stardust' and second version of 'The Supermen' recorded 15 'Five Years' recorded December 17 Album release: *Hunky Dory*	February Promotional tour of USA, including appearances in New York, Philadelphia, Chicago (Quiet Knight Club), Los Angeles, San Francisco and Texas April 29 London, Roundhouse June ? Portsmouth, South Parade Pier 23 Glastonbury, Glastonbury Fayre July 21 Hampstead, Country Club September Promotional tour of Holland and Belgium 25 Aylesbury, Friars October 4 London, Seymour Hall	January 20 Performs 'Holy Holy' on Granada TV
1972	**1972**	**1972**
January 11 BBC radio session for *Sounds Of The 70s* recorded at Kensington House Studios	January London, Tottenham Royal Ballroom *(rehearsals)*	

RECORDING & RELEASES	STAGE	TV & FILM
18 BBC radio session for *Sounds Of The 70s* recorded at Maida Vale Studios February 4 *Ziggy Stardust* sessions conclude with final takes of 'Starman', 'Suffragette City' and 'Rock'n'Roll Suicide'	29 Aylesbury, Friars February 10 London, Tolworth, The Toby Jug *(first date proper of the Ziggy Stardust tour)* 11 High Wycombe, Town Hall 12 London, Imperial College 14 Brighton, Dome *(supporting The Groundhogs)* 18 Sheffield, University 23 Chichester, Chichester College 24 London, Wallington, Public Hall 25 London, Eltham, Avery Hill College 26 Sutton Coldfield, Belfry Hotel 29 Sunderland, Locarno March 1 Bristol, University 4 Portsmouth, Southsea Pier Pavilion 7 Yeovil, Yeovil College 11 Southampton, Guild Hall 14 Bournemouth, Chelsea Village 17 Birmingham, Town Hall 24 Newcastle, Mayfair Ballroom April 20 Harlow, The Playhouse 21 Manchester, Free Trade Hall 29 High Wycombe, Town Hall *(cancelled)* 30 Plymouth, Guild Hall	February 8 'Oh! You Pretty Things', 'Queen Bitch' and 'Five Years' on BBC2's *Old Grey Whistle Test*
May 6 'I Feel Free' from Kingston Polytechnic gig later released on *RarestOneBowie* 14 Mott The Hoople record 'All The Young Dudes' and 'One Of The Boys' at Olympic Studios. *All The Young Dudes* sessions continue at Trident until July 16 BBC radio session for *Sounds Of The 70s* recorded at Maida Vale Studios 22 BBC radio session for *The Johnnie Walker Show* recorded at Aeolian Hall Studio 23 BBC radio session for *Sounds Of The 70s* recorded at Maida Vale Studios June 6 Album release: *The Rise And Fall Of Ziggy Stardust And The Spiders From Mars*	May 5 Aberystwyth, University 6 London, Kingston Polytechnic 7 Hemel Hempstead, Pavilion 11 Worthing, Assembly Hall 12 London, Central Polytechnic 13 Slough, Technical College 19-20 Oxford, Polytechnic *(2 shows)* 25 Bournemouth, Chelsea Village 27 Epsom, Ebbisham Hall June 2 Newcastle, City Hall 3 Liverpool, Stadium 4 Preston, Public Hall 6 Bradford, St George's Hall 7 Sheffield, City Hall 8 Middlesbrough, Town Hall 10 Leicester, Polytechnic	June

RECORDING & RELEASES	STAGE	TV & FILM
	13 Bristol, Colston Hall	15 'Starman' recorded for Granada
	16 Torquay, Town Hall	TV's *Lift Off With Ayshea*
	17 Oxford, Town Hall	
	19 Southampton, Civic Centre	
	21 Dunstable, Civic Hall	21 *Lift Off With Ayshea* transmitted
	24 Guildford, Civic Hall	
	25 Croydon, Greyhound	
26 Original version of 'John, I'm Only	30 High Wycombe, Grammar School	
Dancing' recorded at Olympic Studios	*(cancelled)*	
July-August	July	July
Lou Reed's *Transformer* recorded at	1 Weston-Super-Mare, Winter Gardens	
Trident Studios	Pavilion	
	2 Torquay, Rainbow Pavilion	5 'Starman' performed for
		Top Of The Pops
	8 London, Royal Festival Hall	6 *Top Of The Pops* transmitted
	(Save The Whale charity show organised	
	by Friends Of The Earth; Bowie appears	
	with guest Lou Reed)	
	15 Aylesbury, Friars	
	August	August
	1-14 London, Theatre Royal	
	Stratford East *(rehearsals for Rainbow*	
	Theatre shows)	
	13 Guildford, Civic Hall *(Bowie guests*	
	for the encores at a Mott The Hoople	18 Video of 'John, I'm Only Dancing'
	concert)	filmed during rehearsals at Rainbow
	19-20 London, Rainbow Theatre *(2*	Theatre
	shows)	
	27 Bristol, Locarno Electric Village	
	30 London, Rainbow Theatre	
	31 Boscombe, Royal Ballrooms	
September	September	
	1 Doncaster, Top Rank Suite	
	2-3 Manchester, Hard Rock Club	
	(2 shows)	
	4 Liverpool, Top Rank Suite	
	5 Sunderland, Top Rank Suite	
	6 Sheffield, Top Rank Suite	
	7 Hanley, Stoke-on-Trent, Top Rank	
	Suite	
22 Cleveland show later broadcast by	22 Cleveland, Music Hall *(opening*	
WMMS FM Radio	*date of the first US Ziggy tour)*	
	24 Memphis, Ellis Auditorium	
28 'My Death' from New York gig	28 New York, Carnegie Hall	
later released on *RarestOneBowie*		
October	October	October
1 Live tracks from Boston gig later	1 Boston, Music Hall	
released on *Sound + Vision* box set and		
Aladdin Sane 30th Anniversary Edition	7 Chicago, Auditorium Theater	
6 'The Jean Genie' recorded at RCA	8 Detroit, Fisher Theater	
Studios in New York; the main *Aladdin*	11 St Louis, Kiel Auditorium	
Sane sessions will begin in December	15 Kansas City, Memorial Hall	
	16 Chicago *(cancelled)*	
20 Santa Monica concert recorded for	20-21 Santa Monica, Civic Auditorium	
US radio broadcast; later released as	*(2 shows)*	
Santa Monica '72		
24-25 Bowie mixes Iggy And The	27-28 San Francisco, Winterland	27-28 'The Jean Genie' video filmed
Stooges album *Raw Power* at Western	Auditorium *(2 shows)*	in San Francisco
Sound Studios		

RECORDING & RELEASES	STAGE	TV & FILM
November	November 1 Seattle, Paramount Theater 4 Phoenix, Celebrity Theater 11 Dallas, Majestic Theater 12 Houston, Music Hall 13 Oklahoma City *(cancelled)* 14 New Orleans, Layola University 17 Dania, Fort Lauderdale, Pirate's World 20 Nashville, Municipal Auditorium 22 New Orleans, The Warehouse	
25 'Drive In Saturday' from Cleveland gig later released on *Aladdin Sane 30th Anniversary Edition*	25-26 Cleveland, Public Auditorium *(2 shows)* 28 Pittsburgh, Stanley Theater 29 Philadelphia, Tower Theater *(Bowie joins Mott The Hoople on stage for encores)* 30 Philadelphia, Tower Theater	
December 9 'Drive In Saturday' and 'All The Young Dudes' recorded at RCA, New York. *Aladdin Sane* sessions continue here and at Trident, London until late January	December 1-2 Philadelphia, Tower Theater *(2 shows)* 23-24 London, Rainbow Theatre *(2 shows)* 28-29 Manchester, Hard Rock Club *(2 shows)*	December 'Space Oddity' video shot at RCA Studios, New York
1973	**1973**	**1973**
January 20 Sax version of 'John, I'm Only Dancing' recorded at Trident Studios, along with backing tracks for 'Lady Grinning Soul' and 'Panic In Detroit' 24 *Aladdin Sane* sessions conclude with the recording of lead vocal on 'Panic In Detroit' at Trident Studios	January 5 Glasgow, Green's Playhouse *(2 shows)* 6 Edinburgh, Empire Theatre 7 Newcastle, City Hall 9 Preston, Guild Hall 19-25 Tottenham, Royal Ballroom *(rehearsals)* February 6-13 New York, RCA Studios *(rehearsals)* 14-15 New York, Radio City Music Hall *(2 shows)* 16-19 Philadelphia, Tower Theater *(7 shows)* 23 Nashville, War Memorial Auditorium 26-27 Memphis, Ellis Auditorium *(2 shows)* March 1-2 Detroit, Masonic Temple Auditorium *(2 shows)* 10 Los Angeles, Long Beach Auditorium 12 Los Angeles, Hollywood Palladium	January 17 'Drive In Saturday' and 'My Death' on LWT's *Russell Harty Plus*

RECORDING & RELEASES	STAGE	TV & FILM
April	April	
	8,10-11 Tokyo, Shinjuku Koseinenkin Kaikan *(3 shows)*	
	12 Nagoya, Kokaido	
13 Album release: *Aladdin Sane*	14 Hiroshima, Yubinchokin Kaikan	
	16 Kobe, Kobe Kokusai Kaikan	
	17 Osaka, Koseinenkin Kaikan	
	18, 20 Tokyo, Shibuya Kokaido *(2 shows)*	
	May	May
	12 London, Earls Court Arena	12 'Life On Mars?' video shot during Earls Court rehearsals
	16 Aberdeen, Music Hall *(2 shows)*	
	17 Dundee, Caird Hall	
	18 Glasgow, Green's Playhouse *(2 shows)*	
	19 Edinburgh, Empire Theatre	
	21 Norwich, Theatre Royal *(2 shows)*	
	22 Romford, Odeon Theatre	
	23 Brighton, Dome *(2 shows)*	
	24 London, Lewisham Odeon	
	25 Bournemouth, Winter Gardens	25 BBC's *Nationwide* films backstage interviews and concert footage at Bournemouth gig
	27 Guildford, Civic Hall *(2 shows)*	
	28 Wolverhampton, Civic Hall	
	29 Hanley, Victoria Hall	
	30 Oxford, New Theatre	
	31 Blackburn, King George's Hall	
	June	
	1 Bradford, St George's Hall	
	3 Coventry, New Theatre	
	4 Worcester, Gaumont	
	6 Sheffield, City Hall *(2 shows)*	
	7 Manchester, Free Trade Hall *(2 shows)*	
	8 Newcastle, City Hall *(2 shows)*	
	9 Preston, Guild Hall	
	10 Liverpool, Empire Theatre *(2 shows)*	
	11 Leicester, De Montfort Hall	
	12 Chatham, Central Hall *(2 shows)*	
	13 Kilburn, Gaumont	
	14 Salisbury, City Hall	
	15 Taunton, Odeon *(2 shows)*	
	16 Torquay, Town Hall *(2 shows)*	
	18 Bristol, Colston Hall *(2 shows)*	
	19 Southampton, Guild Hall	
	21-22 Birmingham, Town Hall *(4 shows)*	
	23 Boston, Gliderdrome	
	24 Croydon, Fairfield Halls *(2 shows)*	
	25-26 Oxford, New Theatre *(3 shows)*	
	27 Doncaster, Top Rank	
	28 Bridlington, Royal Spa Ballroom	
	29 Leeds, Rolarena	
	30 Newcastle, City Hall *(2 shows)*	
July	July	July
3 Final Hammersmith gig recorded by RCA, and released ten years later as *Ziggy Stardust: The Motion Picture*	2-3 London, Hammersmith Odeon *(2 shows, of which the second is the famous Ziggy Stardust "retirement" gig)*	3 D A Pennebaker films the final concert, later broadcast on US TV in 1974 and eventually released as *Ziggy Stardust and The Spiders From Mars*
July-August		
Pin Ups sessions at Château		

RECORDING & RELEASES	STAGE	TV & FILM
d'Hérouville Studios, Pontoise October 19 Album release: *Pin Ups* October-December Astronettes and *Diamond Dogs* sessions at Olympic Studios, London	October 18-20 London, Marquee *('The 1980 Floor Show' is recorded over 3 days before a live audience)*	October 18-20 *The 1980 Floor Show* is recorded over 3 days before a live audience at London's Marquee November 16 *The 1980 Floor Show* screened by NBC
1974	**1974**	**1974**
February *Diamond Dogs* sessions conclude at Ludolf Studios, Hilversum April Lulu version of 'Can You Hear Me' and US single version of 'Rebel Rebel' recorded at RCA Studios, New York 24 Album release: *Diamond Dogs* July 8-12 Philadelphia shows recorded for *David Live*	April-May New York, RCA Studios *(rehearsals)* June 8-10 Port Chester, Capitol Theater *(dress rehearsals)* 14 Montreal, Forum *(first date of the Diamond Dogs tour)* 15 Ottawa, Civic Center 16 Toronto, O'Keefe Auditorium *(2 shows)* 17 Rochester, Memorial Auditorium 18-19 Cleveland, Public Hall *(2 shows)* 20 Toledo, Sports Arena 21-22 Detroit, Cobo Arena *(2 shows)* 23 Columbus, Mershon Auditorium 24 Dayton, Harra Arena 25 Akron, Civic Theater 26-27 Pittsburgh, Syria Mosque *(2 shows)* 28 Charleston WV, Civic Center 29 Nashville, Municipal Auditorium 30 Memphis, Mid-South Coliseum July 1 Atlanta, Fox Theater 2 Tampa, Curtis Hixon Convention Hall 3 Casselberry, Orlando, Seminole Jai-Alai Fronton 4 Jacksonville, Exhibition Hall 5 Charlotte NC, Park Center 6 Greensboro NC, Coliseum 7 Norfolk, Scope Convention Hall 8-12 Philadelphia, Tower Theater *(5 shows)* 13 Cape Cod, Coliseum 14 Providence, Palace Theater 15 Waterbury, Palace Theater 16 Boston, Music Hall 17 Hartford, Bushnell Memorial Hall 19-20 New York, Madison Square Garden *(2 shows, closing the Diamond*	February 13 'Rebel Rebel' performance recorded for Dutch TV's *Top Pop* 15 'Rebel Rebel' screened on *Top Pop*

RECORDING & RELEASES	STAGE	TV & FILM
	Dogs tour)	
August 11 *Young Americans* sessions begin at Sigma Sound Studios, Philadelphia		**August** Alan Yentob films interview footage and studio rehearsals for 'Right' during the *Young Americans* sessions in Philadelphia
	September 2-8 Los Angeles, Universal Amphitheater *(7 shows to begin the Philly Dogs tour)* 11 San Diego, Sports Arena 13 Tucson, Convention Center 14 Phoenix, Veterans' Memorial Coliseum 16-17 Los Angeles, Anaheim Convention Center *(2 shows; some doubt exists over these dates)*	**September** 2-8 Live footage is shot by Alan Yentob at Los Angeles concerts for use in *Cracked Actor* documentary
October	**October** 5 St Paul, Civic Center 8 Indianapolis, Indiana Convention Center 10-11 Madison, University of Wisconsin *(2 shows)* 13 Milwaukee, Mecca Arena 16-20 Detroit, Michigan Palace *(5 shows)* 21-23 Chicago, Arie Crown Theater *(3 shows)*	
29 Album release: *David Live*	28-31 New York, Radio City Music Hall *(4 shows)*	
	November 1-3 New York, Radio City Music Hall *(3 shows)* 6 Cleveland, Public Hall 8 Buffalo, Memorial Auditorium 11 Washington, Capital Center 14-16 Boston, Music Hall *(3 shows)* 18-19 Pittsburgh *(2 shows)* 24-25 Philadelphia, Spectrum Arena *(2 shows)* 26 Uniondale, Nassau Coliseum *(some uncertainty surrounds this and the previous Philadelphia dates, which were rescheduled and a third night cancelled. This seems to be the correct version)* 28 Memphis, Mid-South Coliseum 30 Nashville, Municipal Auditorium	**November** 2 Records interview with Dick Cavett and live performances of '1984', 'Young Americans' and 'Footstompin'' for NBC's *Wide World Of Entertainment*
December *Young Americans* sessions resume at Racord Plant Studios, New York	**December** 1 Atlanta, Omni Arena *(last date of the Philly Dogs tour)* 2 Tuscaloosa, University of Alabama *(cancelled)*	**December** 4 NBC's *Wide World Of Entertainment* broadcast
1975	**1975**	**1975**
January *Young Americans* sessions conclude at Record Plant and Electric Lady Studios, New York		**January** 26 BBC2 shows *Cracked Actor*

RECORDING & RELEASES	STAGE	TV & FILM
March 7 Album release: *Young Americans* October *Station To Station* sessions begin at Cherokee Studios, Hollywood December Aborted *The Man Who Fell To Earth* soundtrack sessions at Cherokee Studios, Hollywood	September 8 Los Angeles, venue unknown *(Bowie plays a couple of songs with Bill Wyman and Ron Wood at Peter Sellers's birthday party)*	February 21 BBC1's *Top Of The Pops* shows 'Young Americans' March 1 At the Grammy Awards on US TV, Bowie presents Aretha Franklin with "Best Female Soul Singer" award June *The Man Who Fell To Earth* begins shooting in New Mexico November 4 'Golden Years' and 'Fame' on ABC's *Soul Train* 23 Performs 'Fame' on CBS's *The Cher Show* and duets on 'Can You Hear Me' and 'Young Americans' medley 28 ITV's *Russell Harty Plus* includes live satellite interview with Bowie in LA
1976	**1976**	**1976**
January 23 Album release: *Station To Station*	January Ocho Rios, Jamaica, and New York *(rehearsals)* February 2 Vancouver, PNE Coliseum *(opening night of the Station To Station tour)* 3 Seattle, Center Coliseum 4 Portland, Paramount Theater 6 San Francisco, Cow Palace 8-9,11 Los Angeles, Inglewood Forum *(3 shows)* 13 San Diego, Sports Arena 15 Phoenix, Veterans' Memorial Coliseum 16 Albuquerque, Civic Auditorium 17 Denver, McNichols Sports Arena 20 Milwaukee, Mecca Arena 21 Kalamazoo, Wings Stadium 22 Evansville, Riverfront 23 Cincinatti, Convention Center 25 Montreal, Forum 26 Toronto, Maple Leaf Garden 27-28 Cleveland, Public Auditorium *(2 shows)* 29 Detroit, Olympia Stadium	January 3 CBS's *The Dinah Shore Show* includes 'Stay', 'Five Years' and interview February 3 ABC's *Good Morning America* shows interview with David and Angela

RECORDING & RELEASES	STAGE	TV & FILM
March	March	
	1 Detroit, Olympia Stadium	
	3 Chicago, International Amphitheater	
	5 St Louis, Henry W Kiel Auditorium	
	6 Memphis, Mid-South Coliseum	
	7 Nashville, Municipal Auditorium	
	8 Atlanta, Omni Arena	
	11 Pittsburgh, Civic Arena	
	12 Norfolk, Scope Convention Hall	
	13-14 Washington, Capital Center *(2 shows)*	
	15-16 Philadelphia, Spectrum Arena *(2 shows)*	
	17 Boston, New Boston Garden Arena	
	19 Buffalo, Memorial Auditorium	
	20 Rochester, Memorial Auditorium	
	21 Springfield, Civic Center	
	22 New Haven, Memorial Coliseum	
23 Nassau concert recorded for broadcast on US radio's *The King Biscuit Flower Hour*. 'Stay' and 'Word On A Wing' later released as bonus tracks on *Station To Station*, and 'Queen Bitch' on *RarestOneBowie*	23 Uniondale, Nassau Coliseum	
	26 New York, Madison Square Garden	
	April	
	7 Munich, Olympiahalle	
	8 Düsseldorf, Philipshalle	
	10 Berlin, Deutschlandhalle	
	11-12 Hamburg, Kongress Zentrum *(2 shows)*	
	13 Frankfurt, Festhalle	
	14 Ludwigshafen, Friedrichs-Eberthalle	
	16 Frankfurt, Night Club *(Bowie makes an impromptu appearance at The Linus Band show)*	
	17 Zürich, Hallenstadion *(replaces show in Berne)*	
	24 Helsinki, Nya Masshallen	
	26-27 Stockholm, Kungliga Tennishallen *(2 shows)*	
	28 Gothenburg, Scandinavium	
	29-30 Copenhagen, Falkonerteatret *(2 shows)*	
	May	
	3-8 London, Wembley Empire Pool *(6 shows)*	
	11 Brussels, Vorst Nationaal	
	13-14 Rotterdam, Sport Paleis Ahoy *(2 shows)*	
	17-18 Paris, Pavillon *(2 shows closing the Station To Station tour)*	
	28 Montreux, Casino *(Bowie hires out Casino for his son's fifth birthday party and narrates "Jack And The Beanstalk" for Joe and friends)*	
June *The Idiot* sessions begin at Château d'Hérouville Studios, Pontoise		

RECORDING & RELEASES	STAGE	TV & FILM
September *Low* sessions begin at Château d'Hérouville Studios, Pontoise		
1977	**1977**	**1977**
January 14 Album release: *Low*		
	February Berlin, UFA Studios *(rehearsals for Iggy Pop tour)*	
March	March 1 Aylesbury, Friars *(first show of the Iggy Pop tour on which Bowie plays keyboards)* 2 Newcastle, City Hall 3 Manchester, Apollo Theatre 4 Birmingham, Hippodrome 5,7 London, Rainbow Theatre *(2 shows)* 13 Montreal, Le Plateau Theatre 14 Toronto, Seneca College 16 Boston, Harvard Square Theater 18 New York, Palladium 19 Philadelphia, Tower Theater	
21 'TV Eye', 'Dirt' and 'Funtime' from Cleveland gig later included on *TV Eye*; entire concert released as *Suck On This!*	21-22 Cleveland, Agora Ballroom *(2 shows)* 25 Detroit, Masonic Temple Auditorium 27 Chicago, Riviera Theater	
28 'I Wanna Be Your Dog' from Chicago gig later included on *TV Eye*	28 Chicago, Midnight Mantra Studios 29 Pittsburgh, Leona Theater 30 Columbus, Agora Ballroom	
April-May *Lust For Life* sessions at Hansa By The Wall Studios, Berlin	April 1 Milwaukee, Oriental Theater 4 Portland, Paramount Theater 7 Vancouver, Vancouver Gardens 9 Seattle, Paramount Theater 13 San Francisco, Berkeley Theater 15 Santa Monica, Civic Auditorium 16 San Diego, Civic Auditorium *(last show of the Iggy Pop tour)*	April 15 CBS's *The Dinah Shore Show* interviews David and Iggy, plus 'Funtime' and 'Sister Midnight' with David on keyboards
June-August *"Heroes"* sessions at Hansa By The Wall Studios, Berlin		June 27 Bowie interviewed on French TV shows *Midi Première* and *Actualités* September 9 Records '"Heroes"' and 'Sleeping Next To You' for Granada's *Marc* 11 Records '"Heroes"' and 'Peace On Earth'/'Little Drummer Boy' for *Bing Crosby's Merrie Olde Christmas* 28 *Marc* show broadcast on ITV October 1 Interviews and performances of '"Heroes"' and 'Sense Of Doubt' for Italian TV shows *Odeon* and *L'Altra Domenica*
October		
14 Album release: *"Heroes"*		16 Interview for French TF1 show *Le Rendezvous du Dimanche* 19 BBC1's *Top Of The Pops* features

RECORDING & RELEASES	STAGE	TV & FILM
		'"Heroes"' November 6 Interview on Dutch TV show *Pop Shop* December 24 *Bing Crosby's Merrie Olde Christmas* broadcast on ITV
1978	**1978**	**1978**
		January-February Films *Just A Gigolo* in Berlin
	March Dallas *(rehearsals)* 29 San Diego, Sports Arena *(first date of the Stage tour)* 30 Phoenix, Veterans' Memorial Coliseum	
April	April 2 Fresno, Convention Center 3-4 Los Angeles, Inglewood Forum *(2 shows)* 5 San Francisco, Oakland Coliseum 6 Los Angeles, Inglewood Forum 9 Houston, The Summit 10 Dallas, Convention Center 11 Baton Rouge, LSU Assembly Center 13 Nashville, Municipal Auditorium 14 Memphis, Mid-South Coliseum 15 Kansas City, Municipal Auditorium 17-18 Chicago, Arie Crown Theater *(2 shows)* 20-21 Detroit, Cobo Arena *(2 shows)* 22 Cleveland, Richfield Coliseum 24 Milwaukee, Mecca Auditorium 26 Pittsburgh, Civic Arena 27 Washington, Capital Center	April 3 Interview before LA show featured on *Eyewitness News* on US TV 10 *David Bowie On Stage* recorded for US TV at Dallas show: 21-minute broadcast includes 'What In The World', 'Blackout', 'Sense Of Doubt', 'Speed Of Life', 'Hang On To Yourself' and 'Ziggy Stardust' 21 Interview on NBC's *The Midnight Special*
28-29 Philadelphia gigs recorded for *Stage* album May	28-29 Philadelphia, Spectrum Arena *(2 shows)* May 1 Toronto, Maple Leaf Gardens 2 Ottowa, Civic Center 3 Montreal, Forum	May
5 Providence gig recorded for *Stage* 6 Boston gig recorded for *Stage*	5 Providence, Civic Center 6 Boston, New Boston Garden Arena 7-9 New York, Madison Square Garden *(3 shows)* 14 Frankfurt, Festhalle 15 Hamburg, Kongress Zentrum 16 Berlin, Deutschlandhalle 18 Essen, Grugahalle 19 Cologne, Sporthalle 20 Munich, Olympiahalle 22 Vienna, Stadthalle 24-25 Paris, Pavillon *(2 shows)* 26 Lyon, Palais des Sports 27 Marseilles, Palais des Sports 31 Copenhagen, Falkonerteatret	16 BBC2's *Arena Rock* shows interview and live clips of 'Hang On To Yourself' and 'Ziggy Stardust' from Dallas show recorded April 10 30 *Musikladen Extra* recorded in Bremen studios for ZDF TV: 'Sense Of Doubt', 'Beauty And The Beast',

RECORDING & RELEASES	STAGE	TV & FILM
		'"Heroes"', 'Stay', 'The Jean Genie', 'TVC15', 'Alabama Song', 'Rebel Rebel', 'What In The World'
	June	June
	1 Copenhagen, Falkonerteatret	
	2 Stockholm, Kungliga Tennishallen	
	4 Gothenburg, Scandinavium	
	5 Oslo, Ekebergshallen	
	7-9 Rotterdam, Sport Paleis Ahoy *(3 shows)*	
	11-12 Brussels, Vorst Nationaal *(2 shows)*	
	14-16 Newcastle, City Hall *(3 shows)*	16 Interview on regional TV *Northern Light*
	19-22 Glasgow, Apollo *(4 shows)*	20 Interview on regional TV *Reporting Scotland*, including live clip of 'Hang On To Yourself' shot at Glasgow Apollo the day before
	24-26 Stafford, Bingley Hall *(3 shows)*	
	29-30 London, Earls Court Arena *(2 shows)*	
July	July	July
1 'Be My Wife' and 'Sound And Vision' from Earls Court later included on *RarestOneBowie*	1 London, Earls Court Arena	
2 'Alabama Song' recorded at Good Earth Studio, London		8 LWT's *London Weekend Show* runs 40-minute feature, including clips from Earl's Court ('Star', '"Heroes"', 'Hang On To Yourself')
		August
		4 *Musikladen Extra* show broadcast on German ZDF TV, minus 'What In The World'
September		
Lodger sessions at Mountain Studios, Montreux		
25 Album release: *Stage*	November	November
	11 Adelaide, Oval Cricket Ground *(first show of the Pacific leg of the Stage tour)*	
	14 Perth, Showgrounds	14 Australian TV show *Countdown* includes interview and live clip of 'Alabama Song'
	18 Melbourne, Cricket Ground	
	21 Brisbane, Lang Park	
	24-25 Sydney, Showgrounds	28 Interview on Australian TV show *Willisee At Seven*
	29 Christchurch, QEII Park	December
December	December	
	2 Auckland, Western Springs Speedway	
6 Osaka gig broadcast on Japanese radio	6-7 Osaka, Kouseinenkin Kaikan *(2 shows)*	6 Interview on Japanese TV *Star Sen Ichi Ya*
	9 Osaka, Banpaku Kaikan	
	11-12 Tokyo, NHK Hall *(last 2 shows of the Stage tour)*	12 Tokyo concert filmed for Japanese TV; cut to 60 mins for broadcast: 'Warszawa', '"Heroes"', 'Fame', 'Beauty And The Beast', 'Five Years', 'Soul Love', 'Star', 'Hang On To Yourself', 'Ziggy Stardust', Suffragette City', 'Station To Station', 'TVC15'
1979	**1979**	**1979**
		February
		12 Interviews on ITV's *Afternoon Plus* and BBC1's *Tonight* to coincide with

RECORDING & RELEASES	STAGE	TV & FILM
March *Lodger* sessions conclude at Record Plant Studios, New York May 18 Album release: *Lodger*	March ? New York, Carnegie Hall *(performs 'Sabotage' with John Cale, Philip Glass and Steve Reich)*	premiere of *Just A Gigolo* two days later April 23 Performs 'Boys Keep Swinging' on ITV's *The Kenny Everett Video Show* December 15 Records appearance for NBC's *Saturday Night Live* 31 ITV's *Kenny Everett's New Year's Eve Show* and US TV's *Dick Clark's Salute To The Seventies* both feature new version of 'Space Oddity'
1980	**1980**	**1980**
February-March *Scary Monsters* sessions begin at Power Station Studios, New York April *Scary Monsters* sessions conclude at Good Earth Studios, London September 12 Album release: *Scary Monsters (And Super Creeps)*	April 27 Berlin, Nollendorf Metropol *(Bowie makes guest appearance at Iggy Pop concert to play keyboards on 2 numbers)* July 29 Denver, Centre of Performing Arts *(opening night of The Elephant Man)* August 3 *(The Elephant Man ends its Denver run)* 5-31 Chicago, Blackstone Theater *(The Elephant Man opens for a four-week run in Chicago)* September 23 New York, Booth Theater *(The Elephant Man opens for a three-month run on Broadway)*	January 5 Studio performances of 'The Man Who Sold The World', 'TVC15' and 'Boys Keep Swinging' shown on NBC's *Saturday Night Live* March Films Crystal Jun Rock commercial May 'Ashes To Ashes' video shot at Beachy Head and Hastings, England September 3 'Life On Mars?' and 'Ashes To Ashes' on NBC's *The Tonight Show With Johnny Carson* October *Christiane F.* and 'Fashion' video filmed in Manhattan 10 Interview and live clips from *The Elephant Man* on BBC2's *Friday Night, Saturday Morning*

RECORDING & RELEASES	STAGE	TV & FILM
1981	**1981**	**1981**
	January 3 New York, Booth Theater *(Bowie's final performance in The Elephant Man)*	
		February 24 Bowie receives Best Male Singer award from Lulu at the *Daily Mirror Rock And Pop Awards*, televised by BBC
July 'Cat People (Putting Out Fire)' and 'Under Pressure' recorded at Mountain Studios, Montreux		
		August Rehearses and records *Baal* at BBC Television Centre in London
September *Baal* EP recorded at Hansa Studios, Berlin		
1982	**1982**	**1982**
February 26 Single EP release: *David Bowie In Bertolt Brecht's Baal*		March 1 Begins filming *The Hunger* in London. Shooting will continue until July 2 *Baal* transmitted on BBC2 September Begins filming *Merry Christmas Mr Lawrence* in Rarotonga, Cook Islands. Filming will continue here and in New Zealand until early November
November *Let's Dance* sessions begin at Record Plant Studios, New York. Recording continues into December		
1983	**1983**	**1983**
		January Films *Yellowbeard* cameo in Acapulco 31 Interview on US TV show *Live At Five* February Videos for 'Let's Dance' and 'China Girl' filmed in Carinda and Sydney, Australia March 17 Press conference at Claridge's is filmed by BBC's *Newsnight* and Channel 4's *The Tube*
April 14 Album release: *Let's Dance*	April Dallas, La Colinas *(rehearsals)* May Paris/Brussels *(rehearsals)* 18-19 Brussels, Vorst Nationaal *(first 2 shows of the Serious Moonlight tour)*	May 19 Belgian TV's *Journal* shows live clips of 'The Jean Genie' and '"Heroes"' from the opening Brussels concert

RECORDING & RELEASES	STAGE	TV & FILM
	20 Frankfurt, Festhalle 21-22 Munich, Olympiahalle (2 shows) 24-25 Lyon, Palais des Sports (2 shows) 26-27 Fréjus, Les Arnes (2 shows) 30 Glen Helen Park, San Bernardino, California (US Festival) June 2-4 London, Wembley Arena (3 shows) 5-6 Birmingham, NEC Arena (2 shows) 8-9 Paris, Hippodrome d'Auteuil (2 shows) 11-12 Gothenburg, Ullevi Stadium (2 shows) 15 Bochum, Ruhrland Stadium 17-18 Bad Segeberg, Freilichtbühne (2 shows) 20 West Berlin, Waldbühne 24 Offenbach, Bieberer Berg Stadium 25-26 Rotterdam, Feyenoord Stadium (2 shows) 28 Edinburgh, Murrayfield Stadium 30 London, Hammersmith Odeon	25 Interview and live clip of '"Heroes"' from Frankfurt concert on German TV's Tele Illustrierte June 2 ITV's News At Ten shows clip of '"Heroes"' from the first Wembley gig 6 ITV's Central News shows live clip of '"Heroes"' from Birmingham 9 French TF1's Actualités shows clips of 'The Jean Genie', 'Star' and '"Heroes"' from the first Paris gig 11 Swedish SVT shows Rapport and Aktuellt show clips of 'The Jean Genie' and 'Star' from the first Gothenburg gig 25 Dutch TV's Journaal shows live clip of '"Heroes"' from the first Rotterdam gig 29 BBC's Scotland Today shows live clip of '"Heroes"' from the Edinburgh gig 30 BBC and ITV national news show clips of 'Look Back In Anger' and 'Breaking Glass' from the Hammersmith gig
July 13 Montreal gig broadcast on US radio's Supergroups In Concert, and later on BBC Radio 1; 'Modern Love' later released as B-side	July 1-3 Milton Keynes, Bowl (3 shows) 11 Quebec, Colisee 12-13 Montreal, Forum (2 shows) 15-16 Hartford, Civic Center (2 shows) 18-21 Philadelphia, Spectrum Arena (4 shows) 25-27 New York, Madison Square Garden (3 shows) 29 Cleveland, Richfield Coliseum 30-31 Detroit, Joe Louis Arena (2 shows) August 2-4 Chicago, Rosemont Horizon (3 shows) 7 Edmonton, Commonwealth Stadium 9 Vancouver, BC Place Stadium 11 Seattle, Tacoma Dome 14-15 Los Angeles, Forum (2 shows) 17 Phoenix, Veterans' Memorial Coliseum 19 Dallas, Reunion Arena 20 Austin, Frank Erwin Center 21 Houston, The Summit 24-25 Norfolk, Scope Convention Hall	July 3 LWT's South Of Watford shows clips of 'Breaking Glass' and 'Scary Monsters' from Milton Keynes 20 'Modern Love' video filmed at the third Philadelphia concert 24 Interview and live Philadelphia clips ('What In The World', '"Heroes"', 'Fashion', 'Let's Dance') on CBS's Entertainment Tonight 25 US TV's News 4 New York shows clip of 'Star' from the first Madison Square Garden gig August

RECORDING & RELEASES	STAGE	TV & FILM
	(2 shows)	
	27-28 Washington, Capital Center	
	(2 shows)	
	29 Hershey, Hershey Park Stadium	30 British documentary *The Oshima*
	31 Boston, Sullivan Stadium	*Gang* includes interview and clips
		from *Merry Christmas Mr Lawrence*
		press conference
	September	September
	3-4 Toronto, CNE Grandstand	3 Canadian and US news channels
	(2 shows)	show clips of 'Look Back In Anger'
	5 Buffalo, Memorial Auditorium	from the first Toronto gig
	6 Syracuse, Carrier Dome	6 US TV news channels show clip of
	9 Los Angeles, Anaheim Stadium	'Look Back In Anger' from Buffalo gig
	11-12 Vancouver, PNE Coliseum	11-12 David Mallet shoots the *Serious*
	(2 shows)	*Moonlight* video at the Vancouver
	14 Winnipeg, Stadium	concerts
	17 San Francisco, Oakland Coliseum	17 Documentary *Britons In America*
		includes interview and 'Look Back In
		Anger' clip from San Francisco
October	October	
Album release: *Ziggy Stardust: The*	20-22,24 Tokyo, Budokan Arena	
Motion Picture	*(4 shows)*	
	25 Yokohama, Stadium	
	26-27 Osaka, Funitsu Taikukan	
	(2 shows)	
	29 Nagoya, Kokusai Tenji Kaikan	
	30 Osaka, Expo Memorial Park	
	31 Kyoto, Funitsu Taikukan	
	November	November
	4-6 Perth, Entertainment Center	3 Interviews and press conference for
	(3 shows)	Australian TV's *Newsworld, Morning*
	9 Adelaide, Oval Cricket Ground	*Show* and *Today Show*
	12 Melbourne, VFL Park	
	16 Brisbane, Lang Park	
	19-20 Sydney, RAS Showgrounds	
	(2 shows)	
	24 Wellington, Athletic Park	
	26 Auckland, Western Springs Stadium	
	December	December
	3 Singapore	
	5 Bangkok, Army Stadium	
	7-8 Hong Kong, Coliseum *(last 2*	
	shows of the Serious Moonlight tour)	23 First broadcast of Raymond
		Briggs's *The Snowman* on Channel 4,
		introduced by David
1984	**1984**	**1984**
May-June		
Tonight sessions at Le Studio, Morin		
Heights, Canada		
		August
		Jazzin' For Blue Jean filmed in
		Shepperton and Kensington. Second
		'Blue Jean' video for use at MTV
		Awards filmed in Soho's Wag Club
September		September
24 Album release: *Tonight*		14 Bowie's Wag Club 'Blue Jean'
		promo shown at MTV Awards at

RECORDING & RELEASES	STAGE	TV & FILM
		Radio City Music Hall, where Iggy Pop collects David's award for 'China Girl'
1985	**1985**	**1985**
June *Absolute Beginners* soundtrack songs and 'Dancing In The Street' recorded at Abbey Road Studios, London	March 23 Birmingham, NEC Arena *(Bowie makes guest appearance at Tina Turner concert)* July 13 London, Wembley Stadium *(Live Aid)* November 19 New York, China Club *(Bowie joins Iggy Pop, Ronnie Wood and Stevie Winwood on stage for an impromptu set)*	June 'Dancing In The Street' video shot in London Docklands July 13 Live Aid broadcast worldwide July-August Films *Absolute Beginners* at Shepperton Studios Autumn Films *Labyrinth* at Elstree Studios, Herts
1986	**1986**	**1986**
May *Blah-Blah-Blah* sessions at Mountain Studios, Montreux Autumn *Never Let Me Down* sessions at Mountain Studios, Montreux and Power Station Studios, New York	June 20 London, Wembley Arena *(Bowie and Jagger perform 'Dancing In The Street' at The Prince's Trust concert)*	June 21 Prince's Trust concert broadcast on TV
1987	**1987**	**1987**
April 27 Album release: *Never Let Me Down*	March 17 Toronto, Diamond Club *(first of a short promotional press tour for 'Never Let Me Down' and Glass Spider tour. All March 1987 dates are press shows)* 18 New York, Cat Club 20 London, Player's Theatre 21 Paris, La Locomotive 24 Madrid, Halquera Plateaux 25 Rome, Piper Club 26 Munich, Parkcafe Lowenbrau 28 Stockholm, Ritz 30 Amsterdam, Paradiso May 18-24 Rotterdam, Sport Paleis Ahoy *(rehearsals)*	March-April Interviews and live press conference clips of 'Bang Bang', 'Day-In Day-Out' and '87 And Cry' appear on innumerable international news programmes in America, Holland, France, Italy, Germany, Sweden, Norway and Denmark. UK coverage includes an interview and London press conference clips on SuperChannel's *Coca Cola Rockfile*, and two interviews for Channel 4's *The Tube*, all recorded on 20 March April 29 MTV's *Night Network* screens a half-hour special with interviews, footage from tour rehearsals and European press conferences May David films Pepsi commercial with Tina Turner in Amsterdam

RECORDING & RELEASES	STAGE	TV & FILM
	27-28 Rotterdam, Stadion Feyenoord *(dress rehearsals)* 30-31 Rotterdam, Stadion Feyenoord *(first 2 shows of the Glass Spider tour)* June 2 Werchter, Festival Terreine 6 Berlin, Platz der Republik 7 Koblenz, Nurburgring 9 Florence, Stadio Comunale 10 Milan, Stadio San Siro 13 Hamburg, Festweise Am Stadtpark 15 Rome, Stadio Flaminio	31 Dutch TV's *Countdown* shows 'Glass Spider' clip from the opening night June 6 Live clips of the Berlin concert ('Glass Spider', 'Day-In Day-Out' and the near riots) recorded by German TV shows *Wochenspiegel* and *1500 Jahre Berlin* 13 German TV's *Hamburger Journal* shows 'Glass Spider' clip from Hamburg show
	17-18 London, Wembley Stadium *(rehearsals)* 19-20 London, Wembley Stadium *(2 shows)* 21 Cardiff, Cardiff Arms Park 23 Sunderland, Roker Park Stadium 27 Gothenburg, Eriksberg Festival Site 28 Lyon, Stade Municipal de Gerland July 1 Vienna, Prater Stadion 3 Paris, Parc Departemental de la Courneuve 4 Toulouse, Le Stadium 6 Madrid, Estadio Vicente Calderon 7-8 Barcelona, Mini Estadio CF *(2 shows)* 11 Dublin, Slane Castle 14-15 Manchester, Maine Road *(2 shows)* 17 Nice, Stade de L'Ouest 18 Torino, Stadio Comunale 30-31 Philadelphia, Veterans' Stadium *(2 shows)*	17 Bowie records 'Time Will Crawl' appearance for *Top Of The Pops*; it is dropped and will not be shown until 1989 27 Swedish SVT's *Aktuellt* shows 'Glass Spider' clip from Gothenburg gig July 1 'Glass Spider' from Vienna gig shown on Austrian television 4 French TV's *News Soir 3* shows 'Up The Hill Backwards'/'Glass Spider' clip from Paris gig 10 Irish RTE's *Visual Eyes* shows 30-minute item including interview and 'Up The Hill Backwards'/'Glass Spider' clips from Wembley on 19 June 27-31 US news channels show clips from Bowie's Philadelphia press conference and 'Glass Spider' clips from the first US gig
August	August 2-3 East Rutherford, Giants Stadium *(2 shows)* 7 San Jose, Spartan Stadium 8-9 Los Angeles, Anaheim Stadium *(2 shows)* 12 Denver, Mile High Stadium 14 Portland, Civic Auditorium 15 Vancouver, BC Place Stadium 17 Edmonton, Commonwealth Stadium 19 Winnipeg, Winnipeg Stadium 21-22 Chicago, Rosemont Horizon *(2 shows)* 24-25 Toronto, CNE Stadium *(2 shows)* 28 Ottawa, Lansdowne Park	August
30 Montreal gig broadcast on BBC Radio 1	30 Montreal, Olympic Stadium September 1-2 New York, Madison Square Garden *(2 shows)* 3 Foxboro, Sullivan Stadium	30 MTV Awards screens 'Never Let Me Down' live by satellite from Montreal

RECORDING & RELEASES	STAGE	TV & FILM
	6-7 Chapel Hill, Dean Dome *(2 shows)* 10-11 Milwaukee, Marcus Amphitheater *(2 shows)* 12 Detroit, Pontiac Silverdome 14 Lexington, Rupp Arena 18 Miami, Orange Bowl 19 Tampa, Stadium 21-22 Atlanta, Omni Arena *(2 shows)* 25 Hartford, Civic Center 28-29 Washington, Capitol Center *(2 shows)* October 1-2 Minneapolis, St Paul Civic Center *(2 shows)* 4 Kansas City, Kemper Arena 6 New Orleans, Superdome 7-8 Houston, The Summit *(2 shows)* 10-11 Dallas, Reunion Arena *(2 shows)* 13-14 Los Angeles, Sports Arena *(2 shows)* 27 Sydney, Tivoli Club *(Australian press conference)* 29-30 Brisbane, Boondall Entertainment Centre *(2 shows)* November 3-4, 6-7, 9-10, 13-14 Sydney, Entertainment Centre *(8 shows)* 18, 20-21, 23 Melbourne, Kooyong Stadium *(4 shows)* 28 Auckland, Western Springs Stadium *(last show of the Glass Spider tour)*	October 27-28 Australian news programmes show live clips of 'The Jean Genie', 'Young Americans', 'Time Will Crawl' and 'Bang Bang' from the Sydney press conference November David Mallet shoots the *Glass Spider* video at the Sydney concerts December Bowie shoots *The Last Temptation Of Christ* in Morocco
1988	**1988**	**1988**
August *Tin Machine* sessions begin at Mountain Studios, Montreux; they will later move to Compass Point Studios, Nassau	July 1 Dominion Theatre, London *(Bowie performs 'Look Back In Anger' at the Intruders At The Palace benefit gig)*	July 1 "Intruders At The Palace" gig recorded for BBC broadcast September 10 'Look Back In Anger' performance transmitted from New York's WNET Studios as part of *Wrap Around The World*
1989	**1989**	**1989**
May 22 Album release: *Tin Machine*	May ? Nassau, venue unknown *(warm-up gig for the first Tin Machine tour)*	April Julien Temple films *Tin Machine* video May BBC2's *Def II* shows Tin Machine documentary including interviews,

RECORDING & RELEASES	STAGE	TV & FILM
	31 New York, The Armory (Tin Machine perform 'Heaven's In Here' at the Coca-Cola International Music Awards)	tour rehearsal footage and Julien Temple's Tin Machine videos
	June	June
		3 Interview with Bowie and Gabrels on MTV Europe's Week In Rock
	14 New York, The World (first date of the 1989 Tin Machine tour)	
	16 Los Angeles, Roxy Theater (2 shows)	
	21 Copenhagen, Saga Rockteatre	21 'Sacrifice Yourself' and 'Working Class Hero' shot at Copenhagen for Danish TV2
	22 Hamburg, The Docks	22 'Amazing' shot at Hamburg gig for German RTL TV's Ragazzi Report
	24 Amsterdam, Paradiso	24 'Maggie's Farm' video shot live at Amsterdam concert
25 Paris gig broadcast on Westwood One Radio Nework; 'Maggie's Farm', 'I Can't Read', 'Bus Stop', 'Baby Can Dance' and 'Crack City' later released as singles/B-sides	25 Paris, La Cigale	
	27 London, Town & Country Club	
	29 Kilburn, National Ballroom	
	July	
	1 Newport, Leisure Centre	
	2 Bradford, St George's Hall	
	3 Livingston, The Forum (last night of the Tin Machine tour)	
October		
Tin Machine II sessions begin in Sydney; work continues into December		
	November	
	4 Sydney, Moby Dick's (one-off Tin Machine date)	
1990	**1990**	**1990**
January	January	January
'Pretty Pink Rose' and 'Gunman' recorded for Adrian Belew's Young Lions	23 London, Rainbow Theatre (press conference for the Sound + Vision tour)	23 Clips from the Rainbow Theatre press conference (including 'Space Oddity', 'Panic In Detroit', 'John, I'm Only Dancing' and 'Queen Bitch') are shown on numerous TV channels, including SKY, MTV, CNN and SuperChannel
	March	March
	4 Quebec, Colisee (first date of the Sound + Vision tour)	
	6 Montreal, Forum	
	7 Toronto, Skydome	
	10 Winnipeg, Winnipeg Arena	
	12 Edmonton, Northlands Coliseum	
	13 Calgary, Saddledome	
	15 Vancouver, PNE Coliseum	
	19-20 Birmingham, NEC Arena (2 shows)	20 BBC's Midlands Today shows clip of 'Changes' from first Birmingham concert
	23-24 Edinburgh, Royal Highland Exhibition Centre (2 shows)	
	26-28 London, Docklands Arena (3 shows)	26 'Changes' and 'Fame' from London gig shot by BBC's Rocksteady Report
	30 Rotterdam, Sport Paleis Ahoy	30 'Space Oddity' and 'Changes' from Rotterdam gig shot for Dutch TV show Veronica Countdown

RECORDING & RELEASES	STAGE	TV & FILM
	April	April
	1 Dortmund, Westfalenhalle *(cancelled)*	
	2-3 Paris, Palais Omnisports *(2 shows)*	
	5 Frankfurt, Festhalle	
	7 Hamburg, Alsterdorfer Sportshalle	
	8 Berlin, Deutschlandhalle	
	10 Munich, Olympiahalle	10 'Changes' and backstage interview
	11 Stuttgart, Schleyerhalle	from Munich gig shown on
	13-14 Milan, Palatrussardi *(2 shows)*	Norwegian NRK TV show *I Egne Oyne*
	17 Rome, Palauer *(2nd show on 18th cancelled)*	
	20-21 Brussels, Vorst Nationaal *(2 shows)*	
	22 Dortmund, Westfalenhalle	
	27 Miami, Arena	27 'Space Oddity', 'Rebel Rebel' and
	29 Pensacola, Civic Center	'Suffragette City' from Miami gig shot for *MTV News*
	May	May
	1 Orlando, Arena	
	4 St Petersburg, Suncoast Dome	
	5 Jacksonville, Coliseum	
	7 Atlanta, Omni Arena	
	9 Chapel Hill, Dean Smith Center	
	12 Tokyo, Keio Plaza Hotel *(press conference)*	
	15-16 Tokyo, Dome *(2 shows)*	16 Entire Tokyo gig shot for 90-minute
	20 Vancouver, BC Place Stadium	broadcast on Japanese NHK TV
	21 Seattle, Tacoma Dome	
	23 Los Angeles, Sports Arena	
	24 Sacramento, California Expo	
	26 Los Angeles, Dodger Stadium	
	28-29 San Francisco, Shoreline Amphitheater *(2 shows)*	
	June	
	1-2 Denver, McNichols Arena *(2 shows)*	
	4 Dallas, Starplex Amphitheater	
	6 Austin, Frank Irwin Center	
	7 Houston, Woodlands Pavilion	
	9 Kansas City, Sandstone Amphitheater	
	10 St Louis, Arena	
	12 Indianapolis, Deer Creek	
	13 Milwaukee, Marcus Amphitheater	
	15-16 Chicago, World Music Amphitheater *(2 shows)*	
	19-20 Cleveland, Richfield Coliseum *(2 shows)*	
	22, 24-25 Detroit, Auburn Hills Palace *(3 shows)*	
	27 Pittsburgh, Starlake Amphitheater	
	30 St John's, City Park	
	July	
	2 Moncton, Coliseum	
	4 Toronto, CNE Stadium	
	6 Ottawa, Lansdowne Park	
	7 New York, Saratoga Performing Arts Center	
	9-10, 12-13 Philadelphia, Spectrum Arena *(4 shows)*	
	16 Uniondale, Nassau Coliseum	

RECORDING & RELEASES	STAGE	TV & FILM
	18-19 Columbia, Merriweather Post Pavilion *(2 shows)* 21 Foxboro, Sullivan Stadium 23 Hartford, Civic Center 25 Niagara Falls, Convention & Civic Center 29 East Rutherford, Giants Stadium	
August 5 Milton Keynes gig broadcast on BBC Radio 1	August 4-5 Milton Keynes, Bowl *(2 shows)* 7 Manchester, Maine Road 9-10 Dublin, Point Depot *(2 shows)* 13 Fréjus, Les Arnes 16 Ghent, Flanders Expo 18 Nijmegen, Goffert Park 19 Maastricht, MECC 22 Oslo, Jordal Stadion 24 Stockholm, Olympic Stadion 26 Copenhagen, Indraetsparhen 29 Linz, Linz Stadion 31 East Berlin, Weissensee	August 9 'Rebel Rebel' from Dublin gig shown on German ORF TV show *X-Large*
	September 1 Schuttorf, Veechteweise *(Festival)* 2 Ulm, Baden-Wuerttemburgh *(Festival)* 4 Budapest, MTK Stadium 5 Zagreb, Stadion Dinamo 8 Modena, Festa Nationale *(Festival)* 11 Gijon, Hipodromo las Mestas 12 Madrid, Rockodromo de la Casa de Campo	September
	14 Lisbon, Alvalade Stadium *(Festival)* 16 Barcelona, Estadio Olimpico de Montjuic 20 Rio de Janeiro, Sambodromo de Rio 22-23 Sao Paolo, Estadio de Palmeiras *(2 shows)* 25 Sao Paolo, Olympia	14 Lisbon gig shot for 70-minute broadcast on Portuguese Canal 1 TV 25 Sao Paolo gig shot for edited 60-minute broadcast on Brazilian TV
	27 Santiago, Rock In Chile Festival 29 Buenos Aires, River Plate Stadium *(last date of the Sound + Vision tour)*	27 Santiago gig shot for edited 60-minute broadcast on Chilean TV 29 Buenos Aires gig shot for edited 40-minute broadcast on Argentine TV November-December Films *The Linguini Incident*
1991	**1991**	**1991**
March *Tin Machine II* sessions reconvene in Los Angeles August	February 6 Los Angeles, Inglewood Forum *(David makes guest appearance at Morrissey concert)* July St-Malo, France *(rehearsals)* August	Spring Films *Dream On* Summer Films cameo in *Twin Peaks: Fire Walk With Me* August 3 'You Belong In Rock N'Roll' and 'Baby Universal' on BBC1's *Paramount City*
13 BBC Radio session for *Mark*	10-15 Dublin, Factory Studios *(rehearsals)*	12 Dublin rehearsal footage ('If There Is Something', 'Baby Universal')

RECORDING & RELEASES	STAGE	TV & FILM
Goodier's Evening Session recorded live at Maida Vale Studios; tracks later released as B-sides	16 Dublin, Baggott Inn *(first of 2 warm-up shows)* 19 Dublin, Waterfront Rock Café 25 Los Angeles, Rockit Cargo LAX *(press show for Tin Machine It's My Life tour)*	shown on MTV 14 'You Belong In Rock N'Roll' on BBC1's *Wogan*; rehearsal footage and interviews shown on Channel 4's *6:30 Something* 25 LA gig recorded by ABC TV 29 'You Belong In Rock N'Roll' on BBC1's *Top Of The Pops*
September 2 Album release: *Tin Machine II*	September 7 Minneapolis, Marriott City Center *(this and remaining September gigs are US trade shows)* 10 Los Angeles, Marriott 12 San Francisco, Slim's	September
October	October 5-6 Milan, Teatro Smeraldo *(first 2 dates proper of the Tin Machine It's My Life tour)* 8 Florence, Palazzo Dello Sport 9-10 Rome, Teatro Brancaccio *(2 shows)* 12 Munich, Zirhus Krone 14 Offenbach, Stadthalle 15 Ludwigsburg, Forum Schlosspark 17 Berlin, Neue Welt 19 Copenhagen, Falkonerteatret 21 Stockholm, Cirkus 22 Oslo, Konserthus	October 18 'You Belong In Rock N'Roll' on Danish TV2 show *Elevaern*
24 'Baby Can Dance' from Hamburg gig later released on *Best Of Grunge Rock*	24 Hamburg, Docks 25 Hannover, Musikhalle 26 Cologne, E-Werk 28 Utrecht, Muziekcentrum Vredenburg 29 Paris, Olympia 30 Paris, Le Zenith 31 Brussels, Ancienne Belgique	24 Live pre-recording of 'Baby Universal' shown on BBC1's *Top Of The Pops*; Hamburg gig is filmed for official *Oy Vey, Baby* video. Clips from Hamburg gig also shown on MTV
November	November 2 Wolverhampton, Civic Hall 3 Manchester, International 5 Newcastle, Mayfair 6 Liverpool, Royal Court 7 Glasgow, Barrowlands Ballroom 9 Cambridge, Corn Exchange 10-11 London, Brixton Academy *(2 shows)* 15 Philadelphia, Tower Theater 16 Washington, Citadel Center 17 Philadelphia, Tower Theater 19 New Haven, Toads Place	November
20 'I Can't Read' recorded at Boston gig for *Oy Vey, Baby* 27, 29 'Stateside' and 'Heaven's In Here' recorded in New York for *Oy Vey, Baby*	20 Boston, Orpheum Theater 24 Providence, New Campus Club 25 New Britain, The Sting 27, 29 New York, The Academy *(2 shows)*	23 'Baby Universal' and 'If There Is Something' on NBC's *Saturday Night Live*
December	December 1-2 Montreal, La Brique *(2 shows)* 3 Toronto, Concert Hall 4 Detroit, Clubland 6 Cleveland, Agora Metropolitan	December

RECORDING & RELEASES	STAGE	TV & FILM
7 'Amazing' and 'You Belong In Rock N'Roll' recorded at Chicago gig for *Oy Vey, Baby*	Ballroom 7 Chicago, Riviera 9 Dallas, Bronco Bowl 10 Houston, Back Alley 12 Los Angeles, Hollywood Palladium 13 Los Angeles, Variety Arts Theater 14-15 San Diego, Speckles Theater *(2 shows)* 17-18 San Francisco, Warfield Theater *(2 shows)* 20 Seattle, Paramount Theater 21 Vancouver, Commodore Ballroom	13 Interview, 'A Big Hurt' and 'Heaven's In Here' on US TV's *The Arsenio Hall Show*
1992	**1992**	**1992**
February 5-6 'If There Is Something', 'Goodbye Mr. Ed' recorded in Tokyo for *Oy Vey, Baby* 10-11 'Under The God' recorded live in Sapporo for *Oy Vey, Baby* May *Black Tie White Noise* sessions begin at Mountain Studios, Montreux and The Hit Factory, New York July 27 Album release: *Tin Machine Live: Oy Vey, Baby*	January 29 Kyoto, Kaikan Dai-ichi Hall 30-31 Osaka, Festival Hall *(2 shows)* February 2 Fukuoka, Kyusyu Kouseinenkin Kaikan 3 Hiroshima, Kouseinenkin Kaikan 5-6 Tokyo, NHK Hall *(2 shows)* 7 Yokohama, Bunka Taiikukan 10-11 Sapporo, Kouseinenkin Kaikan *(2 shows)* 13 Sendai, Sunplaza Hall 14 Oumiya, Soniku City Hall 17 Toyko, Budokan Hall *(last date of the Tin Machine It's My Life tour)* April 20 London, Wembley Stadium *(the Freddie Mercury tribute concert)*	April 20 The Freddie Mercury tribute concert is broadcast live by BBC TV May 3 American A&E TV show *Behind The Scenes* has interviews with Bowie and other stars of *The Linguini Incident*
1993	**1993**	**1993**
April 5 Album release: *Black Tie White Noise*		January 5 Bowie's cameo in comedy *Full Stretch* transmitted by ITV May 5 *Black Tie White Noise* promotional video shot at Hollywood Center Studios, Los Angeles 6 Interview and performances of 'Jump They Say', 'Black Tie White Noise' and 'Pallas Athena' on US TV's *The Arsenio Hall Show* 13 Interview and performances of 'Nite Flights' and 'Black Tie White Noise' on NBC's *The Tonight Show*

RECORDING & RELEASES	STAGE	TV & FILM
Summer *The Buddha Of Suburbia* sessions at Mountain Studios, Montreux November 8 Album release: *The Buddha Of Suburbia*		*With Jay Leno*
	December 1 London, Wembley Arena *(Bowie co-hosts Concert of Hope AIDS benefit, but does not perform)*	
1994	**1994**	**1994**
March *1.Outside* sessions begin at Mountain Studios, Montreux April 25 Album release: *Santa Monica '72*		
1995	**1995**	**1995**
January-February Final *1.Outside* sessions in New York June 19 Album release: *RarestOneBowie* September	September New York *(rehearsals)* 14 Hartford, Meadows Amphitheater *(first date of the Outside tour)* 16 Mansfield, Great Woods Center 17 Hershey, Hershey Park Stadium 18 New York *(Bowie and Mike Garson perform 'A Small Plot of Land' and 'My Death' at a private charity function)* 20 Toronto, Sky Dome 22 Philadelphia, Camden Waterfront Center 23 Pittsburgh, Starlake Amphitheater	April 20 MTV Europe's *MTV News* shows interview and footage from *New Afro/Pagan and Work 1975-1995*, Bowie's exhibition at London's Cork Street Gallery September 16 Interview and live clips of 'The Hearts Filthy Lesson' and 'I'm Deranged' filmed at Mansfield gig by *MTV News*
25 Album release: *1.Outside* October	27-28 New York, Meadowlands Arena *(2 shows)* 30 Cleveland, Blossom Music Center October 1 Chicago, World Music Theater 3 Detroit, Auburn Hills Palace 4 Columbus, Polaris Amphitheater 6 Washington, Nissan Stone Ridge 7 Raleigh, Walnut Creek Amphitheater 9 Atlanta, Lakewood Amphitheater 11 St Louis, Riverport Amphitheater 13 Dallas, Starplex Amphitheater 14 Austin, Meadows Amphitheater 16 Denver, McNichols Arena 18 Phoenix, Desert Sky Pavilion	26 'The Hearts Filthy Lesson' on CBS's *The Late Show With David Letterman* 30 German ZDF TV shows documentary *Inside Outside*, including live clips and studio footage of *1.Outside* sessions October 1 CNN's *Showbiz Today* includes 1995 rehearsal footage of 'Look Back In Anger'

RECORDING & RELEASES	STAGE	TV & FILM
	19 Las Vegas, Thomas & Mack Center	
	21 Mountain View, Shoreline Amphitheater	21 Swedish ZTV's *Artistspecial* shows interview, tour rehearsals and behind-
	24 Seattle, Tacoma Dome	the-scenes footage of 'The Hearts
	25 Portland, Rose Garden Arena	Filthy Lesson' video shoot
	28-29 Los Angeles, Great Western Forum *(2 shows)*	27 Interview and 'Strangers When We Meet' on NBC's *The Tonight Show With*
	31 Los Angeles, Hollywood Palladium	*Jay Leno*
November	November	November
	8-13 Elwood Studios, Watford *(rehearsals)*	10 'Strangers When We Meet' on BBC1's *Top Of The Pops*
18 Wembley gig recorded by BBC Radio for edited broadcast	14-15, 17-18 London, Wembley Arena *(4 shows)*	
	20-21 Birmingham, NEC Arena *(2 shows)*	
	23 Dublin, Point Depot	
	24 Paris, Le Zenith	24 'The Man Who Sold The World'
	26 Exeter, Westpoint	performed at MTV's European Music
	27 Cardiff, International Arena	Awards
	29 Aberdeen, Scottish Exhibition & Conference Centre	
	30 Glasgow, Scottish Exhibition & Conference Centre	
December	December	December
	3-4 Sheffield, Arena *(second show cancelled)*	2 Interview, 'Hallo Spaceboy', 'The Man Who Sold The World' and
	5 Belfast, King's Hall	'Strangers When We Meet' on BBC2's
	6 Manchester, Nynex Arena *(cancelled)*	*Later… With Jools Holland*
	7 Newcastle, Newcastle Arena	
	8 Manchester, Nynex Arena	
13 'Under Pressure' and 'Moonage Daydream' from Birmingham gig later released as B-sides	13 Birmingham, NEC Hall 5 *("The Big Twix Mix Show")*	13 'Hallo Spaceboy', The Man Who Sold The World' and 'Under Pressure' recorded at the Birmingham show for TV broadcast
		14 'Hallo Spaceboy', 'The Voyeur', 'Under Pressure', 'Boys Keep Swinging', 'The Man Who Sold The World' and 'Teenage Wildlife' record- ed for Channel 4's *The White Room* (last two not broadcast)
1996	**1996**	**1996**
	January	January
	14-16 Helsinki *(rehearsals)*	
	17 Helsinki, Icehall	
	19 Stockholm, Globe Arena	19 Clips from 'Look Back In Anger' and 'The Motel' recorded at Stockholm gig by MTV and Swedish SVT's *Nöjesrevyn*
	20 Gothenburg, Scandinavium	20 Interview, 'The Man Who Sold The
	22 Oslo, Spektrum	World' and 'Hallo Spaceboy' for Swedish SVT's *Det Kommer Mera*
	24 Copenhagen, Valbyhallen	24 Interview and live clip of 'The
	25 Hamburg, Sportshalle	Motel' from Copenhagen gig on Danish TV2's *Superpuls*
	27 Brussels, Vorst Nationaal	26 Interview, 'The Voyeur', 'Under
	28 Utrecht, Prins Van Oranjehal	Pressure', 'The Man Who Sold The
	30 Dortmund, Westfalenhalle	World', 'Hallo Spaceboy' and

RECORDING & RELEASES	STAGE	TV & FILM
	31 Frankfurt, Festhalle	'Strangers When We Meet' for French TV's *Taratata*
	February	February
	1 Berlin, Deutschlandhalle	
	3 Prague, Sportovini Hala	3 Dutch TV's *Karel* includes interview
	4 Vienna, Stadthalle	and performances of 'The Voyeur',
	6 Ljublijana, Hala Tivoli	'Hallo Spaceboy', 'Under Pressure'
	8 Milan, Palatrussardi	and 'Warszawa'
	9 Bologna, Palasport di Casalecchio	
	11 Lyon, Halle Tony Garnier	
	13 Geneva, Arena	
	14 Zurich, Hallenstadion	
	16 Amneville, Le Galaxie	
	17 Lille, Le Zenith	
	18 Rennes, Salle Expos-Aeroport	
	19 London, Earls Court *(Brit Awards)*	19 Bowie collects "Outstanding
	20 Paris, Palais Omnisports *(last date of the Outside tour)*	Contribution" award from Tony Blair at the Brit Awards, and plays 'Hallo Spaceboy' (with Pet Shop Boys), 'Moonage Daydream' and 'Under Pressure'
		March
		1 'Hallo Spaceboy' with Pet Shop Boys on BBC1's *Top Of The Pops*
	June	June
	4-5 Tokyo, Budokan Hall *(first 2 shows of the "Summer festivals" tour)*	
	7 Nagoya, Century Hall	
	8 Hiroshima, Kouseinenkin Kaikan	
	10 Osaka, Castle Hall	
	11 Kokura, Kyusyu Kouseinenkin Kaikan	
	13 Fukuoka, Sun Palace	
	16 St Petersburg, White Nights Festival *(cancelled)*	
	18 Moscow, Kremlin Palace Concert Hall	18 Edited 50-minute selection from Moscow gig broadcast on Russian OPT
	20 Reykjavik, Laugardalsholl Arena	20 Clips of 'Look Back In Anger' and 'Hallo Spaceboy' from Reykjavik gig later shown on MTV Europe's *Summertime Weekend*
	22 St Goarshausen, Loreley Freilichtbühne	22 Entire Loreley Festival gig broadcast on German TV
	23 Lisbon *(Super Rock Festival)*	
	25 Toulon, Zenith Omega	
	28 Halle, Peissnitzinsel *(Outside Festival)*	
	30 Roskilde *(Roskilde Festival)*	
July	July	July
3 Excerpts from Tel Aviv gig broadcast on FM radio	1 Athens, PAO Stadium	
	3 Tel Aviv, Ha-Yarkron Park	
	5 Torhout *(Torhout Festival)*	5 'Hallo Spaceboy' clip from Torhout Festival gig later shown with interview on MTV Europe's *News Weekend Edition*
	6 Werchter *(Festival Terrein)*	
	7 Belfort *(Eurokennes Festival)*	
	9 Rome, Curva Stadium Olimpico	
	10 Monte Carlo, Espace Fontveille	
	12 Esclarre *(Esclarre Festival)*	
	14 St Polten *(St Polten Festival)*	
	16 Rotterdam, Sport Paleis Ahoy	

RECORDING & RELEASES	STAGE	TV & FILM
18 Six songs from Phoenix Festival gig broadcast live on Radio 1's *Mark Radcliffe* show 20 Excerpts from Ballingen gig broadcast on FM radio August *Earthling* sessions begin at Looking Glass Studios, New York	18 Stratford-upon-Avon *(Phoenix Festival)* 20 Ballingen, Piazzetta del Valle 21 Bellinzona, Piazza del Sol *(last date of the "Summer Festivals" tour)* September 6 Philadelphia, Electric Factory *(first of the "East Coast Ballroom" tour)* 7 Washington, Capitol Ballroom 13 Boston, Avalon Ballroom 14 New York, Roseland Ballroom October 19-20 Mountain View, Shoreline Amphitheater *(Bridge School benefit concerts)* 24 New York, Madison Square Garden *(VH1 Fashion Awards)*	18 Selections from the Phoenix Festival gig ('Scary Monsters', 'The Hearts Filthy Lesson', '"Heroes"', 'Hallo Spaceboy', 'White Light/White Heat', 'Moonage Daydream') recorded for broadcasts on ITV and abroad October 24 'Fashion' and 'Little Wonder' from the VH1 Fashion Awards later screened on VH1
1997	**1997**	**1997**
January BBC Radio session for *ChangesNowBowie* recorded during rehearsals in New York February 3 Album release: *Earthling*	January 3-4 New York, SIR Studios *(rehearsals)* 7 Hartford, Meadows Music Theater *(rehearsals)* 9 New York, Madison Square Garden *(fiftieth birthday concert)*	January 4 BBC2 shows *Changes – David Bowie At Fifty* 8 ITV shows *An Earthling At 50* 9 The fiftieth birthday gig has pay-per-view broadcast on US television; press conference clips and footage appear on countless news channels worldwide 26 Interview and backstage footage from fiftieth birthday gig on BBC2's *The O-Zone* 31 French Canal + TV's *A Part Ca* shows 110-minute Bowie documentary February 8 'Little Wonder' and 'Scary Monsters' on NBC's *Saturday Night Live* 11 Interview and performance of 'Little Wonder' on NBC's *The Tonight Show With Jay Leno* 12 News cameras cover Bowie unveiling his star on the Hollywood Walk Of Fame 17 Interview, 'Little Wonder' and 'Telling Lies' on French Canal + TV's *Nulle Part Ailleurs* 20 'Little Wonder' on Italian RAI Uno's *San Remo Festival* 22 Interview and 'Little Wonder' on German ZDF's *Wetten Dass…?* March 3 Interview, 'Seven Years In Tibet', 'Dead Man Walking', 'Scary Monsters' and 'Rosie Girl' on American TV's *Rosie O'Donnell Show*

RECORDING & RELEASES	STAGE	TV & FILM
		14 'Dead Man Walking' video filmed in Toronto
April	April	April
		4 'Dead Man Walking' on CBS's *The Late Show With David Letterman*
8 Radio sessions for Boston WBCN ('Scary Monsters', 'Dead Man Walking', 'The Jean Genie', 'I Can't Read') and WNNX Atlanta (as above plus 'The Supermen')		10 Interview, 'Dead Man Walking' and 'I'm Afraid Of Americans' on NBC's *Late Night With Conan O'Brien*
	20 Dublin, Factory Studios *(rehearsals)*	18 Interview, 'Dead Man Walking' and 'Scary Monsters' on Channel 5's *The Jack Docherty Show*
		25 'Dead Man Walking' on BBC1's *Top Of The Pops*
May	May	
Bowie records vocals for Goldie track 'Truth' at Trident Studios	17 Dublin, Factory Studios *(warm-up show. Rehearsals continue for the rest of May at the Brixton Academy, London)*	
June	June	June
	2-3 London, Hanover Grand *(2 warm-up shows for the Earthling tour)*	3 Clips of 'Fashion' and 'Fun' from the second Hanover Grand gig are later shown by VH1
	5 Hamburg, Grosse Freiheit *(warm-up show)*	
	7 Lubeck, Flughafen Blankense *(first date proper of the Earthling tour)*	
	8 Offenbach, Bieberer Berg Stadion	
10 'V-2 Schneider' and 'Pallas Athena' from Amsterdam gig later released on *Tao Jones Index* 12" single	10 Amsterdam, Paradiso	
	11 Utrecht, Muziekcentrum Vredenburg	
	13 Dortmund, Westfalenhalle	
	14 Paris, Parc des Princes	
	16 Nantes-Reze, La Trocadiere	
	17 Bordeaux, La Medocquine	
	19 Clermont-Ferrand, Maison des Sports	
	21 Leipzig, AGRA-Gelaende	
	22 Munich, Neu-Biberg Airport	
	24 Vienna, Sommer Arena	24 'Strangers When We Meet' and 'The Man Who Sold The World' from Vienna gig shown on Austrian ORF 2 TV's *Zeit Im Bild*
	25 Prague, Congress Centre	
	28 Oslo, Kalvoeya Festival	
	29 Turku, Ruisrock Festival	
	July	July
	1 Zagreb, Stadium Zagreb	
	2 Pistoia, Piazza del Duomo	
	4 Torhout *(Torhout Festival)*	
	5 Werchter *(Werchter Festival)*	
	6 Ringe *(Midtfyns Festival)*	
	8 Brescia, Stadio Rigamonti	9 'Seven Years In Tibet' video shot in Italy
	10 Napoli, Ilva di Bagnoli	
	11 Arbatax, Rocce Rosse	
	13 Frauenfeld, Out In The Green	
	15 Madrid, Aqua Lung	
	16 Zaragoza, Pebellon de Principe Felipe	
	17 San Sebastian, Velodromo de Anoeta	
	19-20 Stratford-upon-Avon, Phoenix Festival *(first night as "Tao Jones Index" in Radio 1 Tent, second night main stage)*	20 'Little Wonder' from the Phoenix Festival is later broadcast on MTV Europe's *Festivals '97*
	22 Glasgow, Barrowlands Ballroom	
	23 Manchester, Academy	

RECORDING & RELEASES	STAGE	TV & FILM
	25 Malmo, Mulleplatsen	
	26 Stockholm, Lollipop Festival	27 Clips of 'Quicksand' and 'The
	27 Gdansk, venue unknown	Man Who Sold The World' from the
	29 Lyon, Fourviere	previous day's Stockholm gig are
	30 Juan-les-Pins, Pinede Gould	shown on Swedish ZTV's *ZTV På Väg*
		August
	August	
	1 Birmingham, Que Club	
	2 Liverpool, Royal Court Theatre	
	3 Newcastle, Riverside	
	5 Nottingham, Rock City	
	6 Leeds, Town & Country Club	
	8-9 Dublin, Olympia Theatre *(2 shows)*	11 Clips of 'The Jean Genie' and 'I'm
	11-12 London, Shepherds Bush	Afraid Of Americans' recorded at
	Empire *(2 shows)*	Shepherds Bush gig by MTV's *News*
	14 Budapest *(Student Island Festival)*	*Weekend Edition*
September	September	
	6 Vancouver, Plaza of Nations	
8 Acoustic session for Seattle 103.7 FM	7 Seattle, Paramount Theater	
radio's *The Mountain Morning Show*		
('Dead Man Walking', 'Always Crashing		
In The Same Car', 'Scary Monsters')		
9 Acoustic session for San Francisco	9 San Francisco, Warfield Theater	
105 FM radio ('Always Crashing In	10 Los Angeles, Hollywood Athletic	
The Same Car', 'I Can't Read', 'Dead	Club	
Man Walking', 'Scary Monsters')	12-13 Los Angeles, Universal	
	Amphitheater *(2 shows)*	
	15-16 San Francisco, Warfield Theater	
	(2 shows)	
	19 Chicago, Vic Theater	
	21-22 Detroit, State Theater *(2 shows)*	
	24-25 Montreal, Metropolis *(2 shows)*	
26 Acoustic session for CFNY Toronto	27-28 Toronto, Warehouse Docks	
radio ('Always Crashing In The Same	*(2 shows)*	
Car', 'I Can't Read', 'The Supermen')	30 Boston, Orpheum Theater	
October	October	October
1 Boston gig Webcast live on the	1 Boston, Orpheum Theater	
Internet	3-4 Philadelphia, Electric Factory	
	(2 shows)	
	7-8 Fort Lauderdale, Chili Pepper	6 'I'm Afraid Of Americans' video shot
	(2 shows)	in New York
	10 Atlanta, International Ballroom	
	12 Washington, Capitol Ballroom	
	13 New York, The Supper Club	
	14 Port Chester, Capitol Theater	14 Port Chester gig broadcast on
	(special MTV gig)	MTV's *Live At The 10 Spot*
	15 New York, Radio City Music Hall	
	(GQ Awards)	
	17 Chicago, Aragon Ballroom	
	18 St Paul, Roy Wilkins	
	23 Mexico City, Autodromo	
	Hermanos Rodriguez	
	31 Curitiba, Pedreira Paulo Leminski	
November	November	November
	1 Sao Paolo, Pista de Atletismo	1 'Fashion', 'I'm Afraid Of Americans',
	2 Rio de Janeiro, Metropolitan	'Little Wonder' and 'Moonage Day-
	5 Santiago, Estadio Nacional	dream' from the New York GQ Awards
7 Acoustic session for Argentina's 95.9	7 Buenos Aires, Ferrocarril Oeste	gig on 15 October broadcast on VH1

RECORDING & RELEASES	STAGE	TV & FILM
FM *Rock & Pop* radio ('Always Crashing In The Same Car', 'I Can't Read', 'The Supermen')	Stadium *(last date of the Earthling tour)* December 6 Los Angeles, Universal Amphitheater 7 San Francisco, Kezar Pavilion	7 Interview and entire Buenos Aires gig shot for two-part broadcast on Argentine Much Music TV's *Especial*
1998	**1998**	**1998**
	January 29 New York, Hammersmith Ballroom *(Bowie performs at Howard Stern's birthday party)*	February 5 American E!TV broadcasts *Howard Stern Birthday Show* recorded 29 January: 'Fame', 'Hallo Spaceboy' and 'I'm Afraid Of Americans' 21 Begins shooting *Everybody Loves Sunshine* on the Isle of Man June Films *Il Mio West* in Tuscany July Films *Mr Rice's Secret* in Vancouver
August '(Safe In This) Sky Life' and 'Mother' recorded in New York September 1 BowieNet launched in America		September 27 American VH1 TV shows *Legends*, a 45-minute documentary including many rare clips
1999	**1999**	**1999**
March 29 Vocals for Placebo duet 'Without You I'm Nothing' recorded at Looking Glass Studios, New York April *'hours…'* sessions begin at Seaview Studios, Bermuda May 24 'What's Really Happening?' recorded at Looking Glass Studios, New York	February 16 London, Docklands Arena *(performs '20th Century Boy' with Placebo at Brit Awards)* March 29 New York, Irving Plaza *(plays encores at Placebo gig)* May 8 Boston, Hynes Convention Center *(receives honorary doctorate from Berklee College of Music)*	February 17 ITV screens highlights of Brit Awards ceremony, including Bowie's duet with Placebo March Films role in *The Hunger: Sanctuary* 12 Pre-recorded appearance on BBC's Comic Relief Red Nose Day July 29 CNN's *Showbiz Today* includes studio footage from the 'What's Really Happening?' session August 23 Records *VH1 Storytellers* set and three live tracks for *Top Of The Pops*

RECORDING & RELEASES	STAGE	TV & FILM
	September 9 New York City, Metropolitan Opera House *(introduces Lauryn Hill at MTV Awards)*	September 9 MTV *Video Music Awards* 10 *The Hunger – Sanctuary* screened by Showtime TV 23 'The Pretty Things Are Going To Hell' on Canadian *Much Music Awards* 24 *Top Of The Pops* broadcasts 'Thursday's Child' pre-recorded in New York 26 Introduces Eurythmics on NBC's *Saturday Night Live 25 Year Special*
October 4 Album release: *'hours…'*	October	October 2 'Thursday's Child' and 'Rebel Rebel' on NBC's *Saturday Night Live* 4 'The Pretty Things Are Going To Hell' on *The Late Show With David Letterman* 8 'Survive', 'Rebel Rebel' and 'China Girl' taped for Channel 4's *TFI Friday* (only 'Survive' broadcast; 'Rebel Rebel' shown a week later)
9 NetAid broadcast on BBC Radio 1	9 London, Wembley Stadium *(NetAid)* 10 Dublin, HQ *(first date of the 'hours…' promotional tour)*	9 BBC2 shows 'Life On Mars?', 'Survive', 'China Girl' and 'Rebel Rebel' from NetAid; US *Ku-Band Satellite* screens the full set (as above plus 'The Pretty Things Are Going To Hell' and 'Drive In Saturday') 13 'Thursday's Child' on French TF1's *Les Années Tubes*
14 'Survive', 'Thursday's Child' and 'Seven' from Paris gig recorded for release as B-sides	14 Paris, Elysée Montmartre	14 CNN *World News* shows clip from the Paris gig and footage of Bowie receiving Chevalier des Arts et Lettres 16 'Thursday's Child' on German ZDF's *Wetten Dass…?*
17 Vienna gig Webcast live on BowieNet	17 Vienna, Libro Music Hall	17 Austrian stations ORF and W1 screen 'Life On Mars?', 'Thursday's Child' and 'Something In The Air' from Vienna gig 18 Broadcast of *VH1 Storytellers* show recorded in August 19 'Survive' and 'Thursday's Child' on Spanish TVE's *Cosas Que Importan* 20 Eight-song set for French Canal + show *Nulle Part Ailleurs* 21 'Thursday's Child' on Italian Rai Uno's *Francamente Me Ne Infischio*
25 Live session at BBC Maida Vale Studios broadcast on Radio 1's *Mark Radcliffe Show*	28 Las Vegas, Mandalay Bay Casino *(WB Radio Music Awards)*	28 Accepts award and performs 'Thursday's Child' and 'Rebel Rebel' on US Warner Bros *WB Radio Music Awards*
November	November	November 3 BBC2's *TOTP2* includes interview and pre-recorded exclusives 'The Pretty Things Are Going To Hell' and 'Survive' 16 'Thursday's Child' and 'Cracked Actor' on NBC's *Late Night With Conan O'Brien* 17 'Thursday's Child' and 'China Girl' on *The Rosie O'Donnell Show*
19 New York gig Webcast live	19 New York, Kit Kat Club	22 Ten-song session on Canadian

RECORDING & RELEASES	STAGE	TV & FILM
		station Musique Plus 26 Channel 4's *TFI Friday* screens unseen 'Rebel Rebel' performance recorded in October 28 German VIVA's *Jam* shows 50-minute special with interview and studio footage from the *'hours...'* sessions 29 Records 'Ashes To Ashes', 'Something In The Air', 'Cracked Actor', 'Survive' and 'I'm Afraid Of Americans' for BBC2's *Later... With Jools Holland* (last song not broadcast)
	December 2 London, Astoria 4 Milan, Alcatraz 7 Copenhagen, Vega	December 3 Interview on BBC2's *Newsnight* 4 *Later... With Jools Holland* broadcast 8 'Survive' and 'Thursday's Child' for Swedish TV4's *Inte Bara Blix* 11 'Thursday's Child' on Swedish TV4 show *Bingolotto* 30 Guests on Channel 4's *The Big Breakfast*
2000	**2000**	**2000**
	March 31 New York *(rehearsals begin for 2000 live shows)* June 16,19 New York, Roseland Ballroom *(show on 17 June cancelled)* 25 Glastonbury, Glastonbury Festival	June 23 'Wild Is The Wind', 'Starman', 'Absolute Beginners' and 'Cracked Actor' recorded for Channel 4's *TFI Friday* (last two not broadcast) 25 'Wild Is The Wind', 'China Girl', 'Changes', 'Stay', 'Life On Mars?', 'Ziggy Stardust' and '"Heroes"' from Glastonbury screened on BBC2 and BBC Choice 27 BBC concert recorded at Radio Theatre, Broadcasting House
July *Toy* sessions begin at Sear Sound and Looking Glass Studios, New York, continuing on and off until October 24 Live webcast of Yahoo! Internet Life Online Music Awards September 13 Album release: *liveandwell.com* 25 Album release: *Bowie At The Beeb*	July 24 New York, Studio 54 *(Yahoo! Internet Life Online Music Awards)*	 September 24 60-minute compilation of BBC Radio Theatre concert from 27 June shown on BBC2
 December 31 Complete New York gig from 19 November 1999 broadcast on Radio France	October 20 New York, Madison Square Garden *(guest appearance at VH1 Fashion Awards)*	October Films cameo appearance in *Zoolander* December 25 BBC Choice screens live selection from Glastonbury: same as 25 June plus 'Let's Dance'

RECORDING & RELEASES	STAGE	TV & FILM
2001	**2001**	**2001**
January Preliminary *Heathen* sessions begin. Main recording takes place in August and September at Allaire Studios, New York		
	February 26 New York, Carnegie Hall *(Tibet House Benefit Concert)*	February Films interview for *Rutles 2: Can't Buy Me Lunch* March 21 BBC2's *Omnibus* screens Stanley Spencer documentary *Resurrecting Stanley*, narrated by Bowie
July 14,21 BBC Radio 2 broadcasts two-part history of the Marquee Club, narrated by Bowie		
	October 20 New York, Madison Square Garden *(The Concert For New York City)*	October 20 The Concert For New York City screened live on VH1 in America 21 The Concert For New York City screened on VH1 in the UK
2002	**2002**	**2002**
	February 22 New York, Carnegie Hall *(Tibet House Benefit Concert)* May 10 New York, Battery Park City *(MTV Tribeca Film Festival)* 30 New York, Javits Center *(performs 'America' at Robin Hood Foundation charity auction)*	
June	June	June 2 *Top Of The Pops* and *TOTP2* performances recorded at Kaufman Studios, New York 7 'Slow Burn' on BBC1's *Top Of The Pops* (recorded 2 June)
10 Album release: *Heathen*	11 New York, Roseland Ballroom *(BowieNet members' warm-up gig for the Heathen tour)* 14 New York, Rockefeller Plaza *(NBC Today Show's 7th Annual Summer Concert Series)*	10 'Slow Burn' and short interview on CBS's *The Late Show With David Letterman* 14 NBC's *The Today Show* includes live performance from New York 15 Two-hour live concert on A&E's *Live By Request* 18 'Fame' on BBC2's *TOTP2* (recorded 2 June) 19 'Slow Burn', 'Cactus' and interview on NBC's *Late Night With Conan O'Brien*; 'I Took A Trip On A Gemini Spaceship' on BBC2's *TOTP2* (recorded 2 June) 27 Records *Friday Night With Ross And Bowie*, including performances of 'Fashion', 'Slip Away', 'Be My Wife', 'Everyone Says 'Hi'' and 'Ziggy Stardust'
	29 London, Royal Festival Hall *(Meltdown Festival gig, billed as 'The New Heathens Night'; first show proper of the Heathen tour)*	

RECORDING & RELEASES	STAGE	TV & FILM
	July	July
	1 Paris, Olympia	
	3 Odderøya, Kristiansand, Norway *(Quart Festival)*	
	5 FriluftsScenen Lunden, Sundvej, Denmark *(Horsens Festival)*	5 BBC1 screens *Friday Night With Ross And Bowie* ('Be My Wife' not screened)
	7 Ostend, Wellington Race Track *(Seat Beach Rock Festival)*	
	10 Manchester, Lancashire County Cricket Club Ground *(Move Festival)*	11 Interview and 'Everyone Says 'Hi'' on German TV's *Die Harald Schmidt Show*
	12 Cologne, E-Werk	
	14 Nimes, Les Arenes *(Festival de Nimes)*	
	15 Lucca, Tuscany *(Lucca Summer Festival)*	
	18 Montreux, Auditorium Stravinski *(36th Montreux Jazz Festival)*	
	28 Bristow, VA, Nissan Pavilion *(first date of the Area: 2 Festival tour; all subsequent July & August dates are part of Area: 2)*	28 Australian Channel Nine broadcasts *60 Minutes* Bowie documentary
	30 Philadelphia, PA, Tweeter Center	
	31 Holmdel, NJ, PNC Bank Center	
	August	August
	2 Wantagh, New York, Jones Beach	
	3 Boston, MA, Tweeter Center	
	5 Toronto, Molson Amphitheater	
	6 Detroit, DTE Energy Music Center	7 Interview, 'Cactus' and 'Everyone Says 'Hi'' on NBC's *Last Call With Carson Daly* (recorded 1 August)
	8 Chicago, Tweeter Center	
	10 Denver, Pepsi Arena	12 Interview, 'Cactus' and 'Everyone Says 'Hi'' on NBC's *The Tonight Show With Jay Leno*
	13 Los Angeles, Verizon Amphitheater	
	14 San Francisco, Shoreline Amphitheater	18 Feature on Area: Two tour on CNN's *The Music Room*
	16 George, WA, Gorge Amphitheater	25 Interview on CNN's *People In The News*
		30 US station AMC shows documentary *Hollywood Rocks The Movies: The 1970s*, narrated by Bowie
September	September	September
6 Interview on London's Capital FM Radio	3 London, Natural History Museum *(receives Outstanding Achievement prize at GQ Men of the Year Awards)*	12 European station ARTE broadcasts Paris concert from 1 July 2002
		14 'Everyone Says 'Hi'' and 'Slip Away' on Swedish *BingoLotto*
16 Interviews on Radio 1's *Mark And Lard* and XFM's Zoe Ball show		
18 BBC Radio Session recorded at Maida Vale Studios		21 Interview, 'Everyone Says 'Hi'' and 'Life On Mars?' on BBC1's *Parkinson* (recorded 19 September)
	22 Berlin, Max Schmelling Halle	22 Interview on French *Vivement Dimanche* (recorded 10 September)
	24-25 Paris, Zenith *(2 shows)*	
	27 Bonn, Museumsmeile	27 'Everyone Says 'Hi'' on BBC1's *Top Of The Pops* (recorded 2 June)
	29 Munich, Olympiahalle	
October	October	October
5 Maida Vale Session from 18 September broadcast on BBC Radio 2 as *David Bowie – Live And Exclusive*	2 London, Carling Apollo Hammersmith	5 Interview and 'Everyone Says 'Hi'' on German ZDF's *Wetten Dass…?*
		6 'Everyone Says 'Hi'' and 'Cactus' on Italian *Quelli Che Il Calcio*

RECORDING & RELEASES	STAGE	TV & FILM
	11 Staten Island, NY, The Music Hall at Snug Harbor 12 Brooklyn, NY, St Anne's Warehouse 15 New York, Radio City Music Hall (*VH1/Vogue Fashion Awards*) 16 Queens, NY, Colden Center at Queens College 17 Bronx, NY, Jimmy's Bronx Café	10 'Everyone Says 'Hi'' and 'Changes' on ABC's *Live With Regis And Kelli* 15 'Rebel' Rebel' and 'Cactus' from VH1/Vogue Fashion Awards on VH1 18 'Rebel Rebel', '5.15 The Angels Have Gone' and 'Heathen (The Rays)' on BBC2's *Later… With Jools Holland* (recorded 20 September)
	20 Manhattan, NY, Beacon Theater 21 Philadelphia, Tower Theater 23 Boston, Orpheum Theater (*final show of the Heathen tour*)	19 'Afraid' and 'I've Been Waiting For You' on NBC's *Late Night With Conan O'Brien* 30 'Cactus' and 'Rebel' Rebel' on CBS's *The Early Show*
November 4 Album release: *Best Of Bowie* 11 DVD release: *Best Of Bowie*		November 4 *VH1 Reveals* interview on VH1 UK; *David Bowie Biography* on US A&E Channel (later released on DVD as *Sound & Vision*) December 26 A&E's *Live By Request* from 15 June shown on UK's ITV1 31 'Slip Away' and 'Afraid' on CBS's *The Early Show* (held over from 30 October); 'Afraid' from Berlin concert on 22 September shown on ABC's *Dick Clark's Primetime Rockin' New Year's Eve*
2003	**2003**	**2003**
January-May *Reality* sessions at Looking Glass Studios, New York	February 28 New York, Carnegie Hall (*Tibet House Benefit Concert*)	January 8 'Ashes To Ashes' on BBC1's *TOTP2* (recorded 2 June 2002) February 8 90-minute compilation from the Berlin concert on 22 September 2002 broadcast by German SAT1
March 24 Album and DVD release: *Ziggy Stardust And The Spiders From Mars: The Motion Picture* (new version remixed by Tony Visconti)		March 2 *Liquid Assets: Bowie's Millions* shown on BBC3
		May 15 NBC shows 'clay-mation' version of *Late Night With Conan O'Brien* from 19 October 2002
September	August 19 Poughkeepsie, NY, Chance Theater (*BowieNet members' warm-up show for A Reality Tour*) September 8 London, Riverside Studios (*BowieNet show transmitted live to cinemas world-*	September 4 France 2 TV special recorded (see 18 September) 8 Riverside Studios show filmed for cinema transmission and DVD release

RECORDING & RELEASES	STAGE	TV & FILM
15 Album release: *Reality*	*wide and later released on DVD)* 18 New York, Rockefeller Plaza *(NBC Today Show's Annual Summer Concert Series)*	12 Interview, 'New Killer Star' and 'Modern Love' on BBC1's *Friday Night With Jonathan Ross* (recorded 11 September) 18 'New Killer Star', 'Modern Love' and 'Never Get Old' live from the Rockefeller Plaza on NBC's *The Today Show*; Two-hour Bowie special, including interview and 'New Killer Star', 'Never Get Old', 'She'll Drive The Big Car', 'Modern Love', 'Fashion' (with Damon Albarn), 'Days' and 'Fall Dog Bombs The Moon' on French TV's France 2 (recorded 4 September)
23 Exclusive session recorded for AOL Broadband ('New Killer Star', 'I'm Afraid Of Americans', 'Rebel Rebel', 'Fall Dog Bombs The Moon' and 'Days')		22 'New Killer Star' on CBS's *The Late Show With David Letterman* 25 'New Killer Star', 'Never Get Old' and 'Hang On To Yourself' on NBC's *Last Call With Carson Daly* (recorded 17 September) 28 Profile of Bowie on CBS's *60 Minutes*
October	October 7 Copenhagen, Forum *(first show proper of A Reality Tour)* 8 Stockholm, The Globe	October
10 AOL Broadband begins streaming exclusive session recorded on 23 September	10 Helsinki, Hartwall Arena 12 Oslo, Spectrum 15 Rotterdam, Ahoy Arena 16 Hamburg, Color Line Arena	
		15 Performance of 'Fashion' from Rotterdam beamed to 'Fashion Rocks' charity show at London's Royal Albert Hall 17 'Never Get Old' and 'New Killer Star' on German TV's *Die Harald Schmidt Show*
	18 Frankfurt, Festhalle-Messe 20-21 Paris, Palais Omnisports Bercy *(2 shows)* 23 Milan, Palazzetto Dello Sport FilaForum 24 Zürich, Hallenstadion 26 Stuttgart, Hanns-Martin-Schleyer-Halle 27 Munich, Olympiahalle 29 Vienna, Wiener Stadthalle 31 Cologne, Köln Arena	19 UK Channel 4 screens 'Fashion Rocks' charity show from Royal Albert Hall 29 US A&E screens 'Fashion Rocks' charity show from Royal Albert Hall
November	November 1 Hanover, Preussag Arena 3 Berlin, Max Schmelling Halle 5 Antwerp, Sportpaleis 7 Lille, Le Zenith 8 Amneville, Le Galaxie 10 Nice, Zenith 12 Toulouse, Le Zenith *(cancelled)* 14 Marseille, Le Dome 15 Lyon, La Halle Tony Garnier	November
17 Album release: *Reality (Tour Edition)*	17 Manchester, MEN Arena 19-20 Birmingham, NEC *(2 shows)* 22-23 Dublin, The Point *(2 shows)* 25-26 London, Wembley Arena	14 French TV5's *Acoustic* shows 'New Killer Star', 'Fame', 'Cactus' and 'Never Get Old' from Paris concert on 20 October

RECORDING & RELEASES	STAGE	TV & FILM
	(2 shows) 28 Glasgow, SECC	29 Interview, 'Ziggy Stardust' and 'The Loneliest Guy' on BBC1's *Parkinson* (recorded 27 November)
December	December 6-12 *(6: Atlantic City, 7: Washington, 9: Boston, 10: Philadelphia, 12: Toronto; first five US/Canada shows cancelled owing to illness and rescheduled for 2004)* 13 Montreal, Bell Centre 15 New York City, Madison Square Garden 16 Uncasville, Mohegan Sun Arena	
20 Paradise Island concert broadcast by various US radio stations	20 Bahamas, Paradise Island, Atlantis *(promotional concert, not billed as part of A Reality Tour)*	
2004	**2004**	**2004**
	January 7 Cleveland, CSU Convocation Center 9 Detroit, Palace of Auburn Hills 11 Minneapolis, Target Center 13,14,16 Chicago, Rosemont Theatre *(3 shows)* 19 Denver, Fillmore Auditorium 21 Calgary, Pengrowth Saddledome 24 Vancouver, General Motors Place Bowl 25 Seattle, Paramount Theatre 27 San José, HP Pavilion 30 Las Vegas, The Joint 31 Los Angeles, Shrine Auditorium February 2 Los Angeles, Shrine Auditorium 3 Los Angeles, The Wiltern 5 Phoenix, Dodge Theatre 6 Las Vegas, The Joint 7 Los Angeles, The Wiltern 14 Wellington, Westpac Stadium 17 Brisbane, Entertainment Centre 20-21 Sydney, Entertainment Centre *(2 shows)* 23 Adelaide, Entertainment Centre 26-27 Melbourne, Rod Laver Arena *(2 shows)* March 1 Perth, Supreme Court Gardens 4 Singapore, Indoor Stadium 8-9 Tokyo, Nippon Budokan Hall *(2 shows)* 11 Osaka, Castle Hall 14 Hong Kong, Wanchai Convention and Exhibition Centre 29 Philadelphia, Wachovia Center 30 Boston, Fleet Center April 1 Toronto, Air Canada Centre 2 Ottawa, Corel Centre	February 24 Interview, 'The Man Who Sold The World' and 'New Killer Star' on Australian Network Ten's *Rove Live* April

RECORDING & RELEASES	STAGE	TV & FILM
	4 Quebec City, Pepsi Coliseum 7 Winnipeg, Arena 9 Edmonton, Rexall Centre 11 Kelowna, Prospera Place 13 Portland, Rose Garden 14 Seattle, Key Arena 16-17 Berkeley, Community Theatre (2 shows) 19 Santa Barbara, SB Bowl 22 Los Angeles, Greek Theatre 23 Anaheim, Theatre At The Pond 25 Denver, Budweiser Events Center 27 Austin, The Back Yard 29 Houston, Woodlands 30 New Orleans, Saenger Theater May 5 Tampa, Performing Arts Center 6 Miami, James L Knight Center 8 Atlanta, Chastain Park Amphitheatre 10 Kansas City, Starlight Theatre 11 St Louis, Fox Theatre 13 Hershey, Star Pavilion 14 London, Ontario, John Labatt Centre 16 Washington, Fairfax, Patriot Center 17 Pittsburgh, Benedum Center 19 Milwaukee, Milwaukee Theatre 20 Indianapolis, Murat Theatre 22 Moline, The Mark of the Quad Cities 24 Columbus, Veterans Memorial Auditorium 25 Buffalo, Shea's Performing Arts Center 27 Scranton, Ford Pavilion at Montage Mountain 29-30 Atlantic City, The Borgata (2 shows) June 1 Manchester, NH, Verizon Wireless Arena 2 Uncasville, Mohegan Sun 4 Wantagh, Tommy Hilfiger at Jones Beach Theater 5 Holmdel, PNC Bank Arts Center 11 Amsterdam, ArenA 13 Isle of Wight, Medina, Isle of Wight Festival 17 Bergen, Bergen Festival 18 Oslo, Norwegian Wood Festival 20 Seinajoki, Finland, Provinssirock Festival 23 Prague, Park Kolbenova 25 Scheeßel, Hurricane Festival 26 Neuhausen, Southside Festival 29 Vienna, Schloss Schönbrunn 30 Salzburg, Residenzplatz July 2 Roskilde, Roskilde Festival	21 'Never Get Old' on NBC's *The Tonight Show With Jay Leno* 23 'Changes' and 'Never Get Old' on NBC's *The Ellen DeGeneres Show* (recorded 20 April)

RECORDING & RELEASES	STAGE	TV & FILM
	4 Werchter, Werchter Festival 6 Ile de Gaou, Six-Fours Festival 7 Carcassonne, Stade Albert Domec 10 Balado, Perth & Kinross, T In The Park Festival 11 Co Kildare, Punchestown Racecourse, Oxegen Festival 14 Bilbao, Bullring 16 Santiago de Compostela, Xacobeo Festival 20 Nyon, Switzerland, Paleo Festival 21 Monaco, Club du Sporting	

11 SINGLES DISCOGRAPHY

This discography makes no attempt to cover every last picture sleeve, limited-edition green vinyl 12" or exclusive Japanese poster bag. All major UK releases are included, but promos, picture discs and non-UK releases appear only if they feature recordings or mixes unavailable elsewhere.

All singles are UK releases credited to David Bowie unless otherwise indicated in brackets after the release date. Releases featuring remixes and instrumentals of the same track abbreviate secondary titles to 'A' (A-side) or 'B' (B-side). Where applicable, UK chart placings appear in square brackets at the end of each entry. From 1964-1989, all releases are 7" singles unless otherwise indicated. From 1990 onward, all releases are CD singles unless otherwise indicated.

In June 1983, RCA reissued 20 of Bowie's 1970s singles in 7" picture sleeves (numbered BOW 501-520) in its Lifetimes series. Details of these reissues are included in brackets after the original releases. RCA's 1982 Fashions reissue was a compilation pack and is covered in Chapter 2.

June 1964 (*Davie Jones with The King Bees*): 'Liza Jane' (2'18") / 'Louie, Louie Go Home' (2'12") (Vocalion Pop V 9221) (*reissued September 1978 as Decca F13807*)

March 1965 (*The Manish Boys*): 'I Pity the Fool' (2'09") / 'Take My Tip' (2'16") (Parlophone R 5250)

August 1965 (*Davy Jones*): 'You've Got A Habit of Leaving' (2'32") / 'Baby Loves That Way' (3'03") (Parlophone R 5315)

January 1966 (*David Bowie with The Lower Third*): 'Can't Help Thinking About Me' (2'47") / 'And I Say To Myself' (2'29") (Pye 7N 17020)

April 1966: 'Do Anything You Say' (2'32") / 'Good Morning Girl' (2'14") (Pye 7N 17079)

August 1966: 'I Dig Everything' (2'45") / 'I'm Not Losing Sleep' (2'52") (Pye 7N 17157)

December 1966: 'Rubber Band' (2'05") / 'The London Boys' (3'20") (Deram DM 107)

April 1967: 'The Laughing Gnome' (3'01") / 'The Gospel According to Tony Day' (2'48") (Deram DM 123)

July 1967: 'Love You Till Tuesday' (2'59") / 'Did You Ever Have A Dream' (2'06") (Deram DM 135)

July 1969: 'Space Oddity' (4'33") / 'Wild Eyed Boy from Freecloud' (4'52") (Philips BF 1801) [5]

July 1969 (*US*): 'Space Oddity' (3'26") / 'Wild Eyed Boy From Freecloud' (3'14") (Mercury 72949)

January 1970 (*Italy*): 'Ragazzo Solo, Ragazza Sola' (5'15") / 'Wild Eyed Boy From Freecloud' (4'52") (Philips 704 208 BW)

March 1970: 'The Prettiest Star' (3'09") / 'Conversation Piece' (3'05") (Mercury MF 1135)

June 1970: 'Memory Of A Free Festival Part 1' (3'59") / 'Memory Of A Free Festival Part 2' (3'31") (Mercury 6052 026)

December 1970 (*US Promo*): 'All The Madmen' (3'14") / 'A' (3'14") (Mercury DJ-311)

December 1970 (*US, unreleased*): 'All The Madmen' (3'14") / 'Janine' (3'19") (Mercury 73173)

January 1971: 'Holy Holy' (3'13") / 'Black Country Rock' (3'32") (Mercury 6052 049)

May 1971 (*Arnold Corns*): 'Moonage Daydream' (3'52") / 'Hang On To Yourself' (2'51") (B&C CB149)

January 1972: 'Changes' (3'33") / 'Andy Warhol' (3'58") (RCA 2160)

April 1972: 'Starman' (4'16") / 'Suffragette City' (3'25") (RCA 2199), April 1972 [10]

August 1972 (*Arnold Corns*): 'Hang On To Yourself' (2'51") / 'Man in the Middle' (4'08") (B&C CB189)

September 1972: 'John, I'm Only Dancing' (2'43") / 'Hang On To Yourself' (2'38") (RCA 2263) [12] (*reissued June 1983 as BOW 517*)

October 1972: 'Do Anything You Say' (2'32") / 'I Dig Everything' (2'45") (Pye 7NX 8002)

November 1972: 'The Jean Genie' (4'02") / 'Ziggy Stardust' (3'13") (RCA 2302) [2] *(reissued June 1983 as BOW 515)*

April 1973: 'Drive In Saturday' (3'59") / 'Round and Round' (2'39") (RCA 2352) [3] *(reissued June 1983 as BOW 501)*

April 1973: 'John, I'm Only Dancing' (2'41") / 'Hang On To Yourself' (2'38") (RCA 2263)

June 1973: 'Life on Mars?' (3'48") / 'The Man Who Sold the World' (3'55") (RCA 2316) [3] *(reissued June 1983 as BOW 502)*

September 1973: 'The Laughing Gnome' (3'01") / 'The Gospel According to Tony Day' (2'48") (Deram DM 123) *(reissue)* [6]

September 1973: 'Sorrow' (2'48") / 'Amsterdam' (3'19") (RCA 2424) [3] *(reissued June 1983 as BOW 519)*

February 1974: 'Rebel Rebel' (4'20") / 'Queen Bitch' (3'13") (RCA LPBO 5009) [5] *(reissued June 1983 as BOW 514)*

April 1974: 'Rock'n'Roll Suicide' (2'57") / 'Quicksand' (5'03") (RCA LPBO 5201) [22] *(reissued June 1983 as BOW 503)*

May 1974 *(US)*: 'Rebel Rebel' (2'58") / 'Lady Grinning Soul' (3'46") (RCA APBO 0287)

June 1974: 'Diamond Dogs' (5'56") / 'Holy Holy' (2'20") (RCA APBO 0293) [21] *(reissued June 1983 as BOW 504)*

September 1974: 'Knock On Wood' (3'03") / 'Panic In Detroit' (5'52") (RCA 2466) [10] *(reissued June 1983 as BOW 505)*

February 1975: 'Young Americans' (5'10") / 'Suffragette City' (3'45") (RCA 2523) [18] *(reissued June 1983 as BOW 506)*

February 1975 *(US)*: 'Young Americans' (3'11") / 'Suffragette City' (3'45") (RCA JB 10152)

May 1975: 'The London Boys' (3'20") / 'Love You Till Tuesday' (2'59") (Decca F 13579)

August 1975: 'Fame' (3'30") / 'Right' (4'13") (RCA 2579) [17] *(reissued June 1983 as BOW 507)*

September 1975: 'Space Oddity' (4'33") / 'Changes' (3'33") / 'Velvet Goldmine' (3'09") (RCA 2593) [1] *(reissued June 1983 as BOW 518)*

November 1975: 'Golden Years' (3'22") / 'Can You Hear Me' (5'04") (RCA 2640) [8] *(reissued June 1983 as BOW 508)*

April 1976: 'TVC15' (3'43") / 'We Are The Dead' (4'58") (RCA 2682) [33] *(reissued June 1983 as BOW 509)*

July 1976: 'Suffragette City' (3'25") / 'Stay' (3'21") (RCA 2726)

July 1976 *(US)*: 'Stay' (3'21") / 'Word On A Wing' (3'09") (RCA PB 10736)

1977 *(Australia)*: 'Breaking Glass' (2'47") / 'Art Decade' (3'43") (RCA 103295)

February 1977: 'Sound And Vision' (3'00") / 'A New Career In A New Town' (2'50") (RCA PB 0905) [3] *(reissued June 1983 as BOW 510)*

June 1977: 'Be My Wife' (2'55") / 'Speed Of Life' (2'45") (RCA PB 1017) *(reissued June 1983 as BOW 511)*

September 1977: '"Heroes"' (3'35") / 'V-2 Schneider' (3'10") (RCA PB 1121) [24] *(reissued June 1983 as BOW 513)*

September 1977 *(France)*: '"Héros"' (3'35") / 'V-2 Schneider' (3'10") (RCA PB 9167)

September 1977 *(Germany)*: '"Helden"' (3'35") / 'V-2 Schneider' (3'10") (RCA PB 9168)

December 1977 *(US Promo 12")*: 'Beauty And The Beast (Disco Version)' (5'18") / 'Fame' (4'12") (RCA JD 11204)

January 1978: 'Beauty And The Beast' (3'32") / 'Sense Of Doubt' (3'57") (RCA PB 1190) [39] *(reissued June 1983 as BOW 512)*

November 1978: 'Breaking Glass' (3'28") / 'Art Decade' (3'10") / 'Ziggy Stardust' (3'32") (RCA BOW 1) [54] *(reissued June 1983 as BOW 520)*

April 1979: 'Boys Keep Swinging' (3'17") / 'Fantastic Voyage' (2'55") (RCA BOW 2) [7]

1979 *(Netherlands)*: 'Yassassin' (3'03") / 'Fantastic Voyage' (2'55") (RCA PB 9417)

1979 *(Turkey)*: 'Yassassin' (3'03") / 'Red Money' (4'17") (RCA 79014)

June 1979: 'D.J.' (3'20") / 'Repetition' (2'59") (RCA BOW 3) [29] *(reissued June 1983 as BOW 516)*

June 1979 *(David Bowie and the Rebels, Japanese 7")*: 'Revolutionary Song' (3'43") / 'Charmaine' (Overseas Records MA 185V)

December 1979: 'John, I'm Only Dancing (Again)' (3'26") / 'John, I'm Only Dancing' (2'43") (RCA BOW 4) [12]

December 1979 *(12")*: 'John, I'm Only Dancing (Again)' (6'57") / 'John, I'm Only Dancing' (2'43") (RCA BOW 124) [12]

February 1980: 'Alabama Song' (3'51") / 'Space Oddity' (4'57") (RCA BOW 5) [23]

August 1980: 'Ashes to Ashes' (3'34") / 'Move On' (3'16") (RCA BOW 6) [1]

October 1980: 'Fashion' (3'23") / 'Scream Like a Baby' (3'35") (RCA BOW 7) [5]

January 1981: 'Scary Monsters (And Super Creeps)' (3'27") / 'Because You're Young' (4'51") (RCA BOW 8) [20]

March 1981: 'Up The Hill Backwards' (3'13") / 'Crystal Japan' (3'08") (RCA BOW 9) [32]

November 1981 *(Queen and David Bowie)*: 'Under Pressure' (4'09") / 'Soul Brother' *(Queen only)* (EMI 5250) [1]

November 1981: 'Wild is the Wind' (3'34") / 'Golden Years' (3'22") (RCA BOW 10) [24]

November 1981 *(12")*: 'Wild Is The Wind' (5'58") / 'Golden Years' (4'03") (RCA BOW T10) [24]

February 1982: 'Baal's Hymn' (4'00") / 'Remembering Marie A.' (2'04") / 'Ballad of the Adventurers'/ (1'59") / 'The Drowned Girl' (2'24") / 'The Dirty Song' (0'37") (RCA BOW 11) [29]

April 1982: 'Cat People (Putting Out Fire)' (4'08") / 'Paul's Theme (Jogging Chase)' (MCA 770) [26]

April 1982 *(12")*: 'Cat People (Putting Out Fire)' (6'41") / 'Paul's Theme (Jogging Chase)' (MCA MCAT 770) [26]

April 1982 *(Australian 12")*: 'Cat People (Putting Out Fire)' (6'41") / 'A (Remix)' (9'20") (MCA DS12087)

April 1982 *(US Promo)*: 'Cat People (Putting Out Fire) (Edit)' (3'18") (Backstreet 545-17-67)

October 1982 *(David Bowie and Bing Crosby)*: 'Peace On Earth'/'Little Drummer Boy' (2'38") / 'Fantastic Voyage' (2'55") (RCA BOW 12) [3]

October 1982 *(David Bowie and Bing Crosby, 12")*: 'Peace On Earth'/'Little Drummer Boy' (4'23") / 'Fantastic Voyage' (2'55") (RCA BOW T12) [3]

March 1983: 'Let's Dance' (4'07") / 'Cat People (Putting Out Fire)' (5'09") (EMI America EA 152) [1]

March 1983 *(12")*: 'Let's Dance' (7'38") / 'Cat People (Putting Out Fire)' (5'09") (EMI America 12EA 152) [1]

May 1983: 'China Girl' (4'14") / 'Shake It' (3'49") (EMI America EA 157) [2]

May 1983 *(12")*: 'China Girl' (5'32") / 'Shake It (Remix)' (5'07") (EMI America 12EA 157) [2]

September 1983: 'Modern Love' (3'56") / 'A (Live Version)' (3'43") (EMI America EA158) [2]

September 1983 *(12")*: 'Modern Love' (4'46") / 'A (Live Version)' (3'43") (EMI America 12EA 158) [2]

October 1983: 'White Light, White Heat' (4'06") / 'Cracked Actor' (2'51") (RCA 372) [46]

September 1984: 'Blue Jean' (3'10") / 'Dancing With The Big Boys' (3'34") (EMI America EA 181) [6]

September 1984 *(12")*: 'Blue Jean (Extended Dance Mix)' (5'16") / 'Dancing With The Big Boys (Extended Dance Mix)' (7'28") / 'B (Extended Dub Mix)' (7'15") (EMI America 12EA 181) [6]

November 1984: 'Tonight' (3'43") / 'Tumble And Twirl' (4'56") (EMI America EA 187) [53]

November 1984 *(12")*: 'Tonight (Vocal Dance Mix)' (4'29") / 'Tumble And Twirl (Extended Dance Mix)' (5'03") / 'B (Dub Mix)' (4'18") (EMI America 12EA 187) [53]

February 1985 *(David Bowie/Pat Metheny Group)*: 'This Is Not America' (3'51") / 'A (Instrumental)' (3'51") (EMI America EA 190) [14]

May 1985: 'Loving The Alien (Remixed Version)' (4'43") / 'Don't Look Down (Remixed Version)' (4'04") (EMI America EA 195) [19]

May 1985 *(12")*: 'Loving The Alien (Extended Dance Mix)' (7'27") / 'Don't Look Down (Extended Dance Mix)' (4'50") / 'A (Extended Dub Mix)' (7'14") (EMI America 12EAG 195) [19]

August 1985 *(David Bowie and Mick Jagger)*: 'Dancing In The Street' (3'14") / 'A (Dub Version)' (4'41") (EMI America EA 204) [1]

August 1985 *(David Bowie and Mick Jagger, 12")*: 'Dancing In The Street (Steve Thompson Mix)' (4'40") / 'A (Dub Version)' (4'41") / 'A (Edit)' (3'14") (EMI America 12EA 204) [1]

March 1986: 'Absolute Beginners' (5'36") / 'A (Dub Mix)' (5'42") (Virgin VS 838) [2]

March 1986 *(12")*: 'Absolute Beginners (Full Length Version)' (8'00") / 'A (Dub Mix)' (5'42") (Virgin VS 12838) [2]

June 1986: 'Underground' (4'25") / 'A (Instrumental)' (5'54") (EMI America EA 216) [21]

June 1986 *(12")*: 'Underground (Extended Dance Mix)' (7'51") / 'A (Dub)' (5'59") / 'A (Instrumental)' (5'40") (EMI America 12EA 216) [21]

November 1986: 'When The Wind Blows' (3'32") / 'A (Instrumental)' (3'52") (Virgin VS 906) [44]

November 1986 *(12")*: 'When The Wind Blows (Extended Mix)' (5'46") / 'A (Instrumental)' (3'52") (Virgin VS 90612) [44]

January 1987 *(US 12")*: 'Magic Dance (A Dance Mix)' (7'11") / 'A (Dub)' (5'28") / 'Within You' (3'29") (EMI America 19217)

March 1987: 'Day-In Day-Out' (4'14") / 'Julie' (3'40") (EMI America EA 230) [17]

March 1987 *(12")*: 'Day-In Day-Out (Extended Dance Mix)' (7'15") / 'A (Extended Dub Mix)' (7'17") / 'Julie' (3'40") (EMI America 12EA 230) [17]

March 1987 *(12")*: 'Day-In Day-Out (Remix)' (6'30") / 'A (Extended Dub Mix)' (7'17") / 'Julie' (3'40") (EMI America 12EAX 230) [17]

March 1987 *(US Promo 12")*: 'Day-In Day-Out (7" Dance Edit)' (3'35") / 'A (Extended Dance Mix)' (7'15") / 'A (Edited Dance Mix)' (4'30") (EMI America SPRO9996/7)

June 1987: 'Time Will Crawl' (4'18") / 'Girls' (4'13") (EMI America EA 237) [33]

June 1987 *(12")*: 'Time Will Crawl (Extended Dance Mix)' (6'11") / 'A' (4'18") / 'Girls (Extended Edit)' (5'35") (EMI America 12EA 237) [33]

June 1987 *(12")*: 'Time Will Crawl (Dance Crew Mix)' (5'43") / 'A (Dub)' (5'23") / 'Girls (Japanese Version)' (4'06") (EMI America 12EAX 237) [33]

August 1987: 'Never Let Me Down' (3'58") / "87 And Cry' (3'53") (EMI America EA 239) [34]

August 1987 *(12")*: 'Never Let Me Down (Extended Dance Remix)' (7'03") / 'A (Dub)' (3'57") / 'A (A Cappella)' (2'03") (EMI America 12EA 239) [34]

August 1987 *(Japanese CD)*: 'Never Let Me Down (Extended Dance Remix)' (7'03") / 'A (7" Remix Edit)' (3'58") / 'A (Dub)' (3'57") / 'A (A Cappella)' (2'03") / 'A (Instrumental)' (4'02") / "87 And Cry (Single Version)' (3'53") (EMI CP20 5520)

1987 *(US Promo CD)*: 'Bang Bang (Live)' / 'A (LP Version)' (4'02") / 'Modern Love' (4'46") / 'Loving The Alien' (7'10") (EMI America DPRO 31593)

November 1988 *(CD)*: 'Absolute Beginners (Full Length Version)' (8'00") / 'A (Dub Mix)' (5'42") (Virgin CDT20) [2]

November 1988 *(Queen and David Bowie, CD)*: 'Under Pressure' (4'09") / 'Soul Brother' *(Queen only)* / 'Body Language' *(Queen only)* (Parlophone QUE CD9)

June 1989 *(Tin Machine)*: 'Under The God' (4'06") / 'Sacrifice Yourself' (2'08") (EMI USA MT 68) [51]

June 1989 *(Tin Machine, 12" & CD)*: as above plus 'The Interview' (EMI USA 12MT 68 / CDMT 68) [51]

1989 *(Tin Machine, US Promo CD)*: 'Heaven's In Here (Edited Version)' (4'21") / 'A (Album Version)' (6'01") (EMI USA DPRO 4375)

September 1989 *(Tin Machine)*: 'Tin Machine' (3'34") / 'Maggie's Farm (Live)' (4'29") (EMI USA MT 73) [48]

September 1989 *(Tin Machine, 12")*: as above plus 'I Can't Read (Live)' (6'13") (EMI USA 12MTP 73) [48]

September 1989 *(Tin Machine, CD)*: as 12" above plus 'Bus Stop (Live Country Version)' (1'52") (EMI USA CDMT 73) [48]

October 1989 *(Tin Machine)*: 'Prisoner Of Love (Edit)' (4'09") / 'Baby Can Dance (Live)' (6'16") (EMI MT 76)

October 1989 *(Tin Machine, 12" & CD)*: as above plus 'Crack City (Live)' (5'13") / 'A (LP Version)' (4'15") (EMI 12MT 76 & CDMT 76)

March 1990 *(7")*: 'Fame 90 (Gass Mix)' (3'36") / 'A (Queen Latifah's Rap Version)' (3'10") (EMI FAME 90) [28]

March 1990 *(Picture 7")*: 'Fame 90 (Gass Mix)' (3'36") / 'A (Bonus Beat Mix)' (4'51") (EMI PD FAME 90) [28]

March 1990 *(12" & CD)*: 'Fame 90 (House Mix)' (5'58") / 'A (Hip Hop Mix)' (5'58") / 'A (Gass Mix)' (3'36") / 'A (Queen Latifah's Rap Version)' (3'10") (EMI 12 FAME 90 & CDFAME 90) [28]

March 1990 *(US)*: as above plus 'Fame 90 (Absolutely Nothing Premeditated/Epic Mix)' (14'26") (Ryko RCD5 1018)

May 1990 *(Adrian Belew featuring David Bowie, 7")*: 'Pretty Pink Rose' (4'09") / 'Heartbeat' *(Adrian Belew only)* (Atlantic A7904)

May 1990 *(Adrian Belew featuring David Bowie, CD & 12")*: as above plus 'Oh Daddy' *(Adrian Belew only)* (Atlantic A7904CD & 7904T)

August 1991 *(Tin Machine, 7")*: 'You Belong In Rock N'Roll' (3'33") / 'Amlapura (Indonesian Version)' (3'49") (London LON 305) [33]

August 1991 *(Tin Machine)*: as above plus 'Stateside' (5'38") / 'Hammerhead' (3'15") (London LONCD 305) [33]

August 1991 *(Tin Machine, 12" & CD)*: 'You Belong In Rock N'Roll (Extended Mix)' (6'32") / 'You Belong In Rock N' Roll (LP Version)' (4'07") / 'Amlapura (Indonesian Version)' (3'49") / 'Shakin' All Over' (2'49") (London LONX 305 & LOCDT 305) [33]

1991 *(Germany)*: 'One Shot (Edit)' (4'02") / 'Hammerhead' (3'15") (London INT 8695742)

October 1991 *(Tin Machine, 7")*: 'Baby Universal (7")' (3'07") / 'You Belong In Rock N'Roll (Extended Version)' (6'32") (London LON 310) [48]

October 1991 *(Tin Machine)*: 'Baby Universal (7")' (3'07") / 'Stateside (BBC Version)' (6'35") / 'If There Is Something (BBC Version)' (3'25") / 'Heaven's In Here (BBC Version)' (6'41") (London LOCDT 310) [48]

October 1991 *(Tin Machine, 12")*: 'Baby Universal (Extended)' (5'49") / 'A Big Hurt (BBC Version)' (3'33") / 'A (BBC Version)' (3'12") (London LONX 310) [48]

December 1991 *(David Bowie vs 808 State, US)*: 'Sound And Vision (808 Giftmix)' (3'58") / 'A (808 'Lectric Blue Remix Instrumental)' (4'07") / 'A (David Richards Remix '91)' (4'43") / 'A (Original Version)' (3'00") (Tommy Boy TBCD 510)

August 1992 *(7")*: 'Real Cool World (Album Edit)' (4'15") / 'A (Instrumental)' (4'29") (Warner Bros. W0127) [53]

August 1992 *(12")*: 'Real Cool World (12" Club Mix)' (5'28") / 'A (Cool Dub Thing #2)' (6'54") / 'A (Cool Dub Thing #1)' (7'28") / 'A (Cool Dub Overture)' (9'10") (Warner Bros. W0127 T) [53]

August 1992: as above plus 'Real Cool World (Album Edit)' (4'15") / 'A (Radio Remix)' (4'23") (Warner Bros. W0127 CD) [53]

March 1993 *(7")*: 'Jump They Say (7" Version)' (3'53") / 'Pallas Athena (Don't Stop Praying Mix)' (5'36") (Arista 74321 139424) [9]

March 1993 *(12")*: 'Jump They Say (Hard Hands Mix)' (5'40") / 'A (Full Album Version)' (4'22") / 'A (Leftfield 12" Vocal)' (7'42") / 'A (Dub Oddity Mix)' (4'44") (Arista 74321 139421) [9]

March 1993: 'Jump They Say (7" Version)' (3'53") / 'A (Hard Hands

Mix)' (5'40") / 'A (JAE-E Remix)'
(5'32") / 'Pallas Athena (Don't Stop
Praying Mix)' (5'36") (Arista 74321
139422) [9]

March 1993: 'Jump They Say (Brothers
in Rhythm Mix)' (8'28") / 'A (Brothers
in Rhythm Instrumental)' (6'25") / 'A
(Leftfield 12" Vocal)' (7'42") / 'A (Full
Album Version)' (4'22") (Arista 74321
139432) [9]

March 1993 *(Germany)*: 'Jump They
Say (Radio Edit)' (3'53") / 'A (JAE-E
Edit)' (3'58") / 'A (Club Hart Remix)'
(5'05") / 'A (Leftfield Remix)' (7'41") /
'Pallas Athena (Album Version)'
(4'40") / 'B (Don't Stop Praying Mix)'
(5'36") (Arista 74321 136962)

March 1993 *(Promo 12")*: 'Jump They
Say (Leftfield Instrumental)' (Arista
LEFT-1)

March 1993 *(US Promo)*: 'Jump They
Say (Brothers In Rhythm Edit)' (3'54")
/ 'A (Brothers In Rhythm Mix)' (8'24")
/ 'A (Brothers In Rhythm Instrumental)'
(6'20") / 'A (Leftfield Remix)' (7'41") /
'A (Album Version Edit)' (3'58")
(Savage/Arista SADJ500422)

March 1993 *(US Promo)*: 'Jump They
Say (Rock Mix)' (4'22") / 'A (Single
Edit)' (3'53") (Savage/Arista
SADJ500442)

1993 *(Promo 12")*: 'Pallas Athena'
(Meat Beat Manifesto Mix 1)' (7'13") /
'A (Meat Beat Manifesto Mix 2)'
(4'25") / 'A (Don't Stop Praying Mix)'
(5'36") (BMG MEAT 1)

1993 *(Promo 12")*: 'Nite Flights'
(9'55") / '100% Total Success'
(Moodswings) (Arista/Back To Basics
HOME 1)

June 1993 *(David Bowie featuring Al B
Sure!, 7")*: 'Black Tie White Noise
(Radio Edit)' (4'10") / 'You've Been
Around (Dangers Remix)' (4'24")
(Arista 74321 148682) [36]

June 1993 *(David Bowie featuring Al B
Sure!, 12")*: 'Black Tie White Noise
(Extended Remix)' (8'12") / 'A (Trance
Mix)' (7'15") / 'A (Album Version)'
(2'52") / 'A (Club Mix)' (7'33") / 'A
(Extended Urban Remix)' (5'32")
(Arista 74321 14868 1) [36]

June 1993 *(David Bowie featuring Al B
Sure!)*: 'Black Tie White Noise (Radio
Edit)' (4'10") / 'A (Extended Remix)'
(8'12") / 'A (Urban Mix)' (4'03") /
'You've Been Around (Dangers Remix)'
(4'24") (Arista 74321 14868 2) [36]

June 1993 *(David Bowie featuring Al B
Sure!, US)*: 'Black Tie White Noise
(Waddell Mix)' (4'12") / 'A (3rd Floor
Mix)' (3'43") / 'A (Al B Sure! Mix)'
(4'03") / 'A (Album Version)' (4'52") /
'A (Club Mix)' (7'33") / 'A (Digi
Funky's Lush Mix)' (5'44") / 'A (Supa
Pump Mix)' (6'36") (Savage/Arista
74785 50045 2)

June 1993 *(David Bowie featuring Al B
Sure!, US Promo)*: 'Black Tie White
Noise (CHR Mix 1)' (3'43") / 'A (CHR
Mix 2)' (4'12") / 'A (Churban Mix)'
(3'45") / 'A (Urban Mix)' (4'03") / 'A
(Album Edit)' (4'10") (Savage/Arista
SADJ 50046 2)

June 1993 *(David Bowie featuring Al B
Sure!, US Promo)*: 'Black Tie White
Noise (Extended Remix)' (8'12") / 'A
(Club Mix)' (7'33") / 'A (Trance Mix)'
(7'15") / 'A (Digi Funky's Lush Mix)'
(5'44") / 'A (Supa Pump Mix)' (6'36")
/ 'A (Funky Crossover Mix)' (3'45") /
'A (Extended Urban Remix)' (5'32")
(Savage/Arista SADJ500451)

June 1993 *(David Bowie featuring Al B
Sure!, US Promo 12")*: 'Black Tie White
Noise (Extended Remix)' (8'12") / 'A
(Trance Mix)' (7'15") / 'You've Been
Around (Dangers Trance Mix)' (7'03")
/ 'A (Club Mix)' (7'33") / 'A (Here
Comes Da Jazz)' (5'30") / 'A (Dub)'
(4'25") (Savage/Arista/BMG BLACK 1)

October 1993 *(7")*: 'Miracle Goodnight'
(4'14") / 'Looking For Lester' (5'36")
(Arista 74321 162267) [40]

October 1993 *(12")*: 'Miracle
Goodnight (Blunted 2)' (8'12") / 'A
(Make Believe Mix)' (4'14") / 'A (12" 2
Chord Philly Mix)' (6'22") / 'A (Dance
Dub)' (7'50") (Arista 74321 162261)
[40]

October 1993: 'Miracle Goodnight
(Album version)' (4'14") / 'A (12" 2
Chord Philly Mix)' (6'22") / 'A
(Masereti Blunted Dub)' (7'40") /
'Looking For Lester (Album Version)'
(5'36") (Arista 74321 162262) [40]

November 1993 *(7")*: 'Buddha Of
Suburbia' (4'24") / 'Dead Against It'
(5'48") (Arista 74321 177057) [35]

November 1993: 'Buddha Of
Suburbia' (4'24") / 'South Horizon'
(5'26") / 'Dead Against It' (5'48") / 'A
(Rock Mix)' (4'21") (Arista 74321
177052) [35]

April 1994: 'Ziggy Stardust' (3'24") /
'Waiting For The Man' (6'01") / 'The
Jean Genie' (4'02") (Golden Years
GYCDS 002)

September 1995 *(7")*: 'The Hearts
Filthy Lesson (Radio Edit)' (3'32") / 'I
Am With Name (Album Version)'
(4'06") (RCA 74321 307034) [35]

September 1995 *(12")*: 'The Hearts
Filthy Lesson (Alt. Mix)' (5'19") / 'A
(Bowie Mix)' (4'56") / 'A (Rubber
Mix)' (7'41") / 'A (Simple Text Mix)'
(6'38") / 'A (Filthy Mix)' (5'51") (RCA
74321 307031) [35]

September 1995: 'The Hearts Filthy
Lesson (Radio Edit)' (3'32") / 'I Am
With Name (Album Version)' (4'06") /
'A (Bowie Mix)' (4'56") / 'A (Alt. Mix)'
(5'19") (RCA 74321 307032) [35]

September 1995 *(US)*: 'The Hearts
Filthy Lesson (Good Karma Mix)'
(5'00") / 'A (Alt. Mix)' (5'20") /
'Nothing To Be Desired' (2'15")
(Virgin 72438 385182)

November 1995 *(7")*: 'Strangers When
We Meet (Edit)' (4'19") / 'The Man
Who Sold The World (Live Version)'
(3'35") (RCA 74321 329407) [39]

November 1995: as above plus 'A (LP
Version)' (5'06") / 'Get Real' (RCA
74321 329402) [39]

November 1995 *(US Promo)*: 'Strangers
When We Meet (Edit)' (4'19") / 'A
(Buddha Of Suburbia Edit)' (4'10") /
'A (Album Version)' (5'06") (Virgin
DPRO 11062)

February 1996 *(7")*: 'Hallo Spaceboy
(Remix)' (4'23") / 'The Hearts Filthy
Lesson' (3'32") (BMG/RCA 74321
353847) [12]

February 1996: 'Hallo Spaceboy (Remix)' (4'23") / 'Under Pressure (Live Version)' (4'06") / 'Moonage Daydream (Live Version) (5'26") / 'The Hearts Filthy Lesson (Radio Edit)' (3'32") (RCA 74321 353842) [12]

February 1996 (US Promo 12"): 'Hallo Spaceboy (12" Remix)' (6'42") / 'A (7" Remix)' (4'25") / 'A (Lost In Space Mix)' (6'32") / 'A (Double Click Mix)' (7'46") (Virgin SPRO 11513)

November 1996 (CD & 12"): 'Telling Lies' (Feelgood Mix) (5'07") / 'A (Paradox Mix)' (5'10") / 'A (Adam F Mix)' (3'58") (RCA 74321 397412 & 397411)

January 1997 (12"): 'Little Wonder (Junior's Club Mix)' (8'10") / 'A (Danny Saber Dance Mix)' (5'30") / 'Telling Lies (Adam F Mix)' (3'58") (RCA 74321 452071) [14]

January 1997: 'Little Wonder (Edit)' (3'40") / 'A (Ambient Junior Mix)' (9'55") / 'A (Club Dub Junior Mix)' (8'10") / 'A (4/4 Junior Mix)' (8'10") / 'A (Junior's Club Instrumental)' (8'10") (RCA 74321 452072) [14]

January 1997: 'Little Wonder (Edit)' (3'40") / 'Telling Lies (Adam F Mix)' (3'58") / 'Jump They Say (Leftfield 12" Vocal)' (7'40") / 'A (Danny Saber Remix)' (3'06") (RCA 74321 452082) [14]

January 1997 (US Promo): 'Little Wonder (Single Edit)' (3'40") / 'A (Video Edit)' (4'10") / 'Little Wonder Research Hooks 1 & 2' (Virgin DPRO 11595)

February 1997 (French Sampler): 'The Hearts Filthy Lesson (Live)' (5'26") / 'Hallo Spaceboy (Live)' (5'34") / 'Pallas Athena (Don't Stop Praying Mix)' (5'36") (Arista 74321 458262)

April 1997: 'Dead Man Walking (Edit)' (4'01") / 'I'm Deranged (Jungle Mix)' (7'00") / 'The Hearts Filthy Lesson (Good Karma Mix)' (5'00") (RCA 74321 475842) [32]

April 1997: 'Dead Man Walking (Album Version)' (6'50") / 'A (Moby Mix)' (7'31") / 'A (House Mix)' (6'00") / 'A (This One's Not Dead Yet Remix)' (6'28") (RCA 74321 475852) [32]

April 1997 (12"): 'Dead Man Walking (House Mix)' (6'00") / 'A (Vigor Mortis Remix)' (6'29") / 'Telling Lies (Paradox Mix)' (5'10") (RCA 74321 475841) [32]

August 1997 (7"): 'Seven Years In Tibet (Edit)' (4'01") / 'A (Mandarin Version)' (3'58") (RCA 74321 512547) [61]

August 1997: as above plus 'Pallas Athena (Live)' (8'18") (RCA 74321 512542) [61]

August 1997 (Tao Jones Index, 12"): 'Pallas Athena (Live)' (8'18") / 'V-2 Schneider (Live)' (6'55") (RCA 74321 512541)

1997 (US Promo): 'Looking For Satellites (Edit)' (3'51") / 'Seven Years In Tibet (Edit)' (4'01") / 'I'm Afraid Of Americans (Edit)' (4'30") (Virgin DPRO 1257)

October 1997 (US): 'I'm Afraid Of Americans (V1)' (5'31") / 'A (V2)' (5'51") / 'A (V3)' (6'18") / 'A (V4)' (5'25") / 'A (V5)' (5'38") / 'A (V6)' (11'18") (Virgin 73438 3861828)

October 1997 (US Promo): 'I'm Afraid Of Americans (V1 Edit)' (4'30") / 'A (Original Edit)' (4'12") / 'A (V3)' (6'18") / 'A (V1 Clean Edit)' (4'30") (Virgin DPRO 12749)

November 1997 (Various Artists): 'Perfect Day '97' (3'46") / 'A (Female Version)' / 'A (Male Version)' (3'48") (Chrysalis CDNEED 01)

February 1998: 'I Can't Read (Short Version)' (4'40") / 'A (Long Version)' (5'30") / 'This Is Not America' (3'51") (Velvel ZYX 87578) [73]

February 1998 (Netherlands): 'Commercial Ingesproken Door David Bowie' (3 edits of Bowie's War Child Appeal over instrumental version of 'No Control') (War Child K 972321A)

August 1999 (Placebo featuring David Bowie): 'Without You I'm Nothing (Single Mix)' (4'16") / 'A (Unkle Remix)' (5'09") / 'A (The Flexirol Mix)' (9'26") / 'A (Brothers In Rhythm Club Mix)' (10'52") (Hut FLOORCD10)

September 1999: 'Thursday's Child (Radio Edit)' (4'25") / 'We All Go Through' (4'09") / 'No One Calls' (3'51") (Virgin VSCDT 1753) [16]

September 1999: 'Thursday's Child (Rock Mix)' (4'27") / 'We Shall Go To Town' (3'56") / '1917' (3'27") 'Thursday's Child (Video)' (CD-ROM) (Virgin VSCDX 1753) [16]

September 1999 (Australia): 'The Pretty Things Are Going To Hell (Edit)' (3'59") / 'A' (4'40") / 'We Shall Go To Town' (3'56") / '1917' (3'27") (Virgin 72438 9629323)

December 1999 (Queen + David Bowie): 'Under Pressure (Rah Mix Album Version)' (4'11") / 'Bohemian Rhapsody' (Queen only) / 'Thank God It's Christmas' (Queen only) (Parlophone CDQUEEN 28) [14]

December 1999 (Queen + David Bowie): 'Under Pressure (Rah Mix Radio Edit)' (3'46") / 'A (Mike Spencer Mix)' (3'53") / 'A (Knebworth Mix)' (Queen only) (Parlophone CDQUEENS 28) [14]

December 1999 (Queen + David Bowie, Promo 12"): 'Under Pressure (Rah Mix Radio Edit)' (3'46") / 'A (Club 2000 Mix)' (Parlophone QUEENS WL28)

December 1999 (David Bowie and Bing Crosby, US): 'Peace On Earth/Little Drummer Boy' (4'23") / 'A (Video)' (CD-ROM) (Oglio OGL 85001-2)

January 2000: 'Survive (Marius de Vries Mix)' (4'18") / 'A (Album Version)' (4'11") / 'The Pretty Things Are Going To Hell (Stigmata Film Version)' (4'46") (Virgin VSCDT 1767) [28]

January 2000: 'Survive (Live)' (4'10") / 'Thursday's Child (Live)' (5'37") / 'Seven (Live)' (4'07") / 'Survive (Live in Paris)' (CD-ROM) (Virgin VSCDX 1767) [28]

July 2000: 'Seven (Marius de Vries Mix)' (4'12") / 'A (remix by Beck)' (3'44") / 'A (Demo)' (4'05") (Virgin VSCDT 1776) [32]

July 2000: 'Seven (Album Version)' (4'04") / 'I'm Afraid Of Americans (Nine Inch Nails V1 Mix)' (5'31") / 'B (Video)' (CD-ROM) (Virgin VSCDX 1776) [32]

July 2000: 'Seven (Live)' (4'00") / 'Something In The Air (Live)' (4'50") / 'The Pretty Things Are Going To Hell (Live)' (4'10") (Virgin VSCDXX 1776) [32]

April 2002 (The Scumfrog vs Bowie): 'Loving The Alien (Radio Edit)' (3'20") / 'A (8'23") / '8 Days, 7 Hours' (The Scumfrog only) / 'A (Video)' (CD-ROM) (Positiva CDTIV-172) [41]

April 2002 (The Scumfrog vs Bowie, 12"): 'Loving The Alien' (8'23") / '8 Days, 7 Hours' (The Scumfrog only) (Positiva 12TIV-172) [41]

June 2002 (Promo): 'Slow Burn (Edit)' (3'55") / 'Everyone Says 'Hi'' (3'59") / 'I Took A Trip On A Gemini Spaceship' (4'05") / 'Sunday (Moby Remix)' (5'09") (ISO/Columbia SAMPCS 115901)

June 2002 (Austria): 'Slow Burn' (4'43") / 'Wood Jackson' (4'48") / 'Shadow Man' (4'46") (ISO/Columbia 672744 1)

June 2002 (Austria): 'Slow Burn' (4'43") / 'Wood Jackson' (4'48") / 'Shadow Man' (4'46") / 'When The Boys Come Marching Home' (4'46") / 'You've Got A Habit Of Leaving' (4'51") (ISO/Columbia 672744 1)

September 2002: 'Everyone Says 'Hi' (Radio Edit)' (3'31") / 'Safe' (4'44") / 'Wood Jackson' (4'48") (Columbia 673134 2) [20]

September 2002: 'Everyone Says 'Hi' (Radio Edit)' (3'31") / 'When The Boys Come Marching Home' (4'46") / 'Shadow Man' (4'46") (Columbia 673134 3) [20]

September 2002: 'Everyone Says 'Hi' (Radio Edit)' (3'31") / 'Baby Loves That Way' (4'45") / 'You've Got A Habit Of Leaving' (4'51") (Columbia 673134 5) [20]

September 2002 (Canada): 'I've Been Waiting For You' (3'00") / 'Sunday (Tony Visconti Mix)' (4'56") / 'Shadow Man' (4'46") (Columbia 38K 003369)

November 2002 (Solaris vs Bowie, 12"): 'Shout (Original Mix)' / 'A (Phazon Dub)' (Nebula NEBT 038)

January 2003 (US Promo 12"): 'Everyone Says 'Hi' (METRO Remix)' (7'21") / 'A (METRO Remix – Radio Edit)' (3'43") / 'I Took A Trip On A Gemini Spaceship (Deepsky's Space Cowboy Remix)' (7'52") (ISO/Columbia CAS 59068)

June 2003 (David Guetta vs Bowie): 'Just For One Day (Heroes) (Radio Edit)' (3'00") / 'A (Extended Version)' (6'39") / 'Distortion (Main Vocal Mix)' (7'02") (Virgin 72435 479822 8) [73]

June 2003 (David Guetta vs Bowie, 12"): 'Just For One Day (Heroes) (Extended Version)' (6'39") / 'A (Extended Dub)' (6'10") / 'Distortion (Main Vocal Mix)' (7'02") (Virgin 072435 472826 DISNT 263) [73]

August 2003 (Singapore & Hong Kong Promo): 'Let's Dance' (Club Bolly Extended Mix)' (7'55") / 'A (Club Bolly Radio Mix 1)' (5'15") / 'China Girl (Club Mix)' (7'17") / 'B (Club Mix Radio Edit 3 with 'Let's Dance')' (3'56") / 'B (Cinemix)' / 'A (Club Bolly Radio Mix 2)' (4'45") / 'A (Club Bolly Nocturnal Mix)' (5'45") / 'B (Club Mix Radio Edit 1 with 'Major Tom')' / 'B (Club Mix Radio Edit 2 with 'Major Tom'/'Let's Dance')' / 'B (Club Mix Radio Edit 4 with 'Major Tom'/'Let's Dance')' / 'A (Red Shoes Mix Heavy Alt. Club Mix)' / 'A (Bollyclub Mix)' (4'49") / 'A (Bollymovie Mix)' (EMI, no catalogue)

August 2003 (Singapore & Hong Kong Promo): 'China Girl (Riff & Vox – Radio)' (3'52") / 'A – (Riff & Vox – Club)' (7'06") / 'Let's Dance (Club Bolly Extended Mix)' (7'55") / 'B (Club Bolly Radio Mix 1' (5'15") / 'A (Club Mix)' (7'17") 'A (Club Mix Radio Edit)' (3'56") (EMI, no catalogue)

September 2003 (DVD Single): 'New Killer Star (Video Version)' / 'Reality (EPK)' / 'Love Missile F1-11' (ISO/Columbia 674275 9)

September 2003 (Italy): 'New Killer Star' (4'40") / 'Love Missile F1-11' (4'14") (ISO/Columbia 674275 1)

November 2003 (Promo): 'Never Get Old' (3'40") / 'Waterloo Sunset' (3'28") (ISO/Columbia SAMPCS 13495 1)

November 2003 (US Promo): 'Let's Dance' (Club Bolly Extended Mix)' (7'55") / 'A (Bollyclub Mix)' (4'49") (Virgin 70876-18286-2-7)

December 2003 (12" Promo): 'Magic Dance (Danny S Magic Party Mix)' (7'39") / 'A (Danny S Magic Dust Dub)' (EMI 08 53490 20 1A/B1 DBD001)

March 2004 (Japan): 'Never Get Old' (3'40") / 'Love Missile F1-11' (4'14") (Sony SICP-456)

afterword: future legend

As I deliver this manuscript, the second American leg of A Reality Tour is nearing its conclusion and Bowie is preparing to return to Europe for a series of summer festival dates. What the future holds thereafter is, as ever, an exhilarating mystery.

In 2003 David told more than one interviewer that he was working on a novel, or possibly even a series of novels, inspired by the underground history of London's political and artistic avant-garde, and its roots in the early socialist parties. "It needs about a hundred years of research, and it'll never be completed in my lifetime, but I'm having a ball," he told *Word* in August 2003. "I start with the first female trade unionists in the 1890s in the East End of London, and I'm coming right through to Indonesia and the political problems of the South China Seas. I'm picking up these extraordinary things I never knew ... It's something I've been writing for the last 18 months and it's hideously hard. The trouble is my through-line started splintering at some point, because I kept finding so many interesting things and I'd have to go, 'No, come back to the story, stop going off at tangents. Just show that you can write a fucking story that has a beginning, a middle and an end. It's so epic that I'm not sure I'll ever finish. Maybe the notes will emerge after I'm dead. They're interesting notes!"

It seems unlikely that Bowie will stay away from the recording studio for long. Still not forgotten is the elusive *Contamination*, a prospective album to be culled from unreleased material recorded in 1994

during the Montreux sessions for *1.Outside*. "The one thing that I can truly, seriously think about in the future that I would like to get my teeth into – it's just so daunting – is the rest of the work that Eno and I did when we started to do the *Outside* album," David told *Ice* magazine in 2003. "We did improv for eight days, and we had something in the area of 20 hours' worth of stuff that I just cannot begin to get close to listening to. But there are some absolute gems in there." David has also intimated that the once-touted plans for a theatrical extravaganza based on *1.Outside* have not yet been laid to rest, and that he has considered teaming up with artist Tony Oursler to work on "the theatrical presentation of *Outside* and *Contamination* and what hopefully will be a third piece. His visual vocabulary is very similar to my own. And we get on extremely well whenever we do theatrical ventures together." Of the Montreux material itself, David has revealed that he is "very pleasantly surprised at how completely nutty it sounds," and remarked in 2003 that "after we get off the road on this tour, I might bring myself to doing it. Or I'll fail – I'll have written another album."

This last observation seems to indicate the more likely route that Bowie will take, for there is every indication that he is still suffused with the enthusiasm for new writing that brought forth *Heathen* and *Reality* in such rapid succession. "I'm heading for another period of experimentation," he told reporters at a press conference in Tokyo in March 2004. "I'm at a time when I'm collecting myself before I break all my own rules." A month later he was speaking of his intention to return to the studio as soon as the summer festival dates were over, and intimated that he hoped to have another new album completed by the end of the year.

Quite what form the follow-up to *Reality* might take is anybody's guess. "I might get back into the realm of something even more abstract," Bowie pondered in 2003. '"However, I'm not sure, and I hate to paint myself into a corner, because I might have a terrific change of mind. I mean, my ability that's helped me a lot is the ability to change horses mid-stream, and I've never seen that as something that's held me back. In fact, I've seen it as a positive thing, and I don't feel as though I'm obliged to stick to my word. Whereas other people might think they have to stand by what they've said, I don't have that problem. It's only fucking art!"

Undoubtedly not every project will be carried through to a conclusion, as old ideas are adapted or outstripped by new enthusiasms. But one way or another, by the time this updated edition reaches the shelves David Bowie will have ensured that it's already out of date. And while that might be frustrating to a chronicler who has spent the last eight years trying to outrun the man's progress, it is also exactly the reason why Bowie exerts such inextinguishable fascination and respect.

Whatever David Bowie does next, some people are going to love it and others will hate it. The only reliable certainty is that it won't be quite what anyone expected. And three cheers for that.

sources

SELECT BIBLIOGRAPHY

All publications are London unless otherwise stated.

Badman, Keith, *The Beatles After The Break-Up:
1970-2000* (Omnibus Press, 1999)

Barnes, Richard, *The Who: Maximum R&B*
(Plexus, 1982; revised 2000)

Bockris, Victor, *Lou Reed: The Biography* (Vintage, 1995)

Bowie, Angela, with Patrick Carr, *Backstage Passes*
(Orion, 1993)

Bowie, David, and Mick Rock, *Moonage Daydream:
The Life And Times Of Ziggy Stardust*
(Guildford: Genesis Publications, 2002)

Boyd, William, *Nat Tate: An American Artist*
(21, 1998)

Buckley, David, *The Complete Guide To The Music of
David Bowie* (Omnibus Press, 1996)

Buckley, David, *Strange Fascination – David Bowie:
The Definitive Story* (Virgin, 1999; revised 2000)

Buckley, David, and Kevin Cann, sleeve-notes for
Aladdin Sane 30th Anniversary Edition (EMI, 2003)

Buckley, David, and Kevin Cann, sleeve-notes for
Diamond Dogs 30th Anniversary Edition (EMI, 2004)

Buckley, David, and Kevin Cann, sleeve-notes for
*The Rise And Fall Of Ziggy Stardust And The Spiders
From Mars 30th Anniversary Edition* (EMI, 2002)

Cann, Kevin, *David Bowie: A Chronology*
(Vermilion, 1983)

Carr, Roy, and Charles Shaar Murray,
David Bowie: An Illustrated Record (Eel Pie, 1981)

Crowley, Aleister, and Lady Frieda Harris, *The Aleister
Crowley Thoth Tarot* (Neuhausen: A G Müller, 1986)

Currie, David, *The Starzone Interviews*
(Omnibus Press, 1985)

De La Parra, Pimm Jal, *David Bowie: The Concert Tapes*
(Amsterdam: P J Publishing, 1985)

Donne, John, *The Complete English Poems*
(Harmondsworth: Penguin, 1971)

Eno, Brian, *A Year With Swollen Appendices*
(Faber, 1996)

Flippo, Chet, *David Bowie's Serious Moonlight*
(Sidgwick & Jackson, 1984)

Fry, Stephen, and Hugh Laurie, *A Bit Of Fry & Laurie*
(Mandarin, 1990)

Gambaccini, Paul, with Jonathan Rice and Tim Rice,
British Hit Albums (Enfield: Guinness, 1994)

Gambaccini, Paul, with Jonathan Rice, Tim Rice and
Tony Brown, *The Complete Eurovision Song Contest
Companion* (Pavilion Books, 1998)

Gambaccini, Paul, with Jonathan Rice and Tim Rice,
Top 40 Charts (Enfield: Guinness, 1992)

Garner, Ken, *In Session Tonight: The Complete Radio 1
Recordings* (BBC Books, 1993)

Gillman, Peter, and Leni Gillman, *Alias David Bowie*
(Hodder & Stoughton, 1986)

Guiley, Rosemary Ellen, *The Encyclopedia Of Witches
And Witchcraft* (Oxford: Facts On File, 1989)

Hall, James, *Dictionary of Subjects & Symbols in Art*
(John Murray, 1974)

Hardy, Phil, *The Encyclopedia Of Science Fiction Movies*
(Aurum Press, 1986)

Heatley, Michael, with Spencer Leigh,
*Behind The Song: The Stories of 100 Great
Pop & Rock Classics* (Blandford, 1998)

Hopkins, Jerry, *Bowie* (Hamish Hamilton, 1985)

Hoskyns, Barney, *Glam!: Bowie, Bolan and the
Glitter Rock Revolution* (Faber, 1998)

Hutton, Jim, with Tim Wapshott, *Mercury And Me*
(Bloomsbury, 1995)

Juby, Kerry (Ed), *In Other Words ... David Bowie*
(Omnibus, 1986)

Kerouac, Jack, *On The Road*
(Harmondsworth: Penguin, 1991)

Kuipers, Dean (Ed), *I Am Iman*
(New York: Universal Publishing, 2001)

Lawson, Twiggy, *In Black And White*
(Simon & Schuster, 1997)

Mayes, Sean, *We Can Be Heroes: Life On Tour With
David Bowie* (Independent Music Press, 1999)

McGough, Roger, *Penguin Modern Poets 10*
(Harmondsworth: Penguin, 1967)

Naji, Jamilla, and David Bowie, *Musical Storyland* (San Diego: Worlds In Ink, 2004)

Nicholls, Peter, *The World Of Fantastic Films* (New York: Dodd, Mead & Co, 1984)

Opie, Iona, and Peter Opie, *The Oxford Dictionary of Nursery Rhymes* (Oxford: OUP, 1951)

Orwell, George, *Nineteen Eighty-Four* (Harmondsworth: Penguin, 1954)

Paytress, Mark, *Classic Rock Albums: Ziggy Stardust* (New York: Schirmer Books, 1998)

Paytress, Mark, and Steve Pafford, *Bowiestyle* (Omnibus Press, 2000)

Pitt, Kenneth, *Bowie: The Pitt Report* (Omnibus Press, 1985)

Pollack, Rachel, *The New Tarot* (Wellingborough: Aquarian Press, 1989)

Rock, Mick, *Blood And Glitter* (Vision On Publishing, 2001)

Rogan, Johnny, *Starmakers And Svengalis* (Queen Anne Press, 1988)

Sandford, Christopher, *Bowie: Loving The Alien* (Little, Brown, 1996)

Santos-Kayda, Miriam, *David Bowie: Live In New York* (New York: powerHouse Books, 2003)

Strong, M C, *The Great Rock Discography* (Edinburgh: Canongate, 1996)

Taylor, Rod, *The Guinness Book Of Sitcoms* (Enfield: Guinness, 1994)

Thompson, Dave, *David Bowie: Moonage Daydream* (Plexus, 1987)

Thompson, David and Ian Christie (Eds), *Scorsese On Scorsese* (Faber, 1996)

Thomson, Elizabeth and David Gutman (Eds), *The Bowie Companion* (Sidgwick & Jackson, 1993)

Tremlett, George, *The David Bowie Story* (Futura, 1974)

Tremlett, George, *David Bowie: Living On The Brink* (Century Books, 1996)

Vahimagi, Tise, *British Television* (Oxford: Oxford University Press, 1994)

Walker, John (Ed), *Halliwell's Film & Video Guide* (HarperCollins, 1997)

Walker, John (Ed), *Halliwell's Who's Who In The Movies* (HarperCollins, 1999)

Weller, Helen (Ed), *British Hit Singles* (Enfield: Guinness, 1997)

Zanetta, Tony, and Henry Edwards, *Stardust: The Life And Times Of David Bowie* (Michael Joseph, 1986)

Although I may occasionally dispute their facts and conclusions, I am very much indebted to Bowie's biographers. The best life of Bowie is still Peter and Leni Gillman's influential *Alias David Bowie*. It is unusually well written for a rock biography and is exhaustive and brilliant on David's early years; in particular, the colourful account of the MainMan madness of 1972-1975 is second to none. But – and it is a substantial but – the Gillmans' account has a disagreeable tendency to founder on the rocks of sensationalism. The authors display an almost comical amazement at the very thought of drug-taking or homosexuality, and devote acres of space to half-baked psychobabble regarding Bowie's family history. It's not difficult to see why their book gave offence to David at the time.

A more recent contender is David Buckley's 1999 book *Strange Fascination – David Bowie: The Definitive Story*. Buckley's big picture is better than his (occasionally inaccurate) detail, but he approaches his subject from a position that is both knowledgeable and enthusiastic about the music itself, and benefits splendidly from by far the best published interviews with Carlos Alomar, Reeves Gabrels, Adrian Belew, Hugh Padgham and Nile Rodgers. *The Pitt Report*, Kenneth Pitt's 1983 account of his tenure as Bowie's manager on the eve of his breakthrough, is a fascinating and touching curio, definitive on the period it covers and never remotely self-serving. Jerry Hopkins's 1985 book *Bowie* boasts some valuable interviews with figures from David's 1970s American career. Dave Thompson's 1987 work *Moonage Daydream* gives a clear, well-researched account supported by an extensive interview with Tony Visconti.

Christopher Sandford's 1996 biography *Bowie: Loving The Alien* offers worthwhile interviews with the likes of Kenneth Pitt and Keith Christmas, but is hamstrung by some whopping inaccuracies and its author's dogged mission to portray his subject as a ruthless manipulator. George Tremlett's 1996 offering *David Bowie: Living On The Brink* trades on a batch of ancient interviews which the author conducted with Bowie in the 1960s. These are fascinating and valuable in themselves, but Tremlett's facts on later years are shaky and his fondness for Rabelaisian description becomes a little wearing: this is the book to buy if you need to know that the basement flat of Bowie's early manager Ralph Horton "stank of chip grease, cat shit and stale sperm." Angela Bowie's 1993 memoir *Backstage Passes* provokes nothing so much as pity, whereas *The Bowie Companion*, edited by Elizabeth Thomson and David Gutman, is one of the finest Bowie books in print – an excellent compilation of journalism written between 1964 and 1993.

Three recent photo-books are eminently worthy of mention. Mick Rock's *Blood And Glitter* is a superb portfolio of the photographer's work during the heyday of glam rock (accompanied by a foreword from David), while *Bowiestyle* is a lavish large-format compilation of rare photos from every period of Bowie's career, illuminated with text by Mark Paytress and Steve Pafford which, as the title suggests, concentrates on Bowie's status as a musical and sartorial style guru. Finally, *Moonage Daydream: The Life And Times Of Ziggy Stardust* is undoubtedly the most beautiful Bowie book ever published: a lavish and costly release from Genesis Publications, it was limited to 2500 copies signed by Mick Rock, whose photographs appear throughout, and by David Bowie himself, whose accompanying text discusses the influences and experiences of the Ziggy period with warmth, wit and humour.

Although an exhaustive discography appears in Chapter 11, this book makes no attempt to cover every last elusive item of variant overseas packaging. For fuller information on worldwide releases I refer you to Marshall Jarman's *David Bowie's World 7" Discography 1964-81*, to the ongoing scholarship of *Record Collector* magazine, and above all to Ruud Altenburg's peerless *Illustrated db Discography* website (see address below), which is the finest resource of its kind that the Internet has to offer. The late Pimm Jal de la Parra's 1985 labour of love, *David Bowie: The Concert Tapes*, is long since out of print but worth hunting down as an invaluable guide to hundreds of unlicensed live recordings.

MEDIA

The numerous newspapers, journals and periodicals I have consulted are credited in the main text. My researches have been particularly indebted to *Arena, BBC Music Magazine, Billboard, Creem, Disc & Music Echo, Guitar, Guitar Player, Hit Parader, i-D, International Musician, Interview, Melody Maker, Modern Drummer, Mojo, Mojo Collections, New Musical Express, Performing Songwriter, Q, Record Collector, Record Mirror, Rolling Stone, Smash Hits, Sound On Sound, Sounds, Uncut, Vanity Fair* and *Word*. In addition I must give special thanks to the BBC's Written Archives Centre for assisting with information regarding radio and television dates.

INTERNET

I am indebted to the enthusiasm and expertise of the many Bowie-related websites. While writing this book I have found the following particularly valuable:

BowieNet	www.davidbowie.com
Bowie Wonderworld	www.bowiewonderworld.com
Illustrated db Discography	
	www.illustrated-db-discography.nl
Bassman's David Bowie Page	
	www.algonet.se/~bassman
Teenage Wildlife	www.teenagewildlife.com
The Ziggy Stardust Companion	
	www.5years.com
Gail Ann Dorsey	www.gailanndorsey.com
Reeves Gabrels	www.reevesgabrels.com
Mike Garson	www.mikegarson.com
Mark Plati	www.markplati.net
Tony Visconti	www.tonyvisconti.com

'JAN 2005

acknowledgements

My gratitude is due to a number of individuals whose support, encouragement and assistance have made this undertaking both possible and enjoyable. Thanks to John Ainsworth, Alex Alexander, Ruud Altenburg, David Bishop, Tom Bowden, Graham Brown, David Buckley, Paul Cornell, David Darlington, Ricky Gardiner, Gary Gillatt, Paul Gough, Simon Guerrier, David Hankinson, John Harrison, Dan Hogarth, Julia Houghton, Tony Jordan, Paul Kinder, Trey Korte, Phil Lawton, Andrew Lilley, Rob Lines, Claire Longhurst, Mary Longhurst, Alistair McGown, Jonathan Morris, Jamilla Naji, Per Nilsen, Dara O'Kearney, Phil Packer, Steve Pafford, Clare Pegg, Ian Potter, Nigel Reeve, Pascal Reyreau, Paul Rhodes, Gareth Roberts, Jim Sangster, Tom Spilsbury, Tim Sutton, Rob Swain, Evan Torrie, Tragic Youth, Stephen Warnes and Mark Wyman. For patience, faith and perseverance, special thanks to my agent, John McLaughlin, and my publishers, Marcus Hearn and Richard Reynolds.

The biggest thanks go to Gary Russell, Barnaby Edwards and especially Rob Byrne, for unstinting research assistance, proof-reading and rude comments. This book could not have been written without them.

Finally, heartfelt gratitude and admiration to the two B's in my life – one for being such a source of pleasure and passion ever since I bought 'Sound And Vision' (my first ever single), and the other, who is far more important, for tolerating ceaseless alternative versions of 'When I Live My Dream' with almost supernatural equanimity. It's all done; you can have the stereo, and me, back now.